MYCOPLASMAS

Molecular Biology
and Pathogenesis

MYCOPLASMAS

Molecular Biology and Pathogenesis

Editor in Chief

Jack Maniloff

Department of Microbiology and Immunology
University of Rochester
Rochester, New York

Editors

Ronald N. McElhaney

Department of Biochemistry
University of Alberta
Edmonton, Alberta, Canada

Lloyd R. Finch

Russell Grimwade School of Biochemistry
University of Melbourne
Parkville, Victoria, Australia

Joel B. Baseman

Department of Microbiology
University of Texas Health Science Center
San Antonio, Texas

AMERICAN SOCIETY FOR MICROBIOLOGY
Washington, D.C.

Library of Congress Cataloging-in-Publication Data

Mycoplasmas : molecular biology and pathogenesis / editor in chief,
 Jack Maniloff ; editors, Ronald N. McElhaney, Lloyd R. Finch, Joel
 B. Baseman.
   p. cm.
  Includes index.
  ISBN 1-55581-050-0
  1. Mycoplasma diseases. 2. Mycoplasma. 3. Mycoplasma
diseases—Molecular aspects. I. Maniloff, Jack.
  [DNLM: 1. Mycoplasma—genetics. 2. Mycoplasma—pathogenicity.
WC 246 M9953]
QR201.M97M93   1992
589.9—dc20
DNLM/DLC
for Library of Congress   92-49746
                                                                      CIP

CONTENTS

VI. MOLECULAR BASIS OF MYCOPLASMA PATHOGENICITY

VII. EVOLUTION

CONTRIBUTORS

Yoshiki Andachi • Department of Biology, School of Science, Nagoya University, Furo-cho, Chikusa-Ku, Nagoya 464-01, Japan

Michael F. Barile • Laboratory of Mycoplasma, Division of Bacterial Products, Center for Biologics Evaluation and Research, Food and Drug Administration, Bethesda, Maryland 20892

Joel B. Baseman • Department of Microbiology, University of Texas Health Science Center at San Antonio, 7703 Floyd Curl Drive, San Antonio, Texas 78284-7758

Thomas Borén • Department of Medical Biochemistry, University of Göteborg, Medicinareg. 9, S-413 90 Göteborg, Sweden

Michael J. Boyer • Department of Biochemistry, University of Umeå, S-901 87 Umeå, Sweden

Gary H. Butler • Coriell Institute for Medical Research, Camden, New Jersey 08103

Johnny L. Carson • Department of Pediatrics, Department of Cell Biology and Anatomy, and Center for Environmental Medicine and Lung Biology, University of North Carolina School of Medicine, Chapel Hill, North Carolina 27599

Gail H. Cassell • Department of Microbiology, University of Alabama at Birmingham, Birmingham, Alabama 35294

Gunna Christiansen • Institute of Medical Microbiology, University of Aarhus, DK-8000 Aarhus C, Denmark

Albert M. Collier • Department of Pediatrics, Center for Environmental Medicine and Lung Biology, and Frank Porter Graham Child Development Center, University of North Carolina School of Medicine, Chapel Hill, North Carolina 27599

Christopher C. Dascher • Department of Microbiology and Immunology, University of Rochester, Medical Center Box 672, Rochester, New York 14642

Maureen K. Davidson • Department of Comparative Medicine, University of Alabama at Birmingham, and Veterans Administration Medical Center, Birmingham, Alabama 35294

Robert E. Davis • Microbiology and Plant Pathology Laboratory, Agricultural Research Service, U.S. Department of Agriculture, Beltsville, Maryland 20705

Jerry K. Davis • Department of Comparative Medicine and Department of Microbiology, University of Alabama at Birmingham, Birmingham, Alabama 35294

Gang Deng • Department of Molecular Microbiology and Immunology, School of Medicine, University of Missouri–Columbia, Columbia, Missouri 65212

Kevin Dybvig • Department of Comparative Medicine and Department of Microbiology, University of Alabama at Birmingham, Birmingham, Alabama 35294

Jane S. Ellison • Laboratory of Mycoplasma, Division of Bacterial Products, Center for Biologics Evaluation and Research, Food and Drug Administration, Bethesda, Maryland 20892

Rebecca V. Ferrell • Department of Molecular Microbiology and Immunology, School of Medicine, University of Missouri–Columbia, Columbia, Missouri 65212

Lloyd R. Finch • Department of Biochemistry, University of Melbourne, Parkville, Victoria, Australia, 3052

Randy S. Fischer • Department of Microbiology and Cell Science, University of Florida, Gainesville, Florida 32611-0100

Brenda E. Fischer • Department of Microbiology and Cell Science, University of Florida, Gainesville, Florida 32611-0100

Gad Glaser • Department of Cellular Biochemistry, The Hebrew University–Hadassah Medical School, Jerusalem 91010, Israel

Richard Herrmann • Microbiology (ZMBH), University of Heidelberg, Im Neuenheimer Feld 282, 6900 Heidelberg, Germany

Ping-Chuan Hu • Department of Pediatrics, Department of Microbiology and Immunology, and Center for Environmental Medicine and Lung Biology, University of North Carolina School of Medicine, Chapel Hill, North Carolina 27599

Hana C. Hyman • Department of Membrane and Ultrastructure Research, The Hebrew University–Hadassah Medical School, Jerusalem 91010, Israel

Roy A. Jensen • Department of Microbiology and Cell Science, University of Florida, Gainesville, Florida 32611-0100

George E. Kenny • Department of Pathobiology, SC-38, School of Public Health and Community Medicine, University of Washington, Seattle, Washington 98195

Helga Kirchhoff • Institut für Mikrobiologie und Tierseuchen, Tierärztliche Hochschule, D-3000 Hannover, Federal Republic of Germany

Hitoshi Kotani • Genetic Therapy, Inc., 19 Firstfield Road, Gaithersburg, Maryland 20878

Duncan C. Krause • Department of Microbiology, University of Georgia, Athens, Georgia 30602

Jacques Labarère • Laboratoire de Génétique Moléculaire, Université de Bordeaux II–INRA, Centre de Recherches Agronomiques de Bordeaux, BP 81, F-33883 Villenave d'Ornon Cédex, France

Ing-Ming Lee • Microbiology and Plant Pathology Laboratory, Agricultural Research Service, U.S. Department of Agriculture, Beltsville, Maryland 20705

Shyh-Ching Lo • Division of Molecular Pathobiology, Department of Infectious and Parasitic Disease Pathology, Armed Forces Institute of Pathology, Washington, D.C. 20306-6000

Jack Maniloff • Department of Microbiology and Immunology, University of Rochester, Medical Center Box 672, Rochester, New York 14642

Ronald N. McElhaney • Department of Biochemistry, University of Alberta, Edmonton, Alberta, Canada T6G 2H7

Gerard J. McGarrity • Genetic Therapy, Inc., 19 Firstfield Road, Gaithersburg, Maryland 20878

Mark A. McIntosh • Department of Molecular Microbiology and Immunology, School of Medicine, University of Missouri–Columbia, Columbia, Missouri 65212

R. J. Miles • Microbial Physiology Research Group, Division of Life Sciences, King's College, University of London, Campden Hill Road, London W8 7AH, United Kingdom

F. Chris Minion • Veterinary Medical Research Institute, Iowa State University, Ames, Iowa 50011

Alana Mitchell • Baker Institute of Medical Research, Prahran, Australia, 3181

Akira Muto • Department of Biology, School of Science, Nagoya University, Furo-cho, Chikusa-ku, Nagoya 464-01, Japan

Lyn D. Olson • Laboratory of Mycoplasma, Division of Bacterial Products, Center for Biologics Evaluation and Research, Food and Drug Administration, Bethesda, Maryland 20892

Syozo Osawa • Department of Biology, School of Science, Nagoya University, Furo-cho, Chikusa-ku, Nagoya 464-01, Japan

J. Dennis Pollack • Department of Medical Microbiology and Immunology, Ohio State University, 333 West 10th Avenue, Columbus, Ohio 43210

Shmuel Razin • Department of Membrane and Ultrastructure Research, The Hebrew University–Hadassah Medical School, Jerusalem 91010, Israel

Marilyn C. Roberts • Department of Pathobiology, SC-38, School of Public Health and Community Medicine, University of Washington, Seattle, Washington 98195

Ricardo F. Rosenbusch • Veterinary Medical Research Institute, Iowa State University, Ames, Iowa 50011

Renate Rosengarten • Institut für Mikrobiologie und Tierseuchen, Tierärztliche Hochschule Hannover, Bischofsholer Damm 15, 3000 Hannover 1, Federal Republic of Germany

Suzanne E. Ross • Department of Microbiology, University of Alabama at Birmingham, Birmingham, Alabama 35294

Tore Samuelsson • Department of Medical Biochemistry, University of Göteborg, Medicinareg. 9, S-413 90 Göteborg, Sweden

Jerry W. Simecka • Department of Microbiology, University of Alabama at Birmingham, Birmingham, Alabama 35294

Todd L. Sladek • Department of Genetics, School of Medicine, Case Western Reserve University, Cleveland, Ohio 44106

Paul F. Smith • Department of Microbiology, University of South Dakota, Vermillion, South Dakota 57069

Christian T. K.-H. Städtlander • Department of Microbiology, University of Alabama at Birmingham, Birmingham, Alabama 35294

Reiji Tanaka • Aburahi Laboratories, Shionogi Ltd., Kouga, Shiga 520-34, Japan

David Taylor-Robinson • Division of Sexually Transmitted Diseases, Clinical Research Centre, Watford Road, Harrow, Middlesex HA1 3UJ, United Kingdom

Victor V. Tryon • Department of Microbiology, University of Texas Health Science Center at San Antonio, 7703 Floyd Curl Drive, San Antonio, Texas 78284-7758

Åke Wiselander • Department of Biochemistry, University of Umeå, S-901 87 Umeå, Sweden

Kim S. Wise • Department of Molecular Microbiology and Immunology, M642 Medical Sciences Building, University of Missouri–Columbia, Columbia, Missouri 65212

Henri Wróblewski • Université de Rennes I, Centre National de la Recherche Scientifique, Unité de Recherche Associée no. 256, 35042 Rennes Cédex, France

Fumiaki Yamao • National Institute of Genetics, Mishima 411, Japan

David Yogev • Department of Membrane and Ultrastructure Research, The Hebrew University–Hadassah Medical School, P.O. Box 1172, Jerusalem 91010, Israel

Jianhong Zheng • Department of Molecular Microbiology and Immunology, School of Medicine, University of Missouri–Columbia, Columbia, Missouri 65212

PREFACE

The idea for this volume originated from two developments. The first was the maturation of mycoplasma biology in the past 10 to 15 years, made possible both by experimental advances in molecular biology (particularly DNA cloning and sequencing), which allowed investigation of molecular aspects of mycoplasma biology and pathogenicity, and by construction of the mycoplasma phylogenetic tree, which established the relationship of mycoplasmas to the bacteria and made it possible to understand mycoplasmas in the larger perspective of bacterial biology and pathogenicity. The second development was publication of the *Escherichia coli and Salmonella typhimurium: Cellular and Molecular Biology* volumes in 1987 by the American Society for Microbiology (ASM), which served as a model for a single modern comprehensive treatment of a microbial taxon.

The original outline for this book was put together by three of the editors at an outdoor cafe in Baden, Austria, in 1988, and the thirteenth (and last) revision of the table of contents was finally completed in the spring of 1992. During this period, most of the individuals invited to participate in this project graciously accepted, and many made useful suggestions regarding the material to be included in the volume.

This book is the first thorough description of the mycoplasmas in terms of modern cellular and molecular biology. It is designed to provide a single comprehensive reference on mycoplasma molecular biology and pathogenicity for those in the field and to make current information and ideas about mycoplasma pathogenicity available to a wide range of scientists and clinicians. Therefore, in preparing their chapters, authors were requested to incorporate a comprehensive treatment of important data, maps, pathways, structures, and processes from the primary literature into review chapters. The goal of each chapter is to integrate data in a particular area of mycoplasma biology, to place this information in a broader microbiological perspective, and to indicate future areas for investigation.

The Editors thank our approximately 60 fellow authors, and we also thank the members of the ASM Books Division for their advice and patience throughout this project. Particular thanks are due to Patrick Fitzgerald, Senior Editor, ASM, for his suggestions during the pre-production stage and to Eleanor Tupper, Senior Production Editor, ASM, and her staff for their skill and professionalism in the production of this volume.

Jack Maniloff
Ronald N. McElhaney
Lloyd R. Finch
Joel B. Baseman

I. INTRODUCTION

1. Mycoplasma Taxonomy and Ecology

SHMUEL RAZIN

INTRODUCTION

Mycoplasmas as Organisms: A Historical Perspective

The first successful cultivation of a mycoplasma, the bovine pleuropneumonia agent, was reported by Nocard and Roux in 1898 (125). Thus, in a few years, the centennial of mycoplasmology will be celebrated. Yet despite our rather long acquaintance with mycoplasmas, the nature of these organisms has presented a continued enigma to microbiologists. There is, perhaps, no other group of bacteria that caused so much controversy and confusion as to its identity and taxonomic status. In the early days, the minute mycoplasmas were considered to be viruses, since they could pass through filters which blocked the passage of ordinary bacteria. With the elucidation of the true nature of viruses in the 1930s, it became evident that mycoplasmas cannot be defined as viruses. Yet history tends to repeat itself; the mycoplasma found recently in AIDS patients was initially considered by Lo (103) to be a "novel virus."

The isolation by Klieneberger in 1935 (90) of the L form (or L-phase variant) from *Streptobacillus moniliformis* cultures was the first shot in a long battle about the independent taxonomic status of mycoplasmas. Klieneberger considered the L forms to be mycoplasmas, living in symbiosis with the bacterium. It took

years to correct this misconception, since it required advancement in the knowledge of the structure, composition, and biosynthesis of bacterial cell walls. In the late 1950s (98), the definition of L forms as bacteria which had partially or entirely lost their cell walls became available. Unfortunately, clarification of the nature of the bacterial L forms served to increase confusion as to mycoplasma identity. The finding that ordinary bacteria can be induced to grow as stable L forms, devoid of cell walls and morphologically and culturally resembling mycoplasmas, led to the notion that mycoplasmas are no more than stable L-phase variants of common bacteria. Isolation of a variety of walled bacteria from mycoplasma cultures was brought up to support this notion (135). If this view were true, mycoplasmas would not qualify for an autonomous taxonomic status. The mycoplasma literature in the 1950s and 1960s was full of papers supporting or opposing the definition of mycoplasmas as bacterial L forms. The heated controversy came to an end in the late 1960s when the first genomic analysis data (guanine-plus-cytosine content and DNA-DNA hybridization) became available, ruling out any relationship of mycoplasmas to stable L forms of present-day walled bacteria (135). However, misconceptions show a marked tendency to survive and reappear from time to time, the most recent example being the claim that the aster yellows mycoplasmalike organism is an L-phase variant of a mycobacterium (129). Fortunately, the molecular genetic data that have just been

---

Shmuel Razin • Department of Membrane and Ultrastructure Research, The Hebrew University–Hadassah Medical School, Jerusalem 91010, Israel.

reported point out very clearly that the aster yellows agent is a bona fide mycoplasma and not an L form (see chapter 23).

It should, perhaps, be brought up at this point that associating mycoplasmas with L forms is not totally wrong when one considers from the long-range evolutionary perspective. The theme underlying the current evolutionary scheme of mycoplasmas is that of degenerative evolution from walled bacteria (chapter 33). Consequently, the evolutionary history of mycoplasmas appears to include the loss of a cell wall, reminiscent of induction of L forms. The major difference is that in the case of mycoplasmas, loss of the cell wall was apparently only one step in the lengthy process of mycoplasma evolution, involving many more steps resulting in marked diminution of the genome. The present-day L forms are, on the other hand, laboratory artifacts, produced by partial or complete cell wall removal, with minimal changes in the genomic makeup of the parent bacterium.

Advancement in the 1960s and 1970s of our knowledge about the ultrastructure, cell membrane, genome, and metabolic pathways of mycoplasmas has led to the recognition that mycoplasmas are the smallest and simplest self-replicating organisms (139). Naturally, this finding has raised the intriguing question as to the place of mycoplasmas in the evolutionary scheme. The extreme simplicity and compactness of mycoplasma cells led Morowitz and Wallace (118) to propose that mycoplasmas are the most primitive extant organisms, representing the descendants of bacteria that existed prior to the development of a peptidoglycan cell wall. Accordingly, mycoplasmas should be placed at the root of the phylogenetic tree. This notion was challenged by Neimark, who since the 1960s has persistently promoted the thesis that mycoplasmas originated from walled bacteria by degenerative evolution (122). It was only with the introduction of rRNA sequencing data as a phylogenetic measure (216) that the balance of evidence shifted in favor of degenerative evolution of mycoplasmas from walled bacteria, more specifically from the gram-positive branch of eubacteria (chapter 33). This view has been continuously strengthened by molecular biology data accumulating at an exponential rate in recent years (107, 138, 140, 141).

In summing up this brief historical introduction, it appears that only now, nearly 100 years after the discovery of the first mycoplasma, have we reached the stage where mycoplasmas can be defined rather clearly as a group of eubacteria, phylogenetically related to gram-positive bacteria but retaining the rather unique position as the smallest self-replicating procaryotes devoid of cell walls.

Evolution of Mycoplasma Taxonomy

The difficulties and uncertainties accompanying the definition of mycoplasmas as organisms are reflected in the rather frequent and radical changes in their classification and nomenclature. No fewer than nine different names were given between 1910 and 1956 to the bovine pleuropneumonia organism, known now as *Mycoplasma mycoides* subsp. *mycoides* (51). Several organisms isolated subsequently, and considered to be related to *M. mycoides*, were designated by Klienenberger in the 1930s by the letter "L" followed by numbers from 1 to 7 (91), pointing to the ambiguity created by the confusion of mycoplasmas with bacterial L forms. Sabin (164) followed in 1941 with the first classification and nomenclature system, which for some reason did not catch on. Thus, the rather vague and tongue-twisting term "pleuropneumonialike organisms" dominated the field for many years to describe all organisms resembling the bovine pleuropneumonia mycoplasma.

The basis for the current classification system was laid down by Edward and Freundt in 1956 (47). It consisted of a single order, *Mycoplasmatales*, containing a single family, *Mycoplasmataceae*, with a single genus, *Mycoplasma*, and 15 species. The name "mycoplasma" was derived from a combination of the Greek *mykes*, for fungus, and *plasma*, for something formed or molded, to denote the mycelar funguslike morphology of the pleuropneumonia agent *M. mycoides*. This classification system was gradually expanded by adding new genera, families, and orders and by raising the taxonomic status of the group to that of a class, *Mollicutes* (48), a name derived from the Latin *mollis* (soft) and *cutis* (skin) to denote the lack of a rigid cell wall for these organisms. *Mollicutes* is presently the only class in the division *Tenericutes* (wall-less bacteria), forming one of the four divisions of the kingdom *Procaryotae* (120). The other three divisions are *Firmicutes* (the gram-positive bacteria), *Gracilicutes* (the gram-negative bacteria), and *Mendosicutes* (the archaebacteria) (Table 1).

This is the place to mention the policy concerning the naming of new species, adopted by the Subcommittee of the International Committee of Systematic Bacteriology (ICSB) on the Taxonomy of Mollicutes (hereafter referred to as the Subcommittee). The minimal standards for description of new mycoplasma species proposed by the Subcommittee (173) have received wide recognition and have greatly restrained premature publication of binomial names for mycoplasmas with inadequate supporting data. In addition, the fact that almost all of the descriptions of new mycoplasma species have been published during the last decade in the *International Journal of Systematic Bacteriology*, the official publication of the ICSB, considerably helped the implementation of the aforementioned policy, saving the mycoplasma literature from a possible deluge of ill-defined species.

The trivial name "mycoplasmas" has replaced "pleuropneumonialike organisms" and has been rather loosely used to denote any organism in the class *Mollicutes*. However, with the coining of new generic names, trivial names based on the generic names, including acholeplasmas, ureaplasmas, spiroplasmas, anaeroplasmas, and asteroleplasmas, came into wide use to denote specifically organisms in the corresponding genera. This convention has led to the suggestion (174) that a new trivial name, mollicutes, be used to describe any member of the class, retaining the trivial name "mycoplasmas" to describe only members of the genus *Mycoplasma*. Nevertheless, "mycoplasmas" is still widely used in its broader sense and will be used as such in this volume, though it will be replaced by the term "mollicutes" when appropriate.

As mentioned above, history tends to repeat itself,

Table 1. Taxonomy and properties of mycoplasmas (class *Mollicutes*)[a]

Classification	Current no. of recognized species	Genome size[b] (kbp)	Mol% G+C of DNA	Cholesterol requirement	Distinctive properties	Habitat
Order I: *Mycoplasmatales* Family I: *Mycoplasmataceae* Genus I: *Mycoplasma*	92	580–1,300	23–41	+		Humans, animals, plants, insects
Genus II: *Ureaplasma*	5	730–1,160	27–30	+	Urease positive	Humans, animals
Family II: *Spiroplasmataceae* Genus I: *Spiroplasma*	11	1,350–1,700	25–31	+	Helical filaments	Arthropods (including insects), plants
Order II: *Acholeplasmatales* Family I: *Acholeplasmataceae* Genus I: *Acholeplasma*	12	About 1,600	27–36	−		Animals, plants, insects
Order III: *Anaeroplasmatales* Family: *Anaeroplasmataceae* Genus I: *Anaeroplasma*	4	About 1,600[c]	29–33	+	Oxygen-sensitive obligate anaerobes	Bovine-ovine rumen
Genus II: *Asteroleplasma*	1	About 1,600[c]	40	−	Oxygen-sensitive obligate anaerobes	Bovine-ovine rumen
Uncultivated, unclassified MLOs		500–1,185	23–29	Not established	Uncultivated as yet	Plants, insects

[a] Updated and modified from Razin (136).
[b] According to recent data obtained by PFGE except as indicated.
[c] Data obtained by renaturation kinetics.

and the feeling of relief upon discarding the unwieldy term "pleuropneumonialike organisms" did not last for long. The discovery of uncultivated mycoplasmas in plants, insects, and possibly in humans and animals has led to use of the term "mycoplasmalike (or mollicuteslike) organisms" (MLOs), indicating that the problem of naming mycoplasmas is still with us. A detailed picture of the development of mycoplasma taxonomy can be obtained in the reviews of Sabin (163, 164) and Edward and Freundt (47, 52). More recent reviews on mycoplasma taxonomy are included in *Bergey's Manual of Systematic Bacteriology* (53, 143, 157, 182, 184, 205), in *The Mycoplasmas* series (140, 185, 186), and in the second edition of *The Prokaryotes* (141, 194).

Basing Taxonomy on Phylogeny

Bacterial taxonomy, which began as a largely intuitive process, is now on the verge of becoming an exact science as a result of the wide application of molecular approaches both to taxonomy and to bacterial phylogeny. As discussed by Maniloff (chapter 33), major developments in bacterial phylogeny have already found expression in taxonomy; an example is the provision of a class status, *Archaeobacteria*, to the archaebacteria (120), a decision based largely on molecular biology

data and on phylogenetic considerations rather than on traditional phenotypic characteristics. Considering the inherent conservative nature of any classification system, which in order to be effective must resist any hasty and radical changes, there is no wonder that some clashes between the traditional phenetically oriented and the phylogenetically oriented taxonomists have occurred. Still, deep inside, even the most traditional taxonomist, being aware of the deficiencies of the present system, agrees that basing bacterial taxonomy on phylogeny is both inevitable and advantageous. The major disagreement concerns the question of whether the time is ripe for radical changes in bacterial taxonomy.

One should remember that a major reason for establishing bacterial systematics has been to facilitate the identification of bacterial strains. For this purpose, phenotypic characteristics are generally, though not always, adequate. In essence, for the traditional taxonomist and bench worker, classification of a new isolate at the genus and species level has absolute priority, while relationships of higher taxa are of secondary importance. Classification at higher levels has always been a major problem in bacterial taxonomy because of the frequent lack of phenotypic markers and the absence of well-defined and established criteria for higher taxa.

As mentioned above, mycoplasmas have always constituted a puzzle to bacterial taxonomists. The provision of a class status to mycoplasmas in 1967 (48) signified the conviction of mycoplasmologists that these organisms constitute a well-defined and coherent group. In retrospect, this was a most adequate and productive move, as it helped to accommodate, within the broad frame of a class, the many phenotypically and genotypically different mycoplasmas cultivated so far, also taking into account that the 125 established species (Table 1) represent only a portion, most probably a minor one, of the mycoplasmas existing in nature and uncultivated so far. Moreover, the major phenotypic criterion for including an organism in *Mollicutes*—the lack of a cell wall—has failed so far only once, in the case of *Thermoplasma acidophilum*, a wall-less archaebacterium (140). Thus, the phenotypic criteria for defining mycoplasmas appear to have withstood well the test of time.

The phylogenetic data of Woese et al. (216), indicating that mycoplasmas apparently evolved as a branch of low-G + C "clostridial" subdivision, raised the problem of whether mycoplasmas deserve an independent higher-level taxon such as a class or a division. The conclusion of Woese et al. (216) was that mollicutes are not a phylogenetically coherent group in the sense that all derive from a common ancestor, itself a mycoplasma. Accordingly, mollicutes would cluster within the gram-positive bacteria, specifically within the family *Bacillaceae*, which contains the clostridia (107; see also chapter 33). Adoption of this notion, which would have entailed abolishing the class *Mollicutes*, met with opposition by the Subcommittee (174), which feared that the abolition of a taxonomic group for mollicutes without providing an alternative would mean returning to the chaotic taxonomic status existing at the peak of the dispute about mycoplasmas and L forms.

Although the recently accumulated molecular data, in particular the extensive study of Weisburg et al. (202) on 16S rRNA sequences of mollicutes, support the early conclusions of Woese et al. (216) as to the phylogenetic relationship of mollicutes to gram-positive bacteria (chapter 33), the controversy as to the class status of mycoplasmas has subdued, awaiting general policy decisions to be taken by the ICSB as to the weight to be given to phylogenetic considerations in bacterial taxonomy. To progress in this direction, the ICSB established two ad hoc committees consisting of leading taxonomists and bacterial phylogeny experts. The recommendations made by the two committees were published (121, 201). There was general agreement that the complete DNA sequence of the bacterial genome would be the reference standard to determine phylogeny and that phylogeny should determine taxonomy. In other words, nomenclature should agree with and reflect genomic information (201). While this is the agreed goal, given the lack of information on complete genomic sequences, we have to resort to a combination of the best phenotypic and phylogenetic analyses available in order to develop the most effective bacterial grouping (121). It was also stated that rRNA sequences provide the only source so far recognized for both discerning and testing phylogenetic associations that have the appropriate qualities of universality, genetic stability, and conservation of structure. However, it was also emphasized (121) that

differences in the evolutionary rates in various groups of organisms, as well as other considerations, prevent the use of phylogenetic parameters alone in delineating taxa.

The committees' reports also refer to definition of genera and species. Since the first step in the identification of a bacterium consists of the assignment of the organism to a genus, the greatest clarity in circumscription and utility in the choice of characteristics must rest at this taxonomic level. Unfortunately, there is currently no satisfactory phylogenetic definition of a genus. It is completely impractical, therefore, to define genera solely on the basis of phylogenetic data. Genera need to be characterized by using phenotypic properties. In cases in which there is a disparity between phylogenetic and phenotypic data, priority should be provisionally given to the latter (121).

At present, the species is the only taxonomic unit that can be defined in phylogenetic terms. The phylogenetic definition of a species generally would include strains with approximately 70% or greater DNA-DNA relatedness and with 5°C or lower ΔT_m. Phenotypic characteristics should agree with this definition and would be allowed to override the phylogenetic concept of species only in a few exceptional cases (201).

In conclusion, it appears that the current policy adopted by the ICSB proceeds in the direction of construction of a mixed taxonomic system based on available phylogenetic relationships, with many phenetic groups attached or inserted intuitively between known phylogenetic lineages. This policy requires many compromises, especially with respect to ranking. Hence, one would expect an evolution rather than a revolution in bacterial taxonomy, leading to the final goal of basing taxonomy on phylogeny. In the meantime, the Subcommittee, as well as most if not all mycoplasmologists, find it useful to retain the class *Mollicutes* with the present classification system, deeming it essential for the proper identification of isolates.

MOLECULAR TOOLS IN TAXONOMY

Genome Size

For almost 20 years, genome size has served as a major taxonomic criterion distinguishing the *Mycoplasmataceae* from *Acholeplasmataceae*, *Spiroplasmataceae*, and *Anaeroplasmataceae*. The organisms included in *Mycoplasmataceae*, that is, *Mycoplasma* and *Ureaplasma* species, were regarded as having genomes of about 500 MDa (about 750 kbp), while the organisms in the other three families were considered to have genomes double this size (142, 143). The significant apparent gap in genome size between the families generated much speculation, particularly as to its phylogenetic and evolutionary meaning (118, 159, 216). The first indication that the generalization as to two defined genomic size clusters in mollicutes may be wrong came from the study of Pyle et al. (131). They applied pulsed-field gel electrophoresis (PFGE) to measure the size of restriction fragments of genomic DNA of several *Mycoplasma* and *Ureaplasma* species. The sum of sizes of the various fragments yielded values which were considerably higher (900 to 1,330 kbp) than the expected 750 kbp. Consequently, Maniloff (108) expressed concern as to the validity of the data, suggesting that the low-G + C mycoplasmal DNA may exhibit anomalous behavior in PFGE, leading to slower than expected mobilities of the fragments and thus to incorrect calculated genome size values. A subsequent analysis by Neimark and Lange (124) of PFGE data on genome sizes of a large number of mollicutes showed the lack of any correlation between genome size and average G + C content; thus, the aforementioned reservation does not appear to hold.

Extensive studies on mycoplasma genome size were carried out in the last couple of years by using various modifications of PFGE (9, 12, 23, 101, 155, 156). A marked improvement in technique was achieved by preparing linearized full-size genomic DNA by gamma irradiation. The irradiation introduces double-strand breaks in the chromosome, so that it can enter the gel, unlike the circular intact chromosome. The linearized entire chromosome migrates in the gel as a single band, so that its mobility can be conveniently measured and compared with that of DNA size references (124, 226). Physical mapping of mycoplasma genomes and sizing of restriction fragments have served as an additional source of data on genome size (37, 94, 132, 133, 171, 203, 204). The voluminous amount of new genome size data, available for over 40 different mollicutes, led to the far-reaching conclusion that genome sizes of *Mycoplasma* and *Ureaplasma* species, as well as those of the uncultivated plant and insect MLOs, vary within the range of 500 to 1,300 kbp, while genome sizes of the *Acholeplasma* and *Spiroplasma* species fall within the expected range of 1,350 to 1,700 kbp (Table 1). Hence, some *Mycoplasma* and *Ureaplasma* species have genomes close in size to those of *Acholeplasma* and *Spiroplasma* species, while other *Mycoplasma* and *Ureaplasma* species have genomes of intermediate size, between 600 and 1,300 kbp. For more details, see chapter 9.

The gap in genome size appears no longer to exist. This development has important taxonomic implications, as it invalidates the dogma that a genome size of 500 MDa or 750 kbp is a determinative characteristic for a mycoplasma to be included within *Mycoplasmataceae*. We have thus lost a useful taxonomic property but gained in solving the difficult genome gap problem. It is much easier to perceive a gradual reduction in genome size by deletions occurring during evolution than to explain the shortening of the genome by one-half in a single step (159). Still, it is relevant to mention here that many if not most *Mycoplasma*, *Ureaplasma*, and the presumed MLO species carry genomes of 500 to 800 kbp, keeping their status as the organisms with the smallest recorded genomes (117, 139).

Genomic Base Composition and DNA Modification

The moles percent G + C of procaryotic DNA is an effective taxonomic measure. A difference in the G + C content of greater than 1.5 to 2.0 mol% between DNAs of two bacteria is sufficient to rule out their inclusion in the same species (81). Determination of the genomic DNA G + C content has therefore been included among the tests required for the definition of new mollicutes species (173). The values of moles percent G + C of mycoplasma genomes are available for essentially all of the new species defined in the last 10 years or so and for most of the species established earlier (20, 148, 185). With very few exceptions, the G + C content of mycoplasma genomes is within the range of 24 to 33 mol%. Interestingly, the G + C contents of the plant MLO DNAs examined so far fall also within the range of 23 to 29 mol% (79, 100, 166), supporting their inclusion within *Mollicutes*. The much lower G + C content of the MLO DNAs than of the DNAs of their plant or insect hosts has been most effectively exploited to separate the parasite from the host DNA by buoyant density centrifugation.

As in other procaryotes, some of the adenine and cytosine residues in mycoplasma genomes may be methylated (134). Use of the type of base methylated, the extent of methylation, and methylation sequence specificity as taxonomic markers has been suggested (127, 140). A relatively simple way to test methylation sequence specificity is by using pairs of restriction endonucleases (isoschizomers). These isoschizomers recognize the same site, but while one of the pair cleaves the DNA when cytosine or adenine is methylated, the other enzyme does not act. For example, *M. hyopneumoniae* DNA was found to resist digestion by *Mbo*I (recognition site GATC) but to be cleaved by its isoschizomer *Dpn*I (recognition site GmATC), indicating that the adenine at this sequence was methylated. The sensitivity of *M. flocculare* DNA to cleavage by *Mbo*I indicated that in this mycoplasma the GATC sequences are not methylated, suggesting the use of this procedure as a means of differentiating these genotypically related *Mycoplasma* species (25). The same approach was recently used by Bergemann et al. (13) to differentiate 22 strains belonging to the taxonomically problematic *M. mycoides* cluster. Strains of the bovine group 7 and the small-colony-type *M. mycoides* subsp. *mycoides* lacked methylated adenine at the GATC site, whereas the large-colony-type *M. mycoides* subsp. *mycoides* had it at this site. Results were less definite with regards to *M. capricolum* and *M. mycoides*, as some strains exhibited methylated adenine at the GATC site whereas others lacked it.

Spiroplasma species and strains could also be differentiated according to methylation patterns of their DNAs (127). Of special interest was the finding that *Spiroplasma* sp. strain MQ-1, isolated from the *Monobia* wasp, methylates cytosine only when it is 5' to guanine (CpG), a methylation trait considered unique to eucaryotes. The MQ-1 spiroplasma CpG methylase gene has recently been cloned and expressed in *Escherichia coli*. The enzyme product is of use in DNA modification studies on eucaryotic DNAs (153).

Another interesting observation with possible taxonomic implications is that of Cocks and Finch (36), who reported on a restriction endonuclease in *Ureaplasma urealyticum* T-960 (serotype 8) that cleaves at the sequence 5'-GC/NGC-3' and thus is an isoschizomer of *Fnu*4HI. While *Fnu*4HI cleaved DNA of serotypes 1, 3, and 6, it did not cleave DNA of serotypes 2, 4, 5, 7, 8, and 9, indicating that the DNA of the larger serotype cluster of *U. urealyticum* is modified at the sequence noted above. This finding adds an additional property for distinguishing strains belonging to the two genotypically different serotype clusters of *U. urealyticum*.

The data described above, together with the earlier findings showing different methylation patterns in two *Acholeplasma laidlawii* strains (45), support the use of DNA methylation patterns as fine tools for differentiating strains within a species, but they may be too sensitive to differentiate species.

DNA-DNA Hybridization

Complete nucleotide sequences of bacterial genomes would provide the most direct and valuable information for determination of the genetic relatedness among bacterial strains and would serve as the basis for establishing species. Although complete sequencing of the small mycoplasma genomes appears to be in the realm of the possible in the near future, we still have to settle for partial and indirect information derived from DNA-DNA and DNA-RNA hybridization tests, genomic cleavage patterns, and genomic maps, as well as rely on sequence comparison of specific genes and defined chromosomal segments. According to the ICSB's recommended criteria (81, 201), bacterial strains belonging to the same species should exhibit at least 70% DNA homology, while 60 to 70% homology justifies their separation into subspecies. Strains showing 20 to 60% homology can be described as separate but closely related species. Clearly, these criteria are, to a large extent, arbitrary, reflecting the ill-defined species concept as applied to procaryotes. Consequently, there is no reason to follow them blindly. We have examples in the mycoplasma literature of strains showing 60 to 70% DNA homology being placed in different species, mainly for practical reasons such as differences in ecology and pathogenicity. Thus, the honeybee pathogenic spiroplasma strains were given the species status *Spiroplasma melliferum*, although in DNA-DNA hybridization tests they exhibit between 60 and 70% homology to *S. citri* (20). On the other hand, the 14 human *U. urealyticum* serotypes fall within two genotypically distinct clusters, exhibiting over 75% DNA homology within each cluster but only 40 to 60% homology between clusters (29, 67). The two clusters differ also in genome size (156). Despite the formal justification for separating the clusters as two distinct species, or at least subspecies, this step has not yet been taken, given the lack of any definitive evidence that coining a new name will serve a useful purpose.

The taxonomic relationship of *M. capricolum* strains to the so-called F38 strains, the putative etiological agents of caprine pleuropneumonia, presents a similar problem but leads apparently to a different solution. In a collaborative study by several laboratories (R. H. Leach, J. G. Tully, D. L. Rose, F. Bonnet, C. Saillard, and J. M. Bové), DNA-DNA hybridization was applied to DNAs of four recently isolated *M. capricolum* strains and four F38-like isolates. Under high-stringency conditions, the *M. capricolum* isolates shared 84% DNA homology with the type strain of *M. capricolum* used as a probe, compared with values of 68 to 69% homology obtained for the F38 strains with use of the same *M. capricolum* probe. Although these hybridization data show a high degree of genetic homology between the

M. capricolum and F38 strains, approval was given by the Subcommittee at its meeting in 1990 to endow the F38 strains with the status of a subspecies of *M. capricolum*. The major reason for this taxonomic decision was to facilitate distinction of the pathogenic F38 strains from the nonpathogenic *M. capricolum* strains. This case illustrates the need to take into account practical considerations in taxonomic decisions. Taxonomy was required in this instance to refer to pathogenicity, so that veterinarians would be able to distinguish by name the pathogenic F38 strains.

Generally speaking, the DNA homology data support the present largely phenotypic classification of mycoplasmas into species (66, 175). However, DNA hybridization tests carried out on strains of some species, such as *M. hominis* (8), *A. laidlawii*, and *A. axanthum* (169), yielded homology values ranging from 50 to 100% for strains included in the same species. Clearly, we must accept the fact that some of the currently established species comprise strain clusters showing various degrees of relatedness. This is to be expected in light of our largely phenetic classification system and the pronounced genetic drifts brought about by a variety of means, as described below and in other chapters in this volume.

Cleavage Patterns and Genomic Maps

DNA-DNA hybridization tests are laborious and expensive. Consequently, simpler tests for assessing genetic relatedness were sought. Of these, restriction patterns of mycoplasmal DNA digested by restriction endonucleases have gained wide use. The patterns produced by electrophoresis of cleaved chromosomal fragments in agarose gels provide valuable information on the type and number of specific nucleotide sequences in the genome and can be considered genomic fingerprints, known also as restriction fragment length polymorphisms (RFLPs). After viral DNA chromosomes, mycoplasmal chromosomes were probably the first procaryotic genomes to be analyzed in this way. Bové and Saillard proposed the application of this technique to mycoplasmas at the first International Organization of Mycoplasmology meeting in 1976, the rationale being that because of the small size of the mycoplasma genome, the number of restriction fragments produced is relatively small, and even with enzymes like *Eco*RI which cut the mycoplasma genome in many sites, the electrophoretic patterns exhibit well-defined bands rather than smears (21).

The restriction patterns are particularly effective in determining genetic homogeneity or heterogeneity of strains within established mollicutes species (140, 145, 149). Thus, restriction patterns were instrumental in the separation of the *U. urealyticum* serotypes into two genotypic clusters (67, 145), distinguished also by DNA homology values (29, 67), cell protein profiles (119), genome size (156), and DNA modification patterns (36).

Further advancement in use of the genomic cleavage patterns as taxonomic tools was achieved by subjecting the DNA cleavage fragments, separated on an agarose gel, to Southern blot hybridization, with cloned conserved genes as probes. The rRNA genes of *M. capricolum* cloned in plasmid pMC5 (5) were the first to be used and are still the most popular probes. The fact that the rRNA operons of various mycoplasmas differ in restriction sites within the operon and in their flanking sequences (4, 74; also see chapter 10) leads to hybridization patterns peculiar to the different mycoplasma species, a finding used to identify mycoplasmas in infected cell cultures (144). As could be expected, the hybridization patterns with rRNA gene probes were effective in demonstrating genotypic heterogeneity among strains of species such as *U. urealyticum* (150), *M. hominis* (31, 218), *A. laidlawii* (218), *M. capricolum*, *M. mycoides* (32), *M. gallisepticum*, and *M. synoviae* (89, 219). Of special interest is the ability of this technique to distinguish the live vaccine strain F of *M. gallisepticum* from virulent field isolates in areas where vaccination with this strain took place (89, 219), indicating the value of hybridization patterns as epidemiological tools (Fig. 1). In contrast to the genotypic heterogeneity of the above-mentioned species, the hybridization patterns of *M. pneumoniae* strains isolated from pneumonia patients during different epidemics exhibited a remarkable degree of genotypic homogeneity (Fig. 2).

The rRNA genes can be replaced by other conserved genes as probes in the hybridization tests. A cloned segment of the ATPase (*atp*) operon from *E. coli* was effective in showing genotypic heterogeneity of *M. hominis* strains (30). Another conserved gene found useful for this purpose is the *tuf* gene, encoding the elongation factor protein Tu. We could show that the genome of mollicutes species carries only one copy of this important gene, compared with two copies in gram-negative bacteria (167, 224). The cloned *tuf* gene from *M. pneumoniae* exhibited a considerable degree

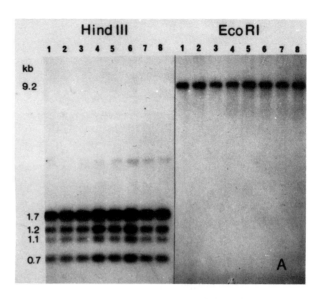

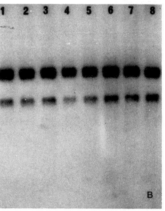

Figure 2. Hybridization patterns of DNAs from eight *M. pneumoniae* strains collected from different epidemics. (A) DNAs digested by *Hin*dIII or by *Eco*RI and hybridized with the rRNA gene probe pMC5 (from Yogev et al. [218]). (B) DNAs of the same strains digested by *Cla*I and hybridized with the elongation factor *tufA* gene of *E. coli* (from Yogev et al. [223]). The marked genotypic homogeneity of the strains can be seen.

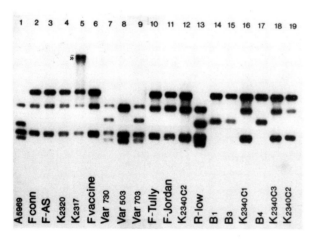

Figure 1. Hybridization patterns (RFLPs) of *Bgl*II-digested DNAs of *M. gallisepticum* strains with the rRNA gene probe pMC5. Four strain clusters can be observed. The largest cluster consists of the vaccine strain F obtained from different laboratories and the K strains isolated from chickens in areas where the F vaccine strain was used. The B cluster consists of strains isolated from hosts other than chickens. The third cluster, designated "Var," consists of atypical *M. gallisepticum* strains, and the fourth consists of the A5969 and pathogenic R-low strains. The extra band in lane 5 (marked by arrowheads) signifies incomplete digestion of the DNA. (From Yogev et al. [219].)

of sequence homology with *tuf* genes of other procaryotes, mitochondria, and chloroplasts (224). This finding enabled the use of the cloned *tufA* gene of *E. coli* as a probe for testing intraspecies genomic homogeneity in mycoplasmas (223). The hybridization patterns obtained revealed genotypic heterogeneity among *M. gallisepticum* strains and a high degree of genotypic homogeneity of the clinical isolates of *M. pneumoniae* (Fig. 2). The distinction among the *M. gallisepticum* strain clusters achieved by the *tuf* gene probe corresponded exactly with that obtained with use of the rRNA gene probe.

The Southern blot technique can also be used to assess for possible genetic relatedness between different species. In this case, labeled total DNA of one organism is hybridized with the electrophoresed digested DNA of the other. The appearance of hybridization bands other than those detected by the rRNA gene probe pMC5 indicates the presence of genomic sequences shared by the two organisms. In this way, the pairs *M. pneumoniae*-*M. genitalium* and *M. gallisepticum*-*M. synoviae* were shown to be genetically related (220, 221), while *M. pirum* showed no relatedness to either *M. pneumoniae* or *M. genitalium* (225).

The patterns produced by electrophoresis of chromosomal segments obtained by restriction enzyme digestion provide valuable information on the type and number of specific nucleotide sequences in the genome. The construction of genomic maps from such segments and the placement of gene loci on the map is the step which brings us closer to the final goal of complete sequencing and functional mapping of the entire genome. Physical genomic maps are now available for a number of mycoplasma species (12, 37, 38, 93, 116, 132, 133, 203, 204), and studies are now in progress to refine the maps by locating additional restriction sites and genes (for details, see chapter 9). The usefulness of genomic maps as taxonomic tools is obvious. For example, Pyle et al. (133) and Whitley et al. (207) constructed genomic maps of strains of the *M. mycoides* cluster. The number and order of all mapped restriction sites were fully conserved in the genomes of the small-colony-type *M. mycoides*, as were the approximate positions of several gene loci. A number of restriction sites appeared to be conserved in the large-colony Y strain of *M. mycoides*, and some but fewer appeared in the genome of the related PG50 strain. Similarly, Herrmann (69) applied as probes the cloned genomic fragments used for the construction of the genomic map of *M. pneumoniae* to compare six *M. pneumoniae* strains by RFLP. In this way, RFLPs were determined on about 150 *Eco*RI-generated DNA fragments. Although the results pointed to the same conclusion as that derived from hybridization experiments with the single-gene probes pMC5 and *tuf* (Fig. 2), they are much more dependable since they are based on comparison of a large number of restriction sites distributed over the entire genome. Nevertheless, use of subclones of the P1 adhesin gene of *M. pneumoniae* as probes in Southern blot analysis of 25 clinical isolates of *M. pneumoniae* revealed minor nucleotide variations in the P1 gene among the strains (39), demonstrating again the potential of RFLP analysis as an epidemiological tool.

Specific Genomic Sequences as Taxonomic Tools

At present, the nucleotide sequences of the highly conserved rRNA genes provide the best basis for determining phylogenetic relationships among bacteria. Their role in mycoplasma phylogeny is discussed in chapter 33. However, the 16S rRNA gene sequences of about 40 mollicutes species stored in GenBank (202) have already proved their effectiveness in the solution of a taxonomic problem. The sterol-requiring mycoplasma known as the PPAV mycoplasma, isolated from apple seeds over 10 years ago, has presented a taxonomic enigma, as it appeared to possess unique properties, precluding its assignment to any of the known genera. The solution came only when the sequence of its 16S rRNA gene was determined and compared with the sequences in GenBank (60). Unexpectedly, the sequence was found to be identical to that of *M. iowae*,

a chicken pathogen. The location from which the PPAV strain was isolated (apple seeds) and its lack of serological response with antiserum to the type strain of *M. iowae* explain the surprise with which the rRNA comparative data were received. Nonetheless, subsequent tests, including determinations of genome size, DNA restriction patterns, and cell protein profiles, have left no doubt about the identification of PPAV as *M. iowae*, an excellent illustration of the taxonomic potential of 16S rRNA gene sequences (60).

The number and arrangement of rRNA genes on the chromosome also have a taxonomic value. Hence, the recent finding that genomes of plant and insect MLOs carry only one or two copies of rRNA operons supports their inclusion in *Mollicutes* (88, 100). Besides, the primary sequence and secondary structure of the 16S rRNA of the MLOs are consistent with those of other mollicutes, the closest being the *Acholeplasma* and *Anaeroplasma* groups. However, the rRNA operons of the few MLOs examined so far carry a single tRNA^{Ile} gene in the spacer region between the 16S and 23S rRNA genes (88, 100), a feature not found so far in rRNA operons of the classical mollicutes (see chapter 10).

A field rapidly expanding is that of DNA probes for identification and diagnosis of mycoplasma infections (75, 126, 146). Considering the great difficulties in cultivating mollicutes and our total failure to cultivate the so-called MLOs, development of DNA probes specific for mycoplasma pathogens forms the most promising approach for rapid and accurate diagnosis of mycoplasma infections. In principle, the DNA probes consist of cloned genomic fragments of different sizes carrying sequences specific for a species or a strain, so that the probe will hybridize only with DNA of the target organism. The number of publications concerning DNA probes for mycoplasma detection and identification is mounting rapidly, particularly with the introduction of the polymerase chain reaction, which increases sensitivity considerably (14, 16, 17). Therefore, no attempt will be made to summarize the literature. Although DNA probes are important primarily as diagnostic means, they can also be used as sensitive taxonomic tools. For example, an oligonucleotide probe prepared by Blanchard (16) from a region upstream of the urease gene of *U. urealyticum* was found to recognize only the DNAs of the strains in one of the two genotypic strain clusters characterizing this species. The DNA probe can be selected in such a way as to distinguish a specific strain, such as the F vaccine strain of *M. gallisepticum*, which is hard to distinguish by routine serological means (85).

A Molecular Basis for Strain Variation

Our understanding of genotypic variability of strains within established mycoplasma species has been considerably advanced by recent studies on variability of mycoplasma surface antigens. Watson et al. (198) were the first to describe an immunodominant surface antigen, named V-1 to denote variability, in *M. pulmonis*, a mycoplasma infecting rats and mice. The antigen was shown to vary at a high rate (2×10^{-3} per cell per generation) among strains and within single subclones of the same strain (200). Analysis of 18 different *M. pulmonis* strains from different animal colonies and geographic locations showed that no two displayed identical immunoblot patterns for V-1 (200). The antigen was shown to be composed of subunits which may aggregate via hydrophobic interaction. The aggregates partially dissociate when exposed to harsh denaturing conditions, resulting in a characteristic ladder pattern in sodium dodecyl sulfate-polyacrylamide gel electrophoresis (199). Colony size variations correlated with changes in the electrophoretic properties of the V-1 surface antigen, indicating that variations in V-1 are reflected in alterations in surface properties of the organism (44). A structural variation in V-1 was the only protein difference detected between a virulent and an avirulent strain of *M. pulmonis*, suggesting the association of V-1 with virulence and disease severity (197). The V-1 antigen carries both conserved and variable epitopes, with the variable epitopes appearing to be immunodominant. The variability of V-1 resembles protein variations reported for other organisms, such as the pilus protein of *Neisseria gonorrhoeae* and the M protein of group A streptococci.

While the findings for the V-1 variable surface protein suggest that the rate of variation is too high to be explained by random mutational events, the genetic mechanism involved has not yet been elucidated. Analyses of antigenic strain variation, including the characterization of the membrane components and of the genetic mechanism governing variation, have recently been reported for *M. hyorhinis* (162). This swine pathogen carries on its surface lipid-modified protein antigens which spontaneously vary in size, contain highly repetitive structures, and are oriented with their carboxyl-terminal regions at the external membrane surface. The proteins are integral amphiphilic membrane lipoproteins, covalently bound to fatty acids through cysteine residues. As in the case of the *M. pulmonis* V-1 protein, the *M. hyorhinis* proteins undergo high-frequency, independent phase variations resulting in a highly diverse set of lipoprotein products. Phase variation of these surface proteins is reflected by changes in colony morphology and opacity (162). The genetic basis for this phase variation has recently been elucidated. It is based on rearrangements, deletions, and insertions into the chromosome of repetitive genetic structures (177, 222).

The highly variable surface protein antigens are apparently rather common in mycoplasmas. Thus, a repeating ladder protein pattern was seen in immunoblots of a *U. urealyticum* strain (24) and in *M. hominis* (33). The ability of a microorganism to rapidly alter its structural and antigenic surface mosaic provides versatility in the interaction of organisms with their environment. This fact may be relevant to an understanding of the survival of mycoplasmas for weeks, months, or even years in an immunocompetent host. As much as these findings are important for our understanding of mycoplasma pathogenicity, they have great relevance to taxonomy, as they define in molecular genetic terms strain variations detected by the variety of molecular tools employed in current taxonomy.

Metabolic Markers, Nutritional Requirements, and Cell Protein Maps

The present tendency to depend on direct genomic analysis, made available by the dramatic advancement of molecular genetics methodology, has put aside further development of classical taxonomic tools based on determination of nutritional requirements and enzymatic activities. Even the more recent cell protein profiles, obtained by one- and two-dimensional polyacrylamide gel electrophoresis (140), are used less frequently now than in the 1970s and early 1980s. The simple reason is that these profiles reflect the expression of specific genes and are thus liable to changes. It is now easier to clone and sequence the genes themselves. Nevertheless, cell protein profiles are still being used and can be effective in determining the genetic relatedness of strains (96, 183).

The same can be said regarding determination of metabolic activities. Glucose catabolism and arginine and urea hydrolysis are obligatory tests in identification of mollicutes. They are easy to perform and are key tests required to place an isolate within a genus or species. Considering the nutritional tests, determination of a cholesterol requirement still holds its key position in determining placement of a strain in the order *Acholeplasmatales* or in the anaerobic genus *Asteroleplasma* (140) (Table 1). Whether this test will retain its importance depends on the development of taxonomy based on phylogeny.

A practical problem arose concerning the current method for determination of a cholesterol requirement. In this method, cholesterol is added to a serum-free medium solubilized in Tween 80 (147). The final concentration of Tween 80 in the medium is 0.01%. Tween 80 serves both as a solubilizer of cholesterol and as a source for oleic acid. *Acholeplasma* species are expected to grow in serum-free medium with 0.01% Tween 80 but without cholesterol. However, the newly characterized *A. florum* and *A. seiffertii* species from flowers and plant surfaces (19, 110) and *A. entomophilum* from insects (188) failed to grow in the presence of 0.01% Tween, with or without cholesterol, and could therefore be mistaken for sterol-requiring mycoplasmas. Only an increase in the Tween 80 concentration to 0.04% enabled their growth in the absence of cholesterol, defining these mollicutes as acholeplasmas. Tween 80 at the higher concentration apparently provides an essential nutrient, most probably a fatty acid that is present as a contaminant. In any case, one should consider this possible pitfall when determining a cholesterol requirement by the standard method.

ECOLOGY

Prevalence of Mycoplasmas in Animals

The list of animals found to harbor mycoplasmas becomes longer each year (78, 79, 185, 186). It appears as though the main factor for adding an animal to the list is the willingness of a mycoplasmologist to invest the effort required to isolate and characterize mycoplasmas from the animal. The laboratory rabbit represents an exception to this rule, as it was found to be free of mycoplasmas. Lack of a natural mycoplasma flora makes the rabbit a preferred animal for production of specific antisera to mycoplasmas.

As the list of animal hosts becomes longer, so does the number of established mollicutes species (Table 1).

In the last report of the International Research Program on Comparative Mycoplasmology Working Team on Zoo and Wild Animals (79), one can find Dall sheep, elephants, lions, pumas, voles, shrews, Chinese hamsters, Norwegian rats, and seals added to the list of hosts harboring mycoplasmas. While in many cases the mycoplasmas isolated from new hosts represent new species, complete characterization of isolates lags behind, as the need to fulfill the minimal requirements for establishing new species (173) involves the performance of many tests. Particularly difficult is the requirement of serological differentiation of the new isolate from the other established species. A large battery of species-specific antisera and seed is needed for this task. For example, establishment of *M. oxoniensis*, a new species isolated from Chinese hamsters, involved, in addition to morphological, biochemical, and genomic characterization, the demonstration that it is serologically distinct from 94 *Mycoplasma* and *Acholeplasma* species (70). The mounting difficulties arising from the need to compare a new isolate serologically with a continuously growing number of antisera or strains of established species will probably be overcome by introduction of genomic sequence comparisons, such as comparison of the 16S rRNA gene sequence of the new isolate with the homologous gene sequences of established species stored in GenBank. This step has already been found very effective in identification of the apple proliferation mycoplasma as *M. iowae* (60).

Of current interest is the topic of aquatic mycoplasmas, that is, mycoplasmas of aquatic animals. The isolation of a motile and apparently pathogenic mycoplasma, named *M. mobile*, from the gills of a diseased tench by Kirchhoff et al. (86, 168) has raised hopes of opening a new field of fish mycoplasmas. Repeated trials by the same laboratory to isolate additional mycoplasma strains from fish have failed so far. Nevertheless, Kirchhoff's group has recently isolated and characterized two new species, *M. phocarhinis* and *M. phocacerebrale*, from harbor seals suffering from an acute and fatal disease (59). The question of whether mycoplasmas inhabit lower forms of aquatic animals cannot be answered as yet. Structures resembling mycoplasmas have been observed in tissues of oysters (68) and bryozoans (228). Boyle et al. (22) went further by reporting the isolation of an acholeplasma from the bryozoan *Waterispora arcuata*. Thin sections of the bryozoan tissues showed the presence of spherical structures larger than and different in ultrastructure from those of a classical acholeplasma. Unfortunately, since no sections of the cultured organism were presented, it cannot be compared with the structures observed in the bryozoan. Furthermore, the isolated organism was not deposited in any culture collection, a step essential for further characterization by mycoplasma laboratories.

Another debatable identification of structures as MLOs is that reported by Feely et al. (50). Transmission and scanning electron microscopy revealed structures resembling mycoplasmas on the surface of *Giardia* trophozoites from mammalian and avian hosts. Although some of the structures may well represent mycoplasmas, as long as no culture is available, one cannot be certain of their true nature.

Mycoplasmas in Nontypical Hosts and Tissues

Mycoplasmas usually exhibit a rather strict host and tissue specificity, probably reflecting their nutritionally exacting nature and obligate parasitic mode of life. However, there are numerous examples of the presence of mycoplasmas in hosts and tissues different from their normal habitats (53, 135). To cite some of the more recent examples, *M. salivarium*, a common human buccal mycoplasma, was detected in swine (49), and *A. oculi*, a goat mycoplasma, was isolated from the amniotic fluid of a woman (196). Strangely enough, a mycoplasma isolated from apple seeds was recently identified as *M. iowae*, an established avian pathogen (discussed above). How *M. iowae* got into the apple seed is open to speculation.

Less anecdotal and more directed is the case developed by Taylor-Robinson and his colleagues, showing that hormonal treatment renders animals susceptible to infection by mycoplasmas which the animals usually resist. Thus, estradiol treatment of female mice renders them susceptible to genital tract infection by the human mycoplasmas *M. hominis*, *M. fermentans*, *M. salivarium*, and *U. urealyticum* (54–56), and progesterone treatment rendered the mice susceptible to vaginal infection by *M. pneumoniae* and *M. genitalium* (180). The mechanism of induction of host susceptibility to infection by foreign mycoplasmas is still unclear. It could be due to abrogation of the local immune response or to a change in the vaginal epithelium. More expected, and with no need of hormonal treatment, is the susceptibility of nonhuman primates to infection with human mycoplasmas. *M. pneumoniae* was shown to infect chimpanzees and produce a respiratory disease, with development of cold agglutinins, respiratory symptoms, and X-ray findings very similar to those of primary atypical pneumonia in humans (7).

As to localization of mycoplasmas in nontypical organs, *M. pneumoniae*, long regarded as a pathogen with strict specificity for the tracheal epithelium of humans, has been recovered from joints of hypogammaglobulinemic patients as well as from joints of immunocompetent patients (40). This mycoplasma was also isolated from blister fluid of children suffering from Stevens-Johnson syndrome (170) and from the central nervous system (3, 195), suggesting that not all post-*M. pneumoniae* pneumonia sequelae affecting organs other than the lungs are due to an abnormal immune response (15). Thus, mycoplasmas and ureaplasmas belonging to the normal urogenital flora have been isolated from the blood of patients suffering from AIDS or treated with immunosuppressive drugs (128). Other reports concerned hypogammaglobulinemic patients who were susceptible to infections by *M. hominis* and *U. urealyticum* spreading into organs such as the respiratory tract and joints (154, 160, 181). The widespread use of immunosuppressive medication in patients undergoing organ transplantation and in immunocompromised AIDS patients has brought to light the possibility of outbreaks of infections by nonpathogenic mycoplasmas of the normal flora.

One of the most baffling riddles in mycoplasma ecology concerns the tissue location of *M. genitalium*. This mycoplasma, first isolated from the urethral discharge of two men with nongonococcal urethritis (NGU) (193), has attracted much attention because of its marked resemblance to *M. pneumoniae* and its apparent pathogenic potential (26, 151, 178). The fact that no *Chlamydia* strain or *U. urealyticum*, known bacterial agents of NGU, could be detected in about 30% of NGU patients responding favorably to tetracyclines pointed to the possibility that *M. genitalium* is responsible for these cases. Efforts invested by many laboratories to isolate more *M. genitalium* strains from the genital tract have met with failure. A possible explanation for this failure has recently been provided by Baseman et al. (10), who succeeded in isolating *M. genitalium* from 4 of 16 preserved throat isolates previously identified as *M. pneumoniae*. In fact, the tested specimens, kept at −70°C for over 15 years, were shown to consist of mixtures of *M. pneumoniae* and *M. genitalium*, so that isolation of single colonies was required prior to identification. Cell protein profiles and a specific monoclonal antibody to the 140-kDa adhesin of *M. genitalium* were used for identification. It should be stressed at this point that conventional serological techniques are not completely adequate to distinguish between *M. genitalium* and *M. pneumoniae*, since the two organisms share genomic sequences and epitopes (221). Consequently, differential diagnosis should employ either species-specific monoclonal antibodies or DNA probes (75).

Although the findings by Baseman et al. (10) suggested that the respiratory tract may be the preferred site of residence of *M. genitalium*, explaining the repeated failures to isolate this mycoplasma from the urogenital tract, the situation still remains blurred, as no additional data are available to support this suggestion. The highly fastidious nature of *M. genitalium* hampers its primary cultivation and indicates the advantage of using DNA probes to search for this mycoplasma. Application of the polymerase chain reaction to 150 genital tract specimens from 100 patients yielded positive results for 10 samples from 8 patients, suggesting the presence of *M. genitalium* DNA in these specimens (80). These studies are now being extended to respiratory tract specimens, and the results may solve the enigma concerning the location of *M. genitalium* in humans (187).

Cell cultures infected by mycoplasmas constitute an artificial unnatural habitat, a problem of great concern to researchers and biotechnology companies. The serious problems created by the persistent and hard to detect infections of cell cultures have produced a voluminous literature (113). Despite the much higher awareness of the need to prevent mycoplasma infections of cell cultures, the problem is still with us. Reports from various countries show that 10 to 87% of cell cultures are infected (18). The percentage of infected cell cultures depends to a large extent on the population of cell cultures assayed, on the control practices used, and on the efficiency of the assay procedure. The mycoplasma species infecting cell cultures have remained essentially the same throughout the years, *M. hyorhinis*, *M. orale*, *M. arginini*, and *A. laidlawii* being the dominant contaminants. Of interest is the relatively high percentage of *M. fermentans* (13% of the infected cultures) reported by Bolske (18), in light of the finding of this mycoplasma in AIDS and other fatal infections (see below). Uncultivable *M. hyorhinis* strains infecting cell cultures still constitute a diagnostic problem, although Kotani et al. (92) claim that the inclusion of freshly prepared yeast extract in mycoplasma media and an atmosphere of 5% CO_2 in air facilitate cultivation of *M. hyorhinis* from cell cultures. In the cell cultures examined by them, *M. hyorhinis* constituted 40% of the total mycoplasma isolates.

MLOs in Humans and Animals

The recent molecular evidence for identification of plant and insect MLOs as bona fide mycoplasmas in the absence of cultivation (see the following section) draws attention to the possibility that uncultivable pathogenic MLOs are also present in humans and animals. Mycoplasmalike structures have been repeatedly observed by electron microscopy in tissues of humans and animals suffering from a variety of diseases. In some cases, as in the AIDS patients examined by Lo et al. (104, 106), a mycoplasma was ultimately cultivated and was first considered a newly discovered species, *M. incognitus*, but later identified as a strain of the established species *M. fermentans* (165). But there is little doubt that not all members of the human mycoplasma flora have been identified. In fact, a new mycoplasma species, *M. spermatophilum*, isolated from the genital tract of patients with infertility problems, has very recently been characterized (71). Of particular interest is the recent finding of a new human mycoplasma in the urine samples of AIDS patients. This mycoplasma is distinct serologically and by DNA analysis from all other human mycoplasmas; it is characterized by being highly invasive and capable of penetrating cells following its attachment by a specialized tip structure (105). It appears that the common statement that human and animal mycoplasmas are exclusive extracellular parasites that cannot penetrate host cells should be revised (179).

Of current interest are the claims by Wirostko et al. (211) that MLOs cause uveitis, an inflammation of the ocular vascular coat in humans. The organisms were observed in the cytoplasm of leukocytes in biopsy specimens from patients with inflammatory orbital disease associated with juvenile rheumatoid arthritis (213) and Crohn's disease (83). In support of their thesis, Wirostko et al. reported the induction of chronic ocular and lethal cardiac vasculitis as well as of cataracts in mice inoculated with human biopsy specimens (82, 212, 214, 215). The lesions exhibited tissue lysis with infiltrates of MLO-parasitized leukocytes. In all cases, cultures from the biopsied material on mycoplasma media remained negative. While one should keep an open mind as to the possible involvement of uncultivable mycoplasmas in disease processes in humans, serious reservations were recently expressed in an editorial in *Lancet* (6a) as to the validity of the conclusions drawn by Wirostko et al. Accordingly, structures identified as MLOs in the sectioned leukocytes may be no more than normal leukocyte organelles. In their rebuttal, Wirostko and Johnson (210) claim that those familiar with bacterial and leukocyte ultrastructure should have no difficulty in distinguishing MLOs from leukocyte organelles. The claim by Wirostko et al. (211) that ocular diseases in humans and mice respond well to rifampin adds to the doubts about the MLO etiology, as all mycoplasmas tested so far are resistant to this drug. In fact, rifampin resistance has been listed as a property distinguishing mollicutes from other eubacteria (Table 2). The argument

Table 2. Molecular properties distinguishing mollicutes from eubacteria[a]

Property	Mollicutes	Eubacteria	Reference(s)
Cell wall	Absent	Present	135, 137
Peptidoglycan	Absent	Present	135
Genome size (kbp)	500–1,700	>1,500	124, 131, 156
Mol% G + C content of genome	23–41	25–75	20, 148
Detectable cell proteins	About 400	>1,000	84, 158
No. of rRNA operons	1–2	1–10	100, 138
5S rRNA length (nucleotides)	104–113	>114	159
No. of *tuf* genes	1	1 or 2	167, 224
RNA polymerase	Rifampin resistant	Rifampin sensitive	57
UGA codon usage	Tryptophan codon in *Mycoplasma*, *Spiroplasma*, and *Ureaplasma* spp. but not in *Acholeplasma* spp.	Stop codon	16, 43, 76, 77, 152, 172, 176, 217
DNA polymerase complex	One enzyme in *Mycoplasma* and *Ureaplasma* spp., three in *Acholeplasma* and *Spiroplasma* spp.	Three enzymes	109, 115

[a] Updated and modified from Razin (140).

brought up by Wirostko and Johnson (210) that rifampin may act in vivo but not in vitro, like sulfonamide, has no experimental support. In light of the recent successful experience gained with plant and insect MLOs (discussed below), an obvious way to solve the problem is to use a molecular approach to prove or disprove the presence of MLOs in the tissues of uveitis patients.

The degenerative central nervous system disorder Creutzfeldt-Jakob (CJ) disease appears to also fall in the category of infectious diseases of unknown etiology in which mollicuteslike structures have been observed. Spiral membranous inclusions were seen in the brain of a patient with CJ disease (61). The resemblance of these structures to spiroplasmas and the spongiform encephalopathy in rats inoculated intracerebrally with *S. mirum* have led to the suggestion that spiroplasmas may be associated with CJ disease. In the early 1980s, however, evidence was obtained that subviral prions are the etiological agents of CJ disease as well as of scrapie (130). It has been suggested that prions contain protease-resistant sialoglycoproteins that form fibrils responsible for the amyloid plaques in the brain. Interestingly, antibodies to the scrapie-associated fibril protein were shown by Bastian et al. (11) to cross-react with fibril protein purified from *S. mirum*. On the other hand, Leach et al. (96) failed to cultivate spiroplasma from CJ-diseased tissues, nor could they detect antibodies to spiroplasmas in patient sera. Similarly, Chastel et al. (27) could not demonstrate antibodies to five mosquito spiroplasmas in sera of patients suffering from CJ disease, multiple sclerosis, and Alzheimer's sclerosis. Moreover, Humphrey-Smith and Chastel (72) have reported that the spiroplasmalike structures observed in brain material from CJ patients are crystalline artifacts. It appears that the balance of evidence is not in favor of a spiroplasma etiology for CJ disease or other degenerative brain diseases.

The grey lung "virus" disease of mice (6) may represent another case of an animal MLO. The disease is a laboratory-induced pneumonia of mice, arising during attempted mouse passage of pneumonia material from other animals. The agent, which has thus far resisted cultivation, resembles mycoplasmas in thin sections of lung material and is sensitive to tetracyclines but not to penicillin. Leach and Mitchelmore (97), by using the commercial Gen-Probe, a DNA probe reacting with rRNA of mycoplasmas infecting cell cultures (114), obtained positive hybridization with lung wash fluids of grey lung-infected, but not control, mice. These positive results, obtained with a DNA probe of low specificity, are inconclusive but justify persistence with attempts to find a culture medium capable of growing the grey lung disease agent.

Mycoplasmas in Arthropods and Plants

Arthropods and plants are major habitats for the greatest variety of mollicutes, including the helical spiroplasmas, sterol-nonrequiring acholeplasmas, sterol-requiring mycoplasmas, and uncultivable MLOs. The rapidly advancing field of arthropod and plant mycoplasmas is extensively covered in volume 5 of *The Mycoplasmas* series (206).

The spiroplasma group is apparently one of the most abundant groups of microbes. About one new cultivable and one uncultivable putative *Spiroplasma* species are found for every 10 species of insects surveyed so far, and the number of insect species is estimated at 30 million (34, 63). Spiroplasmas have been reported from species of six evolutionary advanced insect orders: *Hymenoptera* (honeybees, wasps), *Coleoptera* (beetles), *Diptera* (flies, blood-sucking insects such as mosquitoes, tabanid flies, *Drosophila* spp.), *Lepidoptera* (butterflies, which feed on flower nectar), *Homoptera* (leafhoppers, which transmit the pathogenic spiroplasmas to plants), and *Hemiptera* (leaf bugs). Spiroplasmas have also been isolated from ticks, but we do not know whether spiroplasma occurrence relates to developmental stages of the tick or whether vertebrates play a role in maintaining the spiroplasmas in the ticks (63).

The taxonomy of spiroplasmas, the first of the arthropod and plant mollicutes to be cultivated, is the most advanced. The scheme for classification of spiroplasmas, based on genomic analysis and serology, at present includes 24 groups and 8 subgroups (79, 189, 194). Although each of these groups represents at least one species, taxonomic designation and species naming are lagging behind, following the restrictive policy (173) intended to prevent publishing binomial names with inadequate supporting data. New additions to the list of established *Spiroplasma* species (209) are nevertheless made continuously, with priority usually being given to species of economic importance. Some of the mosquito spiroplasmas have recently been named: *S. culicicola* (73), *S. sabaudiense* (1), and *S. taiwanense* (2). The occurrence of spiroplasmas in blood-sucking arthropods, such as ticks, tabanid flies, and mosquitoes, suggests the potential for their transmission to a variety of vertebrates, including humans. Whether spiroplasmas have any association with vertebrate infections is still unclear, but the question is important enough to receive further study, prompting the characterization and naming of the spiroplasmas isolated from arthropods.

Spiroplasmas are most frequently found in the insect gut, less frequently in the hemolymph, and occasionally in various organs such as the salivary glands. Spiroplasmas in the insect gut are generally acquired by natural feeding, either from plant tissue, from nectar, or from ingestion of other insects (209). Of interest is the frequent intracellular location of spiroplasmas in the gut or salivary gland cells. In contrast, animal mycoplasmas are usually extracellular parasites and can be found intracellularly when phagocytized. Still, it should be stressed that in leafhoppers, most spiroplasmas are in the hemolymph and not in cells.

Some spiroplasmas, like the honeybee spiroplasmas, are pathogenic and may kill their hosts, while others are considered commensals, even when present in large numbers in the hemolymph. Spiroplasmas involved in vector-transmitted plant diseases (citrus stubborn, corn stunt) must pass through a complex biological cycle that involves uptake from the sieve cells of the plant phloem and subsequent passage to or multiplication in the insect alimentary tract, gut epithelium, basement membrane, hemocoel, and possibly some internal organs. The organisms eventually pass from the hemocoel into the salivary cells and salivary duct, from which reinoculation of healthy plants takes place. Induction of disease in the plant is the rule. The symptoms in plants include chlorosis, leaf mottling, proliferation of growing points, and general stunting (194, 209).

Many of the spiroplasmas observed in the hemolymph of insects have resisted cultivation. Only recently, the sex-ratio spiroplasma of *Drosophila* spp., one of the first spiroplasmas to be described, was cultivated in vitro (65) following the principles leading to the successful cultivation of the Colorado potato beetle spiroplasma (64). To isolate this organism, the spiroplasmas were cocultivated with selected coleopteran and lepidopteran cell lines. Later, the spiroplasmas were adapted to grow in broth in the absence of cells (62). Following a similar approach, Yunker et al. (227) cultivated spiroplasma strains in continuous embryonic cell lines from ixodid ticks and mosquitoes. While the use of cocultivation of fastidious spiroplasmas with arthropod cell lines has proved itself in these cases, the choice of an adequate medium for primary isolation and/or subsequent sustained cultivation of these organisms is still much more an art than a science. However, all of the extensive knowledge and

techniques developed in primary isolation and cultivation of spiroplasmas have failed so far when applied to cultivation of the plant and insect MLOs (65a).

Mycoplasmas resembling classical animal mycoplasmas in shape were first reported on vegetable and floral plant surfaces in 1979 (46, 111). Some of these organisms were identified as established animal acholeplasmas (*A. axanthum* and *A. oculi*), while others were subsequently shown to represent new species (e.g., *A. florum*) known only from plant hosts (110). The ecological link between the acholeplasmas on plant surfaces and insect reservoirs was established by Clark et al. (35), who reported the isolation of sterol-nonrequiring mycoplasmas from insect guts. Some of these isolates were identified as *A. florum*, others were shown to belong to new species, *A. entomophilum* (188) and *A. seiffertii* (19), and still others await detailed characterization and taxonomic designation (186).

The insect gut flora also appears to carry sterol-requiring nonhelical mollicutes that by definition should be included in *Mycoplasmataceae*. Tully et al. have isolated a significant number of such strains from the guts and hemolymph of a wide range of insect species (186, 192). Three isolated from the guts and one isolated from the hemolymph of firefly beetles were recently characterized and named: *M. somnilux*, *M. luminosum*, *M. lucivorax* (208), and *M. ellychniae* (190). Two sterol-requiring mycoplasmas isolated from plant surfaces, *M. lactucae* (161) and *M. melaleucae* (191), also have been recently added to the list of established plant and insect mycoplasmas.

In addition to the insect and plant spiroplasmas, acholeplasmas, and mycoplasmas described above, there is a large group of insect and plant mollicutes designated MLOs. Members of this group were the first plant and insect mycoplasmas to be discovered (in the 1960s) (42) and are economically the most important group among the plant mycoplasmas. Over 300 MLO-associated plant diseases transmitted by insects have been described (111), but relatively little was known until recently about the properties of the causative agents, since none has been cultivated thus far.

A breakthrough in the characterization of the plant and insect MLOs was achieved with the recent application of molecular genetic methodology to MLO DNAs, separated physically from host DNA by bisbenzimide-CsCl buoyant density gradient centrifugation. Molecular analysis of the MLO DNAs revealed properties typical of the genome of the classical mollicutes: small size, low G + C content, and low number of rRNA gene copies. These properties, together with the ultrastructural features of MLOs, leave little doubt about the identification of these organisms as bona fide mollicutes. Moreover, the new data provide proof for the diversity of these organisms.

Values for genome sizes vary according to the origin of the MLO (101). The genome sizes of several tree-decline MLOs (western X-disease) and the beet leafhopper-transmitted virescence agent ranged from 640 to 675 kbp, while that of the severe aster yellows agent was about 1,185 kbp (88). Genome sizes of nonphytopathogenic MLOs, which apparently reside as symbionts in the gut of healthy insects, ranged from 500 to 550 kbp (123). The genome size of the maize bushy stunt MLO was estimated at 630 kbp, while genome sizes of the aster yellows and the periwinkle virescence

MLOs were estimated at 850 and 770 kbp, respectively (41).

Southern blot and dot hybridization tests with cloned MLO DNA probes have indicated the multiplicity of MLO species, confirming the diversity suspected from symptom expression, host plant range, vector transmission characteristics, and geographic distribution of MLO diseases. Serological studies with polyclonal and monoclonal antibodies as probes have yielded data that in general agree with the conclusions derived from the DNA hybridization tests (28, 58, 87, 99, 102, 229). Although information is still very limited and fragmentary, it appears that MLOs in woody plants, inducing proliferation and decline symptoms, are usually not closely related to the MLOs infecting herbaceous plants, inducing virescence symptoms (79). As with the classical mollicutes, there seem to be clusters of genotypically related MLOs. The aster yellows group appears to form a relatively large cluster. RFLP analysis is recommended for comparison of strains (99). Three groups were identified in the aster yellows strain clusters, each group with identical or very close RFLP patterns. An apple proliferation MLO DNA probe hybridized only with the homologous DNAs and with DNA of a few strains occurring in stone fruit species in Europe. The probe did not hybridize with DNAs of 16 MLOs from herbaceous hosts (79). Obviously, once the breakthrough in MLO research provided the tools, progress in this field has been extremely rapid; consequently, by the time this chapter is published, it may already be outdated.

CONCLUSION

Molecular genetic tools have provided the means for genotypic determination of strain identity, considerably improving mycoplasma taxonomy at the species level. Although phenotypic characteristics still retain their important role in mycoplasma taxonomy, we have reached the point where a mycoplasma can be identified on the basis of its DNA and rRNA structure. Analysis of genomic DNAs from the uncultivable MLOs was sufficient to provide the proof for their being bona fide mollicutes with great genotypic diversity.

Recent mycoplasma genome size determinations by PFGE have revealed that *Mycoplasma* and *Ureaplasma* species have genomes varying in size from 500 to 1,300 kbp, invalidating the previous doctrine that a genome size of 700 to 800 kbp is a determinative characteristic for a mycoplasma to be included in these genera. Nonetheless, most mycoplasmas can still be considered the organisms with the smallest reported genomes.

The day when complete sequences of the small mycoplasma genomes will be available is not too far away. The complete sequences would be the reference standard to determine phylogeny, leading us to the final goal of basing taxonomy on phylogeny.

REFERENCES

1. **Abalain-Colloc, M. L., C. Chastel, J. G. Tully, J. M. Bové, R. F. Whitcomb, B. Gilot, and D. L. Williamson.** 1987. *Spiroplasma sabaudiense* sp. nov. from mosquitoes collected in France. *Int. J. Syst. Bacteriol.* **37:**260–265.

2. **Abalain-Colloc, M. L., L. Rosen, J. G. Tully, J. M. Bové, C. Chastel, and D. L. Williamson.** 1988. *Spiroplasma taiwanense* sp. nov. from *Culex tritaeniorhynchus* mosquitoes collected in Taiwan. *Int. J. Syst. Bacteriol.* **38:**103–107.

3. **Abramovitz, P., P. Schvartzman, D. Harel, and Y. Naot.** 1987. Direct invasion of the central nervous system by *Mycoplasma pneumoniae:* a report of two cases. *J. Infect. Dis.* **155:**482–487.

4. **Amikam, D., G. Glaser, and S. Razin.** 1984. Mycoplasmas (*Mollicutes*) have a low number of rRNA genes. *J. Bacteriol.* **158:**376–378.

5. **Amikam, D., S. Razin, and G. Glaser.** 1982. Ribosomal RNA genes in mycoplasma. *Nucleic Acids Res.* **10:**4215–4222.

6. **Andrewes, C. H., and R. E. Glover.** 1945. Grey lung virus: an agent pathogenic for mice and other rodents. *Br. J. Exp. Pathol.* **26:**379–387.

6a.**Anonymous.** 1990. Do human MLO exist? *Lancet* **335:**1068–1069. (Editorial.)

7. **Barile, M. F., M. W. Grabowski, C. Graham, P. Snoy, and D. K. F. Chandler.** 1990. Experimentally-induced *Mycoplasma pneumoniae* pneumonia in non-human primates. *IOM Lett.* **1:**158–159.

8. **Barile, M. F., M. W. Grabowski, E. B. Stephens, S. J. O'Brien, J. M. Simonson, K. Izumikawa, D. K. F. Chandler, D. Taylor-Robinson, and J. G. Tully.** 1983. *Mycoplasma hominis*-tissue cell interactions: a review with new observations on phenotypic and genotypic properties. *Sex. Transm. Dis.* **10:**345–354.

9. **Barlev, N. A., and S. N. Borchsenius.** 1990. Gradual distribution of mycoplasma genome sizes. *IOM Lett.* **1:**238–239.

10. **Baseman, J. B., S. F. Dallo, J. G. Tully, and D. L. Rose.** 1988. Isolation and characterization of *Mycoplasma genitalium* strains from the human respiratory tract. *J. Clin. Microbiol.* **26:**2266–2269.

11. **Bastian, F. O., R. A. Jennings, and W. A. Gardner.** 1987. Antiserum to scrapie-associated fibril protein cross-reacts with *Spiroplasma mirum* fibril proteins. *J. Clin. Microbiol.* **25:**2430–2431.

12. **Bautsch, W.** 1988. Rapid physical mapping of the *Mycoplasma mobile* genome by two-dimensional field inversion gel electrophoresis techniques. *Nucleic Acids Res.* **16:**11461–11467.

13. **Bergemann, A. D., J. C. Whitley, and L. R. Finch.** 1990. Taxonomic significance of differences in DNA methylation within the *Mycoplasma mycoides* cluster detected with restriction endonucleases *Mbo*I and *Dpn*I. *Lett. Appl. Microbiol.* **11:**48–52.

14. **Bernet, C., M. Garret, B. de Barbeyrac, C. Bébéar, and J. Bonnet.** 1989. Detection of *Mycoplasma pneumoniae* by using the polymerase chain reaction. *J. Clin. Microbiol.* **27:**2492–2496.

15. **Biberfeld, G.** 1985. Infection sequelae and autoimmune reactions in *Mycoplasma pneumoniae* infection, p. 293–311. *In* S. Razin and M. F. Barile (ed.), *The Mycoplasmas*, vol. 4. *Mycoplasma Pathogenicity*. Academic Press, Inc., Orlando, Fla.

16. **Blanchard, A.** 1990. *Ureaplasma urealyticum* urease genes; use of a UGA tryptophan codon. *Mol. Microbiol.* **4:**669–676.

17. **Blanchard, A., M. Gautier, and V. Mayau.** 1991. Detection and identification of mycoplasmas by amplification of rDNA. *FEMS Microbiol. Lett.* **81:**37–42.

18. **Bolske, G.** 1988. Survey of mycoplasma infections in cell cultures and a comparison of detection methods. *Zentralbl. Bakteriol. Hyg. Reihe A* **269:**331–340.

19. **Bonnet, F., C. Saillard, J. C. Vignault, M. Garnier, P. Carle, J. M. Bové, D. L. Rose, J. G. Tully, and R. F. Whitcomb.** 1991. *Acholeplasma seiffertii* sp. nov., a mol-

licute from plant surfaces. *Int. J. Syst. Bacteriol.* **41**:45–49.

20. **Bové, J. M., P. Carle, M. Garnier, F. Laigret, J. Renaudin, and C. Saillard.** 1989. Molecular and cellular biology of mycoplasmas, p. 243–364. *In* R. F. Whitcomb and J. G. Tully (ed.), *The Mycoplasmas*, vol. 5. *Spiroplasmas, Acholeplasmas, and Mycoplasmas of Plants and Arthropods.* Academic Press, Inc., San Diego, Calif.

21. **Bové, J. M., and C. Saillard.** 1979. Cell biology of spiroplasmas, p. 83–153. *In* R. F. Whitcomb and J. G. Tully (ed.), *The Mycoplasmas*, vol. 3. *Plant and Insect Mycoplasmas.* Academic Press, Inc., New York.

22. **Boyle, P. J., J. S. Maki, and R. Mitchell.** 1987. Mollicute identified in novel association with aquatic invertebrate. *Curr. Microbiol.* **15**:85–89.

23. **Carle, P., O. Grau, C. Bové, and J. M. Bové.** 1990. Reports of consultations. International Research Program on Comparative Mycoplasmology, Istanbul.

24. **Cassell, G. H., H. L. Watson, D. K. Blalock, S. A. Horowitz, and L. B. Duffy.** 1988. Protein antigens of genital mycoplasmas. *Rev. Infect. Dis.* **10**:S391–S398.

25. **Chan, H. W., and R. F. Ross.** 1984. Restriction endonuclease analysis of two porcine mycoplasma deoxyribonucleic acids: sequence-specific methylation in the *Mycoplasma hyopneumoniae* genome. *Int. J. Syst. Bacteriol.* **34**:16–20.

26. **Chandler, D. K. F., M. W. Grabowski, H. Yoshida, R. Harasawa, S. Razin, and M. F. Barile.** 1990. Experimentally-induced *Mycoplasma pneumoniae* and *Mycoplasma genitalium* pneumonias in hamsters. *IOM Lett.* **1**:156–157.

27. **Chastel, C., F. LeGoff, J.-Y. Goas, J. Goaguen, G. Kerdaon, and A. M. Simitzis-LeFlohic.** 1990. Serosurvey on the possible role of mosquito spiroplasmas in central nervous system disorders in man, p. 910–911. *In* G. Stanek, G. H. Cassell, J. G. Tully, and R. F. Whitcomb (ed.), *Recent Advances in Mycoplasmology.* Gustav Fischer Verlag, Stuttgart.

28. **Chen, T. A., J. D. Lei, and C. P. Lin.** 1989. Detection and identification of plant and insect mollicutes, p. 393–424. *In* R. F. Whitcomb and J. G. Tully (ed.), *The Mycoplasmas*, vol. 5. *Spiroplasmas, Acholeplasmas, and Mycoplasmas of Plants and Arthropods.* Academic Press, Inc., San Diego, Calif.

29. **Christiansen, C., F. T. Black, and E. A. Freundt.** 1981. Hybridization experiments with deoxyribonucleic acid from *Ureaplasma urealyticum* serovars I to VIII. *Int. J. Syst. Bacteriol.* **31**:259–262.

30. **Christiansen, C., G. Christiansen, and O. F. Rasmussen.** 1987. Heterogeneity of *Mycoplasma hominis* as detected by a probe for *atp* genes. *Isr. J. Med. Sci.* **23**:591–594.

31. **Christiansen, G., and H. Andersen.** 1988. Heterogeneity among *Mycoplasma hominis* strains as detected by probes containing parts of ribosomal ribonucleic acid genes. *Int. J. Syst. Bacteriol.* **38**:108–115.

32. **Christiansen, G., and H. Erno.** 1990. Ribosomal RNA genes used in diagnosis of caprine mycoplasmas. *IOM Lett.* **1**:176–177.

33. **Christiansen, G., S. Mathiesen, S. Ladefoged, B. Brock, and S. Hauge.** 1990. Surface antigens of *Mycoplasma hominis. IOM Lett.* **1**:111–112.

34. **Clark, T. B.** 1982. Spiroplasmas: diversity of arthropod reservoirs and host-parasite relationships. *Science* **217**:57–59.

35. **Clark, T. B., J. G. Tully, D. L. Ross, R. Henegar, and R. F. Whitcomb.** 1986. Acholeplasmas and similar nonsterol-requiring mollicutes from insects: missing link in microbial ecology. *Curr. Microbiol.* **13**:11–16.

36. **Cocks, B. G., and L. R. Finch.** 1987. Characterization of a restriction endonuclease from *Ureaplasma urealyticum* 960 and differences in the deoxyribonucleic acid modification of human ureaplasmas. *Int. J. Syst. Bacteriol.* **37**:451–453.

37. **Cocks, B. G., L. E. Pyle, and L. R. Finch.** 1989. A physical map of the genome of *Ureaplasma urealyticum* T960 with ribosomal RNA loci. *Nucleic Acids Res.* **17**:6713–6719.

38. **Colman, S. D., P.-C. Hu, W. Litaker, and K. F. Bott.** 1990. A physical map of the *Mycoplasma genitalium* genome. *Mol. Microbiol.* **4**:683–687.

39. **Dallo, S. F., J. R. Horton, C. J. Su, and J. B. Baseman.** 1990. Restriction fragment length polymorphism in the cytadhesin P1 gene of human clinical isolates of *Mycoplasma pneumoniae. Infect. Immun.* **58**:2017–2020.

40. **Davis, C. P., S. Cochran, J. Lisse, G. Buck, A. R. DiNuzzo, T. Weber, and J. A. Reinarz.** 1988. Isolation of *Mycoplasma pneumoniae* from synovial fluid samples in a patient with pneumonia and polyarthritis. *Arch. Intern. Med.* **148**:969–970.

41. **Davis, M. J., M. Konai, and W.-C. Bak.** 1990. Electrophoretic separation of chromosomal DNA of mycoplasma-like organisms. *IOM Lett.* **1**:231–232.

42. **Doi, Y., M. Teranaka, K. Yora, and H. Asuyama.** 1967. Mycoplasma- or PLT group-like microorganisms found in the phloem elements of plants infected with mulberry dwarf, potato witches' broom, aster yellows or Paulownia witches' broom. *Ann. Phytopathol. Soc. Jpn.* **33**:259–266.

43. **Dudler, R., C. Schmidthauser, R. W. Parish, R. E. H. Wetterhal, and T. Schmidt.** 1988. A mycoplasma high-affinity transport system and the *in vitro* invasiveness of mouse sarcoma cells. *EMBO J.* **7**:3963–3970.

44. **Dybvig, K., J. W. Simecka, H. L. Watson, and G. H. Cassell.** 1989. high-frequency variation in *Mycoplasma pulmonis* colony size. *J. Bacteriol.* **171**:5165–5168.

45. **Dybvig, K., D. Swinton, J. Maniloff, and J. Hattman.** 1982. Cytosine methylation of the sequence GATC in a mycoplasma. *J. Bacteriol.* **151**:1420–1424.

46. **Eden-Green, S. J., and J. G. Tully.** 1979. Isolation of *Acholeplasma* spp. from coconut palms affected by lethal yellowing disease in Jamaica. *Curr. Microbiol.* **2**:311–316.

47. **Edward, D. G. ff., and E. A. Freundt.** 1956. The classification and nomenclature of organisms of the pleuropneumonia group. *J. Gen. Microbiol.* **14**:197–207.

48. **Edward, D. G. ff., E. A. Freundt, R. M. Chanock, J. Fabricant, L. Hayflick, R. M. Lemcke, S. Razin, N. L. Somerson, and R. G. Wittler.** 1967. Recommendation on nomenclature of the order *Mycoplasmatales. Science* **155**:1964–1966.

49. **Erickson, B. Z., R. F. Ross, and J. M. Bové.** 1988. Isolation of *Mycoplasma salivarium* from swine. *Vet. Microbiol.* **16**:385–390.

50. **Feely, D. E., D. G. Chase, E. L. Hardin, and S. L. Erlandsen.** 1988. Ultrastructural evidence for the presence of bacteria, viral-like particles, and mycoplasma-like organisms associated with *Giardia* spp. *J. Protozool.* **35**:151–158.

51. **Freundt, E. A.** 1958. *The Mycoplasmataceae (the Pleuropneumonia Group of Organisms): Morphology, Biology and Taxonomy.* Munksgaard, Copenhagen.

52. **Freundt, E. A., and D. G. ff. Edward.** 1979. Classification and taxonomy, p. 1–41. *In* M. F. Barile and S. Razin (ed.), *The Mycoplasmas*, vol. 1. *Cell Biology.* Academic Press, Inc., New York.

53. **Freundt, E. A., and S. Razin.** 1984. Mycoplasma, p. 742–770. *In* N. R. Krieg and J. G. Holt (ed.), *Bergey's Manual of Systematic Bacteriology*, vol. 1. Williams & Wilkins, Baltimore.

54. **Furr, P. M., C. M. Hetherington, and D. Taylor-Robinson.** 1989. The susceptibility of germ-free, oestradiol-treated, mice to *Mycoplasma hominis. J. Med. Microbiol.* **30**:233–236.

55. **Furr, P. M., and D. Taylor-Robinson.** 1989. The establishment and persistence of *Ureaplasma urealyticum* in oestradiol-treated female mice. *J. Med. Microbiol.* **29**:111–114.

56. **Furr, P. M., and D. Taylor-Robinson.** 1989. Ostradiol-induced infection of the genital tract of female mice by *Mycoplasma hominis. J. Gen. Microbiol.* **135:**2743–2749.

57. **Gadeau, A.-P., C. Mouches, and J. M. Bové.** 1986. Probable insensitivity of mollicutes to rifampin and characterization of spiroplasmal DNA-dependent RNA polymerase. *J. Bacteriol.* **166:**824–828.

58. **Garnier, M., G. Martin-Gros, M.-L. Iskra, L. Zreik, J. Gandar, A. Fos, and J. M. Bové.** 1990. Monoclonal antibodies against the MLOs associated with tomato stolbur and clover phyllody, p. 263–269. *In* G. Stanek, G. H. Cassel, J. G. Tully, and R. F. Whitcomb (ed.), *Recent Advances in Mycoplasmology.* Gustav Fischer Verlag, Stuttgart.

59. **Giebel, J., J. Meier, A. Binder, J. Flossdorf, J. B. Poveda, R. Schmidt, and H. Kirchhoff.** 1991. *Mycoplasma phocarhinis* sp. nov. and *Mycoplasma phocacerebrale* sp. nov., two new species from harbor seals (*Phoca vitulina* L.). *Int. J. Syst. Bacteriol.* **41:**39–44.

60. **Grau, D., F. Laigret, P. Carle, J. G. Tully, D. L. Rose, and J. M. Bové.** 1991. Identification of a plant-derived mollicute as a strain of an avian pathogen, *Mycoplasma iowae,* and its implications for mollicute taxonomy. *Int. J. Syst. Bacteriol.* **41:**473–478.

61. **Gray, A., R. J. Francis, and C. L. Scholtz.** 1980. Spiroplasma and Creutzfeld-Jakob disease. *Lancet* **ii:**152.

62. **Hackett, K. J.** 1990. Adaptational biology and spiroplasmas, p. 21–32. *In* G. Stanek, G. H. Cassel, J. G. Tully, and R. F. Whitcomb (ed.), *Recent Advances in Mycoplasmology.* Gustav Fischer Verlag, Stuttgart.

63. **Hackett, K. J., and T. B. Clark.** 1989. Ecology of spiroplasmas, p. 113–200. *In* R. F. Whitcomb and J. G. Tully (ed.), *The Mycoplasmas,* vol. 5. *Spiroplasmas, Acholeplasmas, and Mycoplasmas of Plants and Arthropods.* Academic Press, Inc., San Diego, Calif.

64. **Hackett, K. J., and D. E. Lynn.** 1985. Cell-assisted growth of a fastidious spiroplasma. *Science* **230:**825–827.

65. **Hackett, K. J., D. E. Lynn, D. L. Williamson, A. S. Ginsberg, and R. F. Whitcomb.** 1986. Cultivation of the Drosophila sex-ratio spiroplasma. *Science* **232:**1253–1255.

65a. **Hackett, K. J., and R. F. Whitcomb.** Personal communication.

66. **Harasawa, R., K. Dybvig, H. L. Watson, and G. H. Cassell.** 1991. Two genomic clusters among 14 serovars of *Ureaplasma urealyticum. Syst. Appl. Microbiol.* **14:**393–396.

67. **Harasawa, R., E. B. Stephens, K. Koshimizu, I.-J. Pan, and M. F. Barile.** 1990. DNA relatedness among established *Ureaplasma* species and unidentified feline and canine serogroups. *Int. J. Syst. Bacteriol.* **40:**52–55.

68. **Harshbarger, J. C., S. C. Chang, and S. V. Otto.** 1977. Chlamydiae (with phages), mycoplasmas, and rickettsiae in Chesapeake Bay bivalves. *Science* **196:**666–668.

69. **Herrmann, R.** 1990. Reports of consultations. International Research Program on Comparative Mycoplasmology, Istanbul.

70. **Hill, A. C.** 1991. *Mycoplasma oxoniensis,* a new species isolated from Chinese hamster conjunctivas. *Int. J. Syst. Bacteriol.* **41:**21–24.

71. **Hill, A. C.** 1991. *Mycoplasma spermatophilum,* a new species isolated from human spermatozoa and cervix. *Int. J. Syst. Bacteriol.* **41:**229–233.

72. **Humphrey-Smith, I., and C. Chastel.** 1988. Creutzfeldt-Jacob disease, spiroplasmas and crystalline artifacts. *Lancet* **ii:**1119.

73. **Hung, S. H. Y., T. A. Chen, R. F. Whitcomb, J. G. Tully, and Y. X. Chen.** 1987. *Spiroplasma culicicola* sp. nov. from the salt marsh mosquito *Aedes sollicitans. Int. J. Syst. Bacteriol.* **37:**365–370.

74. **Hyman, H. C., R. Gafny, G. Glaser, and S. Razin.** 1988. Promoter(s) of the *Mycoplasma pneumoniae* rRNA operon *J. Bacteriol.* **170:**3262–3268.

75. **Hyman, H. C., D. Yogev, and S. Razin.** 1987. DNA probes for detection and identification of *Mycoplasma pneumoniae* and *Mycoplasma genitalium. J. Clin. Microbiol.* **25:**726–728.

76. **Inamine, J. M., T. P. Denny, S. Loechel, U. Schaper, C. H. Huang, K. F. Bott, and P. C. Hu.** 1988. Nucleotide sequence of the P1 attachment-protein gene of *Mycoplasma pneumoniae. Gene* **64:**217–229.

77. **Inamine, J. M., K.-C. Ho, S. Loechel, and P. C. Hu.** 1990. Evidence that UGA is read as a tryptophan codon rather than a stop codon by *Mycoplasma pneumoniae, Mycoplasma genitalium,* and *Mycoplasma gallisepticum. J. Bacteriol.* **172:**504–506.

78. **International Research Program on Comparative Mycoplasmology.** 1988. Reports of consultations. Baden, Austria.

79. **International Research Program on Comparative Mycoplasmology.** 1990. Reports of consultations. Istanbul.

80. **Jensen, J. S., S. A. Uldum, J. Sondergard-Andersen, J. Vuust, and K. Lind.** 1991. Polymerase chain reaction for the detection of *Mycoplasma genitalium* in clinical samples. *J. Clin. Microbiol.* **29:**46–50.

81. **Johnson, J. L.** 1984. Nucleic acids in bacterial classification, p. 8–11. *In* N. R. Krieg and J. G. Holt (ed.), *Bergey's Manual of Systematic Bacteriology,* vol. 1. Williams & Wilkins, Baltimore.

82. **Johnson, L., E. Wirostko, and W. Wirostko.** 1988. Mouse lethal cardiovascular disease: induction by human leucocyte intracellular mollicutes. *Br. J. Exp. Pathol.* **69:**265–279.

83. **Johnson, L., E. Wirostko, and W. Wirostko.** 1989. Crohn's disease uveitis. Parasitation of vitreous leukocytes by mollicute-like organisms. *Am. J. Clin. Pathol.* **91:**259–264.

84. **Kawauchi, Y., A. Muto, and S. Osawa.** 1982. The protein composition of *Mycoplasma capricolum. Mol. Gen. Genet.* **188:**7–11.

85. **Khan, M. I., B. C. Kirkpatrick, and R. Yamamoto.** 1989. *Mycoplasma gallisepticum* species and strain-specific recombinant DNA probes. *Avian Pathol.* **18:**135–146.

86. **Kirchhoff, H., P. Beyene, M. Fischer, J. Flossdorf, J. Heitmann, B. Khattab, D. Lopatta, R. Rosengarten, and C. Yousef.** 1987. *Mycoplasma mobile* sp. nov., a new species from fish. *Int. J. Syst. Bacteriol.* **37:**192–197.

87. **Kirkpatrick, B. C., and D. A. Golino.** 1990. DNA characterizations of a plant-pathogenic mycoplasmalike organism for the establishment of evolutionary relationships. *IOM Lett.* **1:**223–224.

88. **Kirkpatrick, B. C., C. R. Kuske, P. O. Lim, and B. B. Sears.** 1990. Phylogeny of plant pathogenic mycoplasma-like organisms. *IOM Lett.* **1:**45–46.

89. **Kleven, S. H., G. F. Browning, D. M. Bulach, E. Ghiocas, C. J. Morrow, and K. G. Whithear.** 1988. Examination of *Mycoplasma gallisepticum* strains using restriction endonuclease DNA analysis and DNA-DNA hybridization. *Avian Pathol.* **17:**559–570.

90. **Klienenberger, E.** 1935. The natural occurrence of pleuropneumonia-like organisms in apparent symbiosis with *Streptobacillus moniliforms* and other bacteria. *J. Pathol. Bacteriol.* **40:**93–105.

91. **Klienenberger, E.** 1939. Studies on pleuropneumonia-like organisms: the L4 organism as the cause of Woglom's pyogenic virus. *J. Hyg.* (Cambridge) **39:**260–265.

92. **Kotani, H., G. H. Butler, D. Tallarida, C. Cody, and G. J. McGarrity.** 1990. Microbiological cultivation of *Mycoplasma hyorhinis. In Vitro Cell Dev. Biol.* **26:**91–96.

93. **Krause, D. C., and C. B. Mawn.** 1990. Physical analysis and mapping of the *Mycoplasma pneumoniae* chromosome. *J. Bacteriol.* **172:**4790–4797.

94. **Ladefoged, S., B. Brock, and G. Christiansen.** 1990. Physical and genetic maps of the genome of five strains of *Mycoplasma hominis. IOM Lett.* **1:**253–254.

95. **Leach, R. H., M. Costas, and D. L. Mitchelmore.** 1989.

Relationship between *Mycoplasma mycoides* subsp. *mycoides* ('large-colony' strains) and *M. mycoides* subsp. *capri*, as indicated by numerical analysis of one-dimensional SDS-PAGE protein patterns. *J. Gen. Microbiol.* **135:**2993–3000.

96. **Leach, R. H., W. B. Matthes, and R. Will.** 1983. Creutzfeldt-Jacob disease: failure to detect spiroplasmas by cultivation and serological tests. *J. Neurol. Sci.* **59:**349–353.

97. **Leach, R. H., and D. L. Mitchelmore.** 1990. Grey lung "virus" of mice—an animal MLO? *IOM Lett.* **1:**393–394.

98. **Lederberg, J., and J. St. Clair.** 1958. Protoplasts and L-type growth of *Escherichia coli. J. Bacteriol.* **75:**143–160.

99. **Lee, I. M., and R. E. Davis.** 1990. Identification of distinct strain clusters among uncultured mycoplasmalike organisms from plants. *IOM Lett.* **1:**234–235.

100. **Lim, P. O., and B. B. Sears.** 1989. 16S rRNA sequence indicates that plant-pathogenic mycoplasmalike organisms are evolutionary distinct from animal mycoplasmas. *J. Bacteriol.* **171:**5901–5906.

101. **Lim, P.-O., and B. B. Sears.** 1991. Genome size of a plant-pathogenic mycoplasmalike organism resembles those of animal mycoplasmas. *J. Bacteriol.* **173:**2128–2130.

102. **Lin, C.-P., and T. A. Chen.** 1985. Monoclonal antibodies against the aster yellows agent. *Science* **227:**1233–1235.

103. **Lo, S.-C.** 1986. Isolation and identification of a novel virus from patients with AIDS. *Am. J. Trop. Med. Hyg.* **35:**675–676.

104. **Lo, S.-C., M. S. Dawson, D. M. Wong, P. B. Newton III, M. A. Sonoda, W. F. Engler, R. Y.-H. Wang, J. W.-K. Shih, H. J. Alter, and D. J. Wear.** 1989. Identification of *Mycoplasma incognitus* infection in patients with AIDS: an immunohistochemical, in situ hybridization and ultrastructural study. *Am. J. Trop. Med. Hyg.* **41:**601–605.

105. **Lo, S.-C., M. M. Hayes, R. Y.-H. Wang, P. F. Pierce, H. Kotani, and J. W.-K. Shih.** 1991. Newly discovered mycoplasma isolated from patients infected with HIV. *Lancet* **338:**1415–1418.

106. **Lo, S.-C., J. W.-K. Shih, P. B. Newton III, D. M. Wong, M. M. Hayes, J. R. Benish, D. J. Wear, and R. Y.-H. Wang.** 1989. Virus-like infectious agent (VLIA) is a novel pathogenic mycoplasma: *Mycoplasma incognitus. Am. J. Trop. Med. Hyg.* **41:**586–600.

107. **Maniloff, J.** 1983. Evolution of wall-less prokaryotes. *Annu. Rev. Microbiol.* **37:**477–499.

108. **Maniloff, J.** 1989. Anomalous values of *Mycoplasma* genome sizes determined by pulse-field gel electrophoresis. *Nucleic Acids Res.* **17:**1268.

109. **Maurel, D., A. Charron, and C. Bébéar.** 1989. Mollicutes DNA polymerases: characterization of a single enzyme from *Mycoplasma mycoides* and *Ureaplasma urealyticum* and three enzymes from *Acholeplasma laidlawii. Res. Microbiol. Inst. Pasteur* **140:**191–205.

110. **McCoy, R. E., H. G. Basham, J. G. Tully, D. L. Rose, P. Carle, and J. M. Bové.** 1984. *Acholeplasma florum*, a new species isolated from plants. *Int. J. Syst. Bacteriol.* **34:**11–15.

111. **McCoy, R. E., A. Caudwell, C. J. Chang, T. A. Chen, L. N. Chiykowski, M. T. Cousin, J. L. Dale, G. T. N. de Leeuw, D. A. Golino, K. J. Hackett, B. C. Kirkpatrick, R. Marwitz, H. Petzold, R. C. Sinha, M. Sugiura, R. F. Whitcomb, I. L. Yang, B. M. Zhu, and E. Seemuller.** 1989. Plant diseases associated with mycoplasma-like-organisms, p. 545–640. *In* R. F. Whitcomb and J. G. Tully (ed.), *The Mycoplasmas*, vol. 5. *Spiroplasmas, Acholeplasmas, and Mycoplasmas of Plants and Arthropods.* Academic Press, Inc., San Diego, Calif.

112. **McCoy, R. E., D. S. Williams, and D. L. Thomas.** 1979. Isolation of mycoplasmas from flowers, p. 75–81. *In* J. Su and R. E. McCoy (ed.), *Proceedings of the Republic of China-United States Cooperative Science Seminar on Mycoplasma Diseases of Plants.* National Science Council Symposium Series no. 1. National Science Council, Taipei, Taiwan.

113. **McGarrity, G. J., and H. Kotani.** 1985. Cell culture mycoplasmas, p. 353–390. *In* S. Razin and M. F. Barile (ed.), *The Mycoplasmas*, vol. 4. *Mycoplasma Pathogenicity.* Academic Press, Inc., Orlando, Fla.

114. **McGarrity, G. J., and H. Kotani.** 1986. Detection of cell culture mycoplasmas by a genetic probe. *Exp. Cell Res.* **163:**273–278.

115. **Mills, L. B., E. J. Stanbridge, W. D. Sedwick, and D. Korn.** 1977. Purification and partial characterization of the principal deoxyribonucleic acid polymerase from *Mycoplasmatales. J. Bacteriol.* **132:**641–649.

116. **Miyata, M., L. Wang, and T. Fukumura.** 1991. Physical mapping of the *Mycoplasma capricolum* genome. *FEMS Microbiol. Lett.* **79:**329–334.

117. **Morowitz, H. J.** 1984. The completeness of molecular biology. *Isr. J. Med. Sci.* **20:**750–753.

118. **Morowitz, H. J., and D. C. Wallace.** 1973. Genome size and life cycle of the mycoplasma. *Ann. N.Y. Acad. Sci.* **225:**63–73.

119. **Mouches, C., D. Taylor-Robinson, L. Stipkovits, and J. M. Bové.** 1981. Comparison of human and animal ureaplasmas by one and two-dimensional protein analysis on polyacrylamide slab gel. *Ann. Microbiol. (Inst. Pasteur)* **132B:**171–196.

120. **Murray, R. G. E.** 1984. The higher taxa, or, a place for everything . . . ?, p. 31–34. *In* N. R. Krieg and J. G. Holt (ed.), *Bergey's Manual of Systematic Bacteriology*, vol. 1. Williams & Wilkins, Baltimore.

121. **Murray, R. G. E., D. J. Brenner, R. R. Colwell, P. De Vos, M. Goodfellow, P. A. D. Grimont, N. Pfennig, E. Stackebrandt, and A. Zvarzin.** 1990. Report of the ad hoc committee on approaches to taxonomy within the proteobacteria. *Int. J. Syst. Bacteriol.* **40:**213–215.

122. **Neimark, H. C.** 1986. Origins and evolution of wall-less prokaryotes, p. 21–42. *In* S. Madoff (ed.), *The Bacterial L-Forms.* Marcel Dekker Inc., New York.

123. **Neimark, H., and B. C. Kirkpatrick.** 1990. Isolation and size estimation of whole chromosomes from mycoplasma-like organisms. *IOM Lett.* **1:**574–575.

124. **Neimark, H. C., and C. S. Lange.** 1990. Pulse-field electrophoresis indicates full-length mycoplasma chromosomes range widely in size. *Nucleic Acids Res.* **18:**5443–5448.

125. **Nocard, E., and E. R. Roux.** 1898. Le microbe de la peripneumonie. *Ann. Inst. Pasteur Paris* **12:**240–262.

126. **Nur, I., A. Reinhartz, H. C. Hyman, S. Razin, and M. Herzberg.** 1989. Chemiprobe™, a nonradioactive system for labeling nucleic acid: principles and applications. *Ann. Biol. Clin.* **47:**601–606.

127. **Nur, I., M. Szyf, A. Razin, G. Glaser, S. Rottem, and S. Razin.** 1985. Procaryotic and eucaryotic traits of DNA methylation in spiroplasmas (mycoplasmas). *J. Bacteriol.* **164:**19–24.

128. **Parides, G. C., J. W. Bloom, N. M. Ampel, and C. G. Ray.** 1988. Mycoplasma and ureaplasma in bronchoalveolar lavage fluids from immunocompromised hosts. *Diagn. Microbiol. Infect. Dis.* **9:**55–57.

129. **Ploaie, P. G.** 1990. Aster Yellows Agent (AYA), a L-phase variant of myxobacteria cultivated on artificial media. *IOM Lett.* **1:**576–577.

130. **Prusiner, S. B.** 1987. Prions and neurodegenerative diseases. *N. Engl. J. Med.* **317:**1571–1581.

131. **Pyle, L. E., L. N. Corcoran, B. G. Cocks, A. D. Bergemann, J. C. Whitley, and L. R. Finch.** 1988. Pulsed-field electrophoresis indicates larger-than-expected sizes for mycoplasma genomes. *Nucleic Acids Res.* **16:**6015–6025.

132. **Pyle, L. E., and L. R. Finch.** 1988. The physical map of the genome of *Mycoplasma mycoides* subspecies *mycoides* Y with some functional loci. *Nucleic Acids Res.* **16:**6027–6039.

133. **Pyle, L. E., T. Taylor, and L. R. Finch.** 1990. Genomic

maps of some strains within the *Mycoplasma mycoides* cluster. *J. Bacteriol.* **172:**7265–7268.

134. **Razin, A., and S. Razin.** 1980. Methylated bases in mycoplasmal DNA. *Nucleic Acids Res.* **8:**1383–1390.

135. **Razin, S.** 1969. Structure and function in mycoplasma. *Annu. Rev. Microbiol.* **23:**317–356.

136. **Razin, S.** 1978. The mycoplasmas. *Microbiol. Rev.* **42:**414–470.

137. **Razin, S.** 1981. The mycoplasma membrane, p. 165–250. *In* B. K. Ghosh (ed.), *Organization of Prokaryotic Cell Membranes*, vol. I. CRC Press, Inc., Boca Raton, Fla.

138. **Razin, S.** 1985. Molecular biology and genetics of mycoplasmas (*Mollicutes*). *Microbiol. Rev.* **49:**419–455.

139. **Razin, S.** 1987. Appealing attributes of mycoplasmas in cell biology research. *Isr. J. Med. Sci.* **23:**318–325.

140. **Razin, S.** 1989. The molecular approach to mycoplasma phylogeny, p. 33–69. *In* R. F. Whitcomb and J. G. Tully (ed.), *The Mycoplasmas*, vol. 5. *Spiroplasmas, Acholeplasmas, and Mycoplasmas of Plants and Arthropods.* Academic Press, Inc., San Diego, Calif.

141. **Razin, S.** 1992. The genera *Mycoplasma, Ureaplasma, Acholeplasma, Anaeroplasma,* and *Asteroleplasma,* p. 1937–1959. *In* A. Balows, H. G. Truper, M. Dworkin, W. Harder, and K.-H. Schleifer (ed.), *The Prokaryotes*, 2nd ed., vol. 2. Springer-Verlag, New York.

142. **Razin, S., M. F. Barile, R. Harasawa, D. Amikam, and G. Glaser.** 1983. Characterization of the mycoplasma genome. *Yale J. Biol. Med.* **56:**357–366.

143. **Razin, S., and E. A. Freundt.** 1984. The *Mollicutes, Mycoplasmatales* and *Mycoplasmataceae,* p. 740–742. *In* N. R. Krieg and J. G. Holt (ed.), *Bergey's Manual of Systematic Bacteriology*, vol. 1. Williams & Wilkins, Baltimore.

144. **Razin, S., M. Gross, M. Wormser, Y. Pollack, and G. Glaser.** 1984. Detection of mycoplasmas infecting cell cultures by DNA hybridization. *In Vitro* **20:**404–408.

145. **Razin, S., R. Harasawa, and M. F. Barile.** 1983. Cleavage patterns of the mycoplasma chromosomes, obtained by using restriction endonucleases as indicators of genetic relatedness among strains. *Int. J. Syst. Bacteriol.* **33:**201–206.

146. **Razin, S., H. C. Hyman, I. Nur, and D. Yogev.** 1987. DNA probes for detection and identification of mycoplasmas (Mollicutes). *Isr. J. Med. Sci.* **23:**735–741.

147. **Razin, S., and J. G. Tully.** 1970. Cholesterol requirement of mycoplasmas. *J. Bacteriol.* **102:**306–310.

148. **Razin, S., and J. G. Tully.** 1983. Appendix, p. 495–499. *In* S. Razin and J. G. Tully (ed.), *Methods in Mycoplasmology*, vol. 1. Academic Press, Inc. New York.

149. **Razin, S., J. G. Tully, D. L. Rose, and M. F. Barile.** 1983. DNA cleavage patterns as indicators of genotypic heterogeneity among strains of *Acholeplasma* and *Mycoplasma* species. *J. Gen. Microbiol.* **129:**1935–1944.

150. **Razin, S., and D. Yogev.** 1986. Genetic relatedness among *Ureaplasma urealyticum* serotypes (serovars). *Pediatr. Infect. Dis.* **5:**S300–S304.

151. **Razin, S., and D. Yogev.** 1989. Molecular approaches to characterization of mycoplasmal adhesins, p. 52–76. *In* L. Switalski, M. Hook, and E. H. Beachy (ed.), *Molecular Mechanisms of Microbial Adhesion.* Springer-Verlag, New York.

152. **Renaudin, J., M. C. Pascarel, C. Saillard, C. Chevalier, and J. M. Bové.** 1986. In spiroplasmas, UGA is not a termination codon but seems to code for tryptophan. *C.R. Acad. Sci. Paris Ser. III* **303:**539–540.

153. **Renbaum, P., D. Abrahamove, A. Fainsod, G. G. Wilson, S. Rottem, and A. Razin.** 1990. Cloning, characterization and expression in *Escherichia coli* of the gene coding for the CpG DNA methylation from *Spiroplasma* sp. strain MQ1 (M.SssI). *Nucleic Acids Res.* **18:**1145–1152.

154. **Roberts, D., A. E. Murray, B. C. Pratt, and R. E. Meigh.** 1989. *Mycoplasma hominis* as a respiratory pathogen in X-linked hypogammaglobulinaemia. *J. Infect.* **18:**175–177.

155. **Robertson, J. A., L. E. Pyle, J. Kakulphimp, G. W. Stemke, and L. R. Finch.** 1990. The genomes of the genus *Ureaplasma. IOM Lett.* **1:**72–73.

156. **Robertson, J. A., L. E. Pyle, G. W. Stemke, and L. R. Finch.** 1990. Human ureaplasmas show diverse genome sizes by pulse-field electrophoresis. *Nucleic Acids Res.* **18:**1451–1455.

157. **Robinson, I. M.** 1984. Genus *Anaeroplasma,* p. 787–790. *In* N. R. Krieg and J. G. Holt (ed.), *Bergey's Manual of Systematic Bacteriology*, vol. 1. Williams & Wilkins, Baltimore.

158. **Rodwell, A. W.** 1982. The protein fingerprints of mycoplasmas. *Rev. Infect. Dis.* **4**(Suppl.):S8–S17.

159. **Rogers, M. J., J. Simmons, R. T. Walker, W. G. Weisburg, C. R. Woese, R. S. Tanner, I. M. Robinson, D. A. Stahl, G. Olsen, R. H. Leach, and J. Maniloff.** 1985. Construction of the mycoplasma evolutionary tree from 5S rRNA sequence data. *Proc. Natl. Acad. Sci. USA* **82:**1160–1164.

160. **Roifman, C. M., C. P. Rao, H. M. Lederman, S. Lavis, P. Quinn, and E. W. Gelfand.** 1986. Increased susceptibility to mycoplasma infection in patients with hypogammaglobulinemia. *Am. J. Med.* **80:**590–594.

161. **Rose, D. L., J. P. Kocka, N. L. Somerson, J. G. Tully, R. F. Whitcomb, P. Carle, J. M. Bové, D. E. Colflesh, and D. L. Williamson.** 1990. *Mycoplasma lactucae* sp. nov., a sterol-requiring mollicute from a plant surface. *Int. J. Syst. Bacteriol.* **40:**138–142.

162. **Rosengarten, R., and K. S. Wise.** 1990. Phenotypic switching in mycoplasmas: phase variation of diverse surface lipoproteins. *Science* **247:**315–318.

163. **Sabin, A. B.** 1941. The filtrable micro-organisms of the pleuropneumonia group. *Bacteriol. Rev.* **5:**1–65.

164. **Sabin, A. B.** 1941. The filtrable micro-organisms of the pleuropneumonia group (appendix on classification and nomenclature). *Bacteriol. Rev.* **5:**331–335.

165. **Saillard, C., P. Carle, J. M. Bové, C. Bébéar, S.-C. Lo, J. W.-K. Shih, R. Y.-H. Wang, D. L. Rose, and J. G. Tully.** 1990. Genetic and serologic relatedness between *Mycoplasma fermentans* strains and a mycoplasma recently identified in tissues of AIDS and non-AIDS patients. *Res. Virol.* **141:**385–395.

166. **Sears, B. B., P. Lim, N. Holland, and K. L. Klomparens.** 1990. DNA characterization of a plant-pathogenic mycoplasmalike organism for the establishment of evolutionary relationships. *IOM Lett.* **1:**233.

167. **Sela, S., D. Yogev, S. Razin, and H. Bercovier.** 1989. Duplication of the *tuf* gene: a new insight into the phylogeny of eubacteria. *J. Bacteriol.* **171:**581–584.

168. **Städtlander, C., and H. Kirchhoff.** 1990. Surface parasitism of the fish mycoplasma *Mycoplasma mobile* 163 K on tracheal epithelial cells. *Vet. Microbiol.* **21:**339–343.

169. **Stephens, E. B., G. S. Aulakh, D. L. Rose, J. G. Tully, and M. F. Barile.** 1983. Intraspecies genetic relatedness among strains of *Acholeplasma laidlawii* and of *Acholeplasma axanthum* by nucleic acid hybridization. *J. Gen. Microbiol.* **129:**1929–1934.

170. **Stutman, H. R.** 1987. Stevens-Johnson syndrome and *Mycoplasma pneumoniae:* evidence for cutaneous infection. *J. Pediatr.* **111:**845–847.

171. **Su, C. J., and J. B. Baseman.** 1990. Genome size of *Mycoplasma genitalium. J. Bacteriol.* **172:**4705–4707.

172. **Su, C. J., V. V. Tryon, and J. B. Baseman.** 1987. Cloning and sequence analysis of cytadhesin P1 gene from *Mycoplasma pneumoniae. Infect. Immun.* **55:**3023–3029.

173. **Subcommittee on the Taxonomy of *Mollicutes*.** 1979. Proposal of minimal standards for descriptions of new species of the class *Mollicutes. Int. J. Syst. Bacteriol.* **29:**172–180.

174. **Subcommittee on the Taxonomy of *Mollicutes*.** 1984.

Minutes of the 1980 meeting in Custer, S. D. *Int. J. Syst. Bacteriol.* **34**:358–360.

175. **Sugino, W. M., R. C. Wek, and D. T. Kingsbury.** 1980. Partial nucleotide sequence similarity within species of *Mycoplasma* and *Acholeplasma. J. Gen. Microbiol.* **121**:333–338.

176. **Tanaka, R., A. Muto, and S. Osawa.** 1989. Nucleotide sequence of tryptophan tRNA gene in *Acholeplasma laidlawii. Nucleic Acids Res.* **17**:5842.

177. **Taylor, M. A., R. V. Ferrell, K. S. Wise, and M. A. McIntosh.** 1988. Reiterated DNA sequences defining genomic diversity within the species *Mycoplasma hyorhinis. Mol. Microbiol.* **2**:665–672.

178. **Taylor-Robinson, D.** 1985. Mycoplasmal and mixed infections of the human male urogenital tract and their possible complications, p. 27–63. *In* S. Razin and M. F. Barile (ed.), *The Mycoplasmas*, vol. 4. *Mycoplasma Pathogenicity.* Academic Press, Inc., Orlando, Fla.

179. **Taylor-Robinson, D., H. A. Davis, P. Sarathchandra, and P. M. Furr.** 1991. Intracellular location of mycoplasmas in cultured cells demonstrated by immunochemistry and electron microscopy. *Int. J. Exp. Pathol.* **72**:705–714.

180. **Taylor-Robinson, D., and P. M. Furr.** 1990. Hormones influence genital mycoplasma infections. *IOM Lett.* **1**:63–64.

181. **Taylor-Robinson, D., P. M. Furr, and A. D. B. Webster.** 1986. *Ureaplasma urealyticum* in the immunocompromised host. *Pediatr. Infect. Dis.* **5**:S236–S238.

182. **Taylor-Robinson, D., and R. N. Gourlay.** 1984. *Ureaplasma*, p. 770–775. *In* N. R. Krieg and J. G. Holt (ed.), *Bergey's Manual of Systematic Bacteriology*, vol. 1. Williams & Wilkins, Baltimore.

183. **Thirkell, D., R. K. Spooner, G. E. Jones, and W. C. Russell.** 1990. Polypeptide and antigenic variability among strains of *Mycoplasma ovipneumoniae* demonstrated by SDS-PAGE and immunoblotting. *Vet. Microbiol.* **21**:241–254.

184. **Tully, J. G.** 1984. Family II. *Acholeplasmataceae*, p. 775–781. *In* N. R. Krieg and J. G. Holt (ed.), *Bergey's Manual of Systematic Bacteriology*, vol. 1. Williams & Wilkins, Baltimore.

185. **Tully, J. G.** 1985. Newly discovered mollicutes, p. 1–26. *In* S. Razin and M. F. Barile (ed.), *The Mycoplasmas*, vol. 4. *Mycoplasma Pathogenicity.* Academic Press, Inc., Orlando, Fla.

186. **Tully, J. G.** 1989. Class Mollicutes: new perspectives from plant and arthropod studies, p. 1–31. *In* R. F. Whitcomb and J. G. Tully (ed.), *The Mycoplasmas*, vol. 5. *Spiroplasmas, Acholeplasmas, and Mycoplasmas of Plants and Arthropods.* Academic Press, Inc., San Diego, Calif.

187. **Tully, J. G., and J. B. Baseman.** 1991. Mycoplasma. *Lancet* **337**:1296.

188. **Tully, J. G., D. L. Rose, P. Carle, J. M. Bové, K. J. Hackett, and R. F. Whitcomb.** 1988. *Acholeplasma entomophilum* sp. nov. from gut contents of a wide range of host insects. *Int. J. Syst. Bacteriol.* **38**:164–167.

189. **Tully, J. G., D. L. Rose, E. Clark, P. Carle, J. M. Bové, R. B. Henegar, R. F. Whitcomb, D. E. Colflesh, and D. L. Williamson.** 1987. Revised group classification of the genus *Spiroplasma* (class *Mollicutes*), with proposed new groups XII to XXIII. *Int. J. Syst. Bacteriol.* **37**:357–364.

190. **Tully, J. G., D. L. Rose, K. J. Hackett, R. F. Whitcomb, P. Carle, J. M. Bové, D. E. Colflesh, and D. L. Williamson.** 1989. *Mycoplasma ellychniae* sp. nov., a sterol-requiring mollicute from the firefly beetle *Ellychnia corrusca. Int. J. Syst. Bacteriol.* **39**:284–289.

191. **Tully, J. G., D. L. Rose, R. E. McCoy, P. Carle, J. M. Bové, R. F. Whitcomb, and W. G. Weisburg.** 1990. *Mycoplasma melaleucae* sp. nov., a sterol-requiring mollicute from flowers of several tropical plants. *Int. J. Syst. Bacteriol.* **40**:143–147.

192. **Tully, J. G., D. L. Rose, R. F. Whitcomb, K. J. Hackett, T. B. Clark, R. B. Henegar, E. Clark, P. Carle, and J. M. Bové.** 1987. Characterization of some new insect-derived acholeplasmas. *Isr. J. Med. Sci.* **23**:699–703.

193. **Tully, J. G., D. Taylor-Robinson, R. M. Cole, and D. L. Rose.** 1981. A newly discovered mycoplasma in the human urogenital tract. *Lancet* **i**:1288–1291.

194. **Tully, J. G., and R. F. Whitcomb.** 1992. The genus *Spiroplasma*, p. 1960–1980. *In* A. Balows, H. G. Truper, M. Dworkin, W. Harder, and K.-H. Schleifer (ed.), *The Prokaryotes*, 2nd ed., vol. 2. Springer-Verlag, New York.

195. **Waits, K. B., N. R. Cox, D. T. Crouse, J. C. McIntosh, and G. H. Cassell.** 1990. Mycoplasma infections of the central nervous system in humans and animals, p. 379–386. *In* G. Stanek, G. H. Cassel, J. G. Tully, and R. F. Whitcomb (ed.), *Recent Advances in Mycoplasmology.* Gustav Fischer Verlag, Stuttgart.

196. **Waits, K. B., J. G. Tully, D. L. Rose, P. A. Marriott, R. O. Davis, and G. H. Cassell.** 1987. Isolation of *Acholeplasma oculi* from human amoniotic fluid in early pregnancy. *Curr. Microbiol.* **15**:325–327.

197. **Watson, H. L., and G. H. Cassell.** 1990. Surface antigens of *Mycoplasma pulmonis. IOM Lett.* **1**:113–114.

198. **Watson, H. L., M. K. Davidson, N. R. Cox, J. K. Davis, K. Dybvig, and G. H. Cassell.** 1987. Protein variability among strains of *Mycoplasma pulmonis. Infect. Immun.* **55**:2838–2840.

199. **Watson, H. L., K. Dybvig, D. K. Blalock, and G. H. Cassell.** 1989. Subunit structure of the variable V-1 antigen of *Mycoplasma pulmonis. Infect. Immun.* **57**:1684–1690.

200. **Watson, H. L., L. S. McDaniel, D. K. Blalock, M. T. Fallon, and G. H. Cassell.** 1988. Heterogeneity among strains and a high rate of variation within strains of a major surface antigen of *Mycoplasma pulmonis. Infect. Immun.* **56**:1358–1363.

201. **Wayne, L. G., D. J. Brenner, R. R. Colwell, P. A. D. Grimont, O. Kandler, M. I. Krichevsky, L. H. Moore, W. E. C. Moore, R. G. E. Murray, E. Stackebrandt, M. P. Starr, and H. G. Truper.** 1987. Report of the ad hoc committee on reconciliation of approaches to bacterial systematics. *Int. J. Syst. Bacteriol.* **37**:463–464.

202. **Weisburg, W. G., J. G. Tully, D. L. Rose, J. P. Petzel, H. Oyaizu, D. Yang, L. Mandelco, J. Sechrest, T. G. Lawrence, J. Van Etten, J. Maniloff, and C. R. Woese.** 1989. A phylogenetic analysis of the mycoplasmas: basis for their classification. *J. Bacteriol.* **171**:6455–6467.

203. **Wenzel, R., and R. Herrmann.** 1988. Physical mapping of the *Mycoplasma pneumoniae* genome. *Nucleic Acids Res.* **16**:8323–8336.

204. **Wenzel, R., and R. Herrmann.** 1989. Cloning of the complete *Mycoplasma pneumoniae* genome. *Nucleic Acids Res.* **17**:7029–7043.

205. **Whitcomb, R. F., and J. G. Tully.** 1984. *Spiroplasmataceae*, p. 781–787. *In* N. R. Krieg and J. G. Holt (ed.), *Bergey's Manual of Systematic Bacteriology*, vol. 1. Williams & Wilkins, Baltimore.

206. **Whitcomb, R. F., and J. G. Tully (ed.).** 1989. *The Mycoplasmas*, vol. 5. *Spiroplasmas, Acholeplasmas, and Mycoplasmas of Plants and Arthropods.* Academic Press, Inc., San Diego, Calif.

207. **Whitley, J. C., A. D. Bergemann, L. E. Pyle, B. G. Cocks, R. Youil, and L. R. Finch.** 1990. Genomic maps of mycoplasmas and Tn916 insertion, p. 47–55. *In* G. Stanek, G. H. Cassel, J. G. Tully, and R. F. Whitcomb (ed.), *Recent Advances in Mycoplasmology.* Gustav Fischer Verlag, Stuttgart.

208. **Williamson, D. L., J. G. Tully, D. L. Rose, K. J. Hackett, R. Henegar, P. Carle, J. M. Bové, D. E. Colfesh, and R. F. Whitcomb.** 1990. *Mycoplasma somnilux* sp. nov., *Mycoplasma luminosum* sp. nov., and *Mycoplasma lucivorax* sp. nov., new sterol-requiring mollicutes from firefly beetles (*Coleoptera*: Lampyridae). *Int. J. Syst. Bacteriol.* **40**:160–164.

209. **Williamson, D. L., J. G. Tully, and R. F. Whitcomb.** 1989. The genus *Spiroplasma*, p. 71–111. *In* R. F. Whitcomb and J. G. Tully (ed.), *The Mycoplasmas*, vol. 5. *Spiroplasmas, Acholeplasmas, and Mycoplasmas of Plants and Arthropods.* Academic Press, Inc., San Diego, Calif.

210. **Wirostko, E., and L. Johnson.** 1990. Mycoplasma-like organisms. *Lancet* **336:**246–247.

211. **Wirostko, E., L. Johnson, and B. Wirostko.** 1989. Chronic orbital inflammatory disease: parasitization of orbital leucocytes by mollicute-like organisms. *Br. J. Ophthalmol.* **73:**865–870.

212. **Wirostko, E., L. Johnson, and W. Wirostko.** 1988. Mouse exophthalmic chronic orbital inflammatory disease. Induction by human leucocyte intracellular mollicutes. *Virchows Arch. A* **413:**349–355.

213. **Wirostko, E., L. Johnson, and W. Wirostko.** 1989. Juvenile rheumatoid arthritis inflammatory eye disease. Parasitization of ocular leukocytes by mollicute-like organisms. *J. Rheumatol.* **16:**1446–1453.

214. **Wirostko, E., L. Johnson, and W. Wirostko.** 1991. Postinflammatory cataracts in the mouse: induction by human mycoplasma like organisms. *Br. J. Ophthalmol.* **75:**671–674.

215. **Wirostko, E., L. Johnson, and W. J. Wirostko.** 1988. Mouse interstitial lung disease and pleuritis induction by human mollicute-like organisms. *Br. J. Exp. Pathol.* **69:**891–902.

216. **Woese, C. R., J. Maniloff, and L. B. Zablen.** 1980. Phylogenetic analysis of the mycoplasmas. *Proc. Natl. Acad. Sci. USA* **77:**494–498.

217. **Yamao, F., A. Muto, Y. Kawauchi, M. Iwami, S. Iwagami, Y. Azumi, and S. Osawa.** 1985. UGA is read as tryptophan in *Mycoplasma capricolum. Proc. Natl. Acad. Sci. USA* **82:**2306–2309.

218. **Yogev, D., D. Halachmi, G. E. Kenny, and S. Razin.** 1988. Distinction of species and strains of mycoplasma (*Mollicutes*) by genomic DNA fingerprints with an rRNA gene probe. *J. Clin. Microbiol.* **26:**1198–1201.

219. **Yogev, D., S. Levisohn, S. H. Kleven, D. Halachmi, and S. Razin.** 1988. Ribosomal RNA gene probes detect intraspecies heterogeneity in *Mycoplasma gallisepticum* and *M. synoviae. Avian Dis.* **32:**220–231.

220. **Yogev, D., S. Levisohn, and S. Razin.** 1989. Genetic and antigenic relatedness between *Mycoplasma gallisepticum* and *Mycoplasma synoviae. Vet. Microbiol.* **19:**75–84.

221. **Yogev, D., and S. Razin.** 1986. Common deoxyribonucleic acid sequences in *Mycoplasma genitalium* and *Mycoplasma pneumoniae* genomes. *Int. J. Syst. Bacteriol.* **36:**426–430.

222. **Yogev, D., R. Rosengarten, R. Watson-McKown, and K. S. Wise.** 1991. Molecular basis of mycoplasma antigenic variation: a novel set of divergent genes undergo spontaneous mutation of periodic coding regions and 5′ regulatory sequences. *EMBO J.* **10:**4069–4079.

223. **Yogev, D., S. Sela, H. Bercovier, and S. Razin.** 1988. Elongation factor (EF-Tu) gene probe detects polymorphism in *Mycoplasma* strains. *FEMS Microbiol. Lett.* **50:**145–149.

224. **Yogev, D., S. Sela, H. Bercovier, and S. Razin.** 1990. Nucleotide sequence and codon usage of the elongation factor Tu (EF-Tu) gene from *Mycoplasma pneumoniae. Mol. Microbiol.* **4:**1303–1310.

225. **Yogev, D., J. G. Tully, D. L. Rose, and S. Razin.** 1988. Genetic and antigenic distinction of *Mycoplasma pirum* from other mycoplasmas with specialized tip structures. *Int. J. Syst. Bacteriol.* **38:**147–150.

226. **Youil, R., and L. R. Finch.** 1990. Genome rearrangements in *Mycoplasma mycoides* subsp. *mycoides. IOM Lett.* **1:**276–277.

227. **Yunker, C. E., J. G. Tully, and J. Cory.** 1987. Arthropod cell lines in the isolation and propagation of tick borne spiroplasmas. *Curr. Microbiol.* **15:**45–50.

228. **Zimmer, R. L., and R. M. Woollacott.** 1983. Mycoplasma-like organisms: occurrence with the larvae and adults of a marine bryozoan. *Science* **220:**208–210.

229. **Zreik, L., J.-L. Danet, A. Fos, J. Gander, J. M. Bové, and M. Garnier.** 1990. Detection of tomato stolbur and clover phyllody MLOs in plants and insects with monoclonal antibodies. *IOM Lett.* **1:**225–226.

2. Cell Nutrition and Growth

R. J. MILES

INTRODUCTION

The mollicutes are among the most nutritionally fastidious groups of microorganisms. Their intimate association with animals and plants, as commensals, parasites, or pathogens, has presumably led to their dependence on the host for a vast array of organic nutrients and for relatively constant environmental conditions. The provision of these nutrients and conditions in vitro has proved difficult to achieve, and many mollicutelike organisms from plants have yet to be grown in culture. In addition, it is to be expected that as our understanding of mollicute nutrition increases, improved isolation media will enable growth of hitherto unsuspected species.

Thus, a primary objective of nutritional studies is the efficient isolation of mollicutes from their diverse natural habitats and the development of media giving high and reproducible yields to enable their subsequent investigation. The aim of this chapter, however, is not merely to describe those factors which influence mollicute growth and isolation but also to demonstrate how nutrient and cultural conditions may critically affect biochemical, physiological, and morphological attributes of mollicutes and influence genetic adaptation of strains. These complex relationships demand a quantitative approach to growth and nutritional studies and the description of mollicute populations used in all aspects of research. The determination of biomass is also discussed, since this may present a particular difficulty in studies of mollicutes as a consequence of their osmotic fragility, their tendency to filament formation, and the characteristically low cell yields obtained during growth.

Frequent reference is made to previous reviews of mollicute growth and nutrition, particularly those of Rodwell (99, 100) and Rodwell and Mitchell (102). Reviews concerning the nutrition of acholeplasmas (124), anaeroplasmas (94, 95), spiroplasmas (12, 15, 54, 130), and ureaplasamas (113, 114) are also available, and a variety of articles on mollicute cultivation are contained in *Methods in Mycoplasmology* (90).

R. J. Miles • Microbial Physiology Research Group, Division of Life Sciences, King's College, University of London, Campden Hill Road, London W8 7AH, United Kingdom.

ESTIMATION OF BIOMASS

"Biomass" is a general term used to refer to the organisms in culture. The biomass parameter measures the extent of growth and is required for the derivation of growth yields and metabolic quotients (i.e., specific rates of substrate utilization or product formation). It is of fundamental importance in describing cultural systems. However, the value of much published work is limited by a failure to include an explicit statement of the amount of biomass formed or to use an appropriate method for biomass determination (79).

A variety of methods have been used to measure biomass: total mass; mass of protein, DNA, or other biomass component; mass of substrate consumed or product formed; metabolic rates; light scattering; and cell counts, either of total or of viable cells. These measures of biomass may increase proportionately during balanced growth in which the specific growth rate is constant and cell viability is close to 100%. However, mollicutes are typically grown in statically incubated cultures (i.e., without shaking or stirring), thus leading to concentration gradients of dissolved gases and perhaps nutrients and toxic products. In addition, mollicute growth is controlled by the availability of a large number of organic substrates, the concentration of which will constantly change in culture as a consequence of their utilization or instability during the often prolonged incubation necessary to achieve growth. Thus, the conditions for balanced growth of mollicutes probably occur only at very low biomass densities, during the early stages of growth, and biomass values determined will be critically dependent on the methods used to obtain them.

Dry Mass

Dry mass is probably the most unequivocal parameter of biomass. Its determination requires separation of the organisms from the medium, usually by centrifugation, and washing and drying at 105°C for 24 h. Washing must be carried out in such a way as to prevent lysis (106), such as by including stabilizing cations (Mg^{2+}, spermine) in the washing solution and carrying out the procedure at 4°C (96). However, the usefulness of dry mass determinations in studies of mollicutes is limited by lack of sensitivity. To determine dry mass with an accuracy of <2%, 50 mg is needed (79), whereas the highest mollicute concentrations achieved in culture are 0.5 mg of dry mass per ml; the vast majority of strains give only a fraction of this value.

Mass of a Cell Component

A number of cell components, including cell nitrogen, protein, DNA, and more recently ATP, have been used as measures of biomass. The underlying assumption is that these components form a constant proportion of dry mass. However, the protein content of bacterial cells may vary with the specific growth rate (37). DNA content varies to a lesser extent (37), though in chemical assays protein determinations are more widely used because of their greater sensitivity. Accurate determination of DNA by colorimetric estimation of deoxyribose requires approximately 1 mg of dry cell mass, whereas protein determinations by the method of Lowry require only 100 μg (79). An alternative approach to the estimation of DNA is to grow cells in the presence of [^{32}P]phosphate or [^{3}H]- or [^{14}C]thymidine and assay the radioactivity of the trichloroacetic acid (TCA)-insoluble material in cultures (103); protein may be similarly determined by using ^{3}H- or ^{14}C-labeled amino acids. When cell growth is determined in undefined media, the specific activities of the precursors will be unknown. Thus, label recovered can be related to an absolute amount of protein or DNA only by reference to a standard curve (chemically determined cell protein or DNA versus label) produced in the same medium. In procedures whereby cells are not separated from the medium before determination of the TCA-insoluble material, recovered activities may remain high after cell death, and presumably cell lysis, has taken place (111), indicating little extracellular hydrolysis of labeled macromolecules. In a recent modification of the DNA-labeling technique, Bastian et al. (3) pulsed cultures of *Spiroplasma mirum* 8 h prior to determining [^{3}H]thymidine uptake. TCA-insoluble material was washed in TCA, dissolved in NaOH, neutralized with HCl, and counted on a scintillation counter. This method measured the rate of DNA synthesis (over the 8-h period) rather than the actual mass of DNA. However, the method readily detected 10^6 CFU/ml and under a variety of conditions gave results which correlated with colony counts.

The ATP content of mollicute cells has been determined by chemical means (4) and by luciferin-luciferase luminometry (5, 111, 119). The latter method is sensitive and rapid and, once operational, relatively simple; culture is added to a chemical nucleotide-releasing agent, and after addition of luciferin-luciferase reagent, light emitted is determined. During the growth of *Ureaplasma urealyticum* cultures, ATP increased in a manner similar to that of color-changing units (CCU) (discussed below), and the assay could detect 10^4 CCU in 100 μl of culture (119). However, after the cessation of active growth, ATP fell dramatically while CCU remained high. In a detailed study of *S. citri*, essentially similar results were obtained (111). Populations of 10^5 CFU/ml were detectable, and during exponential growth, the ATP content of cells correlated well with viable count and [^{14}C]thymidine and [^{3}H]phenylalanine incorporation into cells. However, at the end of exponential growth, there was a rapid fall in the ATP content of cells, which occurred more than 40 h before the viable count started to decline. The fall in ATP content reflected a very sharp decrease in the adenylate nucleotide pool and also a reduction in the adenylate energy charge (EC_A; equal to [ATP + 0.5 ADP]/[ATP + ADP + AMP]) from 0.9 to 0.65. The ATP content and EC_A of a range of *Mycoplasma* and *Acholeplasma* species has also been determined; during exponential growth, the EC_A of mycoplasmas and *Acholeplasma morum* (approximately 0.7) was significantly lower than that of *A. laidlawii* (0.9) (4, 5).

Substrate Utilization and Product Formation

The amount of biomass formed during growth may be estimated from the amount of a substrate utilized or of a product formed, provided that the growth yields are constant. Sources of energy, carbon, nitrogen, or growth factors (e.g., essential amino acids or vitamins) are suitable substrates in bacteria generally, but in mollicutes for which growth media are undefined or contain many potential sources of carbon, energy, and nitrogen, the range of useful substrates is limited. Glucose may be readily assayed via the glucose oxidase reaction and is the principal energy source in media for fermentative *Mycoplasma* species and other mollicutes. However, the amount of glucose utilized during the growth of *M. gallisepticum* in an undefined medium containing serum was poorly correlated with viable count (117).

Analysis of metabolic products formed during mollicute growth is made difficult by the presence of medium components. Acid or alkali production may be qualitatively determined by the incorporation of pH indicator dyes into media, and in a broth medium containing phenol red, Meur et al. (66) have claimed a linear inverse relationship between A_{550} and log CFU (see below) during the early stages of the growth of *M. mycoides* subsp. *capri*. Titratable acidity increases exponentially during the growth phase of most fermentative mollicutes (103). However, the relationship between growth and amount of acid formed may be complex, since acid production may result from the metabolism of not only the principal energy source (usually glucose) but also other medium components such as glycerol. In addition, differences in the products of glucose metabolism under aerobic and anaerobic conditions (102) will be of importance when mollicutes are incubated statically in air (as is usually the case) and oxygen saturation of cultures is not maintained. However, a number of fermentative *Mycoplasma* species that are apparently unable to oxidize glucose to acetate and presumably form lactate under both aerobic and anaerobic conditions have been identified (69); for these organisms, titratable acidity as a measure of growth may be especially applicable. The application of biomass assays based on substrate utilization or product formation may also be limited when these activities (e.g., acid formation) continue during the stationary phase of the growth cycle. However, this problem could be overcome by the use of appropriate nutrient-limited media.

Impedance monitoring (26) is a relatively new technique for detecting metabolism which has apparently received little or no attention from those working with mollicutes. Impedance measures the apparent resistance between two electrodes immersed in a solution when an alternating current is applied. It is dependent on the true resistance of the system and also on its capacitance and the applied frequency. During microbial metabolism, there is generally an increase in the number of ions present in the culture medium. Thus, there is a decrease in resistance and increase in capacitance of the system, and impedance is reduced. The relationship between growth, increase in the number of ions, and impedance is complex. However, commercial and almost fully automated multichannel instruments are available, and although the technique is used predominantly for the rapid detection of microbial growth, it also allows derivation of growth kinetics.

Metabolic Rates

A diverse range of metabolic activities are potentially of value in the determination of biomass, including those of enzymes. There have been few systematic studies of the effect of cultural conditions and phase of growth on enzyme synthesis. However, urease activity in growing cultures of *U. urealyticum* was closely correlated with the number of CCU (119). Similarly, in growing cultures of *M. mycoides*, there was a high correlation (correlation coefficient of 0.97) between the number of CFU and the lactate dehydrogenase activity of lysed cells (7). Lactate dehydrogenase was readily assayed by spectrophotometric assay of NADH oxidation with pyruvate as a substrate (despite the presence of NADH oxidase activity in lysed cells), and the assay was sufficiently sensitive to detect 10^6 CFU/ml. However, the application of this procedure to the determination of viable cells after growth ceased at 37°C, or when cultures were stored at 4°C, was unsuccessful, and the decline in viable count was more rapid than that of lactate dehydrogenase activity (92). Other processes which may be used to determine metabolic activity include dye reduction and oxygen uptake. The rate of reduction of tetrazolium to form the red formazan has been used to estimate the amount of *M. pneumoniae* cells (9), and Rodwell and Whitcomb (103) suggested that the rate of oxygen consumption in sealed reaction vessels could be determined from changes in dissolved oxygen tension measured with a Clarke-type oxygen electrode. Such a method would enable detection of small amounts of oxygen (a few nanomoles per milliliter) and has been used to detect substrate oxidation by glucose- and lactate-oxidizing mollicutes suspended in a salts solution (69, 70).

A universal feature of metabolic activity is the generation of heat, which may be continuously and sensitively monitored with microcalorimeters without the need to disturb or sample culture systems. These instruments, linked to a chart recorder, produce power-time curves, and integration of the area under the curves enables calculation of the total enthalpy (heat) change during growth. Power-time curves for the growth of *M. fermentans*, *M. hominis*, *A. laidlawii*, *A. granularum*, and *U. urealyticum* showed increase in power output to a maximum value (P_{max}) followed by a decline (55). However, the curves for each species were distinguished by the rates of increase and decline in power and by the value of P_{max}. It was suggested that the microcalorimetric technique might therefore be applied to mollicute identification; however, experiments with other microorganisms have shown that substantial differences in power-time curves may occur between strains of the same species and even for the same strain with use of inocula from different sources (77). Microcalorimetry has also been used to study the growth of *M. mycoides*, in sealed ampoules, with different sugar sources (68). With glucose, there were three phases of exponential increase in power (Fig. 1), and gradients of natural log power versus time were 0.32 (the first phase), 0.10, and 0.10/h. Thus, the data suggested that there were three periods of exponential growth with culture doubling times of 2.2, 6.9, and 6.9 h, respectively. The detail observable with use of microcalorimetry is greater than that for other growth-monitoring techniques, and the minimum

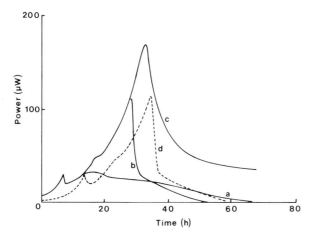

Figure 1. Power-time curves of the growth of *M. mycoides* in a pig serum medium. The medium contained no added sugar (curve a) or 0.1% (curves b and d) or 0.5% (curve c) glucose. The inoculum was 4×10^6 (curves a to c) or 4×10^5 (curve d) CFU/ml.

number of mollicute cells detectable is approximately 10^5 CFU/ml (55, 68). Thus, there may be a considerable potential for microcalorimetry in studies of mollicute growth, though the cost of instruments may be prohibitive.

Light Scattering

Suspensions of organisms scatter light and appear turbid. Turbidity increases with increasing organism concentration and thus provides a means of measuring biomass. The application of turbidity measurements to studies of mollicutes has been described previously (103). Essentially, the degree of light scattering is dependent on the size and shape of particles, the wavelength of the light, and the difference in the refractive index of the particles and the medium (58). Increasing the ratio of particle size to wavelength of light increases scattering; thus, for maximum sensitivity, light of a low wavelength should be used. However, at low wavelengths, absorption of light increases, and so a wavelength of 540 nm is commonly used. The dependence of light scattering on the refractive indices of both the suspending medium and the organisms is of particular significance to studies of mollicutes. Since mollicutes lack a rigid cell wall, osmotic swelling or shrinking may readily occur with changes in the tonicity of the suspending medium. An increase in cell volume is associated with a decline in turbidity as the refractive index of the organism is lowered. It is therefore essential that turbidity be related to a parameter such as dry cell mass or cell protein by using a standard curve and that a separate standard curve be constructed for each organism and suspension medium. The validity of turbidity measurements may still be questioned if there is a significant change in cell morphology during the cell cycle, e.g., in those *Mycoplasma* species that have a marked tendency toward filamentous growth but appear as single cells in stationary-phase cultures. However, despite these

limitations, turbidity measurements are widely used to determine biomass, since measurements are instantaneous and nondestructive of the sample. Also, Snell (117) compared seven methods for estimating growth of *M. gallisepticum* and concluded that turbidity measurements gave the highest reproducibility and correlation with viable count. Unfortunately, turbidity measurements require approximately 100 µg of dry cell mass per ml for accurate biomass determination (79) and are insufficiently sensitive for use with many mollicutes in which these concentrations are not reached even at the end of the growth phase.

Cell Counts

The number of CFU may be determined by plating suitable dilutions of cultures on agar medium and counting the numbers of colonies formed after incubation. Procedures suitable for use with mollicutes have been described previously (103) and are similar to those for other bacteria (82). However, to avoid loss of viability during the preparation of dilutions, the use of a broth medium as the diluent has been recommended (103); salts solutions containing catalase have also been used (67). The importance of the quality of the agar medium used has been discussed by Razin (85); isolated cells are often more exacting nutritionally than are dense populations, and it is usual to include a high concentration of serum (up to 25% [vol/vol]). Colonies of mollicutes are usually observed under a light microscope (85), and Bastian et al. (3) counted the small colonies of *S. mirum* by using dark-field illumination at a magnification of ×200. The inclusion of calcium or manganese salts in the agar gives *Ureaplasma* colonies a dark color, thus enhancing their visualization (113). Colony diameter for a range of *Mycoplasma* species and *A. laidlawii* has been shown to be inversely related to the number of colonies per unit area and might therefore also be used as an indicator of viable count (43).

Viable counts are probably the most sensitive means of assaying biomass. However, in the interpretation of results, it should be remembered that the count is critically dependent on the quality of the agar medium used and is subject to a sampling error. The 95% confidence limits of viable counts are approximately $n \pm 2(n)^{1/2}$, where n is the number of colonies counted; thus, n must be >400 for the confidence limits to be within ±10% (79). Confidence limits of viable counts are often not included in published papers, thus raising doubts about their significance. A further important qualification concerning viable counts is their application to studies of filamentous organisms. In, for example, *M. mycoides*, there may be a substantial increase in the number of viable particles at the end of the growth phase, as a consequence of the fragmentation of filaments, with no corresponding increase in cell mass (102). Also, in *M. mycoides* (see below) and in cell-walled bacteria (37), it has been shown that mean cell mass is a function of growth rate, and in *Aerobacter aerogenes*, this value increased by a factor of more than 3 as the specific growth rate increased from 0.1 to 0.9/h.

The viable count may also be determined in liquid media by using a most probable number (MPN) method (82, 103). A suspension of the organism is diluted to extinction in a broth medium, and after a period of time adequate to allow growth from a single organism, the presence or absence of growth is determined in all dilutions. The reciprocal of the highest dilution in which growth occurs is the estimated population size. In practice, a number of replicate dilutions are usually prepared, and the most probable population size is calculated by using tables (2, 82). In work with mollicutes, detection of growth is usually aided by the presence of a pH indicator in the growth medium, and hence the estimate of the viable number of cells present in the original suspension is often referred to as the number of CCU. The method is convenient, but this advantage should not disguise the inherent inaccuracy of MPN techniques (82). For example, for a 10-fold dilution series with five replicates at each dilution, the 95% confidence limits of counts are between approximately one-third and three times the estimated value (2). Thus, the use of MPN methods may not be appropriate for quantitative studies. An important justification for their use, however, is that CFU counts on agar plates may underestimate the viable count of some mollicute strains, and in a study of *U. urealyticum* and *M. hominis*, cell DNA content gave a higher correlation with the number of CCU than with the number of CFU (118).

Total cell counts may be estimated microscopically for those mollicutes with a readily identifiable morphology and are widely used with spiroplasmas. The technique has been described previously (103) and depends on counts of cells in 5 μl of suspension placed on a microscope slide and covered by a coverslip. It is recommended that the organisms in at least 25 fields of view, in two separate slide preparations, be counted. The sampling error in this technique would be similar to that for colony counts (see above) if there were a uniform thickness of suspension under the coverslip.

However, since this would be most unlikely, it is appropriate that when this technique is used, a sufficiently detailed statistical analysis of counts is undertaken so that the significance of data may be properly evaluated. The technique is less sensitive than colony counts and requires cell densities of 10^6 CFU/ml (103).

In conclusion of this section, it is clear that considerable attention needs to be paid to the choice of parameter used to determine biomass. This choice will be influenced by the magnitude of the cell yield and the sensitivity required and also whether cells are actively growing. In many situations, it may be appropriate to use more than one parameter, for example, viable count and cell mass or cell protein. The recently reported ultrasonic detection of biomass (132) may have particular application to work with mollicutes, though large volumes of culture sample currently are required.

GROWTH REQUIREMENTS OF MOLLICUTES

Organic Requirements

General considerations

The ability to demonstrate specific nutrient requirements for microorganisms generally demands the availability of fully defined growth media, and these have been developed for only a few mollicute species. The components of a minimal defined medium (i.e., a medium containing only those nutrients essential for growth) for *M. mycoides* Y are listed in Table 1. The nutritional requirements of *A. laidlawii* B are also listed; these were established (102) from results from various studies using fully and partly defined media. It should be remembered, however, that the nutritional requirements of microorganisms may vary both quan-

Table 1. Essential components of defined and semidefined media for *M. mycoides* Y and *A. laidlawii* B[a]

Organism	Component(s)					
	Inorganic ions	Amino acids	Saccharide	Lipids and precursors	Nucleic acid precursors	Vitamins and coenzymes
M. mycoides Y	K^+, Mg^{2+}, PO_4^{3-}	Alanine, arginine, asparagine, cysteine, glutamine, glycine, histidine, isoleucine, leucine, lysine, methionine, phenylalanine, proline, serine, threonine, tryptophan, tyrosine, valine	Glucose	Fatty acid, glycerol, sterol	Guanine, uracil, thymine	Coenzyme A, riboflavin, nicotinic acid, thiamine, pyridoxamine, α-lipoic acid
A. laidlawii B	K^+, Mg^{2+}, PO_4^{3-}	Alanine, arginine, asparagine, cysteine, glutamine, glycine, histidine, isoleucine, leucine, lysine, methionine, proline, serine, threonine, tryptophan, valine	Glucose	Unsaturated fatty acid	Adenosine, gluanosine, cytidine	Pantetheine, riboflavin, nicotinic acid, thiamine, pyridoxal, biotin, folinic acid

[a] Revised from Rodwell and Mitchell (102).

titatively and qualitatively with the conditions of culture (79).

In attempting to define organic requirements for growth, interactions between metabolic pathways may cause considerable difficulty. For example, alanine was essential for the growth of *M. mycoides* Y only in the absence of pyridoxal (98), and in *A. laidlawii* B, tyrosine and phenylalanine were not required when alanine was provided (122). Also, Rodwell (98) observed a nutritional antagonism between alanine and glycine, which could be overcome by raising the ratio of glycine to alanine or, interestingly, by providing alanine as L-Ala$_3$ or L-Ala$_4$; alanylalanine inhibited growth. Such antagonisms are widely reported in cell-walled bacteria and may result, for example, from shared transport systems; thus, in the presence of a high concentration of one amino acid, transport of a second amino acid is inhibited.

Amino acids

The large number of amino acids required by *M. mycoides* Y and *A. laidlawii* B reflects the limited synthetic abilities of mollicutes. Strain Y can also obtain amino acids from peptides and by proteolytic degradation of bovine serum albumin (BSA) (100). In spiroplasmas, the number of amino acids required for growth in a defined medium varied with the species; 14 were required for "good growth" in *S. citri*, and only seven were required in *S. apis* (76). In this study, the effect of amino acid deletion on growth rate was determined, and kinetic data were presented which suggested that, in general, saturation constants for amino acid utilization by *Spiroplasma* species are low (about 10 μM). Chang and Chen (13) also showed considerable variation in the amino acid requirements of *Spiroplasma* species. Requirements for individual amino acids may be increased when, in addition to their role in protein synthesis, they are subject to catabolism. Threonine and serine are readily oxidized by *M. mycoides* cells suspended in a salts solution (67, 97). More details of amino acid requirements and metabolism are presented in chapter 12.

Nucleic acid precursors

Requirements for nucleic acid precursors by *M. mycoides* have been explained by elucidation of nucleotide biosynthetic pathways (71); although pathways for de novo synthesis are absent, a number of nucleotide interconversions are possible (71, 73, 74). Thus, in *M. mycoides*, guanine could serve as a source of all purine nucleotides. *M. capricolum*, however, required both guanine and adenine (100). In *A. laidlawii*, reported differences in requirements for nucleic acid precursors may reflect strain differences (102). Sources of nucleotides and nucleotide metabolism are discussed in more detail in chapter 13.

Lipids

The fatty acid and sterol requirements of mollicutes have been discussed by Rodwell (99) and Rodwell and Mitchell (102). Information concerning these requirements is available for those species which will grow in either defined or serum-free medium. Fatty acids are required primarily for phospholipid synthesis, and their uptake in *M. capricolum* is energy linked and protein mediated (22). *M. mycoides* is unable to synthesize or alter the chain length of either saturated or unsaturated fatty acids, which must therefore be provided in the growth medium (102). Palmitic acid plus oleic acid are recommended for use in defined media (100), but any single fatty acid or combination of fatty acids may support growth provided that the fluidity of the membrane lies within certain limits. Fatty acids supporting optimal growth of *M. mycoides* include elaidate, *trans*-vaccentate, *cis*-12-octadecanoate, isopalmitate, isostearate, and anteisoheptadecanoate (102). Palmitic acid plus oleic acid support the growth of *S. melliferum*, *S. floricola*, and *S. apis*. Palmitic acid could be substituted by laevic, myristic, or stearic acid, and oleic acid could be substituted by palmitic, linoleic, or linolenic acid (11).

Acholeplasmas are capable of the biosynthesis of saturated fatty acids and the elongation of exogenously supplied unsaturated acids (116); however, exogenously supplied fatty acids are readily incorporated into membrane lipid. For example, in *A. laidlawii* B, 69% of the membrane lipid fatty acid was palmitic acid when this fatty acid was supplied exogenously, whereas it was only 20% when oleic acid was the supplied fatty acid (6). Ureaplasmas can synthesize both saturated and unsaturated fatty acids from [^{14}C]acetate (104).

Exogenous phospholipid (phosphatidylcholine and sphingomyelin) may also be directly incorporated into mycoplasma and spiroplasma membranes (23, 107). In *M. gallisepticum*, sphingomyelin was required for growth (101), and several phospholipids were required for optimal growth in serum-free medium (19). Using a defined medium, Hackett et al. (33) also showed the importance of sphingomyelin for the growth of *S. mirum*.

Sterol is essential for the growth of all mollicutes except *Acholeplasma* and *Asteroloplasma* species; in *Acholeplasma* species, it is incorporated into the membrane if provided in the medium (6). Cholesterol is usually the sterol provided in defined or serum-free medium but may be replaced for *Mycoplasma* species by cholestanol, stigmasterol, ergosterol, or 7-cholestan-3β-ol (102); 7β-hydroxycholesterol could also substitute for cholesterol in cholesterol-poor medium for *M. capricolum*, but in cholesterol-rich medium, it reduced the growth rate (53). Sterol normally accounts for 20% of the mass of total membrane lipids in mycoplasmas (52, 110); however, when *M. mycoides* (52, 110), *M. capricolum* (17), and *M. gallisepticum* (51) were adapted to growth in the presence of low cholesterol concentrations, membrane sterol decreased by 4- to 10-fold. Adaptation was associated with an increased generation time and reduced cell yield.

Carbohydrates

Glucose was included in the minimal defined medium for *M. mycoides* Y and in media for *A. laidlawii* (Table 1) as a source of energy and is perhaps also used in the synthesis of other sugars and polysaccharides. It may presumably be replaced in defined media by other sugars (discussed below), or perhaps by pyruvate (70), but these components might support lower growth rates (68). Energy sources for the growth of other mollicutes are discussed below.

Glycerol is required by *M. mycoides* for the synthesis of L-α-glycerophosphate (GP) and thus glycerides (97). GP may be oxidized to triose phosphate (dihydroxyacetonephosphate); however, this reaction occurs via a GP oxidase with the consumption of molecular oxygen and is essentially irreversible. The rate of glycerol oxidation was greater than that of glucose in cells suspended in a salts solution (67, 97), and during aerobic growth, only a small quantity (10%) of glycerol metabolized was incorporated into cellular material (principally glycerides). Thus, the quantity of glycerol required for maximum biomass production in aerobic culture will be considerably greater than that for glyceride synthesis (102). Glycerol oxidation, via GP oxidase activity, has also been demonstrated to occur at high rates in other *Mycoplasma* species, including *M. canis*, which does not oxidize glucose (69).

Vitamin and other requirements

The vitamin requirements of *M. mycoides* Y and *A. laidlawii* B (Table 1) have been discussed previously (99, 102). In defined media for spiroplasmas, a large number of vitamins are usually included; however, Chang could demonstrate a requirement for only nicotinic acid or riboflavin by *S. melliferum*, *S. floricola*, and *S. apis*. Maximal growth of all three strains was apparently achieved only in the presence of both vitamins, and high concentrations of vitamins reduced growth yield (11).

The polyamines spermine and spermidine, although not essential, stimulated the growth of *M. mycoides* Y in defined medium, and putrescine and the tripeptide glycyl-L-histidyl-L-lysine are often included in media for ureaplasmas (113).

Energy Sources

A variety of energy-yielding mechanisms exist within mollicutes, some of which are poorly understood. In the genus *Mycoplasma*, ATP may be generated during glycolysis, the oxidation of pyruvate to acetate, and the metabolism of arginine. In *M. mycoides*, glucose is transported by a phosphoenolpyruvate:phosphotransferase system and metabolized by the Embden-Meyerhof pathway (20). Under anaerobic conditions, lactate is the end product and there is a yield of 2 mol of ATP per mol of glucose; however, under aerobic conditions, a partial oxidation occurs and pyruvate is converted via phosphate acetyltransferase and acetate kinase activities to acetate plus CO_2 (40, 72), giving an additional 2 mol of ATP per mol of glucose. *M. mycoides* might be considered typical of those species which produce acid from glucose metabolism and are referred to as fermentative. However, in a number of *Mycoplasma* species, including *M. fermentans* and *M. canis*, lactate may be the end product of glucose metabolism under aerobic and anaerobic conditions (69).

Among the fermentative *Mycoplasma* species, a number of sugars and other substrates may be utilized in addition to glucose, and patterns of substrate utilization are distinctive features of species. It has been reported that all glucose-fermenting mycoplasmas also ferment maltose, starch, and glycogen (88, 102).

However, such reports are based on experiments carried out with media containing serum or serum fractions, which contain saccharolytic enzymes. Maltose is, however, utilized by a number of species, including *M. mycoides* subsp. *capri* (129).

There have been few quantitative studies of carbohydrate utilization by mycoplasmas. In *M. mycoides* subsp. *mycoides* suspended in a salts solution, saturation constants for the metabolism of glucose, fructose, N-acetylglucosamine, and glycerol were low (2 to 5 μM); however, values for glucosamine and mannose were high (130 μM and 1 mM, respectively), suggesting that although these substrates were utilized with maximum rates similar to that of glucose, they were probably not metabolized to a significant extent at the low concentrations found in vivo (67). The ability to use sugars was constitutive except in the case of fructose; the maximum rate of fructose utilization in fructose-grown cells was four times higher than that in glucose-grown cells. In *M. mycoides* subsp. *capri* and in *A. laidlawii*, maltose-utilizing ability was also partly inducible (115, 129).

The growth of *M. mycoides* subsp. *mycoides* in a medium containing serum was markedly affected by the nature of the sugar source (68). Glucose supported higher growth rates than did other sugars, even though these sugars were present in saturating concentrations. Thus, it appeared that glucose had a role in metabolism in addition to that of energy source, a role perhaps associated with metabolic regulation or the synthesis of other sugars.

Arginine is metabolized by the arginine dihydrolase pathway (83):

arginine + H_2O $\xrightarrow{\text{arginine deiminase}}$ citrulline + NH_3

citrulline + P_i $\xleftarrow{\text{ornithine transcarbamylase}}$ ornithine + carbamyl phosphate

carbamyl phosphate + ADP $\xleftrightarrow{\text{carbamate kinase}}$ ATP + CO_2 + NH_3

The net gain of ATP is only 1 mol/mol of arginine. Considering the likely energy requirement for arginine transport, the energetic advantage of this pathway appeared doubtful until the demonstration of an arginine-ornithine antiport system in *S. melliferum* (109a). Arginine appears to be the sole energy source in the majority of *Mycoplasma* species possessing the arginine dihydrolase pathway. However, a number of arginine-utilizing strains also ferment sugars (88), and *M. hominis* (arginine utilizing, nonfermentative) apparently possesses an additional (unknown) energy-yielding mechanism (25).

A number of *Mycoplasma* species neither ferment sugars nor hydrolyze arginine. However, it has been shown that many of these species, including *M. agalactiae*, *M. bovis*, and *M. californicum*, oxidize lactate, pyruvate, α-ketobutyrate, and in some cases ethanol (129a). These substrates may therefore serve as energy sources, and pyruvate was shown to increase the growth yield of *M. agalactiae* (70).

The spiroplasmas, acholeplasmas, and anaeroplasmas appear to be essentially fermentative, and enzymes of the Embden-Meyerhof-Parnas pathway have been found in all groups (20, 24, 78, 81). *Acholeplasma* species ferment a small range of sugars, and patterns of sugar utilization appear to be species specific (88); the sugars utilized include sucrose, maltose, glucose, galactose, fructose, and xylose. Under aerobic conditions, glucose, pyruvate, and lactate are oxidized to acetate and CO_2 (121). Acetate kinase activity has been demonstrated in *A. laidlawii* (40), suggesting that as in fermentative *Mycoplasma* species, aerobic incubation will lead to increased ATP production. *A. parvum* neither ferments glucose nor hydrolyzes arginine.

Spiroplasmas also use a range of sugars for growth (11), and some strains may use glucose 6-phosphate, 3-phosphoglyceraldehyde, and pyruvate (14). Differences in the patterns of carbohydrate utilization occur between species and even among strains of the same species. Some strains have apparently given inconsistent results, which may reflect the use of medium containing serum or serum fractions to determine substrate metabolism (11). In addition to fermenting carbohydrates, a number of strains have been shown to metabolize arginine via the the arginine dihydrolase pathway. However, in arginine-containing medium, some fermentable carbohydrate was necessary for the growth of all strains except *S. floricola* 23-6 (11, 13). Anaeroplasmas use soluble starch, and some strains may also use maltose, galactose, or glucose. The end products of fermentation include ethanol, CO_2, H_2, and acetic, formic, lactic, and propionic acids (94).

In ureaplasmas, the mechanism of energy generation is unclear. The high urease activity shown by members of this group, together with the ability of urea to promote growth (42), invites the suggestion that urea hydrolysis is coupled to ATP synthesis, perhaps through the creation of ionic gradients (63). Putrescine and other diamines also promoted ureaplasma growth in medium containing small quantities of urea (61). The role of urea in *Ureaplasma* growth is discussed by Shepard and Masover (114).

Other potential energy-yielding substrates in mollicutes include glutamine (80). Desantis et al. (24) have also emphasized the importance of 2-deoxyribose 5-phosphate aldolase activity in mollicutes, which may enable the utilization of DNA as a carbon and energy source for growth.

The amount of dry cell mass produced during growth of bacteria in media limited by the concentration of energy substrate is usually about 10.5 g/mol of ATP generated but may vary from 5 to 32 g/mol of ATP (79). Our own calculations, for *M. mycoides* subsp. *mycoides* grown in glucose-limited medium in sealed ampoules with no access to air, give a value of between 9 and 10 g/mol of ATP, though this value might not be typical of the slower-growing mollicutes for which the maintenance energy requirement may be more significant. However, when energy sources for mollicutes are known, it should be possible to calculate whether media are likely to be energy source limited. In media containing, for example, 0.2% arginine (48), the predicted maximum cell yield would be only 120 mg of dry cell mass per liter (assuming 10 g of dry cell mass per mol of ATP and production of 1 mol of ATP per mol of arginine). However, even this yield is substantially greater than that obtained for many mollicutes, and it appears that in general, most commonly used mollicute media (28) are unlikely to be energy source lim-

ited (given that the energy source added is appropriate to the mollicute being cultured). Leach (48) has shown that high concentrations of arginine may inhibit mycoplasma growth.

Inorganic Requirements

The inorganic requirements of mollicutes have been the subject of relatively few studies, and the results are often difficult to interpret when growth yields are low or metal ions and phosphorus, for example, are present in undefined or even in defined medium components (10). However, the inorganic requirements of cell-walled bacteria have been extensively studied, and if the approximate elemental composition of microbial cells is known, media can be quickly assessed for possible deficiencies in mineral ions. The major elements that are present in bacterial cells, and which may be provided by inorganic medium components in mollicutes, are (with their approximate percentage of dry cell mass [93]) P (4.2%), Mg^{2+} (0.6%), K^+ (1.2%), and Fe^{2+} (0.02%). A potentially large number of other elements, principally metals, may also be required in small quantities but are usually considered to be present in adequate amounts as contaminants of glassware and other medium components. K^+, Mg^{2+}, and PO_4^{3-} were essential components of the defined and semidefined media for *M. mycoides* and *A. laidlawii* (100). It is unlikely that there will be substantial differences between the inorganic requirements of mollicutes and other bacteria. However, it has been demonstrated that *M. pneumoniae* binds human lactoferrin, an iron-sequestering glycoprotein, with a binding affinity of 20 nM (123). It is possible that in this organism, iron uptake may occur primarily or exclusively via lactoferrin.

High concentrations of metal ions, particularly divalent metal ions, may inhibit mollicute growth (99); for example, Zn^{2+}, Mn^{2+}, Co^{2+}, and Fe^{2+} were growth inhibiting for *M. mycoides* Y at concentrations ranging from 1 to 100 μM. Also, although KCl was essential for the growth of *M. mycoides* Y and *A. laidlawii* B in defined medium (Table 1), it was inhibitory at concentrations above 0.06 M; however, strain Y could be adapted to growth at higher concentrations (99). The concentrations of inorganic salts may also affect cell growth indirectly by their contribution to medium tonicity (discussed below).

Physical Requirements

In mollicutes, the temperature range over which growth occurs and the optimum temperature for growth (i.e., that supporting the highest growth rate) are species dependent. In general, the temperature range for growth covers about 7 to 40°C, and the optimum temperature is toward the top of the range, reflecting increased metabolic activity with increasing temperature until thermal denaturation of some essential cell component takes place. Optimum temperatures are indicative of natural habitats and for mollicutes associated with mammals and birds are close to 37°C (29); *M. mobile* (from tench) was isolated at 25°C (44). Spiroplasmas from infected plants have temperature optima of 30 to 32°C, whereas *S. mirum*, the suckling mouse cataract agent, is typically cultured at 30°C but also shows good growth at 37°C (131). Anaeroplasmas may grow at temperatures as high as 47°C (29).

Mollicutes generally grow and survive over a fairly narrow pH range. For most species of plant and vertebrate origin, the optimum pH is approximately 7.4 (i.e., similar to that of serum and of mammalian intracellular pH) and growth occurs between about pH 6.5 and 8.0 (102). Ureaplasmas are exceptional, having an optimum pH of 6.0 to 6.5 and being inhibited above pH 7.5 (89). In attempts to isolate mollicutes from new environments, however, pH optima of 7 to 8 should not be assumed. Hackett and Clark (32) considered the possible habitats of invertebrate spiroplasmas to include the lumen of cytolysosomes, in which the pH may be as low as 5.0.

A major problem presented by the relatively narrow pH range for growth is growth inhibition in culture media as a consequence of excessive acid or alkali production. The yield of ATP from energy sources in mollicutes is low (discussed above). Thus, glucose-fermenting and arginine-hydrolyzing species may produce large quantities of acid and NH_3, respectively; NH_3 production also accompanies urea hydrolysis by *Ureaplasma* species. A variety of buffers and conditions have been used in culture media to limit pH change, including phosphate buffer for *M. mycoides*, which was, however, inhibitory for *A. laidlawii* (102); *N*-2 - hydroxyethylpiperazine - *N'* - 2 - ethanesulfonic acid (HEPES), which is widely used (11, 33, 50, 100, 113); and incubation in an atmosphere of 100% CO_2 (89) (discussed below). An increase in the pH of culture media for ureaplasmas was also retarded by L-histidine (1).

The optimum osmotic pressure for the growth of a range of *Mycoplasma* species and *A. laidlawii*, on both solid and fluid media, was found by Leach (47) to be about 10 atm (1 atm = 101.29 kPa). *M. gallisepticum*, the most exacting of the species studied, failed to grow outside the range of 7 to 14 atm, whereas *A. laidlawii* multiplied at up to 27 atm. In spiroplasmas, growth has been reported at osmotic pressures of between 6.5 and 32 atm (54), though the range and optimal values for growth varied widely with the species. *S. citri* had an optimal value of approximately 12 atm, whereas for *S. mirum*, the range was 6.5 to 14 atm and the optimum value was only 7.2 atm. Plant spiroplasmas may be adapted to relatively high osmotic pressures since they inhabit sieve tubes, in which osmotic pressures of 13 to 15 atm prevail (54). These demonstrations of the critical effects of tonicity on mollicute growth rate, and the variability of osmotic requirements for growth in those species studied, are of significance to many aspects of research, including isolation and nutritional studies. However, it is possible to draw examples from the recent literature in which effects attributed to the presence of high concentrations of salts or sugars could not clearly be distinguished from osmotic effects. Medium osmotic pressure may increase during growth as a consequence of metabolism.

Atmospheric Requirements

Atmospheric requirements for the growth of mollicutes have been discussed by Gardella and Del Giudice (29). They made the important point that the gaseous environment of a culture could not be viewed as an independent variable and that interacting factors, including pH and composition of the medium, oxidation and reduction of medium components, and humidity (for growth on agar plates), must be considered. In general, isolation of mollicutes from animal sources is favored by anaerobic conditions; the anaeroplasmas are strict anaerobes and require prereduced media for growth (94). However, *A. laidlawii* was occasionally isolated only aerobically (65), and 5% O_2 in nitrogen was optimal for the isolation of *M. hyorhinis* from cell culture (29). The growth of fastidious *Spiroplasma* strains in a serum-free medium occurred readily in both aerobic and anaerobic conditions, though in a serum-containing medium, growth was better anaerobically (50).

The ability of oxygen to prevent growth may be due to depletion of cellular reducing power, and all mollicutes investigated possess NADH oxidase. Cell death may then occur as a result of the formation of H_2O_2 and possibly other active oxygen intermediates, including superoxide (O_2^-). H_2O_2 is a product of glycerol oxidation in *M. mycoides* and other *Mycoplasma* species (see above) and may also be formed during NADH oxidation (56, 69). Oxygen, though, may also stimulate the growth rate of some mycoplasmas (102, 121), presumably because it may increase the yield of ATP generated during the metabolism of glucose and other carbohydrates (see above). However, the effects of oxygen on mollicute growth may not be seen in many apparently aerobically incubated cultures. The solubility of oxygen in water is low (220 nmol/ml at 37°C), and the maintenance of high dissolved oxygen tensions in cultures which utilize oxygen will be dependent on the rate of oxygen diffusion across the gas-liquid interface; thus, when the ratio of the interface area to culture volume is low, O_2 metabolism may become limited by its concentration. Since mollicute cultures are almost universally incubated statically (i.e., without shaking or stirring; see below), O_2-limited conditions are likely to occur during the growth of the faster-growing O_2-utilizing strains. Thus, gentle aeration increased the growth rate and yield of *M. mycoides* (102), whereas vortex aeration of cultures prevented growth unless large cell populations were present (75). Tourtellotte and Jacobs (121) also found that for a variety of fermentative strains, growth rate and yield under anaerobic conditions (in liquid culture and on agar plates) were poorer than in air and that optimal growth was achieved in an atmosphere of 1 to 8% O_2.

Catalase has been added to *Mycoplasma* cell suspensions to promote survival (67) and has also been used in some culture media (see below). It may be of relevance to studies with fastidious mollicutes that the inability of *Legionella* species to grow in common laboratory media has been ascribed to the accumulation of low levels of H_2O_2 and O_2^-, produced by photochemical oxidation of medium components (38). Such accumulation was prevented by the addition of activated charcoal, or catalase plus superoxide dismutase, which allowed *Legionella* growth.

The concentration of atmospheric CO_2 may also affect mollicute growth, and levels of 5 to 15% (vol/vol) have been advised for the cultivation of ureaplasmas (29). In spiroplasmas, increased CO_2 concentrations (achieved by using a candle jar) improved growth in serum-containing but not serum-free medium (50). An increase in atmospheric CO_2 concentration leads to increased concentrations of dissolved CO_2 and hence HCO_3^-. Thus, CO_2 may act to buffer culture media and prevent or delay an increase in pH as a consequence of, for example, urea hydrolysis (89). CO_2 may also be required for anaplerotic reactions (60).

MEDIA

Undefined Media

Mollicutes are nutritionally exacting and need to be supplied with a large array of precursors for the synthesis of macromolecules. Numerous undefined growth media have been described, and formulations for many of these are listed in *Methods for Mycoplasmology* (28, 95, 113, 130). Media may contain peptone; beef heart infusion; yeast extract; animal serum; DNA; glucose, arginine, or urea; and sodium chloride. Peptones contain polypeptides, dipeptides, and amino acids and vary according to the source of protein used in their preparation. Fresh yeast extract contains labile components not present in commercial preparations of dehydrated, enzymatic digests of yeast cells and may be readily prepared (28); many formulations include both dried and fresh yeast extracts. Animal sera are widely used at 5 to 20% (vol/vol) to provide a nontoxic source of lipids; however, they also provide a range of other nutrients, including inorganic ions, sugars, and urea. DNA supplies nucleic acid precursors but is not included in all media; it is required for the primary isolation of *M. bovigenitalium* and stimulates the growth of many other species (28). Glucose or another suitable carbohydrate, or arginine or urea, may be added as an energy source (discussed above). The role of NaCl is to increase medium tonicity.

In addition to the ingredients listed above, media may contain NADH, which will be present to some extent in other components, including fresh yeast extract; L-cysteine hydrochloride, which at the concentrations used (0.1% [wt/vol]; e.g., Frey medium [28]) will act as a reducing agent and lower the oxidation-reduction potential of the medium, making it more suitable for the growth of anaerobic or microaerophilic organisms; putrescine and glycyl-L-histidyl-L-lysine for ureaplasmas; and sorbitol (up to 70 g per liter) in place of NaCl to adjust the tonicity of media for spiroplasmas. Catalase has also been included in a medium specifically designed for the production of live *M. mycoides* vaccine for contagious bovine pleuropneumonia, for which retention of a high viable count over a long period was required (39).

Media developed for anaeroplasmas are quite different from those for other mollicutes (94, 95). Serum is not used, and clarified rumen fluid (40% [vol/vol]) is included in some media formulations, especially for isolation. However, growth may occur in rumen-fluid-free medium supplemented with cholesterol and lipopolysaccharide. Starch is provided as an energy source.

The use of undefined media, and the inherent variation in such components as serum and meat and yeast extracts, requires that attention be paid to the quality control of culture media. This problem is discussed by Tully and Rose (127), who suggest basic testing procedures that might be followed. Of special importance is the use of appropriate test strains; for example, mycoplasma strains with a minimum passage level on artificial media should be used to test medium quality for primary isolation of that mycoplasma. Serum is a particularly variable component of most media, and its growth-promoting ability may vary with the animal from which it is derived and sometimes also for the same animal when bled at different times (28). Horse serum, not heat inactivated, is most commonly used. However, some media formulations stipulate the use of fetal calf, porcine, or bovine serum and, in some cases, combinations of sera (e.g., horse plus pig serum in FF medium [28]).

Natural antibodies in sera may inhibit mollicute growth but may be avoided by the use of agamma sera. Mollicutes might also be susceptible to lysis by complement, which may be inactivated by heating serum at 56°C for 30 min. The nutritive properties of serum vary markedly with the animal source used, perhaps reflecting variation in the levels and proportions of lipids, which will influence the composition of the mollicute membrane and thus affect many aspects of cell morphology and transport of medium components (discussed below). There may also be other differences; for example, fetal mammalian serum contains a high concentration of fructose (67), and horse serum is relatively rich in urea (114). Thus, the most suitable serum for each mollicute species can be determined only by experimentation.

While in undefined media the major role of serum is to provide the lipids essential for mollicute growth, the presence of serum proteins is also important, since they protect against the toxic effects of other serum and medium components. In particular, serum proteins bind phospholipids and fatty acids which are surface active. Enzymes present in serum may also be significant. Animal sera may be replaced by PPLO serum fraction (Difco) for the cultivation of some mollicutes (28), and egg yolk extract was superior to horse serum for the growth and primary isolation of *M. pneumoniae* (112). Serum may also be replaced by serum albumin-lipid mixtures (discussed below).

The range of possible factors limiting growth rate or growth yield in undefined medium is vast. There is clearly substantial metabolic, nutritional, and ecological diversity among mollicutes. However, for the vast majority of species, optimal physical and atmospheric conditions for growth have not been systematically determined. The diversity of nutrients makes it unlikely that a specific nutrient(s) is absent per se. However, when energy sources are unknown, low growth yields may reflect low concentrations of energy substrates and the small quantities of ATP generated during substrate metabolism. Nutrients may also be available in a form in which they may not be assimilated. For example, *M. pneumoniae* specifically binds lactoferrin but not transferrin, whereas *M. genitalium* binds neither of these iron-sequestering compounds (123). Such differences in iron uptake mechanisms may have important implications for the design of culture media. Lactoferrin is found in mucosal secretions, whereas transferrin is present in serum.

A further possibility is that growth of some mollicutes may be prevented or inhibited by an imbalance of nutrients, such as fatty acids or amino acids which share the same transport system. Although it is known that amino acids may be taken up by an active transport mechanism in *Mycoplasma* species (16), the number of animo acid transport proteins, the organisms' specificities for amino acids, and the variation in specificities among different mollicute species are unknown. Also, while it is known that the lipid composition of growth media affects cell morphology and membrane function, we generally attempt to grow mollicutes from diverse habitats in media with relatively fixed lipid composition. For species that grow well in undefined media and for ureaplasmas, a major factor limiting biomass production may be change in medium pH, which may at least in part be overcome by the use of buffered medium. Another limiting factor may be production of H_2O_2 and other active oxygen intermediates (discussed above). Catalase is present in serum but may be inactivated by O_2^- (45); O_2^- production has been demonstrated in *M. pneumoniae* (57).

Defined Media

Defined media allow precise investigation of the role and effect of individual nutrients on cell yield, growth rate, morphology, and formation of products such as toxic metabolites like H_2O_2 and the galactan capsule of *M. mycoides* subsp. *mycoides*. This information is of crucial importance to the understanding of mollicute-host interactions and may help explain mollicute ecology. It is also of general interest in view of the small genome sizes of mollicutes and their lack of a cell wall and the implications of this feature as regards the mechanism of chromosome separation (following DNA replication), cell division, and maintenance of cell volume. In addition, since defined media allow precise control over medium constituents, it should be possible to optimize concentrations of amino acids, fatty acids, and other components so as to avoid (as far as possible) nutrient antagonisms which may limit growth rate or cell yield in undefined media (discussed above). Inhibitory components of, for example, serum would also be avoided, and problems arising from the adsorption of serum proteins on cell membranes in antigenic studies would be eliminated. Finally, defined media would not be subject to the batch-to-batch variation of media containing such products as serum and meat and yeast extracts. The development of defined media supporting high growth rates and cell yields is thus a significant research objective.

A major difficulty in devising defined media for mollicutes is in providing lipids in a nontoxic but available form. Successful approaches have included the use of mixtures of water-dispersible diacetoxysuccinoyl esters of mono- and diglycerides for *M. mycoides* Y (98) and Tween 80 (120) or low concentrations of free fatty acids (122) for *A. laidlawii*. The use of esters and Tween 80 is presumably dependent on cellular lipase activity (108), resulting in the slow release of free fatty acid. For many mollicute species, serum may also be replaced with lipids bound to serum albumin. Commercial serum albumin contains both fatty acids and cholesterol, which may be removed by mild alkaline

methanolysis or charcoal treatment (100). Lipids for inclusion in growth media (e.g., cholesterol, palmitic and oleic acids, Tween 40, Tween 80, phosphatidic acid, and phospholipids) are dissolved in ethanol and added to an aqueous solution of defatted serum albumin. The BSA may be regarded as a defined medium constituent, since it may be purified and its amino acid sequence is known. However, it may be subject to proteolytic degradation by some mycoplasmas, including *M. mycoides* Y (100), thus making it difficult to determine amino acid requirement and also leading to variable concentrations of free amino acids and peptides. Serum has also been successfully replaced by liposomes for the cultivation of some fermentative mycoplasmas (18, 41); however, in *M. gallisepticum*, the addition of defatted BSA was required to give optimal yields (19). It has been shown that serum albumin enhances the exchange of cholesterol between *M. gallisepticum* cells and phosphatidylcholine and cholesterol vesicles (109).

The provision of amino acids in proportions favorable to growth may also be difficult to achieve; reference to amino acid antagonism has already been made (discussed above). In a defined medium for *M. mycoides* Y, growth rate was increased by the addition of vitamin-free casein digest, leading Rodwell to suggest that the rate of transport of an amino acid limited growth (100). Comparison of the amino acid concentrations required for the growth of *M. mycoides* Y and *M. capricolum* in defined media also suggested that multiple amino acid antagonisms for uptake occurred in the latter organism. One approach to this problem is to provide some amino acids as peptides. Mollicute requirements for energy sources, nucleic acid precursors, and vitamins have been discussed above.

Defined media (C4 and C5) containing BSA, for *M. mycoides* Y and *M. capricolum*, and a partly defined medium containing BSA and (undefined) casein digest, for *A. laidlawii*, are described by Rodwell (100); the latter medium is a modification of that of Razin and Cohen (87). These media are essentially minimal media and, in addition to organic components, contain K^+, PO_4^{3-}, and Mg^{2+} (as $MgSO_4$). Trace elements (e.g., $Fe^{2+/3+}$, Mn^{2+}, and Zn^{2+}) were not included (see above). In media C4 and C5, NaCl was excluded and a high concentration of sodium phosphate buffer (140 mM) was used to adjust tonicity. In the medium for *A. laidlawii*, buffering capacity was provided by HEPES and NaCl was included. This medium also contained $(NH_4)_2SO_4$.

In C4 medium, *M. mycoides* Y grew with a mass doubling time of 2.2 h and gave a yield of 0.3 g of cell protein per liter. In C5 medium, the doubling time of *M. capricolum* was usually 4 h, but after adaptation, clones were isolated with doubling times as low as 2.5 h (100). These media, however, were not suitable for the growth of even closely related strains without the addition of vitamin-free casein digest or, in some cases, adaptation by serial passage. The *A. laidlawii* medium gave yields (0.3 g of cell protein per liter) comparable with those in undefined media, but growth rates were lower.

The media so far described are essentially minimal media. An alternative approach has been to base defined media on existing tissue culture formulations, with the addition of appropriate BSA-lipid mixtures and carbohydrates. This approach has led to the description of defined media suitable for the growth of *A. laidlawii* (30) and particularly spiroplasmas (11, 12, 33), for which growth rates and growth yields comparable to those in undefined media have been obtained. Such defined media contain diverse ranges of nutrients (70 or more), and the significance of the majority of these for mollicute growth is unknown. However, the ability of H-1 medium to support the growth of *S. mirum* (33) demonstrated that the development of defined media was a feasible goal, even for the more fastidious mollicutes. Importantly, the use of H-1 medium enabled demonstration of the sphingomyelin requirement of *S. mirum*, thus providing an insight into its pathology and association with sphingomyelin-rich tissue in vivo. A defined medium for anaeroplasmas has also been described (94, 95).

In conclusion, there appears to be no fundamental reason why defined media should not be developed for all mollicutes capable of growth in vitro, and the use of tissue culture formulations may provide an advanced starting point. The description of defined minimal media, and optimization of the concentrations of lipid and particularly amino acid components, will clearly require substantial work. However, even in the absence of fully defined medium, there would seem no reason why a move should not be made to greater definition of undefined media. In particular, pH might be more closely controlled by using buffers, and inorganic ions required in relatively large amounts for growth (K^+, Mg^{2+}, PO_4^{3-}) might be added to ensure that levels of these ions do not become growth limiting. Serum might also be replaced with advantage. Lee and Davis (50) developed a serum-free medium for fastidious *S. kunkelii* strains in which growth rates and growth yields were similar to those in serum-containing medium. The serum-free medium, however, was less subject to deterioration during storage and gave consistently high growth rates and titers, and less stringent atmospheric conditions were required during incubation. Also, the success rate in primary isolation was equal to (*S. citri*) or better than (*S. kunkelii*) that in serum-containing medium, and Lee and Davis stated that serum-free medium was used routinely in all work in their laboratory.

Isolation Media

The media used for isolation of mollicutes may support the rapid growth of bacteria and fungi also present in material to be sampled. Primary isolation media, therefore, usually contain inhibitors of bacterial and fungal growth. Thallium acetate (0.5 to 1.0 g per liter) prevents the growth of many gram-negative and some gram-positive bacteria. Mollicutes are generally resistant to these concentrations, but notable exceptions include ureaplasmas and *M. genitalium* (125). Benzylpenicillin and ampicillin specifically inhibit cross-linking of peptidoglycan chains in the cell walls of both gram-positive and gram-negative bacteria and are widely used in isolation media at concentrations of up to 2,000 U/ml and 1.0 mg/ml, respectively. Surprisingly, however, a number of mollicutes are susceptible to these antibiotics (88). In contrast, polymyxin B, which acts as a cationic detergent and

binds specifically to the cell membrane, appears to be relatively inactive against a number of mycoplasmas, including *M. genitalium*, and can be used (at 500 U/ml) to suppress gram-negative bacterial contamination in clinical specimens (125). A range of antibiotics inhibiting various stages in bacterial cell wall synthesis, including vancomycin, ristocetin, bacitracin, alafosfalin, D-cycloserine, and fosfomycin, may be suitable alternatives to the bacterial inhibitors in current use. Control of fungal contamination may be achieved by using amphotericin B at a concentration of 2.5 mg/ml (125). This antibiotic binds sterol and is therefore active against the cell membrane of mollicutes which contain sterol; however, it has a higher affinity for ergosterol (the principal membrane sterol of fungi) than for cholesterol.

Selection pressures on populations of mollicutes will differ substantially in vivo and in vitro. Thus, during passage in culture media, pathogenic attributes of strains may be lost, and mutations favoring increased cell yield and higher growth rate in vitro will accumulate. The nutritional and cultural conditions required for mollicute isolation are therefore usually more stringent than those for the growth of high-passage strains; these conditions are described in *Methods in Mycoplasmology* (126). Loss of virulence in in vitro-passaged cultures of the cattle pathogen *M. mycoides* subsp. *mycoides* was noted in the early 1920s and led to the development of attenuated live vaccine strains (39). Repeated subculture in broth medium has subsequently been used to develop attenuated strains of a variety of mollicute species. The biochemical mechanisms of attenuation are largely unknown. However, *M. mycoides* subsp. *mycoides* lost the ability to produce GP oxidase when grown for 100 generations in chemostat continuous culture (128). This enzyme produces H_2O_2 during GP oxidation, and selection against the GP-positive parent strain may have been associated with oxidative damage. Also, amino acid transport mutants may be obtained after serial passage of *M. mycoides* Y in defined medium (discussed above).

EFFECTS OF NUTRITIONAL AND CULTURAL FACTORS ON CELL MORPHOLOGY AND GROWTH

Effects of Culture Age and Medium Components on Cell Morphology

A number of morphological types exist within mollicutes (8, 59). In many species, there is a marked tendency toward filament formation, especially during the early exponential phase, and Rodwell and Mitchell (102) concluded that filamentous growth could occur in most, if not all, mollicutes under appropriate conditions. Increase in the number of viable units takes place by binary fission or the fragmentation of filaments. There is substantial evidence in the literature that pronounced morphological change may occur as culture age increases (8, 59). Morphology may also be markedly affected by the nutritional quality and osmotic strength of the medium (84) and importantly by the lipid content of the membrane (102). This effect is either dependent on or largely influenced by medium lipid composition (discussed above), although the membrane lipid composition of *M. capricolum* and *M. mycoides* was also observed to change with culture age (31, 110). Membrane lipid composition may additionally affect cell volume (105), the kinetics of substrate transport (91), cell permeability (64), susceptibility to osmotic lysis, and the temperature range for growth (110). The appearance of rho forms in *M. mycoides* and *M. capricolum* was also dependent upon medium composition (102). In addition, Hackett and Clark (32) point out that whereas spiroplasmas are generally seen as helical filaments in culture, they are usually spherical inside host cells, and these authors speculate on the possible role of ions in bringing about this transition by their effects on membrane integrity and osmotic regulation. Spiroplasmas lacking a helical morphology in vitro have, however, been reported (49), and alteration in medium lipid composition has been shown to induce change in the characteristic helical morphology of *S. citri* (27).

Growth in Liquid Media

Static and stirred cultures

Typically, mollicutes are grown in statically incubated cultures and there is no attempt to ensure homogeneity within the culture. Thus, gradients of oxygen (discussed above), nutrients, and metabolic products (including dissolved CO_2) are likely to exist. The alternative to this procedure is to grow cells in stirred vessels or to incubate them on shakers. Tourtellotte and Jacobs (121) were able to grow a variety of mollicute species by using 8-liter volumes of medium in 12-liter flasks and shaking the flasks at 60 rpm. Shaking increased cell yield, but whether oxygen saturation was maintained with such a large volume of medium is unclear. The maintenance of high dissolved oxygen concentrations may inhibit growth, especially when H_2O_2 is a by-product of substrate oxidation (discussed above). However, *M. mycoides* was able to grow in stirred and aerated chemostat culture (discussed below), and *M. felis* (which ferments but does not oxidize glucose in salts solution) grew readily in 250-ml flasks containing 25 ml of medium when shaken at 220 rpm under aerobic conditions (75a). It has been suggested that vortex aeration may inhibit growth by the action of shear forces on mycoplasma filaments (75), though effects due to such forces were not distinguishable from the possible effects of increased dissolved oxygen tension.

When homogeneous culture conditions are not maintained, the possibility that cell populations will be heterogeneous must be considered. Gradients of, for example, oxygen within media may lead to differences in growth rate (either stimulation or inhibition). Also, the presence of oxygen has been shown to increase the apparent pyruvate dehydrogenase and pyruvate dehydrogenase complex activities in a number of *Mycoplasma* and *Acholeplasma* species (21). The availability of oxygen in cultures incubated statically in air may also determine substrate utilization (70). In a salts solution, *M. agalactiae* oxidized both pyruvate and lactate. However, whereas pyruvate supported growth in a broth medium, lactate did not, suggesting that the oxygen concentration was limiting metabolism; metabolism of pyruvate to lactate, acetate, and CO_2 may occur in the absence of oxygen.

Heterogeneity among cell populations may be of particular significance for work with those mollicutes, including *M. pneumoniae*, which grow as submerged colonies attached to the walls of glass or plastic culture vessels. Substantial differences in nutrient and toxic product concentration may be expected between the center and edges of colonies. However, it is possible that manipulation of the ionic and glucose concentration of the medium may reduce adhesion (86).

Growth curves of mollicutes in batch culture

In liquid culture, mollicutes show typical bacterial growth curves, with lag, exponential, stationary, and decline phases (59). However, it may be inadequate to describe cells simply as being from the exponential or stationary phase. In the complex media used for mollicute growth, it is rarely possible to establish the nutrient factor(s) limiting growth rate or to determine whether it is the same factor(s) throughout the growth phase, though concentrations of individual amino acids markedly affected the growth rate of *M. capricolum* in defined medium (100). Morphology and cell composition during growth may alter as a direct result of a reduction in the concentration of a nutrient(s), for example, a lipid(s) (discussed above). However, it will also alter as changes in the concentration of nutrients, toxic products, or pH affect growth rate. The importance of growth rate in determining cell structure and function should not be underestimated (37, 79).

There have been few studies from which it is clearly possible to determine whether growth rate is constant during the growth phase of cultures, especially at the higher biomass concentrations at which cells are usually harvested for experimental work. In a serum-containing medium, the specific growth rate of *M. mycoides* started to decline rapidly when a cell concentration of 4×10^8 CFU/ml was reached, though the final cell population was approximately 5×10^9 CFU/ml (7). In an independent study in which the heat output of *M. mycoides* cultures was continuously monitored, marked changes in rates of metabolic activity during growth were also apparent (Fig. 1). In addition, it has shown that in *M. mycoides*, the syntheses of DNA, protein, and lipid are not coordinated (102) and that during the later stages of growth, cell DNA, turbidity, and viable count do not increase uniformly (99).

The composition and metabolic activity of apparently stationary-phase cells may also show considerable variation. At the end of active growth, cellular ATP content and the EC_A (see above) fall rapidly, and there may be marked morphological changes (8, 59). In addition, the viable count may decline rapidly (59), especially if there are substantial pH changes during growth (102). It is also possible that the factor limiting growth yield (either nutrient or toxic product) may vary between experiments as a consequence of variation in the nutritive quality of undefined medium components, particularly serum. The cell yield in liquid culture varies widely with the species; values as high as 500 mg of dry mass per liter have been reported; however, even in the most successful media so far devised, ureaplasmas and a number of fastidious spiroplasmas and mycoplasmas give only a few milligrams of dry cell mass per liter. Cell doubling times vary from 0.34 h (for *A. morum* [5]) to several hours. When toxic products or pH limit growth, yields may be increased by using dialysis bag culture. This technique enabled high populations of ureaplasmas to be maintained for approximately 60 h by delaying the adverse effects of NH_3 production (62).

Some of the difficulties in obtaining reproducible batches of cells for experimental work might be overcome by using defined media or growing cells at known and constant growth rates in chemostat continuous culture (discussed below). It might also be advantageous to use nutrient-limited media, i.e., to reduce the concentration of a medium component, such as the energy source, to a level at which it limits the growth yield, rather than some unknown and perhaps variable factor(s). In addition, improved reproducibility of cell production may be obtained by using liquid nitrogen stored inocula. Suspensions of *M. mycoides*, frozen in liquid nitrogen and thawed under controlled conditions, showed little reduction in metabolic activity or viability (67, 68).

Continuous-culture studies

In chemostat continuous culture, culture fluid is continuously removed from a fermentor and replaced at an equal rate by fresh medium. The fermentor contents are stirred to ensure that the system is homogeneous, and at equilibrium (the steady state), the specific growth rate is equal to the dilution rate (the medium flow rate divided by the fermentor volume). Thus, the specific growth rate may be controlled by manipulation of the dilution rate, allowing effects which are directly dependent on growth rate to be distinguished from those due to other environmental factors; also, cells of constant composition and metabolic activity may be produced over substantial time periods. Chemostat culture has been used to determine the effects of specific growth rate on the morphology and carbohydrate (capsule) content of *M. mycoides* (36). Filaments were observed at all growth rates used (0.010 to 0.0160/h, corresponding to culture doubling times of 69 to 4.3 h, respectively). However, at a very low dilution rate (0.034/h), large aberrant cells were seen and there was evidence of reduced culture viability. The ratio of viable count to cell protein decreased by a factor of 12 as the dilution rate increased from 0.034 to 0.16/h, implying that mean cell size or filament length increased with increasing growth rate. Also, the ratio of cell carbohydrate to protein increased with increasing dilution rate and was higher in glucose-excess than in glucose-limited medium. Since more than 90% of cell carbohydrate in *M. mycoides* is accounted for by the capsule, the results suggested that capsule synthesis increased with increasing growth rate and glucose concentration.

The growth of *M. mobile* and *M. hominis* in continuous culture has also been demonstrated (46). The system used in this study was described as a pH-controlled metabolistat, and the flow of fresh medium into the fermentor was not continuous but dependent on pH change. Thus, no real steady state, as regards growth rate, is achieved in the system. However, the system provided a means of producing a continuous supply of mycoplasma cells. When continuous systems are used for mollicute cell production, the possibility that spontaneous mutants will arise and be selected for should be considered.

Growth on Agar

Mollicutes are usually grown on agar plates for the determination of viable count (see above) or for isolation. The growth characteristics of colonies on agar and factors affecting their development have been discussed previously (54, 85). In isolation media, especially for *M. pneumoniae*, biphasic liquid or agar media may be used (28). Agar media are usually undefined, though a serum-free medium has been described for isolation of spiroplasmas (50). Defined agar media may have application in the study of nutritional requirements in mollicutes and in genetic studies for the enumeration of metabolic mutants. In a serum-free medium for *M. mycoides*, the addition of catalase (400 µg/ml) markedly increased colony count and maximum colony diameter (70a).

Cell-Assisted Culture

Hackett and Lynn (34) have reported the growth of the Colorado potato beetle spiroplasma in tissue culture media in the presence of coleopteran and lepidopteran insect lines. High titers (1.2×10^9/ml after 100 passages) were obtained, and a minimum doubling time of 7.5 h was achieved. The sex-ratio organism from *Drosophila* cells has been similarly cultured (35). Neither the Colorado potato beetle spiroplasma nor the sex-ratio organism has been grown in cell-free medium, and this approach might be successfully applied to the cultivation of other highly fastidious mollicutes.

SUMMARY

The complexity of the nutritional requirements and the variable cell form and osmotic fragility of mollicutes make these organisms a significant challenge in physiological investigations relating to their growth and ecology. However, the conditions under which mollicutes are grown may significantly influence cell structure and function and thus are of importance not only to physiologists but to all mycoplasmologists involved in quantitative studies. The difficulties of working with mollicutes have meant that in the majority of published studies, growth conditions, and in some cases growth yields, have been poorly defined. Therefore, an aim in future studies might be to grow cells under conditions which are as defined as possible, whether the purpose of cell production is to provide inocula for growth or pathogenicity studies or to investigate cell metabolism, structure, or morphology. Improved definition of cell production requires that continued effort be applied to the development of defined media and of minimal defined media. However, the conditions under which cultures are incubated may also be of critical importance. Although for many mollicutes (or for those studying them), it may not yet be feasible to attempt growth in fermentor systems offering control of such parameters as specific growth rate, pH, or dissolved oxygen tension, the limitations of current culture techniques should be recognized.

An additional aim of nutritional studies is to enable efficient and rapid isolation of mollicutes, and for this purpose, the complexity of isolation media and the vagaries of current culture techniques may be of little consequence. However, a more systematic approach to determination of the nutritional and cultural requirements of mollicutes might aid the development of media offering improved isolation rates of fastidious species and the detection or cultivation of new species. It might also be advantageous to consider more carefully the physical and chemical environments of mollicutes in vivo and the extent to which they can be reproduced in culture.

REFERENCES

1. **Ajello, F., and N. Romano.** 1975. Effect of L-histidine on the survival of a T-strain of mycoplasma. *Appl. Microbiol.* **29:**293–294.
2. **Anonymous.** 1983. *The Bacteriological Examination of Drinking Water Supplies 1982.* Her Majesty's Stationery Office, London.
3. **Bastian, F. O., B. S. Baliga, and H. M. Pollack.** 1988. Evaluation of [³H]thymidine uptake method for studying growth of spiroplasmas under various conditions. *J. Clin. Microbiol.* **26:**2124–2126.
4. **Beaman, K. D., and J. D. Pollack.** 1981. Adenylate energy charge in *Acholeplasma laidlawii. J. Bacteriol.* **146:**1055–1058.
5. **Beaman, K. D., and J. D. Pollack.** 1983. Synthesis of adenylate nucleotides by mollicutes (mycoplasmas). *J. Gen. Microbiol.* **129:**3103–3110.
6. **Bhakoo, M., and R. N. McElhaney.** 1988. The effect of variations in growth temperature, fatty acid composition and cholesterol content on the lipid polar headgroup composition of *Acholeplasma laidlawii* B membranes. *Biochim. Biophys. Acta* **945:**307–314.
7. **Boarer, C. D. H., W. C. S. Read, and J. J. Read.** 1971. Estimation of the growth of the T1 strain of *Mycoplasma mycoides* in tryptose broth by the measurement of lactate dehydrogenase. I. *Methods Appl. Microbiol.* **22:**763–768.
8. **Boatman, E. S.** 1979. Morphology and ultrastructure of the Mycoplasmatales, p. 63–102. *In* M. F. Barile and S. Razin (ed.), *The Mycoplasmas*, vol. 1. Academic Press, New York.
9. **Bredt, W.** 1976. Estimation of *Mycoplasma pneumoniae* inoculum size by rate of tetrazolium reduction. *J. Clin. Microbiol.* **4:**92–94.
10. **Chang, C.-J.** 1986. Inorganic salts and the growth of spiroplasmas. *Can. J. Microbiol.* **32:**861–866.
11. **Chang, C.-J.** 1989. Nutrition and cultivation of spiroplasmas, p. 201–243. *In* R. F. Whitcomb and J. G. Tully (ed.), *The Mycoplasmas*, vol. 5. Academic Press, San Diego, Calif.
12. **Chang, C.-J., and T. A. Chen.** 1982. Spiroplasmas: cultivation in chemically defined medium. *Science* **215:**1121–1122.
13. **Chang, C.-J., and T. A. Chen.** 1983. Nutritional requirements of two flower spiroplasmas and honeybee spiroplasma. *J. Bacteriol.* **153:**452–457.
14. **Chang, C.-J., and M. G. Garrett.** 1987. Growth of spiroplasmas in the presence of various nutrients and metabolic inhibitors. *Can. J. Microbiol.* **33:**555–562.
15. **Chen, T. A., and R. E. Davis.** 1979. Cultivation of spiroplasmas, p. 65–84. *In* R. F. Whitcomb and J. G. Tully

(ed.), *The Mycoplasmas*, vol. 3. Academic Press, New York.
16. **Cirillo, V. P.** 1979. Transport systems, p. 323–350. *In* M. F. Barile and S. Razin (ed.), *The Mycoplasmas*, vol. 1. Academic Press, New York.
17. **Clejan, S., R. Bittman, and S. Rottem.** 1978. Uptake, transbilayer distribution, and movement of cholesterol in growing *Mycoplasma capricolum* cells. *Biochemistry* **17:**4579–4583.
18. **Cluss, R. G., J. K. Johnson, and N. L. Somersom.** 1983. Liposomes replace serum for cultivation of fermentative mycoplasmas. *Appl. Environ. Microbiol.* **46:**370–374.
19. **Cluss, R. G., and N. L. Somersom.** 1986. Interaction of albumin and phospholipid:cholesterol liposomes in growth of *Mycoplasma* spp. *Appl. Environ. Microbiol.* **51:**281–287.
20. **Cocks, B. G., F. A. Brake, A. Mitchell, and L. R. Finch.** 1985. Enzymes of intermediary carbohydrate metabolism in *Ureaplasma urealyticum* and *Mycoplasma mycoides* subsp. *mycoides. J. Gen. Microbiol.* **131:**2129–2135.
21. **Constantopoulos, G., and G. J. McGarrity.** 1987. Activities of oxidative enzymes in mycoplasmas. *J. Bacteriol.* **169:**2012–2016.
22. **Dahl, J.** 1988. Uptake of fatty acids by *Mycoplasma capricolum. J. Bacteriol.* **170:**2022–2026.
23. **Davis, P. J., A. Katznel, S. Razin, and S. Rottem.** 1985. Spiroplasma membrane lipids. *J. Bacteriol.* **161:**118–122.
24. **Desantis, D., V. V. Tryon, and D. Pollack.** 1989. Metabolism of mollicutes: the Embden-Meyerhof-Parnas pathway and the hexose monophosphate shunt. *J. Gen. Microbiol.* **135:**683–691.
25. **Fenske, J. D., and G. E. Kenny.** 1976. Role of arginine deiminase in growth of *Mycoplasma hominis. J. Bacteriol.* **126:**501–510.
26. **Firstenberg-Eden, R., and R. Eden.** 1984. *Impedance Microbiology.* John Wiley & Sons, New York.
27. **Freeman, B. A., R. Sissenstein, T. T. McManus, J. E. Woodward, I. M. Lee, and J. B. Mudd.** 1976. Lipid composition and lipid metabolism of *Spiroplasma citri. J. Bacteriol.* **125:**946–954.
28. **Freundt, E. A.** 1983. Culture media for classic mycoplasmas, p. 127–135. *In* S. Razin and J. G. Tully (ed.), *Methods in Mycoplasmology*, vol. 1. Academic Press, New York.
29. **Gardella, R. S., and R. A. Del Giudice.** 1983. Optimal temperature and atmospheric conditions for growth, p. 211–218. *In* S. Razin and J. G. Tully (ed.), *Methods in Mycoplasmology*, vol. 1. Academic Press, New York.
30. **Greenaway, S. D., and D. A. J. Wase.** 1982. Two chemically defined media for the growth of *Acholeplasma laidlawii* strain A. *Biotechnol. Lett.* **4:**217–222.
31. **Gross, Z., and S. Rottem.** 1986. Lipid interconversions in aging *Mycoplasma capricolum* cultures. *J. Bacteriol.* **167:**986–991.
32. **Hackett, K. J., and T. B. Clark.** 1989. Ecology of spiroplasmas, p. 113–200. *In* R. F. Whitcomb and J. G. Tully (ed.), *The Mycoplasmas*, vol. 5. Academic Press, San Diego, Calif.
33. **Hackett, K. J., A. S. Ginsberg, S. Rottem, R. B. Henegar, and R. F. Whitcomb.** 1987. A defined medium for a fastidious spiroplasma. *Science* **237:**525–527.
34. **Hackett, K. J., and D. E. Lynn.** 1985. Cell-assisted growth of a fastidious spiroplasma. *Science* **230:**825–827.
35. **Hackett, K. J., D. E. Lynn, D. L. Williamson, A. S. Ginsberg, and R. F. Whitcomb.** 1986. Cultivation of the *Drosophila* sex ratio spiroplasma. *Science* **232:**1253–1255.
36. **Henderson, C. L., and R. J. Miles.** 1990. Growth of *Mycoplasma mycoides* subsp. *mycoides* in chemostat culture:

effect of growth rate upon cell structure. *Zentralbl. Bakteriol. Suppl.* **20:**945–947.

37. **Herbert, D.** 1961. The chemical composition of microorganisms as a function of their environment. *Symp. Soc. Gen. Microbiol.* **11:**391–416.

38. **Hoffman, P. S., L. Pine, and S. Bell.** 1983. Production of superoxide and hydrogen peroxide in medium used to culture *Legionella pneumophila:* catalytic decomposition by charcoal. *Appl. Environ. Microbiol.* **45:**784–791.

39. **Hudson, J. R.** 1971. *Contagious Bovine Pleuropneumonia.* Food and Agricultural Organization, Rome.

40. **Kahane, I., S. Razin, and A. Muhlrad.** 1978. Possible role of acetate kinase in ATP generation in *Mycoplasma hominis* and *Acholeplasma laidlawii. FEMS Microbiol. Lett.* **3:**143–145.

41. **Kazama, S., T. Yagihashi, and T. Nunoya.** 1986. Properties of *Mycoplasma gallisepticum* grown in a medium supplemented with liposomes as a substitute for serum. *Microbiol. Immunol.* **30:**923–929.

42. **Kenny, G. E., and F. D. Cartwright.** 1977. Effect of urea concentration on the growth of *Ureaplasma urealyticum* (T-strain mycoplasma). *J. Bacteriol.* **132:**144–150.

43. **Kihara, K., S. Ishida, M. Shintani, and T. Sasaki.** 1983. Statistical consideration of using colony diameter as a measure of mycoplasmal growth. *FEMS Microbiol. Lett.* **19:**7–9.

44. **Kirchhoff, H., and R. Rosengarten.** 1984. Isolation of a motile mycoplasma from fish. *J. Gen. Microbiol.* **130:**2439–2445.

45. **Kono, Y., and I. Fridovich.** 1982. Superoxide radical inhibits catalase. *J. Biol. Chem.* **257:**5751–5754.

46. **Krebs, B., M. Schutz, M. Fischer, G. Sommer, and H. Kirchhoff.** 1989. pH-controlled continuous cultivation of mycoplasmas. *Appl. Environ. Microbiol.* **55:**852–855.

47. **Leach, R. H.** 1962. The osmotic requirements for growth of mycoplasma. *J. Gen. Microbiol.* **27:**345–354.

48. **Leach, R. H.** 1976. The inhibitory effect of arginine on growth of some mycoplasmas. *J. Appl. Bacteriol.* **41:**259–264.

49. **Lee, I.-M., and R. E. Davis.** 1989. Defects of helicity and motility in the corn stunt spiroplasma, *Spiroplasma kunkelii. Can. J. Microbiol.* **35:**1087–1091.

50. **Lee, I.-M., and R. E. Davis.** 1989. Serum-free media for cultivation of spiroplasmas. *Can. J. Microbiol.* **35:**1092–1099.

51. **Le Grimellec, C., J. Cardinal, M.-C. Giocondi, and S. Carriere.** 1981. Control of membrane lipids in *Mycoplasma gallisepticum:* effect on lipid order. *J. Bacteriol.* **146:**155–162.

52. **Le Grimellec, C., and G. Leblanc.** 1978. Effect of membrane cholesterol on potassium transport in *Mycoplasma mycoides* var *capri. Biochim. Biophys. Acta* **514:**152–163.

53. **Lelong, I., B. Luu, M. Mersel, and S. Rottem.** 1988. Effect of 7β-hydroxycholesterol on growth and membrane composition of *Mycoplasma capricolum. FEBS Lett.* **232:**354–358.

54. **Liao, C. H., and T. A. Chen.** 1982. Media and methods of culture for spiroplasmas, p. 174–200. *In* M. J. Daniels and P. G. Markham (ed.), *Plant and Insect Mycoplasma Techniques.* Croom Helm Ltd., London.

55. **Ljungholm, K., I. Wadso, and P.-A. Mårdh.** 1976. Microcalorimetric determination of growth of mycoplasmatales. *J. Gen. Microbiol.* **96:**283–288.

56. **Low, I. E., and S. M. Zimkus.** 1973. Reduced nicotinamide adenine dinucleotide oxidase activity and H_2O_2 formation of *Mycoplasma pneumoniae. J. Bacteriol.* **116:**346–354.

57. **Lynch, R. E., and B. C. Cole.** 1980. *Mycoplasma pneumoniae:* a pathogen which manufactures superoxide but lacks superoxide dismutase. *Proc. Fed. Eur. Biochem. Soc. Symp.* **62:**49–56.

58. **Mallette, M. F.** 1969. Evaluation of growth by physical and chemical means. *Methods Microbiol.* **1:**521–566.

59. **Maniloff, J., and H. J. Morowitz.** 1972. Cell biology of the mycoplasmas. *Bacteriol. Rev.* **36:**263–290.

60. **Manolukas, J. T., M. F. Barile, D. K. F. Chandler, and D. Pollack.** 1988. Presence of anaplerotic reactions and transaminations, and the absence of the tricarboxylic acid cycle in mollicutes. *J. Gen. Microbiol.* **134:**791–800.

61. **Masover, G. K., J. R. Benson, and L. Hayflick.** 1974. Growth of of T-strain mycoplasmas in medium without added urea: effect of trace amounts of urea and of a urease inhibitor. *J. Bacteriol.* **117:**765–774.

62. **Masover, G. K., and L. Hayflick.** 1974. Dialysis culture of T-strain mycoplasmas. *J. Bacteriol.* **118:**46–52.

63. **Masover, G. K., S. Razin, and L. Hayflick.** 1977. Localization of enzymes in *Ureaplasma urealyticum* (T-strain mycoplasma). *J. Bacteriol.* **130:**297–302.

64. **McElhaney, R. N., J. De Gier, and E. C. M. van der Neut-Kok.** 1973. The effect of alterations in fatty acid composition and cholesterol content on the nonelectrolyte permeability of *Acholeplasma laidlawii* B cells. *Biochim. Biophys. Acta* **298:**500–512.

65. **McGarrity, G. J., J. Sarama, and V. Vanaman.** 1979. Factors influencing microbiological assay of cell culture mycoplasmas. *In Vitro* **15:**73–81.

66. **Meur, S. K., A. Sikdar, N. C. Srivastava, and S. K. Srivastava.** 1989. Rapid photometric assay of growth of *Mycoplasma mycoides* subsp. *capri. J. Appl. Bacteriol.* **66:**301–302.

67. **Miles, R. J., A. E. Beezer, and D. H. Lee.** 1985. Kinetics of utilisation of organic substrates by *Mycoplasma mycoides* subsp. *mycoides:* a flow-microcalorimetric study. *J. Gen. Microbiol.* **131:**1845–1852.

68. **Miles, R. J., A. E. Beezer, and D. H. Lee.** 1986. The growth of *Mycoplasma mycoides* subsp. *mycoides* in a salts solution: an ampoule microcalorimetric study. *Microbios* **45:**7–19.

69. **Miles, R. J., R. R. Taylor, and H. Varsani.** 1991. Oxygen uptake and H_2O_2 production by fermentative *Mycoplasma* spp. *J. Med. Microbiol.* **34:**219–223.

70. **Miles, R. J., B. J. Wadher, C. L. Henderson, and K. Mohan.** 1988. Increased yields of *Mycoplasma* spp. in the presence of pyruvate. *Lett. Appl. Microbiol.* **7:**149–151.

70a.**Mistry, K., and R. J. Miles.** Unpublished data.

71. **Mitchell, A., and L. R. Finch.** 1977. Pathways of nucleotide biosynthesis in *Mycoplasma mycoides* subsp. *mycoides. J. Bacteriol.* **130:**1047–1054.

72. **Muhlrad, A., I. Peleg, J. A. Robertson, I. M. Robinson, and I. Kahane.** 1981. Acetate kinase activity in mycoplasmas. *J. Bacteriol.* **147:**271–273.

73. **Neale, G. A. M., A. Mitchell, and L. R. Finch.** 1983. Pathways of pyrimidine deoxyribonucleotide biosynthesis in *Mycoplasma mycoides* subsp. *mycoides. J. Bacteriol.* **154:**17–22.

74. **Neale, G. A. M., A. Mitchell, and L. R. Finch.** 1983. Enzymes of pyrimidine deoxyribonucleotide metabolism in *Mycoplasma mycoides* subsp. *mycoides. J. Bacteriol.* **156:**1001–1005.

75. **Newing, C. R., and A. K. MacLeod.** 1956. Magnetically induced vortex for small-scale aerated culture studies. *Nature* (London) **177:**939–940.

75a.**Norman, P. J., and R. J. Miles.** Unpublished data.

76. **Patterson, A., C. Stevens, R. M. Cody, and R. T. Gudauskas.** 1985. Differential amino acid utilisation by spiroplasmas and the effect on growth kinetics. *J. Gen. Appl. Microbiol.* **31:**499–505.

77. **Perry, B. F., R. J. Miles, and A. E. Beezer.** 1989. Calorimetry for yeast fermentation monitoring and control, p. 276–347. *In* J. F. T. Spencer and D. M. Spencer (ed.), *Yeast Technology.* Springer-Verlag, Berlin.

78. **Petzel, J. P., M. C. McElwain, D. DeSantis, J. Manolukas, M. V. Williams, P. A. Hartman, M. J. Allison, and J. D. Pollack.** 1990. Enzymic activities of carbohydrate,

purine, and pyrimidine metabolism in the *Anaeroplasmataceae. Zentralbl. Bakteriol. Suppl.* **20**:677–678.

79. **Pirt, S. J.** 1975. *Principles of Microbe and Cell Cultivation.* Blackwell Scientific Publications, Oxford.

80. **Pollack, J. D.** 1979. Respiratory pathways and energy-yielding mechanisms, p. 188–212. *In* M. F. Barile and S. Razin (ed.), *The Mycoplasmas*, vol. 1. Academic Press, New York.

81. **Pollack, J. D., M. C. McElwain, D. DeSantis, J. T. Manolukas, J. G. Tully, C.-J. Chang, R. F. Whitcomb, K. J. Hackett, and M. V. Williams.** 1989. Metabolism of members of the *Spiroplasmataceae. Int. J. Syst. Bacteriol.* **39**:406–412.

82. **Postgate, J. R.** 1969. Viable counts and viability. *Methods Microbiol.* **1**:611–628.

83. **Razin, S.** 1978. The mycoplasmas. *Microbiol. Rev.* **42**:414–470.

84. **Razin, S.** 1983. Introductory comments, p. 29–30. *In* S. Razin and J. G. Tully (ed.), *Methods in Mycoplasmology*, vol. 1. Academic Press, New York.

85. **Razin, S.** 1983. Identification of mycoplasma colonies, p. 83–88. *In* S. Razin and J. G. Tully (ed.), *Methods in Mycoplasmology*, vol. 1. Academic Press, New York.

86. **Razin, S.** 1985. Mycoplasma adherence, p. 161–203. *In* S. Razin and M. F. Barile (ed.), *The Mycoplasmas*, vol. 4. Academic Press, Orlando, Fla.

87. **Razin, S., and A. Cohen.** 1963. Nutritional requirements and metabolism of *Mycoplasma laidlawii. J. Gen. Microbiol.* **30**:141–154.

88. **Razin, S., and E. A. Freundt.** 1984. The mycoplasmas, p. 740–793. *In* N. R. Krieg and J. G. Holt (ed.), *Bergey's Manual of Systematic Bacteriology*, vol. 1. Williams & Wilkins, Baltimore.

89. **Razin, S., G. K. Masover, M. Palant, and L. Hayflick.** 1977. Morphology of *Ureaplasma urealyticum* (T-mycoplasma) organisms and colonies. *J. Bacteriol.* **130**:464–471.

90. **Razin, S., and J. G. Tully (ed.).** 1983. *Methods in Mycoplasmology*, vol. 1. *Mycoplasma Characterization.* Academic Press, New York.

91. **Read, B. D., and R. N. McElhaney.** 1975. Glucose transport in *Acholeplasma laidlawii* B: dependence on the fluidity and physical state of membranes. *J. Bacteriol.* **123**:47–55.

92. **Read, W. C. S., C. D. H. Boarer, and J. J. Read.** 1971. Estimation of the growth of the T1 strain of *Mycoplasma mycoides* in tryptose broth by the measurement of lactate dehydrogenase. II. Application to vaccine production. *Appl. Microbiol.* **22**:769–771.

93. **Ribbons, D. W.** 1970. Quantitative relationships between growth media constituents and cellular yields and composition. *Methods Microbiol.* **3A**:297–304.

94. **Robinson, I. M.** 1979. Special features of anaeroplasmas, p. 515–528. *In* M. F. Barile and S. Razin (ed.), *The Mycoplasmas*, vol. 1. Academic Press, New York.

95. **Robinson, I. M.** 1983. Culture media for anaeroplasmas, p. 159–162. *In* S. Razin and J. G. Tully (ed.), *Methods in Mycoplasmology*, vol. 1. Academic Press, New York.

96. **Rodwell, A. W.** 1965. The stability of *Mycoplasma mycoides. J. Gen. Microbiol.* **40**:227–234.

97. **Rodwell, A. W.** 1967. The nutrition and metabolism of mycoplasma: progress and problems. *Ann. N.Y. Acad. Sci.* **143**:88–109.

98. **Rodwell, A. W.** 1969. A defined medium for *Mycoplasma* strain Y. *J. Gen. Microbiol.* **58**:39–47.

99. **Rodwell, A. W.** 1969. Nutrition and metabolism of the mycoplasmas, p. 413–449. *In* L. Hayflick (ed.), *The Mycoplasmatales and L-Phase of Bacteria.* Appleton-Century-Crofts, New York.

100. **Rodwell, A. W.** 1983. Defined and partly defined media, p. 163–172. *In* S. Razin and J. G. Tully (ed.), *Methods in Mycoplasmology*, vol. 1. Academic Press, New York.

101. **Rodwell, A. W.** 1983. *Mycoplasma gallisepticum* requires exogenous phospholipid for growth. *FEMS Microbiol. Lett.* **17**:265–268.

102. **Rodwell, A. W., and A. Mitchell.** 1979. Nutrition, growth and reproduction, p. 103–109. *In* M. F. Barile and S. Razin (ed.), *The Mycoplasmas*, vol. 1. Academic Press, New York.

103. **Rodwell, A. W., and R. F. Whitcomb.** 1983. Methods for direct and indirect measurement of mycoplasma growth, p. 185–196. *In* S. Razin and J. G. Tully (ed.), *Methods in Mycoplasmology*, vol. 1. Academic Press, New York.

104. **Romano, N., S. Rottem, and S. Razin.** 1976. Biosynthesis of saturated and unsaturated fatty acids by a T-strain mycoplasma (*Ureaplasma*). *J. Bacteriol.* **128**:170–173.

105. **Romano, N., M. H. Shirvan, and S. Rottem.** 1986. Changes in membrane lipid composition of *Mycoplasma capricolum* affect the cell volume. *J. Bacteriol.* **167**:1089–1091.

106. **Rottem, S.** 1983. Harvest and washing of mycoplasmas, p. 221–224. *In* S. Razin and J. G. Tully (ed.), *Methods in Mycoplasmology*, vol. 1. Academic Press, New York.

107. **Rottem, S., L. Adar, Z. Gross, Z. Ne'eman, and P. J. Davis.** 1986. Incorporation and modification of exogenous phosphatidylcholines by mycoplasmas. *J. Bacteriol.* **167**:299–304.

108. **Rottem, S., and S. Razin.** 1964. Lipase activity of mycoplasma. *J. Gen. Microbiol.* **37**:123–134.

109. **Rottem, S., D. Shinar, and R. Bittman.** 1981. Symmetrical distribution and rapid transbilayer movement of cholesterol in *Mycoplasma gallisepticum* membranes. *Biochim. Biophys. Acta* **649**:572–580.

109a. **Rottem, S., and I. Shirazi.** 1990. An arginine-ornithine exchange system in spiroplasmas. *IOM Lett.* **1**:102–103.

110. **Rottem, S., J. Yashouv, Z. Ne'eman, and S. Razin.** 1973. Composition, ultrastructure and biological properties of membranes from *Mycoplasma mycoides* var *capri* cells adapted to grow with low cholesterol concentrations. *Biochim. Biophys. Acta* **323**:495–508.

111. **Saglio, P. H. M., M. J. Daniels, and A. Pradet.** 1979. ATP and energy charge as criteria of growth and metabolic activity of mollicutes: application to *Spiroplasma citri. J. Gen. Microbiol.* **110**:13–20.

112. **Sasaki, T., M. Shintani, and K. Kihara.** 1985. Comparison of the efficacy of egg yolk extract and horse serum for growth of *M. pneumoniae. Microbiol. Immunol.* **29**:499–507.

113. **Shepard, M. C.** 1983. Culture media for ureaplasmas, p. 137–146. *In* S. Razin and J. G. Tully (ed.), *Methods in Mycoplasmology*, vol. 1. Academic Press, New York.

114. **Shepard, M. C., and G. K. Masover.** 1979. Special features of ureaplasmas, p. 452–494. *In* M. F. Barile and S. Razin (ed.), *The Mycoplasmas*, vol. 1. Academic Press, New York.

115. **Slater, M. L., and C. E. Folsome.** 1971. Induction of α-glucosidase in *Mycoplasma laidlawii* A. *Nature* (London) *New Biol.* **229**:117–118.

116. **Smith, P. F.** 1979. The composition of membrane lipids and lipopolysccharides, p. 231–259. *In* M. F. Barile and S. Razin (ed.), *The Mycoplasmas*, vol. 1. Academic Press, New York.

117. **Snell, G. C.** 1981. A comparison of alternative methods to viable count for indicating growth of *Mycoplasma gallisepticum* in liquid culture. *J. Appl. Bacteriol.* **50**:275–281.

118. **Stemke, G. W., and J. A. Robertson.** 1982. Comparison of two methods for enumeration of mycoplasmas. *J. Clin. Microbiol.* **16**:959–961.

119. **Stemler, M. E., G. W. Stemke, and J. A. Robertson.** 1987. ATP measurements obtained by luminometry provide rapid estimation of *Ureaplasma urealyticum* growth. *J. Clin. Microbiol.* **25**:427–429.

120. **Tourtellotte, M. E.** 1969. Protein synthesis in mycoplas-

mas, p. 451–468. *In* L. Hayflick (ed.), *The Mycoplasmatales and L-Phase of Bacteria.* Appleton-Century-Crofts, New York.

121. **Tourtellotte, M. E., and R. E. Jacobs.** 1960. Physiological and serologic comparisons of PPLO from various sources. *Ann. N.Y. Acad. Sci.* **79:**521–530.

122. **Tourtellotte, M. E., H. J. Morowitz, and P. Kasimer.** 1964. Defined medium for *Mycoplasma laidlawii. J. Bacteriol.* **88:**11–15.

123. **Tryon, V. V., and J. L. Baseman.** 1987. The acquisition of human lactoferrin by *Mycoplasma pneumoniae. Microb. Pathog.* **3:**437–443.

124. **Tully, J. G.** 1979. Special features of acholeplasmas, p. 431–451. *In* M. F. Barile and S. Razin (ed.), *The Mycoplasmas,* vol. 1. Academic Press, New York.

125. **Tully, J. G.** 1983. Bacterial and fungal inhibitors in mycoplasma culture media, p. 205–210. *In* S. Razin and J. G. Tully (ed.), *Methods in Mycoplasmology,* vol. 1. Academic Press, New York.

126. **Tully, J. G., and S. Razin (ed.).** 1983. *Methods in Mycoplasmology,* vol. 2. *Diagnostic Mycoplasmology.* Academic Press, New York.

127. **Tully, J. G., and D. L. Rose.** 1983. Sterility and quality control of mycoplasma culture media, p. 121–126. *In* S. Razin and J. G. Tully (ed.), *Methods in Mycoplasmology,* vol. 1. Academic Press, New York.

128. **Wadher, B. J., C. L. Henderson, R. J. Miles, and H. Varsani.** 1990. A mutant of *Mycoplasma mycoides* subsp. *mycoides* lacking the H_2O_2-producing enzyme L-α-glycerophosphate oxidase. *FEMS Microbiol. Lett.* **72:**127–130.

129. **Wadher, B. J., and R. J. Miles.** 1988. α-Glucosidase activity in *Mycoplasma mycoides* subspecies *capri. FEMS Microbiol. Lett.* **49:**459–462.

129a. **Wadher, B. J., H. Varsani, E. A. Abu-Groun, and R. J. Miles.** 1990. Biochemical characterization of bovine, caprine and ovine mycoplasmas. *IOM Lett.* **1:**517–518.

130. **Whitcomb, R. F.** 1983. Culture media for spiroplasmas, p. 147–158. *In* S. Razin and J. G. Tully (ed.), *Methods in Mycoplasmology,* vol. 1. Academic Press, New York.

131. **Williamson, D. L., J. G. Tully, and R. F. Whitcomb.** 1989. The genus *Spiroplasma,* p. 71–112. *In* R. F. Whitcomb and J. G. Tully (ed.), *The Mycoplasmas,* vol. 5. Academic Press, San Diego, Calif.

132. **Zips, A., and U. Faust.** 1989. Determination of biomass by ultrasonic measurements. *Appl. Environ. Microbiol.* **55:**1801–1807.

3. Mycoplasma Viruses

JACK MANILOFF

INTRODUCTION

Mycoplasma viruses have been reviewed recently (91). Therefore, this chapter will concentrate on the molecular biology of mycoplasma virus infection; much of the data discussed has been published since the 1988 review. In view of the gram-positive eubacterial phylogenetic origin of the mycoplasmas (reviewed in references 90 and 147; see also chapter 33), throughout this chapter mycoplasma virology is discussed in the larger context of bacteriophage biology. For detailed data on mycoplasma virus structure (including morphological variants) and physicochemical properties, the 1988 review (91) should be consulted.

Development of Mycoplasma Virology

Acholeplasma viruses

In 1970, the first isolation of a mycoplasma virus was reported by Gourlay in England, using a bovine mycoplasma isolate as host cells and filtrates of mycoplasma bovine isolates as the virus source (45). The virus was designated mycoplasma virus L1, and the host cells were found to be an *Acholeplasma laidlawii* strain. In the next few years, with these host cells, Gourlay and coworkers isolated and characterized two additional viruses, designated L2 and L3, from *A. laidlawii* strains (46–48, 51). Each of the three viruses was found to be morphologically and serologically different from the others.

Other *Acholeplasma* viruses were subsequently isolated in 1972 by Liska in Czechoslovakia from an unknown *A. laidlawii* strain and designated L172 (78), in 1979 by Kenny and coworkers in the United States from an *A. modicum* strain and designated M1 (21), and in 1983 by Ichimaru and Nakamura in Japan from an *A. oculi* strain and designated O1 (71).

In 1971, Maniloff and coworkers in the United States began studies of the Gourlay viruses, which led to the development of mycoplasma virology and to the description of the molecular biology of mycoplasma virus infections (reviewed in reference 91). These studies initially focused on L1 and later shifted to L2 as the

Jack Maniloff • Department of Microbiology and Immunology, University of Rochester, Medical Center Box 672, Rochester, New York 14642.

unique lysogenic cycle of L2 became apparent. Several years later, studies of *Acholeplasma* virus L3 were begun by Haberer and coworkers in Germany (e.g., reference 59).

Spiroplasma viruses

Spiroplasma viruses were first reported in 1973 as "virus-like" particles in *Spiroplasma* cultures during the original ultrastructural characterization of *Spiroplasma* cells by Cole and coworkers in the United States and France (19, 20). The three different morphological forms were designated *Spiroplasma* viruses C1, C2, and C3. Two of these virus types were subsequently propagated and characterized: C3 in 1977 by Cole and coworkers (17) and SV1, a C1-type virus, in 1981 by Liss and Cole (81). Thus far, no C2-type particle has been propagated. A fourth morphological type of *Spiroplasma* virus was isolated and characterized in 1984 by Bové and coworkers in France and designated SpV4 (129).

In the early 1980s, studies of the molecular biology of C1-type *Spiroplasma* viruses began in Townsend's laboratory in England (reviewed in reference 143) and of the SpV4-type *Spiroplasma* viruses in Bové's laboratory (reviewed in reference 9).

Mycoplasma viruses

Three *Mycoplasma* viruses have been described: (i) in 1980, Gourlay and coworkers isolated a virus from an unknown bovine source that infected *Mycoplasma bovirhinis* host cells and designated this virus Br1 (70); (ii) in 1983, Gourlay and coworkers isolated a virus from spontaneous plaques on an *M. hyorhinis* lawn that could be propagated on *M. hyorhinis* cells and designated this virus Hr1 (54); and (iii) in 1987, Dybvig, Liss, and coworkers in the United States isolated a virus from *M. pulmonis* cells that could be propagated on *M. pulmonis* cells and designated this virus P1 (36). Unfortunately, none of these *Mycoplasma* viruses has been grown in sufficient quantities to allow characterization of their structures or infection cycles.

Distribution of Mycoplasma Viruses

Acholeplasma viruses

L1-type viruses are filamentous virions containing circular single-stranded DNA (Table 1). Over 50 isolates of L1-type viruses have been reported from washes of *Acholeplasma* and *Mycoplasma* lawns (47, 85). There have been questions about the original source of these isolates because of the frequency of spontaneous plaques on *A. laidlawii* host cell lawns and the nature of the persistent infections that characterize L1-type virus infected cells (described below).

L2 viruses are enveloped quasi-spherical virions containing circular double-stranded DNA (Table 2). Several isolates that may be related to L2 have been reported but have not been characterized (46, 47, 117).

L3 viruses morphologically resemble T7 phages and contain linear double-stranded DNA (Table 2). Since the original L3 isolation, only one other L3-type virus has been reported (52).

L172 viruses are enveloped virions containing circular single-stranded DNA (Table 1). The only L172 isolate was originally identified as an L2-type virus (78) but subsequently shown to represent a type of virus that has not been described previously (38).

A. laidlawii strains are host cells for L1, L2, L3, and L172 viruses. In addition, a single *Acholeplasma* virus isolate, designated M1, that infects *A. modicum* (21) and a single isolate, designated O1, that infects *A. oculi* (71) have been reported. Both M1 and O1 are enveloped quasi-spherical virions (Table 3); the nucleic acid of M1 has not been determined (21), and O1 contains DNA (114).

The physicochemical properties of the *Acholeplasma* viruses have been reviewed recently (91).

Spiroplasma viruses

C1-type viruses (like L1-type *Acholeplasma* viruses) are filamentous virions containing circular single-stranded DNA (Table 1). Virions morphologically similar to *Spiroplasma* virus C1 have been found in about

Table 1. Properties of single-stranded DNA mycoplasma viruses[a]

Virus	Host cells	Morphology			DNA size (kb)	Reference(s)
		Symmetry	Virion size (nm)	Envelope		
L1 type	*A. laidlawii*	Filamentous		No		
Strain L1			16 by 90			11
Strain L51			14 by 71		4.3–4.5	86, 94, 112
L172	*A. laidlawii*	Quasi-spherical	60–80	Yes	14.0	38, 78
C1 type	*S. citri*	Filamentous		No		
Strain SpV1			10–15 by 230–280		8.3[b]	81, 82, 127
Strain *aa*			10–15 by 240–260		8.5	30
Strain C1/TS2			7–12 by 150–180		6.6	105
SpV4	*S. melliferum*	Isometric	27	No	4.4[c]	128, 129

[a] All of these viruses contain circular single-stranded DNA molecules.
[b] From DNA sequencing studies, this DNA is 8,272 bases (127).
[c] From DNA sequencing studies, this DNA is 4,421 bases (128).

Table 2. Properties of double-stranded DNA mycoplasma viruses

Virus	Host cells	Morphology			DNA		Reference(s)
		Symmetry	Virion size (nm)	Envelope	Size (kbp)	Structure[a]	
L2	*A. laidlawii*	Quasi-spherical	50–125	Yes	12.0[b]	Circular	94, 111, 123
L3	*A. laidlawii*	Short-tailed phage	Head, 60; tail 10 by 20	No	39.4	Linear, CP, TR	42, 49, 59, 73, 94
C3 type		Short-tailed phage		No			
Strain SpV3	*S. citri*		Head, 40; tail, 6–8 by 13–18		21	Linear, CP, TR	14, 16–18, 32
Strain *ai*	*S. citri*		Head, 43–54; tail, 14		16	Linear, COS	32
SRO viruses	SRO cells		Head, 35–45; tail, 7–9 by 10–12		17, 21.8, >30[c]		13, 115, 116, 146

[a] Abbreviations: CP, circular permutation; TR, terminal redundancy; COS, cohesive ends.
[b] From DNA sequencing studies, this DNA is 11,965 bp (98).
[c] The SRO virus preparations that have been studied appear to contain a mixture of SRO viruses and viral DNAs (13).

60% of spiroplasma strains examined by electron microscopy (81, 97), and C1-type PFU have been isolated from several *Spiroplasma* species (81, 82).

C3-type viruses (like L3-type *Acholeplasma* viruses) morphologically resemble T7 phages and contain linear double-stranded DNA (Table 2). Particles with C3 morphology have been detected in over 60% of *Spiroplasma* strains examined by electron microscopy (97). C3-type viruses have been isolated from *Spiroplasma* species (17, 32) and *Drosophila* strains infected with spiroplasma sex-ratio organisms (SRO) (13).

SpV4 virions are isometric particles containing circular single-stranded DNA (Table 1). The single SpV4 isolate came from an early passage of *Spiroplasma melliferum* B63 (129). However, after SpV4 isolation, the *S. melliferum* was cloned and found to no longer contain virions and to be resistant to SpV4 infection (129).

The physicochemical properties of the *Spiroplasma* viruses have been reviewed recently (9, 91).

Mycoplasma viruses

Single *Mycoplasma* virus isolates have been reported from *M. bovirhinis* (70), *M. hyorhinis* (54), and *M. pulmonis* (36) and designated Br1, Hr1, and P1, re-

spectively. Br1 virions resemble long-tailed phage particles, while Hr1 and P1 resemble short-tailed phages (Table 3). Br1 virions probably contain DNA (53), Hr1 virions do contain DNA (54), and the nucleic acid content of P1 virions has not been determined (36).

The physicochemical properties of the *Mycoplasma* viruses have been reviewed recently (91).

MYCOPLASMA VIRUS TAXONOMY

Classification of Bacteriophages

In virus taxonomy, family names end in *-viridae*, genus names end in *-virus*, and species are designated by the vernacular names of their best-known (or only) member (40). The most important taxonomic properties are virion morphology (including presence or absence of an envelope) and nucleic acid structure.

The International Committee on Taxonomy of Viruses currently groups bacteriophages into 12 families (40): (i) *Myoviridae* (phages with long contractile tails), (ii) *Siphoviridae* (phages with long noncontractile tails), (iii) *Podoviridae* (phages with short tails), (iv) *Microviridae* (isometric phages with single-stranded

Table 3. Properties of mycoplasma viruses with undetermined nucleic acid structure

Virus	Host cells	Morphology			Reference
		Symmetry	Virion size (nm)	Envelope	
Acholeplasma virus M1	*A. modicum*	Quasi-spherical	105–160	Yes	21
Acholeplasma virus O1[a]	*A. oculi*	Quasi-spherical	80–130	Yes	114
Mycoplasma virus Br1	*M. bovirhinis*	Long-tailed phage	Head, 73–77; tail 19 by 104	No	53
Mycoplasma virus Hr1[a]	*M. hyorhinis*	Short-tailed phage	Head, 34; tail, 14	No	54
Mycoplasma virus P1	*M. pulmonis*	Short-tailed phage	Head, 28; short tail	No	36

[a] Contains DNA.

DNA), (v) *Corticoviridae* (PM2 phage group), (vi) *Tectiviridae* (phages with double capsids), (vii) *Leviviridae* (single-stranded RNA phages), (viii) *Cystoviridae* (φ6 phage group), (ix) *Inoviridae* (rod-shaped phages), (x) *Lipothrixviridae* (TTV1 phage family), (xi) *Plasmaviridae* (pleomorphic phages), and (xii) SSV1 phage group (lemon-shaped phage).

Classification of Mycoplasma Viruses

Filamentous mycoplasma viruses

The filamentous bacteriophages have been classified in the family *Inoviridae*, which has been divided into two genera: (i) *Inovirus* (filamentous phages), containing the coliphage fd group, and (ii) *Plectrovirus* (rod-shaped phages), containing the L1-type *Acholeplasma* viruses and the C1-type *Spiroplasma* viruses (Table 1) (40). Both genera contain virus strains with a several-fold range in virion length and a twofold range in DNA size.

Isometric mycoplasma viruses

The isometric bacteriophages with single-stranded DNA have been classified in the family *Microviridae*, which has been divided into three genera: (i) *Microvirus*, containing the coliphage φX174 group, (ii) *Spiromicrovirus*, containing the single *Spiroplasma* SpV4 virus isolate (Table 1), and (iii) the possible genus MAC-1-type phages, containing the *Bdellovibrio* phage MAC-1 group (40).

Enveloped mycoplasma viruses

The family *Plasmaviridae*, containing the single genus *Plasmavirus*, was established for the enveloped quasi-spherical *Acholeplasma* virus L2 (Table 2) (40).

Acholeplasma virus L172 is presently unclassified. However, its virion and nucleic acid structure (Table 1) do not match those of any of the established bacteriophage families, and a new family will probably have to be created for it.

Short-tailed mycoplasma viruses

The bacteriophages with short tails have been classified in the family *Podoviridae*, with a single genus for the coliphage T7 group. *Acholeplasma* virus L3 and the C3-type *Spiroplasma* viruses have been placed in this genus (Table 2) (40). However, there are significant differences in genome size and structure between the members of the coliphage T7 group and the short-tailed mycoplasma viruses. This variation suggests the short-tailed mycoplasma viruses will eventually be reclassified to form several new genera within the *Podoviridae*.

Other mycoplasma viruses

At present, it is inappropriate to attempt to classify the other mycoplasma viruses (Table 3) because of difficulties in propagating them and the absence of data on their nucleic acid structures. It should be noted that *Mycoplasma* virus Br1 has been prematurely classified

in the family *Myoviridae* (40), despite the problems mentioned above and differences in head morphology between Br1 and the other members of the *Myoviridae*.

INFECTION CYCLE: ADSORPTION AND PENETRATION

The first stage of viral infection is adsorption (specific interaction of virion and host cell surface receptors) and penetration (release of viral nucleic acid from the virion and its entry into the host cell). The absence of a cell wall in mycoplasmas means that mycoplasma virus adsorption and penetration must resemble the situation for animal viruses, in which adsorption is to a cell membrane, rather than bacteriophages, in which adsorption is to a cell wall. However, the fact that some mycoplasma viruses have tailed-phage morphology raises questions about the function of phage tail structures in viruses that infect wall-less cells.

This section reviews data on adsorption and penetration of filamentous, short-tailed, and enveloped mycoplasma viruses. No data have been reported on adsorption and penetration of SpV4, the only isometric mycoplasma virus.

Filamentous Mycoplasma Viruses

Adsorption kinetics

Adsorption of *Acholeplasma* L1-type viruses L1 (41) and L51 (100) and *Spiroplasma* C3-type virus SpV1 (81) follows pseudo-first-order kinetics. For all three viruses, the experimentally determined adsorption rate constants are close to the theoretical values calculated from single-hit collision kinetics, indicating that most virus-cell collisions result in adsorption.

Adsorption sites

The only available data on structure of the mycoplasma cell membrane receptor for filamentous viruses are for L1-type viruses. Adsorption of L1-type viruses to *A. laidlawii* cell membranes has been proposed to involve electrostatic interactions between virion and cell membrane proteins, based on the pH optimum (about 6.0), cation dependence, and small temperature dependence of the L1 adsorption rate constant (41). Involvement of protein in the cell membrane receptor is also suggested by studies showing that protease treatment of cell membranes reduces L51 adsorption to about 50% of that of untreated cells (4).

A. laidlawii cell membrane lipoglycan may also be involved in adsorption of L1-type viruses, because L51 infectivity is lost by incubation with host cell membrane lipoglycan (4).

L51 plating efficiency is related to *A. laidlawii* host cell membrane fatty acid composition (139). However, it is not clear whether the effect of fatty acid composition is on virus adsorption or maturation by extrusion through the cell membrane (discussed below). Cell membrane lipid may not form part of the receptor for L51 adsorption, because chloroform-methanol-treated (lipid-extracted) cell membranes adsorb L51 virus as well as do untreated membranes (4).

Interaction of *A. laidlawii* cell membrane proteins, oligosaccharides, and lipids to affect virus adsorption and progeny virus maturation may be in part due to effects of lipid packing on the membrane environment (144), selective fatty acid modification of membrane proteins (22, 113), and lipoglycan heterogeneity (136).

Only a small fraction of L1-type viruses adsorbed to host cell membranes are bound to functional receptors. Adsorption studies found up to about 300 L51 viruses can bind per CFU (85). However, only 10 to 20 functional sites are measured in competition experiments with viable and UV-inactivated L1 virus (41) and by measurement of the multiplicity of infection (MOI) needed to saturate intracellular L51 viral DNA-binding sites (24).

Uncoating and penetration

The mechanisms of filamentous mycoplasma virus uncoating and viral DNA penetration of the cell membrane are unknown. In the single-stranded DNA filamentous coliphages (reviewed in reference 126), these processes involve resorption of viral proteins into the cell membrane and conversion of the infecting single-stranded DNA to double-stranded replicative-form (RF) DNA by host cell enzymes. Uncoating and penetration are probably similar for the filamentous mycoplasma viruses, since (as described below) L51 single-stranded DNA penetration appears to be coupled to its conversion to double-stranded RF DNA (reviewed in reference 96).

Short-Tailed Mycoplasma Viruses

Adsorption kinetics

Adsorption of *Acholeplasma* virus L3 (59, 61), *Spiroplasma* virus *ai* (a C3-type virus) (32), and *Mycoplasma* virus P1 (36) follows pseudo-first-order kinetics. For L3 and *ai*, the experimental adsorption rate constants range from close to the theoretical values calculated from single-hit collision kinetics to about 10-fold less. This finding indicates that a large fraction of collisions between the short-tailed *Acholeplasma* and *Spiroplasma* viruses and their host cell membranes result in adsorption. In contrast, the short-tailed *Mycoplasma* virus P1 experimental adsorption rate constant is 100-fold less than the theoretical rate constant, indicating that only about 1% of virus-cell collisions result in adsorption. The lower adsorption efficiency of P1 virus than of L3 and *ai* viruses may be due to the capsular layer of *Mycoplasma* cells (including *M. pulmonis*), which is absent in *Acholeplasma* and *Spiroplasma* cells (see chapter 5).

Adsorption sites

L3 and *ai* adsorption has been proposed to involve electrostatic interactions between virion and cell membrane proteins, as determined from the pH, temperature, and cation dependence of the adsorption rate constants (32, 61). Adsorption of both viruses requires

Ca^{2+}, which cannot be replaced by Mg^{2+} or monovalent cations.

Treatment of *Acholeplasma* host cell membranes with proteases reduces L3 adsorption to about 10 to 35% of that of untreated cells (4, 61), indicating that the L3 virus cell membrane receptor contains protein. The L3 receptor may not involve lipid, because no reduction in adsorption is measured if membranes are lipid extracted with chloroform-methanol (4), or oligosaccharides, because L3 infectivity is not lost when the virus is incubated with *A. laidlawii* membrane lipoglycan (4) and L3 adsorption is not affected by pretreatment of cells with lectins (61). The latter studies used the only lectins reported to bind *A. laidlawii* membranes: concanavalin A (which binds glucose and mannose), *Ricinus communis* type I lectin (which binds *N*-acetylgalactosamine), and *R. communis* type II lectin (which binds galactose).

P1 adsorption has been found to be affected by changes in the *M. pulmonis* V-1 major surface antigen, which is a multiprotein complex (35). However, it is not known whether V-1 is the receptor or affects adsorption indirectly.

L3 virions have a collar between the isometric head and the tail, with tail fibers attached to the collar (59). The tail fibers must function in adsorption of L3 virions to host cell membranes, because adsorbed L3 particles behave as polyvalent ligands and diffuse along the cell surface (63; described below). It is not known whether other short-tailed mycoplasma viruses also have tail fibers.

Each *A. laidlawii* CFU can bind a maximum of about 350 L3 PFU (61), but because of cell clumping, the number of L3 virus receptors per cell may be several times lower.

Penetration

Adsorbed L3 virions diffuse along the cell surface, cross-linking laterally mobile receptors in the membrane (63), and L3 DNA must then somehow be ejected and transported through the cell membrane.

ai virus adsorbs to purified *Spiroplasma* cell membranes, but the virus DNA remains resistant to DNase I treatment, indicating that *ai* adsorption and DNA penetration are uncoupled (32). This characteristic suggests some component of the cell membrane *ai* receptor may have been lost during membrane purification, similar to observations of in vitro bacteriophage adsorption (reviewed in reference 44).

Mechanisms described for bacteriophage DNA passage through the cell membrane involve either pilot proteins attached to the DNA or membrane pore proteins which allow DNA transport (44). Short-tailed mycoplasma virus DNA penetration could involve either mechanism.

Capping and cell fusion

Adsorbed L3 virions have lateral mobility on the cell surface and act as polyvalent ligands cross-linking cell membrane receptors (57, 61, 63, 65). Electron microscopic studies show that after random adsorption of L3 virions to the cell membrane, there is a temperature-dependent clustering or capping of adsorbed virions on the cell surface (63). At 4°C, only 15% of cell sections show L3 capping, while at 37°C, 52% of sections show capping. When adsorption at 4°C is followed by a shift to 37°C, 55% of the sections show capping, meaning that capping involves surface redistribution of L3 virions already adsorbed to cell receptors. L3 tail fibers probably determine the valency and mediate the cross-linking of laterally mobile cell surface receptors.

Scanning electron microscopy of uninfected and L3-infected cells suggests there are virus-induced changes in the cell membrane (64). The effect of L3 adsorption on cell membrane structure was explicitly investigated by spectroscopic measurements of *A. laidlawii* host cells grown in medium containing fluorescence-labeled lipid molecules (65). The change in fluorescence spectra observed after L3 adsorption could be caused by either changes in membrane fluidity or phase separation. Since these studies also showed that L3 adsorption does not alter membrane fluidity, it has been proposed that L3 capping involves phase separation in the cell membrane, possibly by concentrating membrane receptor proteins in the capping region, thereby generating protein-depleted lipid patches.

L3 capping is dependent on host cell energy metabolism, as shown by studies of capping on cells treated with *N,N'*-dicyclohexylcarbodiimide (DCHCD), an irreversible inhibitor of ATPase in *A. laidlawii*, and carbonyl cyanide *m*-chlorophenylhydrazone (CCCP), an oxidative phosphorylation uncoupler which reversibly breaks down the membrane potential in *A. laidlawii* (62, 65). Capping is found in 43% of sections of untreated cells, 18% of sections of DCHCD-treated cells, and 18% of sections of CCCP-treated cells. Similar energy dependence is seen for DNA transport across the bacterial cell membrane in transformation, conjugation, and bacteriophage DNA penetration (reviewed in references 56 and 76).

Giant cells are observed in L3-infected *A. laidlawii* cultures, which were proposed to have arisen by L3-mediated cell fusion, with tail fibers of polyvalent L3 virions cross-linking receptors on different cells and promoting fusion (63). This proposal was confirmed by studies using solutions of different-size colloidal gold particles coated with antiserum against *A. laidlawii* to label host cell membranes and show that enlarged cells in L3-infected cultures arise by cell fusion (57). Giant cells must be the result of multiple cell fusions.

Enveloped Mycoplasma Viruses

The L2 virion is a nucleoprotein condensation bounded by a lipid-protein membrane (94). Both L2 (55, 123) and *A. laidlawii* host cell membranes (reviewed in reference 107) are lipid bilayers with integral and peripheral proteins. Hence, L2 adsorption presumably involves virus-cell membrane interaction followed by fusion of virus and cell membranes. The limited data available on L2 adsorption do not distinguish between virus-cell membrane interaction and fusion.

Kinetics

L2 adsorption to *Acholeplasma* host cells follows pseudo-first-order kinetics. However, the experimentally determined adsorption rate constant varies with the medium being used and ranges from 10- to 1,000-fold less than the theoretical value calculated from single-hit collision kinetics (3, 84, 124). Therefore, depending on the medium, only about 0.1 to 10% of virus-cell collisions result in L2 adsorption.

The small fraction of virus-cell collisions that lead to infection may be explained by data showing that a maximum of two L2 viruses can bind each CFU (132). This small number may be due to (i) a limiting number of L2 receptors on the cell membrane, (ii) virus-cell membrane fusion being a slow rate-limiting step, or (iii) some type of superinfection exclusion due to a physiological change in infected cells.

Adsorption sites

L2 interaction with the *A. laidlawii* cell membrane is not affected by divalent cations (132), suggesting that ionic interactions are not important in adsorption. Although EDTA decreases L2 adsorption to about 95% of that of untreated controls (132), this effect is probably due to osmotic effects on the cell membrane since the survival fraction of *A. laidlawii* cells in EDTA is about 10^{-4} (124).

The role, if any, of L2 virion and host cell membrane proteins in adsorption is not known, although some involvement of cell membrane proteins in L2 adsorption is suggested by studies showing reduced L2 adsorption to protease-treated *A. laidlawii* cell membranes (4, 132).

Three laboratories have studied L2 virion proteins and found four major proteins, but the size estimates vary (55, 89, 118, 123). From the means of the values of these data, the sizes of the four major L2 virion proteins are about 72, 68, 65, and 17 kDa. The 72- and 68-kDa proteins are probably virion membrane proteins, with the 72-kDa protein being an L2 integral membrane protein and the 68-kDa protein being an L2 peripheral membrane protein (55, 131). Urea treatment, which selectively releases the 68-kDa L2 membrane protein, has little effect on L2 adsorption, indicating that this virus peripheral membrane protein is not involved in adsorption (132). In addition, two minor L2 virion proteins with sizes of about 52 and 21 kDa have been identified (118, 123).

Host cell membrane lipids may not form part of the receptor structure for L2 adsorption, because chloroform-methanol-treated (lipid-extracted) *A. laidlawii* membranes adsorb L2 as well as do untreated membranes (4). However, studies of the effect of fatty acid composition on L2 adsorption show that the physical state of both virus and cell membrane lipids is important for L2 virus adsorption and/or penetration (138, 139). Hence, the effect of virion and cell membrane lipids on L2 adsorption may be indirect, perhaps by modulating fusion of these membranes.

The conclusions of several other studies of the involvement of host cell proteins, lipids, and oligosaccharides in L2 adsorption are in question because of concerns about identity of the cell strains and "persistently infected" cells (which must have been lysogens) used in these studies (reviewed in reference 91).

As noted above for *Acholeplasma* virus L1 adsorption, in addition to whatever specific roles they play in determining the virus receptor structure, *A. laid-*

lawii cell membrane proteins, oligosaccharides, and lipids may interact to affect virus infection and maturation by effects of lipid packing on the membrane environment (144), selective fatty acid modification of membrane proteins (22, 113), and lipoglycan heterogeneity (136).

Penetration

If adsorption involves fusion of virion and host cell membranes, this process would result in entry of the L2 nucleoprotein condensation into the cell, which must be followed by nucleoprotein uncoating.

INFECTION CYCLE: REPLICATION

The second stage of a productive viral infection cycle is intracellular replication; i.e., synthesis of viral proteins and nucleic acid. In general, temporal control is implemented by regulation of viral transcription.

Since replication strategies are, to a large degree, a function of viral nucleic acid structure, mycoplasma virus replication will be reviewed in this section in terms of the single-stranded, circular double-stranded, and linear double-stranded DNA mycoplasma viruses. Unfortunately, by comparison with the well-studied bacteriophages, only limited data are available on the molecular biology of mycoplasma virus replication.

Single-Stranded DNA Mycoplasma Viruses

There are two families of single-stranded DNA bacteriophages: filamentous phages with a noncytocidal infection cycle and isometric phages with a lytic infection cycle (40). Some data are available on the replication of a mycoplasma virus belonging to each family: *Acholeplasma* virus L51, which is a filamentous virion with a noncytocidal infection cycle, and *Spiroplasma* virus SpV4, which is an isometric virion with a cytocidal infection cycle. These data will be reviewed in this section.

In addition, there are two other single-stranded DNA mycoplasma viruses (Table 1): SpV1, a filamentous mycoplasma virus with a genome size about twice those of L51 and SpV4, and L172, an enveloped quasi-spherical mycoplasma virus unlike any other virus that has been described. No data on SpV1 or L172 replication have been reported.

Genome structure

L51 and SpV4 genomes are small circular single-stranded DNA molecules with sizes of 4.3 to 4.5 kb (112, 129), about 20% smaller than genomes of the smallest single-stranded DNA phages. SpV4 DNA has been sequenced and found to be 4,421 bases in size and to contain 32.0 mol% G + C (128).

Analysis of the SpV4 sequence data (128) indicates that the genome contains nine open reading frames (ORFs), all coded in the viral strand. The genome contains several cases of small overlaps between genes and one gene that is completely coded (in a different reading frame) within a larger gene.

The L51 genome must also contain overlapping genes, because the coding capacity required for the L51 structural and nonstructural proteins that have been identified is greater than that of the 4.3- to 4.5-kb L51 genome (27, 93).

DNA replication

The DNA replication cycle of the single-stranded DNA bacteriophages has three stages (reviewed in references 5, 67, 109, and 126): (i) synthesis of a complementary DNA strand by host cell gene products, converting the parental viral strand to parental double-stranded RF DNA (SS→RF), (ii) RF replication to form progeny RF DNA (RF→RF) by a rolling-circle mechanism requiring host cell and viral gene products, and (iii) synthesis of progeny viral single-stranded DNA from RF DNA (RF→SS) by asymmetric DNA replication.

DNA replication of mycoplasma virus L51 has been shown to follow these three stages. For reference in considering L51 DNA replication, the L51 latent period is 10 to 15 min and is followed by a 2- to 3-h rise period. After this rise period, the rate of progeny virus release decreases, although the progeny virus titer continues to increase rather than reaching a plateau (85, 86).

L51 DNA SS→RF replication occurs during or soon after viral DNA strand penetration of the cell (96). This replication stage is not affected by pretreatment of host cells with chloramphenicol (26); hence, as for the small single-stranded DNA bacteriophages, L51 SS→RF replication must be carried out by host cell gene products. The nature of some of these host cell gene products can be inferred from inhibitor studies. (i) Since uptake of L51 single-stranded viral DNA into membrane-associated RF DNA is reduced about two-fold in rifampin-treated host cells (26), primer transcription for L51 SS→RF replication probably involves RNA polymerase rather than primase. (ii) Since L51 production in *A. laidlawii* cells is inhibited by 6-(*p*-hydroxyphenylazo) uracil (91), an inhibitor of DNA polymerase III in gram-positive bacteria, L51 DNA replication apparently requires an *A. laidlawii* DNA polymerase similar to gram-positive bacterial polymerase III.

By 10 min postinfection, 50 to 60% of L51 intracellular parental DNA is membrane associated and the remainder is cytoplasmic (24). Most membrane-associated parental DNA is in RF molecules, and most cytoplasmic parental DNA is in small oligonucleotides. There are a maximum of two to three membrane-associated parental RF molecules per infected cell. Parental RF DNA can be dissociated from the membrane by proteolytic enzymes, so the RF DNA-membrane interaction is protein mediated (24).

L51 RF→RF replication accounts for most viral DNA synthesis during the first 70 min postinfection (23). Viral gene products are required for this replication stage, since RF→RF replication is inhibited by chloramphenicol (28). Although progeny L51 RF synthesis is semiconservative (24), it is not known whether L51 RF→RF replication proceeds through a single-stranded DNA intermediate, as has been found for the single-stranded DNA phages. Pulse-label studies show that L51 RF→RF replication is membrane associated, with progeny RF released into the cytoplasm (24, 94).

L51 RF→SS replication accounts for an increasing fraction of L51 DNA synthesis by about 70 min postinfection, although most synthesis continues to be RF→RF replication (23, 28). At 120 min postinfection, about 40 to 45% of nascent viral DNA is in single-stranded DNA and the remainder is in RF DNA (12). This type of simultaneous RF→RF and RF→SS replication is characteristic of single-stranded DNA filamentous phages but not of single-stranded DNA isometric phages. L51 RF→SS replication is probably by a rolling-circle mechanism, since it involves asymmetric synthesis of viral DNA strands from cytoplasmic RF DNA (24).

Chloramphenicol inhibits L51 RF→SS replication, so viral gene products are needed for this replication stage (28). However, unlike treatment during earlier postinfection times, chloramphenicol treatment during the RF→SS replication stage does not inhibit RF→RF replication (28), indicating that sufficient gene products for RF→RF replication have accumulated by 70 min postinfection to allow continuation of this replication stage. However, RF molecules synthesized in the presence of chloramphenicol are defective in some unknown manner and, after chloramphenicol removal, cannot serve as precursors for progeny viral single-stranded DNA synthesis (28).

Low doses of acriflavine stimulate L51 progeny virus yields two- to threefold when added about 120 min postinfection (12), although these acriflavine doses inhibit A. laidlawii cell DNA repair (43) and replication of Acholeplasma virus L2, a double-stranded DNA virus (12). The acriflavine effect on L51 replication is due to increased turnover of viral DNA intermediates in acriflavine-treated cells relative to untreated control cells (12).

DNA replication of the single-stranded DNA Spiroplasma viruses SpV1, aa, and SpV4 probably also involves the three stages described above, since double-stranded RF DNA has been found in cells infected by these viruses (30, 127, 129).

Transcription

Transcriptional regulation of SpV4 involves promoter and rho-independent termination sequences similar to those described for eubacteria (137). Like transcription of the isometric single-stranded DNA phages (reviewed in reference 67), SpV4 transcription takes place throughout the infection cycle and includes synthesis of an mRNA that is greater than one genome in size (137). Four SpV4 transcripts (with sizes of 2.7, 3.4, 4.4, and 7.8 kb) were detected at all times studied postinfection (137). It has been proposed that these mRNAs start at different promoters and stop at the same rho-independent termination site. The 3.4- and 7.8-kb mRNAs start at the same promoter, but the 7.8-kb mRNA must read through the termination site and transcribe the entire genome before stopping at the termination site when it reaches it again.

Only limited data are available on L51 transcription. In A. laidlawii host cells, which have a rifampin-resistant RNA polymerase, L51 progeny virus yields are not affected by rifampin added up to 60 min postinfection (26). However, at longer infection times, L51 replication becomes increasingly sensitive to rifampin addition, and by 120 min postinfection, rifampin addition completely inhibits the appearance of progeny virus. Rifampin inhibits (but does not completely block) L51 transcription, does not affect RF→RF or RF→SS DNA replication, and blocks maturation of progeny virus single-stranded DNA molecules (26). These data suggest that partial inhibition of RNA polymerase by high concentrations of rifampin in rifampin-resistant cells still allows sufficient transcription of L51 gene products for DNA replication, but the level of gene products may not be sufficient for nucleation or assembly of completed virions.

Translation

Analysis of SpV4 DNA sequence data shows that each of the nine ORFs is preceded by a Shine-Dalgarno sequence (128). Of the nine ORFs, eight start with an ATG codon and one starts with a GTG codon (128).

In vivo translation studies of L51-infected cells show synthesis of 70-, 53-, 30-, and 19-kDa virion structural proteins and nonstructural virus-specific 14- and 10-kDa proteins (27). There is a significant intracellular pool of the four structural proteins by 10 min postinfection, suggesting that, as for the single-stranded DNA filamentous phages (reviewed in references 109 and 126), viral RF molecules are actively transcribed and translated.

Synthesis of the 14-kDa nonstructural protein in L51-infected cells is essentially complete by 10 min postinfection (27). This timing and absence of the 14-kDa protein in REP⁻ host cells (discussed below) indicates the 14-kDa protein is a cell gene product and functions in RF→RF DNA replication.

A small amount of 10-kDa nonstructural protein in L51-infected cells is synthesized at early and intermediate infection times, but maximal synthesis begins at 60 to 110 min postinfection, suggesting that this protein functions in either viral RF→SS replication or virion assembly (27).

Replication in REP⁻ cells

An A. laidlawii REP⁻ clone was isolated from an L51 plaque, and it was found (38, 110) that REP⁻ cells (i) do not propagate single-stranded DNA Acholeplasma viruses (L51 and L172) but continue to propagate double-stranded DNA Acholeplasma viruses (L2 and L3), (ii) exhibit no change in cell growth kinetics or host cell restriction and modification relative to wild-type cells, and (iii) are more sensitive to inactivation by UV irradiation than are wild-type cells.

The block in L51 viral replication in REP⁻ cells is in L51 DNA RF→RF replication: parental L51 single-stranded DNA is converted to RF DNA, but there is no detectable RF→RF replication (110, 134). Parental virus RF is transcribed and translated in REP⁻ cells. The absence of the 14-kDa virus-specific nonstructural protein in infected REP⁻ cells suggests that this protein may be the cell REP gene product (27).

The block in single-stranded DNA virus replication in A. laidlawii REP⁻ cells can be overcome by transfection (38, 134). Transfection with either L51 single- or double-stranded DNA leads to an apparently normal infection, with progeny virus yields similar to those for transfection of wild-type host cells (134). It has been suggested the REP protein may be required for L51 membrane-associated RF replication and that this step may be bypassed by transfection, leading to L51 cytoplasmic RF replication.

Replication in SpV4-resistant cells

Mutants of *Spiroplasma* strains selected for resistance to SpV4 infection can be transfected by SpV4 DNA (8). These mutants may be resistant to infection as a result of a cell surface change affecting adsorption or penetration or a block in intracellular viral replication. It is not known whether the mutants have a REP⁻ phenotype similar to that of *Acholeplasma* REP⁻ cells (described above), in which infection of single-stranded DNA viruses is blocked at the level of RF→RF DNA replication (110).

Circular Double-Stranded DNA Mycoplasma Viruses

Acholeplasma virus L2 has a unique infection cycle in which productive infection is followed by establishment of lysogeny; most, if not all, L2-infected cells become lysogens (37, 124, 125). The fact that L2 productive infection is noncytocidal (described below) makes productive infection and lysogeny possible in the same infected cell, as opposed to the decision between lytic productive infection and lysogeny in temperate phage-infected cells. Hence, there are no phage models for L2 replication, although (as described below) aspects of L2 lysogeny resemble those of phage lysogeny.

Genome structure

The L2 genome is circular double-stranded DNA and is packaged in the virion in the form of a negative superhelical molecule (111, 119). Sequence analysis shows that the genome is 11,965 bp in size and contains 32.0 mol% G + C (98).

Analysis of the L2 sequence data (98, 103) indicates the L2 genome contains 15 ORFs, all coded in the same strand. Most ORFs are clustered in three groups, separated by intergenic regions. Within each cluster, there are small overlaps between ORFs, suggesting that translational coupling or reinitiation is involved in gene expression within each cluster (discussed below). One ORF starts from an initiation codon (in the same reading frame) within a larger ORF; hence, the smaller ORF codes for a protein which is the C-terminal part of the protein coded by the larger ORF. Regulatory sites (i.e., the L2 integration site and the two L2 DNA replication origins) map in intergenic regions.

DNA replication

For reference in considering L2 DNA replication, the L2 latent period is 1 to 2 h (84, 124), viral integration into the cell chromosome is detected by 2 to 4 h postinfection (37), and progeny virus release reaches a plateau at 6 to 10 h postinfection (84, 124).

Data from continuous- and pulse-label studies indicate (34, 37) that (i) L2 DNA replication continues throughout the virus rise period, but not all intracellular L2 progeny DNA is packaged into virions; (ii) L2 DNA replication and progeny virus maturation continue for several hours after integration of a viral genome into the host cell chromosome; and (iii) although L2 DNA replication ceases about 5 to 6 h postinfection, cytoplasmic viral DNA persists for at least 10 h postinfection.

Pulse-labeling of nascent L2 DNA in vivo followed by analysis of the gradient of specific radioactivity as a function of L2 genome map position shows that L2 replicates bidirectionally from two origins, *ori1* and *ori2* (122). These data can be explained by assuming that most DNA molecules replicate simultaneously from both origin sites or that half of the molecules replicate from each site. The approximate positions of both *ori* sites were mapped in these studies (122). Subsequent DNA sequence analysis has precisely mapped and characterized the sequences of both *ori* sites (102); it was found that each L2 origin contains features of phage DNA replication origins, such as a *dnaA* box and a repeated sequence (10).

Intracellular parental L2 DNA is membrane associated and appears to replicate at the membrane (91). L2 production in *A. laidlawii* cells is inhibited by 6-(*p*-hydroxyphenylazo)-uracil (91), suggesting that L2 replication requires an *A. laidlawii* DNA polymerase similar to gram-positive bacterial polymerase III. Other cell gene products must also be required for L2 replication, since induction of the cells' SOS repair (95) and heat shock (29) systems stimulates L2 infection.

L2 DNA replication and progeny virus production are inhibited by novobiocin (120). This effect may be due to novobiocin inhibition of an *A. laidlawii* DNA gyrase activity, because novobiocin treatment during L2 infection leads to the accumulation of some L2 DNA molecules with less negative superhelicity than those produced in untreated cells. L2 DNA molecules with reduced superhelicity are not found when L2-infected novobiocin-resistant cells are treated with novobiocin. However, there is some inhibition of L2 progeny production in novobiocin-treated novobiocin-resistant cells (120), suggesting that L2 replication involves another novobiocin-sensitive process in addition to DNA supercoiling.

Acriflavine reduces the rate of L2 production but has little effect on the final progeny virus yield (12). Since acriflavine is a DNA-intercalating agent, its effect on L2 replication is probably DNA mediated.

Transcription

The L2 DNA sequence contains transcriptional promoter and rho-independent termination sites similar to those described for eubacteria (103). Transcription studies show 11 L2 mRNAs ranging in size from 1.3 to 7.8 kb, with temporal control of transcription (103). DNA sequence analysis and mRNA mapping data indicate several cases of transcriptional read-through, in which two transcripts start at the same promoter but stop at different terminators, and antitermination, in which transcription must be regulated to read through terminators immediately downstream of some promoters (103). The three L2 gene clusters appear to be transcribed as polycistronic mRNAs.

Translation

Each of the 12 L2 ORFs is preceded by a Shine-Dalgarno sequence and starts with an ATG codon (98,

103). Two of the ORFs code for proteins that begin with signal sequences, resembling the signal sequences of gram-positive bacteria which are longer than those of gram-negative bacteria (98, 103). One of these ORFs codes for a 78-kDa protein (after cleavage of the signal sequence), which may be the 72-kDa virion integral membrane protein, and the other codes for a 23-kDa protein (after cleavage of the signal sequence), which may be the minor 21-kDa virion protein.

Within the three L2 gene clusters (two coding for four ORFs and the third coding for five ORFs), the small overlaps between ORFs suggest that translational coupling or reinitiation is involved in translation of the polycistronic mRNA for each cluster (103).

Linear Double-Stranded DNA Mycoplasma Viruses

The short-tailed mycoplasma viruses have been classified in the family *Podoviridae* (short-tailed bacteriophages) (40). The type species for the *Podoviridae* is coliphage T7, which has a 39.9-kbp genome that has a short (about 0.5%) terminally redundant sequence but is not circularly permuted (33). Hence, there are significant differences in genome size and structure between the short-tailed bacteriophages and the short-tailed mycoplasma viruses (Table 2), and the coliphage T7 group cannot be used as a model for replication of the short-tailed mycoplasma viruses.

Although limited data are available on *Acholeplasma* virus L3 replication, essentially nothing is known about replication of the *Spiroplasma* C3-type viruses. The differences in genome size and structure between L3 and the C3-type viruses indicate that differences in DNA replication strategy will be found between the L3- and C3-type viruses.

Genome structure

Three types of linear double-stranded DNA genomes have been found for the short-tailed mycoplasma viruses. (i) An *Acholeplasma* L3 virion contains a 39.4-kbp DNA molecule with limited circular permutation and 8% terminal redundancy, giving a circular map of 36.2 kbp (59, 73); (ii) a *Spiroplasma* SpV3 virion contains a DNA molecule of about 21 kbp which is circularly permuted (14, 16) and has a 5% terminal redundancy (14, 16); and (iii) a *Spiroplasma ai* virion contains a DNA molecule of about 16 kbp with cohesive ends (32). The SRO virus preparations that have been examined thus far have contained virus mixtures, with DNA sizes of 17, 21.8, and >30 kbp (13).

Complementation tests of L3 temperature-sensitive mutants have shown that the 36.2-kbp L3 genome contains at least 21 complementation groups (58). It is interesting that 19 L3-specific proteins (close to the number of complementation groups) have been identified in L3-infected cells (58).

An interesting aspect of *Acholeplasma* virus L3 genome structure has been revealed by studies of mycoplasma virus restriction (135). L3 is not restricted by *A. laidlawii* K2 host cells, although these cells restrict DNA containing GATC sequences and L3 DNA should have about 150 GATC sequences. Hence, L3 has evolved a mechanism for avoiding host cell restriction.

Since L3 DNA is not digested by restriction endonuclease *Mbo*I (which cleaves DNA at GATC and GATmC sites) or *Sau*3AI (which cleaves DNA at GATC and GmATC sites), L3 DNA must not contain GATC sites. This means that, like a number of bacteriophages (e.g., reference 133), *Acholeplasma* virus L3 has evolved under selective pressure that led to the loss of DNA recognition sites for restriction by its host cells.

DNA replication

For reference in considering L3 DNA replication, L3 infection has a 60-min eclipse period and a 90-min latent period, followed by a linear increase in extracellular progeny viruses that continues for about 15 h (59).

In L3-infected cells, during the first 2 h postinfection, the rate of total cellular and viral DNA synthesis decreases to about 10% of the rate before infection (60). The rate continues to decrease slowly with time, but measurable DNA replication continues for at least 17 h postinfection.

Replication of cell DNA gradually shuts down after L3 infection: by 1 h postinfection about 40% of nascent DNA is viral DNA, by 2 h about 60 to 80% is viral DNA, and by 3 h essentially all nascent DNA is viral DNA (60). During infection, the cell folded chromosome is progressively unfolded and possibly fragmented, without release of a significant amount of acid-soluble material.

In addition to the lack of host cell DNA degradation in L3-infected cells, other reasons indicating that L3 must obtain nucleotides for DNA replication by biosynthesis rather than reutilization of host cell DNA nucleotides are (i) no significant amount of cellular DNA in L3-infected host cells is recovered in progeny virus DNA (60) and (ii) if cell DNA nucleotides were the only precursors for L3 DNA, exponentially growing *A. laidlawii* host cells with their 1,700-kbp genome (121) could account for at most about 100 progeny L3 viruses, while many L3-infected cells release >500 progeny viruses (59). The possibility of L3-coded nucleotide synthesis is surprising in view of the relatively limited coding capacity of the L3 genome. Medium-size double-stranded DNA phages, like coliphage T7, with genome sizes similar to that of L3 code for enzymes for host cell DNA degradation and reutilization, while large double-stranded DNA phages, like coliphages T4 and T5, code for enzymes for de novo nucleotide metabolism (references in references 104 and 106). However, mycoplasmas use salvage pathways for nucleotide synthesis, in which medium-supplied free bases or nucleosides are converted to nucleoside mono- and triphosphates (143, 145; also see chapter 13). Since most cell DNA in L3-infected cells remains in a high-molecular-weight form throughout L3 infection, salvage pathway enzymes for L3 nucleotide synthesis could be either cell or virus encoded.

Intracellular parental L3 viral DNA is found in fast-sedimenting viral DNA intermediates, free viral DNA, and virus particles (60). At increasing MOI values, the amount of parental DNA in fast-sedimenting intermediates saturates at about 10 L3 DNA molecules per cell.

L3 DNA replication continues for at least 7 h postinfection and involves intermediates sedimenting faster than free viral DNA (60). The structure of these intermediates has not been determined, but they probably are L3 progeny DNA concatemers (formed by recombination between the terminally redundant ends of linear progeny L3 DNA molecules) involved in viral DNA replication and packaging.

Transcription and translation

The rates of total cellular and viral RNA and protein syntheses in L3-infected cells decrease rapidly during the first hour postinfection and then continue to decrease slowly with time (58). Measurable transcription and translation continue for at least 17 h postinfection.

Protein synthesis during the first hour postinfection is predominantly viral, suggesting both transcriptional and translational regulation (58). Approximately 20 virus-specific proteins (including 10 virion proteins) can be identified by sodium dodecyl sulfate-polyacrylamide gel electrophoresis of L3-infected cells. However, the long labeling times needed in mycoplasma studies have thus far precluded differentiation of early, middle, and late L3 gene expression.

INFECTION CYCLE: MATURATION AND RELEASE

The third stage of a productive viral infection cycle is assembly of intracellular viral components to form completed progeny virions and release of these mature virions from the infected cell. For lytic phages and naked animal viruses, maturation and release are separate processes and are cytocidal. However, for filamentous phages and enveloped animal viruses, maturation and release are coupled and noncytocidal.

The absence of cell walls in mycoplasmas and the morphological types of the mycoplasma viruses make the strategies for maturation and release of mycoplasma viruses different from those of phages and animal viruses. Mycoplasma virus maturation and release can be coupled (as in the filamentous and enveloped mycoplasma viruses) or separate (as in the isometric and short-tailed mycoplasma viruses). However, it should be noted that in all cases studied thus far, progeny mycoplasma virus release is nonlytic. Even the cytocidal isometric and short-tailed mycoplasma viruses apparently use a nonlytic budding release mechanism.

Filamentous Mycoplasma Viruses

Filamentous bacteriophages

Maturation and release of the filamentous mycoplasma viruses resembles maturation and release of filamentous phages, in which assembly of progeny single-stranded DNA molecules and virion proteins occurs at specific membrane assembly sites and is coupled to extrusion of progeny virions through the membrane (reviewed in references 109 and 126).

Acholeplasma virus L51

Growth studies originally indicated that filamentous mycoplasma viruses have a noncytocidal type of

infectious cycle leading to persistently infected cells. One-step growth experiments found that after a rise period, although the rate of progeny *Acholeplasma* virus L51 release decreased, the progeny virus titer continued to increase without reaching a plateau (85, 86). Artificial lysis experiments showed that the latent and eclipse periods of L51 are indistinguishable (86), indicating that virus assembly and release are coupled. Consistent with this model of noncytocidal L51 release, there is no measurable loss of cell viability in *A. laidlawii* cells infected with L51 at MOI values up to 10 (86, 99).

Parental virus single-stranded DNA is not transferred to progeny virions (24, 87). Progeny single-stranded DNA is synthesized by asymmetric replication on cytoplasmic RF DNA (24).

An L51 viral DNA-protein complex has been identified at late times postinfection in infected cells growing in nutritionally limiting medium (25). This complex contains viral single-stranded DNA and two of the virion structural proteins, but in different stoichiometric ratios than in mature L51 virions (93). The complex may be an assembly intermediate or an aberrant structure formed late in infection.

Electron micrographs of infected cells show clusters of extracellular progeny L51 viruses at the membrane surface (86), suggesting that viral assembly and release occur at a limited number of specific sites in each cell. L51 virus maturation and release must involve interactions with the cell membrane which do not affect cell viability.

However, despite the lack of measurable loss of cell titer, there must be some cytoplasmic leakage and release of intracellular DNA, because L51 virion preparations are contaminated with viral DNA replication intermediates (134). Infected cells grow more slowly and make smaller colonies than do uninfected control cells, which probably explains the turbid plaques of L1 and related viruses (50, 86, 99). At MOI values greater than 10, there is some decrease in cell viability (99).

Isometric Mycoplasma Viruses

Isometric bacteriophages

Maturation and assembly of isometric single-stranded DNA phages (reviewed in reference 67) involves (i) association of progeny virus rolling-circle DNA replication complexes with precursor capsids; (ii) completion of DNA synthesis, with nascent progeny viral single-stranded DNA molecules being packaged into capsids and cleaved from the DNA replication complexes; (iii) ligation of linear progeny viral DNA strands to form circular DNA molecules and capsid maturation to form infectious virions; and (iv) mature virion accumulation in the cytoplasm and eventual release by cell lysis.

Spiroplasma virus SpV4

No data are available on maturation of the isometric single-stranded DNA *Spiroplasma* virus SpV4. However, SpV4 release appears to be by a mechanism very different from that of the isometric single-stranded DNA phages.

SpV4 produces clear plaques, indicating a cytocidal type of infection, but SpV4 growth curves show progeny virus release from infected cells release for at least 20 h (129). These data indicate that SpV4 infection resembles that of the short-tailed mycoplasma viruses (described below), with a nonlytic cytocidal infection cycle in which infected cells are no longer viable but continue to release progeny virions over many hours.

Enveloped Mycoplasma Viruses

Acholeplasma virus L2

There are no enveloped phages, so there are no phage models for *Acholeplasma* virus L2 maturation and release.

L2 one-step and artificial lysis growth curves indicate that L2 infection is noncytocidal and that L2 maturation and release are coupled (84, 124).

Since L2 infection leads to establishment of lysogeny (37, 124, 125; also discussed below) and there is no measurable loss of cell titer in cultures infected at an MOI of 30 (124), most if not all infected cells must become lysogens.

L2 DNA is packaged as a superhelical molecule (111), so L2 assembly and maturation may involve a novobiocin-sensitive process (120). Some parental L2 DNA is found in progeny virions (91), which may result from semiconservative replication of infecting parental DNA, with one of the two progeny molecules being packaged into a progeny particle.

The only intracellular L2 assembly form that has been identified is a spherical structure near the cell membrane (92). The presence and location of this structure in infected cells indicate that it may be a viral nucleoprotein intermediate prior to maturation by budding.

L2 maturation by budding from the host cell membrane is shown by data on the lipid composition of cell and virus membranes and by electron microscopy studies. L2 virion proteins are virus specific, but the virus fatty acid composition reflects that of the host cell membrane (55, 123). In addition to budding structures, freeze-etch electron microscopy shows that the cell membrane is structurally different at the budding site and lacks protoplasmic face particles (92).

Uninfected *A. laidlawii* cells are osmotically fragile (124). However, after L2 infection, the cells' osmotic stability increases, reaching a plateau by 2 h postinfection, a time corresponding to beginning of the virus rise period (124). The increase in osmotic stability may reflect an increased cell membrane permeability during the period of viral membrane synthesis and L2 maturation and budding. After establishment of lysogenization, the cells' osmotic fragility is similar to that of uninfected cells (124).

Acholeplasma virus L2 minivirus

Two spontaneous L2 insertion variants, designated L2*ins1* and L2*ins2*, have been isolated from wild-type L2 stocks (39). Both L2*ins1* and L2*ins2* have genomes of about 15 kbp, consisting of the L2 genome with a DNA insert of about 3.3 kbp arising from transpositions of two noncontiguous regions of the L2 genome. L2*ins1* and L2*ins2* differ only in location of the DNA insert.

During serial passages of L2*ins1* and L2*ins2*, minivirus DNA is generated by the sixth passage (39). Minivirus DNA also accumulates during passage of wild-type L2, but it does so more slowly and is not seen until passage 18. The minivirus DNA is the 3.3-kbp insert DNA in the form of superhelical circular molecules and multimers of this 3.3-kbp DNA.

The mechanism of the DNA transpositions that led to generation of L2*ins1* and L2*ins2* is unknown. Since L2*ins1* contains three *ori* sites instead of the two found in L2 (122), one of the two L2 *ori* sites must have been transposed in the generation of L2*ins1*.

Minivirus DNA can be packaged into noninfectious particles which sediment more slowly than do L2 virions (39). In addition, the infectious titers of L2 stocks decrease as minivirus DNA accumulates. Therefore, minivirus particles are defective, and perhaps interfering, particles.

No data are available on the mechanism of minivirus production. The finding of a DNA replication origin in the 3.3-kbp DNA insert (122) indicates that minivirus DNA may be an autonomous replicating unit in the cell, which means that minivirus DNA probably contains those sequences required in *cis* for viral DNA replication and packaging.

Short-Tailed Mycoplasma Viruses

Short-tailed bacteriophages

Maturation and release of short-tailed bacteriophages (the coliphage T7 group) (reviewed in references 7 and 66) involves (i) packaging of a unique end of progeny viral DNA from a replicating concatemeric DNA complex into a prohead, (ii) headful DNA packaging and terminase cleavage at a specific site to generate unique linear progeny DNA molecules with a short terminally redundant sequence, (iii) head maturation and tail assembly to generate an infectious virion, and (iv) accumulation of mature virions in the cytoplasm and subsequent release by cell lysis.

Acholeplasma virus L3

The process of L3 maturation and release differs from that of the coliphage T7 group at least in terms of DNA packaging and the mechanism of progeny virus release.

L3 DNA packaging is probably from concatemers (60). However, L3 DNA is terminally redundant with limited circular permutation, indicating that it is packaged by a *pac* site-cutting mechanism (73). This mechanism has been described for some large DNA phages, in which an initial *pac* site cutting and headful packaging from concatemeric DNA is followed by processive headful packaging and *pac* site cutting (reviewed in reference 7). Linear progeny DNA molecules, which are terminally redundant and have limited circular permutation, are generated by *pac* site cutting.

Although L3 produces clear plaques, indicating that it is a cytocidal virus, L3 does not have a lytic infectious cycle (59). Growth and electron microscopy studies show that although L3-infected cells may not be viable, mature progeny virions accumulate in infected cells and are released continuously over a number of hours rather than in a single burst. To confirm the conclusion that infected cells produce virus over an extended period, virus production from individual infected cells was assayed at several times over 24 h, using a modification of the single-burst experimental protocol (59). The data show that every infected cell that begins to release progeny L3 virus during the first few hours postinfection continues to do so through the 24-h time period of the experiment. The onset and rate of virus release vary from cell to cell, and the total number of viruses released per infected cell varies over a 100-fold range from cell to cell. This nonlytic cytocidal type of L3 infection has been observed in other laboratories but with somewhat different infection cycle times and yields, probably reflecting variations in host cell strains and growth conditions (79, 91).

Electron microscopy shows an accumulation of intracellular L3 virions with increasing times postinfection (63). By 8 h postinfection, the cytoplasmic face of the cell membrane is almost covered with L3 particles, oriented radially with their tails toward the membrane.

Only electron microscopic data are available on the nonlytic release of L3 progeny virions. L3 particles appear be released from infected cells in membrane vesicles enclosing one or more progeny virions (15, 63). Since individual L3-infected cells continue to release progeny virions over many hours (59), release of L3 particles by budding from the cell membrane must not destroy the integrity of the cell. It is not known how virus-containing vesicles form or how they break down after release from the cell membrane to yield mature progeny virions.

Spiroplasma virus ai

The *ai* virus appears to have a nonlytic cytocidal productive infectious cycle similar to that of *Acholeplasma* virus L3 (described above). However, unlike L3, *ai* has both productive and lysogenic cycles.

One-step growth and artificial lysis experiments show that the *ai* infectious cycle has an eclipse period of about 3 h, at which time an intracellular accumulation of mature virions begins, and a latent period of 5 to 6 h, at which time progeny virus release begins (32). Progeny virus release continues for about 5 to 6 h (to about 11 h postinfection), to yield an average of 40 *ai* virions per infectious center. The titer of infected cells is lower than that of uninfected control cells (32). Electron microscopy of plants infected with *S. citri* SP-V3, from which *ai* virus was isolated, shows virions apparently budding from *S. citri* cell membranes (2). These data suggest that, like *Acholeplasma* virus L3 (described above), *ai*-infected cells are not viable, but progeny virions continue to accumulate and be released over a number of hours rather than in a single burst.

Other short-tailed mycoplasma viruses

Electron microscopic studies of SpV3-infected cultures (14, 15) and SRO virus-infected SRO cells (116, 146) show accumulations of intracellular progeny viri-

ons and membrane-bound budding virions. These data suggest that release of these viruses involves budding from infected cell membranes, similar to the type of release described above for other short-tailed mycoplasma viruses.

LYSOGENY AND PERSISTENT INFECTION

Bacteriophages can persist in two types of carrier states: lysogenic and persistent infections (reviewed in references 1 and 6). Both types of carrier states also seem to be frequent in mycoplasma virus-infected cells (described below).

In lysogenized cells, the phage genome persists in a stable prophage state and the cells are immune to superinfection by homologous phages. Lysogenic phages have been found in most, if not all, phylogenetic branches of the eubacteria and archaebacteria.

Persistent infections are chronic infections by nonlysogenic phages. Two types of phage persistent infections have been described. (i) Pseudolysogeny is a type of persistent infection in which only a fraction of cells in a bacterial culture are infected, apparently as a result of mutational (in either phage or host cell genomes) or physiological changes which make phage infection or replication inefficient (e.g., reference 109). (ii) Steady-state infections are a type of persistent infection in which all cells in a culture are infected by noncytocidal phages (e.g., reference 1). Persistent infections, particularly examples of pseudolysogeny, appear to be fairly frequent in bacteriophages.

Filamentous Mycoplasma Viruses

Filamentous bacteriophages

The single-stranded DNA filamentous bacteriophages can have lysogenic and persistent infection carrier states, but both types of carrier states have not been reported for the same phage. The filamentous coliphages cause persistent infections (109). In contrast, several *Xanthomonas* filamentous phages cause lysogenic infections, with phage DNA being integrated into host cell chromosomes and lysogenic cells being immune to infection by homologous phages and inducible for phage production (e.g., references 74 and 75).

L1-type Acholeplasma viruses

The L1-type filamentous mycoplasma viruses appear to be able to have both types of carrier states, persistent and lysogenic infections.

In cultures persistently infected with L1-type mycoplasma viruses, cells cloned from virus plaques or persistently infected cultures are either infected and producing virus or uninfected and sensitive to virus infection (reviewed in references 88 and 130). Infected clones are resistant to superinfection, perhaps because the two to three membrane sites per cell for parental DNA SS→RF replication (24) are occupied. However, the infected state is unstable, and most infected clones convert to uninfected, virus-sensitive cells after a number of passages. The conversion may be due to segregation of uninfected cells with a growth rate faster than that of infected cells. Similar persistent infection has been described for the filamentous coliphages (references in reference 77).

Establishment of persistent infection may also involve viral interference, since L51-infected cells contain small circular double-stranded DNA molecules about a third the size of the L51 genome (112). This form of DNA may be similar to the miniphage DNA found in cells infected by small single-stranded DNA filamentous phages (references in reference 69), which replicates to form defective interfering particles (reviewed in reference 5).

Several *A. laidlawii* strains have been shown to contain genomes of L1-type *Acholeplasma* viruses integrated into host cell chromosomal DNA, and L1 virus production can be induced by transfection of these cells with specific DNA fragments from L1 or L3 *Acholeplasma* viruses (72). It would be interesting to determine whether induction results from an L1 repressor concentration being reduced by binding to specific sequences in the transfecting DNA fragments.

L1-type *Acholeplasma* virus persistent infection and/or lysogeny may explain the frequent isolation of L1-type viruses from *A. laidlawii* strains (reviewed in reference 91), the reports of L1-type virus release from *A. laidlawii* cells after treatment with mitomycin (80, 83), and the resistance to L51 superinfection of a clone selected from an L51-infected *A. laidlawii* culture (140).

C1-type *Spiroplasma* viruses

Preliminary data suggest that two C1-type *Spiroplasma* viruses, SpV1 and *aa*, may be lysogenic. SpV1 and *aa* genomic DNAs are about the same size and have similar, but not identical, restriction endonuclease cleavage maps (9). SpV1 sequences have been identified in the chromosomal DNA of several *Spiroplasma* species, but one *S. citri* strain containing sequences homologous to SpV1 DNA that was studied further was found not to be resistant to SpV1 infection (9). Hence, chromosomal SpV1 sequences may be a cryptic prophage, or the SpV1 phage strain used for the infection and the SpV1 prophage may have different immunity specificities.

Acholeplasma Virus L2

Establishment of lysogeny

L2 infection of *A. laidlawii* cells leads to the establishment of lysogeny (124, 125), with an L2 genome integrated into the cell chromosome at a unique site in both virus and cell DNAs (37). The viral integration site has been mapped to within a 600-bp region in the L2 genome (37, 39). Recent L2 DNA sequence analysis suggests that the viral integration site is a 26-bp sequence with dyad symmetry, within the 600-bp region, which is homologous to the lambda phage integrase binding site that is the lambda integration site (103).

Immunity

L2 lysogens are immune to superinfection by homologous virus but can be infected by heterologous virus (125). There are apparently conflicting data on the mechanism of immunity to superinfection by homologous virus. Little or no L2 adsorption was found in most lysogen clones examined (125), suggesting that immunity may be similar to the situation for some *Salmonella* phages (reviewed in reference 6), in which immunity involves lysogenic conversion and modification of cell surface phage receptors. However, some L2 does adsorb, and since the superinfecting L2 DNA is not replicated or degraded (34), superinfecting L2 DNA must be lost by dilution after a number of cell generations. These latter data imply the existence of an L2 repressor in lysogens.

The question of whether immunity to superinfection in L2 lysogens is caused by a repressor or by a surface effect due to lysogenic conversion in L2 lysogens was investigated by examining L2 transfection frequencies in wild-type and L2 lysogen cells (141). By using transfection rather than infection to introduce L2 DNA into lysogens, any cell surface effect on immunity should be obviated. Since L2 lysogens were also immune to superinfection by transfecting L2 DNA, immunity in L2 lysogens is not a cell surface effect and must be due to an L2 repressor.

Induction

Although most cells in a lysogenic culture do not form infectious centers on host cell lawns, they retain the potential to produce L2 virus and transmit this potential as a stable heritable trait. Mitomycin and UV light induce an increase in infectious centers in lysogens (125).

Regulation of lysogeny

Although the properties of L2 and lambdoid phage lysogens are similar, the regulatory mechanisms involved in the decision between productive and lysogenic infection cycles must be different. Lambdoid phages have a lytic productive infection cycle, so the decision is between a lytic cycle and a lysogenic cycle. *Acholeplasma* virus L2 has a noncytocidal productive infection cycle (described above), so a productive infection cycle can be followed by a lysogenic cycle in the same infected cell. L2 regulation is between an initial productive infection cycle and a final lysogenic cycle. This process cannot simply be temporal with a shut-off of L2 productive infection and a turn-on of lysogeny, because integration occurs during the rise period and productive infection continues for several hours after L2 integration into the host cell chromosome (37).

There seems to be an interesting similarity between L2 and other lysogenic phages in the mechanism of integration into host cell chromosomal DNA. Recent L2 DNA sequence analysis has shown one of the L2 gene products is homologous to the phage integrase family of site-specific recombinases, and as for other lysogenic phages, the L2 integrase maps just upstream of the integration site (103).

Spiroplasma Virus *ai*

The C3-type *Spiroplasma* virus *ai* has a genome of linear double-stranded DNA with cohesive ends (32).

Since *ai* is lysogenic and integrates into host cell chromosomal DNA (described below), *ai* DNA may, like lambda phage DNA, circularize after infection and integrate into the cell genome by crossing-over.

Southern blot analysis has shown that all strains of *S. citri* examined contain an *ai* cryptic prophage, a deleted form of the *ai* genome integrated in the cell chromosome (31). Hence, the occurrence of cryptic *ai* prophages must be widespread in *S. citri* strains, and it has been suggested that integrated *ai* DNA may have arisen by site-specific recombination, followed by loss of immunity and attachment sequences by deletion mutations (31). Integration in *ai* lysogens appears to be by homologous recombination between *ai* and cryptic prophage sequences, leading to *ai* integration in the cell chromosome within the cryptic prophage (31).

Some cells infected by *ai* are lysogenized, and *ai* virus is spontaneously released in these lysogen cultures (31), presumably by spontaneous induction. Lysogens are immune to superinfection by homologous virus but can be infected by heterologous virus. These properties are retained after repeated passage in medium containing antiserum to *ai* virions (31).

Although *ai* plaques are normally turbid, a few clear plaques are found when *ai* is plated on *ai* lysogens. Plating efficiencies of virus from these clear plaques are the same on both control host cells and lysogenized cells (31), suggesting the isolates may be virulent *ai* mutants.

No *ai* virus adsorption can be detected to *ai* lysogens or to isolated lysogen membranes (31). This situation may be similar to that for *Salmonella* phage lysogeny (reviewed in reference 6), in which immunity involves lysogenic conversion and modification of cell surface phage receptors.

Since the *ai* productive infectious cycle is cytocidal (discussed above), regulation of *ai* productive and lysogenic cycles may be similar to that of the lambdoid phages (reviewed in reference 68). Infection of a given cell will lead to either cytocidal productive infection or lysogeny.

Lysogeny by *Spiroplasma* virus *ai* and lysogency by *Acholeplasma* virus L2 (described above) appear to have several significant differences. The L2 noncytocidal productive infection cycle allows both productive L2 infection and lysogeny in the same infected cell, while the cytocidal *ai* productive infection cycle requires a decision between productive infection and lysogeny in each *ai*-infected cell. In addition, the mechanism of immunity to superinfection by homologous virus in L2 lysogens appears to be due to a specific L2 repressor, while in *ai* lysogens it appears to be due to lysogenic conversion and modification of the cell surface.

CONCLUSIONS

From a historical perspective, there are interesting parallels between the development of mycoplasma biology and mycoplasma virology. In the early stages of research on mycoplasmas, only fragmentary data were available, and these were frequently interpreted in terms of models outside the general constructs of microbiology as it was then understood. Eventually, sufficient data on the cellular and molecular biology of mycoplasmas and other microorganisms accumulated to allow the information on mycoplasmas to be reviewed and explained simply as another chapter in the biology of microorganisms (101). To be sure, mycoplasma biology has some unique characteristics, reflecting mycoplasma evolutionary history and adaptation to a limited genetic complexity.

In a similar way, mycoplasma virology has seemed full of confusing data that were difficult to place in the context of bacterial virology. However, this review comes at a time when there are enough new data on the molecular biology of both mycoplasma viruses and bacteriophages to allow an understanding of mycoplasma virology as an extension of bacteriophage infection strategies to the special case of virus infection of wall-less mycoplasma cells. However, as in the case of mycoplasma biology, mycoplasma viruses have some novel properties because the unique ecological niche of mycoplasma host cells has selected for an elaboration of viral infection strategies from those seen in the bacteriophages.

It appears that the cell surface has been the most significant difference between mycoplasmas and eubacteria in terms of evolutionarily possible viral infection strategies. This difference in cell surfaces is seen in the beginning and end of the viral infection cycle, the adsorption/penetration and maturation/release stages, and this is where major differences are seen between mycoplasma virus and bacteriophage infections. In the middle of the infection cycle, the intracellular replication stage, the molecular biology aspects are similar and analogous mycoplasma viruses and bacteriophages follow analogous replication strategies.

The wall-less structure of mycoplasma cells allows virion adsorption to cell membrane receptors, nonlytic productive infectious cycles, and progeny virus release by budding. In some cases, this characteristic appears to have led to the evolution of virion morphology not possible for bacteriophages, such as that of the enveloped *Acholeplasma* L2 virus, while in other cases, bacteriophage virions, such as short-tailed phages, appear to have evolved to infect mycoplasmas. In the latter case, one must wonder at the selective pressure that has kept tailed virion structures for infecting wall-less cells.

An alternate possibility should be noted for the origin of mycoplasma viruses with tailed-phage morphology, particularly those mycoplasma viruses described in Table 3 that appear to be poorly adapted to growth in mycoplasma host cells. Mycoplasma cells must come into contact with bacteriophages both in nature in mycoplasma ecological niches and, in view of the prevalence of bacteriophages in commercial serum (108), in the laboratory in serum-containing media. Hence, the various tailed-phage mycoplasma viruses may represent bacteriophages at different stages of adaptation to infection of mycoplasma host cells.

All mycoplasma virus infectious cycles that have been described, including cytocidal and noncytocidal infection cycles, are nonlytic. The release of all mycoplasma viruses, cytocidal and noncytocidal, studied thus far involves budding of progeny virions from infected cell membranes, except for the filamentous mycoplasma viruses, which appear to be extruded through the cell membrane. For *Acholeplasma* virus

L2, nonlytic progeny release allowed evolution of a unique temperate virus, in which productive infection is followed by lysogeny in the same infected cell.

In summary, sometimes mycoplasma viruses seem to have evolved something new, such as the distinctive type of temperate infection of the enveloped L2 virions, and sometimes they seem to have adapted something from the phages, such as the short-tailed phage structures of some mycoplasma viruses. Some of these viruses (perhaps the enveloped mycoplasma viruses) may have evolved from mycoplasmas, and others (perhaps the short-tailed mycoplasma viruses) may have come along with the mycoplasmas as they evolved from gram-positive bacteria. The unusual phenotypes of mycoplasma viruses may be related to the rapid evolutionary rate that characterizes the mycoplasmas. Both mycoplasma cells and viruses appear to have examined evolutionary alternatives not accessible to other biological systems.

Acknowledgments. I thank the students, postdoctoral fellows, and technicians who, over the past two decades in this laboratory, participated in the development of mycoplasma biology and virology: Stephen P. Cadden, Utpal Chauhuri, Jyotirmoy Das, Christopher C. Dascher, Kevin Dybvig, David Gerling, Amit Ghosh, Angela I. Haberer, Klaus Haberer, George J. Kampo, Alan Liss, Jan A. Nowak, Saibal K. Poddar, Resha M. Putzrath, Todd L. Sladek, and Ruengpung Sutthent.

REFERENCES

1. **Ackermann, H.-W., and M. S. DuBow.** 1987. *Viruses of Prokaryotes* vol. 1, p. 87–101. CRC Press, Inc., Boca Raton, Fla.
2. **Alivizatos, A. S., R. Townsend, and P. G. Markham.** 1982. Effects of infection with a spiroplasma virus on the symptoms produced by *Spiroplasma citri. Ann. Appl. Biol.* **101:**85–91.
3. **Al-Shammari, A. J. N., and P. F. Smith.** 1980. Interaction of mycoplasma virus type 2 with cellular components of *Acholeplasma laidlawii* strain JA1. *J. Virol.* **36:**120–124.
4. **Al-Shammari, A. J. N., and P. F. Smith.** 1982. Receptor sites for mycoplasmal viruses on *Acholeplasma laidlawii. Rev. Infect. Dis.* **4:**S109–S114.
5. **Baas, P. D.** 1985. DNA replication of single-stranded *Escherichia coli* DNA phages. *Biochim. Biophys. Acta* **825:**111–139.
6. **Barksdale, L., and S. B. Arden.** 1974. Persisting bacteriophage infections, lysogeny, and phage conversions. *Annu. Rev. Microbiol.* **28:**265–299.
7. **Black, L. W.** 1988. DNA packaging in dsDNA bacteriophages, p. 321–373. *In* R. Calendar (ed.), *The Bacteriophages,* vol. 2. Plenum Press, New York.
8. **Bové, J. M., T. Candresse, C. Mouches, J. Renaudin, and C. Saillard.** 1984. Spiroplasmas and the transfer of genetic information by transformation and transfection. *Isr. J. Med. Sci.* **20:**836–839.
9. **Bové, J. M., P. Carle, M. Garnier, F. Laigret, J. Renaudin, and C. Saillard.** 1989. Molecular and cellular biology of spiroplasmas, p. 243–364. *In* R. F. Whitcomb and J. G. Tully (ed.), *The Mycoplasmas,* vol. 5. Academic Press, Inc., New York.
10. **Bramhill, D., and A. Kornberg.** 1988. A model for initiation at origins of DNA replication. *Cell* **54:**915–918.
11. **Bruce, J., R. N. Gourlay, R. Hull, and D. J. Garwes.** 1972. Ultrastructure of Mycoplasmatales virus laidlawii 1. *J. Gen. Virol.* **16:**215–221.
12. **Chaudhuri, U., J. Das, K. Haberer, and J. Maniloff.** 1979. Replication of mycoplasmavirus MVL51. VI. Acriflavine stimulates growth of this single-stranded DNA virus. *Biochem. Biophys. Res. Commun.* **89:**643–649.
13. **Cohen, A. J., D. L. Williamson, and K. Oishi.** 1987. SpV3 viruses of *Drosophila* spiroplasmas. *Isr. J. Med. Sci.* **23:**429–433.
14. **Cole, R. M.** 1977. Spiroplasmaviruses, p. 451–464. *In* K. Maramorosch (ed.), *The Atlas of Insect and Plant Viruses.* Academic Press, Inc., New York.
15. **Cole, R. M.** 1979. Mycoplasma and spiroplasma viruses: ultrastructure, p. 385–410. *In* M. F. Barile and S. Razin (ed.), *The Mycoplasmas,* vol. 1. Academic Press, Inc., New York.
16. **Cole, R. M., C. F. Garon, W. O. Mitchell, E. Jablonska, and J. M. Ranhand.** 1978. Spiroplasma viruses: current status, abstr. W8/12. *Abstr. 4th Int. Congr. Virol.*
17. **Cole, R. M., W. O. Mitchell, and C. F. Garon.** 1977. *Spiroplasmavirus citri* 3: propagation, purification, proteins, and nucleic acid. *Science* **198:**1262–1263.
18. **Cole, R. M., J. G. Tully, and T. J. Popkin.** 1974. Virus-like particles in *Spiroplasma citri. Colloq. Inst. Natl. Sante Rech. Med.* **33:**125–132.
19. **Cole, R. M., J. G. Tully, T. J. Popkin, and J. M. Bové.** 1973. Morphology, ultrastructure, and bacteriophage infection of the helical mycoplasma-like organism (*Spiroplasma citri* gen. nov., sp. nov.) cultured from "stubborn" disease of citrus. *J. Bacteriol.* **115:**367–386.
20. **Cole, R. M., J. G. Tully, T. J. Popkin, and J. M. Bové.** 1973. Ultrastructure of the agent of citrus "stubborn" disease. *Ann. N.Y. Acad. Sci.* **225:**471–493.
21. **Congdon, A. L., E. S. Boatman, and G. E. Kenny.** 1979. Mycoplasmatales virus MV-M1: discovery in *Acholeplasma modicum* and preliminary characterization. *Curr. Microbiol.* **3:**111–115.
22. **Dahl, C. E., N. C. Sacktor, and J. S. Dahl.** 1985. Acylated proteins in *Acholeplasma laidlawii. J. Bacteriol.* **162:**445–447.
23. **Das, J., and J. Maniloff.** 1975. Replication of mycoplasmavirus MVL51. I. Replicative intermediates. *Biochem. Biophys. Res. Commun.* **66:**599–605.
24. **Das, J., and J. Maniloff.** 1976. Replication of mycoplasmavirus MVL51. Attachment of MVL51 parental DNA to host cell membrane. *Proc. Natl. Acad. Sci. USA* **73:**1489–1493.
25. **Das, J., and J. Maniloff.** 1976. Replication of mycoplasmavirus MVL51. III. Identification of a progeny viral DNA-protein intermediate. *Microbios* **15:**127–134.
26. **Das, J., and J. Maniloff.** 1976. Replication of mycoplasmavirus MVL51. IV. Inhibition of viral synthesis by rifampin. *J. Virol.* **18:**969–976.
27. **Das, J., and J. Maniloff.** 1978. Replication of mycoplasmavirus MVL51. V. *In vivo* synthesis of virus specific proteins. *Virology* **86:**186–192.
28. **Das, J., and J. Maniloff.** 1982. Replication of mycoplasma virus MVL51. VII. Effect of chloramphenicol on the synthesis of DNA replicative intermediates. *J. Virol.* **44:**877–881.
29. **Dascher, C. C., S. K. Poddar, and J. Maniloff.** 1990. Heat shock response in mycoplasmas, genome-limited organisms. *J. Bacteriol.* **172:**1823–1827.
30. **Dickinson, M. J., and R. Townsend.** 1984. Characterization of the genome of a rod-shaped virus infecting *Spiroplasma citri. J. Gen. Virol.* **65:**1607–1610.
31. **Dickinson, M. J., and R. Townsend.** 1985. Lysogenization of *Spiroplasma citri* by a type 3 spiroplasmavirus. *Virology* **146:**102–110.
32. **Dickinson, M. J., R. Townsend, and S. J. Curson.** 1984. Characterization of a virus infecting the wall-free prokaryote *Spiroplasma citri. Virology* **135:**524–535.
33. **Dunn, J. J., and F. W. Studier.** 1983. Complete nucleotide sequence of bacteriophage T7 DNA and the locations of T7 genetic elements. *J. Mol. Biol.* **166:**477–535.

34. **Dybvig, K.** 1981. Ph.D. thesis. University of Rochester, Rochester, N.Y.

35. **Dybvig, K., J. Alderete, H. L. Watson, and G. H. Cassell.** 1988. Adsorption of mycoplasma virus P1 to host cells. *J. Bacteriol.* **170:**4373–4375.

36. **Dybvig, K., A. Liss, J. Alderete, R. M. Cole, and G. H. Cassell.** 1987. Isolation of a virus from *Mycoplasma pulmonis*. *Isr. J. Med. Sci.* **23:**418–422.

37. **Dybvig, K., and J. Maniloff.** 1983. Integration and lysogeny by an enveloped mycoplasma virus. *J. Gen. Virol.* **64:**1781–1785.

38. **Dybvig, K., J. A. Nowak, T. L. Sladek, and J. Maniloff.** 1985. Identification of an enveloped phage, mycoplasma virus L172, containing a 14-kilobase single-stranded DNA genome. *J. Virol.* **53:**384–390.

39. **Dybvig, K., T. L. Sladek, and J. Maniloff.** 1986. Isolation of mycoplasma virus L2 insertion variants and miniviruses. *J. Virol.* **59:**584–590.

40. **Francki, R. I. B., C. M. Fauquet, D. L. Knudson, and F. Brown.** 1991. *Classification and Nomenclature of Viruses: Fifth Report of the International Committee on Taxonomy of Viruses.* Springer-Verlag, New York.

41. **Fraser, D., and C. Fleischmann.** 1974. Interaction of mycoplasma with viruses. I. Primary adsorption of virus is ionic in mechanism. *J. Virol.* **13:**1067–1074.

42. **Garwes, D. J., B. V. Pike, S. G. Wyld, D. H. Pocock, and R. N. Gourlay.** 1975. Characterization of Mycoplasmatales virus-laidlawii 3. *J. Gen. Virol.* **29:**11–24.

43. **Ghosh, A., J. Das, and J. Maniloff.** 1978. Effect of acriflavine on ultraviolet inactivation of *Acholeplasma laidlawii*. *Biochim. Biophys. Acta* **543:**570–575.

44. **Goldberg, E.** 1980. Bacteriophage nucleic acid penetration, p. 115–41. *In* L. L. Randall and L. Philipson (ed.), *Receptors and Recognition*, series B, vol. 7, part 1. Chapman & Hall, London.

45. **Gourlay, R. N.** 1970. Isolation of a virus infecting a strain of *Mycoplasma laidlawii*. *Nature* (London) **225:**1165.

46. **Gourlay, R. N.** 1971. Mycoplasmatales virus-laidlawii 2, a new virus isolated from *Acholeplasma laidlawii*. *J. Gen. Virol.* **12:**65–67.

47. **Gourlay, R. N.** 1972. Isolation and characterization of mycoplasma viruses. *CIBA Found. Symp.* **6:**145–156.

48. **Gourlay, R. N.** 1973. Mycoplasmatales viruses. *Ann. N.Y. Acad. Sci.* **225:**144–148.

49. **Gourlay, R. N.** 1974. Mycoplasma viruses: isolation, physicochemical, and biological properties. *Crit. Rev. Microbiol.* **3:**315–331.

50. **Gourlay, R. N., and S. G. Wyld.** 1972. Some biological characteristics of Mycoplasmatales virus-laidlawii 1. *J. Gen. Virol.* **14:**15–23.

51. **Gourlay, R. N., and S. G. Wyld.** 1973. Isolation of Mycoplasmatales virus-laidlawii 3, a new virus infecting *Acholeplasma laidlawii*. *J. Gen. Virol.* **19:**279–283.

52. **Gourlay, R. N., S. G. Wyld, and A. P. Bland.** 1979. Demonstration by electron microscopy of intracellular virus in *Acholeplasma laidlawii* infected with either MV-L3 or a similar but serologically distinct virus (BN1 virus). *J. Gen. Virol.* **42:**315–322.

53. **Gourlay, R. N., S. G. Wyld, and D. J. Garwes.** 1983. Some properties of mycoplasma virus Br1. *Arch. Virol.* **75:**1–15.

54. **Gourlay, R. N., S. G. Wyld, and M. E. Poulton.** 1983. Some characteristics of mycoplasma virus Hr1, isolated from and infecting *Mycoplasma hyorhinis*. *Arch. Virol.* **77:**81–85.

55. **Greenberg, N., and S. Rottem.** 1979. Composition and molecular organization of lipids and proteins in the envelope of mycoplasmavirus MVL2. *J. Virol.* **32:**717–726.

56. **Grinius, L.** 1982. Protonmotive-force-dependent DNA transport across bacterial membranes, p. 129–132. *In* A. N. Martonosi (ed.), *Membranes and Transport*, vol. 2. Plenum Press, New York.

57. **Haberer, K., and D. Frosch.** 1982. Lateral mobility of membrane-bound antibodies on the surface of *Acholeplasma laidlawii:* evidence for virus-induced cell fusion in a procaryote. *J. Bacteriol.* **152:**471–478.

58. **Haberer, K., A. I. Haberer, S. P. Cadden, and J. Maniloff.** 1990. Isolation and characterization of mycoplasma virus L3 temperature-sensitive mutants. *Microbios* **64:**111–125.

59. **Haberer, K., G. Klotz, J. Maniloff, and A. K. Kleinschmidt.** 1979. Structural and biological properties of mycoplasmavirus MVL3: an unusual virus-prokaryote interaction. *J. Virol.* **32:**268–275.

60. **Haberer, K., and J. Maniloff.** 1980. Virus and host cell DNA syntheses during infection of *Acholeplasma laidlawii* by MVL3, a nonlytic cytocidal mycoplasmavirus. *J. Virol.* **33:**671–679.

61. **Haberer, K., and J. Maniloff.** 1982. Adsorption of the tailed mycoplasma virus L3 to cell membranes. *J. Virol.* **41:**501–507.

62. **Haberer, K., and J. Maniloff.** 1982. Active diffusion of adsorbed mycoplasma virus L3 on *Acholeplasma laidlawii* cell membranes. *Rev. Infect. Dis.* **4:**S105–S108.

63. **Haberer, K., J. Maniloff, and D. Gerling.** 1980. Adsorption, capping, and release of a complex bacteriophage by mycoplasma cells. *J. Virol.* **36:**264–270.

64. **Haberer, K., and M. Pfisterer.** 1981. Altered surface structure of *Acholeplasma laidlawii* induced by mycoplasmavirus L3 infection. *Eur. J. Cell Biol.* **25:**10–12.

65. **Haberer, K., M. Pfisterer, and H.-J. Galla.** 1982. Virus capping on mycoplasma cells and its effect on membrane structure. *Biochim. Biophys. Acta* **688:**720–726.

66. **Hausmann, R.** 1988. The T7 group, p. 259–289. *In* R. Calendar (ed.), *The Bacteriophages*, vol. 1. Plenum Press, New York.

67. **Hayashi, M., A. Aoyama, D. L. Richardson, and M. N. Hayashi.** 1988. Biology of the bacteriophage ϕX174, p. 1–71. *In* R. Calendar (ed.), *The Bacteriophages*, vol. 2. Plenum Press, New York.

68. **Hendrix, R. W., J. W. Roberts, F. W. Stahl, and R. A. Weisberg (ed.).** 1983. *Lambda II*. Cold Spring Harbor Laboratory, Cold Spring Harbor, N.Y.

69. **Horiuchi, K.** 1983. Co-evolution of a filamentous bacteriophage and its defective interfering particles. *J. Mol. Biol.* **169:**389–407.

70. **Howard, C. J., R. N. Gourlay, and S. G. Wyld.** 1980. Isolation of a virus MVBr1, from *Mycoplasma bovirhinis*. *FEMS Microbiol. Lett.* **7:**163–165.

71. **Ichimaru, H., and M. Nakamura.** 1983. Biological properties of a plaque-inducing agent obtained from *Acholeplasma oculi*. *Yale J. Biol. Med.* **56:**761–763.

72. **Just, W., M. da Silva Cardoso, A. Lorenz, and G. Klotz.** 1989. Release of mycoplasmavirus L1 upon transfection of *Acholeplasma laidlawii* with homologous and heterologous viral DNA. *Arch. Virol.* **107:**1–13.

73. **Just, W., and G. Klotz.** 1990. Terminal redundancy and circular permutation of mycoplasma virus L3 DNA. *J. Gen. Virol.* **71:**2157–2162.

74. **Kuo, T.-T., Y.-S. Chao, Y.-H. Lin, B.-Y. Lin, L.-F. Liu, and T. Y. Feng.** 1987. Integration of the DNA of filamentous bacteriophage Cflt into the chromosomal DNA of its host. *J. Virol.* **61:**60–65.

75. **Kuo, T.-T., Y.-H. Lin, C.-M. Huang, S. F. Chang, H. Dai, and T.-Y. Feng.** 1987. The lysogenic cycle of the filamentous bacteriophage Cflt from *Xanthomonas campestris* pv. *citri*. *Virology* **156:**305–312.

76. **Labedan, B., and E. B. Goldberg.** 1982. DNA transport across bacterial membranes, p. 133–138. *In* A. N. Martonosi (ed.), *Membranes and Transport*, vol. 2. Plenum Press, New York.

77. **Lerner, T. J., and P. Model.** 1981. The "steady state" of coliphage f1: DNA synthesis late in infection. *Virology* **115:**282–294.

78. **Liska, B.** 1972. Isolation of a new Mycoplasmatales virus. *Stud. Biophys.* **34:**151–155.

79. **Liss, A.** 1977. *Acholeplasma laidlawii* infection by group 3 mycoplasmavirus. *Virology* **77:**433–436.

80. **Liss, A.** 1981. Release of a group 1 mycoplasma virus from *Acholeplasma laidlawii* after treatment with mitomycin C. *J. Virol.* **40:**285–288.

81. **Liss, A., and R. M. Cole.** 1981. Spiroplasmavirus group 1: isolation, growth, and properties. *Curr. Microbiol.* **5:**357–362.

82. **Liss, A., and R. M. Cole.** 1982. Spiroplasmal viruses: group 1 characteristics. *Rev. Infect. Dis.* **4:**S115–S119.

83. **Liss, A., K. Hakkarainen, and E. Jansson.** 1985. *Acholeplasma laidlawii* retains sensitivity to exogenous virus while releasing endogenous, mitomycin C induced virus. *Arch. Virol.* **85:**165–170.

84. **Liss, A., and R. A. Heiland.** 1983. Characterization of the enveloped plasmavirus MVL2 after propagation on three *Acholeplasma laidlawii* hosts. *Arch. Virol.* **75:**123–129.

85. **Liss, A., and J. Maniloff.** 1971. Isolation of Mycoplasmatales viruses and characterization of MVL1, MVL52, and MVG51. *Science* **173:**725–727.

86. **Liss, A., and J. Maniloff.** 1973. Infection of *Acholeplasma laidlawii* by MVL51 virus. *Virology* **55:**118–126.

87. **Liss, A., and J. Maniloff.** 1974. Intracellular replication of mycoplasmavirus MVL51. *J. Virol.* **13:**769–774.

88. **Liss, A., and B. E. Ritter.** 1985. *Acholeplasma laidlawii* cells acutely and chronically infected with group 1 acholeplasmavirus. *J. Gen. Microbiol.* **131:**1713–1718.

89. **Lombardi, P. S., and B. C. Cole.** 1978. Induction of a pH-stable interferon in sheep lymphocytes by *Mycoplasmatales* virus MVL2. *Infect. Immun.* **20:**209–214.

90. **Maniloff, J.** 1983. Evolution of wall-less prokaryotes. *Annu. Rev. Microbiol.* **37:**477–499.

91. **Maniloff, J.** 1988. Mycoplasma viruses. *Crit. Rev. Microbiol.* **15:**339–389.

92. **Maniloff, J., S. P. Cadden, and R. M. Putzrath.** 1981. Maturation of an enveloped budding phage: mycoplasmavirus L2, p. 503–513. *In* M. S. DuBow (ed.), *Bacteriophage Assembly.* Alan R. Liss, Inc., New York.

93. **Maniloff, J., and J. Das.** 1975. Replication of mycoplasmaviruses, p. 445–450. *In* M. Goulian, P. Hanawalt, and C. F. Fox (ed.), *DNA Synthesis and Its Regulation.* W. A. Benjamin, Inc., Reading, Mass.

94. **Maniloff, J., J. Das, and J. R. Christensen.** 1977. Viruses of mycoplasmas and spiroplasmas. *Adv. Virus Res.* **21:**343–380.

95. **Maniloff, J., J. Das, and J. A. Nowak.** 1977. Mycoplasmaviruses: virus-cell interactions. *Beltsville Symp. Agric. Res.* **1:**221–231.

96. **Maniloff, J., J. Das, and J. A. Nowak.** 1978. Single-stranded DNA mycoplasmaviruses, p. 177–184. *In* D. T. Denhardt, D. H. Dressler, and D. S. Ray (ed.), *Single-Stranded DNA Phages.* Cold Spring Harbor Laboratory, Cold Spring Harbor, N.Y.

97. **Maniloff, J., K. Haberer, R. N. Gourlay, J. Das, and R. Cole.** 1982. Mycoplasma viruses. *Intervirology* **18:**177–188.

98. **Maniloff, J., G. J. Kampo, C. C. Dascher, and R. L. Sutthent.** 1991. Sequence analysis of mycoplasma virus L2 DNA, abstr. 288. *Abstr. 91st Gen. Meet. Am. Soc. Microbiol.*

99. **Maniloff, J., and A. Liss.** 1973. The molecular biology of mycoplasma viruses. *Ann. N.Y. Acad. Sci.* **225:**149–158.

100. **Maniloff, J., and A. Liss.** 1974. Comparative structure, chemistry and evolution of mycoplasmaviruses, p. 583–604. *In* E. Kurstak and K. Maramorosch (ed.), *Viruses, Evolution and Cancer.* Academic Press, Inc., New York.

101. **Maniloff, J., and H. J. Morowitz.** 1972. Cell biology of the mycoplasmas. *Bacteriol. Rev.* **36:**263–290.

102. **Maniloff, J., and S. K. Poddar.** 1991. Analysis of a mycoplasma DNA replication origin, abstr. M-Pos382. *Abstr. 35th Annu. Meet. Biophys. Soc. Microbiol.*

103. **Maniloff, J., R. L. Sutthent, C. C. Dascher, and G. J. Kampo.** Unpublished data.

104. **Mathews, C. K., and J. R. Allen.** 1983. DNA precursor biosynthesis, p. 59–70. *In* C. K. Mathews, E. M. Kutter, G. Mosig, and P. B. Berget (ed.), *Bacteriophage T4.* American Society for Microbiology, Washington, D.C.

105. **McCammon, S., and R. E. Davis.** 1987. Transfection of *Spiroplasma citri* with DNA of a new rod-shaped spiroplasmavirus, p. 458–464. *In* E. L. Civerolo, A. Collmer, R. E. Davis, and A. G. Gillaspie (ed.), *Plant Pathogenic Bacteria.* Martinus Nijhoff Publishers, Boston.

106. **McCorquodale, D. J.** 1975. The T-odd bacteriophages. *Crit. Rev. Microbiol.* **4:**101–159.

107. **McElhaney, R. N.** 1989. The influence of membrane lipid composition and physical properties of membrane structure and function in *Acholeplasma laidlawii. Crit. Rev. Microbiol.* **17:**1–32.

108. **Merril, C. R., T. B. Friedman, A. F. M. Attallah, M. R. Geier, K. Krell, and R. Yarkin.** 1972. Isolation of bacteriophages from commercial sera. *In Vitro* **8:**91–93.

109. **Model, P., and M. Russel.** 1988. Filamentous bacteriophage, p. 375–456. *In* R. Calendar (ed.), *The Bacteriophages,* vol. 2. Plenum Press, New York.

110. **Nowak, J. A., J. Das, and J. Maniloff.** 1976. Characterization of an *Acholeplasma laidlawii* variant with a REP⁻ phenotype. *J. Bacteriol.* **127:**832–836.

111. **Nowak, J. A., and J. Maniloff.** 1979. Physical characterization of the superhelical DNA genome of an enveloped mycoplasmavirus. *J. Virol.* **29:**374–380.

112. **Nowak, J. A., J. Maniloff, and J. Das.** 1978. Electron microscopy of single-stranded mycoplasmavirus DNA. *FEMS Microbiol. Lett.* **4:**59–61.

113. **Nystrom, S., K.-E. Johansson, and .Å Wieslander.** 1986. Selective acylation of membrane proteins in *Acholeplasma laidlawii. Eur. J. Biochem.* **156:**85–94.

114. **Ogawa, H. I., and M. Nakamura.** 1985. Characterization of a mycoplasma virus (MV-01) derived from and infecting *Acholeplasma oculi. J. Gen. Microbiol.* **131:**3117–3126.

115. **Oishi, K.** 1971. Spirochaete-mediated abnormal sex-ratio (SR) condition in *Drosophila:* a second virus associated with spirochaetes and its use in the study of the SR condition. *Genet. Res.* (Cambridge) **18:**45–56.

116. **Oishi, K., and D. F. Poulson.** 1970. A virus associated with SR-spirochetes of *Drosophila nebulosa. Proc. Natl. Acad. Sci. USA* **67:**1565–1572.

117. **Phillpotts, R. J., K. K. T. Patel, and D. G. ff. Edward.** 1977. Heterogeneity among strains of Mycoplasmatales virus-laidlawii-2. *J. Gen. Virol.* **36:**211–215.

118. **Poddar, S. K., S. P. Cadden, J. Das, and J. Maniloff.** 1985. Heterogeneous progeny viruses are produced by a budding enveloped phage. *Intervirology* **23:**208–221.

119. **Poddar, S. K., and J. Maniloff.** 1984. Measurement of DNA superhelix density by dye titration-slab gel electrophoresis. *Electrophoresis* **5:**172–173.

120. **Poddar, S. K., and J. Maniloff.** 1984. Effect of novobiocin on mycoplasma virus L2 replication. *J. Virol.* **49:**283–286.

121. **Poddar, S. K., and J. Maniloff.** 1986. Chromosome analysis by two-dimensional fingerprinting. *Gene* **49:**93–102.

122. **Poddar, S. K., and J. Maniloff.** 1987. Mapping mycoplasma virus DNA replication origins and termini. *J. Virol.* **61:**1909–1912.

123. **Putzrath, R. M., S. P. Cadden, and J. Maniloff.** 1980. Effect of cell membrane composition on the growth and composition of a nonlytic enveloped mycoplasmavirus. *Virology* **106:**162–167.

124. **Putzrath, R. M., and J. Maniloff.** 1977. Growth of an enveloped mycoplasmavirus and establishment of a carrier state. *J. Virol.* **22:**308–314.

125. **Putzrath, R. M., and J. Maniloff.** 1978. Properties of a persistent viral infection: possible lysogeny by an enveloped nonlytic mycoplasmavirus. *J. Virol.* **28:**254–261.

126. **Rasched, I., and E. Oberer.** 1986. Ff coliphages: structural and functional relationships. *Microbiol. Rev.* **50:**401–427.

127. **Renaudin, J., P. Aullo, J. C. Vignault, and J. M. Bové.** 1990. Complete nucleotide sequence of the genome of *Spiroplasma citri* virus SpV1-R8A2 B. *Nucleic Acids Res.* **18:**1293.

128. **Renaudin, J., M. C. Pascarel, and J. M. Bové.** 1987. Spiroplasma virus 4: nucleotide sequence of the viral DNA, regulatory signals, and proposed genome organization. *J. Bacteriol.* **169:**4950–4961.

129. **Renaudin, J., M. C. Pascarel, M. Garnier, P. Carle-Junca, and J. M. Bové.** 1984. SpV4, a new spiroplasma virus with circular, single-stranded DNA. *Ann. Virol.* **135E:**343–361.

130. **Roger, A.** 1983. Instabilité de la liaison hôte-virus lors de l'infection d'*Acholeplasma laidlawii* par un mycoplasmavirus du groupe L1 de Gourlay. *Zentralbl. Bakteriol. Parasitenkd. Infektionskr. Hyg. Abt. 1 Orig. Reihe A* **254:**139–145.

131. **Rottem, S., and N. Greenberg.** 1982. Molecular organization and selective solubilization of lipids and proteins in the envelope of mycoplasmal virus L2. *Rev. Infect. Dis.* **4:**S99–S104.

132. **Rottem, S., and N. Greenberg.** 1983. Binding of MVL-2 virus to *A. laidlawii* cells. *Yale J. Biol. Med.* **56:**765–769.

133. **Sharp, P. M.** 1986. Molecular evolution of bacteriophages: evidence of selection against the recognition sites of host restriction enzymes. *Mol. Biol. Evol.* **3:**75–83.

134. **Sladek, T. L., and J. Maniloff.** 1985. Transfection of REP⁻ mycoplasmas with viral single-stranded DNA. *J. Virol.* **53:**25–31.

135. **Sladek, T. L., J. A. Nowak, and J. Maniloff.** 1986. Mycoplasma restriction: identification of a new type of restriction specificity for DNA containing 5-methylcytosine. *J. Bacteriol.* **165:**219–225.

136. **Smith, P. F.** 1977. Homogeneity of lipopolysaccharides from *Acholeplasma*. *J. Bacteriol.* **130:**393–398.

137. **Stamburski, C., J. Renaudin, and J. M. Bové.** 1990. Characterization of a promoter and a transcription terminator of *Spiroplasma melliferum* virus SpV4. *J. Bacteriol.* **172:**5586–5592.

138. **Steinick, L. E., and A. Christiansson.** 1986. Adsorption of mycoplasmavirus MV-L2 to *Acholeplasma laidlawii:* effects of changes in the acyl-chain composition of membrane lipids. *J. Virol.* **60:**525–530.

139. **Steinick, L. E., and .Å Wieslander.** 1984. Effects of acyl chain composition on production of mycoplasmavirus MV-L2 by *Acholeplasma laidlawii*. *Isr. J. Med. Sci.* **20:**788–792.

140. **Steinick, L. E., .Å Wieslander, K.-E. Johansson, and A. Liss.** 1980. Membrane composition and virus susceptibility of *Acholeplasma laidlawii*. *J. Bacteriol.* **143:**1200–1207.

141. **Sutthent, R. L., and J. Maniloff.** Unpublished data.

142. **Townsend, R.** 1983. Viruses of *Spiroplasma citri* and their possible effects on pathogenicity. *Yale J. Biol. Med.* **56:**771–776.

143. **Tryon, V. V., and J. D. Pollack.** 1985. Distinctions in *Mollicutes* purine metabolism: pyrophosphate-dependent nucleoside kinase and dependence on guanylate salvage. *Int. J. Syst. Bacteriol.* **35:**497–501.

144. **Wieslander, .Å, L. Rilfors, and G. Lindblom.** 1986. Metabolic changes of membrane lipid composition in *Acholeplasma laidlawii* by hydrocarbons, alcohols, and detergents: arguments for effects on lipid packing. *Biochemistry* **25:**7511–7517.

145. **Williams, M. V., and J. D. Pollack.** 1985. Pyrimidine deoxyribonucleotide metabolism in *Acholeplasma laidlawii* B-PG9. *J. Bacteriol.* **161:**1029–1033.

146. **Williamson, D. L., K. Oishi, and D. F. Poulson.** 1977. Viruses of *Drosophila* sex-ratio spiroplasma, p. 465–472. *In* K. Maramorosch (ed.), *The Atlas of Insect and Plant Viruses*. Academic Press, Inc., New York.

147. **Woese, C. R.** 1987. Bacterial evolution. *Microbiol. Rev.* **51:**221–271.

II. MOLECULAR ARCHITECTURE

4. Cell Structural and Functional Elements

JOHNNY L. CARSON, PING-CHUAN HU, and ALBERT M. COLLIER

Nature abounds with little round things.

Lewis Thomas

INTRODUCTION

Mycoplasmas are derived from morphologically, biochemically, and genetically more complex eubacterial forms. It is hypothesized that cell wall genes were lost during evolution, with a reduction in genome size to that of present-day mycoplasmas. All of the mycoplasmas apparently arose by degenerative evolution in the *Bacillus-Lactobacillus-Streptococcus* subgroup of gram-positive sporeforming eubacteria (43).

The order *Mycoplasmatales* further differentiates the members of the class into three representative families, each of which exhibits distinctive structural or biochemical attributes. Although they differ in genome size, the *Mycoplasmataceae* and *Spiroplasmataceae* both require sterol supplementation for growth (15, 18, 58, 67). The helical organization of the cell body and rotational or undulating motility are further distinguishing features of the spiroplasmas (11, 16). Members of the third family, *Acholeplasmataceae*, do not require exogenous sterol for growth and possess a genome size similar to that of the *Spiroplasmataceae*. This chapter will outline the approaches that have been used to study the morphology of mycoplasmas and place these observations in the context of functional and biochemical characteristics of these organisms.

LIGHT MICROSCOPIC STUDIES OF MYCOPLASMAS

The small size of mycoplasmas and the limits of resolution of the light microscope pose problems for light microscopic studies of these organisms. Further, since mycoplasmas lack a cell wall, they are uniformly gram negative. The size of most mycoplasmas lies at the threshold of resolution for light microscopy. Bright-field optics can resolve approximately 0.2 μm, and phase and dark-field optics can resolve approximately 0.1 μm. Thus, the applications of immunofluorescence, dark-field, and phase-contrast optics have provided useful perspectives on cell morphology, motility, and cell division at the light microscopic level. In general, light microscopic examination of mycoplasmas reveals organisms approximately 0.3 μm in diameter and up to 98 μm in length (5–7). The shape of mycoplasmas is often pleomorphic, although coccoidal, diploform, and filamentous patterns have been documented (5–7). Light microscopy of these species also has shown that cell division may occur by binary fission, fragmentation of filaments, and budding. Some mycoplasmas exhibit characteristic shapes visible by light microscopy. Among these are the spiroplasmas, which appear as spiral filaments under dark-field optics. Additionally, several pathogenic mycoplasmas, i.e., *Mycoplasma pneumoniae*, *M. gallisepticum*, *M. pulmonis*, and *M. genitalium*, exhibit a filamentous or flask-shaped polarity of the cell body when viewed by light microscopy. This polarity appears to be involved in mediating the ability of these organisms to undergo a gliding motility (7, 8).

GENERAL ULTRASTRUCTURAL FEATURES OF MYCOPLASMAS

Except for a few notable specializations, ultrathin sections of mycoplasmas viewed by electron micros-

Johnny L. Carson • Department of Pediatrics, Department of Cell Biology and Anatomy, and Center for Environmental Medicine and Lung Biology, University of North Carolina School of Medicine, Chapel Hill, North Carolina 27599. Ping-Chuan Hu • Department of Pediatrics, Department of Microbiology and Immunology, and Center for Environmental Medicine and Lung Biology, University of North Carolina School of Medicine, Chapel Hill, North Carolina 27599. Albert M. Collier • Department of Pediatrics, Center for Environmental Medicine and Lung Biology, and Frank Porter Graham Child Development Center, University of North Carolina School of Medicine, Chapel Hill, North Carolina 27599.

copy are generally unrevealing (Fig. 1). However, cytochemical studies (46, 70) using indium trichloride as a specific cytochemical stain for nucleic acids found cytoplasmic staining of nuclear and ribosomal elements in *M. gallisepticum* and *M. pneumoniae* but no staining of the bleb or terminal organelle of these organisms. The trilaminar membrane delimiting the cell body is typical in its organization and dimensions (17) and can be visualized easily by electron microscopy. Reaction with ruthenium red, which stains specifically for mucopolysaccharides, also has revealed the presence of an extracellular fibrillar matrix in *M. pneumoniae* (70) (Fig. 2). Similar extracellular staining of mucopolysaccharide substances also has been documented in *M. meleagridis* (25), *M. dispar* (28), and other bovine mycoplasmas (4) as well as in *Ureaplasma urealyticum* (56).

Freeze-fracture preparations of *M. pneumoniae* and *M. gallisepticum* reveal a particle-studded PF face containing particle-free zones and EF faces containing few particles (Fig. 3). Other freeze-fracture studies by Wall et al. (66) have imaged the core of the terminal organelle of *M. pneumoniae;* however, the relationship between this structure and the particle-free areas of the membrane is not well characterized.

The cytoplasm of mycoplasmas appears granular, with ribosomes and nuclear material. In *M. gallisepticum*, the ribosomes may be tightly packed into helical configurations (46). Although the cytoplasm of most mycoplasmas is nondescript, that of three *Acholeplasma* species exhibits a distinct spiral protein of molecular weight 100,000 (36). This protein is not found in other mycoplasma species and does not appear to be actinlike.

Several mycoplasmas which are pathogenic for humans, birds, and fish exhibit a flasklike or bullet-shaped polarity (37) (Fig. 4); these include *M. pneumoniae*, *M. pulmonis*, *M. genitalium*, *M. gallisepticum*, *M. mobile*, *M. alvi*, and *M. sualvi*. Cytoskeletal elements with chemical properties of actin have been identified in these species, and all exhibit the ability to attach to glass and demonstrate a gliding motility, although these characteristics are attenuated in *M. alvi* and *M. sualvi*. Despite their morphological, adherent, and kinetic similarities, G + C ratios as well as serological differences suggest that except for *M. pneumoniae* and *M. genitalium*, most of the flask-shaped mycoplasmas are not closely related (32, 34, 42).

UNIQUE ULTRASTRUCTURAL FEATURES OF THE *MYCOPLASMATALES*

Attachment Organelles

Several human, avian, and animal mycoplasmal pathogens possess unique ultrastructural features which constitute considerable specializations for procaryotes. As noted previously, *M. pneumoniae*, *M. genitalium*, *M. pulmonis*, and *M. gallisepticum* have a characteristic cell shape and polarity. Except in *M. pulmonis*, cell polarity is governed by the presence of well-organized terminal organelles or blebs. Because the mycoplasmas in which these structures appear are both motile and capable of attachment to substrates, it has been theorized that such structures govern motility or host-pathogen interaction and ultimately pathogenicity.

In *M. pneumoniae*, the terminal organelle appears in

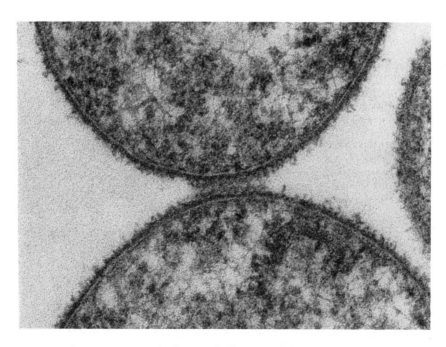

Figure 1. Transmission electron micrograph of two *A. laidlawii* cells illustrating the unit membrane and absence of a cell wall, one of the characteristic identifying features of the *Mycoplasmatales*. Note also the amorphous nature of the cytoplasm containing ribosomes and some fibrous components. Magnification, × 172,200.

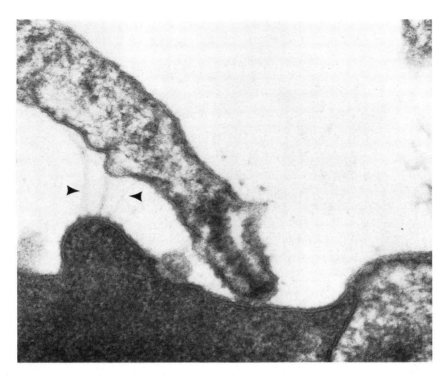

Figure 2. *M. pneumoniae* attached to host epithelial cell by the specialized terminal organelle and fibrillar elements (arrows). Magnification, ×132,200.

ultrathin sections as an electron-dense core surrounded by an electron-lucent zone (12) (Fig. 5a). Cytochemical studies (70) have shown that the terminal organelle, including the central filament and the terminal "button," stains intensely with ethanolic phosphotungstic acid (Fig. 4a). The organisms are able to orient and attach to host cells at this site. Studies by Hu et al. (29, 30) have characterized a protein, identified as P1, that is localized in the tip region and mediates this attachment. It was found that mild protease

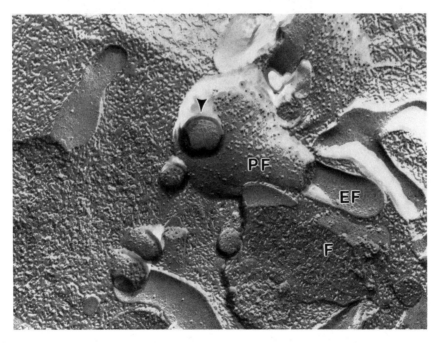

Figure 3. Freeze-fracture preparation of *M. pneumoniae* illustrating PF and EF faces. Note the particle-free bleb (arrow) and the greater abundance of particles on the PF face than on the EF face. Magnification, ×76,200.

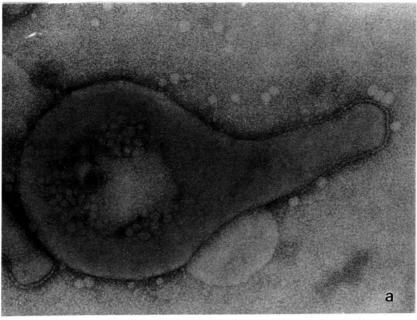

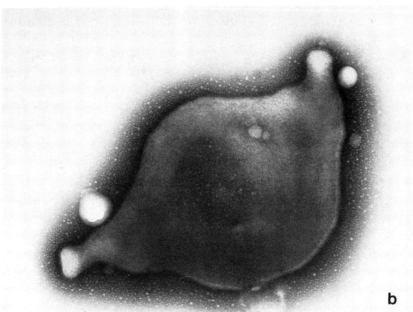

Figure 4. (a) Negative staining of *M. pneumoniae* illustrating flask-shaped morphology. Similar preparations also may reveal a more filamentous appearance. Note the "nap" of particulate material visible around the extended tip structure. Magnification, ×130,000. (b) Negative staining of *M. gallisepticum* illustrating dual terminal structures with nape of particulate material. Magnification, ×74,300.

Figure 5. Patterns of host-pathogen interaction among pathogenic mycoplasmas. Note the similarity of ultrastructure and attachment pattern among the three different species. (a) Transmission electron micrograph of *M. pneumoniae* attached by specialized terminal organelle to host mammalian ciliated epithelium. Compare the filamentous appearance of these cells with the flasklike appearance of the organism in Fig. 4a. Note that the cytoplasm of the mycoplasma cell body is unremarkable except for the area comprising the specialized terminal organelle. Magnification, ×52,100. (b) Transmission electron micrograph of *M. genitalium* attached to human fallopian tube epithelium. Magnification, ×57,000. (c) Transmission electron micrograph of *M. gallisepticum*, a pathogen of poultry, attached to chicken tracheal epithelium. Magnification, ×61,000.

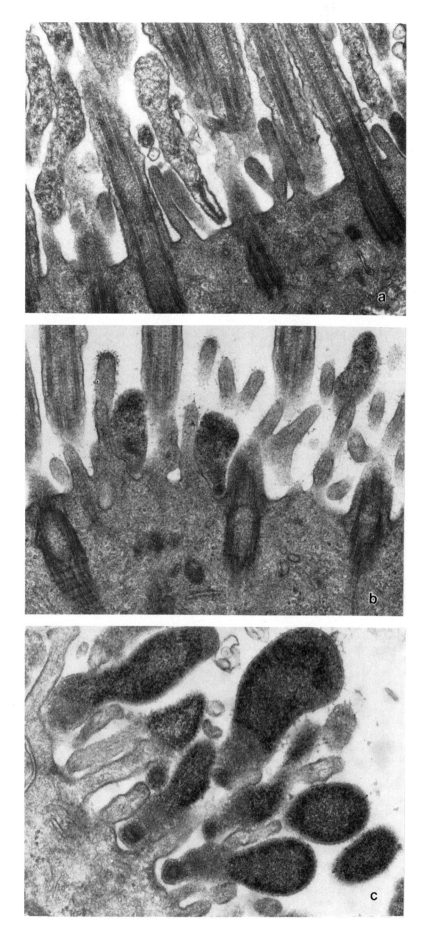

treatment of *M. pneumoniae* cells nullified their ability to attach to respiratory epithelium (29, 30). The attachment ability could be restored by incubating the treated organisms in fresh growth medium. Because the disappearance of P1 protein and its regeneration on sodium dodecyl sulfate (SDS)-gels were directly associated with the loss and restoration of attachment capability, respectively, Hu et al. (30) proposed that P1 is required for the attachment process. It has been confirmed that a monoclonal antibody specific to P1 inhibits the attachment of *M. pneumoniae* to respiratory epithelium (3, 29).

While P1 protein is probably the major component responsible for *M. pneumoniae* attachment, evidence exists that additional proteins also may be involved in this process. Characterization of *M. pneumoniae* hemadsorption-negative mutants revealed that as many as seven proteins were missing on one- or two-dimensional SDS-gels (26, 27, 39). Hemadsorption-positive revertants isolated from spontaneous hemadsorption-negative mutants simultaneously reacquired specific proteins missing in their homologous mutants and restoration of attachment ability and virulence in experimental animals (38). In addition, comparison of protein profiles of the virulent *M. pneumoniae* M129-B7 and its avirulent derivative M129-B169 revealed that a 45-kDa protein is missing in the isogenic avirulent strain and that two protein bands are nonreactive with monoclonal antibodies against corresponding protein bands of the parent virulent strain (31). These findings suggest that the attachment of *M. pneumoniae* is a complex process, although the other proteins are less well characterized.

A similar pattern of attachment has been identified in human fallopian tube organ cultures experimentally infected with *M. genitalium* (13) (Fig. 5b). Ultrastructural studies indicated that *M. genitalium* also possesses a differentiated terminal bleb structure similar to that of *M. pneumoniae* (65). This observation suggested that *M. genitalium* may possess an attachment mechanism similar to that of *M. pneumoniae*. Extensive serological cross-reactivity has been demonstrated between *M. pneumoniae* and *M. genitalium* (31, 42). Using a monoclonal antibody specific to the P1 protein of *M. pneumoniae*, Clyde and Hu (10) identified a surface protein of *M. genitalium* which appears to be a counterpart of the P1 protein of *M. pneumoniae*. This 140-kDa protein, named MgPa, is trypsin sensitive and is clustered over the surface of the terminal structure of *M. genitalium* (32). In a recent study, Collier et al. (13) demonstrated that attachment of *M. genitalium* to the ciliated epithelium of human fallopian tube in organ culture is mediated via the terminal structure. The attachment of *M. genitalium* to the human oviductal epithelium could be inhibited by either treatment of the organisms with trypsin or preincubation of the organisms with monoclonal antibodies specific to MgPa protein. These data suggested that the MgPa protein of *M. genitalium* plays a role in attachment similar to that of the P1 protein of *M. pneumoniae*.

Genes encoding both the P1 protein of *M. pneumoniae* and the MgPa protein of *M. genitalium* have recently been cloned and sequenced (14, 20, 34, 35). Further studies from our laboratory showed that both the P1 gene of *M. pneumoniae* and the MgPa gene of *M. genitalium* are part of an operon. The organizations of

the P1 operon and the MgPa operon are very similar inasmuch as each is composed of three genes, with the P1 gene and the MgPa gene in the middle (33, 35). The deduced amino acid sequences of the 29-kDa, MgPa (160-kDa), and 114-kDa proteins encoded by the MgPa operon (33) show extensive homologies with those of the 28-kDa, P1 (170-kDa), and 130-kDa proteins, respectively, encoded by the P1 operon (34, 35). The common features and homology of these two operons are consistent with earlier observations that the MgPa and P1 proteins share cross-reactive epitopes as well as having similar functions.

In *M. gallisepticum*, polar bleb structures appear prior to division (49). Isolation of the blebs showed that they contain sites of DNA replication and that the chromosome origin remains attached to the bleb throughout the cell cycle (45). On the basis of these observations, it was hypothesized that *M. gallisepticum* blebs might function as a primitive mitotic structure-like apparatus for chromosome organization and segregation. Other studies of chicken tracheal organ cultures infected with *M. gallisepticum* have suggested that the bleb also may serve a role in the attachment of the organism to the target host tissue (40) (Fig. 5c). Further, Clyde and Hu (10) demonstrated that rabbit antiserum raised against the P1 protein of *M. pneumoniae* reacted with a similar-size protein of *M. gallisepticum*, suggesting that this protein may have a function similar to that of P1. Further studies will be necessary to prove whether this protein has a role in the attachment of *M. gallisepticum* to host tissues.

Although *M. pulmonis* is motile (52), the bleb structure lacks the ultrastructural specialization of other mycoplasmas with attachment organelles (9), and it is serologically very different from *M. pneumoniae* and *M. genitalium*. The lack of significant serological cross-reactivity between *M. pulmonis* and other flask-shaped mycoplasmas, including *M. pneumoniae*, *M. genitalium*, and *M. gallisepticum*, also appears to disprove the possibility that *M. pulmonis* adheres to the lung tissue by a mechanism similar to the attachment mechanism of the other three species. Previous studies have shown that other mycoplasmas exhibiting cellular polarity and terminal organelles exhibit trypsin-sensitive attachment (30). Additionally, this group of mycoplasmas presumably attach to sialoglycoproteins on the host cell surface, since treatment of the host tissue with neuraminidase can block attachment to host cells (54). In contrast, treatment of *M. pulmonis* with trypsin or sialic acid, or of the target tissue with neuraminidase, appears not to affect attachment (1). Studies by Minion et al. (48) suggest a multiphasic pattern of *M. pulmonis*-host cell interaction in which the initial recognition phase is nonspecific, but followed by surface molecule reorganization to uncover binding sites which are recognized by the mycoplasma hemagglutinin.

Rodwell et al. (57) identified a specialized structure called the rho form in caprine and bovine mycoplasmas. Mycoplasmal rho forms possess an intracytoplasmic striated fiber that extends axially throughout the cell, terminating at one or both ends in a knoblike structure. Rho forms are seen only under conditions of high medium tonicity and nonlimiting energy source (53). The significance and function of the rho structure are not known.

Spiroplasmas have no flagella or axial filaments such as those found in spirochetes (11) (Fig. 6). However, they possess fibrils composed of a protein of molecular weight 55,000 specific to this family and highly conserved. It is not actinlike and is unrelated to eucaryotic cytoskeletal components. There is a consistent association of the fibrils with DNA filaments (61). Large numbers of fibrils can be obtained from the honeybee spiroplasma BC-3 by treatment of the organism with Triton X-100. The fibrils are associated with two proteins of molecular weights 39,000 and 59,000 and another of 26,000 antigenically related to spiralin, the major membrane protein of *S. citri* (2). Townsend et al. (63) have reported a nonhelical mutant of *S. citri* in which the 39-kDa protein is absent. The fibrils are 3.5 nm in diameter, are flexuous and of indeterminate length, and have an axial repeat of 8.5 nm. They make up approximately 1% of total cell protein and are de-

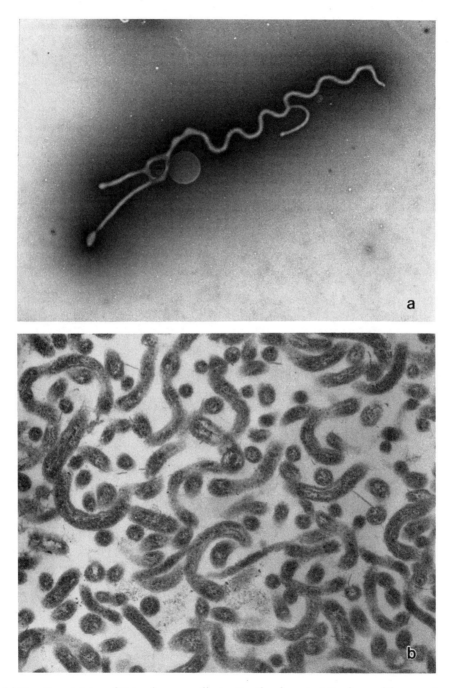

Figure 6. (a) Negative staining of *Spiroplasma* sp. illustrating the characteristic shape of the organism. Magnification, ×20,000. (b) Transmission electron micrograph of ultrathin section of *Spiroplasma* sp. Although less obvious, the spiral form remains evident. The micrograph also suggests fibrillar elements within the cell body. Magnification, ×42,700.

graded by pronase but not trypsin (62). The gene encoding the 55-kDa spiroplasma fibrillar protein has recently been cloned and sequenced (69). Although the fibril monomer molecular weight is similar to that of tubulin subunits present in eucaryotic cells (19), spiroplasma fibrils do not dissociate when cooled to 0°C in the presence of colchicine, conditions which would cause dissociation of microtubules and prevent their reassembly. Helicity and motility are related in the spiroplasmas, but the molecular basis of this relationship is not known (64). From these observations, it has been hypothesized that the fibrils of spiroplasmas may function in the maintenance of cell shape, in the segregation of chromosomes during cell division, and/or in cellular motility, although no shortening or extension of the fibrils has been identified.

Contractile Proteins

The identification and characterization of contractile proteins among the *Mycoplasmatales* has been confounding. Studies undertaken by several groups have isolated actinlike proteins from several mycoplasmas. Göbel et al. (22, 24), Neimark (51), and Meng and Pfister (47) reported the presence of such proteins and a highly organized cytoskeleton in *M. pneumoniae*. The microfilaments were reported to be detergent resistant and similar in structure to eucaryotic actin. The fibers polymerized in buffers containing $MgCl_2$ and/or KCl, were relatively trypsin resistant, were destroyed by KI, cross-reacted with antiactin, and specifically reacted with phalloidin, although they did not react with myosin subfragment 1. Similar findings have been reported for *M. gallisepticum* (21, 44) and for *S. citri*: antisera against denatured invertebrate actin coupled to horseradish peroxidase elicited staining (68). Although mycoplasmas contain filaments with structural and chemical similarities to actin (50) in addition to immunocytochemical cross-reactivity (59), no protein sharing homology with muscle actin has been identified. Additionally, DNA hybridization studies in *M. genitalium* using actin-specific probes indicated hybridization (23), although sequencing of hybridizing fragments did not reveal an open reading frame.

The studies of Ghosh et al. (21) and Maniloff and Chadhuri (44) applied the use of cytochalasins to study mycoplasmas. Cytochalasins are fungal metabolites that interfere with the uptake of small metabolites and cellular processes that involve actin (41, 55, 60). Cytochalasin B was found to inhibit cell division in *M. gallisepticum* but not to inhibit glucose or macromolecule precursor uptake. Additionally, it stops cellular DNA synthesis, although RNA and protein synthesis continue at a reduced level. The studies of Ghosh et al. (21) suggested that the ability of cytochalasin B to inhibit cell division may derive from the disruption of actinlike protein structures required at the time mitotic structures are formed and at the point of actual cell division. Several attempts have been made to demonstrate the existence of contractile proteins in the mycoplasmas. However, discrepancies in analysis of biochemical properties are evident by the lack of homology to other proven contractile proteins.

Taken individually, none of these approaches has been wholly satisfactory in proving the presence of actin in the mycoplasmas. However, they do point to the presence of contractile actinlike proteins which may share a common epitope due to a common evolutionary constraint. Thus, given these similarities as well as the noteworthy differences, future studies of contractile proteins in the *Mycoplasmatales* must be interpreted with caution.

SUMMARY

To those unfamiliar with them, the mycoplasmas may appear overtly dull and uninteresting from a structural point of view. However, discoveries and investigations by many investigators have demonstrated that a number of these microorganisms possess a remarkable degree of structural specialization. The rapid development of molecular biology techniques and their application by mycoplasmologists already have contributed much to our knowledge of the structure of this group. There can be little doubt that future investigations applying imaging techniques and biotechnology to the study of mycoplasmas will further confirm the biological significance of form as it relates to function.

Acknowledgments. We thank Wallace A. Clyde, Jr., for review and helpful comments in the preparation of this chapter. We also acknowledge the excellent technical assistance of Nancy Hu and Todd Gambling. This work was supported by grant HL-19171 from the National Institutes of Health and by cooperative agreement CR812738 from the U.S. Environmental Protection Agency.

REFERENCES

1. **Araake, M., M. Yayoshi, and M. Yoshioka.** 1985. Attachment of *Mycoplasma pulmonis* to rat and mouse synovial cells cultured *in vitro*. *Microbiol. Immunol.* **29**:601–607.
2. **Archer, D. B., and R. Townsend.** 1981. Immunoelectrophoretic separation of spiroplasma antigens. *J. Gen. Microbiol.* **123**:61–68.
3. **Baseman, J. B., M. Banai, and I. Kahane.** 1982. Sialic acid residues mediate *Mycoplasma pneumoniae* attachment to human and sheep erythrocytes. *Infect. Immun.* **38**:389–391.
4. **Boatman, E. S.** 1979. Morphology and ultrastructure of the Mycoplasmatales, p. 63–102. *In* M. F. Barile and S. Razin (ed.), *The Mycoplasmas*, vol. 1. Academic Press, New York.
5. **Bredt, W.** 1969. Filamentous growth of some mycoplasma species of man. *Experientia* **25**:1118–1119.
6. **Bredt, W.** 1970. Experimental studies on the morphology and multiplication of human mycoplasma with special reference to *Mycoplasma homonis*. *Z. Med. Mikrobiol. Immunol.* **155**:248–274.
7. **Bredt, W.** 1973. Motility of mycoplasmas. *Ann. N.Y. Acad. Sci.* **225**:246–250.
8. **Bredt, W., and U. Radestock.** 1977. Gliding motility of *Mycoplasma pulmonis*. *J. Bacteriol.* **130**:937–938.
9. **Cassell, G. H., W. H. Wilborn, S. H. Silvers, and F. C. Minion.** 1981. Adherence and colonization of *Mycoplasma pulmonis* to genital epithelium and spermatozoa. *Isr. J. Med. Sci.* **17**:593–598.
10. **Clyde, W. A., Jr., and P. C. Hu.** 1986. Antigenic determinants of the attachment protein of *Mycoplasma pneumon-*

iae shared by other pathogenic *Mycoplasma* species. *Infect. Immun.* **50**:690–692.

11. **Cole, R. M., J. G. Tully, T. J. Popkin, and J. M. Bové.** 1973. Morphology, ultrastructure, and bacteriophage infection of the helical mycoplasma-like organisms (*Spiroplasma citri* gen. nov., sp. nov.) cultured from "stubborn" disease of citrus. *J. Bacteriol.* **115**:367–386.

12. **Collier, A. M.** 1972. Pathogenesis of *Mycoplasma pneumoniae* infection as studied in the human foetal trachea in organ culture, p. 307–327. *In Pathogenic Mycoplasmas: CIBA Foundation Symposium.* Elsevier, New York.

13. **Collier, A. M., J. L. Carson, P. C. Hu, S. S. Hu, C. H. Huang, and M. F. Barile.** 1990. Attachment of *Mycoplasma genitalium* to the ciliated epithelium of human fallopian tubes. *Zentralbl. Bakteriol. Suppl.* **20**:730–732.

14. **Dallo, S. F., A. Chavoya, C.-J. Su, and J. B. Baseman.** 1989. DNA and protein sequence homologies between the adhesins of *Mycoplasma genitalium* and *Mycoplasma pneumoniae. Infect. Immun.* **57**:1059–1065.

15. **Daniels, M. J.** 1983. Mechanisms of spiroplasma pathogenicity. *Annu. Rev. Phytopathol.* **21**:29–43.

16. **Davis, R. E., and J. F. Worley.** 1973. Spiroplasma: motile, helical microorganism associated with corn stunt disease. *Phytopathology* **63**:403–408.

17. **Domermuth, C. H., M. H. Nielsen, E. A. Freundt, and A. Birch-Andersen.** 1964. Ultrastructure of mycoplasma species. *J. Bacteriol.* **88**:727–744.

18. **Edward, D. G. ff., and E. A. Freundt.** 1970. Amended nomenclature for strains related to *Mycoplasma laidlawii. J. Gen. Microbiol.* **62**:1–2.

19. **Erickson, H. P.** 1975. The structure and assembly of microtubules. *Ann. N.Y. Acad. Sci.* **253**:60–77.

20. **Frydenberg, J., K. Lind, and P. C. Hu.** 1987. Cloning of *Mycoplasma pneumoniae* DNA and expression of P1-epitopes in *Escherichia coli. Isr. J. Med. Sci.* **23**:759–762.

21. **Ghosh, A., J. Maniloff, and D. A. Gerling.** 1978. Inhibition of mycoplasma cell division by cytochalasin B. *Cell* **13**:57–64.

22. **Göbel, U.** 1983. Supramolecular structures in mycoplasmas. *Yale J. Biol. Med.* **56**:695–700.

23. **Göbel, U. B., M. M. Müller, and R. Maas.** 1990. Actin-related DNA sequences and proteins from motile mycoplasmas: a molecular puzzle. *Zentralbl. Bakteriol. Suppl.* **20**:337–344.

24. **Göbel, U., V. Speth, and W. Bredt.** 1981. Filamentous structures in adherent *Mycoplasma pneumoniae* cells treated with non-ionic detergents. *J. Cell Biol.* **91**:537–543.

25. **Green, F., and R. P. Hanson.** 1973. Ultrastructure and capsule of *Mycoplasma meleagridis. J. Bacteriol.* **116**:1011–1018.

26. **Hansen, E. J., R. M. Wilson, and J. B. Baseman.** 1979. Two-dimensional gel electrophoretic comparison of proteins from virulent and avirulent strains of *Mycoplasma pneumoniae. Infect. Immun.* **24**:468–475.

27. **Hansen, E. J., R. M. Wilson, W. A. Clyde, Jr., and J. B. Baseman.** 1980. Characterization of hemadsorption-negative mutants of *Mycoplasma pneumoniae. Infect. Immun.* **32**:127–136.

28. **Howard, C. J., and R. N. Gourlay.** 1974. An electron-microscopic examination of certain bovine mycoplasma stained with ruthenium red and the demonstration of a capsule on *Mycoplasma dispar. J. Gen. Microbiol.* **83**:393–398.

29. **Hu, P. C., R. M. Cole, Y. S. Huang, J. A. Graham, D. E. Gardner, A. M. Collier, and W. A. Clyde, Jr.** 1982. *Mycoplasma pneumoniae* infection: role of a surface protein in the attachment organelle. *Science* **216**:313–315.

30. **Hu, P. C., A. M. Collier, and J. B. Baseman.** 1977. Surface parasitism by *Mycoplasma pneumoniae* of respiratory epithelium. *J. Exp. Med.* **145**:1328–1343.

31. **Hu, P. C., A. M. Collier, and W. A. Clyde, Jr.** 1984. Serological comparison of virulent and avirulent *Mycoplasma*

pneumoniae by monoclonal antibodies. *Isr. J. Med. Sci.* **20**:870–873.

32. **Hu, P. C., U. Schaper, A. M. Collier, W. A. Clyde, Jr., and M. Horikawa.** 1987. A *Mycoplasma genitalium* protein resembling the *Mycoplasma pneumoniae* attachment protein. *Infect. Immun.* **55**:1126–1131.

33. **Inamine, J. M., K. C. Ho, S. Loechel, and P. C. Hu.** 1990. Evidence that UGA is read as a tryptophan codon rather than a stop codon by *Mycoplasma pneumoniae, Mycoplasma genitalium,* and *Mycoplasma gallisepticum. J. Bacteriol.* **172**:504–506.

34. **Inamine, J. M., S. Loechel, A. M. Collier, M. F. Barile, and P. C. Hu.** 1989. Nucleotide sequence of the MgPa (*mgp*) operon of *Mycoplasma genitalium* and comparison to the P1 (*mpp*) operon of *Mycoplasma pneumoniae. Gene* **82**:259–267.

35. **Inamine, J. M., S. Loechel, and P. C. Hu.** 1988. Analysis of the nucleotide sequence of the P1 operon of *Mycoplasma pneumoniae. Gene* **73**:175–183.

36. **Kessel, M., I. Peleg, A. Muhlrad, and I. Kahane.** 1981. Cytoplasmic helical structure associated with *Acholeplasma laidlawii. J. Bacteriol.* **147**:653–659.

37. **Kirchhoff, H., R. Rosengarten, W. Lotz, M. Fischer, and D. Lopatta.** 1984. Flask-shaped mycoplasmas: properties and pathogenicity for man and animals. *Isr. J. Med. Sci.* **20**:848–853.

38. **Krause, D. C., D. K. Leith, and J. B. Baseman.** 1983. Reacquisition of specific proteins confers virulence in *Mycoplasma pneumoniae. Infect. Immun.* **39**:830–836.

39. **Krause, D. C., D. K. Leith, R. M. Wilson, and J. B. Baseman.** 1982. Identification of *Mycoplasma pneumoniae* proteins associated with hemadsorption and virulence. *Infect. Immun.* **35**:809–817.

40. **Levisohn, S., and M. J. Dykstra.** 1987. A quantitative study of single and mixed infection of the chicken trachea by *M. gallisepticum. Avian Dis.* **31**:1–12.

41. **Lin, S., and J. A. Spudich.** 1974. Biochemical studies on the mode of action of cytochalasin B. *J. Biol. Chem.* **249**:5778–5783.

42. **Lind, K.** 1982. Serological cross-reactions between *Mycoplasma genitalium* and *M. pneumoniae. Lancet* **ii**:1158–1159.

43. **Maniloff, J.** 1981. Cytoskeletal elements in mycoplasmas and other prokaryotes. *BioSystems* **14**:305–312.

44. **Maniloff, J., and U. Chadhuri.** 1979. Gliding mycoplasmas are inhibited by cytochalasin B and contain a polymerizable protein fraction. *J. Supramol. Struct.* **12**:299–304.

45. **Maniloff, J., and D. C. Quinlan.** 1974. Partial purification of a membrane-associated deoxyribonucleic acid complex from *Mycoplasma gallisepticum. J. Bacteriol.* **120**:495–501.

46. **Maniloff, J. H., H. J. Morowitz, and R. J. Barrnett.** 1965. Ultrastructure and ribosomes of *Mycoplasma gallisepticum. J. Bacteriol.* **90**:193–204.

47. **Meng, K. E., and R. M. Pfister.** 1980. Intracellular structures of *Mycoplasma pneumoniae* revealed after membrane removal. *J. Bacteriol.* **144**:390–399.

48. **Minion, F. C., G. H. Cassell, S. Pnini, and I. Kahane.** 1984. Multiphasic interaction of *Mycoplasma pulmonis* with erythrocytes defined by adherence and hemagglutination. *Infect. Immun.* **44**:394–400.

49. **Morowitz, H. J., and J. Maniloff.** 1966. Analysis of the life cycle of *Mycoplasma gallisepticum. J. Bacteriol.* **91**:1638–1644.

50. **Neimark, H.** 1983. Mycoplasma and bacterial proteins resembling contractile proteins: a review. *Yale J. Biol. Med.* **56**:419–423.

51. **Neimark, H. C.** 1977. Extraction of an actin-like protein from the prokaryote *Mycoplasma pneumoniae. Proc. Natl. Acad. Sci. USA* **74**:4041–4045.

52. **Nelson, J. B., and M. J. Lyons.** 1965. Phase-contrast and

electron microscopy of murine strains of mycoplasma. *J. Bacteriol.* **90:**1750–1763.

53. **Peterson, J. E., A. W. Rodwell, and E. S. Rodwell.** 1973. Occurrence and ultrastructure of a variant (rho) form of mycoplasma. *J. Bacteriol.* **115:**411–425.

54. **Powell, D. A., P.-C. Hu, M. Wilson, A. M. Collier, and J. B. Baseman.** 1976. Attachment of *M. pneumoniae* to respiratory epithelium. *Infect. Immun.* **13:**959–966.

55. **Rampal, A. L., H. B. Pinkofsky, and C. Y. Jung.** 1980. Structure of cytochalasin and cytochalasin B binding sites in human erythrocyte membranes. *Biochemistry* **19:**679–683.

56. **Robertson, J., and E. Smook.** 1976. Cytochemical evidence of extramembranous carbohydrates on *Ureaplasma urealyticum* (T-strain mycoplasma). *J. Bacteriol.* **128:**658–660.

57. **Rodwell, A. W., J. E. Petersen, and E. S. Rodwell.** 1972. Macromolecular synthesis and growth of mycoplasmas, p. 123–140. *In Pathogenic Mycoplasmas: CIBA Foundation Symposium.* Elsevier, New York.

58. **Saglio, P., M. L'Hospital, D. Laflèche, G. Dupont, J. M. Bové, J. G. Tully, and E. A. Freundt.** 1973. *Spiroplasma citri* gen. and sp. n.: a mycoplasma-like organism associated with "stubborn" disease of citrus. *Int. J. Syst. Bacteriol.* **23:**191–204.

59. **Simoneau, P., and J. Laberère.** 1990. Immunochemical identification of an actin-like protein from *Spiroplasma citri. Zentralbl. Bakteriol. Suppl.* **20:**927–931.

60. **Tanenbaum, S. W. (ed.).** *Cytochalasins.* North Holland Publishing Co., New York.

61. **Townsend, R.** 1983. Spiroplasma fibrils. *Yale J. Biol. Med.* **56:**447–452.

62. **Townsend, R., D. B. Archer, and K. A. Plaskitt.** 1980. Purification and preliminary characterization of *Spiroplasma* fibrils. *J. Bacteriol.* **142:**694–700.

63. **Townsend, R., J. Burgess, and K. A. Plaskitt.** 1980. Morphology and ultrastructure of helical and nonhelical strains of *Spiroplasma citri. J. Bacteriol.* **142:**973–981.

64. **Townsend, R., P. G. Markham, K. A. Plaskitt, and M. J. Daniels.** 1977. Isolation of a nonhelical strain of *Spiroplasma citri. J. Gen. Microbiol.* **100:**15–21.

65. **Tully, J. G., D. Taylor-Robinson, D. L. Rose, R. M. Cole, and J. M. Bové.** 1983. *Mycoplasma genitalium,* a new species from the human urogenital tract. *Int. J. Syst. Bacteriol.* **33:**387–396.

66. **Wall, F., R. M. Pfister, and N. L. Somerson.** 1983. Freeze-fracture confirmation of the presence of a core in the specialized tip structure of *Mycoplasma pneumoniae. J. Bacteriol.* **154:**924–929.

67. **Whitcomb, R. F.** 1980. The genus *Spiroplasma. Annu. Rev. Microbiol.* **34:**677–709.

68. **Williamson, D. L., D. I. Blanstein, R. J. C. Levine, and M. J. Elfvin.** 1979. Anti-actin peroxidase staining of the helical wall-free prokaryote *Spiroplasma citri. Curr. Microbiol.* **2:**143–145.

69. **Williamson, D. L., J. Renaudin, and J. M. Bové.** 1990. Spiroplasma fibrillar protein gene isolation. *IOM Lett.* **1:**306–307.

70. **Wilson, M. H., and A. M. Collier.** 1976. Ultrastructural study of *Mycoplasma pneumoniae* in organ culture. *J. Bacteriol.* **125:**332–339.

5. Cell Envelope: Morphology and Biochemistry

RICARDO F. ROSENBUSCH and F. CHRIS MINION

INTRODUCTION

Many procaryotes are covered by envelope materials, polymeric substances that are endowed with a multiplicity of properties and functions (13). This envelope material, or capsule, is usually attached to the cell surface, but is distinct from and extraneous to the bilayer membrane (60). In bacteria, the term "capsule" is reserved for high-molecular-weight polymers which are attached to the bacterial surface; slime, in contrast, is not intimately attached (3). In addition, most procaryotes are surrounded by a monomolecular extracellular polymer that provides the shape of the organism. This structure, called the murein sacculus, is composed of peptidoglycan, a polymer of carbohydrates and amino acids (58). Among the mollicutes, the peptidoglycan layer is absent (36). Capsules or capsulelike structures have been described among several mollicute species, and these descriptions will constitute the basis for the review presented in this chapter. The chapter focuses on the morphology, biochemistry, and biological role of mycoplasmal envelopes, excluding from discussion all aspects that relate to the cell membrane such as asymmetries of the external component of the trilamellar membrane (3). Other aspects related to envelopes, such as the polysaccharides and lipopolysaccharides that are an integral part of the mycoplasmal membrane, are presented in chapter 8, and the role of mycoplasma envelopes as immunogens is discussed in chapter 29.

ENVELOPE MORPHOLOGY

Studies of procaryotic capsules have benefited from information obtained by light microscopy, particularly when combined with the India ink contrast technique (14). This type of methodology has not proven useful with mollicutes because of their smaller size and the complex nature of background components provided by the media or animal tissue environment in which capsule is being expressed. The use of interference (Nomarski) microscopy has allowed the visualization of capsular material in clumps of mycoplasma cells (15), but the majority of the morphological information available has arisen from electron microscopy observations. Mycoplasma capsules may be highly hydrated layers, as has been observed in other procaryotes (51). This possibility is suggested by the lack of electron density obtained in the space external to mycoplasma cells fixed with osmium tetroxide prior to examination by electron microscopy (21). Stabilization of these structures by appropriate fixation prior to dehydration is therefore required. In addition, most mycoplasma capsules have been visualized with the aid of polycationic compounds such as ruthenium red, which complexes with osmium tetroxide to stain polyanionic compounds (34). This finding raises the question of whether capsular structures that are not polyanionic (or at least not reactive with polycations) exist among mycoplasmas but have not been reported. It is possible to detect capsular structures with the aid of specific antibodies, since the proteinaceous antibody molecules provide the required stabilization and contrast (4). An ideal antibody preparation would be that which is obtained from the mucosal site of animals exposed to the mycoplasma infection. This approach has been used successfully by us with *Mycoplasma dispar* in studies in which bronchoalveolar lavage fluid from infected calves was used as a source of antibody (2a). To enhance contrast, the antibody reagents can be tagged with electron-dense markers such as colloidal gold (2a, 42).

With the aid of ruthenium red staining, capsules could be seen as amorphous layers with thickness of up to 30 nm in *M. mycoides* subsp. *mycoides* and up to 24 nm in *M. dispar* when both of these mycoplasmas were grown in vitro (21). In general, the electron density of ruthenium red-stained capsules appeared to diminish as distance from the membrane increased.

Ricardo F. Rosenbusch and F. Chris Minion • Veterinary Medical Research Institute, Iowa State University, Ames, Iowa 50011.

Capsules of up to 40 nm in thickness were seen surrounding *M. hyopneumoniae* in infected porcine lung tissue (54). These investigators also reported that in preparations not stained with ruthenium red, fibrillar material of 5 nm in diameter and up to 200 nm in length was seen external to the mycoplasma membrane. A strain expressing prominent capsule also had extracellular fibrillar material, while strains with thinner capsule did not have fibrillar material. Fibrillar structures are associated with capsules of many bacteria (11).

Capsular polymers are generally viscous, and a similar property has been reported in *M. mycoides* subsp. *mycoides*. Broth cultures of this organism commonly exhibit "comets" or "threads" associated with filamentous growth of this highly capsulated mollicute, whereas noncapsulated strains do not (17).

The species of mycoplasmas described as capable of expressing capsule include *M. mycoides* subsp. *mycoides* (10), *M. dispar* (21), *M. gallisepticum* (55), *M. hominis* (15), *M. hyopneumoniae* (54), *M. meleagridis* (18), *M. pneumoniae* (61), *M. pulmonis* (55), and *M. synoviae* (2). Among the ureaplasmas, the human pathogen *Ureaplasma urealyticum* expresses capsule (40), but there is great variation among strains. In contrast, *U. diversum* has been described to have only a very thin exopolymer (6). An extracellular polysaccharide described for *M. capricolum* may also be capsular in nature in view of its reported size (over 200 kDa by size exclusion chromatography), although no morphological data are available (41).

Capsules have not been described among acholeplasmas or among spiroplasmas, anaeroplasmas, or asteroleplasmas. Lipoglycans have commonly been found in members of these mollicute families, but these structures are considered integral to the mycoplasmal membrane, do not provide any significant extracellular electron microscopic image when stained with ruthenium red, are of lower molecular weight than capsules, and require hot phenol extraction for their separation from other membrane components (49). A discussion of these components can be found in chapter 8.

An extracellular structure that requires additional characterization is the thin capsule, an 11-nm layer that has most commonly been described as an electron-lucent space separating many mycoplasma organisms from the parasitized eucaryotic cells. Spacing of these dimensions has been observed in many mycoplasmas contaminating cell cultures and in *M. arginini*, the bovine mycoplasma PG50 (5), bovine ureaplasmas (6), and *M. bovoculi* (42).

CAPSULE PURIFICATION

Purification of the extracellular capsule fraction is an essential first step prior to chemical and structural analysis. Several workers have used hot phenol extraction procedures followed by ethanol precipitation or ion-exchange chromatography (10, 41); capsule material can also be extracted by proteinase K digestion. However, both of these extraction methods also result in removal of lipoglycans from the membrane. Prolonged exposure to buffered saline can be used to extract capsular material from *M. dispar* (2a). Additionally, methods suitable for the extraction of polysaccharide capsules of gram-positive bacteria may be useful in mycoplasmas (12).

The binding of mycoplasma polysaccharide fractions to specific lectins (29, 44, 45) can also be explored as a component of purification protocols. Examples of such reactivity are the affinity of the capsule of *U. urealyticum* for concanavalin A (40, 59) and that of the capsule of *M. dispar* for *Ricinus communis* I (2a). When lectin affinity is used as part of a purification protocol, elution of the bound polysacharide must be effected by competition (28) with a disaccharide or monosaccharide at fairly high concentrations (usually 0.2 M), and a gel filtration step is necessary to separate the polysaccharide from the mono- or disaccharide.

CHEMICAL COMPOSITION

Two presumably divergent lines of evidence provide some information on the chemical composition of capsules of mycoplasmas. A common method used to visualize capsules of mycoplasmas consists of a polycationic, electron-dense reagent together with the osmium tetroxide fixative. Common choices are ruthenium red (34) and cationized ferritin (43). The results obtained suggest that most of the mycoplasma capsules described are polyanionic in nature and are thus composed at least in part of acidic carbohydrates or lipids.

Direct chemical analysis of few mycoplasma capsules has been reported. The capsule of *M. mycoides* subsp. *mycoides* is a galactan, composed of polymers of the neutral monosaccharide galactose (10) which are linked in a β(1–6) configuration (7, 37). In contrast, the capsule of *M. dispar* has been shown to be composed of a polymer of galacturonic acid (40a). Polysaccharides isolated from *M. mycoides* subsp. *capri* (27) and from a bovine mycoplasma of unknown species causing arthritis (38) were recognized as glucan, a polymer of glucose, but their relationship with capsular structures is unclear.

BIOSYNTHESIS OF CAPSULAR POLYSACCHARIDES

In direct correlation with the scant information available on the chemical composition of mycoplasma capsules, little is known about their synthesis and catabolism. Electron microscopy observations of capsules stained with polycationic compounds are in some cases suggestive of an asymmetric export of capsular polymers at localized sites on the surface of the mycoplasma (21, 40), but it cannot be excluded that the clustering of electron-dense, polycationic compounds is due to artifacts in fixation or binding. Asymmetric export or translocation of polymer has been shown to occur in *Escherichia coli* (3). Some neutral polysaccharides produced by gram-positive cocci, such as the levans and glucans, are synthesized from sucrose on the outer surface of the procaryotic membrane (52). It is improbable that the galactan of *M. mycoides* subsp. *mycoides* is similarly produced, since lactose is not available on the respiratory mucosa.

Capsule production is an energy-demanding synthesis, since monosaccharides have to be coupled with one or, more commonly, two phosphate groups prior to polymerization (56). In addition, polysaccharide synthesis requires that one of the ends of the chain be attached to a specialized carrier lipid. The final polymer may then be transferred to an anchoring molecule on the membrane. Diacylglycerols may act as carrier lipids, but it cannot be excluded that mycoplasmas use other lipids, including complex lipids scavenged from eucaryotic cell membranes, as carriers or anchors for capsular polysaccharides (49). The galactan of *M. mycoides* subsp. *mycoides* was found to be linked to a diacylglycerol containing palmitic and stearic acids (10).

Some mycoplasmas synthesize capsular polysaccharide only in vivo or when cocultured in vitro with eucaryotic cells. Increases in the thickness of the capsule have been shown to occur with cocultured *M. gallisepticum* (62) and *M. hyopneumoniae* (53), and capsule synthesis was induced by coculture of *M. dispar* with bovine lung fibroblasts (2a). The nature of the interaction occurring between eucaryotic cells and mycoplasmas is still undefined, but in the *M. dispar* model, it has been shown that a 14-kDa-pore-size dialysis membrane can be interposed between cells and mycoplasmas without interfering with capsule synthesis induction.

The synthesis of capsular polysaccharide, whether as an intracellular polymer that is exported or as an exopolysaccharide, requires several distinct enzymes. Thus, a branched polysaccharide will require additional enzymes not needed for the synthesis of the linear homolog (52). Synthesis of the K1 capsule of *E. coli*, which is composed only of polymerized sialic acid, requires 15 kb of genome DNA coding for 12 proteins (48). The group B streptococcus capsule contains four different monosaccharides in repeating units and requires over 30 kb of genomic DNA to code for the necessary complement of proteins (31). Knowledge about the nature and regulation of capsule-associated enzymes in mycoplasmas will be forthcoming only once a detailed chemical and structural analysis of several mycoplasma capsules has been obtained. Information related to the genes involved in capsule expression in mollicutes will provide insight into the assembly of similar structures in other bacteria. Some of the enzymes may be membrane associated, which will be of interest since mollicutes have undergone large genome losses in their evolution from gram-positive bacteria (35). Significant among these genome losses are the deficiencies in envelope structural genes. In this context, information about those envelope structural genes that remain functional may have important implications for the study of procaryote phylogenetics.

BIOLOGIC AND PATHOGENIC ROLE OF CAPSULES

Capsular polysaccharides of bacteria can bind irreversibly to negatively charged surfaces by a latch effect provided by the multiple binding sites from repeating units in the polysaccharide (39). Association of the mycoplasma capsule with attachment has been suggested (18, 23, 61). Attachment of *M. dispar* to erythrocytes appeared to be mediated by ruthenium red-stainable capsular material and fine extracellular threads bridging gaps between membranes (23). Similar observations were made with *M. hyopneumoniae* attaching to porcine respiratory epithelium (54). Strains of *M. hyopneumoniae* that were extensively passaged in vitro did not exhibit these fibrillar structures and were less pathogenic to pigs.

Capsular polysaccharides have antiphagocytic properties associated with their electronegative charges and with their capacity to nonspecifically bind factor H, a normal inhibitor of the alternative pathway of complement activation (30). In addition, capsules prevent the nonspecific deposition of immunoglobulin G on bacterial surfaces (1). Additional protection against phagocytosis is afforded by the formation of microcolonies surrounded by a glycocalyx of joined individual exopolysaccharides which are resistant to enzymatic degradation (26). In mycoplasmas, the production of capsule does not appear to be required to avoid phagocytosis. All but 1 of 15 mycoplasma strains tested were resistant to killing by gnotobiotic calf serum, and this finding was attributed to lack of activation of the alternative complement pathway (19). The ability to attach and multiply on the surface of cultured macrophages and neutrophils without stimulation of ingestion was also described for mycoplasmas pathogenic for the respiratory tract of cattle (24). Both the capsulated *M. dispar* and the noncapsulated *M. bovis* were capable of exerting an inhibitory effect on the ability of bovine neutrophils to phagocytose *E. coli*. Thus, capsular polysaccharides do not appear per se to enhance or diminish the antiphagocytic properties exhibited by mycoplasmas.

The galactan of *M. mycoides* subsp. *mycoides* does not induce antibody responses in immunized animals unless combined with Freund's adjuvant (25). It has been suggested that the mycoplasmal galactan possesses serological similarity to pneumogalactan, a product of normal lung epithelial cells (16, 47). A similar immunological anergy may be associated with the capsule of *M. dispar*, since cattle may have low antibody titers against this species (20). In addition, immune responses to capsular polysaccharides are normally T cell independent and absent in the very young (50). These features are also seen in immune responses against *M. dispar* (22).

Mycoplasma capsules may have toxic effects on specific eucaryotic cells in the body. These effects are expressed as capillary thrombosis and pulmonary edema in calves given purified galactan intravenously (9). Lethal effects for chicken embryos inoculated in the chorioallantoic cavity included hemorrhagic lesions, but this toxic effect was significantly reduced with more purified galactan preparations (57). Impurities of concern include nucleic acids and lipoglycans, since these latter compounds from acholeplasmas have been shown to elicit pyrogenic responses in rabbits and clotting of *Limulus* amoebocyte lysates (46). Another effect ascribed to the galactan of *M. mycoides* subsp. *mycoides* is the deposition of fibrin around chronic lung lesions in cattle (8); this effect is mimicked by placing the organism within diffusion chambers in the peritoneal cavity or tissues of calves and rabbits (8, 32). Cattle given galactan developed persistent mycoplasmemia when concurrently infected by subcutaneous injection, and polyarthritis was seen in calves similarly infected (33).

CONCLUDING REMARKS AND OUTLOOK

The capsules of mycoplasmas have been incompletely studied, and only for one species (*M. mycoides* subsp. *mycoides*) is there enough information to warrant attempts at understanding the biological and pathogenic role of these extracellular polymers. The first requirement is the chemical characterization of the capsules of several additional species of mycoplasmas. The chemical composition of these capsules may vary among species, but the capsules may be generally homopolymeric, as opposed to lipoglycans, in which a large variety of monosaccharides are represented. Because of this potential simplicity, exploration of the capsule genes of mycoplasmas may prove to be relatively straightforward. Development of knowledge about the molecular biology of capsule biosynthesis and regulation of expression may provide important background for further understanding of the biology and pathogenesis of mycoplasma infections.

An area that needs further study is that of the toxic and immunomodulatory effects of mycoplasma capsules, in particular with expansion to the capsules of species other than *M. mycoides* subsp. *mycoides*. The role of capsules as immunogens also warrants further study, particularly within the context of the development of conjugated polysaccharide subunit vaccines.

REFERENCES

1. **Absolom, D. R.** 1988. The role of bacterial hydrophobicity in infection: bacterial adhesion and phagocytic ingestion. *Can. J. Microbiol.* **34:**287–298.
2. **Ajufo, J. C., and K. G. Whithear.** 1978. Evidence for a ruthenium red-staining extracellular layer as the haemagglutinin of the WVU 1853 strain of *Mycoplasma synoviae. Aust. Vet. J.* **54:**502–504.
2a. **Almeida, R., and R. F. Rosenbusch.** 1991. Capsulelike surface material of *Mycoplasma dispar* induced by in vitro growth in culture with bovine cells is antigenically related to similar structures expressed in vivo. *Infect. Immun.* **59:**3119–3125.
3. **Bayer, M. E.** 1979. The fusion sites between outer membrane and cytoplasmic membrane of bacteria: their role in membrane assembly and virus infection, p. 167–202. *In* M. Inouye (ed.), *Bacterial Outer Membranes.* John Wiley & Sons, Inc., New York.
4. **Bayer, M. E.** 1990. Visualization of the bacterial polysaccharide capsule. *Curr. Top. Microbiol. Immunol.* **150:**129–157.
5. **Boatman, E. S.** 1979. Morphology and ultrastructure of the mycoplasmatales, p. 63–101. *In* M. F. Barile and S. Razin (ed.), *The Mycoplasmas*, vol. 1. *Cell Biology.* Academic Press, New York.
6. **Boatman, E. S., F. Cartwright, and G. Kenny.** 1976. Morphology, morphometry and electron microscopy of HeLa cells infected with bovine mycoplasma. *Cell Tissue Res.* **170:**1–16.
7. **Buttery, S. H.** 1970. Hapten inhibition of the reaction between *Mycoplasma mycoides* polysaccharide and bovine antisera. *Immunochemistry* **7:**305–310.
8. **Buttery, S. H., G. S. Cottew, and L. C. Lloyd.** 1980. Effect of soluble factors from *Mycoplasma mycoides* subsp. *my-*
coides on the collagen content of bovine connective tissue. *J. Comp. Pathol.* **90:**303–314.
9. **Buttery, S. H., L. C. Lloyd, and D. A. Titchen.** 1976. Acute respiratory, circulatory and pathological changes in the calf after intravenous injections of the galactan from *Mycoplasma mycoides* subsp. *mycoides. J. Med. Microbiol.* **9:**379–391.
10. **Buttery, S. H., and P. Plackett.** 1960. A specific polysaccharide from *Mycoplasma mycoides. J. Gen. Microbiol.* **23:**357–368.
11. **Cagle, G. D.** 1975. Fine structure and distribution of extracellular polymer surrounding selected aerobic bacteria. *Can. J. Microbiol.* **21:**395–408.
12. **Chomarat, M., Y. Ichiman, and K. Yoshida.** 1989. Protection of mice by a pseudodiffuse strain of *Staphylococcus aureus* possessing polyvalent capsular type antigen. *J. Med. Microbiol.* **28:**129–136.
13. **Costerton, J. W., and R. T. Irvin.** 1981. The bacterial glycocalyx in nature and disease. *Annu. Rev. Microbiol.* **35:**299–324.
14. **Domermuth, C. H., M. H. Nielsen, E. A. Freundt, and A. Birch-Andersen.** 1964. Ultrastructure of *Mycoplasma* species. *J. Bacteriol.* **88:**727–744.
15. **Furness, G., J. Whitescarver, M. Trocola, and M. DeMaggio.** 1976. Morphology, ultrastructure, and mode of division of *Mycoplasma fermentans, Mycoplasma hominis, Mycoplasma orale,* and *Mycoplasma salivarium. J. Infect. Dis.* **134:**224–229.
16. **Gourlay, R. N., and M. Shifrine.** 1966. Antigenic cross-reactions between the galactan from *Mycoplasma mycoides* and polysaccharides from other sources. *J. Comp. Pathol.* **76:**417–425.
17. **Gourlay, R. N., and K. J. Thrower.** 1968. Morphology of *Mycoplasma mycoides* thread-phase growth. *J. Gen Microbiol.* **55:**155–159.
18. **Green, F., III, and R. P. Hanson.** 1973. Ultrastructure and capsule of *Mycoplasma meleagridis. J. Bacteriol.* **116:**1011–1018.
19. **Howard, C. J.** 1980. Variation in susceptibility of bovine mycoplasmas to killing by the alternative complement pathway in bovine serum. *Immunology* **41:**561–568.
20. **Howard, C. J.** 1983. Mycoplasmas and bovine respiratory disease: studies related to pathogenicity and immune response—a selective review. *Yale J. Biol. Med.* **56:**789–797.
21. **Howard, C. J., and R. N. Gourlay.** 1974. An electron-microscopic examination of certain bovine mycoplasmas stained with ruthenium red and the demonstration of a capsule on *Mycoplasma dispar. J. Gen. Microbiol.* **83:**393–398.
22. **Howard, C. J., and R. N. Gourlay.** 1983. Immune response of calves following the inoculation of *Mycoplasma dispar* and *Mycoplasma bovis. Vet. Microbiol.* **8:**45–56.
23. **Howard, C. J., R. N. Gourlay, and J. Collins.** 1974. Serological comparison and hemoagglutinating activity of *Mycoplasma dispar. J. Hyg.* (Cambridge) **73:**457–466.
24. **Howard, C. J., R. N. Gourlay, and G. Taylor.** 1980. Immunity to mycoplasma infections of the calf respiratory tract. *Adv. Exp. Med. Biol.* **137:**711–726.
25. **Hudson, J. R., S. Buttery, and G. S. Cottew.** 1967. Investigations into the influence of the galactan of *Mycoplasma mycoides* on experimental infection with that organism. *J. Pathol. Bacteriol.* **94:**257–273.
26. **Isenberg, H. D.** 1988. Pathogenicity and virulence: another view. *Clin. Microbiol. Rev.* **1:**40–53.
27. **Jones, A. S., J. R. Tittensor, and R. T. Walker.** 1965. The chemical composition of nucleic acids and other macromolecular constituents of *Mycoplasma mycoides* var. *capri. J. Gen Microbiol.* **40:**405–411.
28. **Kahane, I., and H. G. Schiefer.** 1983. Characterization of carbohydrate components of mycoplasma membranes, p. 285–294. *In* S. Razin and J. G. Tully (ed.), *Methods in Mycoplasmology*, vol. 1. *Mycoplasma Characterization.* Academic Press, New York.

29. **Kahane, I., and J. G. Tully.** 1976. Binding of plant lectins to mycoplasma cells and membranes. *J. Bacteriol.* **128**:1–7.

30. **Kasper, D. L.** 1986. Bacterial capsules. Old dogmas and new tricks. *J. Infect. Dis.* **153**:407–415.

31. **Kuypers, J. M., L. M. Heggen, and C. E. Rubens.** 1989. Molecular analysis of a region of the group B streptococcus chromosome involved in type III capsule expression. *Infect. Immun.* **57**:3058–3065.

32. **Lloyd, L. C.** 1966. Tissue necrosis produced by *Mycoplasma mycoides* in intraperitoneal diffusion chambers. *J. Pathol. Bacteriol.* **92**:225–229.

33. **Lloyd, L. C., S. H. Buttery, and J. R. Hudson.** 1971. The effect of the galactan and other antigens of *Mycoplasma mycoides* var. *mycoides* on experimental infection with that organism in cattle. *J. Med. Microbiol.* **4**:425–439.

34. **Luft, J. H.** 1964. Electron microscopy of cell extraneous coats as revealed by ruthenium red staining. *J. Cell Biol.* **23**:54a.

35. **Neimark, H.** 1983. Evolution of mycoplasmas and genome losses. *Yale J. Biol. Med.* **56**:377–383.

36. **Plackett, P.** 1959. On the probable absence of "mucocomplex" from *Mycoplasma mycoides. Biochim. Biophys. Acta* **35**:260–262.

37. **Plackett, P., and S. H. Buttery.** 1964. A galactofuranose disaccharide from the galactan of *Mycoplasma mycoides. Biochem. J.* **90**:201–205.

38. **Plackett, P., S. H. Buttery, and G. S. Cottew.** 1963. Carbohydrates of some mycoplasma strains. *Rec. Prog. Microbiol.* **8**:535–547.

39. **Robb, I. D.** 1984. Stereo-biochemistry and functions of polymers in microbial adhesion and aggregation, p. 39–49. *In* K. C. Marshall (ed.), *Microbial Adhesion and Aggregation.* Springer-Verlag, Berlin.

40. **Robertson, J., and E. Smook.** 1976. Cytochemical evidence of extramembranous carbohydrates on *Ureaplasma urealyticum* (T-strain mycoplasma). *J. Bacteriol.* **128**:658–660.

40a. **Rosenbusch, R. F., et al.** Unpublished data.

41. **Rurangirwa, F. R., T. C. McGuire, N. S. Magnuson, A. Kibor, and S. Chema.** 1987. Composition of a polysaccharide from mycoplasma (F-38) recognized by from goats with contagious pleuropneumonia. *Res. Vet. Sci.* **42**:175–178.

42. **Salih, B. A., and R. Rosenbusch.** 1988. Attachment of *Mycoplasma bovoculi* to bovine conjunctival epithelium and lung fibroblasts. *Am. J. Vet. Res.* **49**:1661–1664.

43. **Schiefer, H. G., H. Krauss, H. Brunner, and U. Gerhardt.** 1976. Ultrastructural visualization of anionic sites on mycoplasma membranes by polycationic ferritin. *J. Bacteriol.* **127**:461–468.

44. **Schiefer, H. G., H. Krauss, U. Schummer, H. Brunner, and U. Gerhardt.** 1978. Cytochemical localization of surface carbohydrates on mycoplasma membranes. *Experientia* **34**:1011–1012.

45. **Schiefer, H. G., H. Krauss, U. Schummer, H. Brunner, and U. Gerhardt.** 1978. Studies with ferritin-conjugated concanavalin A on carbohydrate structures of mycoplasma membranes. *FEMS Microbiol. Lett.* **3**:183–185.

46. **Seid, R. C., Jr., P. F. Smith, G. Guevarra, H. D. Hochstein, and M. F. Barile.** 1980. Endotoxin-like activities of mycoplasma lipopolysaccharides (lipoglycans). *Infect. Immun.* **29**:990–994.

47. **Shifrine, M., and R. N. Gourlay.** 1965. Serologic relationship between galactans from normal bovine lung and from *Mycoplasma mycoides. Nature* (London) **208**:498–499.

48. **Silver, R. P., W. F. Vann, and W. Aaronson.** 1984. Genetic and molecular analyses of *Escherichia coli* K1 antigen genes. *J. Bacteriol.* **157**:568–575.

49. **Smith, P. F.** 1984. Lipoglycans from mycoplasmas. *Crit. Rev. Microbiol.* **11**:157–185.

50. **Stein, K. E.** 1985. Network regulation of the immune response to bacterial polysaccharide antigens. *Curr. Top. Microbiol. Immunol.* **119**:57–74.

51. **Sutherland, I. W.** 1972. Bacterial exopolysaccharides. *Adv. Microb. Physiol.* **8**:143–213.

52. **Sutherland, I. W.** 1982. Biosynthesis of microbial exopolysaccharides. *Adv. Microbiol. Physiol.* **23**:79–150.

53. **Tajima, M., T. Nunoya, and T. Yagihashi.** 1979. An ultrastructural study on the interaction of *Mycoplasma gallisepticum* with the chicken tracheal epithelium. *Am. J. Vet. Res.* **40**:1009–1014.

54. **Tajima, M., and T. Yagihashi.** 1982. Interaction of *Mycoplasma hyopneumoniae* with the porcine respiratory epithelium as observed by electron microscopy. *Infect. Immun.* **37**:1162–1169.

55. **Taylor-Robinson, D., P. M. Furr, H. A. Davies, R. J. Manchee, and J. M. Bové.** 1981. Mycoplasmal adherence with particular reference to the pathogenicity of *Mycoplasma pulmonis. Isr. J. Med. Sci.* **17**:599–603.

56. **Troy, F. A.** 1979. The chemistry and biosynthesis of selected bacterial capsular polymers. *Annu. Rev. Microbiol.* **33**:519–560.

57. **Villemot, J. M., A. Provost, and R. Queval.** 1962. Endotoxin from *Mycoplasma mycoides. Nature* (London) **193**:906–907.

58. **Weidel, W., and H. Pelzer.** 1964. Bag shaped macromolecules: a new outlook on bacterial cell walls. *Adv. Enzymol.* **26**:193–232.

59. **Whitescarver, J., F. Castillo, and G. Furness.** 1975. The preparation of membranes of some human T-mycoplasmas and the analysis of their carbohydrate content. *Proc. Soc. Exp. Biol. Med.* **150**:20–22.

60. **Whitfield, C.** 1988. Bacterial extracellular polysaccharides. *Can. J. Microbiol.* **34**:415–420.

61. **Wilson, M. H., and A. M. Collier.** 1976. Ultrastructural study of *Mycoplasma pneumoniae* in organ culture. *J. Bacteriol.* **125**:332–339.

62. **Yagihashi, T.** Unpublished data.

6. Membrane Lipid and Lipopolysaccharide Structures

PAUL F. SMITH

INTRODUCTION

The lipids of the mollicutes are as diverse as the genera and species that make up this class of microorganisms. They are located exclusively in the cytoplasmic membrane and constitute 25 to 35% of the dry weight of the membrane (67). Several unique lipids occur. Some of these lipids are derived from the culture medium and represent absolute nutritional requirements; most are synthesized de novo. Although mollicutes appear capable of incorporating many diverse lipids, only those which are absolute growth requirements or become radiolabeled from biosynthetic precursors are discussed in this chapter. Preformed lipids are restricted to planar 3-hydroxy sterols required by species of the genera *Mycoplasma*, *Spiroplasma*, and *Ureaplasma* and by some *Anaeroplasma* species and to fatty acids required by all of the named genera but not by some *Acholeplasma* species. An exception is *Mycoplasma gallisepticum*, which has a growth requirement for phospholipid which can be satisfied with phosphatidylcholine or sphingomyelin (46), both of which appear intact in the organism (51, 94).

Three general classes of lipids, neutral lipids, glycolipids, and phospholipids, occur in most species. Glycolipids are notably absent from many *Mycoplasma* species. Generally, the percentage by weight of phospholipids equals the combined percentages of neutral and glycolipids. Among the sterol-nonrequiring acholeplasmas, the neutral lipids, composed of carotenoids, represent only 5% or less of the total, while glycolipids constitute about 45% (2, 13, 22, 27, 34, 39, 48, 57, 59, 67, 72, 85, 92). If glycolipids are absent, the neutral lipid content equals the phospholipid content. These distributions apply to organisms grown in normal medium to the late exponential phase. Quantitative variation does occur during the growth cycle (24, 42, 52, 59, 85, 89). Exogenously supplied lipids can modulate the proportions of polar lipids, glycolipids, and sterols (57, 91, 96–98) but not the qualitative nature of the essential lipids.

Table 1 lists the types of lipids currently known to occur in various species of mollicutes. For some the exact chemical structures have been elucidated, while for others they have been resolved only in part.

NEUTRAL LIPIDS

Sterols

The sterol content ranges from 4 to 20% of the total lipid among those species having this growth requirement (2, 44, 48, 70, 91, 92). Exogenously supplied sterol does not undergo structural modification by the or-

Paul F. Smith • Department of Microbiology, University of South Dakota, Vermillion, South Dakota 57069.

Table 1. Lipids of mollicutes[a]

Organism	Neutral lipids	Glycolipids	Polar lipids	Reference(s)
Acholeplasma axanthum S743	Carotenoids; free fatty acids; long-chain bases of dihydrosphingosine type; 3-hydroxyacyl ceramides; cholesterol	α-D-Gal$f$-(1→3)-1,2-diacyl-sn-glycerol; α-D-Glc$p$-(1→3)-(O-acyl)-α-D-Glc$p$-(1→3)-cholesterol; α-D-Glc$p$-(1→3)-α-D-Glc$p$-(1→3)-cholesterol; α-D-Glc$p$-(1→3)-cholesterol; 2′3′-di-O-acyl-α-D-Gal$f$-(1→3)-1,2-diacyl-sn-glycerol	PG; acylPG; DPG; lysoPG; ceramide phosphoglycerol; acylceramide phosphoglycerol; polyprenol phosphate	26, 28, 39, 76, 89, 93
A. equifetale C1	Carotenoids; acylglycerols	Monoglucosyldiacylglycerol; diglucosyldiacylglycerol	PG; lysoPG; DPG; lysoDPG	1a
A. granularum BTS-39	Carotenoids; acylglycerols	α-D-Glc$p$-(1→1)-2,3-diacylglycerol; α-D-Glc$p$-(1→2)-α-D-Glc$p$-(1→1)-2,3-diacylglycerol; β-D-Glc$p$-(1→3)-α-D-Glc$p$-(1→2)-α-D-Glc$p$-(1→1)-2,3-diacylglycerol	PG; DPG; [β-D-glucopyranosyl-(1-1)-x-glycerol-2-O-] [D-glyceraldehyde-3-O-] [1,2-diacyl-x-glycerol-3-O-kojibiosyl = 6 = O)-]-phosphate; polyprenol phosphate	76, 90
A. hippikon C112	Carotenoids; acylglycerols	Monoglucosyldiacylglycerol; diglucosyldiacylglycerol	PG; lysoPG; DPG; lysoDPG; phosphoglycolipid	1a
A. laidlawii A	Carotenoids; carotenyl esters; acylglycerols	α-D-Glc$p$-(1→3)-1,2-diacyl-sn-glycerol; 3-O-acyl-α-D-Glc$p$-(1→3)-1,2-diacyl-sn-glycerol; α-D-Glc$p$-(1→2)-α-D-Glc$p$-(1→3)-1,2-diacyl-sn-glycerol; carotenyl-α-D-glucopyranoside	PG; DPG; 6-O-glycerophosphoryl-α-D-Glc$p$-(1→2)-α-D-Glc$p$-(1→3)-1,2-diacyl-sn-glycerol; glycerophosphoryl-monoglucosyl-diacylglycerol	30, 65, 80, 98
A. laidlawii B	Carotenoids; carotenyl esters; acylglycerols	α-D-Glc$p$-(1→2)-α-D-Glc$p$-(1→2)-2,3-diacylglycerol; α-D-Glc$p$-(1→1)-2,3-diacylglycerol; carotenyl-β-D-glucopyranoside; 2-O-acyl-α-D-Glc$p$-polyisoprenol	PG; DPG; D- and L-alanylPG; 6-O-glycerophosphoryl-α-D-Glc$p$-(1→2)-α-D-Glc$p$-(1→1)-2,3-diacylglycerol; phosphatidyl-α-D-Glc$p$-(1→2)-α-D-Glc$p$-(1→1)-2,3-diacylglycerol	4, 59, 65, 73, 86
A. modicum PG49	Carotenoids; acylglycerols	α-D-Glc$p$-(1→2)-α-D-Glc$p$-(1→1)-2,3-diacylglycerol; α-D-Glc$p$-(1→1)-2,3-diacylglycerol; α-D-Glc$p$-(1→2)-α-D-Gal$p$-(1→3)-β-D-glycero-D-manno-heptose$p$-(1→3)-α-D-Glc$p$-(1→2)-α-D-Glc$p$-(1→1)-2,3-diacylglycerol	PG; aminoacylPG; DPG; acylDPG; lysoDPG	28

(Continued)

Table 1. Lipids of mollicutes[a] (*Continued*)

Organism	Neutral lipids	Glycolipids	Polar lipids	Reference(s)
A. oculi 19L	Carotenoids; acylglycerols	α-D-Glc$p$-(1→2)-α-D-Glc$p$-(1→1)-2,3-diacylglycerol; α-D-Glc$p$-(1→1)-2,3-diacylglycerol	PG; lysoPG; DPG; lysoDPG	2
Anaeroplasma abactoclasticum 6-1	Cholesterol; unidentified	Unidentified	PG; aminoacylPG; DPG	22, 43
A. bactoclasticum 7LA	Unidentified	Unidentified	PG; aminoacylPG; DPG	22, 43
Mycoplasma arthritidis 07	Cholesterol; cholesteryl esters	None	PG; aminoacylPG; DPG	50, 85
M. capricolum 14	Cholesterol; cholesteryl esters; acylglycerols	None	PG; aminoacylPG; DPG; acylDPG	10, 80a
M. gallinarum J	Cholesterol; cholesteryl esters	Cholesterol-β-D-glucopyranoside; 3,4,6-tri-O=acyl-β-D-glucopyranose	PGP; lysoPGP; DPG	50, 85, 89
M. gallisepticum S-6	Cholesterol; cholesteryl esters; acylglycerols	None	PG; DPG; PC	53, 80a, 94
M. hominis ATCC 15056	Cholesterol; cholesteryl esters; acylglycerols; free fatty acids	None	PG; lysoPG; PA	57
M. hyorhinis BTS-7	Cholesterol; cholesteryl esters; acylglycerols	None	PG; DPG	80a
M. mycoides V5	Cholesterol; acylglycerols	β-D-Gal$f$-(1→1)-2,3-diacylglycerol; unidentified	PG; DPG	35
M. neurolyticum PG28 and PG39	Cholesterol; acylglycerols	β-D-Glc$p$-(1→6)-β-D-Glc$p$-(1→1)-2,3-diacylglycerol; β-D-Glc$p$-(1→1)-2,3-diacylglycerol; triglucosyldiacylglycerol	PG; aminoacylPG; DPG; acylDPG; PA	72, 93
M. pneumoniae FH	Cholesterol	Digalactosyldiacylglycerol; trigalactosyldiacylglycerol; glucosylgalactosyldiacylglycerol	PG; DPG	38
Spiroplasma citri Morocco	Cholesterol; cholesteryl esters; acylglycerols; free fatty acids	Cholesterol glucosides	PG; DPG; lysoDPG	11, 13, 34
Ureaplasma urealyticum	Cholesterol; cholesteryl esters; acylglycerols; free fatty acids	Glucosyldiacylglycerols	PA; PG; DPG; PE; diaminohydroxy compound with adjacent fatty acid ester and N-acyl groups	48, 56

[a] Abbreviations: PC, phosphatidylcholine; PG, phosphatidylglycerol; DPG, diphosphatidylglycerol; PGP, phosphatidylglycerophosphate; PA, phosphatidic acid; PE, phosphatidylethanolamine.

ganisms (50, 64). Any sterol containing an aliphatic side chain can be incorporated (66). Many other lipoidal compounds not necessary for growth, e.g., bilirubin (31) and chlorophyll *a* (100), can be incorporated. However, only planar 3-hydroxy sterols with an aliphatic side chain permit growth (66). Therefore, proper orientation and function are prerequisites for the suitability of the sterol molecule in the membrane. Sterols which fulfill functional requirements are cholesterol, cholestanol, ergosterol, and β-sitosterol (66). Lanosterol can substitute for cholesterol in part (9), leading to the conclusion that sterol in the membrane is bifunctional—a bulk component and a regulator of unsaturated fatty acid uptake (10). A hopanoid, diplopterol, also permits limited growth (20). Appropriate 3,3'-dihydroxypolyterpenes, i.e., sarcinaxanthin, lutein, and the carotenol from *Acholeplasma laidlawii*, can substitute for sterol (16). Functionally, these polyterpenes serve the same purpose in membranes as do sterols (55, 68, 69). Uptake of sterol or polyterpenol is a first-order physical adsorption process mediated by a micelle composed of sterol or polyterpenol, an amphipath such as the salt of a long-chain unsaturated fatty acid, and the protein moiety of an appropriate lipoprotein (91). Sterol apparently is bound by hydrophobic interaction with apolar regions of phospholipids and glycolipids, since only depletion of membrane lipids interferes to any degree with sterol uptake (14, 81). Some species contain esterified cholesterol which is taken up from the culture medium. A few species, i.e., *A. laidlawii*, *M. arthritidis*, and *M. gallinarum*, reportedly are capable of esterifying sterol or carotenol with short-chain fatty acids, e.g., acetic and butyric (67, 70). Unesterified cholesterol also can be derived from exogenous cholesterol esters through the action of cholesterol esterase.

Carotenoids

All *Acholeplasma* species contain carotenoid pigments, as determined from spectral analyses and the incorporation of radiolabeled precursors, i.e., acetic and mevalonic acids (1a, 2, 50, 65, 87). These polyterpenes constitute about 2 to 5% of the total lipids. The exact structures of these compounds have not been established. However, spectral properties and chromatographic behavior suggest the existence of phytoene, phytofluene, neurosporene (Fig. 1, compound I) and their hydroxylated derivatives (67). Recent data (22a) reveal that the carotenoids of all *Acholeplasma* species are C_{30} compounds, i.e., apocarotenoids. Total reduction of purified hydrocarbon polyterpenes from

A. laidlawii A, *A. laidlawii* B, *A. modicum*, *A. axanthum*, *A. granularum*, and *A. oculi* yields only squalane, as identified by gas chromatography/mass spectrometry. The hydrocarbon carotenoid possesses absorption maxima at 414, 438, and 468 nm, and the hydroxylated carotenoid exhibits maxima at 402, 422, and 446 nm, characteristic of neurosporene and its dihydroxy derivative. These carotenoids appear to predominate in all *Acholeplasma* species except *A. axanthum*, in which z-carotene occurs (87). The existence and the nature of polyterpenes in sterol-nonrequiring *Anaeroplasma* species have not been examined. Carotenoids appear to replace, both physically and functionally, the sterols found in genera of mollicutes other than *Acholeplasma* (50, 65, 67). Evidence favoring this hypothesis arises from a variety of experimental approaches. The sterol requirement of *Mycoplasma* species can be satisfied by all-*trans*-3,3'-dihydroxycarotenes, including the carotenol from *A. laidlawii* (16). These compounds can be recovered unchanged, except for esterification, from the organisms. Cholesterol is incorporated into the membranes of acholeplasmas (50) and spares the biosynthesis of carotenoids (65). Compounds which block various enzymatic steps in the biosynthesis of phytoene inhibit the growth of acholeplasmas. This inhibition can be relieved by the addition of exogenous cholesterol, which is incorporated (84). *M. gallinarum*, which lacks three enzymes for the conversion of mevalonic acid into isopentenyl pyrophosphate (82), synthesizes polyterpenes similar to phytoene when supplied with exogenous isopentenyl pyrophosphate (68). Carotenoid pigments have been demonstrated to rigidify the acholeplasmal membrane and to maintain fluidity in a narrow range by modifying the fatty acyl composition of complex membrane lipids (19, 55) in a fashion similar to that for sterols.

Glycerides

No concerted analyses of glycerides have been performed, although all species of mollicutes contain small amounts of triacylglycerol and 1,2- and 1,3-diacylglycerols. These glycerides have been detected as radiolabeled compounds arising from growth of the organisms in the presence of radiolabeled fatty acids. Since de novo synthesis must occur, these glycerides are considered natural lipids of the organisms (2, 13, 34, 48, 57, 72, 85). Identification has been based primarily on mobility on thin-layer chromatograms.

Long-Chain Bases

A. axanthum is distinctive from all other known mollicutes by the possession of dihydrosphingosine-type bases (Fig. 1, compound II), which occur as segments of complex polar lipids and as the free bases. When existing as the free bases, they are accompanied by a molar equivalent of free fatty acids (26, 39). Bases with chain lengths 16:0 and 20:1 make up over 90% of the total amount. Precursor-product studies indicate that the organism synthesizes these bases by a two-carbon addition to fatty acids, except for fatty acids of chain length greater than 20 carbon atoms, in which case no elongation occurs. Unsaturated fatty acids give rise to unsaturated long-chain bases; saturated fatty acids give rise to saturated long-chain bases.

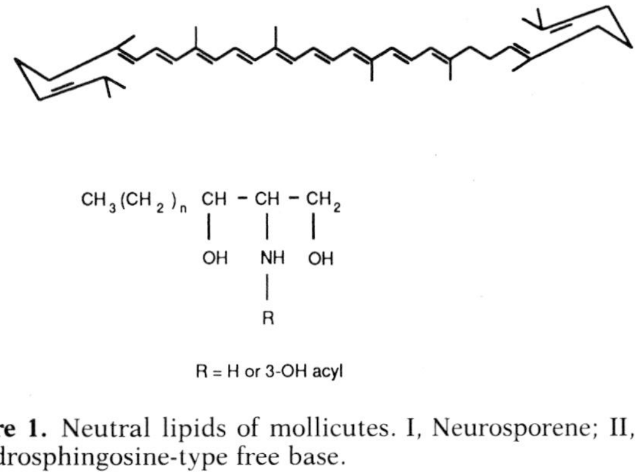

Figure 1. Neutral lipids of mollicutes. I, Neurosporene; II, dihydrosphingosine-type free base.

Free Fatty Acids

Free fatty acids frequently are found in small amounts in all mollicutes and usually are considered to arise from deacylation of complex lipids during processing. Exceptions are the large amounts of fatty acids found in *A. axanthum* (39), *Ureaplasma urealyticum* (48), and *M. pneumoniae* when grown in a palmitate-supplemented medium (23). Except in this apparently special case of *M. pneumoniae*, the free fatty acids are indistinguishable from the acyl fatty acids of complex lipids. Although it was believed originally that all *Acholeplasma* species could synthesize saturated fatty acids de novo (17, 41), that *U. urealyticum* could synthesize both saturated and unsaturated fatty acids (47), and that *Mycoplasma* and *Spiroplasma* species were incapable of forming either (13, 22), recent studies showed that only some *Acholeplasma* species could synthesize only saturated fatty acids and all other mollicutes could not (46). *Anaeroplasma* species have not been studied. These biosynthetic deficiencies have led to the use of these organisms in membrane studies because of the ease of manipulation of fatty acid composition (33, 62, 63).

GLYCOLIPIDS

Three classes of glycolipids, namely, glycosylacylglycerols, polyterpenol glycosides, and acylated sugars, occur in certain *Acholeplasma*, *Mycoplasma*, *Spiroplasma*, and *Ureaplasma* species. Glycolipids also are found in *Anaeroplasma* species, but their structures have not been elucidated. When present, glycolipids can account for almost 50% of the total lipids.

Glycosylacylglycerols

The presently known structures of glycosylacylglycerols in species of mollicutes are shown in Fig. 2. Their distribution among species is listed in Table 1. Glycosylacylglycerols are the most ubiquitous of the glycolipids. The monoglycosyldiacylglycerol predominates, in contrast to bacteria, in which diglycosyldiacylglycerol is found in greater quantity. *A. axanthum* is unique in possessing a galactofuranose residue (26). Variation in the ratio of mono- to diglycosyl lipid occurs during the growth cycle (59, 98). Monoglucosyldiacylglycerol synthesis is stimulated in *A. laidlawii* A by exogenously supplied saturated or *trans*-unsaturated fatty acids (98). The ratio of mono- to diglucosyl lipid at any given stage of growth depends upon the optimal physical state of the lipid bilayer compatible with physiological function (97, 99). Glycosyldiacylglycerols containing three, four, and five sugar residues have been found in mollicutes. A pentaglycosyldiacylglycerol predominates in *A. modicum*, with one of the sugars being D-glycerol-D-mannoheptose (25, 27). *A. granularum* contains a structurally identified triglucosyldiacylglycerol (90). A triglycosyldiacylglycerol with glucose and galactose residues also has been isolated from *M. pneumoniae* (38). Sugar residues of the glycosyldiacylglycerols sometimes carry *O*-acyl groups, e.g., in *A. axanthum* (26) and *A. laidlawii* A (80). All sugars in these lipids are glycosidically linked but vary as to anomeric configuration and the carbon atoms involved. The nature and number of sugar residues and their anomeric linkages provide great diversity and are responsible for imparting antigenic specificity to many species (93).

The fatty acids associated with glycosyldiacylglycerols mimic the total fatty acid composition of the organisms. The distribution of total fatty acids is dependent upon the nature of the exogenous fatty acids of the culture medium. Almost 90% are 14:0, 16:0, and 18:1 (9) when organisms are grown in crude culture medium without specific fatty acid supplementation. Hydroxy fatty acids occur only in *A. axanthum*, which synthesizes D-(−)-3-hydroxyhexadecanoate and its analogs by elongation of preformed saturated fatty acids (28).

Polyterpenol Glycosides

Carotenyl and steryl glycosides occur in *Acholeplasma* species (26, 70), *M. gallinarum* (50, 71), and *Spiroplasma citri* (34). Although the usual glycoside in *M. gallinarum* is cholesteryl-β-D-glucopyranoside (Fig. 3, compound XI), this organism also is capable of biosynthesis of cholesteryl galactoside (71). Acholeplasmas synthesize carotenyl glucosides when grown in the absence of exogenous sterols. The anomeric configuration of the glucose moiety of this lipid in *A. laidlawii* A is α, while in *A. laidlawii* B it is β (65). Growth of acholeplasmas in the presence of cholesterol results in the formation of cholesteryl glucosides. *A. axanthum* also forms a diglucosylcholesterol (Fig. 3, compound XII) in addition to monoglucosylcholesterol. Acyl groups are found esterified to the sugar hydroxyl groups of the diglycosyl lipid (26). Limiting the glucose concentration in the culture medium stimulates the formation of a polyprenyl-α-D-glucoside with a long-chain fatty acid esterified to the 2-hydroxyl group of the sugar residue (4) in *A. laidlawii* B. As for the glycosyldiacylglycerols, the amount of polyterpenol glycosides varies with age, being the greatest in aged cells and lowest during exponential growth (26, 59, 89).

Acylated Sugars

M. gallinarum contains a 3,4,6-triacyl-β-D-glucopyranose in addition to the steryl glucoside (Fig. 3, compound X). The acyl groups are exclusively *cis*-18:1 (9, 89). The concentration of this lipid remains constant during the growth cycle. Acylated glucose also occurs in *S. citri*, although its exact structure has not been determined (34).

POLAR LIPIDS

The polar lipids of mollicutes make up about 50% of the total lipids and exhibit a rather wide diversity. Although glycerophospholipids predominate, nitrogen-containing phospholipids, phosphoglycolipids, and prenol phosphates appear in certain species (Fig. 4).

Phospholipids

Phosphatidylglycerol and diphosphatidylglycerol occur in all species examined (Table 1). Phosphatidic

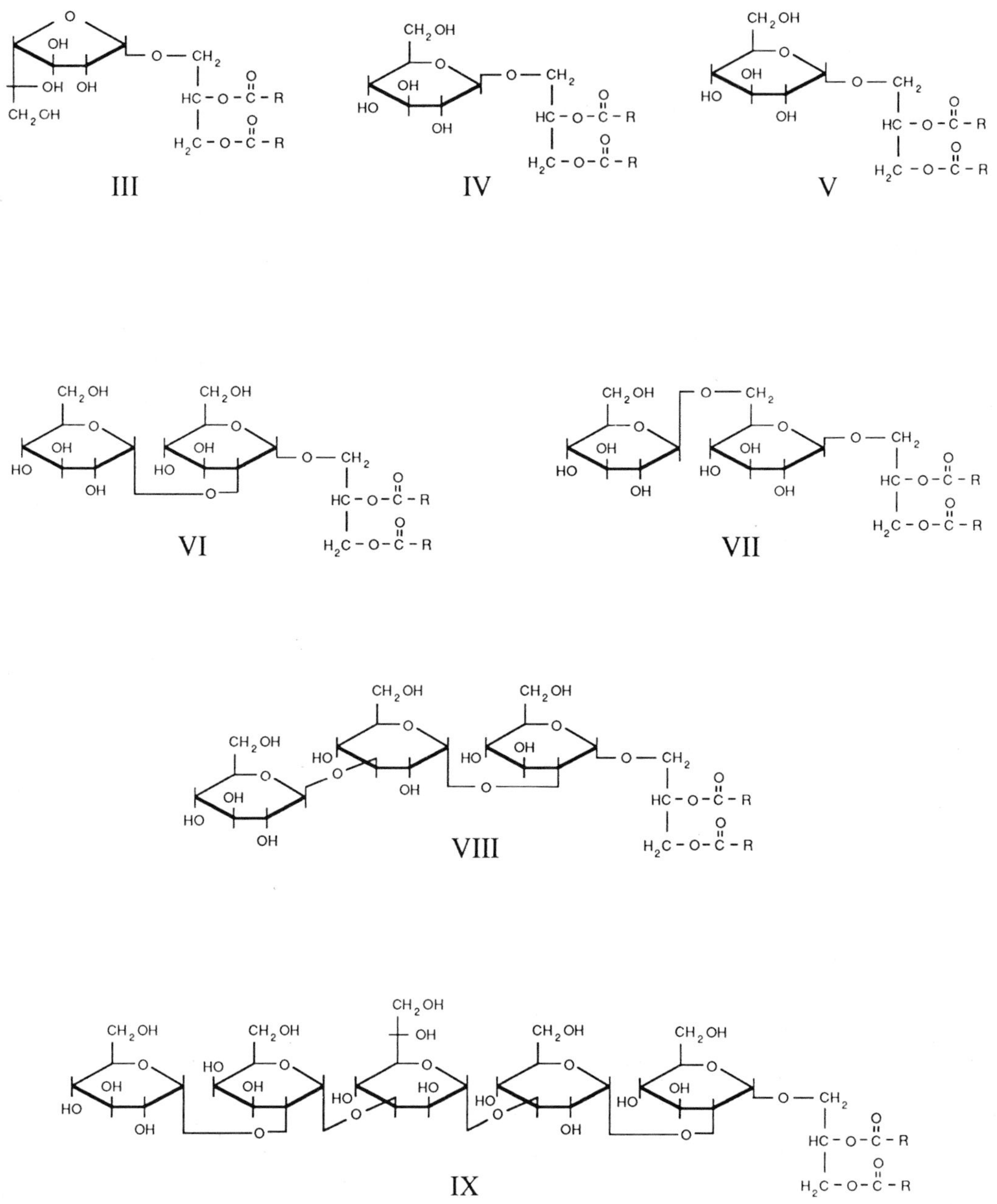

Figure 2. Glycosyldiacylglycerols of mollicutes. III, α-D-galactofuranosyldiacylglycerol; IV, β-D-glucopyranosyldia-cylglycerol; V, α-D-glucopyranosyldiacylglycerol; VI, α-D-glucopyranosyl-(1→2)-α-D-glucopyranosyldiacylglycerol; VII, β-D-glucopyranosyl-(1→6)-β-D-glucopyranosyldiacylglycerol; VIII, β-D-glucopyranosyl-(1→3)-α-D-glucopyran-osyl-(1→2)-α-D-glucopyranosyldiacylglycerol; IX, α-D-glucopyranosyl-(1→2)-α-D-galactopyranosyl-(1→3)-β-D-glyce-ro-D-mannoheptopyranosyl-(1→3)-α-D-glucopyranosyl-(1→2)-α-D-glucopyranosyldiacylglycerol.

acid appears to be a natural lipid in *M. neurolyticum* (72), *M. hominis* (57), and *U. urealyticum* (48). *M. galli-narum* is unique in possessing phosphatidylglycero-phosphate (85). Both lyso and more fully acylated de-rivatives of these glycerophospholipids occur in small amounts. The lyso forms are thought to arise as the result of deacylation during isolation. Fatty acyl groups exist as esters in all genera except *Anaer-oplasma*, in which alk-1-enyl residues of chain length C_{16} and C_{18} replace one-third of the total acyl content (22). Plasmalogens are restricted to the polar lipids of

this genus. The amounts of lipids vary with species and age of culture. Diphosphatidylglycerol accumulates in aged organisms at the expense of phosphatidylglycerol (69, 73). Aminoacylphosphatidylglycerols, which con-tain an amino acid esterified through its carboxyl group to one of the free hydroxyl groups of glycerol, are found in some species of *Acholeplasma* (21), *Myco-plasma* (72, 85), and *Anaeroplasma* (22). Proof of struc-ture has been established only for the alanylphosphati-dylglycerol from *A. laidlawii* B (Fig. 4, compound XIV). Both D and L isomers of alanine exist in a nonracemic

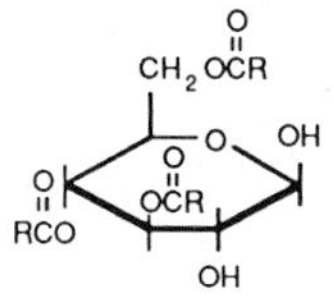

Figure 3. Glycolipids of mollicutes. X, 3,4,6-tri-*O*-acyl-β-D-glucopyranose; XI, β-D-glucopyranosyl-(1→3)-cholesterol; XII, α-D-glycopyranosyl-(1→3)-α-D-glucopyranosyl-(1→3)-cholesterol.

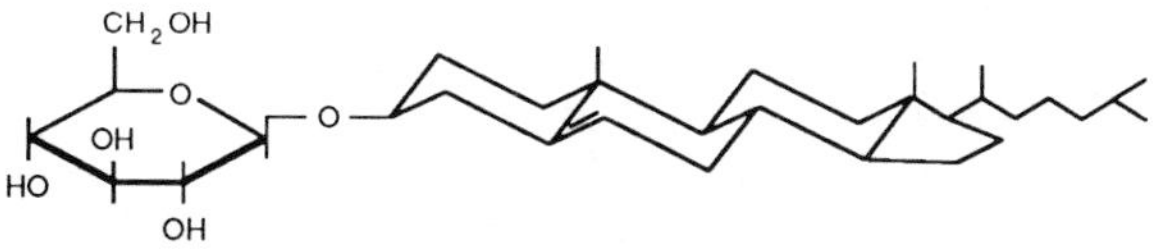

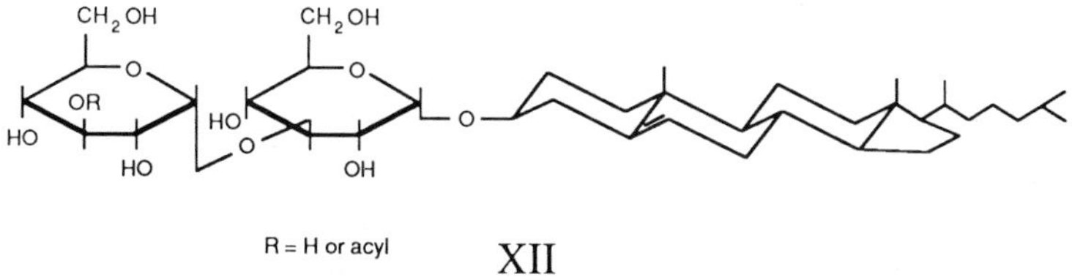

mixture of 2:1. This nonracemic content reflects different modes of biosynthesis. The D isomer is derived from an AMP-D-alanyl–enzyme complex; the L isomer derives from L-alanyl-tRNA (21). Smaller amounts of other amino acids, i.e., glutamic acid, glycine, leucine, lysine, and tyrosine, also are covalently linked to phosphatidylglycerol.

N-containing lipids have been found in *M. gallisepticum*, *U. urealyticum*, and *A. axanthum*. Like many other members of the mollicutes, *M. gallisepticum* incorporates exogenous phospholipids. However, in the case of this organism, phospholipids are required for growth (46). It is possible that the phosphatidylcholine and sphingomyelin found in *M. gallisepticum* (94) are necessary lipid components. Credence is given to this conclusion by the changes carried out on the fatty acyl residues. Transesterification of phosphatidylcholine appears to occur, since the acyl groups of the lipid isolated from the organism are fully saturated in contrast to this lipid in the culture medium (53). A similar alteration of phosphatidylcholine occurs in *M. pulmonis* and *M. pneumoniae* (51). *U. urealyticum* is the only member of the mollicutes thus far shown to contain phosphatidylethanolamine (48). This organism also contains an unidentified amino lipid which appears to be a diaminohydroxy compound with adjacent *O*-acyl and *N*-acyl groups. It is not identical to any known lipid. Ceramide lipids are restricted to *A. axanthum* among the mollicutes (39). An *O*-acyl ceramide-1-phosphoglycerol and its deacyl derivative, ceramide-1-phosphoglycerol, are found (Fig. 4, compound XVI), with the acyl form predominating (39). The chain length of the dihydrosphingosine-type base is

governed by the exogenous fatty acids supplied in the culture medium. This chain length is two carbon atoms longer than the precursor fatty acid, as with the free bases. The fatty acid in *N*-acyl linkage to the long-chain base is predominantly D-(−)-3-hydroxyhexadecanoate, but analogs of different chain lengths occur in smaller quantities (28). The *O*-acyl-linked fatty acid, esterified to the hydroxyl group of the hydroxy fatty acid, is either saturated or unsaturated but nonhydroxylated.

Distribution of the fatty acids of these phospholipids mimics the distribution of fatty acids in the culture medium. As with the glycolipids, over 90% consist of chain lengths 14:0, 16:0, and *cis*-18:1 (9). Except for *Anaeroplasma* species, in which one-third of the hydrocarbon chains of the glycolipids are alk-1-enyl residues, and *A. axanthum*, which contains 3-hydroxy fatty acids, all mollicutes normally possess only straight-chain saturated and unsaturated fatty acids (15, 62). The nutritional requirement for fatty acids permits the manipulation of both their content and their positional distribution. In *A. laidlawii* A, *cis*-18:1 can be replaced by *cis*-9,10-methylene-hexadecanoic acid, but not *cis*-16:1 (33). Growth with equimolar amounts of 16:0 and 18:0 fatty acids together with *trans*-18:1, *cis*-18:1, *cis,cis*-18:2, all-*cis*-18:3, or all-*cis*-20:4 results in decreasing incorporation of the more unsaturated fatty acids (49). The unsaturated fatty acids usually occupy position 2 on the glycerol residue (49). However, all *Mycoplasma* species examined (*M. capricolum*, *M. fermentans*, *M. gallinarum*, *M. gallisepticum*, *M. mycoides*, and *M. pneumoniae*), as well as *S. citri*, exhibit a preference for placing the unsaturated resi-

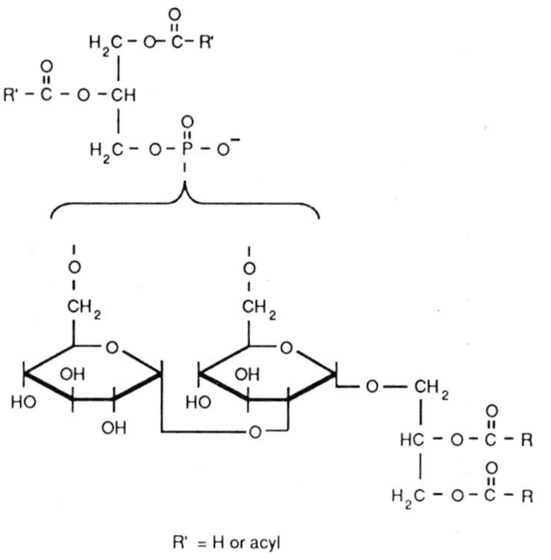

Figure 4. Polar lipids of mollicutes. XIII, 6-*O*-glycerophosphoryl-α-D-glucopyranosyl-(1→2)-α-D-glucopyranosyldiacylglycerol; XIV, phosphatidylglycerol and *O*-alanyl derivative; XV, [β-D-glucopyranosyl-(1→1)-x-glycerol-3-*O*-] [glyceraldehyde-3-*O*-][1,2-diacyl-x-glycerol-3-*O*-kojibiosyl-6-*O*-]-phosphate; XVI, ceramide phosphoglycerol.

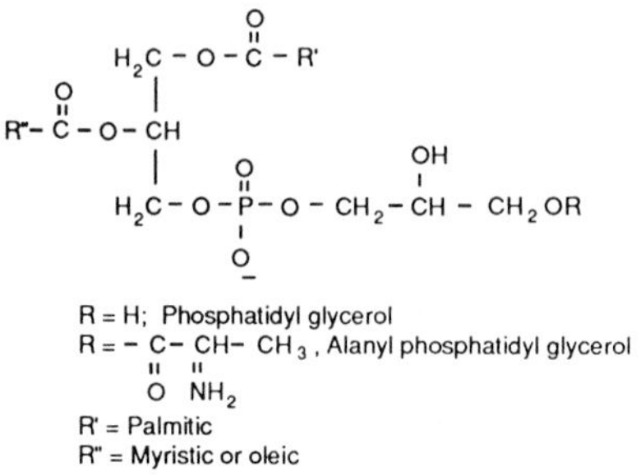

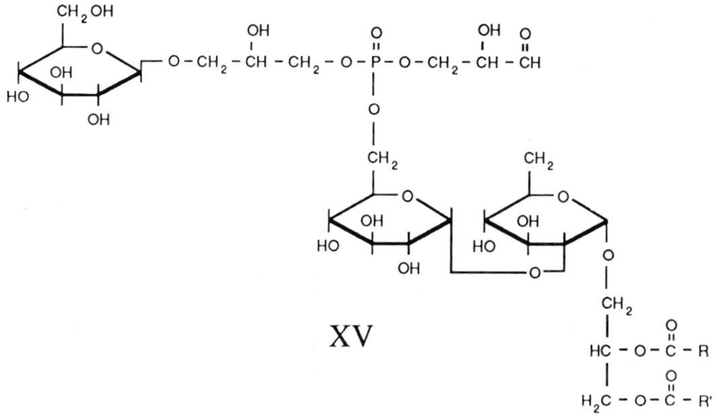

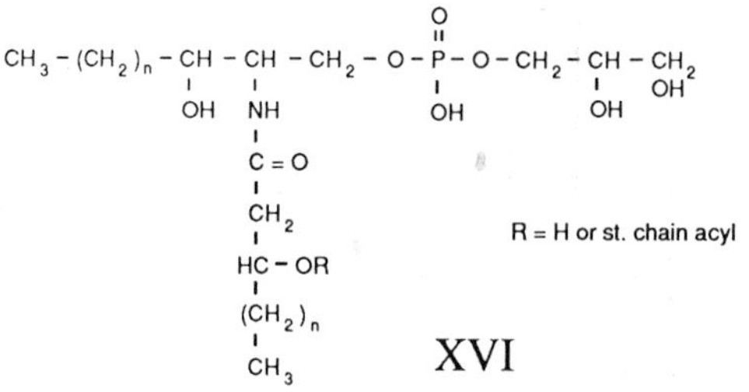

due on position 1 (11, 54) of phosphatidylglycerol. All of the phosphatidylglycerol is not homogeneous. Growth of *A. laidlawii* on *cis*-18:1 results in 16% of the phosphatidylglycerol containing two residues of this fatty acid and 84% with one unsaturated and one saturated fatty acid (3). Growth of *Mycoplasma* sp. strain Y on *trans*-18:1 (9) results in the formation of lipids containing 97% of the acyl residues as this fatty acid (44). Using inhibitors, a homogeneous fatty acid composition also has been obtained in *A. laidlawii* B without any obvious effect on growth (63).

Phosphoglycolipids

Phosphoglycolipids occur in *A. granularum*, in *A. hippikon*, and in *A. laidlawii* A and B. The structure of this type of lipid in *A. granularum*, which accounts for 15% of the total lipids, is unique in being a phosphotriester and containing a glyceraldehyde substituent (Fig. 4, compound XV) (90). The phosphoglycolipid of *A. laidlawii* B occurs both as a glycerophosphoryldiglucosyldiacylglycerol (60, 61) and as a phosphatidyldiglucosyldiacylglycerol (73) (Fig. 4, compound XIII).

Table 2. Occurrence of lipoglycans in mollicutes

Species containing lipoglycans	Species lacking lipoglycans
Acholeplasma axanthum	*Mycoplasma arthritidis*
A. granularum	*M. capricolum*
A. laidlawii	*M. gallinarum*
A. modicum	*M. gallisepticum*
A. oculi	*M. hyorhinis*
Anaeroplasma abactoclasticum	*M. pulmonis*
A. bactoclasticum	*Spiroplasma citri*
Mycoplasma mycoides	
M. neurolyticum	
Ureaplasma urealyticum	

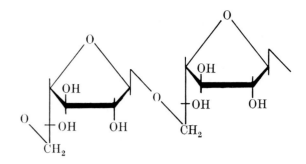

Figure 5. Disaccharide repeating unit of galactan from *M. mycoides*.

The glycolipid moiety is identical to the kojibiosyldiacylglycerol of the organism. *sn*-Glycerophosphate or its 1,2-diacyl derivative is attached to the six-carbon atom of glucose through a phosphodiester bond. It has been presumed, but not well established, that the terminal glucose is the site of the glycerophosphate. Only in *A. laidlawii* A has the stereochemical configuration of the glycolipid moiety been firmly established to be an α-D-glucopyranosyl-(1 → 2)-α-D-glucopyranosyl-(1 → 3)-*sn*-1,2-diacylglycerol (30). A glycerophosphoryl-monoglucosyldiacylglycerol is suspected to exist in both strains A (98) and B (83). The structure of the phosphoglycolipid in *A. hippikon* has not been determined (1a). Glycerophosphoryl glycolipids are found in many gram-positive bacteria, in which they are covalently linked to membrane teichoic acids (12). The relatively large amounts of these lipids in *Acholeplasma* species suggest that they accumulate as a result of attempts to synthesize wall components, reflecting a biosynthetic defect (90). Generally, the fatty acids of these lipids are similar to those of the phospholipids. However, the phosphatidyldiglucosyldiacylglycerol of *A. laidlawii* B contains significantly more short-chain saturated fatty acids (C_8 to C_{11}) in the phosphatidyl residue than in the glycolipid moiety (73).

Polyprenol Phosphates

All *Acholeplasma* species examined contain polyprenol phosphates. Their existence is mandated by the need for biosynthesis of lipoglycans. Although their structures have not been defined, they behave as bactoprenols by chromatographic techniques and become labeled with both [^{14}C]mevalonic acid and ^{32}P (76).

Trace amounts of naphthoquinones have been detected in *Acholeplasma*, *Mycoplasma*, and *Spiroplasma* species (18). Their formation by the organisms and their physiological role are suspect. Nevertheless, the NADH oxidases of some *Mycoplasma* species are stimulated by the naphthoquinone MK-7 (95). Benzoquinones have not been detected in mollicutes.

Table 3. Properties of lipoglycans from mollicutes[a]

Organism	% Dry wt	Sugar composition	Monomer size (Da)	Other components
Acholeplasma axanthum	0.9	Glc:Gal:FucN:QvN, 8:2:6:3	100,000	Gly, FA, P
A. granularum	1.3	Glc:Gal:GlcN:FucN, 3:3:2:1	20,000	Gly, FA
A. laidlawii	0.7	Glc:Man:FucN:QvN, 66:1:14:7	150,000	Gly, FA
A. modicum	0.7	Glc:Gal:GalN:FucN:QvN, 3:27:5:3:1	36,000	Gly, FA
A. oculi	2.3	Glc:Gal:Fuc, 3:19:2	30,000	Gly, FA
Anaeroplasma abactoclasticum	1.8	Glc:Gal:Man:FucN:GlcN, 32:3:1:35:7	ND	Gly, FA
A. bactoclasticum	2.5	Glc:Gal:Man:GlcN:GalN:FucN:QvN, 2:1:1:2:2:1:1	ND	Gly, FA
Mycoplasma neurolyticum	0.9	Gal:Glc:GalN:FucN, 15:1:4:4	ND	Gly, FA
M. mycoides	10.0	Gal	>100,000	Gly, FA
Mycoplasma sp. bovine arthritis strain	ND	Glc	ND	ND
Mycoplasma sp. strain F38	ND	Glc:Man:GlcN:GalN, 6:2:3:1	190,000	Gly, FA
Ureaplasma urealyticum	ND	Type 3: Man:Glc, 3:5 Type 4: Man:Glc:Gal, 15:15:2 Type 8: Man:Glc:Gal, 3:44:1	ND	Gly, FA, P

[a] Data compiled from references 1, 2, 6, 36, 58, 74, 75, 77, 78, 79, 88, and 92a. Abbreviations: Glc, glucose; Gal, galactose; Man, mannose; Fuc, fucose; FucN, fucosamine; QvN, quinovosamine (2-amino-6-deoxyglucose); GlcN, glucosamine; GalN, galactosamine; Gly, glycerol; FA, fatty acid esters; P, phosphorus; ND, not done.

Glc$p$(β1→2)-Glc$p$(α1→4)-Glc$p$(α1→3,4)-FcNAc(β1→3)-Gal$p$(α1→3)-Gal$p$(α1→3)-Gal$p$(α1→3,4)-GlcNAc(β1→3,4)-

GlcNAc(β1→4)-[Glc$p$(β1→2)-Glc$p$(α1→4)-Glc$p$(α1→3,4)-FcNAc(β1→3)-Gal$p$-

(α1→3)-Gal$p$(α1→3)-Gal$p$(α1→3,4)-GlcNAc(β1→3,4)-GlcNAc(β1→4)]$_{10}$-Glc$p$(β1→2)-Glc$p$(α1→4)-Glc$p$(α1→3,4)-

FcNAc(β1→3)-Gal$p$(α1→3)-Gal$p$(α1→3)-Gal$p$(α1→3,4)-GlcNAc(β1→3,4)-GlcNAc-diacylglycerol

Figure 6. Repeating unit of oligosaccharide of lipoglycan from *A. granularum*.

CONJUGATED LIPIDS

Lipoglycans

A class of compounds termed lipoglycans is found associated with the membranes of some species of the mollicutes (Table 2). Although they are extractable into hot aqueous 45% phenol, similar to bacterial lipopolysaccharides, they are distinguishable from these polymers with respect to both molecular structure and biological activity. All *Acholeplasma*, *Anaeroplasma*, and *Ureaplasma* species examined and a few *Mycoplasma* species contain these polymers. The lipoglycans form opalescent suspensions in water and clear upon addition of alkali, a reflection of their dual polymeric and lipoidal nature. Morphologically, they appear as fibrous structures by scanning electron microscopy. Transmission electron micrographs of negatively stained preparations exhibit ribbonlike structures 5 nm in width. Treatment with detergent results in the formation of vesicles (29).

Properties of the known lipoglycans are listed in Table 3. They make up 0.7 to 10% of the cellular dry weight and about 10% of the dry weight of membranes. When purified, they aggregate into large particles of several million daltons. Disaggregation by a variety of methods yields monomers varying in size from 20,000 to 190,000 Da. Each species has a distinctive polymer homogeneous as to size and structure (2, 74). The lipoglycans are firmly attached to the membranes, presumably by insertion of fatty acyl residues into the lipid bilayer. Exceptions to this condition are the polymers of *M. mycoides* and related strains, which shed large quantities of deacylated polysaccharides into the culture medium (6). Both amino and neutral sugars are found in all lipoglycans except those from *A. oculi*, *U. urealyticum*, and *M. mycoides* and the related

bovine arthritis strain (6, 37). All amino sugars of those polymers containing them are N acylated except for strain F-38, in which half are free amino groups (92a). Glycerol and fatty acid esters are found in all of the lipoglycans isolated from the organisms. Phosphorus occurs only in the polymers of *A. axanthum* (77) and *U. urealyticum* (79).

Structural characterization of only two lipoglycans has been accomplished. Some pertinent structural features of three others have been elucidated. The polymers from *M. mycoides* and *Mycoplasma* sp. bovine arthritis strain are homopolysaccharides. The major repeating structural unit of the galactan from *M. mycoides* has been identified as β-D-galactofuranosyl-(1 → 6)-D-galactopyranose (36) (Fig. 5). The predominant structural unit of the glucan from the bovine arthritis strain is β-D-glucopyranosyl-(1 → 2)-D-glucopyranose (37). The polymer from strain F-38 appears to consist of a 36-sugar repeat, every other unit containing a glucose branch attached to a mannose residue. All sugars, both neutral and amino, are linked in the β-anomeric configuration. Half of the amino sugars carry an N-acetyl group (92a). The polymer from *A. granularum* consists of 12 repeating units of 9 sugars terminating in a 2,3-diacylglycerol (1, 75) (Fig. 6). N-Acetyl groups are found on all amino sugars. The polymer from *A. axanthum* is an oligosaccharide chain consisting of 24 repeating units of 19 sugar residues (77) (Fig. 7). One galactose phosphate and two glycerophosphate residues are attached to position 6 of the three glucose units sandwiched by the amino sugars. No terminal diacylglycerol exists, nor are the glycerophosphate residues acylated. Rather, one of every four amino sugars contains an N-acyl fatty acid, 14:0 or 16:0 or 3-hydroxy 14:0 or 3-hydroxy 16:0. The remaining amino sugars are N acetylated.

Glc$p$(β1→2)-Glc$p$(β1→2)-Glc$p$(β1→6)-Gal$p$(β1→4)-Glc$p$(α1→4)-Glc$p$(α1→4)-FcNAc(β1→4)-FcNAc(β1→4)-FcNAc(β1→4)-FcNAc(β1→4)-FcNAc(β1→4)-FcNAc(β1→3)-


```
Gly-P      Gal-P       Gly-P
|(3→6)     |(α1→6)      |(3→6)
  Glcp(β1→3)-Glcp(β1→3)-Glcp(β1→4)-QvNAc(β1→4)-QvNAc(β1→4)-QvNAc(β1→4)-
```

Figure 7. Repeating unit of oligosaccharide of lipoglycan from *A. axanthum*.

Acylated Proteins

Acylated proteins have been detected in *A. laidlawii* (8, 32), *M. capricolum* (7), *M. hyopneumoniae* (101), *M. hyorhinis* (5), and *Spiroplasma* species (102). Thirty of fifty membrane polypeptides in *A. laidlawii* contain covalently bonded 18:0 but not 18:1 (9) fatty acid (8). This preference for saturated fatty acid is reflected in the ratio of 16:0 to 18:1 (9) fatty acids in individual proteins. This ratio was found to be 12 to 14 times larger than in the polar lipids of this organism (32). A similar number of acylated proteins appear in *M. capricolum*. However, this organism possesses the capability of incorporation of 18:1 (9) fatty acid into two major and four minor polypeptides (7). Twenty or more proteins of *M. hyopneumoniae*, *M. hyorhinis*, and *S. citri* exist in acylated form, with 16:0 fatty acid predominating. The number of acylated proteins in mollicutes exceeds by twofold the number in bacteria (32). Both exogenous phosphatidylglycerol and phosphatidylcholine serve as 16:0 fatty acid donors in *M. capricolum* (7). Glycerol is incorporated into the same proteins as is the 18:1 (9) fatty acid, suggesting a protein-bound diacylglycerol. Other sites, in addition to the diacylglycerol, along the polypeptide chain bind 16:0 fatty acid in this organism. The nature and significance of these proteins are covered in chapter 7.

REFERENCES

1. **Al-Samarrai, T. H., P. F. Smith, and R. J. Lynn.** 1983. Identification of the major antigenic determinants on lipoglycans from *Acholeplasma granularum* and *A. axanthum*. *Infect. Immun.* **40**:629–632.

1a. **Al-Shammari, A. J. N., and A. S. A. Al-Safar.** Unpublished data.

2. **Al-Shammari, A. J. N., and P. F. Smith.** 1979. Lipid and lipopolysaccharide composition of *Acholeplasma oculi*. *J. Bacteriol.* **139**:356–361.

3. **Bevers, E. M., J. A. F. OpdenKamp, and L. L. M. van Deenen.** 1978. The distribution of molecular classes of phosphatidyl glycerol in the membrane of *Acholeplasma laidlawii*. *Biochim. Biophys. Acta* **511**:509–512.

4. **Bhakoo, M., R. N. A. H. Lewis, and R. N. McElhaney.** 1987. Isolation and characterization of a novel monoacylated glucopyranosyl neutral lipid from the plasma membrane of *Acholeplasma laidlawii* B. *Biochim. Biophys. Acta* **922**:34–45.

5. **Bricker, T. M., M. J. Boyer, J. Keith, R. Watson-McKown, and K. S. Wise.** 1988. Association of lipids with integral membrane surface proteins of *Mycoplasma hyorhinis*. *Infect. Immun.* **56**:295–301.

6. **Buttery, S. H., and P. Plackett.** 1960. A specific polysaccharide from *Mycoplasma mycoides*. *J. Gen. Microbiol.* **23**:357–368.

7. **Dahl, C. E., and J. S. Dahl.** 1984. Phospholipids as acyl donors to membrane proteins of *Mycoplasma capricolum*. *J. Biol. Chem.* **259**:10771–10776.

8. **Dahl, C. E., N. C. Sacktor, and J. S. Dahl.** 1985. Acylated proteins in *Acholeplasma laidlawii*. *J. Bacteriol.* **162**:445–447.

9. **Dahl, J. S., C. E. Dahl, and K. Bloch.** 1980. Sterols in membranes: growth characteristics and membrane properties of *Mycoplasma capricolum* cultured on cholesterol and lanosterol. *Biochemistry* **19**:1467–1472.

10. **Dahl, J. S., C. E. Dahl, and K. Bloch.** 1981. Effect of cholesterol on macromolecular synthesis and fatty acid uptake by *Mycoplasma capricolum*. *J. Biol. Chem.* **256**:87–91.

11. **Davis, P. J., A. Katznel, S. Razin, and S. Rottem.** 1985. Spiroplasma membrane lipids. *J. Bacteriol.* **161**:118–122.

12. **Fischer, W., R. A. Laine, and M. Nakano.** 1978. On the relationship between glycerophosphoglycolipids and lipoteichoic acids in gram-positive bacteria. II. Structure of glycerophosphoglycolipids. *Biochim. Biophys. Acta* **528**:298–308.

13. **Freeman, B. A., R. Sissenstein, T. T. McManus, J. E. Woodward, I. M. Lee, and J. B. Mudd.** 1976. Lipid composition and lipid metabolism of *Spiroplasma citri*. *J. Bacteriol.* **125**:946–954.

14. **Gershfeld, N. L., M. Wormser, and S. Razin.** 1974. Cholesterol in mycoplasma membranes. I. Kinetics and equilibrium studies of cholesterol uptake by the cell membrane of *Acholeplasma laidlawii*. *Biochim. Biophys. Acta* **352**:371–384.

15. **Henrikson, C. V., and C. Panos.** 1969. Fatty acid composition, distribution, and requirements of two nonsterol-requiring mycoplasma from complex but defatted growth media. *Biochemistry* **8**:646–650.

16. **Henrikson, C. V., and P. F. Smith.** 1966. Growth response of *Mycoplasma* to carotenoid pigments and carotenoid intermediates. *J. Gen. Microbiol.* **45**:73–82.

17. **Herring, P. K., and J. D. Pollack.** 1974. Utilization of [1-¹⁴C] acetate in the synthesis of lipids by acholeplasmas. *Int. J. Syst. Bacteriol.* **24**:73–78.

18. **Holländer, R., G. Wolf, and W. Mannheim.** 1977. Lipoquinones of some bacteria and mycoplasmas, with consideration on their functional significance. *Antonie van Leeuwenhoek J. Microbiol. Serol.* **43**:177–185.

19. **Huang, L., and A. Haug.** 1974. Regulation of membrane lipid fluidity in *Acholeplasma laidlawii:* effect of carotenoid pigment content. *Biochim. Biophys. Acta* **352**:361–370.

20. **Kannenberg, E., and K. Poralla.** 1982. The influence of hopanoids on growth of *Mycoplasma mycoides*. *Arch. Microbiol.* **133**:100–102.

21. **Koostra, W. L., and P. F. Smith.** 1969. D- and L-alanyl phosphatidyl glycerols from *Mycoplasma laidlawii*. *Biochemistry* **8**:4794–4806.

22. **Langworthy, T. A., W. R. Mayberry, P. F. Smith, and I. M. Robinson.** 1975. Plasmalogen composition of *Anaeroplasma*. *J. Bacteriol.* **122**:785–787.

22a. **Langworthy, T. A., and P. F. Smith.** Unpublished data.

23. **Leon, O., and C. Panos.** 1981. Long-chain fatty acid perturbations in *Mycoplasma pneumoniae*. *J. Bacteriol.* **146**:1124–1134.

24. **Lynn, R. J., and P. F. Smith.** 1960. Chemical composition of PPLO. *Ann. N.Y. Acad. Sci.* **79**:493–498.

25. **Mayberry, W. R., T. A. Langworthy, and P. F. Smith.** 1976. Structure of the mannoheptose-containing pentaglycosyl diglyceride from *Acholeplasma modicum*. *Biochim. Biophys. Acta* **441**:115–122.

26. **Mayberry, W. R., and P. F. Smith.** 1983. Structures and properties of acyl diglucosyl cholesterol and galactofuranosyl diacylglycerol from *Acholeplasma axanthum*. *Biochim. Biophys. Acta* **752**:434–443.

27. **Mayberry, W. R., P. F. Smith, and T. A. Langworthy.** 1974. A heptose-containing pentaglycosyl diglyceride among the lipids of *Acholeplasma modicum*. *J. Bacteriol.* **118**:898–904.

28. **Mayberry, W. R., P. F. Smith, T. A. Langworthy, and P. Plackett.** 1973. Identification of amide-linked fatty acids of *Acholeplasma axanthum* S743 as D(−)-3-hydroxyhexadecanoate and its homologs. *J. Bacteriol.* **116**:1091–1095.

29. **Mayberry-Carson, K. J., I. M. Roth, and P. F. Smith.** 1975. Ultrastructure of lipopolysaccharide isolated from *Thermoplasma acidophilum*. *J. Bacteriol.* **121**:700–703.

30. **Michelsen, P.** 1985. A facile method for the determina-

tion of the absolute configuration of monoglucosyldiacyl-*sn*-glycerol. *Chem. Scr.* **25**:217–218.

31. **Nur, I., S. Razin, and S. Rottem.** 1984. Bilirubin incorporation into spirosplasma membrane and methylation of spiroplasmal DNA. *Isr. J. Med. Sci.* **20**:1019–1021.

32. **Nyström, S., K.-E. Johansson, and .Å Wieslander.** 1986. Selective acylation of membrane proteins in *Acholeplasma laidlawii.* *Eur. J. Biochem.* **156**:85–94.

33. **Panos, C., and O. Leon.** 1974. Replacement of the octadecenoic acid growth requirement for *Acholeplasma laidlawii* A by cis-9,10-methylene-hexadecanoic acid, a cyclopropane fatty acid. *J. Gen. Microbiol.* **80**:93–100.

34. **Patel, K. R., P. F. Smith, and W. R. Mayberry.** 1978. Comparison of lipids from *Spiroplasma citri* and corn stunt spiroplasma. *J. Bacteriol.* **136**:829–831.

35. **Plackett, P.** 1967. The glycerolipids of *Mycoplasma mycoides.* *Biochemistry* **6**:2746–2754.

36. **Plackett, P., and S. H. Buttery.** 1964. A galactofuranose disaccharide from the galactan of *Mycoplasma mycoides.* *Biochem. J.* **90**:201–205.

37. **Plackett, P., S. H. Buttery, and G. S. Cottew.** 1963. Carbohydrates of some mycoplasma strains. *Recent Prog. Microbiol.* **8**:533–547.

38. **Plackett, P., B. P. Marmion, E. J. Shaw, and R. M. Lemcke.** 1969. Immunochemical analysis of *Mycoplasma pneumoniae.* 3. Separation and chemical identification of serologically active lipids. *Aust. J. Exp. Biol. Med. Sci.* **47**:171–195.

39. **Plackett, P., P. F. Smith, and W. R. Mayberry.** 1970. Lipids of a sterol nonrequiring mycoplasma. *J. Bacteriol.* **104**:798–807.

40. **Pollack, J. D., K. D. Beaman, and J. A. Robertson.** 1984. Synthesis of lipids from acetate is not characteristic of *Acholeplasma* or *Ureaplasma* species. *Int. J. Syst. Bacteriol.* **34**:124–126.

41. **Pollack, J. D., and M. E. Tourtellotte.** 1967. Synthesis of saturated long chain fatty acids from sodium acetate-1-^{14}C by mycoplasma. *J. Bacteriol.* **93**:636–641.

42. **Razin, S.** 1974. Correlation of cholesterol to phospholipid content in membranes of growing mycoplasmas. *FEBS Lett.* **47**:81–85.

43. **Robinson, I. M., M. J. Allison, and P. A. Hartman.** 1975. *Anaeroplasma abactoclasticum* gen. nov., sp. nov.: an obligately anaerobic mycoplasma from the rumen. *Int. J. Syst. Bacteriol.* **25**:173–181.

44. **Rodwell, A. W.** 1963. The steroid growth requirement of *Mycoplasma mycoides.* *J. Gen. Microbiol.* **32**:91–101.

45. **Rodwell, A. W.** 1968. Fatty acid composition of mycoplasma lipids: biomembrane with only one fatty acid. *Science* **160**:1350–1351.

46. **Rodwell, A. W.** 1983. *Mycoplasma gallisepticum* requires exogenous phospholipid for growth. *FEMS Microbiol. Lett.* **17**:265–268.

47. **Romano, N., S. Rottem, and S. Razin.** 1976. Biosynthesis of saturated and unsaturated fatty acids by T-strain mycoplasma (*Ureaplasma*). *J. Bacteriol.* **128**:170–173.

48. **Romano, N., P. F. Smith, and W. R. Mayberry.** 1972. Lipids of a T-strain of *Mycoplasma.* *J. Bacteriol.* **109**:565–569.

49. **Romijn, J. C., L. M. G. van Golde, R. N. McElhaney, and L. L. M. van Deenen.** 1978. Some studies on the fatty acid composition of total lipids and phosphatidylglycerol from *Acholeplasma laidlawii* B and their relation to the permeability of intact cells of this organism. *Biochim. Biophys. Acta* **280**:22–32.

50. **Rothblat, G. H., and P. F. Smith.** 1961. Nonsaponifiable lipids of representative pleuropneumonia-like organisms. *J. Bacteriol.* **82**:479–491.

51. **Rottem, S., L. Adar, Z. Gross, Z. Ne'eman, and P. J. Davis.** 1986. Incorporation and modification of exogenous phosphatidylcholines by mycoplasmas. *J. Bacteriol.* **167**:299–304.

52. **Rottem, S., and A. S. Greenberg.** 1975. Changes in composition, biosynthesis, and physical state of membrane lipids occurring upon aging of *Mycoplasma hominis* cultures. *J. Bacteriol.* **121**:631–639.

53. **Rottem, S., and O. Markowitz.** 1979. Membrane lipids of *Mycoplasma gallisepticum:* a disaturated phosphatidylcholine and a phosphatidylglycerol with an unusual positional distribution of fatty acids. *Biochemistry* **18**:2930–2935.

54. **Rottem, S., and O. Markowitz.** 1979. Unusual positional distribution of fatty acids in phosphatidylglycerol of sterol-requiring mycoplasmas. *FEBS Lett.* **107**:370–382.

55. **Rottem, S., and O. Markowitz.** 1979. Carotenoids act as reinforcers of the *Acholeplasma laidlawii* lipid bilayer.*J. Bacteriol.* **140**:944–948.

56. **Rottem, S., E. A. Pfendt, and L. Hayflick.** 1971. Sterol requirements of T-strain mycoplasmas. *J. Bacteriol.* **105**:323–330.

57. **Rottem, S., and S. Razin.** 1973. Membrane lipids of *Mycoplasma hominis.* *J. Bacteriol.* **113**:565–571.

58. **Rurangirwa, F. R., T. C. McGuire, N. S. Magnuson, A. Kibor, and S. Chema.** 1987. Composition of a polysaccharide from *Mycoplasma* (F-38) recognized by antibodies from goats with contagious pleuropneumonia. *Res. Vet. Sci.* **42**:175–178.

59. **Shaw, N., P. F. Smith, and W. L. Koostra.** 1968. The lipid composition of *Mycoplasma laidlawii*, strain B. *Biochem. J.* **107**:329–333.

60. **Shaw, N., P. F. Smith, and H. M. Verheij.** 1970. The structure of 'phosphatidyl-glucose.' *Biochem. J.* **120**:439–441.

61. **Shaw, N., P. F. Smith, and H. M. Verheij.** 1972. The structure of a glycerophosphoryl-diglucosyl diglyceride from the lipids of *Acholeplasma laidlawii* strain B. *Biochem. J.* **129**:167–173.

62. **Silvius, J. R., and R. N. McElhaney.** 1978. Lipid compositional manipulation in *Acholeplasma laidlawii* B. Effect of exogenous fatty acids on fatty acid composition and cell growth when endogenous fatty acid production is inhibited. *Can. J. Biochem.* **56**:462–469.

63. **Silvius, J. R., and R. N. McElhaney.** 1978. Growth and membrane lipid properties of *Acholeplasma laidlawii* B lacking fatty acid heterogeneity. *Nature* (London) **272**:645–647.

64. **Smith, P. F.** 1962. Fate of ergosterol and cholesterol in pleuropneumonia-like organisms. *J. Bacteriol.* **84**:534–538.

65. **Smith, P. F.** 1963. The carotenoid pigments of *Mycoplasma. J. Gen. Microbiol.* **32**:307–319.

66. **Smith, P. F.** 1964. Relation of sterol structure to utilization in pleuropneumonia-like organisms. *J. Lipid Res.* **5**:121–125.

67. **Smith, P. F.** 1968. The lipids of mycoplasma. *Adv. Lipid Res.* **6**:69–105.

68. **Smith, P. F.** 1968. Nature of unsaponifiable lipids of a *Mycoplasma* strain grown with isopentenyl pyrophosphate as a substitute for sterol. *J. Bacteriol.* **95**:1718–1720.

69. **Smith, P. F.** 1969. The role of lipids in membrane transport in *Mycoplasma laidlawii. Lipids* **4**:331–336.

70. **Smith, P. F.** 1971. *The Biology of Mycoplasma.* Academic Press, London.

71. **Smith, P. F.** 1971. Biosynthesis of cholesterol glucoside by *Mycoplasma gallinarum. J. Bacteriol.* **108**:986–991.

72. **Smith, P. F.** 1972. Lipid composition of *Mycoplasma neurolyticum. J. Bacteriol.* **112**:554–558.

73. **Smith, P. F.** 1972. A phosphatidyl diglucosyl diglyceride from *Acholeplasma laidlawii* B. *Biochim. Biophys. Acta* **280**:375–382.

74. **Smith, P. F.** 1977. Studies on the homogeneity of lipopolysaccharides from *Acholeplasma. J. Bacteriol.* **103**:393–398.

75. **Smith, P. F.** 1981. Structure of the oligosaccharide of

lipoglycan from *Acholeplasma granularum. Biochim. Biophys. Acta* **665**:92–99.

76. **Smith, P. F.** 1982. Polyprenol phosphate in *Acholeplasma. Rev. Infect. Dis.* **4**:S266.

77. **Smith, P. F.** 1983. Structural characteristics of the lipoglycans from *Acholeplasma axanthum. Biochim. Biophys. Acta* **752**:271–276.

78. **Smith, P. F.** 1984. Lipoglycans from mycoplasmas. *Crit. Rev. Microbiol.* **11**:157–186.

79. **Smith, P. F.** 1985. Detection of lipoglycans in ureaplasmas. *J. Bacteriol.* **162**:611–614.

80. **Smith, P. F.** 1986. Structures of unidentified lipids in *Acholeplasma laidlawii* strain A-EF22. *Biochim. Biophys. Acta* **879**:107–112.

80a. **Smith, P. F.** Unpublished data.

81. **Smith, P. F., and J. E. Boughton.** 1960. Role of protein and phospholipid in growth of pleuropneumonia-like organisms. *J. Bacteriol.* **80**:851–860.

82. **Smith, P. F., and C. V. Henrikson.** 1965. Comparative biosynthesis of mevalonic acid by *Mycoplasma. J. Bacteriol.* **89**:146–153.

83. **Smith, P. F., and C. V. Henrikson.** 1965. Glucose containing phospholipids in *Mycoplasma laidlawii. J. Lipid Res.* **6**:106–111.

84. **Smith, P. F., and C. V. Henrikson.** 1966. Growth inhibition of *Mycoplasma* by inhibitors of polyterpene biosynthesis and its reversal by cholesterol. *J. Bacteriol.* **92**:1854–1858.

85. **Smith, P. F., and W. L. Koostra.** 1967. Phospholipids and glycolipids of sterol-requiring mycoplasma. *J. Bacteriol.* **93**:1853–1862.

86. **Smith, P. F., W. L. Koostra, and C. V. Henrikson.** 1965. Diphosphatidyl glycerol in *Mycoplasma laidlawii. J. Bacteriol.* **90**:282–283.

87. **Smith, P. F., and T. A. Langworthy.** 1979. The existence of carotenoids in *Acholeplasma axanthum. J. Bacteriol.* **137**:185–188.

88. **Smith, P. F., T. A. Langworthy, and W. R. Mayberry.** 1976. Distribution and composition of lipopolysaccharides from mycoplasmas. *J. Bacteriol.* **125**:916–922.

89. **Smith, P. F., and W. R. Mayberry.** 1968. Identification of the major glycolipid from *Mycoplasma* sp., strain J as 3,4,6-triacyl-β-D-glucopyranose. *Biochemistry* **7**:2706–2710.

90. **Smith, P. F., K. R. Patel, and A. J. N. Al-Shammari.** 1980. An aldehydo-phosphoglycolipid from *Acholeplasma granularum. Biochim. Biophys. Acta* **617**:419–429.

91. **Smith, P. F., and G. H. Rothblat.** 1960. Incorporation of cholesterol by pleuropneumonia-like organisms. *J. Bacteriol.* **80**:842–850.

92. **Smith, P. F., and G. H. Rothblat.** 1962. Comparative lipid composition of pleuropneumonia-like organisms and L-type organisms. *J. Bacteriol.* **83**:500–506.

92a. **Smith, P. F., F. R. Rurangirwa, and T. C. McGuire.** Unpublished data.

93. **Sugiyama, T., P. F. Smith, T. A. Langworthy, and W. R. Mayberry.** 1974. Immunological analysis of glycolipids and lipopolysaccharides derived from mycoplasmas. *Infect. Immun.* **10**:1273–1279.

94. **Tourtellotte, M. E., R. G. Jensen, G. W. Gander, and H. J. Morowitz.** 1963. Lipid composition and synthesis in the pleuropneumonia-like organism *Mycoplasma gallisepticum. J. Bacteriol.* **86**:370–379.

95. **VanDemark, P. J., and P. F. Smith.** 1964. Respiratory pathways in *Mycoplasma.* II. Pathway of electron transport during oxidation of reduced nicotine adenine dinucleotide by *Mycoplasma hominis. J. Bacteriol.* **88**:122–129.

96. **Wieslander, Å., A. Christiansson, L. Rilfors, A. Khan, L. B.-A. Johansson, and G. Lindblom.** 1981. Lipid phase structure governs regulation of lipid composition in membranes of *Acholeplasma laidlawii. FEBS Lett.* **124**:273–278.

97. **Wieslander, Å., A. Christiansson, L. Rilfors, and G. Lindblom.** 1980. Lipid bilayer stability in membranes. Regulation of lipid composition in *Acholeplasma laidlawii* as governed by molecular shape. *Biochemistry* **19**:3650–3655.

98. **Wieslander, Å., and L. Rilfors.** 1977. Qualitative and quantitative variations of membrane lipid species in *Acholeplasma laidlawii* A. *Biochim. Biophys. Acta* **446**:336–346.

99. **Wieslander, Å., L. Rilfors, L. B.-A. Johansson, and G. Lindblom.** 1981. Reversed cubic phase with membrane glucolipids from *Acholesplasma laidlawii*, ¹H, ²H and diffusion nuclear magnetic resonance measurements. *Biochemistry* **20**:730–735.

100. **Wieslander, Å., and E. Selstam.** 1987. Acyl-chain-dependent incorporation of chlorophyll and cholesterol in membranes of *Acholeplasma laidlawii. Biochim. Biophys. Acta* **901**:250–254.

101. **Wise, K. S., and M. F. Kim.** 1987. Major membrane surface proteins of *Mycoplasma hyopneumoniae* selectively modified by covalently bound lipid. *J. Bacteriol.* **169**:5546–5555.

102. **Wroblewski, H., S. Nyström, A. Blanchard, and Å. Wieslander.** 1989. Topology and acylation of spiralin. *J. Bacteriol.* **171**:5039–5047.

7. Membrane Protein Structure

ÅKE WIESLANDER, MICHAEL J. BOYER, and HENRI WRÓBLEWSKI

INTRODUCTION

Membrane proteins are usually divided into two categories (191). The majority, integral proteins, are intercalated more or less deeply into or even through the lipid double layer and are held in position by strong, mostly hydrophobic interactions between hydrophobic amino acid side chains and lipid hydrocarbon chains. They require disruption of the membrane bilayer by detergents, protein denaturants, or organic solvents in order to be released from the membrane. Peripheral proteins are bound to protein or lipid surfaces by mostly electrostatic interactions and are easily released by mild treatments such as changes in the ionic strength or pH of the medium or by the presence of a chelating agent.

Features of Mollicutes

Mollicutes possess four important properties that one must consider when analyzing and discussing the abundance, sequence, structure, organization, and function of their membrane proteins. (i) They are structurally simple, lacking a cell wall, periplasmic space, and outer membrane typical of eubacteria for the entrapment of a variety of extracellular proteins. Hence, the cytoplasmic membrane is exposed to the surrounding environment, except for a few species that have a well-developed capsule (see chapter 5). However, several species have a thin polysaccharide coat on the membrane outer surface (see chapters 5 and 6), as do most bacteria and eucaryotic cells. (ii) The genome has little coding capacity. For the mollicutes with the smallest genome sizes (see chapter 9), most genes must code for housekeeping proteins needed for the structure and basal metabolism of the cells. Even for mycoplasma species with larger genomes, the genome sizes are still approximately only one-third that of *Escherichia coli*. Hence, the fraction of housekeeping genes must be large and the ability to respond and adapt to environmental and metabolic conditions must be small, a view supported by the complex nutritional demands of most mollicutes. This notion suggests that many, perhaps even most, mollicute membrane proteins should be analogous to typical membrane and envelope proteins involved in transport and basal metabolism in common eubacteria. (iii) Mollicutes have small cell size, which gives them a substantially larger surface area-to-volume ratio. In combination with the thickness of membrane (see chapter 8) and space demand for the DNA chromosome, this yields a larger-volume fraction of the cells

Åke Wieslander and Michael J. Boyer • Department of Biochemistry, University of Umeå, S-901 87 Umeå, Sweden. **Henri Wróblewski** • Université de Rennes I, Centre National de la Recherche Scientifique, Unité de Recherche Associée no. 256, 35042 Rennes Cédex, France.

occupied by the membrane. This, in turn, suggests that a greater number (and amount) of the different cellular proteins should be of membrane origin than in common larger eubacteria. (iv) Mollicutes occupy specific ecological niches. All currently known species seem to live in close association with eucaryotic hosts, many as membrane surface parasites (see chapter 1). To do so, they must have the means to protect themselves from the various defensive mechanisms of their hosts, such as the immune system in higher animals and antibacterial peptides in insects (16).

Functions of Membrane and Envelope Proteins

The functions associated with membrane and envelope proteins in bacteria can be divided into several characteristic groups. Many proteins in these groups have typical features that are easily discerned at the amino acid sequence level. First, there are the structural and enzyme proteins for the synthesis and assembly of the peptidoglycan mesh, outer membrane, and polysaccharide coat of the envelopes. Second, many bacteria have more or less elaborate electron transport chains in which metabolic free energy is converted through several redox reactions into a chemiosmotic potential difference across the membrane. The potential can be transferred into ATP through the activities of membrane-associated ATPases; this reaction can also occur in the opposite direction. Third, a large number of typical transport and channel proteins are responsible for the uptake and excretion of precursors and metabolites. Outer membrane barriers usually contain more or less selective molecular-sieving pore proteins. Fourth, in addition to the components of the protein secretory apparatus, several export proteins need the assistance of specific helper proteins in order to be secreted. Fifth, bacteria have the means to sense a number of parameters in their immediate surroundings such as the concentrations of certain metabolites. Several of these systems involve both typical binding and sensor proteins. Sixth, motility devices such as flagella and filaments are usually of unique composition. Seventh, several types of receptors and pili for the attachment of bacteria to surfaces have been characterized. In addition to these proteins, many bacteria have proteins with different variable surface regions to escape the immunological surveillance of their eucaryotic hosts.

STRUCTURAL PROPERTIES OF MEMBRANE AND SECRETED PROTEINS

Integral Membrane Proteins

Peripheral proteins have no unique sequence or structural properties, except for a temporary export signal in secreted proteins, but seem in all aspects to be similar to soluble globular proteins. The present structural classifications of soluble proteins were clear only after high-resolution structures were available for over 100 different proteins (183). By contrast, high-resolution three-dimensional (3-D) structures are available only for a small group of intergral membrane proteins. The best known are (i) the photosynthetic reaction center from *Rhodopseudomonas viridis* (41), (ii) the light-driven proton pump bacteriorhodopsin from *Halobacterium halobium* (69), (iii) the plant light-harvesting complex (109), and (iv) an outer membrane porin from *Rhodobacter capsulatus* (221). In a second group containing an increasing number of membrane proteins, 2-D crystals are yielding high-resolution data but at a substantially lower level of detail. For the vast majority of membrane proteins, the primary amino acid sequence, derived from the DNA sequence, is currently the only source of structural information. However, these data are usually complemented with biochemical, genetic, and spectroscopic analyses. Together with an array of methods for computer analysis of amino acid sequences (51, 66), one can often obtain a rough estimate of the possible function and orientation in the membrane of a certain protein.

It was predicted before the structures noted above were solved that the membrane-spanning parts of many integral proteins should consist of one or several α helices containing approximately 18 to 25 mostly hydrophobic and uncharged amino acid residues. For certain proteins like porin, a hydrophobic or amphiphilic β-sheet structure of 8 to 10 amino acid residues has been proposed. Analyses of the few 3-D structures known (see above) have so far verified these predictions. The number and type of membrane-spanning segments are currently used to classify integral membrane proteins, and they are obtained as described above. Monotopic proteins are hydrophobically associated with the membrane but do not pass all the way across the bilayer. Bitopic proteins cross the membrane once, and polytopic proteins cross more than once (85). The hydrophilic loops connecting these hydrophobic segments must be properly localized to the correct side of the membrane in order for the protein to function. It has been shown that the apolar segments are parts of clearly definable sequence elements (topogenic signals) that help to localize the polar loops (reviewed in references 211 and 215). Such hydrophobic segments are usually called signal peptides when localized at an N-terminal position (see next section), whereas the segments that hold the hydrophilic loops in position are called stop transfer or anchor sequences. The bitopic and polytopic proteins can be divided into four classes according to their topology in the membrane (Fig. 1). Class I proteins have a cleavable N-terminal signal peptide followed by hydrophilic loop and a hydrophobic anchor sequence. The latter is followed by a cluster of positively charged amino acids, and the final orientation of processed proteins is N terminus out/C terminus in. Class II proteins have an uncleaved signal peptide acting as an anchor, giving the proteins an N terminus in/C terminus out topology. Class III proteins are similar but have an N terminus out/C terminus in orientation due to a positive cluster after the anchor segment, opposite the class II proteins. Class IV proteins have multiple hydrophobic regions spanning the membrane. For all of these hydrophobic protein segments, an enrichment of positive amino acids in the closely flanking regions is observed on the cytoplasmic side in comparison with the outer side, especially in bacterial proteins—the so-called positive-inside rule (19, 212).

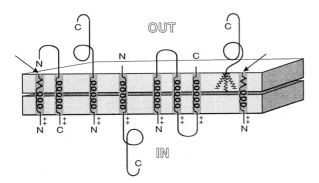

Figure 1. Classification of integral membrane proteins. Cleavable signal peptides are removed (arrows) after initiation of translocation. Classes I to IV refer to the different transmembrane topologies of the proteins. Most bacterial lipoproteins lack transmembrane segments and are anchored in the membrane by three fatty acid chains. (Modified from references 152, 212, and 215.)

Export Signals

The mechanisms whereby proteins are transported across the plasma membrane are evolutionarily highly conserved processes (152, 209). Proteins are allowed entry into a secretory pathway only if they possess specific targeting signals. The majority of proteins destined for export contain an N-terminal extension of 15 to 35 mainly hydrophobic amino acid residues called a signal peptide (212). In eubacteria, most periplasmic, outer membrane, and secreted proteins have cleavable signal peptides, a feature not usually associated with cytoplasmic or inner membrane proteins (130, 152, 192). Analyses of bacterial signal peptides reveal that they display little amino acid sequence similarity despite their common role in mediating protein transport (157). However, they do have some features in common: (i) a positively charged amino-terminal region, (ii) a central hydrophobic core, (iii) a polar carboxy-terminal region containing a recognizable cleavage site (145, 210), and (iv) a net-plus-to-minus-charge dipole around the hydrophobic segment (137). Apart from these similar characteristics, differences are apparent. For example, gram-positive bacteria normally have signal peptides longer than those from gram-negative bacteria (213), whereas signal peptides from lipoproteins are shorter and more hydrophobic (106). In *E. coli*, the composition and properties of signal peptides from proteins destined for different cellular compartments vary in a typical fashion (192). Hence, signal peptides cannot always be interchanged between exported proteins and still promote the export of the heterologous protein (110). Certain proteins are also translocated by the help of noncleaved N- and C-terminal hydrophobic or amphiphilic peptide segments (103, 214, 235).

In *E. coli*, the translocation machinery of the inner membrane contains several different proteins, i.e., SecA, -B, -E, and -Y and leader peptidases I and II, that act upon the preproteins in a stepwise manner during the translocation pathway (222). The process demands ATP and a proton gradient across the membrane and can occur both co- and posttranslationally. Several different chaperons, including SecB, may be involved, imposing upon the preproteins a folding competent for translocation. Several membrane and export proteins are known to have a translocation independent of the Sec proteins, but the structural reasons for this are not established. At present, it is not known whether the translocation machinery has a similar general composition in all bacteria. The only protein found so far that seems to be widespread is SecY, the gene of which is found also in *Mycoplasma capricolum* (107). Secretion beyond the outer membrane in gram-negative bacteria seems to need the assistance of specific helper or accessory proteins, sometimes also those of the translocation machinery (see above). Examples are hemolysins, enterotoxins, colicins, pili, and certain extracellular enzymes (73, 153, 195). Many secreted proteins in gram-positive bacteria have a two-step processing: removal of the signal peptide and, sometimes at a later stage, removal of an extra propeptide between the signal peptide and the mature protein (218). Several gram-positive membrane surface proteins have a conserved sequence motif adjacent to the hydrophobic region important for the anchoring of these proteins (53).

Lipid Modification

A small but significant fraction of the proteins in most biological membranes that have been investigated are covalently modified with various lipid tails. These include proteins with a variety of different functions normally associated with membranes. In procaryotes, structural and enzyme proteins are common (67), whereas in eucaryotes, receptor and signaling proteins have dominated (125).

Typically, bacterial cells contain up to ten different lipid-modified proteins. A unifying feature of most known bacterial lipoproteins is that they are synthesized as precursors with signal peptides which are processed by a specific lipoprotein signal peptidase (leader peptidase II). The latter recognizes a short consensus sequence at the C-terminal region of the signal sequence in the preprotein and leaves a diacylglycerol-modified cysteine residue as the N terminus of the cleaved mature protein (67). This step is specifically inhibited by the drug globomycin. A third acyl chain is later bound to the free amino group of the cysteine residue by an amide bond. The lipoproteins can be metabolically labeled by radioactive glycerol and fatty acids or by native phospholipid acyl chains (67). For Braun's lipoprotein in *E. coli* as well as for several other bacterial lipoproteins, the acyl chain composition is similar to the acyl chain composition of the membrane lipids, perhaps with a slight enrichment of saturated species (23, 140). In *E. coli*, the lipoprotein signal peptidase has a transmembrane topology with the active side on the outer face of the cytoplasmic (inner) membrane similar to the general signal peptidase (leader peptidase I) (129). The overwhelming majority of all known bacterial lipoproteins are devoid of potential membrane-anchoring sequences other than the fatty acyl groups (67, 152). According to the described consensus mechanism, bacterial lipoproteins should contain three N-terminal acyl chains as originally determined for Braun's lipoprotein in *E. coli* (reviewed in reference 23). However, this feature has been established chemically for a surprisingly small number of proteins. For several others, the extent of modification is less than three chains per polypeptide (reviewed in reference 140). It should be noted that several mechanisms other than the consensus one for lipid modification of bacterial proteins exist. For example, a mechanism involving a modification with amide-linked acyl chains in the C-terminal region of the mature protein was recently described in *E. coli* (77).

Recent data suggest that most lipoproteins in *E. coli* and other gram-negative bacteria are anchored by their lipid moiety in the outer membrane and facing the periplasmic space (18, 154). In gram-positive bacteria, certain enzymatic lipoproteins, anchored at the outer surface of the membrane after signal peptide cleavage, can be released to the surroundings by a protease-dependent mechanism, leaving the lipid moiety plus a small peptide in the membrane (126). A similar two-step release process has recently been found in a gram-negative bacterium, but translocation across the outer membrane demands the presence of helper proteins (72). Proteolytic release of lipid-modified membrane proteins is a common phenomenon in eucaryotes (47).

At least four different mechanisms exist for the modification of eucaryotic proteins with lipid tails. One group of proteins found in both the cytosol and plasma membrane contain an amide-linked myristic acid (14:0) at the N-terminal glycine, which is added cotranslationally and has no turnover (125). Another group of proteins, predominantly membrane associated, have an ester-linked (S or O) palmitic acid at an internal residue, most often a cysteine. The fatty acid is most often added posttranslationally and can show turnover (182). Yet other proteins may change location from the cytosol to the membrane dependent upon the addition of an S-ether-linked isoprenoid chain to an internal or C-terminal cysteine residue (118). Lastly, a large group of proteins are anchored, most often at the outer surface of the plasma membrane, by a C-terminal glycosylphosphatidylinositol lipid anchor (116). Many of these proteins may be released by proteolytic processing after, e.g., a hormone signal (47). So far, none of these eucaryotic mechanisms have been observed in procaryotes. Likewise, the consensus lipoprotein modification in procaryotes has not been found in eucaryotes. For the recently observed isoprenoid-modified proteins in archaebacteria (50) and *Acholeplasma laidlawii* (141), the chemical structures of the isoprenoid chains are not yet known.

OCCURRENCE OF MOLLICUTE MEMBRANE PROTEINS

Electrophoretic patterns of mollicute membrane proteins are highly reproducible and species specific. Moreover, membrane protein composition is usually not affected by variations in growth conditions (164). The fraction of proteins in the membranes (50 to 60% by weight) is similar to that in many other bacterial and eucaryotic membranes (161). In *A. laidlawii*, the number of membrane proteins, as estimated by 2-D gel electrophoresis, has been reported to be approximately 140 or 200 (9, 140). The first figure was 44% of the total number of proteins in the cell, i.e., 320 (9). This percentage is similar to the weight fraction of membrane protein in relation to the total cell protein, as determined by colorimetric methods. 2-D gel electrophoretic analysis has revealed 300 and 355 cellular proteins in *M. mycoides* and *M. capricolum* (102, 173). A simultaneous analysis revealed approximately 1,100 proteins in *E. coli* and *Bacillus subtilis* (102). Recent analyses have revealed approximately 1,800 polypeptides in *E. coli*, at least 200 of which are of membrane origin (6, 134, 181). However, the genome of 4,720 kbp in *E. coli* has a substantially larger coding capacity, but only a fraction of these genes are expressed under any given conditions. Most likely, *E. coli* codes for well over 3,000 different peptides. Many of these peptides probably occur at extremely low numbers, perhaps a few dozen per cell (134), and are thus difficult to analyze.

Membranes constitute slightly less than 10% of *E. coli* on a weight basis (134), which makes 300 different membrane proteins a reasonable estimate. For *A. laidlawii*, with a genome size of 1,600 kbp (see chapter 9), a larger fraction of the cellular proteins localized to the membrane, and perhaps a larger fraction of constitutively expressed genes, the number of membrane proteins is probably at least 200. *M. mycoides* and *M. capricolum* should contain fewer membrane proteins because of their smaller genomes, as observed for their estimated numbers of cellular proteins (see above). However, the 40 to 50 membrane proteins resolved by 2-D gel electrophoresis from *Spiroplasma citri* and *M. gallisepticum* are most likely substantially below the true values (8, 189). The same holds for the more than 50 polypeptides resolved from membranes of *M. pneumoniae* and *M. fermentans* by high-resolution 1-D gel electrophoresis (55).

SOLUBILIZATION, PURIFICATION, AND RECONSTITUTION

Full structural and functional characterization of a protein requires its purification to homogeneity. In the case of membrane proteins, it is generally necessary to isolate the relevant membrane, to detach or extract proteins under a soluble form from the membrane, and to eventually separate them by appropriate techniques. When one deals with mollicutes, the preliminary step of the procedure, the isolation of a pure membrane fraction, is in principle much easier than with other bacteria or with eucaryotic cells, the mammalian erythrocyte being one exception. The permanent absence of a cell wall in mollicutes considerably facilitates the lysis of the cells. Furthermore, the fact that the plasma membrane is the only membrane present in the cell leads de facto to obtaining homogeneous membrane preparations (164, 165).

Cell Lysis and Membrane Isolation

The great structural simplicity and the absence of a cell wall facilitate the lysis of mollicute cells by gentle methods such as hypo-osmotic shock (164, 165, 167). Osmotic lysis is thus often the most appropriate method for disrupting these bacteria. However, it should be stressed that though the cells of some species are very sensitive to osmotic shock, others are much more resistant. *A. laidlawii* and *M. gallisepticum* exemplify the two extremes which may be encountered, the former being much more tractable than the latter. Mollicutes are indeed capable of resisting osmotic lysis by both passive and active mechanisms. Because of its small size, the mollicute cell exhibits a high surface-to-volume ratio, which facilitates the quick lowering of the intracellular osmotic pressure by fast leakage of cytoplasmic solutes (164). Furthermore, the plasma membrane possesses a high tensile strength which may be further increased by the presence of large amounts of cholesterol. The abundance of glycolipids provides an additional means of strengthening the membrane by the formation of a network of hydrogen bonds (34). The situation is complicated by the fact that osmotic sensitivity is also dependent on the physiological state of the cells. Stationary-phase cells are much more resistant than exponentially growing ones (158, 159), and the lipid composition of the membrane markedly affects the sensitivity of the cells (170). In addition to the above-mentioned effect of cholesterol, fatty acid composition contributes to the molecular ordering and subsequently the elasticity of the membrane. For example, enrichment of membrane lipids with palmitoyl and stearoyl chains enhances the osmotic sensitivity of *A. laidlawii* cells (170). It is also likely that mollicutes can resist osmotic lysis by active permeability mechanisms dependent on membrane ATPases. For example, dicyclohexylcarbodiimide, an ATPase inhibitor, enhances swelling and subsequent lysis of *M. gallisepticum* cells placed in an iso-osmotic NaCl solution (176a). Some species of mollicutes might also possess a type of intracellular cytoskeleton (119) conferring on them an additional means of resisting lysis.

To overcome these difficulties, alternative methods may be used to lyse mollicute cells. An improvement of the standard osmotic shock method consists of preloading the cells with glycerol to increase internal osmotic pressure (178). Osmotic lysis of *M. gallisepticum* cells has been enhanced by treatment with dicyclohexylcarbodiimide (176a, 188), a procedure which also was found to work with different spiroplasma species (238, 240). Lysis may also be enhanced by incorporation of digitonin into the membrane of mollicutes containing large amounts of cholesterol (177). In this case, digitonin modifies the membrane architecture by forming complexes with cholesterol: the asymmetrical incorporation of digitonin into the membrane induces the formation of hemitubules, with subsequent disruption of the cell envelope (127). The use of alkali is another simple means of lysing wall-less bacteria (166), a method which proved efficient with *M. gallisepticum* (63, 187).

In case of failure of these gentle procedures, one may rely on mechanical methods, notably ultrasonic oscillation or treatment with a French pressure cell or an X press. Sonic oscillation is usually very efficient on mollicutes but has the drawback of breaking the membrane into small pieces which are difficult to recover by centrifugation, especially if the irradiation time has been unduly prolonged (100, 101, 150, 151). However, this method offers the advantage of breaking the chromosome into small fragments which are easy to wash out. Otherwise, it is necessary to hydrolyze the DNA, *A. laidlawii* being an exception because in this species endogenous nucleases are highly active. When commercial nucleases are used, it is of utmost importance that phospholipase-free preparations be used if unaltered membranes are to be obtained (11). In some cases, the presence of active peptidases may also be a problem (29). Cell coating with concanavalin A was used to stabilize *S. citri* membranes against excessive fragmentation by ultrasonic irradiation (189). However, because of the introduction of high levels of the lectin in the preparations, this method seems of little value for purifying membrane proteins. Finally, alternate freezing and thawing (56) has also been used to disrupt mollicute cells. Though this method is quite simple, it has been much less used than the methods mentioned above because of protein denaturation.

Once cells are lysed, membranes can be recovered by the simple means of centrifugation. Repeated sedimentations and dispersions in an appropriate buffer may then be used to wash out contaminating material of cytoplasmic or culture medium origin. At this stage of membrane preparation, it is often difficult to find a good compromise between elimination of undesirable nonmembrane molecules and involuntary removal of loosely bound peripheral membrane proteins (see below). To assess the purity of the preparations, the more commonly used criteria are homogeneity in isopycnic ultracentrifugation, ultrastructure, chemical composition, and enzyme markers (162, 169). ATPase activity is exclusively associated with the plasma membrane in mollicutes and therefore constitutes a good marker of this compartment, whereas enzymes such as hexokinase for fermentative mollicutes or urease for ureaplasmas may be used as markers of the cytoplasm (165).

For detailed coverage of mollicute cell lysis and membrane preparation, the reader is referred to references 162 and 165.

Solubilization and Analysis

Essentially two distinct cases must be considered for the solubilization of membrane proteins: (i) peripheral proteins which have to be detached from the membrane to which they are adsorbed and (ii) integral membrane proteins which have to be extracted from the lipid bilayer in which they are more or less deeply embedded or anchored by covalently attached acyl chains.

Since peripheral proteins are adsorbed to the membrane by weak forces such as ionic bonds and divalent cation bridges (191), they may be detached by transferring the membranes in buffers of appropriate pH and ionic strength. In the case of mollicutes, low-ionic-strength buffers are the most effective, but EDTA must be used to achieve the release of some peripheral proteins which are more tightly bound to the membrane. According to different estimations, 8 to 14% of the proteins are released by EDTA treatment of *A. laidlawii* and *M. hominis* membranes obtained from cells lysed by osmotic shock (4, 131, 132). In the case of *S. citri*, use of the method developed to detach spectrin and other peripheral proteins from the membrane of human erythrocytes (120) permits desorption of about 15% of the spiroplasma membrane protein fraction (229). In fact, these values should be considered as a minimum since it is generally assumed that a fraction of the peripheral proteins is lost during membrane isolation (162, 163). In *A. laidlawii*, for example, these components probably represent about 50% of the membrane protein fraction, corresponding to approximately 60 polypeptides out of 140 resolved by 2-D electrophoresis (9). In the case of sealed membrane vesicles, it may prove necessary to disrupt the vesicles with low concentrations of mild surfactants to bring about desorption of peripheral proteins. The risk is then that some integral membrane proteins may also be extracted.

Thus, given the operational definition of most peripheral membrane proteins of mollicutes, it is difficult to rigorously describe this fraction. At the extremes, one finds tightly bound proteins which may be released only if divalent cations are chelated and loosely bound proteins which are sometimes difficult to distinguish from cytoplasmic proteins or serum proteins from the culture medium. Contamination of membrane preparations by adsorption or precipitation and cosedimentation of serum proteins most frequently happens with fast-growing fermentative mollicutes (22), and with fastidious mollicutes such as ureaplasmas and some mycoplasmas such as *M. hyopneumoniae* (135, 144). Adsorption of serum proteins to the cell surface is enhanced by low pH (176), which occurs at the end of the growth of fermentative mollicutes. Some of these exogenous proteins are so tightly bound to the membrane that they may easily be confused with true membrane proteins. Metabolic radiolabeling is one effective way to discriminate cell proteins from exogenous contaminants in mollicutes (128, 190).

In contrast to peripheral proteins, integral membrane proteins are bound to the membrane not only by ionic bonds but also by hydrophobic interactions. Though ethanol and sodium diiodosalicylate have been used to extract NADH oxidase and a glycoprotein from the membranes of, respectively, *A. laidlawii* (84) and *M. gallisepticum* (64), the use of surfactants is a much more effective and general procedure. Sodium dodecyl sulfate (SDS) is a powerful anionic surfactant capable of completely dissolving the membrane of mollicutes (168). It is thus widely used for analytical purposes, chiefly in SDS-polyacrylamide gel electrophoresis and the 2-D method of O'Farrell (142), in which SDS-polyacrylamide gel electrophoresis constitutes the second-dimension electrophoresis. High-resolution 1-D SDS-polyacrylamide gel electrophoresis techniques are capable of detecting about 50 distinct polypeptides in mollicute membranes, whereas at least three times more components are evidenced by 2-D methods. Full dissociation of the proteins necessitates, in both cases, reduction of disulfide bonds. It should be noted, however, that when silver is used to reveal proteins, staining artifacts must be taken into account for accurate estimation of the number of polypeptides (46). Furthermore, the information obtained by 2-D techniques may be redundant in the sense that the same polypeptide may contribute to the formation of several distinct spots in the gel. This is the case for *S. citri* spiralin, which is resolved into four spots differing in their isoelectric points, which probably reflects heterogeneity in posttranslational modifications of the protein (13).

Nondenaturing surfactants have also been used for analytical purposes, specifically in 2-D immunoelectrophoresis (crossed immunoelectrophoresis) (1–3, 88, 89, 93, 96, 97, 104, 105, 202, 226, 233). The advantage of these surfactants is that they extract membrane proteins in a nondenatured form, identical or nearly identical to the native structure, with the possible retention of activity. Their drawback is that in principle, they do not completely dissolve membranes but instead selectively extract a more limited number of proteins. As discussed below, this differential extraction may be exploited for the purification of integral membrane proteins. The first analysis of a mollicute membrane by crossed electrophoresis was performed by Johansson and Hjertén (91) after extraction of *A. laidlawii* membrane proteins with Tween 20. About 20 distinct antigens, amounting to 70% of the whole membrane protein, could be detected by this method. Membrane lipid composition may have an influence on the extractability of membrane proteins. Indeed, the extractabilities of several membrane proteins of *A. laidlawii* are dependent on the fatty acyl chain and polar headgroup composition of the lipids, although the total amounts of these proteins in the membrane are independent of the lipid composition (94). One exception is the flavoprotein T_{4a}, whose total amount in the membrane increases with the fraction of ionic lipids. Furthermore, increasing the fraction of unsaturated acyl chains increases the extractability of this protein.

In one study, *A. laidlawii* and *S. citri* membrane protein extractabilities by different types of surfactants were compared to find the most suitable surfactant for crossed immunoelectrophoresis (230). The effects of three ionic surfactants (SDS, Sarkosyl, and sodium deoxycholate [DOC]) and of three nonionic surfactants (Triton X-100, Tween 20, and Brij 58) were analyzed. As expected, because of its denaturing effect on proteins (68), SDS proved unsuitable for use in crossed immunoelectrophoresis though it very effectively solubilized both membranes. Of the five other detergents, the best compromise was obtained with DOC, which proved most effective with both membranes with respect to the amount of protein extracted, the retention of antigenicity, and the resolution which could be achieved in crossed immunoelectrophoresis. It was concluded from this investigation that it is preferable to use DOC as a membrane protein-solubilizing agent in standardized procedures of antigen analysis by crossed immunoelectrophoresis. The use of DOC also proved efficient with *M. hyopneumoniae* (155) and with several avian mycoplasmas, including *M. gallisepticum* (15). The extraction of proteins by Triton X-100 from the membranes of some mollicutes is improved by the addition of EDTA and of anionic detergents such as DOC and SDS (113).

It should be noted that in the case of mollicutes, as for other organisms, blotting techniques, particularly electroblotting (205), have now superseded crossed immunoelectrophoresis for the routine analysis of antigens, whether they are of membrane origin or not.

This is because electroblotting (often called Western immunoblotting) takes advantage of the great efficacy of SDS for the solubilization of membrane proteins and of the high resolving power of SDS-polyacrylamide gel electrophoresis or of 2-D polyacrylamide gel electrophoresis, notably the O'Farrell method. Another important advantage of these techniques is that they require much less serum than does crossed immunolectrophoresis. However, comparisons of antigens by blotting techniques are less informative than comparisons performed by crossed immunoelectrophoresis since in the first case, a positive reaction may be obtained with a single epitope, whereas in the second case, to obtain an immunoprecipitate, at least three distinct epitopes, simultaneously accessible to antibodies, should in principle be involved. Therefore, it is wise to use both techniques for analysis of the antigenic properties of proteins, particularly in comparative studies (54, 238, 239). Finally, it should be noted that resolution of crossed immunoelectrophoresis of mollicute membrane proteins may be improved by the use of SDS-polyacrylamide gel electrophoresis or isoelectrofocusing in the first direction (14, 156).

Some authors have also used the Triton X-114 phase fractionation method (17) for identification of amphiphilic membrane antigens. Thus, 20 acylated proteins have been identified in the membrane of M. hyorhinis (24), including p23, a polypeptide that mediates complement-dependent mycoplasmacidal monoclonal antibody activity (172). In the same way, the lower-molecular-weight species of the variable V-1 antigen of M. pulmonis partitioned into the hydrophobic phase of Triton X-114, whereas the higher-molecular-weight variants were found in the aqueous phase (219).

Extraction and Purification of Membrane Proteins

So far, 20 proteins have been purified from the membrane of mollicutes (Table 1): 4 enzymes, 3 adhesins, and 13 proteins whose functions are still unknown or hypothetical.

A. laidlawii membrane antigens

Hjertjén and Johansson (71, 91) have taken advantage of the selectivity of protein extraction by Tween 20 to purify six integral membrane polypeptides from the plasma membrane of A. laidlawii (87, 90), t_{1a} (140 kDa), t_{1b} (>100 kDa), T_2 (52 kDa), T_3 (110 kDa), the flavoprotein T_{4a} (34 kDa), and T_{4b} (52 kDa). The proteins were first extracted with 2.5% Tween 20 from membranes of cells grown in a cholesterol-containing medium and subsequently separated into three main fractions (t_1, $T_2 + T_3$, and T_4) by agarose suspension electrophoresis in the presence of the same surfactant. Polypeptides t_{1a} and t_{1b} were purified from fraction t_1 by dextran-gel electrophoresis in the absence of Tween 20. Polypeptides T_2 and T_3 were purified from fraction $T_2 + T_3$ by preparative polyacrylamide gel electrophoresis also in the absence of surfactant. Finally, polypeptides T_{4a} and T_{4b} were purified from fraction T_4 by agarose suspension electrophoresis in the presence of 1% Tween 20 and 6 M urea. The bulk of Tween 20 was removed from T_{4a} and T_{4b} preparations by preparative polyacrylamide gel electrophoresis. Removal of Tween 20 from the different preparations could also be achieved by agarose suspension electrophoresis (44). Purified protein recoveries ranged from 4 to 18%, de-

Table 1. Purified membrane proteins of mollicutes

Protein	Organism	Scale[a] (mg)	Reference(s)
$t_{1a}(D_{12})$	A. laidlawii	0.3	87, 90, 96
t_{1b}		0.3	
T_2		0.1	
T_3		0.1	
T_{4a}		0.1	
T_{4b}		0.1	
Spiralin	S. citri	1	13, 231, 234
	S. melliferum	1	232, 234
Fibril protein	S. melliferum	?	207
NADH oxidase	A. laidlawii	6.6	171
$(Na^+ + Mg^{2+})$-ATPase	A. laidlawii	6.5	115
		Micro[b]	26
Aminopeptidase My	M. salivarium	1.4	185
Carboxypeptidase My	M. salivarium	1	186
Cytadhesin P1	M. pneumoniae	Micro	113
		Micro	80
		0.3	81
MgPa adhesin	M. genitalium	0.3	117
75-kDa adhesin	M. gallisepticum	?	99
60-kDa glycoprotein	M. pneumoniae	?	98
84-kDa glycoprotein	S. citri	?	190
54-kDa cytopathic factor	M. hyopneumoniae	Micro	56
p37	M. hyorhinis	Micro	45
V-1 antigen	M. pulmonis	?	219

[a] Approximate amount of protein obtained in a single run of the last purification step.
[b] Micro, microscale purification (1 μg to several micrograms).

pending on the protein considered (Table 1). It should be noted that in the extraction procedure, the protein/Tween 20 ratio is quite critical and the surfactant should be used well in excess to obtain a good yield (42). Furthermore, separation of the three fractions t_1, $T_2 + T_3$, and T_4 is improved by performing the agarose suspension electrophoresis in the presence of Tween 20 at a concentration slightly above its critical micelle concentration (43). Polypeptide t_{1a} was later identified as being D_{12}, a major band in SDS-polyacrylamide gel electrophoresis of *A. laidlawii* membrane proteins. A more effective procedure was subsequently developed for the purification of D_{12}, based on extraction of the protein with 5% DOC from the material insoluble in Tween 20 and fractionation by size exclusion chromatography on Bio-Gel P-200 in the presence of 0.5% DOC to prevent protein aggregation (94).

Spiroplasma spiralin and fibril protein

The systematic study of membrane protein solubility and extractability by surfactants proved very rewarding for the purification of spiralin (231), the major membrane protein of *S. citri* and *S. melliferum* (234, 239). This protein is very poorly extracted from the spiroplasma membrane by the nonionic surfactants Tween 20, Triton X-100, and Brij 58 and by the anionic detergent Sarkosyl, even when high surfactant concentrations are used (227–231). In contrast, the extraction of spiralin by high-critical-micelle-concentration nondenaturing detergents such as DOC, alkylsulfobetaines, or 6-O-(N-heptylcarbamoyl)methyl-α-D-glucopyranoside (Hecameg) is efficient and selective (12, 148, 226, 230, 231). In the case of the two latter detergents, efficacy and selectivity are both increased with increasing surfactant concentration. Incidentally, it was shown in the course of these studies that the inefficacy of a surfactant to extract a protein from a membrane is not an indication that this protein is not soluble in this surfactant. Indeed, once purified, spiralin is quite soluble in many if not all detergents, including those like Sarkosyl which are unable to extract it from the membrane (227). Spiralin was originally purified by selective extraction with surfactants from *S. citri* membranes depleted of extrinsic proteins and fractionation by agarose suspension electrophoresis (231). The extraction was performed with 0.2 M DOC from the material insoluble in Tween 20, and because of the simplicity of the procedure, the recovery was higher than 70%. This purification method was later improved by performing the first membrane extraction with 20 mM Sarkosyl instead of Tween 20. This modification allowed the overall purification time to be reduced from 72 to 48 h without loss in yield (232, 234). Furthermore, the new method proved more general since it was quite effective for the purification of spiralin from a nonhelical mutant of *S. citri* (13) and from *S. melliferum* strains (232, 234), whereas it was difficult to obtain a perfectly pure spiralin preparation from these strains by using the original procedure.

The spiroplasma cell contains a bundle of fibrils which are attached to the cytoplasmic face of the plasma membrane (25, 208) and composed of a single type of protein exhibiting an apparent polypeptide mass of approximately 55 kDa in SDS-polyacrylamide gel electrophoresis (207). The fibrils are stable in the presence of mild surfactants, and they are solubilized only by treatment with SDS or by maleylation (206, 208). These fibrils were purified from *S. melliferum* by ultracentrifugation of the Triton X-100-insoluble cell material in Urografin gradients containing 0.1% Triton X-100 (207). Purification was improved by the addition of 1 M KCl and 10 mM EDTA to the surfactant-insoluble material.

Membrane enzymes

In contrast to the proteins mentioned above, whose functions remain to be discovered, four enzymes of known activity, NADH oxidase, $(Na^+ + Mg^{2+})$-ATPase, aminopeptidase My, and carboxypeptidase My, have been purified from the membrane of mollicutes.

NADH oxidase is a multimeric metalloflavoprotein optimally extracted from the membrane of *A. laidlawii* under nondenaturing conditions by 3% Triton X-100. Purification could be achieved by three successive chromatographic steps: size exclusion chromatography on Sephadex G-150, ion-exchange chromatography on DEAE–Sepharose CL-6B, and finally size exclusion chromatography on Sephacryl S-300 (171). The enzyme prepared by this procedure retained its original activity, in contrast to the ethanol-extracted protein (86), which was no longer able to catalyze electron transfer from NADH to oxygen and was thus designated NADH dehydrogenase.

The membrane $(Na^+ + Mg^{2+})$-ATPase of *A. laidlawii* B, which is distinct from all other bacterial or mitochondrial ATPases studied to date, has been purified by a combination of size exclusion and ion-exchange chromatographies after solubilization with a mixture of Brij 58 and DOC in the presence of 16% ethylene glycol (115). In brief, the membrane extract was subjected to size exclusion chromatography on Sepharose 6B, ion-exchange chromatography on DEAE-Sephacel, and finally size exclusion chromatography on Sepharose 6B. All of these steps were performed in the presence of Brij 58, DOC, and ethylene glycol but at much lower concentrations than in the extraction step. The enzyme obtained by this procedure is partially delipidated, and its kinetic properties are similar to those of the membrane-bound enzyme, suggesting that the native structure is retained. However, its specific activity is enhanced upon the addition of exogenous phospholipids. Chen et al. (26) have described an alternative, small-scale purification procedure for this ATPase that is based on extraction with 2% Triton X-100, fractionation by polyacrylamide gradient electrophoresis in the presence of the same detergent to prevent protein aggregation, and elution from the gel.

M. salivarium membrane aminopeptidase was purified by Shibata and Watanabe (185) in a water-soluble form. In summary, isolated membranes were treated with Triton X-100, and aminopeptidase activity was recovered in the insoluble fraction. The enzyme (named aminopeptidase My) was released in solution by treatment with papain and purified by three successive chromatographic steps: ion-exchange chromatography on DEAE–Sephadex A-50, affinity chromatography on L-leucylglycine–AH-Sepharose 4B, and size exclusion chromatography on Sepharose CL-6B. Thus, this purification procedure permits a functional complex to be obtained in a water-soluble form by cleaving off the membrane-anchoring part of the protein.

Shibata and Watanabe (186) have also purified, from *M. salivarium*, an arginine-specific carboxypeptidase (carboxypeptidase My) which seems to be present exclusively in nonfermentative mycoplasmas (184). This 218-kDa enzyme was extracted very effectively by Trition X-100 from the membrane of the mycoplasma and purified after four chromatographic steps in the presence of 0.5% Triton X-100: ion-exchange chromatography on DEAE-Sephacel, affinity chromatography on arginine-Sepharose 4B, chromatofocusing, and again affinity chromatography on arginine-Sepharose 4B. The purification yield was 15%, and the specific activity was increased 45-fold.

Membrane adhesins

M. pneumoniae cytadhesin P1 (168 kDa) is another integral membrane protein of known function which has been purified to homogeneity. The first published purification procedure for this protein was that of Leith and Baseman (112). The protein was extracted from the plasma membrane with a mixture of three detergents (DOC, SDS, and Triton X-100) in the presence of EDTA and purified in a single step by immunoaffinity chromatography, using a combination of four anti-P1 monoclonal antibodies. Elution of the bound protein was achieved with 50% ethylene glycol. Jacobs and Clad (79) and Jacobs et al. (80) have proposed an alternative small-scale purification procedure based on the electroelution of the adhesin from SDS-polyacrylamide gels. More recently, Jacobs et al. (81) have developed a milder and faster purification procedure. *M. pneumoniae* cells were treated with 1% 3-[(3-cholamidylpropyl)dimethylammonio]-1-propanesulfonate, and the adhesin was extracted from the insoluble residue with 1% β-octylglucoside. Purification was achieved by size exclusion chromatography on a Superose-6 column in the presence of 0.1% SDS.

The same procedure was used for the purification of the MgPa adhesin of *M. genitalium*. Sequence comparison revealed that this 153-kDa membrane protein is closely related to cytadhesin P1 of *M. pneumoniae* (117).

An adhesin has also been partially purified by affinity chromatography from *M. gallisepticum* membranes after extraction with 1% DOC (99). In this case, human erythrocyte sialoglycopeptides conjugated to Sepharose 4B were used as the affinity matrix.

Glycoproteins

A 60-kDa glycoprotein was purified by extraction with lithium diiodosalicylate from the membrane of two strains of *M. pneumoniae* (98). However, it remains to be demonstrated that this protein is a true component of the mycoplasma membrane and not a serum glycoprotein from the culture medium tightly adsorbed to the cell surface. Indeed, this has been shown to a critical problem with some mycoplasma species (144, 155, 164).

A protein which is also believed glycosylated has recently been purified from the membrane of *S. citri* by affinity chromatography on concanavalin A-Sepharose after extraction with a mixture of SDS and Triton X-100 (190). Unfortunately, the preparation was only partially pure, being contaminated by a small amount of another protein of the membrane and also by an exogenous polypeptide tentatively identified as a concanavalin A subunit.

Miscellaneous membrane proteins

To complete this survey, two other proteins which have been purified from the plasma membrane of mycoplasma and a third one isolated from mouse fibrosarcoma cells should be mentioned.

The first protein in this group is a 54-kDa cytopathic factor extracted from *M. hyopneumoniae* membranes with Triton X-100 and eluted from gels after separation by isoelectric focusing (56). This protein has not been characterized at the molecular level, and it remains to be shown that it is not a cytoplasmic protein contaminating membrane preparations.

One intriguing case is that of the V-1 antigen of *M. pulmonis*. This component is exposed on the surface of the mycoplasma and gives rise to a characteristic ladder pattern in the 21- to 131-kDa range when analyzed by SDS-polyacrylamide gel electrophoresis (220). This behavior is indicative of a polydisperse entity with a discrete size variability. The investigations performed by using trypsin treatment and extraction with Triton X-114 suggest that V-1 antigen is attached to the mycoplasma membrane via a lipophilic anchor (219). Some of the size variants of this protein have been purified by selective extraction with aqueous phenol (219).

p37 was first evidenced as being associated with the surface of cultured mouse fibrosarcoma cells and found to be a component of *M. hyorhinis* (45). This protein has been purified in two steps from fibrosarcoma cells solubilized with 1% Triton X-100 (45). The cell extract was subjected to immunoaffinity chromatography using monoclonal antibodies, and p37 was subsequently purified by SDS-polyacrylamide gel electrophoresis. This protein is mentioned because the gene in the *M. hyorhinis* chromosome encoding p37 is part of an operon coding for three proteins highly similar to the components of the periplasmic binding protein-dependent transport systems of gram-negative bacteria. It was thus suggested that p37 is part of a homologous, high-affinity transport system in *M. hyorhinis* (45, 62) (see below). It is now necessary to purify p37 from the mycoplasma cell and verify whether or not it is a true membrane protein in this bacterium.

Reconstitution

Studies on the reconstitution of membranes from mollicutes started in the mid-1960s with the solubilization of the *A. laidlawii* membrane with SDS and its reconstitution upon detergent removal by dialysis (168). In fact, this work was the first to describe the anticipated reconstruction of a plasma membrane from SDS-solubilized components. The conclusions which could be drawn from that work and subsequent publications (see reference 160 for a review) were that the lipoprotein subunit theory of biomembrane structure (65) was wrong and that the structure of membranes obtained by reassembly of components solubilized with SDS was different from the native architecture (see chapter 8).

Reconstitution experiments with purified membrane proteins of mollicutes were hampered by the difficulties encountered in their purification. Proteoliposomes were obtained by the association of spiralin with lecithin upon removal of DOC by dialysis (227). The use of spiralin in this form permitted the demonstration that the extraction of this protein into a soluble form by different mild detergents was much easier than when *S. citri* membrane was used as the starting material. It was also shown that once lyophilized, pure spiralin cannot be solubilized by any surfactant unless strongly denaturing conditions are employed. In contrast, protein micelles of pure spiralin or lecithin-spiralin proteoliposomes (227, 232) are easy to solubilize with most types of mild detergents. Probing of epitopes with antispiralin antibodies on the surface of spiralin-lecithin proteoliposomes obtained by the dialysis method leads to the conclusion that incorporation of spiralin into the liposomes is symmetrical, in contrast to the asymmetrical disposition of the protein in the *S. melliferum* membrane (232).

The membrane $(Na^+ + Mg^{2+})$-ATPase from *A. laidlawii*, which appears to function in vivo as an ATP-driven sodium pump (see chapter 15), is the only mollicute membrane protein of known activity which has been used in a pure form for reconstitution experiments. The protein was associated with dimyristoylphosphatidylcholine by the cholate dialysis method (58, 59). The formation of sealed vesicles occurred only at low protein-to-lipid ratios. The incorporation of the enzyme into phospholipid bilayers enhanced its specific activity and restored its lipid phase state-dependent properties which were lost during solubilization and purification. The reconstituted ATPase proved relatively resistant to cold inactivation, oxidative degradation, and thermal denaturation. It has also been shown in earlier studies with proteoliposomes that the α subunit bears the nucleotide-binding site (60, 114) and penetrates into or traverses the hydrophobic core of the phospholipid bilayer, since this polypeptide could be labeled by phospholipids containing a photosensitive fatty acyl group (58). This ATPase has also been reconstituted with different phospho- and glycolipids to evaluate the ability of these lipids to support the function of the enzyme (57). The conclusion of these studies (see also references 122 and 123) is that a lipid bilayer of low to moderate negative surface charge, predominantly liquid-crystalline and of a minimal thickness, is required for the enzyme to be fully active. When these requirements are met, the enzyme exhibits considerable flexibility with respect to the nature of the phospholipids which can effectively support its function.

MOLECULAR PROPERTIES AND FUNCTION

Composition and Disposition

Important features of the *A. laidlawii* membrane contributed to the development of the fluid mosaic model for the organization of membrane proteins in biological lipid bilayers (191). The composition, properties, and a few known functions of mollicute membrane proteins have been reviewed elsewhere (7, 88, 89, 163, 164). The molecular weights of mollicute membrane proteins are within a range similar to that found for other biological membranes. Approximately 85% of the membrane proteins in *A. laidlawii* are of the integral type (131). Early amino acid analyses revealed only a slightly higher percentage of nonpolar amino acids than in water-soluble globular proteins (reviewed in references 163 and 164). However, the nonionic detergent Tween 20 selectively solubilizes the integral proteins enriched in hydrophilic amino acids, leaving the more hydrophobic proteins behind (71, 95, 139). Many of the Tween 20-soluble proteins are covalently modified by fatty acid tails (see below). According to the translated DNA sequences of known *E. coli* proteins, 2-D gel electrophoresis gives correct estimates of protein molecular weights and pI values (133). 2-D gel analysis of mollicute membrane proteins reveals that most are acidic, with pI values ranging from pH 4 to 7 (9, 140, 189), similar to values for *E. coli* membrane proteins (181). Interestingly, the majority of the acyl proteins in *A. laidlawii* and individual acyl proteins in *M. hyorhinis* and *S. melliferum* are very acidic, having isoelectric points in the range of pH 4 to 5 (24, 140), analogous to the negative surface potential of the membrane lipids (30).

A transbilayer asymmetry for the membrane proteins has been established for several species of mollicutes (reviewed in references 163 and 164). The majority of the proteins are exposed on the inner, cytoplasmic side of the membrane. This has been shown by several different techniques, such as lactoperoxidase-mediated iodination (9), selective proteolytic degradation of proteins exposed (or accessible) on the outside, analysis of protein antigenic exposure by crossed immunoelectrophoresis (89), and freeze fracture electron microscopy (204). A bilayer-spanning topology has been established for just a few mollicute membrane proteins, although the translated amino acid sequences from several recently cloned genes strongly suggest this topology for several more proteins (see Table 3). For membrane proteins D_{12} in *A. laidlawii*, cytadhesin P1 in *M. pneumoniae*, and spiralin in *S. melliferum*, adsorption with monospecific or monoclonal antibodies indicates the presence of different epitopes on the two sides of the bilayer (61, 78, 89, 232). However, D_{12} and spiralin are both modified with acyl chains, and a transmembrane topology of such proteins seems to be very rare in bacteria (152).

A change in the vertical disposition of bulk membrane integral proteins was anticipated as a function of changes in the molecular ordering of lipid chains. However, no consistent correlation could be found between the molecular ordering and the exposure of *A. laidlawii* membrane proteins to lactoperoxidase-mediated iodination (reviewed in reference 164). The changes in the lipid-protein matrix were brought about by specific acyl chain supplementation, growth temperature changes, aging of cultures, and treatment with antibiotics (164). The observed changes in protein disposition were suggested to be correlated with the energy status of the cell or membrane. However, changes in the extent of protein iodination after treatment of cells with uncouplers and ionophores (5) do not correlate with recorded changes in the transmembrane electric potential and pH gradient (31). One possibility is that the observed effects in protein disposition or conformation depend on changes in the intracellular concentrations of important ions such as K^+, Na^+ and H^+. The sequence and length of protein segments crossing a membrane must be genetically determined and match the thickness of the lipid bilayer. However, *A. laidlawii* can tolerate a substantial variation in lipid acyl chain length and still grow well (49, 223).

In mollicute membranes containing cholesterol, freeze fracture electron microscopy has revealed that the proteins (i.e., particles on the fracture faces) are randomly distributed in the plane of the membrane (reviewed in reference 164). For cholesterol-poor cells or the bleb organelle in *M. gallisepticum*, patches of proteins can be observed. In *A. laidlawii*, this patching is correlated with the extent of the gel phase in the lipids (84) and with lowering of the pH of the medium (32). Most likely, the proteins are randomly dispersed in the liquid-crystalline lipid matrix due to protein charge repulsion (see the low pI values described above). A low solubility of the proteins in gel phases, or decreased charge repulsion by low pH, must cause the patching in the remaining liquid lipid phase.

In addition to the purified membrane proteins listed in Table 1, many membrane-associated enzyme activities have been described for mollicutes (reviewed in references 163, 164, 193, and 194). Prominent among these are transport activities for K^+ and glucose, phosphatase, peptidase, thioesterase, nucleases, and enzymes in membrane lipid metabolism (see also chapters 6, 11, 14, and 15). Several of these enzymes are dependent upon a specific lipid environment for proper function, as demonstrated recently for the synthesis of the two major membrane glucolipids in *A. laidlawii* (38).

Proteins Modified with Fatty Acids

A prominent feature of several mollicutes is the large number of membrane proteins that contain covalently attached fatty acyl chains (Table 2). With one excep-

tion, all investigated species contain a substantially larger number of acyl proteins than has been found in cell wall-containing bacteria. The latter seem to contain 10 different lipoproteins at most (18, 67, 136). Most other mollicutes will probably reveal numbers of membrane acyl proteins similar to those in Table 2. Surprisingly, the numbers found for different species do not correlate with the coding capacity (i.e., genome sizes) of the cells (see chapter 9). This finding may imply that mollicute cells, lacking other protective surface layers, need this minimum number of otherwise soluble protein functions secured to the membranes (see below). The sizes of these proteins (Table 2) seem to coincide with the size range of all of the membrane proteins as resolved by SDS-gels. A survey of the literature (data not shown) shows that lipoproteins with a molecular mass larger than 65 kDa occur in just a few bacteria of the many shown to have lipoproteins. Hence, large acyl proteins are more common in mollicutes (Table 2).

For several of the species in Table 2, practically all acyl proteins are found in the detergent-rich bottom phase after solubilization and phase partitioning in the detergent Triton X-114, as modified from Bordier (17). Dominant surface antigens of certain other mollicutes also partition this way. This selective enrichment (24, 140) can probably be attributed to certain packing preferences between the detergent aggregates and the fatty acyl chains of the proteins and is not affected by changes in protein acyl chain length (140). Of the species in Table 2, only *A. laidlawii* can synthesize (saturated) fatty acids (194), and these are preferred over those exogenously supplied (140). The fatty acid preferences have not been extensively investigated for other species except *S. melliferum*, but most likely the strong enrichment of saturated chains in these two species are valid for all others. It should be pointed out that this enrichment does not occur for the membrane lipid acyl chains in *A. laidlawii* (140) and probably not for *S. melliferum* lipids (232). The chain lengths of the protein acyl chains are kept more constant than the lipid acyl chain lengths when *A. laidlawii* cells are fed different fatty acids (138). Cholesterol affects the fraction of saturated and unsaturated chains in both *M. capricolum* and *A. laidlawii* proteins

Table 2. Membrane lipoproteins in mollicutes

Organism	Acylated proteins[a]	Molecular mass (kDa)[b]	Fatty acids[c]	Glycerol labeling[d]	Reference(s)
A. laidlawii B	~30	17–100	16:0 (no 18:1c)[e]	NA	37
A. laidlawii A	~25	15–130	14:0 > 16:0 > 18:0 > 18:1c > 18:2c[e]	–	139, 140
S. melliferum	>20	15–85	16:0 > 14:0 > 18:2c > 18:0 > 18:1c	–	232
M. capricolum	25–30	15–100	16:0 > 18:1c	+ (not all)	35, 36
M. hyopneumoniae	4	44–65	16:0 > ? (also 18:1c)[e]	NA	225
M. hyorhinis	~20	23–120	16:0[e]	NA	21, 24
M. arginini	~15	14–105	16:0 > 14:0	NA	179, 223
U. urealyticum	~25	16–126	16:0	NA	203

[a] Estimated numbers of membrane proteins in slab gels labeled by radioactive fatty acids.
[b] Range of acyl protein molecular masses estimated from gel photos.
[c] Fatty acids tested and preferences of incorporation. 14:0, myristic acid; 16:0, palmitic acid; 18:0, stearic acid; 18:1c, oleic acid; 18:2c, linoleic acid.
[d] Incorporation of radioactive glycerol in acyl chain-labeled proteins. NA, not analyzed.
[e] Acyl chain composition verified after release from proteins.

(36, 139). According to the consensus mechanism for acyl chain modification of bacterial lipoproteins (see above), the latter should have two acyl chains attached by ester bounds to a glycerol moiety on an N-terminal cysteine residue plus one amide-linked chain at the N terminus. Glycerol incorporation could not be demonstrated in *A. laidlawii* and *S. melliferum* and was observed for only a few of the acyl proteins in *M. capricolum* (Table 2). In addition, labeling was not achieved from uniformly labeled glucose in *A. laidlawii* (140). More than two-thirds of the proteins acyl chains in *M. capricolum* and *A. laidlawii* A and B are linked by ester bonds. The drug globomycin did not decrease the extent of acylation in *A. laidlawii* (139). This finding indicates that these proteins do not contain an amide-linked chain or that many proteins are not fully acylated, i.e., do not contain three acyl chains per peptide. Both of these features have been observed for a number of other bacterial lipoproteins (reviewed in reference 140). The maximum extent of modification found in *A. laidlawii* is two acyl chains per peptide, whereas most proteins had just one chain. In *A. laidlawii* and *M. capricolum*, these acyl chains can be donated by both polar lipids and free fatty acids, but the latter was most efficient in *A. laidlawii* (35, 140).

The DNA sequences of the genes for three acyl proteins from *M. hyorhinis* (236) and the acylated spiralin from *S. melliferum* (28) have revealed that these four proteins have typical bacterial amino acid consensus sequences for lipoprotein signal peptide cleavage (67) and a potential cysteine residue for acyl chain attachment at the N terminus of the processed, mature proteins. This consensus sequence was also found in the translated gene for another *M. hyorhinis* protein (45), but in this case, as for spiralin from *S. citri* (27), acylation has not been verified. None of these *M. hyorhinis* proteins contain any hydrophobic, putative transmembrane amino acid segments and are most likely attached to the membrane by their lipid tails. These features are thus similar to properties of corresponding proteins in cell wall-containing bacteria, and these few selected *M. hyorhinis* and *S. melliferum* proteins should therefore be termed mollicute or mycoplasma membrane lipoproteins. However, a full chemical characterization will reveal whether they contain three acyl chains and glycerol as does the reference Braun's lipoprotein (23).

What are the functions of these fatty acid-modified proteins? The DNA sequences for three size-variant membrane surface lipoproteins (Vlps) from *M. hyorhinis* show (236) that they all encode conserved N-terminal signal peptides and lipoprotein processing sites, but divergent external domains undergo size variations by loss or gain of repetitive intragenic coding sequences while retaining a motif with a characteristic negative charge (see also chapter 28). This is obviously a system for antigenic variation used for host adaptation and for maintenance of diversity in the populations (236). The fourth sequenced *M. hyorhinis* protein, named p37, exhibits the same N-terminal features as do the three proteins mentioned above (45) but probably does not undergo size variation (175). This surface protein constitutes the binding or receptor part in an operon belonging to the large periplasmic or ATP-binding cassette (ABC) superfamily of transport systems (70), (see below). The proposed function is most likely not compatible with extensive size and antigenic variation as for the Vlps. Appearance of p37 on fibrosarcoma cells correlates with increasing invasiveness of these cell lines, which obviously are infected with *M. hyorhinis* (45). The DNA sequences of the spiralin protein genes from *S. citri* and *S. melliferum* show the typical N-terminal features of bacterial lipoproteins, but there are no hints as to the function of these very numerous membrane proteins (28). No size variations occur. A transmembrane topology has been suggested on the basis of antigen epitope exposure and a putative transmembrane amphiphilic segment in the otherwise hydrophilic amino acid sequence (28, 232).

The *A. laidlawii* proteins D_{12}, T_2, T_3, T_{4a} and T_{4b} (Table 1) are all acylated (140). Analyses with monospecific antibodies on protein gel blots have shown that these proteins have not undergone any size variations, at least not over the last 8 years (223). However, comparisons among different *A. laidlawii* strains (A-EF22, B-PG9, B-JU, JA1, and K2) reveal slight differences in molecular masses for these proteins except for protein T_3, which shows large variations between strains. Several of the proteins also appear as doublets on gels, and the relative proportions within these pairs may vary as a function of strain or growth conditions (82, 223). A possible explanation for these differences may be that *A. laidlawii* is a cluster of various strains with different extents of relatedness (196). Protein T_{4a} (Table 1), exposed on the inside of the membrane (89), can be covalently labeled with fatty acids, phosphorus, and riboflavin (83, 140) and is most likely an acylated flavin redox cofactor protein. Acyl protein T_3 (Table 1) is also labeled by phosphorus (83) and may be identical to the high-molecular-mass acylphosphate protein showing phosphorus turnover (216). Another type of function is the lymphokinelike activity of *M. arginini* TUH-14 (180), which stimulates growth of lipopolysaccharide preactivated B cells. This activity withstands extraction with organic solvents and hot phenol and was tentatively localized to four high-molecular-mass acylated (16:0 and 14:0) membrane proteins (179). Two of the proteins are probably related according to protease V8 peptide maps. *M. arginini* G 230 is similar in number of membrane acyl proteins to strain TUH-14 (Table 2) but has no lymphokine activity. One possibility is that this stimulating activity of the four TUH-14 proteins involves spontaneous mutations like those for the antigenic Vlps on the *M. hyorhinis* membrane surface.

Cloned and Sequenced Membrane Proteins

The mollicute membrane proteins that have been cloned and sequenced are listed in Table 3. Note that there is only a partial overlap with the list of solubilized and purified membrane proteins in Table 1. This repertoire of proteins can roughly be divided into two groups. One contains the structural and enzyme proteins of *A. laidlawii*, *Spiroplasma* species, and *M. capricolum*; the other contains the adhesin-related and antigenic-variable proteins of the pathogenic species *M. genitalium*, *M. hyorhinis*, and *M. pneumoniae*. This division is a reflection of the research on mollicutes; i.e.,

Table 3. Cloned and sequenced mollicute membrane proteins

Organism	Proteins	Signal peptide[a]	Transmembrane segments[a]	Reference(s)
A. laidlawii A	D_{12}[b]	—	—	201
	T_3[b]	—	—	201
	31 kDa	—	—	201
	E2 subunit of PDHC[c]	No	0	217
	42 kDa	No	0	20
	ABC transport protein[d]	?	Several	20
S. citri	Spiralin[b]	Yes	1?	27, 111
	Fibril protein	No	0	224
S. melliferum	Spiralin[b]	Yes	1?	28
M. capricolum	SecY	No	Several	143
M. genitalium	MgPa Adhesin	Yes	Several	40, 75
	114 kDa	Yes	Several	40, 75
	29 kDa	?	1	40, 75
M. hyorhinis	p37[b]	Yes	0	45
	p69	No	Several	45
	p101	?	1?	237
	VlpA,[b] -B,[b] and -C[b]	Yes	0	236
M. pneumoniae	Cytadhesin P1	Yes	Several	74, 200
	130 kDa	Yes	Several	76
	P30	?	1	39, 40
	HMW1 and 3	—	—	108

[a] Deduced from the translated DNA sequence. —, sequence not available; ?, presence of a *cleavable* signal peptide or a transmembrane hydrophobic segment not clear from sequence. The numbers of transmembrane segments are estimates.
[b] Proteins covalently modified with fatty acids according to chemical analysis and/or consensus lipoprotein DNA sequence.
[c] PDHC, pyruvate dehydrogenase enzyme complex.
[d] Belongs to the same superfamily as does p69 in *M. hyorhinis*.

they are interesting and structurally simple models for membrane studies and are also of increasing importance as surface parasites and pathogens. The structural properties of these proteins, as deduced mostly from the translated DNA sequences, reveal no unique features but show the characteristics of membrane proteins described earlier. There are several soluble proteins without hydrophobic segments. These are typically peripheral proteins or anchored to the membrane bilayers by their lipid tails. For the integral membrane proteins, there is a range of hydrophobicities, from those having only one putative hydrophobic transmembrane segment to those having several (e.g., SecY and P1) to many segments (e.g., p69 and the ABC transport protein), in relation to the lengths of the proteins and their hydrophilic parts. Several of these hydrophobic segments (e.g., in P1, p69, and the ABC protein; Table 3) reveal a distribution of charged residues around the segments which appears similar to that of other transmembrane proteins, according to the positive-inside rule (see above).

Several of the proteins have typical bacterial signal peptides, including lipoprotein ones. The presence, and especially the cleavage processing, have been verified chemically for only spiralin, p37, and P1 (Table 3). The very long signal peptide of protein P1 may have a two-step processing (76), typical of certain gram-positive preproenzymes (218). Still others (p101) have signal peptides that are probably not cleaved but act as hydrophobic anchors (237). Such signal peptides were also obtained from *A. laidlawii* by using a specific export signal selection vector (20). For an *E. coli* hydrophobic membrane protein (MalF) related to p69 and the ABC transport protein (Table 3), insertion into the membrane can occur independently of the bacterial

secretion machinery even after deletion of the first transmembrane, noncleaved signal peptide segment (48, 124). Since these proteins have similar hydrophobicity profiles, and most likely also membrane topologies (70), an analogous membrane insertion probably can occur in the mollicutes. Although p69 and the ABC transport protein belong to the same superfamily of transport proteins and are both mollicute proteins, their sequences (Table 3) revealed only a low percentage identity at the amino acid sequence level (20, 45). However, the latter *A. laidlawii* protein has significant sequence identity and similarity to a *B. subtilis* dipeptide transport protein (20, 121). In analogy with other operons of this type (70) in gram-positive bacteria (62), which contain one lipoprotein-binding protein at the membrane outer surface, *A. laidlawii* probably contains a corresponding lipoprotein fulfilling a function similar to that of p37 (Table 3) in *M. hyorhinis*.

The characteristic properties and variation of the Vlps (Table 3) were discussed above. A variation also occurs for the cytadhesin P1, since two-thirds of the P1 gene is found in multiple copies on the chromosome (see chapters 27 and 28). However, the signal sequence region and one membrane-anchoring domain are conserved in different clinical isolates which contain significant variations in amino acid sequence in other regions (199). Parts of the P1 sequence are homologous to certain viral, cytoskeletal, and fibrinogen sequences (200). Sequence similarities between short regions of the MgPa adhesin (Table 3) and key proteins in the human immune system have also been reported (174). The basic pI value of P1 might prevent electrostatic repulsion between P1 and its supposedly negatively charged target membrane.

Phosphorus, Iron, and Isoprenoid Contents

Protein phosphorylation is an important covalent modification in the regulation of adaptive responses in bacteria (198). A recent estimate listed at least 130 different phosphoprotein species in *E. coli* (33). However, only some of these are phosphorylated under any given condition, and very few are associated with the membranes. Fewer endogenous proteins are also phosphorylated in vitro than in vivo (33). In vivo labeling of mollicute proteins with radioactive phosphorus has been observed in *A. laidlawii* and *M. gallisepticum* (97, 147). In *A. laidlawii*, only two specific membrane proteins were labeled (83) (see above). In vitro, several proteins can be phosphorylated, most typically a 55- to 57-kDa soluble protein in *M. mobile*, *M. gallisepticum*, and *S. melliferum* (52, 146, 147). These species have a defined cell morphology with organellelike structures, which may involve a cytoskeleton or fibrillar network. The presence of the former has been proposed (119), but it is most clearly visualized for the cytoskeleton in *M. pneumoniae* (197) and the fibril assembly of spiroplasmas (208). Indeed, the 57-kDa phosphoprotein of *S. melliferum* was found associated with the fibrillar and membrane fractions when dephosphorylated (146). A similar protein does not occur in *A. laidlawii*, as indicated from the molecular masses of membrane proteins phosphorylated in vitro (216).

Mollicutes lack cytochrome pigments and most probably obtain the majority of their ATP from substrate-level phosphorylation (see chapter 11). Analysis of 11 different species revealed that they all contain significant amounts of iron in their membranes (10, 149). This iron may be involved with flavins, participating in various redox reactions. *A. laidlawii* membranes contain at least eight different flavoproteins, as visualized by riboflavin labeling (140). Several iron-containing proteins, including the membrane-associated NADH oxidase flavoprotein (171), have also been identified in *A. laidlawii* (83).

In eucaryotes, isoprenoid-modified proteins have key positions in signal-transducing pathways across membranes, especially involving GTP binding and hydrolysis (118). The membrane attachment of these proteins is also sometimes enhanced by ester-linked 16:0 acyl chains. So far, isoprenoid-modified proteins have been found only in archaebacteria (50), not in eubacteria. Recently, such proteins were found in *A. laidlawii*. Labeling with radioactive mevalonate, a precursor to isoprenoids (194), revealed several membrane-associated isoprenoid proteins of 17 to 45 kDa and two soluble ones of 23 to 25 kDa (141). None of the membrane acyl proteins (Table 2) or polar membrane lipids became labeled. The isoprenoid is attached most likely by an ether (or amide) bond and gives the proteins a hydrophobic character; all isoprenoid proteins are found in the detergent-containing bottom phase upon partitioning in Triton X-114 (see above). Like most other mollicutes, *A. laidlawii* can live on eucaryotic membrane surfaces and even exchange metabolites, such as lipid components, with its host. An exchange of isoprenoids or isoprenoid protein may interfere with the signaling pathways in the eucaryotic hosts.

Another important covalent modification of proteins is glycosylation. As discussed above, this has been reported for several supposedly mollicute membrane proteins. However, as pointed out above, proof for glycosylation is best achieved by metabolic incorporation of radioactive sugars, and this has not been done. In *A. laidlawii*, despite claims for the existence of glycosylated proteins, no membrane proteins were uniqely labeled by five different radioactive sugars. However, one small cytosolic protein, also labeled with biotin, was labeled with glucose (140).

CONCLUSIONS

Mollicutes lack a bacterial cell wall, periplasmic space, and outer membrane for the entrapment of proteins needed close to their cell surfaces. The coding capacities of their small genomes are probably used to a larger extent than in other bacteria, for basal housekeeping functions, and membrane protein patterns are little affected by changes in growth conditions. Because of the small dimensions of most mollicute cells, a larger fraction of the cellular protein contents is in the membranes. This view is corroborated by the maximum numbers of different membrane proteins recorded. Another typical feature of most mollicutes investigated is substantially larger numbers of fatty acid-modified membrane proteins than in other bacteria, e.g., threefold those of *E. coli* and bacilli. These numbers seem not to correlate with the coding capacities (genome sizes) of different mollicutes. Most likely, many of these proteins function as otherwise soluble proteins which are anchored to the mollicute membranes by their fatty acid tails.

Essentially two groups of mollicute membrane proteins have been solubilized, purified and analyzed, or cloned and sequenced. The first group consists of structural and enzyme proteins, and the second consists of adhesin-related and antigen-variable proteins of pathogenic mollicutes. These studies have been hampered by the lack of established genetics and suitable tools and vectors adapted for the mollicutes. Chemical, immunological, and genetic analyses of this limited set have revealed that the mollicute membrane proteins exhibit the same structural features as established for membrane proteins in general. Hence, with respect to the basic membrane feature of hydrophobicity, a range from typical peripheral (i.e., hydrophilic) proteins to proteins with one or more hydrophobic, putatively transmembrane segments has been described. Likewise, sequence analysis has indicated the presence of typical cleavable signal peptides as well as noncleaved signal anchor segments. Many of the fatty acid-modified membrane proteins have pI values lower than the average for membrane proteins, as visualized from gel migration and a few gene sequences. Besides certain amino acid sequence similarities for a few membrane proteins, no obvious close relationships to the gram-positive relatives of the mollicutes have been found. This lack of identified relationship may be attributed not only to the wealth of information about gram-negative bacteria, especially *E. coli*, but also to the unique cellular structure and organization of the mollicutes.

REFERENCES

1. **Alexander, A. G., and G. E. Kenny.** 1977. Characterization of membrane and cytoplasmic antigens of *Mycoplasma arginini* by two-dimensional (crossed) immuno-electrophoresis. *Infect. Immun.* **15:**313–321.

2. **Alexander, A. G., and G. E. Kenny.** 1978. Application of charge shift electrophoresis to antigenic analysis of mycoplasma membranes by two-dimensional (crossed) immunoelectrophoresis. *Infect. Immun.* **20:**861–863.

3. **Alexander, A. G., and G. E. Kenny.** 1980. Characterization of the strain specific and common surface antigens of *Mycoplasma arginini*. *Infect. Immun.* **29:**442–451.

4. **Amar, A.** 1977. Protein disposition in the mycoplasma membrane. Ph. D. thesis. The Hebrew University, Jerusalem, Israel.

5. **Amar, A., S. Rottem, and S. Razin.** 1978. Disposition of membrane proteins as affected by changes in the electrochemical gradient across mycoplasma membranes. *Biochem. Biophys. Res. Commun.* **84:**306–312.

6. **Ames, G. F.-L., and K. Nikaldo.** 1976. Two-dimensional gel electrophoresis of membrane proteins. *Biochemistry* **15:**616–623.

7. **Archer, D. B.** 1981. The structure and functions of the mycoplasma membrane. *Int. Rev. Cytol.* **69:**1–44.

8. **Archer, D. B., and A. W. Rodwell.** 1982. Membrane proteins of *Mycoplasma gallisepticum*. *J. Bacteriol.* **159:**1598–1601.

9. **Archer, D. B., A. W. Rodwell, and A. S. Rodwell.** 1978. The nature and location of *Acholeplasma laidlawii* membrane proteins investigated by two-dimensional gel electrophoresis. *Biochim. Biophys. Acta* **513:**268–283.

10. **Bauminger, E. R., S. G. Cohen, F. Labenski de Kanter, A. Levy, S. Ofer, M. Kessel, and S. Rottem.** 1980. Iron storage in *Mycoplasma capricolum*. *J. Bacteriol.* **141:**378–381.

11. **Bayer, M. H.** 1982. Phospholiphase A activity in commercial nucleases. Implications for membrane vesicle isolation. *Biochim. Biophys. Acta* **692:**498–500.

12. **Blanchard, A., G. Baffet, and H. Wroblewski.** 1985. Highly selective extraction of spiralin from the *Spiroplasma citri* cell membrane with alkly-N-sulfobetaines. *Biochimie* **67:**1251–1256.

13. **Blanchard, A., L. Quillien, C. Fontenelle, K.-E. Johansson, and H. Wroblewski.** 1986. Combinasion de l'immunoelectrophorèse croisée et de l' immunodétection avec l'électrophorèse bidimensionelle d'O'Farrell pour l'analyse des protéines membranaires, p. 309–315. *In* M.-M. Galteau and G. Siest (ed.), *Recent Progresses in Two-Dimensional Electrophoresis.* Presses Universitaires de Nancy, Nancy, France.

14. **Blanchard, A., L. Quillien, and H. Wroblewski.** 1984. *Spiroplasma citri* membrane protein analysis by sodium deoxycholate-crossed immunoelectrophoresis with a sieving first directional gel. *Protides Biol. Fluids Proc. Colloq.* **32:**1005–1008.

15. **Blot, M.-F.** 1989. Spécificité des antigènes protéiques membrainaires de *Mycoplasma gallisepticum* et mise au point de deux techniques sérologiques de diagnostic. Ph.D. thesis. The University of Rennes I, Rennes, France.

16. **Boman, H. G., I. Faye, G. H. Gudmundsson, J.-Y. Lee, and D.-A. Lidholm.** 1991. Cell-free immunity in Cecropia. A model system for antibacterial proteins. *Eur. J. Biochem.* **201:**23–31.

17. **Bordier, C.** 1980. Phase separation of integral membrane proteins in Triton X-114 solution. *J. Biol. Chem.* **256:** 1604–1607.

18. **Bouvier, J., A. P. Pugsley, and P. Stragier.** 1991. A gene for a new lipoprotein in the *dapA-purC* interval of the *Escherichia coli* chromosome. *J. Bacteriol.* **173:**5523–5531.

19. **Boyd, D., and J. Beckwith.** 1990. The role of charged amino acids in the localization of secreted and membrane proteins. *Cell* **62:**1031–1033.

20. **Boyer, M. J., T. K. Sundström, V. Tegman, and Å. Wieslander.** Sequence regions from *Acholeplasma laidlawii* which restore export of β-lactamase in *Escherichia coli*. Submitted for publication.

21. **Boyer, M. J., and K. S. Wise.** 1989. Lipid-modified surface protein antigens expressing size variation within the species *Mycoplasma hyorhinis*. *Infect. Immun.* **57:**245–254.

22. **Bradbury, J. M., and F. T. W. Jordan.** 1972. Studies on the adsorption of certain medium proteins to *Mycoplasma gallisepticum* and their influence on agglutination and hemagglutination reactions. *J. Hyg.* **70:**267–278.

23. **Braun, V.** 1975. Covalent lipoprotein from the outer membrane of *Escherichia coli*. *Biochim. Biophys. Acta* **415:**335–377.

24. **Bricker, T. M., M. J. Boyer, J. Keith, R. Watson-McKown, and K. S. Wise.** 1988. Association of lipids with integral membrane surface proteins of *Mycoplasma hyorhinis*. *Infect. Immun.* **56:**295–301.

25. **Charbonneau, D. L., and W. C. Ghiorse.** 1984. Ultrastructure and localization of fibrils in *Spiroplasma floricola* OBMG. *Curr. Microbiol.* **10:**65–72.

26. **Chen, J. W., Q. Sun, and F. Hwang.** 1984. Properties of the membrane-bound Mg^{2+}-ATPase isolated from *Acholeplasma laidlawii*. *Biochim. Biophys. Acta* **777:**151–154.

27. **Chevalier, C., C. Saillard, and J. M. Bové.** 1990. Organization and nucleotide sequences of the *Spiroplasma citri* genes for ribosomal protein S2, elongation factor Ts, spiralin, phosphofructokinase, pyruvate kinase, and an unidentified protein. *J. Bacteriol.* **172:**2693–2703.

28. **Chevalier, C., C. Sailard, and J. M. Bové.** 1990. Spiralins of *Spiroplasma citri* and *Spiroplasma melliferum*: amino acid sequences and putative organization in the cell membrane. *J. Bacteriol.* **172:**6090–6097.

29. **Choules, G. L., and W. R. Gray.** 1971. Peptidase activity in the membranes of *Mycoplasma laidlawii*. *Biochem. Biophys. Res. Commun.* **45:**849–855.

30. **Christiansson, A., L. E. G. Eriksson, J. Westman, R. Demel, and Å. Wieslander.** 1985. Involvement of surface potential in regulation of polar membrane lipids in *Acholeplasma laidlawii*. *J. Biol. Chem.* **260:**3984–3990.

31. **Clementz, T., A. Christiansson, and Å. Wieslander.** 1986. Transmembrane electrical potential affects the lipid composition of *Acholeplasma laidlawii*. *Biochemistry* **25:**823–830.

32. **Copps, T. P., W. S. Chelack, and A. Petkau.** 1976. Variation in distribution of membrane particles in *Acholeplasma laidlawii* B with pH. *J. Ultrastruct. Res.* **55:**1–3.

33. **Cozzone, A. J.** 1988. Protein phosphorylation in prokaryotes. *Annu. Rev. Microbiol.* **42:**97–125.

34. **Curatolo, W.** 1987. Glycolipid function. *Biochim. Biophys. Acta* **906:**137–160.

35. **Dahl, C. E., and J. S. Dahl.** 1984. Phospholipids as acyl donors to membrane proteins of *Mycoplasma capricolum*. *J. Biol. Chem.* **259:**10771–10776.

36. **Dahl, C. E., J. S. Dahl, and K. Bloch.** 1983. Proteolipid formation in *Mycoplasma capricolum*. Influence of cholesterol on unsaturated fatty acid acylation of membrane proteins. *J. Biol. Chem.* **258:**11814–11818.

37. **Dahl, C. E., N. C. Sactor, and J. S. Dahl.** 1985. Acylated proteins in *Acholeplasma laidlawii*. *J. Bacteriol.* **162:**445–447.

38. **Dahlqvist, A., S. Andersson, and Å. Wieslander.** 1992. The enzymatic synthesis of membrane glucolipids in *Acholeplasma laidlawii*. *Biochim. Biophys. Acta*, **1105:**131–140.

39. **Dallo, S. F., A. Chavoya, and J. B. Baseman.** 1990. Characterization of the gene for a 30-kilodalton adhesin-related protein of *Mycoplasma pneumoniae*. *Infect. Immun.* **58:**4163–4165.

40. **Dallo, S. F., A. Chavoya, C.-J. Su, and J. B. Baseman.** 1989. DNA and protein sequence homologies between

the adhesins of *Mycoplasma genitalium* and *Mycoplasma pneumoniae*. *Infect. Immun.* **57**:1059–1065.

41. **Deisenhofer, J., and H. Michel.** 1989. The photosynthetic reaction center from the purple bacterium *Rhodopseudomonas viridis*. *Science* **245**:1463–1473.

42. **Dresdner, G.** 1978. Efficiency and specificity of the sequential extraction of membrane proteins of *Acholeplasma laidlawii* with the neutral detergent Tween 20. *FEBS Lett.* **89**:69–72.

43. **Dresdner, G., and H. Cid-Dresdner.** 1976. Tween 20-soluble membrane proteins of *Acholeplasma laidlawii*. Fractionation in the presence of a Tween 20 concentration slightly above its critical micelle concentration and in the absence of detergent by means of agarose-suspension electrophoresis. *FEBS Lett.* **72**:243–246.

44. **Dresdner, G., and H. Cid-Dresdner.** 1977. The removal of the neutral detergent Tween 20 from solubilized membrane proteins of *Acholeplasma laidlawii* and other proteins by agarose suspension electrophoresis. *Anal. Biochem.* **78**:171–181.

45. **Dudler, R., C. Schmidhauser, R. W. Parish, R. E. H. Wettenhall, and S. Thomas.** 1988. A mycoplasma high-affinity transport system and the *in vitro* invasivness of mouse sarcoma-cells. *EMBO J.* **7**:3963–3970.

46. **Dunbar, B. S.** 1987. Protein detection in polyacrylamide gel electrophoresis, p. 67–76. *In* B. S. Dunbar (ed.), *Two-Dimensional Electrophoresis and Immunological Techniques*. Plenum Press, New York.

47. **Ehlers, M. R. W., and J. F. Riordan.** 1991. Membrane proteins with soluble counterparts: role of proteolysis in the release of transmembrane proteins. *Biochemistry* **30**:10065–10074.

48. **Ehrmann, M., and J. Beckwith.** 1991. Proper insertion of a complex membrane protein in absence of its amino-terminal export signal. *J. Biol. Chem.* **266**:16530–16533.

49. **Engelman, D. M.** 1971. Lipid bilayer structure in the membrane of *Mycoplasma laidlawii*. *J. Mol. Biol.* **58**:153–165.

50. **Epstein, W. P., D. Lever, L. M. Leining, E. Bruenger, and H. C. Rilling.** 1991. Quantitation of prenylcysteines by a selective cleavage reaction. *Proc. Natl. Acad. Sci. USA* **88**:9668–9670.

51. **Fasman, E. D. (ed.).** 1989. *Prediction of Protein Structure and Principles of Protein Conformation*. Plenum Press, New York.

52. **Fischer, M., M. H. Shirvan, M. W. Platt, H. Kirchoff, and S. Rottem.** 1988. Characterization of membrane components of flask-shaped mycoplasma *Mycoplasma mobile*. *J. Gen. Microbiol.* **134**:2385–2392.

53. **Fischetti, V. A.** 1991. Strepococcal M. protein *Sci. Am.* **264**:32–39.

54. **Fontenelle, C., A. Zaarla, M. F. Blot, and H. Wroblewski.** 1987. Conjugasion de l'immunoélectrophorèse bidimensionnelle et de la technique de 'Western blotting' pour l'evalation de la similarité antigénique entre protéines membranaires. *Rev. Inst. Pasteur Lyon* **20**:127–132.

55. **Gabridge, M. G., S. E. Singer, and R. A. Esposito.** 1976. Gradient, polyacrylamide gel electrophoresis of proteins from cytotoxic mycoplasma membranes. *Biochem. Biophys. Res. Commun.* **70**:271–279.

56. **Geary, S. J., and E. M. Walczak.** 1985. Isolation of a cytopathic factor from *Mycoplasma hyopneumoniae*. *Infect. Immun.* **48**:576–578.

57. **George, R., R. N. A. H. Lewis, S. Mahajan, and R. McElhaney.** 1989. Studies on the purified, lipid-reconstituted $(Na^+ + Mg^{2+})$-ATPase from *Acholeplasma laidlawii* B membranes. Dependence of enzyme activity on lipid headgroup and chain structure. *J. Biol. Chem.* **264**:11598–11604.

58. **George, R., R. N. A. H. Lewis, and R. N. McElhaney.** 1987. Reconstitution of the purified $(Na^+ + Mg^{2+})$-ATPase from *Acholeplasma laidlawii* B membranes into lipid vesicles and a characterization of the resulting proteoliposomes. *Biochim. Biophys. Acta* **903**:283–291.

59. **George, R., R. N. A. H. Lewis, and R. N. McElhaney.** 1987. Lipid modulation of the activity and temperature dependence of the purified $(Na^+ + Mg^{2+})$-ATPase from *Acholeplasma laidlawii* B membranes. *Isr. J. Med. Sci.* **23**:374–379.

60. **George, R., and R. N. McElhaney.** 1985. Affinity labeling of the $(Na^+ + Mg^{2+})$-ATPase in *Acholeplasma laidlawii* B membranes by the 2',3'-dialdehyde derivative of adenosine 5'-triphosphate. *Biochim. Biophys. Acta* **813**:161–166.

61. **Gerstenecker, B., and E. Jacobs.** 1990. Topological mapping of the P1-adhesin of *Mycoplasma pneumoniae* with adherence-inhibiting monoclonal antibodies. *J. Gen. Microbiol.* **136**:471–476.

62. **Gilson, E., G. Alloing, T. Schmidt, J.-P. Claverys, R. Dudler, and M. Hofnung.** 1988. Evidence for high affinity binding-protein dependent transport systems in Gram-positive bacteria and *Mycoplasma*. *EMBO J.* **7**:3971–3974.

63. **Goel, M. C.** 1973. New method for the isolation of membranes from *Mycoplasma gallisepticum*. *J. Bacteriol.* **116**:994–1000.

64. **Goel, M. C., and R. M. Lemcke.** 1975. Dissociation of *Mycoplasma gallisepticum* membranes with lithium diiodosalicylate and isolation of a glycoprotein. *Ann. Microbiol. Inst. Pasteur* **126B**:299–312.

65. **Green, D. E., and J. F. Perdue.** 1966. Membranes as expressions of repeating units. *Proc. Natl. Acad. Sci. USA* **55**:1295–1302.

66. **Gribskov, M., and J. Devereux (ed.).** 1991. *Sequence Analysis Primer*. Stockton Press, New York.

67. **Hayashi, S., and H. C. Wu.** 1990. Lipoproteins in bacteria. *J. Bioenerg. Biomembr.* **22**:451–471.

68. **Helenius, A., and K. Simons.** 1975. Solubilization of membrane proteins by detergents. *Biochim. Biophys. Acta* **415**:29–79.

69. **Henderson, R., J. M. Baldwin, T. A. Ceska, F. Zemlin, E. Beckman, and K. H. Downing.** 1990. Model for the structure of bacteriorhodopsin based on high-resolution electron cryo-microscopy. *J. Mol. Biol.* **213**:899–929.

70. **Higgins, C. F., M. P. Gallagher, S. C. Hyde, M. L. Mimmack, and S. R. Pearce.** 1990. Periplasmic binding protein-dependent transport systems: the membrane-associated components. *Phil. Trans. R. Soc. London Ser. B* **326**:353–365.

71. **Hjertén, S., and K.-E. Johansson.** 1972. Selective solubilization with Tween 20 of membrane proteins from *Acholeplasma laidlawii*. *Biochim. Biophys. Acta* **288**:312–325.

72. **Huang, J., and M. A. Schell.** 1990. Evidence that extracellular export of endoglucanase encoded by *egl* of *Pseudomonas solanacearum* occurs by a two-step process involving a lipoprotein intermediate. *J. Biol. Chem.* **265**:11628–11632.

73. **Hultgren, S. J., S. Normark, and S. N. Abraham.** 1991. Chaperone-assisted assembly and molecular architecture of adhesive pili. *Annu. Rev. Microbiol.* **45**:383–415.

74. **Inamine, J. M., T. P. Denny, S. Loechel, U. Schaper, C.-H. Huang, K. F. Bott, and P.-C. Hu.** 1988. Nucleotide sequence of the P1 attachment-protein gene of *Mycoplasma pneumoniae*. *Gene* **64**:217–229.

75. **Inamine, J. M., S. Loechel, A. M. Collier, M. F. Barile, and P.-C. Hu.** 1989. Nucleotide sequence of the MgPa (*mgp*) operon of *Mycoplasma genitalium* and comparision to the P1 (*mpp*) operon of *Mycoplasma pneumoniae*. *Gene* **82**:259–267.

76. **Inamine, J. M., S. Loechel, and P.-C. Hu.** 1988. Analysis of the nucleotide sequence of the P1 operon of *Mycoplasma pneumoniae*. *Gene* **73**:175–183.

77. **Issartel, J.-P., V. Koronakis, and C. Hughes.** 1991. Activation of *Escherichia coli* prohaemolysin to the mature toxin by acyl carrier protein-dependent fatty acylation. *Nature* (London) **351**:759–761.

78. **Jacobs, E.** 1991. *Mycoplasma pneumoniae* virulence factors and the immune response. *Rev. Med. Microbiol.* **2:**83–90.

79. **Jacobs, E., and A. Clad.** 1986. Electroelution of fixed stained membrane proteins from preparative sodium dodecyl sulfate-polyacrylamide gel into a membrane trap. *Anal. Biochem.* **154:**583–589.

80. **Jacobs, E., K. Fuchte, and W. Bredt.** 1987. Amino acid sequence and antigenicity of the amino-terminus of the 168kDa adherence protein of *Mycoplasma pneumoniae*. *J. Gen. Microbiol.* **133:**2233–2236.

81. **Jacobs, E., K. Fuchte, and W. Bredt.** 1988. Isolation of the adherence protein of *Mycoplasma pneumoniae* by fractionated solubilization and size exclusion chromatography. *Biol. Chem. Hoppe-Seyler* **369:**1295–1299.

82. **Jägersten, C.** 1984. Membrane antigens of *Acholeplasma laidlawii*. Ph. D. thesis. The University of Uppsala, Uppsala, Sweden.

83. **Jägersten, C., L. Odelstad, and K.-E. Johansson.** 1982. Identification of iron- and phosphorus-containing antigens of the *Acholeplasma laidlawii* cell membrane. *FEBS Lett.* **144:**130–134.

84. **James, R., and D. Branton.** 1973. Lipid and temperature-dependent structural changes in *Acholeplasma laidlawii* cell membranes. *Biochim. Biophys. Acta* **323:** 378–390.

85. **Jennings, M. L.** 1989. Topography of membrane proteins. *Annu. Rev. Biochem.* **58:**999–1027.

86. **Jinks, D. C., and L. L. Matz.** 1976. Purification of the reduced nicotinamide adenine dinucleotide dehydrogenase from membranes of *Acholeplasma laidlawii*. *Biochim. Biophys. Acta* **452:**30–41.

87. **Johansson, K.-E.** 1974. Fractionation of membrane proteins from *Acholeplasma laidlawii* by preparative agarose-suspension electrophoresis. *Protides Biol. Fluids Proc. Colloq.* **21:**151–156.

88. **Johansson, K.-E.** 1982. Membrane components of mycoplasmas. *Ann. Clin. Res.* **14:**278–288.

89. **Johansson, K.-E.** 1983. Characterization of the *Acholeplasma laidlawii* membrane by electroimmunochemical analysis methods, p. 321–346. *In* O. J. Bjerrum (ed.), *Electroimmunochemical Analysis of Membrane Proteins.* Elsevier Science Publishers, Amsterdam.

90. **Johansson, K.-E., I. Blomqvist, and S. Hjertén.** 1975. Purification of membrane proteins from *Acholeplasma laidlawii* by agarose suspension electrophoresis in Tween 20 and polyacrylamide and dextran gel electrophoresis in detergent-free media. *J. Biol. Chem.* **250:**2463–2469.

91. **Johansson, K.-E., and S. Hjertén.** 1974. Localization of the Tween 20-soluble membrane proteins of *Acholeplasma laidlawii* by crossed immunoelectrophoresis. *J. Mol. Biol.* **86:**341–348.

92. **Johansson, K.-E., and C. Jägersten.** 1982. Elucidation of the antigenic architecture of the *Acholeplasma laidlawii* cell membrane by immunoadsorption in combination with crossed immunoelectrophoresis. *Rev. Infect. Dis.* **4:**S73–S79.

93. **Johansson, K.-E., and C. Jägersten.** 1982. Vibrations in the antigenic architecture of the *Acholeplasma laidlawii* cell membrane. *Protides Biol. Fluids Proc. Colloq.* **29:** 251–254.

94. **Johansson, K.-E., C. Jägersten, A. Christiansson, and Å. Wieslander.** 1981. Protein composition and extractibility of lipid-modified membranes from *Acholeplasma laidlawii*. *Biochemistry* **20:**6073–6079.

95. **Johansson, K.-E., H. Pertoft, and S. Hjertén.**. 1979. Characterization of the Tween 20-soluble membrane proteins of *Acholeplasma laidlawii*. *Int. J. Biol. Macromol.* **1:**111–118.

96. **Johansson, K.-E., and H. Wroblewski.** 1978. Crossed immunoelectrophoresis, in the presence of Tween 20 or sodium deoxycholate, of purified membrane proteins from *Acholeplasma laidlawii*. *J. Bacteriol.* **136:**324–330.

97. **Johansson, K.-E., and H. Wroblewski.** 1983. Characterization of membrane proteins by crossed immunoelectrophoresis, p. 257–267. *In* S. Razin and J. G. Tully (ed.), *Methods in Mycoplasmology*, vol. 1. Academic Press, New York.

98. **Kahane, I., and Brunner.** 1977. Isolation of a glycoprotein from *Mycoplasma pneumoniae* membranes. *Infect. Immun.* **18:**273–277.

99. **Kahane, I., J. Granek, and A. Reisch-Saada.** 1984. The adhesins of *Mycoplasma gallisepticum* and *M. pneumoniae*. *Ann. Microbiol.* **135A:**25–32.

100. **Kahane, I., and S. Razin.** 1969. Synthesis and turnover of membrane protein and lipid in *Mycoplasma laidlawii*. *Biochim. Biophys. Acta* **183:**79–89.

101. **Kahane, I., and S. Razin.** 1969. Immunological analysis of mycoplasma membranes. *J. Bacteriol.* **100:**187–194.

102. **Kawauchi, Y., A. Muto, and S. Osawa.** 1982. The protein composition of *Mycoplasma capricolum*. *Mol. Gen. Genet.* **188:**7–11.

103. **Kenny, B., R. Haig, and I. B. Holland.** 1991. Analysis of the haemolysin transport process through the secretion from *Escherichia coli* PCM, CAT or β-galactosidase fused to the Hly C-terminal signal domain. *Mol. Microbiol.* **5:**2557–2568.

104. **Kenny, G. E.** 1979. Antigenic determinants, p. 351–384. *In* M. F. Barile and S. Razin (ed.), *The Mycoplasmas*, vol. 1. Academic Press, New York.

105. **Kenny, G. E.** 1983. Agar precipitin and immunoelectrophoretic methods for detection of mycoplasmic antigens, p. 441–456. *In* S. Razin and J. G. Tully (ed.), *Methods in Mycoplasmology*, vol. 1. Academic Press, New York.

106. **Klein, P., R. L. Somorjai, and P. C. K. Lau.** 1988. Distinctive properties of signal sequences from bacterial lipoproteins. *Protein Eng.* **2:**15–20.

107. **Koivula, T., I. Palva, and H. Hemilä.** 1991. Nucleotide sequence of the *sec*Y gene from *Lactococcus lactis* and identification of conserved regions by comparison of four SecY proteins. *FEBS Lett.* **288:**114–118.

108. **Krause, D. C., and K. K. Lee.** 1991. Juxtaposition of the genes encoding *Mycoplasma pneumoniae* cytadherence-accessory protein HMW1 and HMW3. *Gene* **107:**83–89.

109. **Kuhlbrandt, W., and D. N. Wang.** 1991. Three-dimensional structure of plant light-harvesting complex determined by electron microscopy. *Nature* (London) **350:**130–134.

110. **Laforet, G. A., E. T. Kaiser, and D. A. Kendall.** 1989. Signal peptide subsegments are not always functionally interchangeable. *J. Biol. Chem.* **264:**14478–14485.

111. **Le Hénaff, M., C. Brenner, C. Fontenelle, C. Delamarche, and H. Wroblewski.** 1991. Does spiralin possess a cleavable N-terminal signal sequence? *C. R. Acad. Sci.* **312:**189–195.

112. **Leith, D. K., and J. B. Baseman.** 1984. Purification of *Mycoplasma pneumoniae* adhesin by monoclonal antibody affinity chromatography. *J. Bacteriol.* **157:** 678–680.

113. **Leith, D. K., L. B. Trevino, J. G. Tully, L. B. Senterfit, and J. B. Baseman.** 1983. Host discrimination of *Mycoplasma pneumonia* proteinaceous antigens. *J. Exp. Med.* **157:**502–514.

114. **Lewis, R. N. A. H., R. George, and R. N. McElhaney.** 1986. Structure-function investigations of the membrane $(Na^+ + Mg^{2+})$-ATPase from *Acholeplasma laidlawii* B: studies of reactive amino acid residues using group-specific reagents. *Arch. Biochem. Biophys.* **247:** 201–210.

115. **Lewis, R. N. A. H., and R. N. McElhaney.** 1983. Purification and characterization of the membrane $(Na^+ + Mg^{2+})$-ATPase from *Acholeplasma laidlawii*. *Biochim. Biophys. Acta* **735:**113–122.

116. **Low, M. G.** 1989. The glycosyl-phosphatidylinositol anchor of membrane proteins. *Biochim. Biophys. Acta* **988:**427–454.

117. **Mader, B., P.-C. Hu, C.-H. Huang, E. Schiltz, and E. Jacobs.** 1991. The mature MgPa-adhesin of *Mycoplasma genitalium. Zentralbl. Bakteriol.* **274:**507–513.

118. **Maltese, W. A.** 1990. Posttranslational modification of proteins by isoprenoids in mammalian cells. *FASEB J.* **4:**3319–3328.

119. **Maniloff, J.** 1981. Cytoskeletal elements in mycoplasmas and other procaryotes. *BioSystems* **14:**305–312.

120. **Marchesi, J. L., E. Steers, V. T. Marchesi, and T. W. Tillack.** 1970. Physical and chemical properties of a protein isolated from red cell membranes. *Biochemistry* **9:**50–57.

121. **Mathiopoulos, C., J. P. Mueller, F. J. Slack, C. G. Murphy, S. Patankar, G. Bukusoglu, and A. L. Sonenshein.** 1991. A *Bacillus subtilis* dipeptide transport system expressed early during sporulation. *Mol. Microbiol.* **5:**1903–1913.

122. **McElhaney, R. N.** 1984. The structure and function of the *Acholeplasma laidlawii* plasma membrane. *Biochim. Biophys. Acta* **779:**1–42.

123. **McElhaney, R. N.** 1989. The influence of membrane lipid composition and physical properties of membrane structure and function in *Acholeplasma laidlawii. Crit. Rev. Microbiol.* **17:**1–32.

124. **McGovern, K., and J. Beckwith.** 1991. Membrane insertion of *Escherichia coli* MalF protein in cells with impaired secretion machinery. *J. Biol. Chem.* **266:**20870–20876.

125. **McIlhinney, R. A. J.** 1990. The fats of life: the importance and function of protein acylation. *Trends Biochem. Sci.* **15:**387–391.

126. **Mézes, P. S. F., and J. O. Lampen.** 1985. Secretion of proteins by bacilli, p. 151–183. *In* D. A. Dubnau (ed.), *The Molecular Biology of the Bacilli*, vol. II. Academic Press, Orlando, Fla.

127. **Miller, R. G.** 1984. Interactions between digitonin and bilayer membranes. *Biochim. Biophys. Acta* **774:**151–157.

128. **Mouches, C., J. C. Vignault, J. G. Tully, R. F. Whitcomb, and J.-M. Bové.** 1979. Characterization of spiroplasmas by one- and two-dimensional protein analysis on polyacrylamide slab gels. *Curr. Microbiol.* **2:**69–74.

129. **Munoa, F. J., K. W. Miller, R. Beers, M. Graham, and H. C. Wu.** 1991. Membrane topology of *Escherichia coli* prolipoprotein signal peptidase (signal peptidase II). *J. Biol. Chem.* **266:**17667–17672.

130. **Nakai, K., and M. Kanehisa.** 1991. Expert system for predicting protein localization sites in Gram-negative bacteria. *Proteins* **11:**95–110.

131. **Ne'eman, Z., I. Kahane, and S. Razin.** 1971. Characterization of the mycoplasma membrane proteins. II. Solubilization and enzyme activities of *Acholeplasma laidlawii* membrane proteins. *Biochim. Biophys. Acta* **249:**169–176.

132. **Ne'eman, Z., and S. Razin.** 1975. Characterization of the mycoplasma membrane proteins. V. Release and localization of membrane-bound enzymes in *Acholeplasma laidlawii. Biochim. Biophys. Acta* **375:**54–68.

133. **Neidhardt, F. C., D. B. Appleby, P. Sankar, M. E. Hutton, and T. Phillips.** 1989. Genomically linked cellular protein databases derived from two-dimensional polyacrylamide gel electrophoresis. *Electrophoresis* **10:**116–122.

134. **Neidhardt, F. C., J. L. Ingraham, and M. Schaechter.** 1990. *Physiology of the Bacterial Cell: A Molecular Approach.* Sinauer Associates, Sunderland, Mass.

135. **Nicolet, J., P. H. Paroz, and B. Kristensen.** 1980. Growth medium constituents contaminating mycoplasma preparations and their role in the study of membrane glycoproteins in porcine mycoplasmas. *J. Gen. Microbiol.* **119:**17–26.

136. **Nielsen, J. B. K., and J. O. Lampen.** 1982. Glyceride-cysteine lipoproteins and secretion by gram-positive bacteria. *J. Bacteriol.* **152:**315–322.

137. **Nilsson, I., and G. von Heijne.** 1990. Fine-tuning the topology of a polytopic membrane protein: role of positively and negatively charged amino acids. *Cell* **62:**1135–1141.

138. **Nyström, S.** 1991. Modification of Mycoplasma membrane proteins with fatty acid and isoprenoid chains. Ph.D. thesis. The University of Umeå, Umeå, Sweden.

139. **Nyström, S., K.-E. Johansson, and Å. Wieslander.** 1986. Selective acylation of membrane proteins in *Acholeplasma laidlawii. Eur. J. Biochem.* **156:**85–94.

140. **Nyström, S., P. Wallbrandt, and Å. Wieslander.** 1992. Membrane protein acylation. Preference for exogenous myristic acid or endogenous saturated chains in *Acholeplasma laidlawii. Eur. J. Biochem.* **204:**231–240.

141. **Nyström, S., and Å. Wieslander.** 1992. Isoprenoid modification of proteins distinct from membrane acyl proteins in the prokaryote *Acholeplasma laidlawii. Biochim. Biophys. Acta* **1107:**39–43.

142. **O'Farrell, P. H.** 1975. High resolution two-dimensional electrophoresis of proteins. *J. Biol. Chem.* **250:**4007–4021.

143. **Ohkubo, S., A. Muto, Y. Kawauchi, F. Yamao, and S. Osawa.** 1987. The ribosomal protein gene cluster of *Mycoplasma capricolum. Mol. Gen. Genet.* **210:**314–322.

144. **Paroz, P. H., and J. Nicolet.** 1978. Glycoproteins in mycoplasmas. Contamination with serum aggregates from growth media. *Experientia* **34:**1668.

145. **Perlman, D., and H. O. Halvorson.** 1983. A putative signal peptidase recognition site and sequence in eukaryotic and prokaryotic signal peptides. *J. Mol. Biol.* **167:**391–409.

146. **Platt, M. W., J. Reizer, and S. Rottem.** 1990. A 57-kilodalton protein associated with *Spiroplasma melliferum* fibrils undergoes reversible phosphorylation. *J. Bacteriol.* **172:**2808–2811.

147. **Platt, M. W., S. Rottem, Y. Milner, M. F. Barile, A. Peterkofsky, and J. Reizer.** 1988. Protein phosphorylation in *Mycoplasma gallisepticum. Eur. J. Biochem.* **176:**61–67.

148. **Plusquellec, D., G. Chevalier, R. Talibart, and H. Wroblewski.** 1989. Synthesis and characterization of 6-O-(N-heptylcarbamoyl)-methyl-α-D-glucopyranoside, a new surfactant for membrane studies. *Anal. Biochem.* **179:**145–153.

149. **Pollack, J. D., A. J. Merola, M. Platz, and R. L. Booth, Jr.** 1981. Respiration-associated components of Mollicutes. *J. Bacteriol.* **146:**907–913.

150. **Pollack, J. D., S. Razin, and R. C. Cleverdon.** 1965. Localization of enzymes in *Mycoplasma. J. Bacteriol.* **90:**617–622.

151. **Pollack, J. D., S. Razin, M. E. Pollack, and R. C. Cleverdon.** 1965. Fractionation of *Mycoplasma* cells for enzyme localization. *Life Sci.* **4:**973–977.

152. **Pugsley, A. P.** 1989. *Protein Targeting.* Academic Press, New York.

153. **Pugsley, A. P., C. d'Enfert, I. Reyss, and M. G. Kornacker.** 1990. Genetics of extracellular protein secretion by Gram-negative bacteria. *Annu. Rev. Genet.* **24:**67–90.

154. **Pugsley, A. P., and M. G. Kornacker.** 1991. Secretion of the cell surface lipoprotein pullulanase in *Escherichia coli. J. Biol. Chem.* **266:**13640–13645.

155. **Quillien, L.** 1987. Antigènes protéiques membranaires de *Mycoplasma hyponeumoniae.* Ph.D. thesis. The University of Rennes I, Rennes, France.

156. **Quillien, L., A. Zaaria, C. Fontenelle, and H. Wroblewski.** 1986. The combination of isoelectric focusing and crossed immunoelectrophoresis for the analysis of membrane proteins of spiroplasmas, with special reference to spiralin. *Protides Biol. Fluids Proc. Colloq.* **34:**921–924.

157. **Randall, L. L., and S. J. S. Hardy.** 1989. Unity in function in the absence of consensus in sequence: role of leader peptides in export. *Science* **243:**1156–1159.

158. **Razin, S.** 1963. Osmotic lysis of mycoplasma. *J. Gen. Microbiol.* **33:**471–475.

159. **Razin, S.** 1964. Factors influencing osmotic fragility of mycoplasma. *J. Gen. Microbiol.* **36:**451–459.

160. **Razin, S.** 1972. Reconstitution of biological membranes. *Biochim. Biophys. Acta* **265:**241–296.

161. **Razin, S.** 1975. The mycoplasma membrane. *Prog. Surf. Membr. Sci.* **9:**257–312.

162. **Razin, S.** 1979. Isolation and characterization of mycoplasma membranes, p. 213–229. *In* M. F. Barile and S. Razin (ed.), *The Mycoplasmas*, vol. 1. Academic Press, New York.

163. **Razin, S.** 1979. Membrane proteins, p. 289–322. *In* M. F. Barile and S. Razin (ed.), *The Mycoplasmas*, vol. 1. Academic Press, New York.

164. **Razin, S.** 1981. The mycoplasma membrane, p. 165–250. *In* B. K. Ghosh (ed.), *Organization of Prokaryotic Cell Membranes*, vol. 1. CRC Press, Boca Raton, Fla.

165. **Razin, S.** 1983. Cell lysis and isolation of membranes, p. 225–233. *In* S. Razin and J. G. Tully (ed.), *Methods in Mycoplasmology*, vol. 1. Academic Press, New York.

166. **Razin, S., and M. Argaman.** 1962. Susceptibility of mycoplasma (pleuropneumonia-like organisms) and bacterial protoplast to lysis by various agents. *Nature* (London) **193:**502–503.

167. **Razin, S., and M. Argaman.** 1963. Lysis of mycoplasma, bacterial protoplasts, spheroplasts and L-forms by various agents. *J. Gen. Microbiol.* **30:**155–172.

168. **Razin, S., H. J. Morowitz, and T. M. Terry.** 1965. Membrane subunits of *Mycoplasma laidlawii* and their assembly to membrane-like structures. *Proc. Natl. Acad. Sci. USA* **54:**219–225.

169. **Razin, S., and S. Rottem.** 1976. Techniques for the manipulation of mycoplasma membranes, p. 20–36. *In* A. H. Maddy (ed.), *Biochemical Analysis of Membranes.* Chapman & Hall, London.

170. **Razin, S., M. E. Tourtellotte, R. N. McElhaney, and J. D. Pollack.** 1966. Influence of lipid components of *Mycoplasma laidlawii* membranes on osmotic fragility of cells. *J. Bacteriol.* **91:**609–616.

171. **Reinards, R., J. Kubicki, and H.-D. Ohlenbusch.** 1981. Purification and characterization of NADH oxidase from membranes of *Acholeplasma laidlawii*, a copper-containing iron-sulfur flavoprotein. *Eur. J. Biochem.* **120:**329–337.

172. **Riethman, H. C., M. J. Boyer, and K. S. Wise.** 1987. Triton X-114 phase fractionation of an integral membrane surface protein mediating monoclonal antibody killing of *Mycoplasma hyorhinis*. *Infect. Immun.* **56:**1094–1100.

173. **Rodwell, A. W., and E. S. Rodwell.** 1978. Relationships between strains of *Mycoplasma mycoides* subspp. *mycoides* and *capri* studied by two-dimensional gel electrophoresis of cell proteins. *J. Gen. Microbiol.* **109:**259–263.

174. **Root-Bernstein, R. S., and S. H. Hobbs.** 1991. Homologies between mycoplasma adhesion peptide, CD4 and class II MHC proteins: a possible mechanism for HIV-mycoplasma synergism in AIDS. *Res. Immunol.* **142:**519–523.

175. **Rosengarten, R., and K. S. Wise.** 1991. The Vlp system of *Mycoplasma hyorhinis*: combinatorial expression of distinct size variant lipoproteins generating high-frequency surface antigenic variation. *J. Bacteriol.* **173:**4782–4793.

176. **Rottem, S., M. Hasin, and S. Razin.** 1973. Binding of proteins to mycoplasma membranes. *Biochim. Biophys. Acta* **298:**876–886.

176a.**Rottem, S., C. Linker, and T. H. Wilson.** 1981. Proton motive force across the membrane of *Mycoplasma gallisepticum* and its possible role in cell volume regulation. *J. Bacteriol.* **145:**1299–1304.

177. **Rottem, S., and S. Razin.** 1972. Isolation of mycoplasma membranes by digitonin. *J. Bacteriol.* **110:**699–705.

178. **Rottem, S., O. Stein, and S. Razin.** 1968. Reassembly of mycoplasma membranes disaggregated by detergents. *Arch. Biochem. Biophys.* **125:**46–56.

179. **Ruuth, E.** 1988. Murine B lymphocyte growth regulation. A study of host defence factors and their mimicry by *Mycoplasma arginini*. Ph.D. thesis. The University of Umeå, Umeå, Sweden.

180. **Ruuth, E., Å. Wieslander, H. Persson, B. Friedrich, and E. Lundgren.** 1984. Lymphokine-like activity of a strain of *Mycoplasma arginini*. *Isr. J. Med. Sci.* **20:**886–890.

181. **Sato, S., K. Ito, and T. Yura.** 1977. Membrane proteins of *Escherichia coli* K-12: two-dimensional polyacrylamide gel electrophoresis of inner and outer membranes. *Eur. J. Biochem.* **78:**557–567.

182. **Schmidt, M. F. G.** 1989. Fatty acylation of proteins. *Biochim. Biophys. Acta* **988:**411–426.

183. **Schulz, G. E., and R. H. Schirmer.** 1979. *Principles of Protein Structure.* Springer-Verlag, New York.

184. **Shibata, K.-I., and T. Watanabe.** 1986. Carboxypeptidase activity in human mycoplasmas. *J. Bacteriol.* **168:**1045–1047.

185. **Shibata, K.-I., and T. Watanabe.** 1987. Purification and characterization of an aminopeptidase from *Mycoplasma salivarium*. *J. Bacteriol.* **169:**3409–3413.

186. **Shibata, K.-I., and T. Watanabe.** 1988. Purification and characterization of an arginine-specific carboxypeptidase from *Mycoplasma salivarium*. *J. Bacteriol.* **170:**1795–1799.

187. **Shirvan, M. H., Z. Gross, Z. Ne'eman, and S. Rottem.** 1982. Isolation of *Mycoplasma gallisepticum* membranes by a mild alkaline-induced lysis of nonenergized cells. *Curr. Micobiol.* **7:**367–370.

188. **Shirvan, M. H., S. Rottem, Z. Ne'eman, and R. Bittman.** 1982. Isolation of mycoplasma membranes by dicyclohexylcarbodiimide-induced lysis. *J. Bacteriol.* **142:**1124–1128.

189. **Simoneau, P., and J. Labarère.** 1988. Isolation of *Spiroplasma citri* membranes and characterization of membrane proteins by two-dimensional gel electophoresis. *Curr. Microbiol.* **16:**229–235.

190. **Simoneau, P., and J. Labarère.** 1989. Detection of Concanavalin A binding protein in the mollicute *Spiroplasma citri* and purification from the plasma membrane. *Arch. Microbiol.* **152:**488–491.

191. **Singer, S. J., and G. J. Nicolson.** 1972. The fluid mosaic model of the structure of cell membranes. *Science* **175:**720–731.

192. **Sjöström, M., S. Wold, Å. Wieslander, and L. Rilfors.** 1987. Signal peptide amino acid sequences in *Escherichia coli* contain information related to final protein localization. A multivariate data analysis. *EMBO J.* **6:**823–831.

193. **Smith, P. F.** 1979. The composition of membrane lipids and lipopolysaccharides, p. 231–257. *In* M. F. Barile and S. Razin (ed.), *The Mycoplasmas*, vol. 1. Academic Press, New York.

194. **Smith, P. F.** 1990. Diversity and similarities of lipid metabolism among the mollicutes. *Int. J. Med. Microbiol. Suppl.* **20:**155–161.

195. **Stader, J. A., and T. J. Silhavy.** 1990. Engineering *Escherichia coli* to secrete heterologous gene products. *Methods Enzymol.* **185:**166–187.

196. **Stephens, E.B., G. S. Aulakh, D. L. Rose, J. G. Tully, and M. F. Barile.** 1983. Intraspecies genetic relatedness among strains of *Acholeplasma laidlawii* and of *Acholeplasma axanthum* by nucleic acid hybridization. *J. Gen. Microbiol.* **129:**1929–1934.

197. **Stevens, M. K., and D. C. Krause.** 1991. Localization of the *Mycoplasma pneumoniae* cytadherence-accessory proteins HMW1 and HMW4 in the cytoskeletonlike triton shell. *J. Bacteriol.* **173:**1041–1051.

198. **Stock, J. B., A. J. Ninfa, and A. M. Stock.** 1989. Protein phosphorylation and regulation of adaptive response in bacteria. *Microbiol. Rev.* **53:**450–490.

199. **Su, C. J., A. Chavoya, S. F. Dallo, and J. B. Baseman.** 1990. Sequence divergency of the cytadhesin gene of *Mycoplasma pneumoniae. Infect. Immun.* **58:** 2669–2674.

200. **Su, C. J., V. Tryon, and J. Baseman.** 1987. Cloning and sequence analysis of cytadhesin P1 gene from *Mycoplasma pneumoniae. Infect. Immun.* **55:**3023–3029.

201. **Tegman, V., P. Wallbrandt, S. Nyström, K.-E. Johansson, B.-H. Jonsson, and Å. Wieslander.** 1987. Cloning and expression of *Acholeplasma laidlawii* membrane acyl proteins in *Escherichia coli. Isr. J. Med. Sci.* **23:**408–413.

202. **Thirkill, C. E., and G. E. Kenny.** 1974. Serological comparision of five arginine-utilizing *Mycoplasma* species by two-dimensional immunoelectrophoresis. *Infect. Immun.* **10:**624–632.

203. **Thirkill, D., A. D. Myles, and W. C. Russell.** 1991. Palmitoylated proteins in *Ureaplasma urealyticum. J. Bacteriol.* **59:**781–784.

204. **Tourtellotte, M. E., and J. S. Zupnik.** 1973. Freeze-fractured *Acholeplasma laidlawii* membranes: nature of particles observed. *Science* **179:**84–86.

205. **Towbin, H., T. Staehelin, and J. Gordon.** 1979. Electrophoretic transfer of proteins from polyacrylamide gels to nitrocellulose sheets: procedure and some applications. *Proc. Natl. Acad. Sci. USA* **76:**4350–4354.

206. **Townsend, R, and D. B. Archer.** 1983. A fibril protein antigen specific to *Spiroplasma. J. Gen. Microbiol.* **129:**199–206.

207. **Townsend, R., D. B. Archer, and K. A. Plaskitt.** 1980. Purification and characterization of spiroplasma fibrils. *J. Bacteriol.* **142:**694–700.

208. **Townsend, R., and K. A. Plaskitt.** 1985. Immunogold localization of p55-fibril protein and p25-spiralin in spiroplasma cell. *J. Gen. Microbiol.* **131:**983–992.

209. **Verner, K., and G. Schatz.** 1988. Protein translocation across membranes. *Science* **241:**1307–1313.

210. **von Heijne, G.** 1985. Signal sequences. The limits of variation. *J. Mol. Biol.* **184:**99–105.

211. **von Heijne, G.** 1988. Transcending the impermeable: how proteins come to terms with membranes. *Biochim. Biophys. Acta* **947:**307–333.

212. **von Heijne, G.** 1990. The signal peptide. *J. Membr. Biol.* **115:**195–201.

213. **von Heijne, G., and L. Abrahamsen.** 1989. Species-specific variation in signal peptide design: implications for protein secretion in foreign hosts. *FEBS Lett.* **244:** 439–446.

214. **von Heijne, G., and Y. Gavel.** 1988. Topogenic signals in integral membrane proteins. *Eur. J. Biochem.* **174:** 671–678.

215. **von Heijne, G., and C. Manoil.** 1990. Membrane proteins: from sequence to structure. *Protein Eng.* **4:** 109–112.

216. **Walderhaug, M. O., R. L. Post, G. Saccomani, R. T. Leonard, and D. P. Briskin.** 1985. Structural relatedness of three ion-transport adenosine triphosphatases around their active sites of phosphorylation. *J. Biol. Chem.* **260:**3852–3859.

217. **Wallbrandt, P., V. Tegman, B.-H. Jonsson, and Å. Wieslander.** 1992. Identification and analysis of the genes for the putative pyruvate dehydrogenase enzyme complex in *Acholeplasma laidlawii. J. Bacteriol.* **174:**1388–1396.

218. **Wandersman, C.** 1989. Secretion, processing and activation of bacterial extracellular proteases. *Mol. Microbiol.* **3:**1825–1831.

219. **Watson, H. L., K. Dybvig, D. K. Blalock, and G. H. Cassell.** 1989. Subunit structure of the variable V-1 antigen of *Mycoplasma pulmonis. Infect. Immun.* **57:**1634–1690.

220. **Watson, H. L., S. McDaniel, D. K. Blalock, M. T. Fallon, and G. H. Cassell.** 1988. Heterogeneity among strains and a high rate of variation within strains of a major surface antigen of *Mycoplasma pulmonis. Infect. Immun.* **56:**1358–1363.

221. **Weiss, M. S., U. Abele, J. Weckesser, W. Welte, E. Schiltz, and G. E. Schulz.** 1991. Molecular architecture and electrostatic properties of a bacterial porin. *Science* **254:**1627–1630.

222. **Wickner, W., A. J. M. Driessen, and F.-U. Hartl.** 1991. The enzymology of protein translocation across the *Escherichia coli* plasma membrane. *Annu. Rev. Biochem.* **60:**101–124.

223. **Wieslander, Å.** Unpublished data.

224. **Williamson, D. L., J. Renaudin, and J. M. Bové.** 1991. Nucleotide sequence of the *Spiroplasma citri* fibril protein gene. *J. Bacteriol.* **173:**4353–4362.

225. **Wise, K. S., and M. F. Kim.** 1987. Major membrane surface proteins of *Mycoplasma hyopneumoniae* selectively modified by covalently bound lipid. *J. Bacteriol.* **169:**5546–5555.

226. **Wroblewski, H.** 1975. Dissolution sélective de protéines de la membrane de *Spiroplasma citri* par le désoxycholate de sodium. *Biochimie* **57:**1095–1098.

227. **Wroblewski, H.** 1979. The amphilic nature of spiralin, the major protein of the *Spiroplasma citri* cell membrane. *J. Bacteriol.* **140:**738–741.

228. **Wroblewski, H., R. Burlot, and K.-E. Johansson.** 1978. Solubilization of *Spiroplasma citri* cell membrane proteins with the anionic detergent sodium lauroyl-sarcosinate (Sarkosyl). *Biochimie* **60:**389–398.

229. **Wroblewski, H., R. Burlot, and D. Thomas.** 1981. Adsorption of proteins from the *Spiroplasma citri* cell membrane by magnesium lauroyl-sarcosinate crystals. *Biochimie* **63:**177–186.

230. **Wroblewski, H., K.-E. Johansson, and R. Burlot.** 1977. Crossed immunoelectrophoresis of membrane proteins from *Acholeplasma laidlawii* and *Spiroplasma citri. Int. J. Syst. Bacteriol.* **27:**97–103.

231. **Wroblewski, H, K.-E. Johansson, and S. Hjertén.** 1977. Purification and characterization of spiralin, the main protein of the *Spiroplasma citri* membrane. *Biochim. Biophys. Acta* **465:**275–289.

232. **Wroblewski, H., S. Nyström, A. Blanchard, and Å. Wieslander.** 1989. Topology and acylation of spiralin. *J. Bacteriol.* **171:**5039–5047.

233. **Wroblewski, H., and D. Ratanasavanh.** 1976. Etude par immunoélectrophorèse bidimensionnelle de la composition antigénique de la membrane de quelques souches de mycoplasmes. *Can. J. Microbiol.* **22:**1048–1053.

234. **Wroblewski, H., D. Robic, D. Thomas, and A. Blanchard.** 1984. Comparison of the amino acid compositions and antigenic properties of spiralins purified from the plasma membranes of different spiroplasmas. *Ann. Inst. Pasteur Microbiol.* **135A:**73–82.

235. **Yamada, Y., Y.-Y. Chang, G. A. Daniels, L.-F. Wu, J. M. Tomich, M. Yamada, and M. H. Saier, Jr.** 1991. Insertion of the mannitol permease into the membrane of *Escherichia coli*. Possible involvement of an N-terminal amphiphilic sequence. *J. Biol. Chem.* **266:**17863–17871.

236. **Yogev, D., R. Rosengarten, R. Watson-McKown, and K. S. Wise.** 1991. Molecular basis of *Mycoplasma* surface antigenic variation: a novel set of divergent genes undergo spontaneous mutation of periodic coding regions and 5′ regulatory sequences. *EMBO J.* **10:**4069–4079.

237. **Yogev, D., R. Watson-McKown, M. A. Mcintosh, and K. S. Wise.** 1991. Sequence and Tn*phoA* analysis of a *Mycoplasma hyorhinis* protein with membrane export function. *J. Bacteriol.* **173:**2035–2044.

238. **Zaaria, A.** 1989. Antigénicité de la spiraline. Ph.D. thesis. The University of Rennes I, Rennes, France.

239. **Zaaria, A., C. Fontenelle, M. Le Hénaff, and H. Wroblewski.** 1990. Antigenic relatedness between spiralins of *Spiroplasma citri* and *Spiroplasma melliferum. J. Bacteriol.* **172:**5494–5496.

240. **Zaaria, A., and H. Wroblewski.** Unpublished data.

8. Membrane Structure

RONALD N. McELHANEY

INTRODUCTION

The mycoplasmas are a diverse group of procaryotic microorganisms that lack a cell wall. Since the mycoplasmas are genetically and morphologically the simplest organisms capable of autonomous replication, they provide useful models for the study of a number of problems in molecular and cellular biology. Mycoplasmas are particularly valuable for studies of the structure and function of cell membranes. Being nonphotosynthetic procaryotes as well as lacking a cell wall or outer membrane, mycoplasma cells possess only a single membrane, the limiting or plasma membrane. This membrane contains essentially all the cellular lipid and, because these cells are small, a substantial fraction of the total cellular protein as well. Because of the absence of a cell wall, substantial quantities of highly pure membranes can usually be easily prepared by gentle osmotic lysis followed by differential centrifugation, a practical advantage not offered by other procaryotic microorganisms. For a thorough discussion of the isolation and characterization of mycoplasma membranes, the reader is referred to a previous review by Razin (144).

Another useful property of mycoplasmas is the ability to induce dramatic yet controlled variations in the fatty acid composition of their membrane lipids. Thus, relatively large quantities of a number of exogenous saturated, unsaturated, branched-chain, or alicyclic fatty acids can be biosynthetically incorporated into the membrane phospho- and glycolipids of these organisms. In cases in which de novo fatty acid biosynthesis is either inhibited or absent, fatty acid-homogeneous membranes (membranes whose glycerolipids contain only a single species of fatty acyl chain) can sometimes be produced. Moreover, by growing mycoplasmas in the presence or absence of various quantities of cholesterol or other sterols, the amount of these compounds present in the membrane can be dramatically altered. The ability to manipulate membrane lipid fatty acid composition and cholesterol content, and thus to alter the phase state and fluidity of the membrane lipid bilayer, makes these organisms ideal for studying the roles of lipids in biological membranes (145).

The unique advantages of mycoplasmas for membrane studies, especially for studies of membrane lipid organization and dynamics, have induced a large number of investigators to study these microorga-

Ronald N. McElhaney • Department of Biochemistry, University of Alberta, Edmonton, Alberta, Canada T6G 2H7.

nisms by using a wide variety of physical techniques. For this reason, we probably know more about the roles of lipids in mycoplasma membranes in general, and in the *Acholeplasma laidlawii* membrane in particular, than in any other biological membrane. The aim of this chapter is to provide a comprehensive and up-to-date summary of these studies and to offer a critical analysis of their validity and significance.

This review will focus on the molecular aspects of membrane structure and certain of their functional correlates. A more detailed treatment of mycoplasma membrane function is presented in chapter 15. Since, to the best of my knowledge, no detailed molecular studies of the structure of membranes from *Anaeroplasma*, *Spiroplasma*, and *Ureaplasma* species have been published, I deal here only with the membrane of *A. laidlawii* and with the membranes of several *Mycoplasma* species. Although preliminary studies of membrane structure in several *Thermoplasma* species have been reported (89), these members of the archaebacteria are beyond the scope of this review. For a more comprehensive and general coverage of both *Acholeplasma* and *Mycoplasma* membrane structure and function, the reader is referred to earlier reviews by Rottem (155) and by Razin (143, 145); for more detailed summaries of investigations of the *A. laidlawii* membrane, the reader is referred to earlier reviews by McElhaney (118, 120).

CHEMICAL COMPOSITION OF MYCOPLASMA MEMBRANES

General Composition

The gross chemical compositions of mycoplasma membranes are generally similar to those of other procaryotic plasma membranes, consisting primarily of proteins and lipids. Typically, *Acholeplasma* and *Mycoplasma* membranes contain 50 to 60 wt% protein and 30 to 40 wt% lipid. From the average molecular weights of the lipid and protein components, this represents a molar ratio of lipid to protein of approximately 60:1 to 65:1. It should be noted, however, that fairly large variations in lipid/protein ratios can be induced by variations in culture conditions, particularly by changes in the type and amount of exogenous fatty acid or sterol added to the growth medium. As well, the lipid/protein ratio often decreases markedly with the age of the cultures (144, 145). Carbohydrate, present as either a polysaccharide or lipopolysaccharide "fuzzy coat," may account for as much as 10 to 15% of membrane dry weight in *A. laidlawii* and in some *Mycoplasma* species (see chapter 5). Considerable quantities of Mg^{2+} and small amounts of Ca^{2+} are associated with mycoplasma membranes and probably play a role in the stabilization of the lipid bilayer and the binding to it of peripheral membrane proteins (81).

Lipid Composition

The major endogenous membrane polar lipids in most mycoplasmas are the acidic glycerophospho-lipids phosphatidylglycerol (PG) and diphosphatidylglycerol (DPG) and the neutral glyceroglycolipids monoglucosyldiacylglycerol (MGDG) and diglucosyldiacylglycerol (DGDG), although a wide variety of other minor lipids may be present as well (see chapter 6). The neutral glycolipids predominate in *Acholeplasma* species whereas the acidic phosphatides predominate in *Mycoplasma* species. Many *Mycoplasma* species can also take up appreciable exogenous phosphatidylcholine (PC) or sphingomyelin from the growth medium. *Acholeplasma* species neither synthesize nor require cholesterol or related steroids for growth. However, these organisms will incorporate moderate quantities of cholesterol into their membranes if the cholesterol is supplied in the growth medium. Although *Mycoplasma* species are also incapable of synthesizing sterols, they require exogenous cholesterol (or a closely related sterol) for growth, a property unique among procaryotic microorganisms. *Mycoplasma* species usually incorporate large amounts of cholesterol into their membranes, reaching levels comparable to those found in eucaryotic plasma membranes. However, some *Mycoplasma* species can be adapted to grow on rather low levels of exogenous cholesterol, making it possible to markedly vary the amount of cholesterol and other sterols in their membranes (90, 157, 165).

All *A. laidlawii* strains studied to date have been found to be capable of the de novo biosynthesis only of even-chain, saturated fatty acids of 12 to 18 carbon atoms when grown in a lipid-free medium. No unsaturated, branched-chain, or other fatty acid types can be produced under these conditions. However, these organisms will take up large amounts of a wide variety of exogenous fatty acids if the fatty acids are supplied in proper form in the growth medium, and it is thus possible to produce cells whose membranes contain from 50 to 85 mol% of a number of saturated, unsaturated branched-chain, and alicyclic fatty acids, as well as background levels of lauric, myristic, palmitic, and stearic acids. Although the B strain of *A. laidlawii* will readily incorporate exogenous fatty acids, these are not required for growth, at least at temperatures above 20°C. The A strain, however, appears to have a growth requirement for at least small amounts of *cis*-unsaturated or other low-melting-point fatty acids (see chapter 14).

Silvius and McElhaney have shown that it is also possible to selectively inhibit the de novo biosynthesis of saturated fatty acids, and also the associated exogenous fatty acid chain elongation activity, by several means, the most suitable being the use of avidin to complex all of the available biotin in the undefined growth medium (183). Under these conditions, *A. laidlawii* is completely dependent on exogenous fatty acid incorporation for growth. With this technique, it is possible to produce membranes whose lipids contain essentially only a single fatty acyl group. Although not all single exogenous fatty acids will support growth (polyunsaturated and many saturated, *cis*-unsaturated, and *cis*-cyclopropane fatty acids, for example, are unsuitable), a surprisingly wide variety of branched-chain and *trans*-monounsaturated or *trans*-cyclopropane fatty acids, as well as some positional isomers of *cis*-octadecanoic acid and one linear saturated fatty acid, will support fair to good growth.

Moreover, binary combinations of relatively high- and low-melting-point fatty acids (for example, stearic and oleic acids, respectively) often support growth when added together, although neither will do so when added separately to the growth medium. One can therefore produce membranes whose gel/lipid-crystalline phase transition temperature and cooperativity can be markedly yet controllably varied (180, 182, 183). As well, by varying the chain length of suitable classes of exogenous fatty acids, appreciable alterations in the thickness of the hydrophobic core of the lipid bilayer can be obtained (180, 182, 183). The resultant ability to greatly manipulate the fluidity and phase state of the membrane lipid bilayer and its thickness, through fatty acid as well as cholesterol compositional alterations, makes this organism an ideal one for studying the role of lipids in biological membranes (118, 120).

All of the *Mycoplasma* species tested thus far lack the ability to synthesize fatty acids de novo and are thus totally dependent upon exogenous fatty acids for growth. For this reason, marked alterations in the membrane lipid fatty acid composition can be induced in this group of organisms as well. However, only in *Mycoplasma* sp. strain Y (serologically and biochemically related to *Mycoplasma mycoides*) has the manipulation of membrane lipid fatty acid composition been studied systematically. Rodwell and Peterson (152) have shown that in a fatty acid-poor growth medium, *Mycoplasma* sp. strain Y will grow well only in the presence of a relatively small number of exogenous fatty acids, including several *trans*-unsaturated and methyl iso- and anteiso-branched fatty acids. Single linear saturated or *cis*-unsaturated fatty acids will not support growth, but a large number of binary combinations of saturated, branched-chain, and unsaturated fatty acids will support good growth, just as with *A. laidlawii*. The total incorporation of single exogenous fatty acids into the membrane lipids of this organism ranges from 96 to 99 mol%. Thus, relatively large alterations in the fluidity and phase state of the membrane lipids of many *Mycoplasma* species can also be obtained (145, 155).

The reader is referred to chapter 14 for a full account of the biosynthesis and metabolism of mycoplasma fatty acids and membrane lipids and of the biosynthetic incorporation of exogenous lipids and lipid precursors from the growth media.

Protein Composition

The application of two-dimensional electrophoresis to isolated *A. laidlawii* membranes by Archer et al. (7) has revealed the presence of about 140 different polypeptides. In one sense, this number can be considered a minimum value, since peripheral membrane proteins weakly associated with the membrane may be lost even with the gentle osmotic lysis and washing procedures used to isolate these membranes. On the other hand, complex membrane proteins may dissociate into their component subunits during solubilization and electrophoresis, thus producing multiple bands. This has, in fact, recently been shown to be the case with the major ATPase of the *A. laidlawii* membrane, which can dissociate in the presence of deter-

gents into at least five subunits (96). The electrophoretic patterns of *A. laidlawii* membrane proteins are largely invariant with even marked alterations in the fatty acid composition of the membrane lipids (137, 180), although changes in fatty acid composition have been reported to produce a quantitative change in one membrane protein (137), and a reduction in growth temperature from 37 to 25°C was reported to result in the complete disappearance of two other membrane proteins (5). Highly glycosylated membrane proteins, at least, seem to be absent in this organism (5, 96, 137), since none of the protein bands stain with the periodic acid-Schiff reagent and cells grown in the presence of radiolabeled amino sugars do not exhibit significant levels of radioactivity in their membrane proteins (193). However, one deoxycholate-solubilized protein isolated from the *A. laidlawii* membrane has been reported to contain small amounts of amino sugars, mannose, galactose, and glucose (145). The molecular weights of the *A. laidlawii* membrane proteins range from 15,000 to over 200,000, similar to those of many other bacterial membranes. The majority of the membrane proteins are acidic, having pI values of between 4 and 7 (7). A significant number of the membrane proteins in this organism (~25) are fatty acylated (132), perhaps because of a need to anchor normally peripheral membrane proteins, which are located in the periplasmic space of conventional bacteria, to the membrane.

Peripheral membrane proteins are proteins which are not embedded in the hydrophobic core of the lipid bilayer but instead are bound to the membrane primarily by ionic bonds and divalent cation salt bridges, either between the peripheral protein and the lipid polar headgroups or between charged amino acids on other membrane protein constituents. Peripheral proteins usually can be released in water-soluble, lipid-free form by extraction with low-ionic-strength buffer with or without the addition of a divalent cation-chelating agent such as EDTA. Initial reports indicated that only a small fraction (<10%) of the proteins in the membrane of *A. laidlawii* appeared to behave as peripheral proteins (131). However, it now appears that a much larger proportion of the total membrane protein may fall into this category. Archer et al. (7) have demonstrated that about 60 of the 140 membrane protein species, representing about one-half of the total membrane protein, can be solubilized by exhaustive washing with low-ionic-strength, EDTA-containing buffers. One group of peripheral membrane proteins can be released by washing in low-ionic-strength buffer without EDTA, while another group requires EDTA treatment for release. The reason for the apparently lower proportion of peripheral membrane protein originally reported was probably the loss of some of the peripheral proteins during the isolation and washing of *A. laidlawii* membranes in deionized water or dilute buffer. The observation that the two-dimensional electrophoresis of the soluble and membrane-associated proteins of this organism reveals a number of proteins common to both fractions may indicate that the cell lysis and washing procedures do indeed remove at least some loosely bound peripheral membrane proteins (7). The only two enzyme activities to be demonstrated thus far in the peripheral membrane protein fraction are RNase and DNase activities (145).

Integral membrane proteins are bound to membranes by a combination of ionic and hydrophobic forces. To liberate such tightly bound proteins, which penetrate into or completely traverse the lipid bilayer, detergents or organic solvents must usually be used. Moreover, solubilized integral membrane proteins often remain associated with polar lipid and will precipitate in aqueous solution when the solubilizing agent is removed. In the *A. laidlawii* membrane, about 80 integral membrane proteins, constituting about one-half of the total membrane protein, are present (7). Among the integral membrane proteins identified thus far in this organism are a $(Na^+ + Mg^{2+})$-ATPase, a *p*-nitrophenylphosphatase, an NADH oxidase, an NADH dehydrogenase, an aminopeptidase, a lysophospholipase, and an acyl coenzyme A thioesterase (145). Several of these enzymes (the ATPase, NADH oxidase, and NADH dehydrogenase) have been isolated and partially characterized. The ATPase, the acyl coenzyme A thioesterase, and possibly the aminopeptidase are lipid-requiring enzymes whose activities can be modified by the physical state of the membrane lipids (see chapter 15). Unfortunately, the detailed molecular arrangement of these integral proteins in the *A. laidlawii* membrane remains largely unknown.

Johansson et al. (79) have studied the influence of membrane lipid composition on the total amounts and extractability of a number of membrane proteins in *A. laidlawii* B. The total amount of each individual protein present in the membrane was determined by crossed immunoelectrophoresis of a detergent extract containing the totally solubilized membrane proteins, while the extractability was determined by the treatment of the isolated membrane with one of several neutral detergents which produced a selective protein (and lipid) extraction. The extractability of several membrane proteins is dependent on the fatty acid and polar headgroup composition of the membrane lipids, although the total amounts of these proteins present in the membrane are not correlated with the lipid composition. The total amount of one flavoprotein present, however, was found to increase with an increase in the content of ionic membrane lipids. Moreover, the extractability of this flavoprotein was found to increase with an increase in unsaturated fatty acid content. These results were taken to support the view that the extractability of at least some membrane proteins, and thus their interaction with lipids in the membrane, is at least partly dependent on the molecular shapes and charges of the membrane lipid molecules. This point will be discussed further in a later section of this chapter.

In general, the membrane proteins of the various mycoplasma species are much less well studied than in *A. laidlawii* (144, 145). Again, changes in the membrane lipid fatty acid composition or cholesterol content seem not to be accompanied by significant alterations in the electrophoretic patterns of the membrane proteins of these organisms, and aging of the cultures causes only minor changes in the membrane protein profiles (2, 6, 165). Interestingly, in some mycoplasma species, a very high proportion of the membrane proteins contain covalently attached fatty acids (47, 48).

The reader is referred to chapter 7 for a more complete discussion of mycoplasma membrane proteins.

SPATIAL DISPOSITION AND MOBILITY OF MEMBRANE COMPONENTS

Lipids

Transbilayer distribution

Transbilayer lipid asymmetry, the unequal distribution of different membrane lipids in the outer and inner halves of the lipid bilayer, has been convincingly demonstrated in the erythrocyte membrane and less convincingly so in a number of other biological membranes (134). As discussed by Op den Kamp (134), great care must be taken in studies of lipid transbilayer distribution in order to avoid the many artifacts which can easily result from the uncritical use of the enzymatic and chemical labeling techniques usually applied in such studies. It appears that the results of the studies performed thus far with *A. laidlawii* are equivocal with regard to the existence of transbilayer lipid asymmetry in the native, intact membrane.

The transbilayer distribution of PG, often the only major phosphatide of the *A. laidlawii* membrane, has been extensively investigated by Bevers and coworkers by using phospholipase A_2 digestion (9–13). These workers demonstrated that the susceptibility of PG to phospholipase A_2 attack depends on the physical state of the membrane lipids and on the temperature of incubation. In intact cells and in isolated membranes, hydrolysis of PG can occur only at temperatures above the lower boundary of the gel/liquid-crystalline phase transition temperature, indicating that this enzyme can attack only fluid lipid. Membranes enriched in methyl iso- and anteiso-branched fatty acids are an exception to this rule, since the apparently more loosely packed gel-state bilayer formed by lipids containing these fatty acyl groups can be attacked by this enzyme (22). Moreover, even in cells and isolated membranes in which all the lipids are fluid, phospholipase A_2 hydrolysis is strongly temperature dependent. Thus, in intact cells or isolated membranes enriched in low-melting-point unsaturated fatty acids, incubation at 37°C results in a rapid and total hydrolysis of the PG. On the other hand, use of incubation temperatures of 0 to 25°C results in a biphasic hydrolysis pattern. In intact cells, about 50% of the PG is instantaneously hydrolyzed at low temperature, about 20% is hydrolyzed more slowly in a highly temperature-dependent fashion, and about 30% is resistant to attack by phospholipase A_2. Incubation of isolated membranes at low temperature results in a rapid hydrolysis of about 70% of the total PG, with the hydrolysis of the remaining 30% again taking place more slowly and in a highly temperature-dependent manner. These results led Bevers and coworkers to postulate the existence of three separate PG pools in the membranes of intact cells. One pool, comprising about 50% of the total PG, is exposed on the external surface; a second pool, consisting of about 20%, is exposed on the inner surface; and a third pool, comprising the remaining 30%, is in an unknown location, but one in which it is protected from the enzyme attack, at least at low temperatures. These workers also presented evidence that this latter pool of PG is shielded from enzymatic attack by its interaction with integral rather than peripheral membrane proteins. They further suggested that exposure to high temperature results in the exchange of protein-bound PG with other lipids, in turn resulting in the slow, temperature-dependent hydrolysis observed above 25°C. They also found that, in general, the fatty acid compositions of these three pools are identical. It should be noted that all of the experiments described above involving intact cells were done under conditions in which the cells were at least partially deenergized.

Bevers et al. (9) later reported that the susceptibility of PG to phospholipase A_2 attack in the membranes of intact cells, and also possibly its transbilayer distribution, is dependent on the energy state of the cell. As discussed above, cells incubated with phospholipase in the absence of glucose at 37°C undergo a rapid and eventually total hydrolysis of PG. However, if the cells are incubated under the same conditions in the presence of glucose, only about 40% of the PG can be hydrolyzed in intact cells, and that at a much slower rate than in energy-depleted cells. Nigericin, a Na^+-for-H^+ exchanger which normally collapses the ΔpH component of the transmembrane electrochemical potential, abolishes the protective effect of glucose addition, while valinomycin, a K^+ ionophore which should selectively collapse the $\Delta \Psi$ component of the transmembrane electrochemical potential, is without effect. Puzzlingly, carbonyl cyanide p-trifluoromethoxyphenylhydrazone, a proton carrier which should abolish both components of the transmembrane electrochemical potential gradient, also fails to reverse the protective effect of glucose addition. Although the data obtained with the uncouplers and ionophores are open to a number of interpretations, it is clear that the disposition of PG in the native A. laidlawii membrane is dramatically altered by changes in the state of energization of the cell. It is also clear that no definite conclusions about the transbilayer distribution of PG in normally growing cells can be drawn from this work, since it is possible to interpret the experiments discussed above to indicate that as little as 40% or as much as 80% of the total PG may reside in the outer monolayer.

Gross and Rottem (65) have applied the lactoperoxidase-mediated radioiodination technique, normally used to study the transbilayer distribution of membrane proteins, to investigate phospho- and glycolipid symmetry in A. laidlawii. A comparison of the labeling intensities of the various lipid species in intact cells and isolated membranes indicated that essentially all of the neutral glycolipids, MGDG and DGDG, are localized in the outer half of the lipid bilayer, as are about 60% of the phosphatides, PG and DPG, whereas the glycerophosphorylglucosyldiacylglycerols GPMGDG and GPDGDG are about equally distributed between the two halves of the bilayer. If these results are correct, it means that more than two-thirds of the total membrane lipid molecules reside in the outer monolayer and that the inner monolayer is composed essentially exclusively of negatively charged, phosphate-containing lipids! These findings, in addition to being physically implausible, are at variance with all other lipid distribution studies reported thus far, since in erythrocytes and other biological membranes, roughly equal amounts of lipid are found in both halves of the bilayer, and neutral phospho- and glycolipids predominate over charged lipids in both monolayers (134).

Op den Kamp (134) has set out a number of criteria which must be fulfilled by chemical techniques used to study lipid transbilayer distribution in order to produce reliable results. Among these criteria are that the reagent used to chemically label the lipid be totally impermeable to the lipid bilayer, that the chemical specificity of the reagent used be known with certainty, and that the reaction in question be quantitative. None of these criteria are fulfilled by the lactoperoxidase-mediated radioiodination technique used by Gross and Rottem. Although it is certain that the lactoperoxidase enzyme molecule itself does not permeate through or penetrate into the lipid bilayer, the same cannot be said of the reactive iodine species generated in this reaction, which, being rather hydrophobic, could well enter into the hydrophobic core of the lipid bilayer. Also, the chemical specificity of labeling by this technique, as applied to membrane lipids, is completely unknown. It is clear, however, that the various lipids are not randomly labeled, since about 40% of the total radioactivity is found in the several neutral lipids, which constitute only a tiny fraction of the total membrane lipid. It may well be, then, that the differences in the amount of radiolabeling observed in intact cells and isolated membranes may in part reflect the extent of iodination of the various lipids in these two systems rather than differences in the number of lipid molecules being labeled. Finally, it is doubtful that all, or even most, of the membrane lipid molecules are being labeled by this technique, since only 5% of the label is found in the membrane lipids and 95% is found in the membrane proteins. Since the lipid/protein molar ratio in the A. laidlawii membrane is about 60:1 to 65:1, it seems that only a small fraction of the total lipid could be radiolabeled, even assuming large numbers of exposed labeling sites on the membrane proteins. In this regard, it should be noted that when this technique was applied to the plasma membranes of chicken embryo cells (127), which have a lipid/protein ratio similar to that of the A. laidlawii plasma membrane, more than 50% of the total counts were found in the lipid fraction. When one considers further that the energy state of the cells used in this procedure was not controlled, it seems best to consider the results obtained by Gross and Rottem as tentative at this point, pending their confirmation by an independent technique.

The phospho- and glycolipid transbilayer distribution in the membranes of Mycoplasma species has not been studied in a rigorous and quantitative manner, so no definite conclusions concerning the existence of membrane lipid asymmetry are possible at present. For a review of the qualitative studies performed to date on the transbilayer distribution of membrane glycerolipids in various Mycoplasma species, the reader is referred to a review by Razin (145).

In contrast to the glycerolipids, the transbilayer distribution of cholesterol and other sterols has been extensively studied in two Mycoplasma species by Bittman and coworkers. In one series of studies, the polyene antibiotic filipin, which binds fairly specifically to 3β-hydroxysterols, was used to estimate sterol distribution. Since the formation of a filipin-sterol complex is accompanied by a change in the absorbance or fluorescence of the filipin molecule, the initial rapid rate of filipin-sterol association can be monitored in a stopped-flow spectrophotometer. The ratio of the rate constants for filipin-sterol association in intact *Mycoplasma* cells (where presumably only the sterol in the outer monolayer is available for complex formation) to that in isolated, unsealed membranes (where the sterol in both monolayers is exposed to filipin) should reflect the initial transbilayer distribution of that sterol. To minimize the membrane perturbations induced by filipin, which can lead to the formation of pores in the membrane and cell lysis, measurements were conducted at low temperatures using high sterol/filipin ratios and very short times. This latter feature ensures that only the initial transmembrane distribution of sterols will be estimated but precludes a direct determination of the rates of sterol exchange between monolayers (19).

The filipin-binding technique was initially applied to determine the transbilayer distribution of cholesterol in *M. gallisepticum* (chosen because of its high osmotic stability) and *M. capricolum* (chosen for its ability to incorporate exogenous phospho- and sphingolipids and to grow in the presence of low levels of cholesterol). In exponentially growing *M. gallisepticum*, cholesterol is distributed symmetrically in the membrane lipid bilayer, whereas in *M. capricolum*, about 66% of the free cholesterol is localized in the outer monolayer (20). On aging of the cultures, the amount of cholesterol in the *M. gallisepticum* outer monolayer increases from 50 to 60%, whereas it remains unchanged in the *M. capricolum* membrane (16, 41). The amount of cholesterol in the outer leaflet of the *M. gallisepticum* membrane is also increased by cross-linking the surface membrane proteins of intact cells with dimethyl suberimidate. However, variations in the fatty acid composition of the endogenous phospho- and glycolipids, the incorporation of substantial quantities of exogenous PC and sphingomyelin, or the proteolytic treatment of intact cells does not alter cholesterol distribution in *M. capricolum* membranes (16, 42).

The uptake, transbilayer distribution, and movement of cholesterol in growing *M. capricolum* cells was also investigated by the filipin-binding technique. If cells adapted to grow with low cholesterol levels are shifted to a growth medium containing high levels of cholesterol, cell growth is stimulated and about a sixfold increase in total membrane cholesterol concentration occurs within 4 h (two to three cell doublings). However, the transbilayer distribution of cholesterol is invariant from 1 h onward, indicating that exogenous cholesterol is translocated rapidly from the outer monolayer, where it is presumably initially bound, to the inner monolayer in growing cells. Interestingly, when cell growth is inhibited by various ion-translocating antibiotics, exogenous cholesterol incorporation is partially inhibited and cholesterol remains localized predominantly in the outer half of the membrane lipid bilayer of this organism (41).

The distribution and movement of a variety of different sterols were investigated in *M. gallisepticum* (39) and *M. capricolum* (42). In both organisms, alterations in the degree of saturation of the sterol ring system do not alter the characteristic transbilayer distribution of these analogs relative to cholesterol itself, nor do

changes in the length of the alkyl side chain. However, the introduction of a alkyl branch at C-24 or of unsaturation at C-22 results in 85 to 95% of the exogenous sterol remaining in the outer monolayer. Bittman and coworkers suggest that these latter chemical modifications may inhibit the transbilayer movement of the sterol molecule by increasing the bulk of the alkyl side chain, resulting in a steric hindrance effect.

The distribution and movement of cholesterol in *M. gallisepticum* was also investigated by monitoring cholesterol exchange between intact cells or isolated membranes and high-density lipoproteins (163) or unilamellar egg PC vesicles (17, 18, 38, 40, 162). Using both techniques, Bittman and coworkers demonstrated that more than 90% of the cellular cholesterol could be exchanged. However, in intact cells, the kinetics of exchange are biphasic, with about half of the cholesterol exchanging with a half-time of about 4 h and half exchanging with a half-time of 9 h to 18 days. However, the rate of exchange of the rapidly exchanging cholesterol pool with vesicles increases as the cholesterol/phospholipid ratio of the cell membranes decreases, presumably because lowering cholesterol levels decreases the order of the lipid bilayer. Moreover, the rate of exchange of the rapidly exchanging cholesterol pool is lower in cells enriched in sphingomyelin than in those enriched in PC, presumably for the same reason. As well, extensive chemical crosslinking of the surface proteins decreases cholesterol exchange rates whereas depletion of membrane protein by growth in chloramphenicol increases exchange rates, suggesting that the membrane proteins can modulate lipid exchange. These authors interpret their results to indicate that cholesterol is equally distributed between the two halves of the membrane lipid bilayer of this organism and that the transbilayer movement of cholesterol is slow.

Bittman et al. (17) recently studied the effects of modification of the endogenous PG and DPG content of the *M. capricolum* membrane on the kinetics of spontaneous cholesterol and phospholipid exchange between intact cells or isolated membranes and lipid vesicles. The PG/DPG ratio in membranes increases upon the addition of calcium to the growth medium and decreases upon the addition of egg PC. As well, the ratio of palmitate to oleate in both PG and DPG decreases upon supplementation with PC or with PC and Ca^{2+}. These changes in the relative amounts and fatty acid compositions of the PG (a bilayer-forming lipid) and DPG (which can form nonbilayer phases in the presence of Ca^{2+}) were interpreted as an attempt (apparently unsuccessful) to maintain the relative bilayer/nonbilayer phase preference constant upon the addition and incorporation of egg PC (which would tend to stabilize the lamellar phase) and Ca^{2+} (which would tend to promote the formation of nonlamellar phases). However, trypsin-treated membranes from cells grown with Ca^{2+} or with both exogenous egg PC and Ca^{2+} exhibit lipidic particles or actual nonlamellar lipid structures, respectively, indicating that portions of their membrane lipid exist in nonlamellar forms at 37°C, while those supplemented only with egg PC do not. Similarly, the rates of both cholesterol and phospholipid exchange are higher in cells grown in Ca^{2+} alone or in egg PC and Ca^{2+} than in unsupplemented cells. This enhancement in exchange rates was postulated to result from structural defects in the *M. capricolum* membranes due to the instability of their lipid bilayer structures. However, the addition of egg PC alone, which showed no evidence of promoting the formation of nonbilayer structures in trypsin-treated membranes and which should stabilize the lipid bilayer, also enhances exchange rates, although to a lesser degree. Thus, the question of whether or not Ca^{2+} and egg PC exert their characteristic effects on cholesterol and phospholipid exchange via an influence on the formation of nonbilayer structures remains open, as does the relative role of the change in the membrane PG/DPG ratio induced by the addition of these agents to the growth medium.

The slow rate of cholestrol transbilayer movement apparently observed in *M. gallisepticum* cells is surprising in view of the rapid transbilayer movement of cholesterol reported for lipid vesicles (135), *M. capricolum* (41), and human erythrocytes (88). In this regard, Davis and coworkers (53) have reported that a similar, rather slow biphasic exchange of cholesterol is observed in isolated membranes as well as in intact cells in *M. gallisepticum* (also mentioned earlier in passing by Rottem and coworkers) and in *A. laidlawii*. These observations confirm that there exist in *M. gallisepticum* and *A. laidlawii* membranes two pools of cholesterol with marked differences in their kinetics of exchange with lipoproteins or vesicles, but they indicate that these differences in exchange kinetics are not simply the result of a particular transbilayer distribution of cholesterol or of a slow exchange of cholesterol between the inner and outer lipid monolayers of these membranes. Instead, these workers suggest that differences in the exchange kinetics result from the fact that cholesterol is associated with two different pools of lipids, one with a high affinity for cholesterol (the phospholipids) and one with a low affinity for cholesterol (the glycolipids). Evidence in support of this hypothesis includes the generally lower levels of incorporation of cholesterol by the glycolipid-rich *Acholeplasma* species as opposed to the phospholipid-rich *Mycoplasma* species and the negative correlation between cholesterol binding and glycolipid content in various *A. laidlawii* strains (59), the more rapid exchange of cholesterol in *A. laidlawii* once incorporated, and the presence of a single cholesterol exchange rate in *A. laidlawii* treated with phospholipase A_2, which attacks only the phospholipids (53). However, this hypothesis does not explain the fact that in both *A. laidlawii* and *M. gallisepticum*, about 50% of the cholesterol exists in each pool, whereas glycolipids account for 65 to 70% of the *A. laidlawii* membrane lipids but only 10 to 20% of the *M. gallisepticum* membrane lipids. Also, in phospholipase A_2-treated *A. laidlawii* cells or membranes, cholesterol exchange rates are intermediate between those of the rapid and slow rates observed in untreated controls, indicating that phospholipase A_2 treatment must have resulted in more than just the selective removal of the phospholipid pool. Moreover, the existence of separate pools of lipid at temperatures about the gel/liquid-crystalline phase transition temperature is unlikely (118, 120).

It should be noted that there do not appear to be two kinetically distinct pools of cholesterol in isolated membranes from *M. capricolum* (53), as there are in *M. gallisepticum* and *A. laidlawii*. Thus, the earlier work of Bittman and coworkers on the transbilayer distribution of cholesterol in this particular organism may be valid (but see below).

The only information available about the transbilayer distribution of cholesterol in the *A. laidlawii* membrane comes from a study by de Kruijff and coworkers (55), who found that about twice as much filipin was bound by isolated membranes than by intact cells when this organism was grown in the presence of exogenous cholesterol, implying an approximately equal distribution in the two halves of the bilayer. Although this seems a reasonable result, it is difficult to rationalize if Rottem and coworkers (53, 59) are correct in their assertion that the glycolipids do not bind cholesterol well and if the report by Gross and Rottem (65) that most glycolipids are located primarily or exclusively in the outer monolayer of the lipid bilayer of this organism is valid. In this case, one would expect a markedly asymmetric transbilayer distribution of cholesterol favoring the inner monolayer.

Lelong et al. (92) have compared the rate and extent of exchange of both cholesterol and 7β-hydroxycholesterol between *M. capricolum* cells and sterol-containing egg PC vesicles. Although the hydroxylated sterol is incorporated from the growth medium into the *M. capricolum* membrane to almost the same extent as is cholesterol, only about 25% of the incorporated hydroxycholesterol can be exhanged with lipid vesicles. Since the aqueous solubility, and thus the exchange rate between lipid vesicles, is higher for the hydroxylated sterol than for cholesterol itself, these workers postulate that the majority of the incorporated 7β-hydroxycholesterol must interact strongly with the membrane lipids and/or proteins, thus rendering it unexhangeable. However, no direct evidence in support of this suggestion was presented. Although Lelong and coworkers confirm that almost all of the cholesterol incorporated into *M. capricolum* cells can be exchanged with biphasic kinetics, these workers now report that 80 to 85% of the cholesterol pool undergoes rapid exchange. This contrasts with the results of the earlier studies of Bittman and coworkers on this organism indicating that only 66% of the total cholesterol incorporated into intact cells undergoes rapid exchange. Thus, the study of Lelong et al. (92) not only calls into question the earlier result that two-thirds of the incorporated cholesterol resides in the outer monolayer of the *M. capricolum* membrane but also raises further doubts about whether cholesterol exchange kinetics alone are a valid indicator of cholesterol transbilayer distribution.

Lateral mobility

Although there exists a great deal of direct and indirect evidence that the phospho- and glycolipids of the *A. laidlawii* and various *Mycoplasma* membranes diffuse rapidly in the plane of the membrane, at least in the liquid-crystalline state (for example, see reference 63), no rigorous quantitative measurements of lipid lateral diffusion coefficients have been made. This is unfortunate, since the ability to drastically alter the membrane lipid fatty acid composition, and to some extent the cholesterol content and polar headgroup composition as well, would make these ideal biological membrane systems in which to study the relationship between lipid structure and the rates of lateral diffusion.

Proteins

Transbilayer distribution

The *A. laidlawii* membrane exhibits the absolute asymmetry of transbilayer distribution of membrane proteins which has been observed in many other membrane systems, in particular the human erythrocyte membrane (for a review, see reference 153). Early studies using the lactoperoxidase-mediated iodination technique indicated that more proteins, or at least a greater proportion of these proteins, are exposed on the inner than on the outer membrane surface, since the uptake of label was found to be more than threefold higher in isolated membranes than in intact cells (2). Moreover, one-dimensional analysis revealed that only a portion of the proteins resolved are labeled in intact cells, but almost all of the proteins are labeled in isolated membranes. Similarly, the differential fluorescence labeling observed with intact cells and isolated membranes of *A. laidlawii* indicates either that in intact cells only a few high-molecular-weight proteins are exposed on the cell surface or that the carbohydrate polymers present on the membrane surface shield any other membrane proteins present there (170). More recent experiments in which two-dimensional gel electrophoresis was used indicate that only about 40 of the 140 membrane protein bands can be labeled in intact cells, whereas 90 to 100 bands can be labeled in isolated membranes (7). The finding that a substantial fraction of the membrane proteins cannot be labeled from either side of the membranes probably indicates that many *A. laidlawii* membrane proteins lack exposed, iodine-binding tyrosine residues in their native conformations, since it is unlikely that many membrane proteins could be completely buried in the lipid bilayer. Less extensive proteolytic digestion (3) and immunologic experiments (78) on intact cells and isolated membranes seem generally to confirm the lactoperoxidase-catalyzed iodination results just discussed (for a review, see reference 145).

Some qualitative indication of the transbilayer distribution of integral membrane proteins can also be derived from freeze-fracture electron microscopy. This technique is capable of cleaving biological membranes through the center of the lipid bilayer, thus revealing their hydrophobic interiors. The *A. laidlawii* membrane bilayer interior, like that of most membranes, is studded with particles 50 to 100 Å (1 Å = 0.1 nm) in diameter, which have been shown in most instances to be due to the presence of proteins which are embedded into or which traverse the hydrophobic bilayer core (196). The distribution of particles on the two fracture faces of the *A. laidlawii* membrane is asymmetric (194, 195), with more particles observed on the convex fracture face (the inner half of the lipid bilayer) than on the concave face (the outer half of the bilayer). Similar results have been reported for several *Mycoplasma* species (64, 108, 165). This result would thus appear to support the suggestion that more integral membrane proteins face the cytoplasmic surface than the outer surface of the cell membrane.

Lateral mobility

Although no quantitative measurements of protein lateral mobility in *A. laidlawii* membranes have thus far been made, it is clear that some proteins (probably all proteins) undergo relatively rapid lateral diffusion in the plane of the membrane, at least when the membrane lipids exist in the liquid-crystalline state. Thus, anionic sites on the external surface of the *A. laidlawii* membrane, visualized by electron microscopy using cationized ferritin as an electron-dense marker, are randomly dispersed at 0°C but will progressively cluster if maintained at 37°C (169). A similar behavior has been reported for undefined membrane antigens, using immunoelectron microscopy and colloidal gold-labeled anti-*A. laidlawii* antibodies as electron-dense markers (67). Moreover, the temperature-dependent phenomena of mycoplasma virus lateral aggregation and capping have recently been described in this organism (67). These results are to be expected, since *A. laidlawii* does not appear to contain a cytoskeletal system which would retard or completely inhibit the lateral diffusion of membrane proteins, as is the case for most eucaryotic cells (145).

It is well established that the differential crystallization of lipids in the bilayer plane can influence the distribution of intramembranous particles, which correspond to proteins partially or wholly immersed within the membrane bilayer (for a review, see reference 145). The original observation was made by Tourtellotte et al. (195), who demonstrated by freeze-fracture electron microscopy that *A. laidlawii* cells enriched in stearic acid contain areas of tightly aggregated intramembranous particles separated by large, particle-free domains when quick-frozen from room temperature, whereas oleic acid-enriched cells exhibit a uniform, random distribution of particles. Verkleij et al. (197) later studied cells grown with myristic, elaidic, and oleic acids and compared the freeze-fracture electron microscopic patterns with the phase state of the membrane lipids as monitored by differential scanning calorimetry (DSC). The membranes from all three cell types give identical random or lacelike intramembranous particle distributions when rapidly quenched from 37°C, and in all cases the membrane lipids are predominantly (myristate- and elaidic-grown cells) or exclusively (oleate-grown cells) in the liquid-crystalline state at this temperature. In contrast, if cells are maintained at 5°C, the oleate-enriched membranes, which remain in the fluid state at this temperature, continue to exhibit the 37°C pattern, whereas the fracture faces of the myristate- or elaidate-enriched membranes, which exist in the gel state at this temperature, are composed of particle-rich and particle-free domains. These workers suggested that integral membrane proteins are being squeezed out of the tightly packed gel-state lipid domains, thus giving the two-domain pattern noted below the lipid phase transition temperature. These observations were extended by James and Branton (75), who grew *A. laidlawii* cells in a variety of different exogenous fatty acids to produce membranes having lipid hydrocarbon chain motional discontinuities at temperatures of between 10 and 35°C. Molecular motion in these membranes was probed by electron spin resonance (ESR) spectroscopy using a 12-nitroxide stearic acid intercalated probe, and the structure of the membranes was examined by using a quantitative statistical analysis of intramembranous particle aggregation of freeze-fracture electron micrographs. Although these authors found that in general the aggregation of intramembranous proteins into particle-rich and particle-poor regions is correlated with the lipid phase transition temperature, as monitored by ESR spectroscopy, aggregation could begin at temperatures well above the ESR-determined discontinuity and continue at temperatures below this discontinuity. McElhaney (114) subsequently demonstrated that the appearance of particle-free domains in freeze-fracture electron micrographs correlates with the upper boundary of the gel/liquid-crystalline phase transition region, as determined by differential thermal analysis (DTA), and that particle aggregation is complete at the lower phase transition boundary. Similar conclusions were reached by Wallace et al. (199), who used X-ray diffraction and DSC to monitor the membrane lipid phase transition. McElhaney also showed that incubation of plasma membranes at 55°C for 30 min, a treatment resulting in extensive membrane protein denaturation, does not alter the density or (random) distribution of intramembranous protein particles. The gel state-induced aggregation of intramembranous protein particles, however, is not observed in membranes enriched in methyl iso- or anteiso-branched fatty acids (184), presumably because of the more loosely packed gel state existing below the phase transition temperature (37, 83, 105).

In addition to changes in temperature, Copps et al. (45) have reported that changes in medium pH can affect the distribution of intramembranous particles in *A. laidlawii* membranes. Particle distribution in fatty acid-unsupplemented membranes was found to be more heterogeneous and the particles more closely packed at pH 6.0 than at pH 7.5 or 9.0. James and Branton (75), however, previously reported that variations in pH from 6.2 to 8.2 have no effect on intramembranous particle distribution in membranes enriched in a variety of different fatty acids. The basis for this discrepancy in results is not clear.

Wallace and Engelman (198) have studied the planar distribution of proteins exposed on the surface of the *A. laidlawii* membrane by electron microscopy, using a biotin-avidin-ferritin reagent which specifically links to free amino groups on exposed membrane proteins. The surface distribution of the ferritin-containing complex was studied in membranes enriched in several different fatty acids at a variety of temperatures, and the gel/liquid-crystalline membrane lipid phase transition was monitored by X-ray diffraction and DSC. These workers found that the label sites are homogeneously dispersed at temperatures both above and below the lipid phase transition, whereas patches of high and low density are observed in membranes labeled from within the phase transition. In addition, the patching phenomenon was found to be freely reversible in experiments in which the temperature was shifted after labeling. Evidently, freeze fracturing and avidin-ferritin labeling focus on two different classes of membrane proteins whose distributions are differentially affected by the physical state of the membrane lipid. In contrast to the integral transmembrane proteins presumably visualized by the freeze-fracture technique (196), the surface proteins apparently labeled by the avidin-ferritin technique are mobile in the gel as well as in the liquid-crystalline state! Several models have been put forward to account for the behavior of this latter class of proteins.

In my view, the conclusions derived from the avidin-ferritin studies summarized above should be accepted with caution. The electron micrographs presented show only minor, in some cases imperceptible, differences between the surface protein distributions of membranes labeled from above, within, and below the purported lipid phase transition temperatures. In particular, the dramatic differences noted in the previous freeze-fracture studies are not seen. Moreover, the intensity as well as the density of labeling appears to decrease toward the center of these low-density patches, suggesting that technical problems in label visualization may be responsible for the reported observations. Furthermore, the lipid phase transitions reported by X-ray diffraction in this paper are much narrower than those given by DSC, or indeed by the X-ray technique used in previous studies from Engelman's laboratory (60, 61). Thus, considerable fluid lipid in fact remains at temperatures reported by these workers as being "below the lipid phase transition." Thus, the conclusion that these surface proteins are mobile even when the membrane lipids exist entirely in the gel state is questionable.

Vertical displacement

Borochov and Shinitzky (21) have proposed that changes in the microviscosity of the lipid bilayer in a biological membrane can influence the vertical disposition of proteins embedded therein. In particular, these workers have postulated that a decrease in lipid fluidity will diminish lipid-protein hydrophobic interactions, which will in turn result in a partial squeezing out of the hydrophobic domain of the integral membrane protein, and vice versa. Amar et al. (4, 5) have thoroughly tested this hypothesis in *A. laidlawii* by altering membrane fluidity in a variety of ways, including varying the fatty acid composition of the membrane lipids, changing the growth temperature and age of the culture, and inducing alterations in the lipid/protein ratio of the membrane by treatment of growing cells with chloramphenicol, an inhibitor of protein but not lipid biosynthesis. No correlation could be found between membrane lipid fluidity and the degree of exposure of membrane proteins as determined by the extent of lactoperoxidase-mediated iodination. Interestingly, even conversion of the membrane lipid to the gel state, which is known to substantially increase the thickness of the bilayer, does not affect protein iodination, suggesting that this technique may not be a sensitive one for measuring protein penetration. The iodination values for intact cells, however, consistently decrease upon exposure of the organisms to any procedure resulting in suboptimal growth. The iodination values for isolated membranes, in contrast, are invariant regardless of the growth conditions of the cells from which they are derived. Amar et al. (4, 5) provided evidence that the variations observed in the exposure of cell surface proteins in intact cells are the result of changes in the energized state of the cell rather than in membrane lipid fluidity per se. Thus, exposure of cells to the ionophore valinomycin, which dissipates the transmembrane K^+ gradient, or to carbonyl cyanide *m*-chlorophenylhydrazone, which dissipates the transmembrane proton gradient, results in a rapid drop in the iodination values of cell surface proteins. Treatment of isolated membranes with comparable levels of these agents is without effect. It thus appears that the conformation, if not the vertical displacement, of at least some membrane proteins is affected by the transmembrane electrochemical ion gradient, as has also been demonstrated for the Lac carrier protein of *Escherichia coli* (172). As noted earlier, an increased susceptibility of membrane PG to phospholipase A_2 attack also accompanies a deenergization of intact *A. laidlawii* cells (9). Whether or not this increased exposure of PG is due to a membrane protein conformation change induced by an alteration in the transmembrane electrochemical gradient remains to be determined.

Le Grimellec and coworkers (91) have also studied the effects of cellular energization on membrane organization in *M. capricolum* subsp. *capri*. Fluorescence polarization and ESR experiments using various probes demonstrated that addition of glucose to resting cells has a very limited effect, if any, on the physical state of their membrane lipids. Under the same conditions, the degree of exposure of primary amino groups of membrane proteins to the aqueous surroundings, estimated from fluorescence labeling by fluorescamine and the cycloheptaamylose-fluorescamine complex, is significantly increased. This energy-dependent increase is blocked by dicyclohexylcarbodiimide, an inhibitor of the membrane-bound, Mg^{2+}-stimulated ATPase of mycoplasma, and by carbonyl cyanide *p*-trifluoromethoxyphenylhydrazone, which in mycoplasmas affects only the chemical component of the proton motive force. Variations in the proton activity gradient across the membrane, induced by changing the pH of the labeling medium, result in parallel variations in the ratio of the relative intensities of labeling of energized to resting cells. The values taken by this ratio are up to 2 for a maximal proton gradient of 0.9 pH units and tend to unity when the intracellular and extracellular pH values equalize. These authors conclude that upon mycoplasma cell energization, membrane proteins undergo a conformational change resulting in the exposure of new free amino groups. This conformational change is primarily dependent on the existence of a ΔpH across the membrane and occurs in the absence of important modifications in the physical state of membrane lipids.

PHYSICAL STUDIES OF LIPID ORGANIZATION AND DYNAMICS

A wide variety of physical techniques have been applied to the *A. laidlawii* plasma membranes, particularly to investigate the organization and dynamics of the lipid bilayer found therein. The results obtained

by these various techniques are summarized and critically evaluated in the following section. The more circumscribed physical studies of the membranes of various *Mycoplasma* species are also reviewed.

DSC and DTA

The unique properties of the *A. laidlawii* membrane were utilized by Steim et al. (189) to show for the first time that biological membranes can undergo a gel/liquid-crystalline lipid phase transition similar to that previously reported for lamellar phospholipid-water systems. These workers demonstrated that when whole cells or isolated membranes were analyzed by DSC, two relatively broad endothermic transitions are observed on the initial heating scan. The lower-temperature transition is fully reversible, varies markedly in position with changes in the chain length and degree of unsaturation of the membrane lipid fatty acyl chains, is broadened and eventually abolished by cholesterol incorporation, and exhibits a transition enthalpy characteristic of the mixed-acid synthetic phospholipids. Moreover, an endothermic transition having essentially identical properties is observed for the protein-free total membrane lipid extract dispersed in excess water or aqueous buffer, indicating that the presence of membrane proteins has little effect on the thermotropic phase behavior of most of the membrane lipids. The higher-temperature transition, in contrast, is irreversible, is independent of membrane lipid fatty acid composition or cholesterol content, and is absent in total membrane lipid extracts, indicating that it is due to an irreversible thermal denaturation of the membrane proteins. A comparison of the enthalpies of transition of the lipids in the membrane and in water dispersions indicates that at least 75% of the total membrane lipid participates in this transition. Evidence was also presented that the membrane lipids must be predominantly in the fluid state to support normal cell growth. These results were later confirmed and extended by Reinert and Steim (148) and by Melchior et al. (123), who showed that the gel/liquid-crystalline lipid phase transition is a property of living cells. The former authors also demonstrated that the enthalpy of only the higher-temperature transition is reduced by protease treatment of isolated membranes and that changes in the circular dichroism spectra in the 200 to 300 nm range accompany this transition, confirming that it is indeed due to protein denaturation. They also presented more extensive data on the relative transition enthalpies of the lipid in the membrane and in aqueous dispersion, concluding that about 90% of the lipid participates in the gel/liquid-crystalline phase transition. Although this latter interpretation was challenged by Chapman and Urbina (32), its correctness has subsequently been confirmed by a number of other studies using a variety of other techniques. These studies provided perhaps the first strong, direct experimental evidence for the hypothesis that lipids are organized as a liquid-crystalline bilayer in biological membranes, a basic feature of the currently well-accepted fluid-mosaic model of membrane structure (186).

The thermotropic phase behavior of the lipids of the *A. laidlawii* membrane was subsequently investigated by McElhaney (114, 115), using DTA. He demonstrated that the phase transition midpoint temperature of the gel/liquid-crystalline lipid phase transition could be varied from −20°C to greater than +37°C in membranes enriched (50 to 80%) in a variety of exogenous fatty acids. Under such conditions, the lipid phase transitions observed are relatively broad, typically 20 to 30°C in width. Subsequent studies by Silvius and McElhaney (182) and by Silvius et al. (180) have shown that about one-half of this broadness can be attributed to fatty acid heterogeneity, since fatty acid-homogeneous membranes exhibit transition ranges of only 10 to 15°C. The remaining broadness has been shown to be due to polar headgroup heterogeneity. These workers also demonstrated that the thermotropic behavior of the individual membrane lipids varies considerably. Comparing the phospho- and glycolipids of fatty acid-homogeneous membranes, it was found that isolated PG exhibits comparatively simple phase behavior that is nearly identical to that of the total membrane lipids dispersed in water, while the total phosphate-containing lipids (containing small amounts of O-amino acid esters of PG and a GPDGDG as well as PG) exhibit a similar single endotherm but centered at a slightly lower temperature. In contrast, the isolated neutral glycolipids, MGDG and DGDG, show complex thermotropic behavior, with multiple endotherms all centered at higher temperatures than observed for the total membrane lipids. Interestingly, however, mixtures of MGDG and DGDG exhibit a much simpler behavior than does each component separately; in fact, the total neutral glycolipid fraction gives a single major endotherm (with a low-temperature shoulder) which is centered at a temperature similar to that observed for the total membrane lipids and for isolated PG. Thus, although the individual polar lipids of the *A. laidlawii* membrane can exhibit somewhat different thermotropic phase behavior, mixtures of these lipid components nevertheless appear to exhibit an appreciable amount of mutual miscibility in both the gel and liquid-crystalline states. Another interesting finding made in this study was the lack of a measurable effect of the presence of carotenoids or Mg^{2+} on the thermotropic phase behavior of aqueous dispersions of the total membrane lipids.

These early DSC studies of the lipid thermotropic phase behavior in *A. laidlawii* membranes utilized cells whose membrane lipids were only moderately enriched in various exogenous fatty acids, and low-sensitivity calorimeters were used. The resultant broad lipid phase transitions (due primarily to fatty acid compositional heterogeneity) and the relative poor quality of the DSC traces obtained (due to baseline instability and noise) could have obscured subtle differences in lipid thermotropic phase behavior in intact cells, isolated membranes, and total membrane lipid dispersions. Indeed, Mantsch and coworkers, using Fourier transform infrared (FT-IR) spectroscopy, recently reported that the gel/liquid-crystalline phase transition in intact cells highly enriched in saturated fatty acids occurs some 5 to 10°C below that of isolated membranes derived from them, suggesting that the organization of the lipids in the membranes of living cells differs from that of the isolated membranes

(25, 26, 111). This result is in contrast to the finding of the earlier DSC studies, which showed that the lipid chain-melting transition in living cells, isolated membranes, and lipid dispersions is essentially identical, except that in the former systems about 10% of the lipids are prevented from participating in this cooperative phase transition by their interaction with membrane proteins.

To resolve this apparent discrepancy in results and to confirm or to refute the original DSC findings, Seguin and coworkers (176) recently repeated the experiments of Steim et al. (189) by using fatty acid-homogeneous *A. laidlawii* B cells (to remove fatty acid compositional heterogeneity) and a modern, high-sensitivity calorimeter (to improve the quality of the DSC traces obtained). These workers found that the fully reversible gel/liquid-crystalline lipid phase transitions observed in elaidic acid-homogeneous cells and membranes have essentially identical phase transition temperatures, enthalpies, and degrees of cooperativity, suggesting that membrane lipid organizations in these two samples are very similar or identical. In contrast, the midpoint of the chain-melting transition of the membrane lipid dispersion is shifted to a higher temperature, exhibits a greater enthalpy, and is considerably less cooperative than in cells or membranes, suggesting that native membrane lipid organization has been perturbed during extraction and resuspension of the membrane lipid in water. Seguin and coworkers also find that the thermal denaturation of the proteins in the cells and membranes has absolutely no effect on the peak temperature or cooperativity of the lipid phase transition but does increase the transition enthalpy, suggesting some decrease in the number of lipid molecules interacting with denatured membrane proteins. However, about 15% of the lipids do not participate in the cooperative gel/liquid-crystalline phase transition in both the cells and native membranes, presumably because their cooperative phase behavior is abolished by interaction with the transmembrane regions of integral membrane proteins. Alternatively, a larger proportion of the membrane lipids may interact with the membrane proteins but have their cooperative melting behavior only partially perturbed, thereby leading to the 15% reduction in the transition enthalpy observed. The fact that the gel/liquid-crystalline lipid phase transition in cells and membranes exhibits a similar temperature maximum but a higher cooperativity than does the membrane lipid dispersion favors the former interpretation. In general, the results obtained with intact cells and membranes support the earlier DSC studies, which reported a nearly identical lipid thermotropic phase behavior in both systems, and not the FT-IR spectroscopic results of Mantsch and coworkers, who reported significantly different phase behaviors in these systems. We feel that this difference in results may be due at least in part to the existence of a thermal history-dependent gel-state lipid polymorphism (see below).

When similar calorimetric experiments are performed with isopalmitic acid-homogeneous *A. laidlawii* B cells, membranes, and lipids, two well-resolved endotherms are observed in all three systems (176). The properties of the lower-enthalpy lipid transition centered at 8 to 9°C are dependent on the heating scan rate and the thermal history of the sample. In particular, the apparent transition temperature increases with increasing scan rate, and annealing the sample at 0°C for 24 h before beginning the DSC run results in a two- to threefold increase in the observed calorimetric enthalpy. Since similar hysteresis is typically observed in the formation and interconvetions of highly ordered gel phases in bilayers of synthetic phospholipids, the lower-temperature endotherm was tentatively identified as a phase transition between a more highly ordered and a less highly ordered gel state. In contrast, the properties of the higher-enthalpy transition centered at 21 to 22°C exhibit no dependence on heating scan rate or on thermal history, indicating that this is the typical gel/liquid-crystalline or chain-melting transition previously observed in this organism by a variety of techniques.

The structural changes associated with each of the two lipid phase transitions detected by DSC were investigated by FT-IR and ^{31}P nuclear magnetic resonance (NMR) spectroscopy. These spectroscopic techniques confirm that the lower-temperature endotherm is due to a transition from a highly ordered gel phase (in which the all-*trans* lipid hydrocarbon chains are very closely packed, the bilayer interfacial region is partly dehydrated, and the phospholipid polar headgroups are undergoing slow axially asymmetric motion) to a disordered gel phase (in which the lipid hydrocarbon chains, while still largely extended, are more loosely packed, the interfacial region is fully hydrated, and the phospholipid polar headgroups are undergoing fast, axially symmetric motion). These spectroscopic techniques also confirm that the higher-temperature transition corresponds to a conversion from a loosely packed gel state to the liquid-crystalline state, in which the lipid hydrocarbon chains are conformationally disordered and contain a number of *gauche* conformers. All three physical techniques indicate that at least 80% of the total membrane lipid participates in both the gel/gel and gel/liquid-crystalline phase transitions (176).

The finding that gel-phase polymorphism can exist in A. *laidlawii* B membranes is quite surprising in view of the fact that most binary mixtures of synthetic phospholipids do not exhibit multiple gel states even when they contain identical fatty acyl chains. Thus, the ability of the A. *laidlawii* membrane lipids to form a highly ordered gel phase seems all the more remarkable, since this organism contains three major and two minor lipid classes, including both phospho- and glycoglycerolipids. These results thus imply that the A. *laidlawii* B membrane lipid classes are highly miscible in all three lipid phase states detected, a result compatible with the earlier DTA study of mixtures of the individual membrane lipid classes. Moreover, gel-state polymorphism in this organism is not restricted to membranes containing a single methyl iso-branched fatty acid, as A. *laidlawii* B membranes made homogeneous with members of most fatty acid classes tested, or containing two different classes of fatty acids, may also exhibit multiple gel-state phase transitions. It thus seems clear the gel-state polymorphism is not restricted to single-component lipid model membranes but can occur in lipid bilayers and in biological membranes containing appreciable polar

headgroup and fatty acyl chain compositional heterogeneity as well.

The effect of the incorporation of cholesterol into the A. *laidlawii* membrane on lipid thermotropic phase behavior was studied by de Kruyff and coworkers (56, 57) by using low-sensitivity DSC. In membranes enriched with several different fatty acids, the incorporation of cholesterol was reported to reduce the T_m slightly, to reduce the enthalpy markedly, and to have little effect on the cooperativity or the temperature range of the gel/liquid-crystalline phase transition. Very similar results were reported when cholesterol was incorporated into vesicles made from the synthetic phospholipid 1-stearoyl-2-oleoylphosphatidyl-choline. A puzzling aspect of these studies was the rather high transition enthalpy values reported, which ranged from 9.8 ± 06 to 11.3 ± 2.4 cal (1 cal = 4.184 J)/ g, depending on fatty acid supplementation. Previous DSC studies of aqueous dispersions of A. *laidlawii* total membrane lipids have all yielded values of 3.8 to 4.0 ± 0.2 cal/g of lipid.

Macdonald and Cossins (99) examined the effect of hydrostatic pressure and of alcohols on the lipid phase transition temperature of isolated A. *laidlawii* membranes by using turbidimetric, fluorescence, and DTA methods. These workers found that increases in pressure increase the T_m by 16 to 17°C/1,000 atm (1 atm = 101.29 kPa), values in broad agreement with those for both model lipid bilayers (17 to 24°C/1,000 atm) and other biological membranes (18 to 27°C/1,000 atm) (208). In contrast, the presence of 100 mM pentanol or benzyl alcohol decreases the T_m by 8.4 or 9.2°C, respectively, again in agreement with studies on pure phospholipid vesicles. These authors conclude that the lipid bilayer of the A. *laidlawii* membranes responds to pressure and alcohol incorporation, in agreement with thermodynamic theory, and that the presence of lipid fatty acid or polar headgroup heterogeneity and membrane protein has little if any effect on the response of the weakly cooperative gel/liquid-crystalline phase transition to these variables.

In contrast to A. *laidlawii* membranes, there have been only a few preliminary thermal analytical studies of the membranes of *Mycoplasma* species. Rottem and coworkers (157) studied lipid thermotropic phase behavior in isolated membranes from M. *mycoides* subsp. *capri* cells grown at 37°C with high and low levels of exogenous cholesterol. In membranes containing 20 to 25 wt% cholesterol, no cooperative lipid phase transition could be detected by low-sensitivity DSC, presumably because the high levels of cholesterol present either abolished the cooperative gel/liquid-crystalline phase transition entirely or broadened it beyond detectability, as occurs in model phospholipid bilayers containing large amounts of cholesterol. In membranes containing 3 to 4 wt% cholesterol, a reversible endothermic phase transition occurring over the range 22 to 29°C and centered at about 25°C was reported. The unexpectedly small range over which the lipid phase transition appeared to occur is probably due to the poor quality of the DSC trace, which makes accurate detection of the onset and completion temperatures difficult. Although no enthalpy values are reported, these authors state that the energy content of the lipid transition in cholesterol-poor M. *mycoides* subsp. *capri* is very low compared with that of A. *laid-*

lawii membranes. Rottem (156) has also studied the thermotropic phase behavior of an aqueous dispersion of the total membrane lipid extract from *M. arginini*, grown in the presence of high levels of exogenous cholesterol, with the same lipid extract from which the cholesterol component has been removed chromatographically. The total membrane lipid dispersion, which contains 25 to 30 wt% cholesterol, exhibits no detectable cooperative thermotropic phase transition by conventional DSC. In contrast, the cholesterol-free lipid extract exhibits a broad, ramp-like phase transition occurring over the range 35 to 54°C and centered at about 45°C. This means that in the absence of high levels of incorporated cholesterol, the phospho- and glycolipids in *M. arginini* membranes would exist almost exclusively in the gel state at the optimal growth temperature of 37°C. Since mycoplasma and bacterial cells cannot grow properly when most of their membrane lipid exists in the gel state (117), cholesterol is presumably required by this organism in order to fluidize the otherwise solidlike membrane glycerolipids, thus permitting a reasonable level of membrane function to occur at normal growth temperatures (119).

Differential Scanning Dilatometry

Melchior and coworkers (124) utilized differential scanning dilatometry to measure the change in volume of isolated *A. laidlawii* membranes as a function of temperature. These workers found a differential increase in the specific volume of aqueous membrane dispersions of about 2.1% over the temperature 20 to 45°C, a temperature corresponding to the gel/liquid-crystalline phase transition monitored by DSC. Since synthetic lipid bilayers typically exhibit volume increases of 3.5 to 4.0% at their chain-melting phase transitions, and since membrane lipids account for only about one-third by weight of the *A. laidlawii* membranes, a volume increase of this magnitude for the membrane as a whole seems reasonable, although perhaps a bit larger than expected. It is unfortunate that an aqueous dispersion of the total membrane lipids was not also examined by this technique.

X-Ray Diffraction

The X-ray diffraction studies of Engelman (60, 61) provided direct structural confirmation of the conclusions of the DSC studies just discussed. In these studies, the X-ray diffraction patterns from intact, isolated *A. laidlawii* membranes enriched in several different fatty acids were collected over a range of temperatures. At temperatures below the lower boundary of the calorimetrically determined gel/liquid-crystalline phase transition, membranes exhibit a sharp, wide-angle diffraction at 4.15 Å. This diffraction line, which arises from parallel hydrocarbon chains packed in a close hexagonal array with an axis-to-axis spacing of 4.80 Å, had previously been observed in lamellar gel phases of phospholipid-water mixtures. At temperatures within the phase transition range, the sharp diffraction at 4.15 Å gradually gives way to a diffuse reflection at 4.6 Å, which is characteristic of the more widely spaced, more disordered hydrocarbon chain

packing occurring in liquid-crystalline lamellar phospholipid-water phases. At temperatures above the phase transition upper boundary, only the diffuse 4.5-Å reflection is observed. Similar changes in hydrocarbon chain packing were noted in *A. laidlawii* membranes and in the isolated total membrane lipids dispersed in water, and in isolated membranes at least 80% of the lipids participate in the transition. Furthermore, the diffracting regions giving rise to the 4.15-Å reflection are comparatively large, about 400 Å in extent, indicating that relatively large domains of well-ordered lipid exist below the transition temperature, as shown also by freeze-fracture electron microscopy. Above the phase transition temperature, the diffracting regions are much smaller, indicating a loss of long-range order.

Useful information was also obtained from the low-angle X-ray scattering patterns from randomly dispersed and partially oriented membranes. In both cases, the electron density profile obtained is that characteristic of a lipid bilayer, with only a minor contribution from the membrane protein, indicating that the majority of the membrane protein is not present in a regular, repeating structural arrangement. The thickness of the lipid bilayer varies in the expected way with the chain length and structure of the lipid fatty acyl chains, in all cases decreasing substantially in the liquid-crystalline state. In palmitate-enriched membranes below the phase transition temperature, the hydrocarbon chains appear to be oriented perpendicular to the plane of the membrane, while in oleate-enriched membranes, the hydrocarbon chains seem to be tilted about 20°C from perpendicular, presumably because of the presence of a kink produced by the *cis*-double bond. The area per lipid molecule in the membrane is 40 to 45 Å² in the gel state and 60 to 70 Å² in the liquid-crystalline state, just as in the lipid-water dispersions. These results indicate that the bilayer is the predominant or exclusive lipid structure in the *A. laidlawii* membrane and that lipid-protein interactions have little effect on the average spacing and orientation of the lipid molecules.

It has been reported that *A. laidlawii* membranes, which have been solubilized by detergent and separated into their lipid and protein components, can reaggregate under appropriate conditions to form structures which appear similar to the native membranes (145). Metcalfe et al. (129, 130) have studied native and reaggregated membranes by X-ray diffraction and by several other physical techniques (see later sections). These workers report that lipid bilayer structures of similar thickness are present in both systems and that these bilayers undergoes a gel/liquid-crystalline phase transition over the same temperature range in both native and reaggregated membranes. However, in the reaggregated membranes, the size of the coherently reflecting regions of the lipid bilayer is smaller than in the native membranes, and the broad diffraction band due to the presence of membrane protein is altered in position and intensity. These and other results led Metcalfe and coworkers to conclude that although native and reaggregated membranes are indistinguishable in terms of composition, density, electron microscopic appearance, and basic structure, the lipid bilayer is less extensive and the organization and disposition of the membrane proteins are considerably different in the reaggregated compared with the native membranes.

NMR Spectroscopy

The technique of NMR spectroscopy has proven of great value in studies of lipid orientation and dynamics in lipid bilayers and natural membranes (for reviews, see references 51, 102, 174, 175, and 188). Unlike the nitroxide-containing ESR probes and the probes usually used in fluorescence polarization studies, most NMR probes do not significantly perturb their microenvironments. Moreover, the theoretical analyses of NMR spectra are generally more rigorous and based on sounder theoretical frameworks than is usually the case for ESR and fluorescence polarization spectrosopy. Finally, NMR spectroscopy is responsive to relatively slow molecular motions, generally in the range 10^3 to 10^6/s. Motions in this time domain are most likely to have direct biological relevance.

The technique of ^{2}H NMR spectroscopy has been widely used to study lipid hydrocarbon chain orientational order in model and biological membranes, particularly the membrane of A. laidlawii. In addition to being relatively nonperturbing, the deuterium nucleus, having a low natural abundance, can be selectively placed at various positions in the lipid molecule or in the fatty acyl chain. Furthermore, the electric quadruple moment of deuterium allows a direct measurement of the molecular order parameter, a measure of the time-averaged orientation relative to the bilayer normal, from the observed quadruple splittings. Direct measurements of the rates of motion (relaxation times) of the hydrocarbon chains of the A. laidlawii membrane lipids, the other component of fluidity, have not yet been made by ^{2}H NMR spectroscopy. The only significant disadvantage of deuterium is its low sensitivity, which until recently required the presence of relatively high probe levels (typically 50 mol% or more) in the membrane of interest (51, 174, 175).

Oldfield and coworkers (133) were the first to apply ^{2}H NMR spectroscopy to the A. laidlawii membrane. These workers selectively labeled the membrane lipid hydrocarbon chains by growing this organism in the presence of exogenous, fully deuterated lauric or palmitic acid. The ^{2}H NMR spectra obtained from isolated membranes, recorded at the growth temperature of 37°C, consist of a broad, unstructured envelope of numerous overlapping resonances. Nevertheless, the spectral shape observed is qualitatively that expected from the simultaneous presence of both gel and liquid-crystalline lipid phases, in agreement with previous DSC, DTA, and X-ray diffraction studies for A. laidlawii membranes enriched in saturated fatty acids.

Stockton et al. (190) pioneered the use of specifically deuterated fatty acids in NMR studies of biological membranes. A. laidlawii membranes were highly enriched by the biosynthetic incorporation of exogenous palmitic acid labeled only at the terminal methyl group with deuterium, and ^{2}H NMR spectra were recorded at a variety of temperatures. Although instrumental limitations precluded direct observation of the broad gel-phase signal present at lower temperatures, the intensity of the liquid-crystalline spectra, which first appears at 20°C, increases with increasing tem-perature from 20 to 44°C, leveling off at temperatures above 44°C. At 37°C, about half of the lipid appears to exist in the fluid state. Above 44°C, the orientational order decreases fairly rapidly with increasing temperature. Interestingly, the ESR order parameter, derived from the spectra of the intercalated 5-doxylstearic acids in these same membranes, exhibits a sharp jump discontinuity at 37°C, the midpoint of the broad lipid phase transition detected by ^{2}H NMR spectroscopy and other physical techniques. The ESR probe, however, is insensitive to the boundaries of the gel/liquid-crystalline transition.

Stockton et al. (191) later extended their study to include palmitic acid probes labeled at a variety of positions from C-2 through C-16 of the hydrocarbon chain. In this study, both the gel and liquid-crystalline spectra could be observed directly and the phase boundaries assigned in the previous study could thus be confirmed. In addition, the orientational order parameter profile for lipids existing just above the upper boundary of the lipid phase transition could be determined. It was found that a plot of order parameter versus the position of the deuteron in the chain reveals a plateau region of roughly constant order extending from C-2 through C-10, after which the order parameter declines progressively more rapidly toward the methyl terminus, just as observed with model membranes composed of dipalmitoylphosphatidylcholine above its phase transition temperature (175). By using the fully deuterated palmitic acid probe, it was also shown that the effect of cholesterol on the liquid-crystalline membrane lipids is to increase orientational order, particularly in the plateau region.

The spectrum of membranes enriched in 2,2-dideuteropalmitate differed from all other probes tested in revealing an unusual line shape which appears to consist of three overlapping powder doublets, whereas all other positions produce single doublet signals. These authors suggested that these multiple signals, which are also observed in C-2-labeled synthetic phospholipid liquid-crystalline bilayer systems, could be due to differences in the initial conformation of the two acyl chains, to differences in the polar lipid headgroups, or to the presence of membrane protein. This first suggestion has since been confirmed by ^{2}H NMR spectroscopy and by X-ray and neutron diffraction studies of model membranes, which have revealed that the fatty acyl chain at position 1 of the glycerol backbone projects directly downward toward the bilayer core, while the chain esterified at position 2 begins nearly parallel to the bilayer plane before binding to become perpendicular to the bilayer plane at the C-2 position of the hydrocarbon chain (for a review, see reference 51). Three signals are observed because the C-2 chain may exist in one of two forms within the generally preferred conformation, the orientational orders of these two forms being significantly different. Subsequent studies by Rance et al. (141) demonstrated that the conformations of the membrane lipids in the region of the C-2 position are qualitatively similar for all of the various lipid classes and that the presence of membrane protein has little if any effect on these conformations.

The properties of the gel and liquid-crystalline lipid domains of the A. laidlawii membrane were subsequently studied in more detail by Smith et al. (187).

Membranes enriched in 13,13-dideuteropalmitic acid at 45°C, just above the calorimetrically determined upper phase transition boundary, exhibit an almost perfect powder pattern characteristic of fluid lipid with only a single quadruple splitting, just as in the case of the total membrane lipids dispersed in water. This finding means that the presence of the membrane protein does not perturb the average orientational order of the lipid hydrocarbon chains. It also means that lipid molecules must be exchanging rapidly on the NMR time scale between the bulk and protein boundary lipid domains. These results are in contrast to those obtained by ESR using nitroxide fatty acid probes; in the latter studies, the presence of membrane protein appears to immobilize and disorder the lipid hydrocarbon chains, and the exchange between bulk and boundary lipid domains is slow on the ESR time scale (80, 112). Within the calorimetrically determined phase transition boundaries, separate gel and liquid-crystalline spectral components coexist, indicating that the lipids of these domains are in slow exchange (<10,000 times per s). At the lower boundary of the phase transition, the gel-state spectrum indicates a distribution of order parameters, the average being about one-half of the theoretical maximum for totally immobilized chains in the all-*trans* extended conformation. As the temperature is lowered still further, the observed quadruple splitting eventually approaches its theoretical maximum, but only at temperatures well below the phase transition lower boundary. These authors suggested that the membrane lipid hydrocarbon chains exist in the all-*trans* extended conformation as they enter the gel state but continue to undergo rapid rotational motion about their long axes, this rotational motion being slowly decreased with further decreases in temperature. However, this interpretation has been challenged by Pink and Zuckerman (136), who have presented theoretical and reviewed experimental data indicating that transitions between different chain conformational states, through the formation of *gauche* bonds, do occur in gel-state lipids, although on a time scale rapid compared with the ^{2}H NMR time scale. However, the early Raman spectroscopic studies of model membranes on which this argument is based, which indicate substantial numbers of *gauche* conformers in the gel, are not correct, and recent FT-IR spectroscopic studies indicate that few if any *gauche* conformers are present below the T_m (30, 126). Thus, the original ^{2}H NMR interpretations appear to be correct. Both groups agree, however, that rapid rotational motion does occur in the gel state until quite low temperatures are reached.

Generally similar results were reported by Jarrell et al. (76) for a ^{2}H NMR study of *A. laidlawii* membranes highly enriched (≥90 mol%) in myristic acid, except that the length of the plateau region of the order parameter profile appeared to be somewhat shorter than for membranes enriched in palmitic acid. In addition, although the average order parameters of liquid-crystalline hydrocarbon chains were the same in intact membranes and in an aqueous dispersion of membrane lipids, an increase in linewidth of about 20% was detected in the membrane, indicating that the presence of membrane proteins increases the heterogeneity of order distribution without affecting its average value. Furthermore, in the gel state, a small frac-

tion of lipid hydrocarbon chains in the membrane (but not in the lipid-water dispersion) remain disordered near their methyl-terminal region, even at very low temperatures, indicating a small membrane protein-disordering effect. Finally, the gel state of membranes highly enriched in myristic acid was found to be more highly ordered than previously observed for membranes less highly enriched in myristic acid, suggesting that fatty acid heterogeneity may affect lipid gel-state organization more than does the presence of protein.

Rance et al. (139) have also investigated the orientational order of *A. laidlawii* membranes enriched in unsaturated instead of saturated fatty acids, using biosynthetically incorporated, specifically deuterated oleic acid. The orientational order of the oleoyl chain was determined at a variety of temperatures from −50 to +41°C. Above 10 to 15°C, a single, sharp quadrupolar powder pattern was observed for all C^2H_2 segments except the C-9 and C-10 positions (and of course the C-2 segment). The C-9–C-10 spectra appear to consist of two overlapping powder patterns of equal integrated intensity, indicating motional inequivalence of the C-9 and C-10 deuterons. This could occur only if the double bond is not parallel to the bilayer normal but instead is slightly tilted. Below 10 to 15°C, a second, broader spectral component, due to gel-phase lipid, begins to appear and grow at the expense of the liquid-crystalline component as the temperature is reduced. These spectra indicate that the center of the solid/fluid phase transition is about 12°C, in good agreement with DSC studies. As noted in previous ^{2}H NMR studies, some relatively rapid hydrocarbon chain rotation, at least in the terminal half of the chain, persists down to −30 to −35°C, well below the lower boundary of the calorimetrically detectable phase transition, and this was again ascribed to a disordering effect of the membrane protein.

A plot of orientation order parameter versus oleoyl chain position revealed a profile parameter somewhat different from that previously observed with palmitate-enriched *A. laidlawii* membranes. Instead of a plateau region extending from C-2 to C-10, the oleate-enriched membranes exhibit a shortened plateau region extending only to about C-7, followed by a dip in the profile with a local minimum at C-10, after which the order parameters again increase before falling off toward the methyl terminus of the oleoyl chain. Although this profile would appear to indicate a markedly decreased order in the center of the oleoyl chain compared with palmitate, in fact this behavior is due largely to the geometry of the double bond and its tilted alignment with respect to the bilayer normal. Actually, the fluctuations about the average orientation of this segment of the oleoyl chain appear to be rather similar to the corresponding region of the palmitoyl chain if the two are compared at the same reduced temperature (i.e., at the same temperature relative to the phase transition temperature). The major effect of the presence of the double bond then seems to be to cause a local organizational perturbation in its immediate vicinity, which, although not profound, is sufficiently strong to cause the formation of predominantly fluid rather than predominantly gel-state lipid at physiological temperatures.

The temperature dependence of the order parameters of the various C^2H_2 segments of the oleoyl chains was also determined in the study summarized above. The temperature dependence in the liquid-crystalline state is approximately linear, with order decreasing with increasing temperature. In absolute terms, the change in order parameter with temperature was greatest in the plateau region (here C-2 to C-6 or C-7) and smallest at the methyl end of the hydrocarbon chain. The opposite is true, however, if the change in order parameter with temperature is expressed as a percentage change in the quadrupolar splittings observed. Similar findings were also made for *A. laidlawii* membranes highly enriched in fully perdeuterated palmitic acid (52).

Jarrell and coworkers (77) studied the orientational order and dynamics of *A. laidlawii* membranes enriched with a cyclopropyl-containing fatty acid by ^2H NMR. Specifically, dihydrosterculic acid (*cis*-9,10-methyleneoctadecanoic acid), specifically deuterated at several positions along the chain, was biosynthetically incorporated into the membrane lipids of this organism. The transition from the gel to the liquid-crystalline phase was determined to occur from −15 to 0°C, a range somewhat narrower than, but with a midpoint similar to, that found for membranes enriched in oleic acid. The acyl chains of dihydrosterculate-containing membranes are less mobile in the gel and in the liquid-crystalline state than are those of oleic acid-containing membranes. Above 0°C, the lipids are in the liquid-crystalline phase and give rise to powder spectra characteristic of axially symmetric motion. The overall ordering is greater everywhere than that in the case of oleoyl chains and features a maximum at the cyclopropyl moiety, in sharp contrast to the plateau found with saturated chains. Detailed analysis of the data for the cyclopropane ring indicates that the C-9–C-10 bond is inclined at 89° relative to the director of motional averaging, in sharp contrast to the 3° estimated for oleic acid in the same membranes. These authors suggest that the replacement of a *cis*-double bond by a *cis*-cyclopropane ring in the lipid fatty acyl chains of eubacterial membranes gives rise to a less fluid lipid bilayer with generally similar but not identical physical properties.

It should be noted that in all of the ^2H NMR studies reviewed thus far, the *A. laidlawii* membranes highly enriched in palmitic acid residues behaved in all respects quite similarly to dipalmitoylphosphatidylcholine model membranes, while the *A. laidlawii* membranes enriched in palmitate and oleate were very similar in behavior to bilayers of 1-palmitoyl-2-oleoylphosphatidylcholine (for reviews, see references 51 and 175). This finding supports the suitability of simple phospholipid bilayer membranes as reasonable models for more complex biological membranes, at least as far as hydrocarbon chain orientation and dynamics are concerned. Moreover, Kang and coworkers (82) showed that the ^2H NMR spectra of freshly isolated or lyophilized membranes (enriched with specifically deuterated myristic or palmitic acid) and aqueous dispersions of the total membrane lipids are identical. Together, these findings emphasize that the presence of membrane proteins has only a small effect on the average organization of membrane lipid fatty acyl chains, at least on the NMR time scale.

The effect of the presence of cholesterol on the orientational order of palmitate-enriched, oleate-enriched, and dihydrosterculate-enriched *A. laidlawii* membranes has been studied in some detail by Davis et al. (52), Rance et al. (140), and Jarrell et al. (77), respectively. In fully perdeuterated palmitate-containing membranes, the incorporation of relatively large amounts of cholesterol (reported as about 39 mol%) essentially abolishes a discrete gel/liquid-crystalline phase transition, as detected by both ^2H NMR and DSC studies. Between 20 and 45°C, the normal boundaries of the lipid phase transition in palmitate-enriched membranes not containing cholesterol, the cholesterol-enriched membranes exhibit an order parameter profile qualitatively similar to that normally observed for the liquid-crystalline phase in the absence of cholesterol. However, the cholesterol-containing membranes have a higher average order and an extended plateau region. In absolute terms, the increase in order is greatest in the plateau region and smallest at the methyl end of the chains, although the reverse is true if the increase in order is expressed in percentage terms. Below 20°C, the ^2H NMR spectra of cholesterol-enriched membranes are multicomponent, suggestive of complex motional and/or phase behavior. In oleate-enriched and dihydrostertulate-enriched *A. laidlawii* membranes, the order parameters of the various segments of the oleoyl or dihydrosterculoyl chain increase more or less linearly with cholesterol concentration from 0 to 27 mol%. The effect of cholesterol on the liquid-crystalline order parameter profile is quite similar to that just described for palmitate-enriched membranes. Interestingly, the temperature dependence of the ^2H NMR spectra, and the NMR-determined phase transition position and width characteristic of oleic acid-enriched and dihydrosterculic acid-enriched membranes lacking cholesterol, is very little affected by the presence of up to 27 mol% cholesterol. This is in contrast to the ^2H NMR-determined and calorimetrically determined behavior of palmitate-enriched membranes and to the behavior of cholesterol in dipalmitoylphosphatidylcholine model membranes as determined by DSC and other techniques, in which similar amounts of cholesterol significantly broaden the gel/liquid-crystalline phase transition and may also alter the phase transition midpoint temperature (for a review, see reference 116).

In contrast to the many ^2H NMR studies of *A. laidlawii* membranes, this technique has only recently been applied to the membrane of a *Mycoplasma* species. Huang et al. (72) used ^2H NMR spectroscopy to study the effect of cholesterol and lanosterol on the orientational order and dynamics of the lipid hydrocarbon chains of the *M. capricolum* membrane. As reported previously for *A. laidlawii*, the incorporation of increasing quantities of cholesterol increases the order of the lipid hydrocarbon chain at the optimal growth temperature of 37°C and abolishes the formation of gel-state lipid at lower temperatures. As well, the presence of high levels of cholesterol abolishes the temperature dependence of the spin lattice and transverse relaxation times. In contrast, the incorporation of comparable amounts of lanosterol is much less effective in this regard, as reported earlier by Dahl et al. (46, 50) using fluorescence polarization spectroscopy. Also, as reported earlier for *A. laidlawii*, the average order and spin lattice relaxation times of the hydrocarbon chains in isolated membranes and total membrane lipid dispersions are comparable at a given temperature and cholesterol level, indicating that the presence of membrane protein has little effect on the average orientation or on the rates of the fast motions of the lipid hydrocarbon chains. In contrast, the transverse relaxation times of the isolated membranes are much smaller than those of the total membrane lipid dispersions, indicating that the presence of membrane proteins introduces a slow motion of the phospholipid molecules not present in their absence. Huang and coworkers also report that the growth rates of *M. capricolum* cells are positively correlated with the relatively more ordered and less dynamic state of the membrane lipid hydrocarbon chains induced by the incorporation of increasing quantities of cholesterol, results again in agreement with the earlier studies of Dahl et al. (46, 50).

Eriksson et al. (62) recently studied the hydrocarbon chain orientational order and dynamics of the major glucoglycerolipids of the *A. laidlawii* A membrane, using ^{2}H NMR spectroscopy and biosynthetically incorporated perdeuterated palmitic acid. The hydrocarbon chains of the MGDG in lipid-water dispersions were found to exhibit a higher degree of orientational order than did those of the DGDG, but the MGDG chains appeared to undergo a larger amplitude of slow reorientational motion than did the DGDG chains, perhaps because of an increased rate of bilayer fluctuation or lateral diffusion over a curved bilayer surface. Interestingly, similar results have been reported for aqueous dispersions of synthetic phosphatidylethanolamines (PEs) and PCs, with the former exhibiting the larger degree of hydrocarbon chain order and slow-motion fluctuation. Since both MGDG and PE are membrane lipids with relatively small, poorly hydrated but strongly interacting polar headgroups which tend to form nonlamellar phases at higher temperatures, these authors suggest that the relatively high orientational order of the MGDG hydrocarbon chains and their greater amplitude of collective motions may be related to the tendency of this lipid to induce curvature and instability into the liquid-crystalline bilayer phase, as a result of its inverted cone shape (see later discussion). Wieslander et al. (204, 207) had previously used ^{2}H NMR (and ^{1}H NMR) spectroscopy to show that MGDG (or mixtures of MGDG and DGDG), isolated from *A. laidlawii* membranes enriched in oleic acid, can form reversed cubic as well as reversed hexagonal phases when dispersed in water, and they used ^{2}H NMR spectroscopy (and X-ray diffraction) to study the phase structures and water-binding capacities of individual membrane lipids.

The technique of ^{19}F NMR spectroscopy has recently been applied to the *A. laidlawii* membranes by McDonough et al. (113) and Macdonald et al. (100). In these studies, small amounts of palmitic acid probes containing a single fluorine atom at various positions along the hydrocarbon chain were biosynthetically incorporated into the membrane lipids. The much greater sensitivity of the ^{19}F than of the ^{2}H nucleus in the NMR experiment allows usable information to be collected with only small incorporations of probe (5 to 10 mol%), thus allowing the study of membranes which are very highly enriched in a variety of other exogenous fatty acids. This technique also avoids the laborious and expensive synthesis of a complete series of specifically deuterated fatty acids for each exogenous fatty acid to be studied, which has been necessary in ^{2}H NMR studies. Other potential advantages include the ability to determine order parameters in the gel state and to study the rates of motion of various segments of the hydrocarbon chains via relaxation measurements. Physical, biochemical, and biological evidence was presented that the biosynthetic incorporation of these monofluoropalmitic acids does not perturb the structure or function of the *A. laidlawii* membrane.

The orientational order parameters of *A. laidlawii* membranes highly enriched in pentadecanoic, methyl isopalmitic, methyl anteisopalmitic, and palmitelaidic acids were studied by ^{19}F NMR as a function of temperature in the liquid-crystalline state (100). In this series of fatty acids, which have nearly the same effective chain lengths, the effect of the presence of a methyl group substitution or of a *trans*-double bond on chain order could be determined. At all temperatures, the *n*-saturated and methyl branched fatty acid-enriched membranes exhibit the typical plateau profile already described for palmitic acid-containing membranes, whereas the palmitelaidic acid-enriched membranes show a progressive decrease in order from near to carbonyl function toward the methyl terminus without a clear-cut plateau region. At the growth temperature of 37°C, the chain-average order parameter values decrease in the order pentadecanoic > isopalmitic > anteisopalmitic > palmitelaidic acid-enriched membranes, which is also the order of decreasing phase transition temperatures as determined by DTA. Thus, at a constant physiological temperature (37°C), the introduction of a methyl iso branch, a methyl anteiso branch, or a *trans*-double bond into an *n*-saturated fatty acyl chain results in progressively more disorder of the liquid-crystalline bilayer hydrocarbon core. Interestingly, however, if the chain-average order parameters are compared at comparable reduced temperatures, then the results are exactly opposite those obtained at 37°C.

Experimental and theoretical results indicate that the rotation of the membrane lipid hydrocarbon chains in the gel state remains sufficiently rapid to allow for a complete motional averaging and thus axially symmetric spectra on the ^{19}F NMR but not the ^{2}H NMR time scale (101, 102). This permits a detailed determination of the orientational order of the C-F bond in fluoropalmitic acid-labeled gel-state lipid in model and biological membranes, which is not possible with ^{2}H NMR spectroscopy. Macdonald and coworkers (103–107) thus determined the orientational order parameter profiles of *A. laidlawii* membranes highly enriched in a number of linear saturated, methyl iso- and anteiso-branched, and *cis*- and *trans*-monounsaturated and cyclopropyl fatty acids. As well, the effect of the position of the *cis*- or *trans*-double bond within the membrane lipid hydrocarbon chain on gel-state order was determined (104, 107). These workers found that at temperatures below the T_m, all types of hydrocarbon chains are relatively highly ordered but that there are much larger differences between the chain-average order of different classes of fatty acids in the gel than in the liquid-crystalline state. At comparable reduced temperatures in the gel state, order parameter values decrease in the order pentadecanoic > isopalmitic > palmitelaidic > anteisopalmitic > palmitoleic acid. This decreasing sequence of orientational order correlates well with the decreasing phase transition temperatures for the membrane lipids determined by DSC. Thus, membrane lipids whose hydrocarbon chains can pack in the most highly ordered array exhibit the most stable, highest-melting-point gel states, as expected. What was not expected, however, was the finding that membrane lipids with the highest phase transition temperature form the least ordered liquid-crystalline states once melting occurs (i.e., at comparable reduced temperatures in the liquid-crystalline state). This is probably because at the higher temperatures necessary to induce melting of the more stable gel phases, the increased thermal energy possessed by the fluid hydrocarbon chains produces higher rates of motion and lower orientational order than is the case for lower-melting-point membranes. Although the detailed chemical structure of the fatty acyl group also has an effect on chain order, the lipid phase transition is the prime determinant of this parameter. For a more detailed summary of ^{19}F NMR studies of the relationship between fatty acyl chain structure, orientational order, and lipid phase state in *A. laidlawii* membranes, the reader is referred to reviews by Macdonald et al. (102, 103).

Macdonald and coworkers (100) also compared the orientational order parameter profiles and the chain-average order values for intact *A. laidlawii* cells, isolated membranes, and total membrane lipid dispersions having the same lipid polar headgroup and fatty acid compositions. They found that all three systems behave identically within the experimental error of their determinations. Thus, the presence of cytoplasmic or membrane protein does not appear to significantly perturb membrane lipid hydrocarbon chain organization in either the gel or liquid-crystalline state, a result in agreement with those of the ^{2}H NMR studies reviewed earlier.

Metcalfe et al. (128) have conducted a preliminary ^{13}C NMR study of *A. laidlawii* membranes biosynthetically enriched in [1-^{13}C]palmitic acid. The carboxyl carbon resonance consists of a doublet of equal intensity, presumably arising from the two conformationally nonequivalent fatty acyl chains, since a similar doublet spectrum was observed for aqueous dispersions both of the total membrane lipids and of synthetic dipalmitoylphosphatidylcholine. At temperatures below about 30 to 35°C, where the membrane lipid exists predominantly in the gel state, no carboxyl spectrum is observed for either the intact membranes or the membrane lipid dispersion. The intensity of this resonance progressively increases with temperature until 45 to 50°C, where the lipid exists entirely in the liquid-crystalline state. No change in either the position or the intensity of the carboxyl resonance occurs upon exposure of the membranes to a temperature of 65°C, which thermally denatures the membrane proteins. These results thus agree with those from subsequent ^{2}H NMR studies of the lipid hydrocarbon chains, indicating that the membrane proteins have only very minor effects on lipid organization in the *A. laidlawii* membrane.

De Kruijff et al. (54) have utilized ^{31}P NMR spectroscopy to study the behavior of the phosphate headgroups in the PG and GPDGDG of the *A. laidlawii* membrane and in aqueous dispersions of the total membrane lipids. The ^{31}P NMR spectra of both the intact membranes and aqueous membrane lipid dispersions were reported to be essentially identical. Both systems exhibit a typical solid-state spectrum, characteristic of a phospholipid bilayer, in which the major contribution to the linewidth is made by the chemical shift anisotropy. Complete degradation of the PG by phospholipases does not change the nature but only reduces the intensity of the ^{31}P NMR spectrum, indicating that the phosphate groups in PG and GPDGDG in native membranes have similar orientations and motions. This observation is somewhat surprising in view of the quite different chemical environments and probable locations in the bilayer of these two phosphate groups; in fact, Lindblom et al. (98) report different ^{31}P NMR chemical shift anisotropy values for these two phospholipids when separated and purified. In both intact membranes and lipid dispersions, a broadening of the ^{31}P resonance is observed below the lipid phase transition temperature, indicating that some restriction in the motion of the phosphate groups occurs in the gel state. Interestingly, pronase digestion of up to 60% of the protein of the intact membrane, and the subsequent binding of cytochrome *c* to these deproteinated membranes, does not affect the ^{31}P NMR spectrum, suggesting that no strong lipid polar headgroup-protein interactions occur, or at least that these lipid-protein complexes undergo fast rotation about an axis perpendicular to the membrane plane. However, these workers also report that Ca^{2+} binding either to isolated membranes or to membrane lipid dispersions also does not affect the ^{31}P NMR spectrum. This is a surprising result, since Ca^{2+} has been reported to bind tightly to negatively charged phospholipids, even inducing the formation of solidlike phospholipid-calcium clusters in model membranes by a process of isothermal lateral phase separation (116). However, as discussed earlier, Silvius et al. (180) also report that the addition of Mg^{2+} or Ca^{2+} to *A. laidlawii* membrane lipid dispersions does not increase the T_m as measured by DTA. Perhaps these anionic lipids, as isolated, already contain bound cations. Alternatively, the neutral glycolipids present may inhibit the binding of Mg^{2+} and Ca^{2+} by the anionic lipid components.

The only other ^{31}P NMR study of *A. laidlawii* membranes is that of Seguin et al. (176), discussed earlier. In this study, the lipids of isopalmitic acid-homogeneous membranes were shown to undergo two phase transitions, a lower-temperature transition from a more highly ordered to a less highly ordered gel state and a higher-temperature transition from a less highly ordered gel state to the liquid-crystalline state, by DSC and FT-IR spectroscopy. Below the temperature of the first phase transition, proton-decoupled ^{31}P NMR spectra have a basal linewidth of about 120 ppm and are nearly symmetrical. Broad, powder-pattern spectra of this type are indicative of a relatively slow, axially asymmetric motion of the phosphate headgroup and have been observed in the so-called subgel (L$_c$) phases of some synthetic phospholipid bilayers. Upon warming to a temperature above the gel/gel phase transition temperature, the basal linewidth narrows to about 90 ppm and the spectra becomes slightly asymmetric. Spectra of this sort are characteristic of the gel (L_β or P_β) phases of synthetic lipid bilayers. Finally, at temperatures above the gel/liquid-crystalline phase transition temperature, the ^{31}P NMR spectrum narrows further to about 70 ppm and becomes markedly asymmetric, exhibiting an up-field peak and a down-field shoulder. Spectra of this type indicate that the phosphate headgroup is undergoing fast, axially symmetric motion on the NMR time scale and is characteristic of synthetic phospholipid bilayers in the liquid-crystalline (l_α) phase. These workers also report that the ^{31}P NMR spectra of isolated membranes and of vesicles generated from the total membrane lipid are almost identical. However, in this study, some evidence for a separate spectral component due to the phosphate resonance from GPDGDG was presented. These observations indicate that ^{31}P NMR spectroscopy is sensitive to both the gel/gel and gel/liquid-crystalline phase transition of the membrane lipid bilayer and that the presence of proteins has little effect on the motion and orientations of the phosphate headgroup in the membrane.

Metcalfe et al. (129) utilized ^1H NMR spectroscopy of the phenyl protons of a benzyl alcohol probe to study native and reaggregated *A. laidlawii* membranes. These workers report that there are extensive lipid-protein interactions in both membrane systems which exclude some of the binding sites for the probe molecules that are exposed on the detergent-solubilized and separated lipid and protein components. As well, the mobility of the benzyl alcohol molecules in both systems increases with increasing alcohol concentration, implying that both membrane components become more fluid. However, the lipid-associated probe exhibits small differences and the protein-associated probe exhibits larger differences in mobility between the reaggregated and native membranes, indicating that these structures, although generally similar, are not structurally identical, supporting the X-ray diffraction results discussed earlier and the fluorescence spectroscopic results to be discussed below.

Kinsey et al. (85) have reported the first observations of amino acid side chain dynamics in membrane proteins by using high-field ^2H NMR spectroscopy. Although this study concentrated on the spectra of an individual membrane protein, bacteriorhodopsin, in the purple membrane of the bacteria *Halobacterium halobium*, some preliminary data on [γ-$^2H_6$]valine-labeled *A. laidlawii* B membranes were also presented. Similar ^{19}F NMR studies of the environment, exposure, and mobility of membrane proteins that have been biosynthetically labeled with specifically fluorinated amino acids also appear to be feasible in this organism. Thus, it should be possible in the future to observe in some detail the locations and motions of amino acid side chains in various portions of membrane proteins and to study the effects of lipid composition on protein structure and dynamics generally. Needless to say, this would be extremely valuable, since at present we have almost no data on protein structure and dynamics in the *A. laidlawii* membrane, despite a relative wealth of information on the lipids of this membrane.

ESR Spectroscopy

A number of groups have applied ESR spectroscopy to study the fluidity and phase state of the lipids of the *A. laidlawii* membrane. The most common ESR probes used in these studies were free fatty acids containing a nitroxide radical (usually the doxyl group) substituted at a particular position on the hydrocarbon chain. The fatty acid probes can be physically incorporated (intercalated) as such into isolated membranes by simply allowing them to partition into the lipid bilayer, or they can be added to the growth medium, where they are biosynthetically incorporated into the membrane polar lipids by growing cells. The latter technique is, of course, preferable, as the ESR probes are present as fatty acyl groups rather than as free acids and are presumably distributed relatively evenly among the various membrane glyco- and phospholipids. The fluidity of the membrane lipids is usually expressed as a motional parameter, related to the rotational correlation time of the nitroxide group, or as an apparent order parameter, which is related to the time-averaged orientation. However, there is some question as to whether this technique can effectively resolve the static orientational and dynamic motional contributions which determine membrane lipid fluidity. The ESR technique is sensitive to relatively fast motions on a time scale of 10^7 to 10^9/s. Arrhenius plots of the motional or order parameters often show breaks (changes in slope) at a particular temperature, and these are assumed to be related to the gel/liquid-crystalline phase transition temperature of the membrane lipids. Another group of ESR probes, which can be used only to monitor membrane lipid phase transitions, are small, relatively nonpolar nitroxide molecules such as 2,2,6,6-tetramethylpiperidine-*N*-oxyl (TEMPO). These ESR probes will preferentially partition into liquid-crystalline lipid domains in preference to water but are largely excluded from the gel-state regions of lipid bilayers. Since probes like TEMPO have quite different ESR spectra in lipid and in water, the relative partitioning between the membrane and its aqueous environment as a function of temperature can be determined spectroscopically, thus allowing one to monitor the progress of the entire gel/liquid-crystalline phase transition. For a good recent review of the scope and limitations of ESR spectroscopy as applied to membranes, the reader is referred to reference 171.

The TEMPO partitioning technique has been applied to *A. laidlawii* membranes by Metcalfe et al. (128). Palmitic acid-enriched membranes undergo a temperature-dependent increase in TEMPO partitioning over the temperature range of 20 to about 50°C, the latter temperature being an estimate since the nitroxide group is chemically reduced at higher temperatures, leading to a loss of resonance intensity. Aqueous dispersions of the total membrane lipids exhibit essentially identical behavior and moreover bind the same amount of TEMPO at all temperatures above 30°C, although isolated membranes bind about twice as much TEMPO as do the lipid dispersions at temperatures below 20°C. These workers concluded that palmitate-enriched *A. laidlawii* membranes undergo a gel/liquid-crystalline phase transition over the temperature range of 20 to about 50°C in which essentially all of the lipid participates and which is little influenced by the presence of membrane proteins. Similar results were, of course, obtained with the DSC, X-ray diffraction, and NMR studies already reviewed. Although very little TEMPO was found to bind to *n*-butanol-extracted membrane proteins, it could not be definitely determined whether the excess TEMPO bound to isolated membranes at low temperature was due to the presence of membrane proteins in their native state or to a somewhat more disordered gel state than exists in membrane lipid dispersions. Alternatively, some TEMPO might have preferentially partitioned into the somewhat disordered boundary lipid domain thought to surround integral membrane proteins (80, 112). The TEMPO partitioning technique has also been applied to *A. laidlawii* membranes from cells grown without fatty acid supplementation by Grant and McConnell (63). Although these investigators claim that no phase transition could be detected by this technique, a careful inspection of their data indicates the presence of a broad phase transition commencing at about 20°C. Since data were collected only until about 45°C, which is the upper boundary of the calorimetrically determined gel/liquid-crystalline phase transition, one cannot ascertain whether this ESR technique would have accurately detected the completion of the gel/liquid-crystalline lipid phase transition in the membranes of this organism. Lindblom et al. (98) successfully used the TEMPO partitioning technique to monitor the gel/liquid-crystalline phase transition of aqueous dispersions of the *A. laidlawii* total membrane lipids containing various proportions of palmitic and oleic acids.

The first ESR study of the *A. laidlawii* membrane in which a fatty acid spin probe was used was that of Tourtellotte et al. (195), who used biosynthetically incorporated 12-doxylstearic acid to probe the fluidity and phase state of membranes enriched in either stearic or oleic acid. These workers found that the doxyl group of the fatty acid probe is present in a hydrophobic, semiviscous environment in the isolated membranes, just as in aqueous dispersions of the extracted membrane lipids. However, the spin label in the isolated membranes is slightly but significantly less mobile than that in membranes generated from the protein-free lipid extract. However, heat denaturation of the membrane proteins does not affect the mobility of the spin label in the membrane. These workers concluded that the mobility of at least a portion of the hydrocarbon chains in the native *A. laidlawii* membranes is slightly reduced by a weak association with integral membrane proteins. Although the effect of the proteins on the orientational order of the membrane lipids was not determined, studies in model systems using fatty acid spin probes have shown that the boundary lipids surrounding at least some integral membrane proteins are more orientationally disordered and motionally restricted than are the liquid-crystalline lipids not in contact with these proteins (80, 112).

The rotational correlation time of the nitroxide radical of the fatty acid spin probe was found to be a decreasing exponential function of temperature over the range of 20 to 60°C. However, at all temperatures, the values of the stearate-enriched membranes are nearly twice those of the oleate-enriched membranes, indicating that membranes containing stearic acid are less fluid than those containing oleate. The constant ratio of rotational correlation times with temperature is curious, since at 55°C the lipids of both membranes exist exclusively in the liquid-crystalline state, whereas at 20°C the lipids of the stearate-containing membranes are entirely solid while those of the oleate-containing membranes remain completely fluid. These results suggest that the lipids containing the fatty acid spin probe are excluded from gel-state domains, since the mobility of solid-state lipids should be much lower than that observed. An Arrhenius plot gave a straight line for oleate-enriched membranes but yielded a slight break at 40°C with stearate-enriched membranes. The apparent activation energy of probe motion for oleate-enriched membranes was 4.1 to 4.2 kcal/mol, while that for stearate-enriched membranes was 3.9 kcal/mol above and 5.0 kcal/mol below the break temperature of 40°C.

Rottem et al. (158) studied the motion of a variety of intercalated spin labels in isolated *A. laidlawii* membranes enriched in several different fatty acids. In this study, spin label mobility was expressed as the hyperfine splitting ($2T_\parallel$), a spectral motion parameter whose units are in gauss. In the isolated membranes from unsupplemented cells, $2T_\parallel$ exhibits an inverse temperature dependence, indicating that molecular motion increases with increasing temperature. In addition, at any given temperature, the $2T_\parallel$ value progressively decreases as the nitroxide radical is moved away from the carbonyl function, indicating that molecular motion increases toward the methyl-terminal end of the fatty acyl chain. Membranes enriched with elaidic acid exhibit a greater $2T_\parallel$ than do those enriched in oleic acid at low temperatures, as expected, but the values for both membranes nearly converge at temperatures above 30°C. Interestingly, membranes from cells grown without fatty acid supplementation were found to be intermediate in mobility between elaidate- and oleate-enriched membranes at temperatures below 30°C, despite the greater proportion of gel-state lipid present in the unsupplemented membranes. However, the membranes derived from unsupplemented cells did exhibit a lower mobility than did elaidate- or oleate-enriched membranes at higher temperatures. Although the variation in $2T_\parallel$ with temperature was described as steep by these authors, the temperature dependence of this parameter was actually much less than that reported for the rotational correlation time in the study by Tourtellotte et al. (195).

Rottem and Samuni (161) subsequently investigated the effect of proteins on the motion of several fatty acid spin probes intercalated into the *A. laidlawii* membrane. The digestion of up to 75 to 80% of the protein of isolated membranes results in a small but significant increase in probe mobility, as indicated by a progressive decrease in the $2T_\parallel$ value. The addition of the soluble, positively charged proteins lysozyme and cytochrome *c* to the pronase-treated isolated membranes partially reverses the observed increase in the mobility of the spin-labeled fatty acids, and the subsequent removal of these extrinsic proteins by extraction with 1 M NaCl restores the increased probe mobility characteristic of protein-depleted membranes. These workers concluded that membrane proteins, including those bound electrostatically to the membrane surface, restrict the mobility of the lipid fatty acyl chains in native *A. laidlawii* membranes.

Askarova et al. (8) have studied the effect of the aging of *A. laidlawii* cultures on the mobility of both the lipids and proteins in isolated membranes by ESR spectroscopy. Membrane lipid fluidity was probed with the intercalated spin probe 5-nitroxylstearic acid, and membrane protein mobility was probed by a nitroxyl group bound covalently to the exposed sulfhydryl groups of membrane proteins. These workers found that the rotational mobilities of both the lipid and protein probes decrease throughout the logarithmic phase of growth but remain constant in the stationary phase. Since the presence of membrane proteins is known to decrease the rate of motion of adjacent lipid and protein molecules in model systems (112), the decrease in the lipid/protein ratio known to occur upon the aging of *A. laidlawii* cultures can probably explain both of these results. However, the saturated/unsaturated fatty acid ratio of the membrane lipids of this organism can also increase during the logarithmic phase of growth, and this could have contributed to the observed decrease in membrane lipid and protein mobility with culture age.

Huang and coworkers (70, 71) investigated the effect of changes in fatty acid composition on the mobility of intercalated 5- and 12-nitroxide stearic acids in *A. laidlawii* membranes enriched in arachidic, lauric, or oleic acid. When the relative mobilities of these membranes were compared on the basis of the $2T_\parallel$ values of the 5-nitroxide probe, it was found that at the growth temperature (28 or 37°C), the relative mobilities of all membranes were nearly identical. However, at lower temperatures, relative mobilities decreased in the order oleic > arachidic > lauric acid-enriched membranes, while at higher temperatures the order was either arachidic > lauric > oleic acid-enriched membranes (28°C growth temperature) or arachidic > oleic > lauric acid-enriched membranes (37°C growth temperature). These results are at variance with results of other experiments carried out by these workers. For example, at 22°C the relative mobilities, as determined by the values of the 12-nitroxide stearic acid probe, decrease in the order oleic > lauric > arachidic acid-enriched membranes, in contrast to the low-temperature 5-nitroxide stearate results. Moreover, osmotic fragility and glycerol permeability experiments indicate that the relative fluidities should be oleic > lauric > arachidic acid-enriched membranes at all temperatures, which is the same order which would be predicted on the basis of the relative phase transition temperatures as determined by DSC or DTA, for example. The ESR results of Huang and coworkers are thus somewhat suspect, as is their conclusion that *A. laidlawii* maintains a constant membrane lipid fluidity at its growth temperature in the face of marked changes in the chain length and degree of unsaturation of the hydrocarbon chains in its membrane lipids.

Butler et al. (24), using intercalated 5- and 12-nitroxide fatty acid probes, studied the effect of alterations in fatty acid composition and cholesterol content on the molecular order of *A. laidlawii* membranes. Plots of order parameter versus temperature for the 5-nitroxide probe reveal that palmitate- and stearate-enriched membranes have similar degrees of order within the physiological temperature range and that the temperature dependence of the order parameter is relatively steep in both systems. In contrast to the results of Huang et al. (70, 71), the order parameter of this probe in oleate-enriched membranes is less temperature dependent and the degree of orientational order is significantly lower than is the case for membranes enriched in *n*-saturated fatty acids, particularly at lower temperatures. Plots of order parameter versus temperature are linear in both oleate- and palmitate-containing membranes, thus revealing no evidence that the 5-nitroxide probe is sensitive to the gel/liquid-crystalline phase transition which is known to take place in the membranes enriched with palmitate. Evidence suggestive of a phase transition was, however, obtained in stearate-enriched membranes. Both probes also reveal a slightly but significantly lower average order in aqueous dispersions of the total membrane lipids than in the isolated membranes, indicating that the presence of membrane protein produces a small increase in the order of these unoriented systems, in contrast to the results observed in lipid-protein model systems (112). Both probes reveal that the incorporation of cholesterol produces an increase in the degree of order of palmitate-enriched membranes at all temperatures, although the effect is greatest at higher temperatures. It is interesting to note that the presence of cholesterol reduces the temperature dependence of the order parameter in palmitate-containing membranes, making it quite similar to that of oleate-containing membranes. Since the incorporation of cholesterol is known to broaden and eventually abolish a cooperative gel/liquid-crystalline phase transition, it is tempting to speculate that the presence of a phase transition may sometimes manifest itself as an increased temperature dependence of ESR probe motion or order rather than as an abrupt change in that dependence at some discrete temperature.

Two groups have studied the effect of the presence of carotenoid pigment on lipid fluidity of *A. laidlawii* membranes by using ESR spectroscopy. Huang and Haug (69) utilized intercalated 12-nitroxide stearic acid to investigate the fluidity of arachidic acid-supplemented cells whose carotenoid pigment contents had been varied over 50-fold by adding either acetate or propionate to the growth medium. Acetate has been shown to stimulate carotenoid biosynthesis in this organism, whereas propionate inhibits carotenoid production. When cells are cultured in the presence of acetate, a small decrease in membrane lipid mobility is observed by ESR spectroscopy. Membranes isolated from cells grown in acetate are also characterized by a slightly higher buoyant density, a slightly higher fragility, and a slightly lower glycerol permeability. From these results, Huang and Haug concluded that carotenoid pigments rigidify the lipids of the *A. laidlawii* membrane. A similar conclusion was later reached by Rottem and Markowitz (159), who used intercalated 5- and 12-nitroxide stearic acids to study membrane lipid mobility in oleate-supplemented cells cultured with or without exogenous propionate. Both probes reveal much less motional restriction in membranes derived from cells grown in the presence of oleate and propionate than in those cultured in oleic acid alone, especially at higher temperatures. Moreover, as had been observed earlier for cholesterol, the presence of higher levels of carotenoids also decreases the temperature dependence of the motional parameters monitored. In addition, the selective removal of carotenoids from the *A. laidlawii* membranes by incubation with egg PC vesicles induces a restricted probe mobility in that artifical membrane system.

Rottem (154) has used ESR spectroscopy to suggest that the fluidities of the exterior and interior regions of *A. laidlawii* (and *M. hominis*) membranes may be different. When intact cells were spin labeled by incubation with 12-nitroxide stearic acid, the rotational correlation time at 37°C measured from the ESR spectrum was calculated to be 4.25 ns, whereas when isolated membranes were labeled by the same technique, the value was 4.55 ns. When intact cells were labeled but then the membranes were isolated in the absence of probe, the rotational correlation time was determined to be 4.30 ns. If it is assumed that the 12-nitroxide stearic acid does not flip-flop across the lipid bilayer of the *A. laidlawii* membrane, then when intact cells are labeled, the probe should be localized in the outer half of the bilayer, while when isolated membranes are labeled, the probe should be incorporated into both the inner and outer halves of the bilayer. The results presented above thus suggest that a higher degree of fluidity exists in the outer half than in the inner half of the *A. laidlawii* membrane and that the differences in the observed behavior of intact cells and isolated membranes are not due to alterations in membrane structure produced by the isolation procedure. It was further suggested that the presence of a larger amount of protein in the inner region of the membrane of this organism may be responsible for the lower mobility of the probe in the inner half of the bilayer.

The validity of Rottem's study is difficult to assess. The differences between the measured rotational correlation times are quite small and may not be statistically significant. Furthermore, no evidence for the assumption that free fatty acid spin probes do not flip-flop in these membranes was presented. Finally, it should be noted that the results obtained in this study are the opposite of what might be predicted from the lipid transbilayer distribution study of Gross and Rottem (65) reviewed earlier, which suggested that the neutral glycolipids are located essentially exclusively in the outer monolayer of the *A. laidlawii* membrane, whereas the phospholipids are located predominantly in the inner monolayer. Since these glycolipids have higher phase transition temperatures than do the corresponding phospholipids (180) and since membranes formed from synthetic glycolipids have both higher phase transition temperatures and higher viscosities than do those formed from synthetic phospholipids of similar fatty acid composition (74, 109, 110, 178), one might expect that the outer region of the lipid bilayer of the membrane of this organism would have a lower rather than a higher fluidity relative to the inner region.

Burke et al. (23) studied the interaction of amine local anesthetics with the *A. laidlawii* membrane by ESR spectroscopy. Spin-labeled anesthetics and intercalated 5-doxylstearic acid were used to probe both the effect on the anesthetic molecule of binding to the membrane and the effect on the membrane lipid bilayer of the bound anesthetic. These workers found that although both cationic and neutral forms of the anesthetic partition strongly into the membrane, the positively charged, membrane-associated form is considerably more motionally restrained than is the neutral form. However, only the neutral form of the local anesthetic appears to fluidize the membrane lipid bilayer at the concentration tested. Since both cationic and neutral amine local anesthetics are thought to intercalate into lipid bilayers with the polar amine headgroup at the bilayer surface and the hydrophobic tail penetrating into the hydrocarbon region of the bilayer, it is not clear why only the uncharged form appears to fluidize the lipid hydrocarbon chains in the *A. laidlawii* membrane.

As stated earlier, a number of groups have used ESR spectroscopy and nitroxide fatty acid probes to determine apparent phase transition temperatures through the identification of breaks in the Arrhenius plots of some motional or orientational spectral parameter. The agreement between the transition temperature as determined by ESR and by other nonperturbing physical techniques such as DSC, NMR spectroscopy, or FT-IR spectroscopy ranges from good to poor (Table 1). In particular, the ESR-determined transition temperatures, while always falling within the phase transition boundaries as determined by these other techniques, can range from well below to somewhat above the actual midpoint of the gel/liquid-crystalline phase transition as determined by calorimetry and by other physical techniques. Also, the ESR-determined phase transition always appears to be rather sharp, whereas in fact the actual transitions are quite broad, occurring over a range of 25 to 30°C. Finally, in several ESR studies, no breaks in the Arrhenius plots of spectral motional or orientational parameters were observed in *A. laidlawii* membranes in which lipid phase transitions have been detected by DTA and other techniques. It is thus clear that ESR spectroscopic techniques utilizing nitroxide fatty acid probes are not the methods of choice for accurately characterizing lipid phase transitions in biological membranes. On the other hand, TEMPO partitioning may be a more suitable ESR technique for monitoring the gel/liquid-crystalline phase transitions of biological membranes, provided that technical limitations can be overcome. Generally speaking, however, the simplest, quickest, least expen-

Table 1. Some gel/liquid-crystalline phase transition temperatures observed in *A. laidlawii* membranes by ESR spectroscopy and DTA

Fatty acid supplementation	ESR-determined T_m (°C)	DTA-determined T_m (°C) (range)
12:0	25[a]	31 (15–42)[b]
14:0	34[c]	34 (18–45)
16:0	35,[d] ND[e,f]	38 (20–50)
18:0	40[g]	41 (25–55)
20:0	25[a]	40 (20–56)
18:1$_{trans}$	22,[c] 26[d]	21 (5–32)
18:1$_{cis}$	ND (<0°C?)[d,e,g]	−13 (−22 to −4)

[a] From Huang et al. (70).
[b] From McElhaney (114, 115, 120a).
[c] From James and Branton (75).
[d] From Rottem et al. (157).
[d] From Butler et al. (24).
[g] From Tourtellote et al. (195).

sive, and most reliable method for accurately determining the course of the chain-melting transition in model or biological membranes is DSC (116).

A few ESR studies of the membranes of several *Mycoplasma* species have also been carried out. Rottem and Verkleij (164) used ESR spectroscopy to study the orientational order of 5- and 12-doxylstearic acid probes intercalated into *M. gallisepticum* membranes. According to these workers, only single-component, bulk bilayer-type ESR spectra are observed despite the fact that these membranes are unique among the mycoplasmas in having a very high protein/lipid ratio (about 4:1 by weight). The apparent absence of a measurable boundary lipid component was ascribed to the fact that the intramembranous protein particles in these membranes are largely clustered even at 37°C, as revealed by freeze-fracture electron microscopy. This clustering, suggested to be due to the formation of patches of gel-state disaturated PC, was in turn postulated to minimize lipid-protein interactions. Indeed, the order parameter values and their temperature dependencies are essentially identical in 5-doxylstearate-labeled membranes and membrane lipid dispersions, as predicted. However, the order parameter values of isolated membranes are considerably lower, and their temperature dependence is greater, than in membrane lipid dispersions when the 12-doxylstearic acid is used as a probe. Moreover, a similar result is seen by fluorescence polarization spectroscopy using 1,6-diphenyl-1,3,5-hexatriene (DPH) as a probe. These latter results clearly indicate that in fact the membrane protein does interact with the membrane lipids, disordering the hydrophobic core of the lipid bilayer of this organism. Clearly, additional experimental work is required to clarify these apparently contradictory results. Moreover, it seems unlikely that patches of gel-state lipid could form in a membrane which is reported to contain 0.9 mol of cholesterol per mol of phospholipid, since cholesterol has been shown to fluidize lipid below its characteristic gel/liquid-crystalline phase transition temperature (58).

Leon and Panos (93), in their study of the effect of exogenous fatty acid supplementation on the growth, osmotic fragility, membrane lipid composition, and physical properties of *M. pneumoniae*, carried out ESR studies on isolated membranes by using both 5- and 12-doxylstearic acid probes. Not surprisingly, the orientational order revealed by both molecules when intercalated into the membrane decreased with increasing temperature and increased with the saturated/unsaturated ratio of the membrane lipid fatty acids. Also, at all temperatures, order was higher at the 5 position than at the 12 position, as expected, since a gradient of decreasing orientational order and increasing motional rates has been observed in many previous ESR studies of model and biological membranes (80, 112).

Rottem et al. (157), using an intercalated 5-doxylstearic probe, studied the relative fluidities of isolated membranes of *M. mycoides* subsp. *capri* containing high and low levels of exogenous cholesterol. In both membranes, the motional rates of the nitroxide fatty acid probe increase with temperature, as expected. However, in the high-cholesterol membranes, this increase follows a smooth if slightly curvilinear form, whereas in the low-cholesterol membranes, a definite

change in slope is noted at about 20°C, with the slope being greater at the lower temperatures. Since, as discussed earlier, a cooperative gel/liquid-crystalline lipid centered at about 25°C is detected by DSC only in the case of the cholesterol-poor membranes, the change in the temperature dependence of the ESR motional rate presumably occurs at the lower boundary of that phase transition. In the liquid-crystalline state, motional rates decrease slightly even though the saturated/unsaturated fatty acid ratio of the membrane lipids is elevated, indicating that cholesterol decreases the motional freedom of the hydrocarbon chains in fluid bilayers. However, below the calorimetrically determined phase transition temperature, cholesterol increases motional rates, indicating that it fluidizes gel state bilayers. These results are in accord with those of the NMR and ESR studies of the effect of cholesterol on *A. laidlawii* and *M. capricolum* membranes reviewed earlier.

FT-IR Spectroscopy

Casal et al. (27, 28, 31) have used FT-IR spectroscopy to investigate lipid organization and dynamics in *A. laidlawii* membranes. This atomic vibrational spectroscopic technique yields information on the conformation and on the rates and amplitudes of translational and rotational motion of the lipid hydrocarbon chains on a very short time scale (29). Some information about membrane protein conformation can also be obtained by using this technique (192).

Casal et al. (28, 31) initially studied isolated membranes from *A. laidlawii* cells biosynthetically enriched in fully perdeuterated palmitic acid and compared their behavior with that of aqueous dispersions of the total membrane lipids. The temperature dependence of the frequency shift of the symmetric and antisymmetric CD_2 stretching modes, which provide information about the distribution of *trans* and *gauche* conformers in the hydrocarbon chain, and the half-bandwidth of the CD_2 stretching mode, which is related primarily to the rates and amplitudes of motion of the chain, were measured in both systems. The former parameter is primarily a measure of orientational order, and the second parameter is primarily a measure of motion; together, they should provide a reasonable description of membrane lipid fluidity. Both in the isolated membranes and in the aqueous lipid dispersions, a broad, ramplike transition is detected over the temperature range of 15 to 40°C, as expected from earlier physical studies of palmitate-enriched membranes. However, by FT-IR spectroscopy, this transition is shown to occur in two overlapping stages. In the lower temperature range, the principal change is an increase in the rates and amplitudes of hydrocarbon chain motion without a concomitant increase in the number of *gauche* conformers, which are essentially absent in the gel state. In the upper portion of the phase transition, only a small additional increase in chain motion is observed, but a large increase in the *gauche/trans* conformer ratio occurs. Thus, the broad lipid phase transition in the membranes and in the isolated lipids appears to proceed in two stages, the first consisting primarily of a reduction in the packing density and rigidity of the lipid matrix and the second consisting primarily of the actual melting of the hydro-carbon chains. This broad, two-stage phase transition may in fact actually be due to partially overlapping gel/gel and gel/liquid-crystalline lipid phase transitions, as discussed earlier (176).

A comparison of the isolated membrane with the membrane lipid dispersion reveals that the presence of membrane protein had only a minor effect on the lipid phase transition. The membrane proteins produce a slight decrease in the rate of acyl chain motion in the liquid-crystalline state, which could be interpreted as a decrease in membrane lipid fluidity. On the other hand, the membrane proteins also increase the population of *gauche* conformers in both the gel and liquid-crystalline lipid phases, which could be interpreted as a decrease in orientational order and thus as an increase in fluidity. It thus appears that lipid hydrocarbon chain mobility and orientational order do not always vary in parallel, and one must carefully define the term "membrane lipid fluidity" if confusion is to be avoided. Incidentally, the protein amide band patterns reveal that the membrane proteins are predominantly in the α-helical conformation with some random coil structure also being present, but little or no β structure is observed.

The results of a later FT-IR spectroscopic study by Cameron et al. (26) of live *A. laidlawii* cells do not appear to be completely in accord with the studies of Casal and coworkers just described. In particular, the later study found that the onset of the formation of *gauche* conformers in the membrane lipid hydrocarbon chains with heating preceded the increase in the motional rates and amplitudes of these chains, a result opposite that reported by Casal et al. (28). Although in principle this difference could be due to intrinsic differences between the isolated membranes used in the former study and the live cells used in the latter study, it is difficult to rationalize this qualitative difference on these grounds alone. In my view, the results reported by Cameron et al. appear to be less reasonable, since it is difficult to see how even a partial chain melting could be accomplished without an increase in the motion of the lipid hydrocarbon chains.

Casal et al. (27) also studied the phase transition behavior in *A. laidlawii* membranes made nearly homogeneous in fully perdeuterated pentadecanoic acid. Except for the expected increase in the sharpness of the gel/liquid-crystalline lipid phase transition, the results obtained were generally similar to those already reported for the palmitate-enriched membrane and membrane lipid dispersion. However, in contrast to the earlier study, the mobility and the orientational disorder were both reported to be slightly greater in the isolated membranes than in the membrane lipid dispersions above the phase transition temperature, whereas the presence of membrane proteins appeared to decrease the rate and amplitude of hydrocarbon chain motion in the liquid-crystalline phase in their earlier study. The reason for this difference in results is not clear.

Cameron et al. (25, 26) have investigated both "live" *A. laidlawii* cells and isolated membranes by FT-IR spectroscopy. Although in general the lipid phase transition behaviors of these two systems are similar, the gel/liquid-crystalline phase transition, and in particular the rise in the *gauche/trans* conformer ratio, occurs at a lower temperature in the live cells than in the isolated membranes, so that at a comparable temperature within the phase transition boundaries, the proportion of fluid lipid is always higher in the live cells than in isolated membranes. Thus, it appears that the process of membrane isolation may alter somewhat the properties of the lipid phase transition. However, the comparative DSC studies of the thermotropic phase behavior of viable *A. laidlawii* cells and of isolated membranes discussed earlier did not reveal any detectable differences between the two systems. Whether this discrepancy in results is due to the different physical techniques used in these studies or to different methods of membrane isolation remains to be determined.

Mantsch et al. (111) recently reinvestigated the differences in the gel/liquid-crystalline lipid phase transition in intact cells and isolated membranes of *A. laidlawii* by FT-IR spectroscopy, using a wider variety of exogenous fatty acids and growth conditions than were used in the previous studies from this laboratory. Although these workers confirm that the midpoint temperature of the lipid chain-melting phase transition as monitored by this technique is indeed always lower in cells than in membranes, the difference in midpoint temperature was found to decrease as the chain length of the incorporated fatty acid decreases or as the degree of unsaturation increases. As well, the difference in phase transition temperature midpoints between the two systems seems to depend on the method of isolation and treatment of the membranes. Membranes prepared by the mechanical fracture of cells in a French press show a smaller elevation of the midpoint phase transition temperature than do those prepared by osmotic lysis. Moreover, aqueous dispersions of the total membrane lipids exhibit an even more pronounced increase in transition midpoint temperature than do either of the isolated membrane preparations.

Some insight into the molecular basis of this phenomenon may be provided by the data presented by this group on the effect of temperature on the lipid gel/liquid-crystalline phase transition in (initially at least) intact cells. Simply storing cells at −20°C for 1 week was itself found to increase the phase transition midpoint temperature slightly. Also, incubation of cells for 60°C for 1 or 18 h results in progressively larger elevations in transition temperature. The former result is compatible with the suggestion of Seguin et al. (176), based on their DSC studies, that low-temperature incubation may elevate the T_m by inducing the formation of higher-melting-point subgel-like lipid domains in *A. laidlawii* cells but especially in the membranes and isolated lipid dispersions, thus producing differences in their phase transition temperatures. The latter result, and the comparative studies of the lipid thermotropic phase behavior of the total membrane lipids to membranes and cells, suggest that the presence of membrane protein, especially in its undenatured form, tends to lower the phase transition midpoint temperature. This interpretation is partially compatible with the DSC results of Seguin et al., in that the phase transition temperature of aqueous dispersions of the total membrane lipids was found to be slightly higher than in cells or membranes (176).

However, the DSC results for intact cells and isolated membranes were identical (176).

Mantsch and coworkers (111) also studied membrane protein conformation and thermal denaturation in intact cells and isolated membranes by FT-IR spectroscopy, utilizing the conformationally sensitive amide-I and amide-II bands of the polypeptide chain (192). At the optimal growth temperature of 37°C, both membrane and total cellular proteins were found to be predominantly in the α-helical conformation, but with a substantial amount of β-sheet and random coil structures also being present. The finding of a relatively high α-helical content and some random structure in the *A. laidlawii* membrane proteins was also made in an earlier study from this laboratory (28); however, the earlier study indicated little or no β structure to be present. Only small changes in protein conformation were noted over the physiological temperature range, including that over which the membrane lipid gel/liquid-crystalline phase transition occurred. However, for both cells and membranes, major changes in protein conformation occur over the temperature range 40 to >75°C, presumably corresponding to the thermal denaturation of these proteins detected in the earlier DSC studies already discussed.

The accessibility of membrane proteins to water was also probed in this study by replacing H_2O with D_2O and monitoring the exchange of NH to ND by the change in frequency of the amide-I and amide-II bands. At room temperature, no more than 25% of the amide protons could be exchanged, indicating that most peptide bonds are buried in hydrophobic domains, either in the globular portions of proteins on the bilayer surface or in transmembrane α helices. At temperatures between 40 and 50°C, NH-to-ND exchange begins to increase markedly, but only above 90°C does the NH band become negligible. These results confirm that the thermal denaturation of the membrane proteins does indeed involve an unfolding of the polypeptide chain and an exposure of hydrophobic regions of that chain to water (192).

Fluorescence Spectroscopy

Several different fluorescence spectroscopic techniques have been applied to *A. laidlawii* cells or membranes. Metcalfe et al. (130) carried out a study of native and detergent-reaggregated membranes by using the probe 1-anilinonaphthalene-8-sulfonic acid (ANS), whose fluorescence intensity varies with the polarity of its environment. In both membrane systems, the fluorescence intensities of the lipid-associated ANS molecules are similar, whereas those of the protein-associated ANS molecules differ significantly. These workers concluded that the lipid bilayer is a major structural feature in both native and detergent-reaggregated membranes, that the organizations of the membrane proteins differ in the two systems, and that lipid bilayer organization is relatively insensitive to the presence or to the conformational state of the membrane proteins. However, as the exact locations of the probe molecules were not determined and because ANS fluorescence can vary with factors other than polarity, little quantitative molecular information can be derived from this study.

Haberer et al. (68) studied the effect of mycoplasma virus L3 adsorption and capping on membrane structure in intact *A. laidlawii* cells by using the excimer fluorescene technique. In this method, small amounts of the probe pyrene lecithin are intercalated into the cell membrane and the fluorescence intensities of monomers and dimers, which fluoresce at different wavelengths, are measured. From this ratio, the association constant of probe molecules can be determined, and since the association constant is dependent on the lateral mobility of the pyrene lecithin molecules in the plane of the membrane, it is also a measure of the fluidity of the membrane lipid bilayer. These workers observe a decrease in dimer formation upon virus association, which could result either from a rigidification of the hydrophobic core of the lipid bilayer or from an increase in the area of the membrane lipid in which the probe is free to diffuse. Because DPH fluorescence polarization spectroscopic measurements indicate no change in membrane lipid bilayer viscosity upon virus binding, these authors favor the latter interpretation. Their view is that the capping or aggregation of some of the membrane proteins induced by virus binding, which was observed by freeze-fracture electron microscopy, decreases the amount of lipid interacting with the membrane protein, and that this in turn permits additional numbers of lipid molecules to interact with the fluorescent probe, in effect decreasing dimer formation by an effective decrease in probe concentration in the bulk lipid phase. This result implies that mycoplasma virus L3 binds to proteins on the surface of the cell membrane rather than inserting into the lipid bilayer.

Finally, as discussed earlier, Macdonald and Cossins (99) used DPH fluorescence polarization spectroscopy, in conjunction with optical transmission and DSC, to demonstrate that pressure increases and alcohol decreases the gel/liquid-crystalline phase transition temperature of the lipids of isolated *A. laidlawii* membranes.

The technique of DPH fluorescence polarization spectroscopy (179) has also been applied in a number of studies of the role of cholesterol or other sterols in the membranes of several *Mycoplasma* species. The first application of this technique was that of Rottem et al. (157), who investigated lipid bilayer organization in isolated membranes of *M. mycoides* subsp. *capri* containing high or low levels of cholesterol. In cholesterol-enriched membranes, Arrhenius plots of lipid microviscosity (actually primarily lipid orientational order rather than motional rates) are linear over the temperature range of 10 to 45°C with an apparent activation energy of 4.5 kcal/mol. In contrast, in cholesterol-poor membranes, the Arrhenius plots are biphasic linear with a break at about 24°C, very near the calorimetrically determined lipid phase transition midpoint. Above 24°C, the apparent activation energy for probe movement is 3.7 kcal/mol, and below 24°C, it is 10.5 kcal/mol. As well, lipid orientational order in the cholesterol-poor membranes is higher at lower temperatures and lower at higher temperatures than in cholesterol-rich membranes. These authors conclude that the incorporation of high levels of cholesterol into the *M. mycoides* subsp. *capri* membranes abolishes a cooperative gel/liquid-crystalline phase transition by increasing order in the liquid-crystalline phase and decreasing it in the gel phase of the lipid bilayer, thus producing a state of intermediate fluidity. This interpretation is in accord with that of a number of other studies of the role of cholesterol in model and biological membranes (58).

Dahl and coworkers (46) utilized DPH fluorescence polarization spectroscopy to study the effect of alkyl-substituted precursors of cholesterol on the organization of model membranes and on the growth and membrane organization of *M. capricolum*. In both the model and *M. capricolum* membranes, the effectiveness of various sterols in ordering the lipid bilayer above its phase transition temperatures increases in the order lanosterol < 4,4-dimethyl cholestanol ≤ 4β-methyl cholestanol < 4α-methyl cholestanol < cholestanol < cholesterol. Significantly, this is also the order of the effectiveness of these sterols in promoting the growth of this sterol auxotrophic organism and the order in which these compounds are formed in the cholesterol biosynthetic pathway. These authors conclude that the sequential biosynthetic removal of the three methyl groups from the lanosterol ring nucleus and the introduction of a double bond into ring B serve to improve the membrane function of the sterol molecule. The removal of the 14-methyl group, and to a lesser extent the 4β-methyl group, is particularly important in this regard, as their presence decreases the planarity of the α and β faces of the sterol ring nucleus and increases the bulk of the sterol molecule, which in turn disrupts the interactions between the sterol ring nucleus and the fatty acyl chains of adjacent membrane glycerolipid molecules.

Dahl et al. (50) subsequently studied the growth characteristics and membrane lipid organization of *M. capricolum* cultured on cholesterol and lanosterol, again using DPH fluorescence polarization spectroscopy. They found that progressive increases in the cholesterol content, but not in the lanosterol content, of the membrane results in a progressive increase in microviscosity (orientational order) when measured at 37°C, the optimal growth temperature of this organism. Moreover, in cholesterol-rich membranes, Arrhenius plots of microviscosity are linear whereas those from lanosterol-rich membranes exhibit pronounced discontinuities in slope at 20 and 25°C. Moreover, the microviscosities are considerably higher in cholesterol-containing than in lanosterol-containing membranes, especially at higher temperatures. In fact, the microviscosity values of lanosterol-enriched membranes and cholesterol-poor membranes are quite similar. These workers conclude that only cholesterol is able to completely abolish the cooperative gel/liquid-crystalline lipid phase transition in *M. capricolum* membranes and to order the fluid lipid bilayer at the growth temperature.

Dahl et al. (50) also found in this study that the provision of exogenous cholesterol allowed *M. capricolum* cells to grow on media containing a wider variety of exogenous fatty acids than did lanosterol, a finding compatible with the greater effectiveness of cholesterol in regulating membrane lipid fluidity. An unexpected finding, however, was that low levels of cholesterol, which on their own are unable to support cell growth, are able to support good growth when high levels of lanosterol are also present, despite the fact that the microviscosity values of the membrane lipid

remain low in these circumstances. These workers suggest that lanosterol may fulfill one of the more primitive functions of sterols in membranes, namely, to separate polar lipid headgroups and decrease surface charge density, even though it cannot effectively regulate the fluidity of the lipid hydrocarbon chains. Alternatively, small amounts of cholesterol were suggested to serve other, more specialized cellular functions (47–49), a suggestion later confirmed by subsequent studies from this laboratory (reviewed in chapter 15).

Lala et al. (87) investigated the role of the free sterol hydroxyl group of cholesterol on cell growth and membrane lipid organization of *M. capricolum*, again using DPH fluorescence polarization spectroscopy. They found that cholesterol methyl ether or cholesterol acetate is relatively effective at supporting the growth of this organism, although not as effective as cholesterol itself. However, the microviscosity values at 25°C of all three membranes were reported to be essentially identical, indicating that a free hydroxyl group at C-3 of the cholesterol molecule is not required for ordering the lipid bilayer in the membrane of this organism. In model membrane systems, however, it has been reported that the free hydroxyl group is required to produce the maximum reduction in phospholipid cross-sectional area and passive permeability associated with cholesterol incorporation (58).

Le Grimellec et al. (90) studied the effect of variations in membrane lipid fatty acid composition and cholesterol content on lipid orientational order in *M. gallisepticum* by using DPH fluorescence polarization. In isolated membranes containing high amounts of cholesterol, increasing the chain length of the exogenous saturated fatty acid present in the growth medium increases the apparent lipid order parameter almost imperceptibly, while replacing stearic acid with oleic acid decreases order slightly. In all cases, orientational order decreases almost linearly with temperature, with no abrupt changes in slope. In cholesterol-poor membranes, changes in fatty acid composition produce larger changes in lipid orientational order, and plots of orientational order versus temperature exhibit abrupt changes in slope at temperatures of 28, 25, and 23°C for cells enriched in palmitate, palmitate and oleate, and oleate, respectively. Although these changes in slopes were interpreted as membrane lipid gel/liquid-crystalline phase transitions, it seems highly unlikely that cells containing relatively high levels of oleic acid would melt above 0°C. At low temperatures, low-cholesterol membranes exhibit a higher lipid ordering, and at high temperatures, a lower degree of lipid ordering, than do high-cholesterol membranes. These results confirm earlier findings in other organisms that cholesterol modulates the effect of lipid fatty acid composition variations on membrane fluidity by disordering gel and ordering liquid-crystalline lipid domains so as to produce a state of intermediate fluidity (58). Interestingly, the lipid order parameter values obtained for the *M. gallisepticum* membranes are about twice as high as those obtained for *M. mycoides* subsp. *capri* membranes grown under similar conditions (157). This higher degree of ordering of the DPH probe may be due to the presence of larger amounts of protein in the *M. gallisepticum* membrane, since the presence of integral, transmembrane proteins has been shown to decrease the degree of wobble (increase the degree of order) of the rigid DPH molecule in model and other biological membranes (179). Rottem and Verkleij (164), however, report that the apparent microviscosity (actually orientational order) of *M. gallisepticum* membranes is actually slightly lower than in aqueous dispersions of the membrane lipids over the physiological temperature range, a finding at odds with DPH fluorescence polarization studies in other membrane systems. Clearly, additional experimental work is required to resolve these apparently contradictory results. However, since other spectroscopic techniques indicate that the integral, transmembrane membrane proteins disorder the flexible hydrocarbon chains of adjacent membrane lipids in model membrane systems, the results of Le Grimellec et al. (90), even if valid, do not necessarily mean that the lipid molecules themselves are more ordered in *M. gallisepticum* membranes.

Rottem (156) used the DPH fluorescence polarization technique to compare lipid microviscosity (orientational order) in dispersions of the total membrane lipids from *M. arginini*, both with their normal high levels of cholesterol and when the cholesterol had been removed chromatographically. When cholesterol is present, Arrhenius plots of microviscosity are linear over the physiological temperature range and lipid microviscosity is relatively high. When cholesterol is absent, similar Arrhenius plots show changes in slope at 35 and 40°C and lipid microviscosity values are lower, particularly at higher temperatures. The breaks in the Arrhenius plot of the cholesterol-free lipid dispersion correspond to the lower region of the gel/liquid-crystalline phase transition detected by DSC only in the cholesterol-free dispersions. These results support the earlier findings that high levels of cholesterol abolish the cooperative chain-melting transition of the membrane lipids and increase order in the liquid-crystalline state. However, in this study cholesterol appears to increase order in the gel state as well, a result at odds with previous work on mycoplasma and model membranes (58).

The results of the fluorescence polarization and ESR spectroscopic studies of Le Grimellec et al. (91) of the effects of energization on membrane organization in *M. mycoides* subsp. *capri* and *M. capricolum* were discussed earlier. Briefly, these workers found that cellular energization resulting from the addition of glucose to resting cells did not alter membrane lipid order or dynamics in a significant way, although it did affect the conformation of at least some membrane proteins.

Other Physical Techniques

Abramson and Pisetsky (1) used light-scattering measurements to study the phase behavior of isolated *A. laidlawii* membranes and of aqueous dispersions of the total membrane lipids. As the temperature increases, the turbidity values of palmitate- and stearate-enriched membranes and lipid dispersions exhibit a decrease with temperature, which correlates reasonably well with the gel/liquid-crystalline phase transition detected by calorimetry and other techniques. Oleate-enriched membranes, which do not undergo a phase transition within the physiological temperature range, exhibit a relatively constant de-

gree of light scattering over the temperature range of 10 to 45°C. These authors suggested that this technique may be a convenient and relatively sensitive method to measure phase transitions in biological membranes. Indeed, Macdonald and Cossins (99) used this technique (along with DSC and DPH fluorescence polarization) in their studies of the effects of pressure and alcohols on the lipid phase transition in *A. laidlawii* membranes (discussed earlier). A major disadvantage of thermal-turbidimetric studies, however, is that they provide no direct thermodynamic or structural information about the phenomenon which is monitored.

REGULATION OF LIPID FLUIDITY AND PHASE STATE

A consideration of the regulation of membrane lipid fluidity and phase state, by appropriate alterations in membrane lipid fatty acid and polar headgroup composition or cholesterol or carotenoid content, might seem more appropriate for chapter 14. However, we currently know very little about the biochemical mechanisms for the regulation of the uptake of exogenous fatty acids and cholesterol or of membrane lipid biosynthesis in general in this group of organisms. In contrast, we know a considerable amount about the biophysical aspects of membrane lipid compositional regulation. This topic will thus be reviewed here.

Various workers have proposed that *A. laidlawii* and, to a lesser extent, several *Mycoplasma* species are capable of regulating in a coherent way the fluidity and phase state of their membrane lipids by altering their fatty acid compositions or by altering the cholesterol or carotenoid content of the plasma membrane. Other groups have proposed that *A. laidlawii* maintains an optimal lipid bilayer stability by coherently regulating the membrane lipid polar headgroup distribution in response to changes in fatty acid composition, cholesterol incorporation, and growth temperature. Evidence for and against these proposals will be discussed in the following three sections.

Regulation of Lipid Fatty Acid Composition

Melchior and Steim (125) studied the temperature dependence of the relative biosynthetic incorporation of palmitate and oleate into the membrane lipids of *A. laidlawii* B as a function of the physical state of the membrane lipids. Late-log-phase cells, grown with either exogenous palmitate or oleate or without fatty acid supplementation, were incubated for 7.5 min (about 0.1 generation or less) at various temperatures in growth medium containing [^{14}C]palmitate and [^{3}H]oleate, and the incorporation of radioactivity into the total membrane polar lipid fraction was monitored. The ratio of palmitate to oleate incorporated was found to be independent of incubation temperature in unsupplemented and palmitate-enriched membranes below the calorimetrically determined phase transition lower boundaries (about 15 and 20°C, respectively). However, this ratio was found to increase dramatically over the temperature range encompassing most of the gel/liquid-crystalline phase transition (20 to 37°C) (higher temperatures were not examined).

A similar increase in palmitate/oleate ratio over the temperature range of 20 to 40°C was observed when these radioactive fatty acids were simply incubated with aqueous dispersions of the total membrane lipids. Moreover, a sharp increase in the palmitate/oleate binding ratio was also observed to accompany the phase transition of an aqueous dispersion of 25% egg PC and 75% dipalmitoylphosphatidylcholine. These workers thus suggested that the selective binding of palmitic acid by lipid bilayers, which accompanies the gel/liquid-crystalline phase transition, may provide a means of regulating the fatty acid composition of the membrane lipids, by increasing the biosynthetic incorporation of palmitic acid relative to oleic acid without the need to invoke an enzymatic mechanism.

A careful examination of the data presented by Melchior and Steim (125) indicates that the real situation may be more complex than their conclusions would imply. For example, cells grown in the presence of exogenous oleic acid exhibit only a slight increase in their palmitate/oleate ratio over the temperature range of 0 to 10°C but show a more marked increase in this ratio at higher temperatures. Since the gel/liquid-crystalline phase transition in oleate-enriched membranes occurs over the temperature range of −20 to +20°C, it appears that a phase transition need not be accompanied by an abrupt increase in the palmitate/oleate ratio and also that this ratio can increase substantially (albeit less abruptly) over a temperature range during which no phase change occurs. Moreover, the total increase in the palmitate/oleate ratio of the oleic acid-supplemented cells taken over the entire 0 to 37°C temperature range is almost comparable to that observed in the palmitate-supplemented and unsupplemented cells. Finally, one should remember that oleate-supplemented cells are capable of normal growth over the temperature range of 8 to 40°C, whereas fatty acid-unsupplemented and palmitate-supplemented cells exhibit impaired growth below 25 and 30°C, respectively, and cannot grow at all at temperatures below 18 and 22°C (see chapter 15). It is thus quite possible that the variable temperature dependencies of palmitate incorporation, which are the major determinants of the palmitate/oleate ratio, may at least in part simply reflect the different temperature dependencies of growth rates, and thus also rates of membrane lipid biosynthesis, characteristic of cells grown in the presence of these different fatty acids. In fact, the rate-temperature profiles for palmitate incorporation observed in the study of Melchior and Steim parallel very closely the rate-temperature profiles previously reported by McElhaney (114, 115) for the growth of A. laidlawii B cells of similar fatty acid composition.

Perhaps the best evidence that the physical state of the membrane lipids does not determine the specificity of fatty acid incorporation, in A. laidlawii B at least, comes from studies of the fatty acid composition of cells grown in the presence of a variety of fatty acids at a variety of temperatures. In these long-term studies, the equilibrium levels of biosynthetically incorporated fatty acids, rather than the short-term kinetics of the incorporation of radiolabeled fatty acids, were determined. In all cases, the levels of biosynthetic incorporation of single exogenous fatty acids, or of pairs of exogenous acids, do not vary significantly with growth temperature (114, 115, 166). Moreover, a number of studies have shown that the average chain length of the de novo-biosynthesized saturated fatty acids produced by this organism is temperature invariant (115, 167, 183), as is the output spectrum from the exogenous fatty acid chain elongation system also present in this organism (168). Moreover, the incorporation of cholesterol does not alter endogenous or exogenous fatty acid spectra in this strain (121, 122). It is clear, therefore, that A. laidlawii B completely lacks the ability to regulate the fluidity and physical state of its membrane lipids through temperature-induced alterations in fatty acid composition, either by enzymatic or by other means. It is, in fact, precisely the lack of such regulatory ability which permits the wide variations in fatty acid composition, and thus in membrane lipid fluidity and phase state, that makes this organism such an ideal one for studying membrane structural-functional correlates. The absence of a temperature-dependent "homeoviscous" (185) or "homeophasic" (181) adaptation mechanism in this animal mycoplasma is perhaps not too surprising, since this organism is not usually exposed to significant temperature variations in its homeothermic host.

There have been several reports that A. laidlawii B cells grown at lower temperatures have somewhat lower membrane lipid phase transition temperatures or higher degrees of fluidity than do cells grown at higher temperatures under the same conditions (for example, see reference 111). These results would seem to imply that this organism does possess at least some ability to regulate de novo fatty acid biosynthesis and/or exogenous fatty acid incorporation in response to environmental temperature. Two points should be noted, however. The first is that the observed changes in phase transition temperature are in all cases much less than the changes in growth temperature, so that full compensation for the thermal shift is not obtained. The second point relates to the fact that A. laidlawii cells grown at suboptimal temperatures grow more slowly than do those grown at 37°C (114, 115). Thus, cultures grown at a lower temperature for the same period of time as those grown at a higher temperature will be in an earlier stage of growth. Since the fatty acid composition of the membrane lipids of this organism changes with the stage of growth, with these changes generally favoring an increase in the higher-melting-point fatty acids with age, great care is necessary in controlling for the effect of growth stage when growth temperature is varied. Thus, the results discussed above could be due, in part at least, to an effect of culture age rather than to a true homeoviscous or homeophasic regulatory mechanism.

Other strains of A. laidlawii may be able to regulate to some degree their fatty acid compositions by altering the amount of exogenous fatty acid taken up from the growth medium. Thus, Rottem et al. (158) have reported that the oral strain of A. laidlawii biosynthetically incorporates larger amounts of exogenous unsaturated fatty acids when grown at lower temperatures and that membranes derived from these cells are slightly more fluid at 37°C, as determined by ESR spectroscopy. However, Huang et al. (71) found no significant changes in membrane lipid fatty acid composition in oleate-supplemented cells of this same strain when grown at different temperatures, although cells enriched in oleate or other fatty acids and grown at lower temperatures did exhibit a slightly lower fluidity at all temperatures, as measured by ESR spectroscopy. Christiansson and Wieslander (35) have reported that a temperature shift-down in *A. laidlawii* A results in an increased incorporation of unsaturated fatty acids into all of the membrane lipids except DGDG. However, Christiansson et al. (34) reported that growth in the presence of the anesthetics tetracaine and diethyl ether does not alter membrane lipid fatty acid composition in this strain, suggesting that a mechanism for actually sensing the fluidity of the membrane lipids is absent in this organism. In most cases, moreover, the magnitude of the fatty acid compositional change, when observed, was not of sufficient magnitude to maintain the fluidity or phase of the membrane lipids constant when the growth temperature was lowered from 37°C, so that membrane lipid fluidity still decreased and in some cases the proportion of gel-state lipid still increased somewhat at the reduced growth temperatures studied (71, 158). Thus, if a mechanism capable of regulating membrane lipid fluidity and phase state does exist in some *A. laidlawii* strains, it does not seem capable of maintaining either variable constant in the face of changing temperature.

Regulation of Cholesterol and Carotenoid Content

As discussed above, several studies have shown that *A. laidlawii* B does not alter the fatty acid composition of its membrane lipids in response to changes in growth temperature or cholesterol content, implying the absence of a homeoviscous or homeophasic regulatory mechanism in this organism. Further support for this view has come from the work of Koblin and Wang (86), who grew *A. laidlawii* B cells in cholesterol-containing medium with and without the anesthetics halothane and cyclopropane. These workers found that continuous exposure of this organism to these lipid bilayer-fluidizing agents does not alter the membrane lipid fatty acid composition, either when cells are cultured without fatty acid supplementation or when they are cultured in the presence of several exogenous fatty acids. However, cells grown in the presence of halothane or cyclopropane incorporate significantly higher levels of cholesterol into their membranes than do cells grown in the absence of anesthetic. Moreover, membranes from halothane-exposed cells are more ordered at 37°C (in the absence of anesthetic) than are the membranes of cells not exposed to anesthetic, as determined by ESR spectroscopy using an intercalated 5-nitroxide stearic acid probe. These results suggest that *A. laidlawii* B may be able to alter its degree of cholesterol incorporation in a coherent manner in order to maintain an approximately constant degree of membrane lipid fluidity or order.

There is, however, a disturbing feature about the study of Koblin and Wang just summarized. The amounts of cholesterol incorporated into the membrane appear to be much different, even in cells grown in the absence of anesthetic, than have been reported previously for *A. laidlawii* B. Thus, cholesterol/protein weight ratios ranging from about 37 to 92 µg/mg are reported by these authors for isolated membranes, but

cholesterol/phospholipid molar ratios were reported to range from about 1.0 to 2.3. Several earlier studies also showed maximum levels of cholesterol incorporation of about 0.1 mg cholesterol per mg of membrane protein but cholesterol/phospholipid molar ratios of only 0.3 for this organism (145). There is clearly a problem with the experiments of Koblin and Wang, either in terms of the chemical quantitation of lipid and protein or with the nonspecific absorption of cholesterol to the isolated plasma membranes, or both. Until this problem is resolved, the conclusion that *A. laidlawii* B can regulate its degree of cholesterol incorporation in response to alterations in membrane lipid fluidity must be considered tentative.

Razin and coworkers (142, 146) have demonstrated, however, that both the rate and extent of cholesterol uptake into the *A. laidlawii* (oral strain) membrane does depend markedly on the phase state of the membrane lipids. The transfer of elaidate-enriched cells grown at 37 to 4°C virtually abolishes exogenous cholesterol incorporation, while cholesterol uptake continues, although at a slower rate and to a lesser extent, in oleate-enriched cells subjected to a similar temperature shift-down. Since elaidate-enriched membranes exist almost exclusively in the gel state at 4°C while oleate-enriched membranes are largely in the liquid-crystalline state at this temperature, it was concluded that a fluid lipid bilayer is necessary for effective cholesterol incorporation. The physiological significance of this observation is not clear, however, since growth of this organism is inhibited when more than about one-half of the membrane lipid exists in the gel state, and it ceases entirely when the proportion of fluid lipid falls to about 10% (see chapter 15). The effect of variations in membrane lipid fluidity, within the liquid-crystalline state, on the rate and extent of cholesterol uptake was not rigorously investigated.

The ESR results of Huang and Haug (69) and of Rottem and Markowitz (159) discussed earlier indicate that the presence of carotenoids can rigidify the lipid bilayer of the *A. laidlawii* membrane. It is not clear, however, that carotenoid levels are regulated in a coherent manner by this organism so as to maintain an optimal degree of membrane lipid fluidity. This would seem unlikely to be the case, in strain B at least, since carotenoid levels are quite low and the removal of carotenoids from an aqueous dispersion of the total membrane lipids has no detectable influence on the gel/liquid-crystalline phase transition as monitored by DTA (180). Certainly carotenoid content modulation cannot perform an essential regulatory function, since *A. laidlawii* appears to be capable of normal growth in the absence of carotenoid biosynthesis (35, 147, 160).

Regulation of Lipid Polar Headgroup Composition

Lindblom, Rilfors, and Wieslander demonstrated nearly a decade ago that *A. laidlawii* A is able to regulate the polar headgroup composition of its membrane lipids in a coherent manner in response to changes in environmental temperature, fatty acid composition, or cholesterol content, so as to maintain the stability of its lipid bilayer within certain limits (see reference 150 for a review). These investigators have now shown that *A. laidlawii* also possesses a mechanism for regulating the surface potential of the membrane lipid bilayer by altering the proportion of charged and uncharged lipid polar headgroups synthesized in response to changes in membrane lipid fatty acid composition and the ionic strength of the growth medium. Interestingly, studies by McElhaney and coworkers on the closely related B strain revealed significant differences in lipid polar headgroup regulation in comparison with strain A (118, 120). The work from both laboratories is reviewed below.

Regulation of membrane lipid polymorphic phase behavior

The phase preference of different membrane lipids can be related to the overall shape of the lipid molecules under various environmental conditions. The molecular shape is in turn dependent on the relative effective sizes of the polar and nonpolar regions of the rodlike amphiphilic lipid molecules, in particular on the relative cross-sectional area occupied by the polar headgroup and nonpolar hydrocarbon chains. The effective cross-sectional area of the polar headgroup depends on its charge and degree of hydration as well as on its intrinsic bulkiness and is only modestly affected by changes in temperature. The effective cross-sectional area of the apolar region of the lipid molecule depends on the volume occupied by the hydrocarbon chains, which in turn depends on their length and degree of unsaturation. In the case of the nonpolar region of the lipid molecule, temperature is an important variable, since the effective volume occupied by the hydrocarbon chains increases more markedly with temperature, particularly when a change in temperature induces a gel/liquid-crystalline phase transition.

If the effective cross-sectional area occupied by the polar headgroup significantly exceeds that occupied by the nonpolar region of the lipid molecule, as is the case for lysophospholipids above their phase transition temperature, then these wedge-shaped molecules aggregate in water to form spherical or elliptical micelles. If the relative areas occupied by the polar headgroup and the hydrocarbon chains are roughly equal, then these cylindrically shaped molecules form lamellar phases. This is the phase formed, for example, by PC and most other diacylglycerolipids. Finally, if the relative cross-sectional area of the polar headgroup is less than that of the hydrocarbon chains, as is the case for some PEs, for example, then these inverted wedge-shaped molecules may aggregate in water to form a reversed hexagonal phase. It should be noted that cholesterol molecules also have an inverted wedge shape, since the area occupied by the small polar headgroup is much less than that occupied by the steroid ring system. The relationship between molecular shape and lipid phase structure is illustrated schematically in Fig. 1. For a more detailed discussion of this relationship, the reader is referred to excellent reviews by Rilfors et al. (150) and Gruner et al. (66).

In an extensive series of papers, the laboratories of Lindblom, Rilfors, and Wieslander (34–36, 200–202) have demonstrated that changes in growth temperature, fatty acid composition, and cholesterol content can induce substantial variations in the quantitative distribution of the polar lipids of the plasma membrane of *A. laidlawii* A. In certain circumstances, in fact, variations in fatty acid composition can even induce the formation of small amounts of new polar lipid species in this organism (202) and in the closely related *A. laidlawii* B (14). The most important alteration ob-

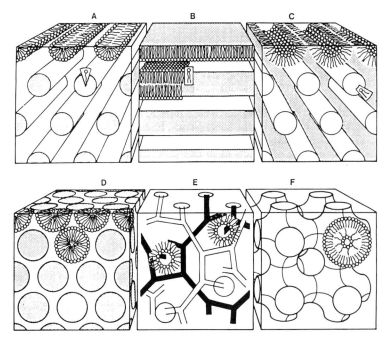

Figure 1. Structure of different liquid-crystalline phases of membrane lipids. (A) Normal hexagonal phase (H_1); (B) lamellar phase (L); (C) reversed hexagonal phase (H_{II}); cubic structures consisting of spherical aggregates (D), rod-shaped aggregates (E), and lamellar aggregates (F). Note the various shapes of the lipid molecules inserted in panels A to C. The hydrocarbon regions are shaded, and the hydrophilic parts are in white. (From Rilfors et al. [149].)

served, however, is generally in the ratio of the two major neutral glycolipids, MGDG and DGDG. The MGDG/DGDG ratio is found to decrease with an increase in growth temperature, with the degree of unsaturation of the membrane lipid fatty acyl chains, or with an increase in the level of exogenous cholesterol incorporation.

Wieslander et al. (204, 207) have also studied the phase structure of the various individual membrane polar lipids of the A. laidlawii A membrane by NMR spectroscopy and X-ray diffraction as well as the effect of cholesterol on the phase preferences of the neutral glycolipids (84). In contrast to all of the other membrane polar lipids, aqueous dispersion of MGDG was found to prefer the reverse hexagonal phase structure at physiological temperatures rather than the lamellar phase preferred by DGDG and the other membrane lipids, particularly if the fatty acid chains were unsaturated. In addition, mixtures of MGDG and DGDG can form either lamellar or reversed cubic phases at physiological temperatures, the formation of the cubic phase being favored by high levels of MGDG and by an increased degree of cis unsaturation in the fatty acyl chains. Moreover, the presence of cholesterol was found to increase the tendency of unsaturated MGDG/DGDG mixtures to form nonbilayer phases. MGDG presumably can form reversed phases because its small, uncharged, and poorly hydrated headgroup may occupy a smaller cross-sectional area than do its hydrocarbon chains.

To explain the changes in polar headgroup distribution observed in the A. laidlawii A membrane, Wieslander et al. have postulated that in all biological membranes, a certain mixture of bilayer-preferring and reversed hexagonal phase-preferring lipids must be maintained in order to preserve an optimal degree of stability and functionality (200, 201). Specifically for this organism, this means maintaining an optimal balance between the level of MGDG and the level of other membrane lipids, including DGDG. However, since the tendency of MGDG to form the reversed hexagonal phase depends markedly on temperature, fatty acid composition, and cholesterol content, one might expect that the MGDG/DGDG ratio would be regulated in a coherent manner in response to these variables. In particular, since a decrease in temperature or a decrease in the degree of unsaturation of the hydrocarbon chains reduces the tendency of MGDG to form a reversed hexagonal phase, favoring instead a lamellar arrangement, then the increased MGDG/DGDG ratio observed in cells growing at low temperature, or with high levels of exogenous saturated fatty acids, could be seen as an attempt by this organism to maintain the proper nonbilayer-forming tendency of its membrane lipid mixture. Similarly, the decreased MGDG/DGDG ratio observed with increasing amounts of cholesterol incorporation could be viewed in a similar way, since cholesterol increases the tendency of MGDG to form reversed, nonbilayer phases. Thus, it was proposed that A. laidlawii A cells actively avoid lipid compositions resulting in a nonlamellar arrangement of the bulk lipids, since this would destroy the integrity of the plasma membrane. On the other hand, since local regions forming nonlamellar structures may be advantageous for certain membrane functions (66, 150), the levels of MGDG were also suggested to be maintained

above a certain level. An optimal mixture of bilayer- and nonbilayer-preferring lipids is thus maintained in the face of variations in temperature, fatty acid composition, and cholesterol content by appropriate variations in the MGDG/DGDG ratio (150).

More recently, Lindblom et al. (98) have studied in more detail the phase behavior of all the individual A. laidlawii A membrane lipids, as well as several lipid mixtures, by using different NMR techniques. In this study, the phase preferences of the various membrane lipids were investigated as a function of temperature and degree of hydration as well as fatty acid composition, and phase diagrams of the various lipid-water systems were constructed. A. laidlawii A membrane lipids highly enriched in oleic acid were studied in greatest detail, but some data on lipids highly enriched in elaidic acid or containing equal amounts of palmitic and oleic acids were also presented.

The phase preference of dioleoyl MGDG varies in a complex manner with hydration and temperature. A notable feature of the dioleoyl MGDG-water system, however, is that at temperatures above about 10°C, only nonlamellar phases are formed. Moreover, in the fully hydrated state, only the reversed hexagonal phase exists at physiological temperatures, although a lamellar gel phase is formed below about −15°C. Also notable is the relatively small amount of water bound by this MGDG, about 11 water molecules per molecule of lipid. As the fatty acid composition of this glycolipid becomes more saturated, the temperature at which the reversed hexagonal phase is formed increases markedly, so that the lamellar liquid-crystalline rather than the reversed hexagonal phase exists at physiological temperatures. The maximum hydration of the MDGD also decreases considerably as the fatty acid composition becomes more saturated. It is interesting to note that the nonbilayer-forming glycolipid, MGDG, and the nonbilayer-forming phospholipid, PE, both possess small, poorly hydrated polar headgroups that interact strongly with one another, as evidenced by the relatively high gel/liquid-crystalline phase transition temperatures of their more highly saturated molecular species (66, 150).

The phase preferences of the dioleoyl species of all of the other membrane lipids were also investigated in this study. The other major glycolipid, DGDG, and the only phospholipid of the A. laidlawii membrane, PG, form only lamellar phases at all temperatures and hydrations studied, as do the minor phosphorylated glycolipids. Thus, the MGDG is the only lipid class present in the membrane of this organism that can, under certain conditions, exist as a nonlamellar form.

Lindblom et al. (98) also investigated the phase behavior of mixtures of dioleoyl MGDG and DGDG in water. They found that mixtures of these two lipids exhibit an increasing tendency to form the reversed hexagonal phase as the ratio of MGDG/DGDG increases, as the temperature increases, and as the hydration decreases. These authors emphasize the fact that at a water content of 5 mol/mol of lipid, mixtures of MGDG/DGDG in ratios above 1.0 form almost exclusively nonlamellar phases at temperatures of 0 to 50°C and that the MGDG component seems to play a dominant role in determining the overall phase structure formed by this system. It should be noted, however, that the binary glycolipid mixtures studied were highly unsaturated, were not fully hydrated, and did not contain the other bilayer preferring glyco- and phospholipids, all conditions that tend to favor the formation of cubic and reversed hexagonal phases.

Finally, the phase equilibria of the total membrane lipids from *A. laidlawii* A grown at 37°C were studied by these workers. In this case, the hydration was maintained constant at 10 mol of water per mol of lipid, but the relative amounts of palmitic and oleic acids in the membrane lipids were varied by altering the relative proportions of these two fatty acids in the growth medium. Lindblom and Wieslander conclude that one of the most striking observations from this study of the in vivo lipid mixtures is that cubic and reversed hexagonal phases can be formed at high temperatures, despite the fact that most of the lipids present prefer to form only bilayer phases in the absence of MGDG. However, the total membrane lipids form only lamellar phases over the physiological temperature range, which is probably about 10 to 45°C (114, 115). Perhaps more noteworthy, however, is the variation in the lamellar gel/liquid-crystalline and the lamellar liquid-crystalline/nonlamellar phase transition temperatures of the total membrane lipids with the increasing degree of unsaturation of the membrane lipids. The lamellar chain-melting phase transition decreases by 15 to 20°C as the oleic acid content of the membrane lipids increases from less than 20 to greater than 95 mol%, as expected. However, the bilayer/nonbilayer phase transition, which would be expected to exhibit a similar decrease in temperature, in fact decreases by only 4 to 5°C. This smaller than expected decrease in the lamellar/nonlamellar phase transition is attributed to the decrease in the MGDG/DGDG ratio that accompanies the increasing biosynthetic incorporation of oleic acid into the membrane lipids. This result provides strong support for the hypothesis presented by Lindblom, Rilfors, and Wieslander, namely, that this organism possesses a biochemical mechanism that maintains the relative bilayer- and nonbilayer-forming tendencies of its membrane lipid at least relatively constant. More specifically, this regulatory mechanism appears to maintain the lipid bilayer as the exclusive, long-term structure in the *A. laidlawii* A membrane but may permit the facile, transient conversion of certain regions of the membrane to nonlamellar structures that may be involved in certain biological functions (66, 150). Alternatively, rather than actually forming nonlamellar structures, the function of nonbilayer-forming lipids in biological membranes may be to impart special properties to the lipid bilayer (73, 177).

Support for the idea that *A. laidlawii* A regulates the polar headgroup composition of its membrane lipids so as to maintain a certain lipid-packing geometry is also provided by a recent study by Wieslander et al. (205), who investigated the effects of the presence of exogenous hydrocarbons, alcohols, and detergents on membrane lipid composition and physical properties. In this study, *A. laidlawii* A cells highly enriched in oleic acid were grown for 6 to 8 h in the presence of one of the above-mentioned additives at a concentration of additive that did not adversely affect cell growth. At the end of this period, cells were harvested, the amount of additive in the lipid phase of the membrane

was estimated, and the MGDG/DGDG ratios were determined.

All of the solvents tested produced a decrease in the MGDG/DGDG ratio. For cyclohexane and benzene, the magnitude of the decrease in MGDG/DGDG ratio increases with an increasing concentration of solvent in the growth medium. Since all four of these organic solvents substantially and progressively decrease the lamellar/nonlamellar phase transition temperature of the *A. laidlawii* A membrane lipids, these workers interpret the observed decrease in the MGDG/DGDG ratio as an attempt to counteract the nonbilayer-promoting tendency of these organic solvent molecules by reducing the fraction of the membrane lipids able to form a nonbilayer phase. A similar good correlation between the magnitude and direction of the shift in the MGDG/DGDG ratio and the effect of various alcohols and detergents on the equilibrium between lamellar and nonlamellar phase was also observed. In contrast, no consistent correlation was found between the effect of these various additives on the gel/liquid-crystalline phase transition temperature or on the order parameter of the lipid hydrocarbon chains and the membrane lipid polar headgroup composition. Thus, it does not appear that the change in MGDG/DGDG ratios observed in these studies here represents an attempt by this organism to regulate the fluidity of its membrane lipids. Instead, it appears that effects of these additives on the effective geometry and packing of the membrane lipids, and thus on the equilibria between lamellar and nonlamellar phases, is the important criterion for lipid metabolic regulation in this organism.

Wieslander and Selstam (206) recently studied the relative abilities of chlorophyll and cholesterol to effect cell growth and membrane lipid polar headgroup composition in *A. laidlawii* A cells supplemented with palmitic acid or with various unsaturated fatty acids. In the absence of chlorophyll or cholesterol, growth yields decreased in the order palmitic > oleic > linoleic acid-enriched cells, and no growth occurred in the linolenic acid-supplemented medium. However, the addition of either chlorophyll or cholesterol increased growth yields in linoleic acid-supplemented cells and permitted some growth to occur in the linolenic acid-supplemented medium. Thus, in the highly unsaturated linoleic and linolenic acid-enriched growth media, *A. laidlawii* A is dependent on these additives for optimal growth and survival, respectively. Moreover, the amount of chlorophyll, and to a lesser extent cholesterol, incorporated into the membrane increases markedly with an increase in the degree of unsaturation of the lipid hydrocarbon chains. These authors attribute the growth-promoting effects of incorporated cholesterol molecules in highly unsaturated membranes to their well-known ability to increase the orientation order and the closeness of packing of lipid hydrocarbon chains in model and *A. laidlawii* membranes. Whether or not chlorophyll also promotes cell growth in cells enriched in highly unsaturated fatty acids by a similar mechanism remains to be determined.

Wieslander and Selstam (206) also studied the effect of chlorophyll and cholesterol incorporation on the MGDG/DGDG ratio and the ratio of charged to uncharged lipids in *A. laidlawii* A cells enriched in these various fatty acids. With palmitic acid-supplemented cells, the incorporation of either on these additives has little effect on the MGDG/DGDG ratio. However, chlorophyll incorporation modestly increases and cholesterol incorporation substantially decreases this ratio in the more highly unsaturated membranes. These authors attribute these results to the reported bilayer-stabilizing effect of chlorophyll in highly unsaturated plant MGDG-water systems and to the well-known bilayer-destabilizing effect of cholesterol in PE-water systems. However, if the MGDG/DGDG ratio is coherently regulated by A. laidlawii A to maintain an optimal bilayer stability, the lack of any additive effect of cholesterol or chlorophyll on this ratio in palmitic acid-enriched cells is not explained, nor is the increase in the MGDG/DGDG ratio that occurs when chlorophyll is incorporated into oleic acid-enriched membranes. The incorporation of cholesterol also results in an increase in the fraction of charged lipids, particularly in cells enriched in unsaturated fatty acids. This is the result expected from the earlier work of Christiansson et al. (33), since the incorporation of the unchanged cholesterol molecule into the membrane lipid bilayer would tend to decrease the surface charge density. Interestingly, however, the incorporation of the neutral chlorophyll molecule into the A. laidlawii membranes has little if any effect on the ratio of charged to uncharged lipids. Although the authors attribute this to the smaller and less bulky hydrophobic portion of the chlorophyll molecule, the isoprenoid side chain of chlorophyll nevertheless should also act as a neutral spacer in the lipid bilayer, resulting in at least some decrease in the surface charge density.

Rilfors and coworkers (151) have recently carried out a very detailed study of the effects of the incorporation of various sterols on A. laidlawii A membranes highly enriched in a variety of fatty acids. The abilities of 12 sterols to affect cell growth, lipid headgroup composition, the order parameter of the acyl chains, and the phase equilibria of in vivo lipid mixtures were studied. The following two effects were observed with respect to cell growth: (i) with a given acyl chain composition of the membrane lipids, growth is stimulated, unaffected, reduced, or completely inhibited (lysis), depending on the sterol structure, and (ii) the effect of a certain sterol depends on the acyl chain composition (most striking for epicoprostanol, cholest-4-en-3-one, and cholest-5-en-3-one, which stimulate growth with saturated acyl chains but cause lysis with unsaturated chains). The three lytic sterols were the only sterols that cause a marked decrease in the ratio between the major lipids MGDG and DGDG and hence a decrease in bilayer stability when the membranes are enriched in saturated (palmitoyl) chains. With these chains, correlations were found for several sterols between the glucolipid ratio and the order parameter of the acyl chains, as well as the lamellar/reversed hexagonal phase transition, in model systems. A shift experiment revealed a marked decrease in the MGDG/DGDG ratio with the lytic sterols in unsaturated (oleoyl) membranes. The two cholestenes induce nonlamellar phases in vivo mixtures of oleoyl A. laidlawii lipids. The order parameters of the oleoyl chains are almost unaffected by the sterols. Generally, the observed effects cannot be explained by an influence of the sterols on the gel/liquid-crystalline phase transition, but they show some correlation with the effects of these sterols on the bilayer/nonbilayer phase preference of the membrane lipids.

Although the work of Lindblom, Rilfors, and Wieslander is interesting and provocative, it should be pointed out that there are some data on A. laidlawii A, and a considerable amount of data on the closely related B strain, that are not fully compatible with their hypothesis of lipid shape regulation by polar headgroup compositional alterations. One example is the effect of altering the chain length of a given type of fatty acid on the MDGD/DGDG ratio. In A. laidlawii A, Rilfors (149) has shown that increases in the chain length of biosynthetically incorporated methyl iso- and anteiso-branched fatty acids leads to a decrease in the MGDG/DGDG ratio, and Silvius et al. (180) report similar observations for the B strain. Since in PEs, the most widely studied nonbilayer-forming lipid, increases in fatty acid chain length reduce the lamellar liquid-crystalline/reversed hexagonal phase transition temperature (95, 173), this result would seem to agree with the predictions of the hypothesis, since this organism would be expected to reduce the proportion of its only nonbilayer-forming lipid component, MGDG, in response to conditions that promote the formation of nonlamellar phases. However, we have recently found that the lamellar liquid-crystalline/reversed hexagonal phase transition temperature of various synthetic MGDGs is essentially independent of fatty acid chain length, especially in the case of glycolipids containing methyl iso- or anteiso-branched fatty acids (94, 109, 110, 178). Therefore, the observed reduction in the MGDG/DGDG ratio, particularly the marked reduction observed in A. laidlawii B, is not explained by this hypothesis.

The dependence of the MGDG/DGDG ratios on the chemical structure of biosynthetically incorporated fatty acids is also not fully accounted for on the basis of their relative nonbilayer-forming tendencies. For example, at a constant effective chain length, the lamellar liquid-crystalline/reversed hexagonal phase transition temperatures of a series of synthetic PEs and MGDGs decrease in the following order: n-saturated > methyl iso-branched > methyl anteiso-branched > trans-monounsaturated > cis-monounsaturated (94, 95). However, in A. laidlawii B, the MGDG/DGDG ratios decrease in the following order: methyl iso-branched > methyl anteiso-branched > n-saturated > trans-unsaturated > cis-unsaturated (15, 210). Moreover, many of the alicyclic fatty acids also do not fit the predictions of this hypothesis either. For example, ω-cyclohexyl fatty acids, which fall between the methyl iso- and anteiso-branched fatty acids in their nonbilayer-forming tendencies, nevertheless produce in A. laidlawii B MGDG/DGDG ratios nearly as low as those produced by the cis-monounsaturated fatty acids, whose nonbilayer-forming tendencies are quite strong (210). Similarly, the trans-cyclopropane fatty acids, which produce PEs and MGDGs with intermediate lamellar/reversed hexagonal phase transition temperatures, induce in A. laidlawii B MGDG/DGDG ratios lower than those of the cis-monounsaturated fatty acids of similar effective chain length (210). Although a more restricted range of fatty acids has been examined in the A strain, it appears that the methyl iso-branched fatty acids may produce higher and the methyl anteiso-branched fatty acids may produce lower MGDG/DGDG ratios than predicted (149).

Bhakoo and McElhaney (15) have also studied the effect of variations in growth temperature and cholesterol content on the MGDG/DGDG ratio of *A. laidlawii* B biosynthetically enriched in various exogenous fatty acids. In palmitate-enriched cells, the MGDG/DGDG ratio was found to decrease substantially with an increase in either the growth temperature or the cholesterol content of the membrane, in agreement with the results of Wieslander and coworkers on the A strain of this organism. Interestingly, however, the effect of variations in growth temperature and cholesterol content on the glycolipid ratio was much less in elaidic acid-enriched cells, and essentially no effect of these variables on the MGDG/DGDG ratio was noted in oleic acid-enriched cells. These results imply that the lamellar/nonlamellar phase preference of the membrane lipids of this organism is not being consistently regulated in strain B in response to changes in growth temperature and cholesterol content.

Yue et al. (210) have recently carried out a more rigorous study of the effect of fatty acid compositional variations on lipid polar headgroup composition in *A. laidlawii* B membranes. In this study, fatty acid-homogeneous membranes were used so that independent variations in fatty acyl chain length and structure could be obtained, since both of these variables affect bilayer/nonbilayer phase transitions (94, 95). Moreover, the authors quantitated all of the membrane lipids, rather than simply the MGDG/DGDG ratio as was done in earlier studies. This distinction is important because Yue and coworkers found that in some cases, changes in the MGDG/DGDG ratio are due to variations in the DGDG content only, such that the MGDG content (and thus the total amount of nonbilayer-forming lipid) remains constant despite large changes in the ratio of these two lipids. When the total amount of nonbilayering-forming lipid was plotted against the bilayer/nonbilayer phase transition temperature of the MGDG component itself, these workers found only a weak correlation between these two variables, whether or not the lamellar/nonlamellar lipid phase transition was varied by changes in fatty acyl chain length or chemical structure. These results strongly suggest that *A. laidlawii* B does not biochemically regulate the bilayer/nonbilayer phase preference of its membrane lipids in a coherent manner.

Yue et al. (210) have also used ^{2}H NMR to investigate the actual thermotropic phase behavior of *A. laidlawii* B membranes and total membrane lipid dispersions from cells grown in perdeuterated palmitic acid with either elaidic, oleic, or linoleic acid with or without cholesterol. As expected from earlier DSC and ^{2}H NMR studies, these workers confirm that in both membranes and lipid dispersions, the gel/liquid-crystalline lipid phase transition temperature decreases in the order elaidic > oleic > linoleic acid and that cholesterol increases hydrocarbon chain orientational order above that phase transition temperature. However, the bilayer/nonbilayer phase behaviors of these two systems differ markedly. Lipid bilayers generated from the total membrane lipids exhibit lamellar/nonlamellar phase transitions at experimentally accessible temperatures. However, the bilayer/nonbilayer phase transition temperatures varied considerably

with fatty acid composition and cholesterol content, in contrast to the results of Lindblom et al. (98) for the A strain. In contrast, isolated membranes do not exhibit bilayer/nonbilayer phase transitions, except perhaps at very high temperatures where membrane lipid degradation occurs. This first result clearly confirms the inability of strain B to effectively regulate the lamellar/nonlamellar phase preference of its membrane lipids, while the second result establishes that nonbilayer lipid phases do not actually form in cells and membranes of this organism. The probable reason for this latter finding is that the nonlamellar cubic and reversed hexagonal phases are three-dimensional structures formed from the interactions of adjacent lipid bilayers. In the real *A. laidlawii* membrane, the presence of protein (and carbohydrate) on the membrane surfaces probably prevents the lipid bilayers in adjacent membranes from interacting to form these three-dimensional structures.

Wieslander et al. (203) have recently carried out a multivariate data analysis of membrane lipid composition alterations in *A. laidlawii* A and B in response to variations in growth temperature and fatty acid and cholesterol supplementation, among other variables. These workers find that when cultured under identical conditions, these two strains often respond in quantitatively or even qualitatively different manners to these and other variables, despite their very similar membrane protein profiles. These results clearly establish that these two strains differ considerably in the regulation of membrane lipid biosynthesis in response to changes in temperature, fatty acid composition, cholesterol content, and other variables and that the differences in biochemical and biophysical behavior reported by Wieslander and coworkers and McElhaney and coworkers for these two strains of *A. laidlawii* are due, at least in part, to intrinsic strain differences. Although in one sense these strain differences were unfortunate, as they generated some controversy in the literature, their existence does offer an opportunity to determine whether the coherent regulation of lipid phase preference and bilayer surface charge density found only in the A strain provides it with a significant growth advantage when adapting to changing growth temperature, fatty acid and cholesterol supplementation, or other variables that tend to alter the properties of the membrane lipid bilayer. If it does, then these lipid biosynthetic polar headgroup alterations will be established as adaptive regulatory responses, perhaps comparable in importance to the fatty acid composition-based homeoviscous (185) and homeophasic (181) lipid regulatory responses already well established in other organisms.

Regulation of glycolipid composition by alterations in the glucose level and the fatty acid composition of the growth medium

Bhakoo et al. (14) have recently reported that the level of a normally minor lipid component of the *A. laidlawii* B membrane is increased significantly when the glucose supplement to the growth medium is reduced from its normal level. Under such glucose-limiting conditions, the proportion of this component in the membrane is markedly dependent on the fatty acid supplement provided and increases in rough proportion to the decrease in the levels of glucose present. With oleic and elaidic acid-enriched cells, the quantity of this minor lipid increases from trace levels to 3 and 10 mol%, respectively, under conditions of severe glucose limitations; however, in palmitic acid-enriched cells, the proportion of this minor lipid increases from 2 to 60 mol%. Interestingly, although the levels of DGDG and PG decrease more than 50% when the levels of this minor lipid component are maximally elevated, the MGDG decreases by over 80%. Thus, the increase of this minor lipid component in the *A. laidlawii* B membranes occurs mainly at the expense of the MGDG constituent.

The chemical composition of this minor lipid component was also determined in this study. The minor lipid was found to consist of one molecule each of glucose, fatty acid, and a polyprenyl alcohol. A number of physical measurements, along with specific chemical and enzymatic degradation studies, provided a tentative identification of this lipid as a polyprenyl-α-D-glucoside with a long-chain fatty acid esterified to the 2-hydroxyl group of the sugar moiety. The relatively large cross-sectional area of the hydrocarbon chain portion of this molecule, due to the presence of the tetramethyl branched isoprenoid alcohol chain, and the very small polar headgroup region of this lipid suggested that it might be capable of forming nonlamellar lipid phases under biologically relevant conditions. In this respect, it may be significant that this neutral glycolipid replaces primarily the nonbilayer-forming MGDG component under glucose-limiting conditions. Lewis et al. (97) subsequently studied the thermotropic phase behavior of this monoacylated neutral glucolipid (2-*O*-acyl,polyprenyl-α-D-glucopyranoside), isolated from palmitate-enriched *A. laidlawii* B membranes, by DSC, FT-IR spectroscopy, and X-ray diffraction. When equilibrated at low temperatures, aqueous dispersions of this lipid form an ordered, crystal-like lamellar gel phase which transforms to an inverted hexagonal phase at temperatures near 65°C upon heating. However, if not annealed at low temperatures (the biologically relevant situation), this lipid forms a metastable gel phase which undergoes a gel/liquid-crystalline phase transition at temperatures near 33°C. These results indicate that this monoacylated glucolipid exhibits its gel/liquid-crystalline phase transition and its lamellar/nonlamellar phase transition at considerably lower temperatures than does the MGDG formed under the same conditions. When cultured in media enriched in high-melting-point fatty acids, *A. laidlawii* B synthesizes large quantities of the 2-*O*-acyl,polyprenyl-α-D-glucopyranoside (up to 60 mol%) mainly at the expense of the MGDG (the only other nonbilayer-forming liquid normally found in the cell membrane of this organism). These workers thus suggest that the biosynthesis of this novel glucolipid, in response to the biosynthetic incorporation of high-melting-point exogenous fatty acids, is an adaptive response designed to maintain a predominantly liquid-crystalline membrane lipid bilayer at the growth temperature while retaining the high proportion of nonbilayer-forming glucolipid species characteristic of *A. laidlawii* B cells cultured under these conditions.

Although the results discussed above lend qualitative support to the lipid phase preference hypothesis of Wieslander and coworkers, it should be noted that the total amount of nonbilayer lipid present varies markedly with the fatty acid composition of this organism (14, 15, 97). For example, palmitate-enriched *A. laidlawii* B membranes contain more than 70 mol% of the two nonbilayer-forming glycolipids (predominantly the monoacylated glycolipid with a small amount of MGDG), while oleate-enriched membranes contain only about 30 mol% (almost exclusively MGDG). Moreover, the isolated membrane lipids from palmitate-enriched cells still exhibit a higher bilayer/nonbilayer phase transition temperature than do those from oleate-enriched cells, despite their enrichment in the monoacylated neutral lipid. Thus, from a quantitative viewpoint, a full compensatory regulation of membrane lipid phase preference is not achieved.

In summary, although the data are not completely consistent, the general weight of evidence favors the view that *A. laidlawii* A does indeed possess at least a relatively effective biochemical regulatory mechanism for adjusting the phase preference of its membrane lipids in response to changes in fatty acid composition, cholesterol content, and temperature, whereas *A. laidlawii* B does not. It is possible that such regulatory mechanisms once existed in the B strain but have somehow been lost or become at least partially defective upon culturing of this organism under laboratory conditions over many years. It is also possible that other, unrecognized factors may be modulating or overriding the normal membrane lipid polar headgroup regulatory response of this particular strain to variations in growth temperature and lipid composition. However, in view of the fact that *A. laidlawii* B appears to grow well under as wide a variety of environmental conditions as does the A strain, it is also possible that the phase preference regulatory mechanisms described by Wieslander and colleagues are not required for successful membrane functions in all organisms. Clearly, additional work will be required to resolve these important questions. It is interesting, however, that these two apparently very closely related strains should differ so fundamentally in their regulation of the biophysical properties of their membrane lipids.

Regulation of lipid bilayer surface potential

The mechanisms that regulate the lipid polar headgroup ratios in biological membranes are not well understood (138). There is evidence that in several bacteria, however, a critical balance between zwitterionic and anionic lipids is maintained, suggesting that the lipid bilayer surface charge density may be regulated within certain limits. Recently, evidence has been presented that *A. laidlawii* A also possesses regulatory mechanisms to maintain the surface potential of its membrane lipids relatively constant in response to variations in either the fatty acid composition or the ionic composition of the growth medium.

Christiansson et al. (33) grew *A. laidlawii* A cells in the presence of different ratios of palmitic and oleic acids so as to vary the degree of unsaturation of the membrane lipids. This organism responds by decreasing its MGDG/DGDG ratio in response to increases in oleic acid content as previously discussed; this variation in ratio is presumably related to maintenance of the bilayer/nonbilayer phase preference of the membrane lipids. However, an increasing degree of unsaturation also results in an increase in the ratio of charged lipids (primarily PG) to uncharged lipids (primarily MGDG plus DGDG). Since an increase in the oleic acid content of the membrane lipids also results in an increase in the molecular area occupied by the total membrane lipids, the surface density of the membrane lipids would be expected to remain relatively constant. In fact, the measured zeta potentials of liposomes prepared from the total membrane lipids of *A. laidlawii* A cells grown at various palmitic/oleic acid ratios are relatively constant. Therefore, this organism can maintain a constant surface potential or surface charge density in response to differences in the cross-sectional areas of its membrane lipids induced by variations in fatty acid composition.

In addition to responding to variations in the lateral packing of the membrane lipids induced by changes in fatty acid composition, *A. laidlawii* A can also alter its membrane lipid polar headgroup composition in response to changes in the NaCl content of the growth medium. Specifically, an increase in the content of charged lipids with an increasing concentration of NaCl in the growth medium is observed. As before, the zeta potentials of liposomes made from the membrane lipids are relatively constant when measured at the NaCl concentration present in the growth medium. These authors conclude that this organism possesses a mechanism to overcome the Na^+-induced decrease in the mutual repulsion of its negatively charged polar headgroups, and thus the decrease in lipid molecular cross-sectional areas, by increasing the biosynthesis of its charged lipids, thereby restoring the effective surface charge density and lateral packing properties of its membrane lipid bilayer (33).

Christiansson et al. (33) also investigated the ability of the chloride salts of a number of monovalent cations and Mg^{2+} to screen negatively charged lipid species and to induce an increase in the proportion of charged lipids species by *A. laidlawii* A. Although the results varied somewhat with the relative proportions of palmitic and oleic acids present in the growth medium, in general there is a negative correlation between the ability of a monovalent cation to bind to negatively charged lipids, thereby reducing their zeta potential, and the amount of negatively charged lipid synthesized by this organism. Moreover, the addition of Mg^{2+}, which is more efficient than monovalent cations at reducing the zeta potentials of anionic lipids, has little effect on the proportion of charged lipids present. These results imply that the mechanism utilized by *A. laidlawii* A to coherently regulate the surface charge density of its membrane lipids in response to variations in fatty acid composition and NaCl content does not involve a direct sensing of the surface potential of its lipid bilayer but must function in some other way.

Clementz and coworkers (43, 44) have also shown that the MGDG/DGDG ratio itself is sensitive to the transmembrane electrical potential in growing *A. laidlawii* A cells. In cells whose membrane lipids are enriched in various fatty acids, a transmembrane electrical potential of about −50 mV (inside negative) is maintained, but no transmembrane pH difference is present. Addition of the K^+ ionophore valinomycin

causes a rapid and dose-dependent hyperpolarization that remains for at least 7 h. Simultaneously, a rapid and lasting metabolic decrease in the MGDG/DGDG ratio occurs. The increase in potential and the decrease in the lipid ratio are both reversed in a dose-dependent manner by extracellular KCl. Likewise, the lipophilic cation tetraphenylphosphonium causes a dose-dependent decrease in membrane potential and an increase in MGDG/DGDG ratio. The ionophores monensin and particularly nigericin have effects on the potential and lipid ratios similar to but less pronounced than the effect of valinomycin. The uncoupler carbonyl cyanide *m*-chlorophenylhydrazone has no effect on cell growth, membrane potential, or lipid regulation at 10 μM. The dissimilar structures and the low concentrations used make a direct disturbance of these drug molecules on lipid packing in membranes unlikely. The coherent variation of lipid composition with the membrane potential supports an effect of the electrical potential on lipid packing and lamellar stability similar to what can be observed in model lipid systems. Specifically, since an increase in the potential difference across a lipid bilayer can compress it, thus presumably shortening and broadening the hydrophobic core of the bilayer, these authors argue that the decrease in the MGDG/DGDG ratio observed may represent an attempt by *A. laidlawii* A to stabilize its lipids in a lamellar arrangement. However, since it has been shown experimentally that the compression of egg PE/water systems by hydrostatic pressure increases the lamellar/inverted hexagonal phase transition temperature, i.e., stabilizes the lipid bilayer (209), one could argue that an increase rather than a decrease in the MGDG/DGDG ratio would have been the more appropriate response of this organism to an increase in transmembrane electrical potential.

Bhakoo and McElhaney (15) have also studied the effect of variations in growth temperature, fatty acid composition, and cholesterol content on the ratio of charged to uncharged lipids in *A. laidlawii* B membranes. In contrast to the results of Clementz et al. (43, 44) with the A strain, the relative proportion of anionic lipid is actually higher in palmitic acid-enriched than in elaidic or oleic acid-enriched membranes, despite the fact that the lipids from palmitate-enriched membranes already occupy a smaller cross-sectional area. Although the incorporation of cholesterol does increase the proportion of charged lipids in palmitic acid-enriched membranes, as predicted, it has no effect in elaidic acid- or oleic acid-enriched membranes. Decreases in growth temperature below 37°C do produce the predicted decrease in anionic lipid content in all cases, but increasing the growth temperature to 40°C results in a decline in charged lipids. These workers conclude that *A. laidlawii* B, unlike strain A, does not possess a coherent regulatory mechanism for regulating the surface charge density of its membrane lipids.

CONCLUSIONS AND OUTLOOK

Although a great deal has been learned about the structure and some of the functions of the mycoplasma membranes in the last two decades, clearly much work remains to be done before a reasonably complete understanding of this system at the molecular level is at hand. With reference to the lipid portion of the membrane, the structure and dynamics of which are relatively well understood, uncertainties still exist about the transbilayer distribution of the glyco- and phospholipids and about their lateral and rotational mobilities in the native membrane. As well, the transbilayer distribution and localization within the membrane of cholesterol are still not known with certainty in some *Acholeplasma* and *Mycoplasma* species. Also, the concept of membrane lipid fluidity must be refined and quantitated, and the relationship between orientational order and rates of motion must be better understood. To do so, the current discrepancies between some of the results obtained, for example, by the various spectroscopic techniques, must be resolved. In particular, the nature of the boundary lipid surrounding integral membrane proteins requires further study. Moreover, the basis for the apparently different regulation of lipid surface charge density and bilayer/nonbilayer phase preference in *A. laidlawii* A and B remains to be elucidated. Finally, we need to know a great deal more about almost every aspect of the structure, organization, and dynamics of the many proteins which compose the bulk of this membrane and which perform most of its specific functions. However, the many natural advantages of mycoplasma membranes for most types of biochemical and biophysical investigations should permit the steady progress in our understanding of this complex supramolecular structure which has characterized the recent past to continue well into the future.

Acknowledgments. The work described in this review that emanated from my laboratory was generously supported by operating and major equipment grants from the Medical Research Council of Canada and by major equipment and personnel support grants from the Alberta Heritage Foundation for Medical Research.

REFERENCES

1. **Abramson, M. B., and D. Pisetsky.** 1972. Thermal-turbidimetric studies of membranes from *Acholeplasma laidlawii*. *Biochim. Biophys. Acta* **282**:80–84.
2. **Amar, A., S. Rottem, I. Kahane, and S. Razin.** 1976. Characterization of the mycoplasma membrane proteins. VI. Composition and disposition of proteins in membranes from aging *Mycoplasma hominis* cultures. *Biochim. Biophys. Acta* **426**:258–270.
3. **Amar, A., S. Rottem, and S. Razin.** 1974. Characterization of the mycoplasma membrane proteins. IV. Disposition of proteins in the membrane. *Biochim. Biophys. Acta* **352**:228–244.
4. **Amar, A., S. Rottem, and S. Razin.** 1978. Disposition of membrane proteins as affected by changes in the electrochemical gradient across mycoplasma membranes. *Biochem. Biophys. Res. Commun.* **84**:306–312.
5. **Amar, A., S. Rottem, and S. Razin.** 1979. Is the vertical disposition of mycoplasma membrane proteins affected by membrane fluidity? *Biochim. Biophys. Acta* **552**:457–467.
6. **Archer, D. B.** 1975. Modification of the membrane composition of *Mycoplasma mycoides* subspecies *capri* by the growth medium. *J. Gen. Microbiol.* **88**:329–338.
7. **Archer, D. B., A. W. Rodwell, and E. S. Rodwell.** 1978. The nature and location of *Acholeplasma laidlawii* membrane proteins investigated by two-dimensional gel electrophoresis. *Biochim. Biophys. Acta* **513**:268–283.
8. **Askarova, E. A., A. B. Kapitanov, V. K. Kol'tover, and O. S. Tatishchev.** 1987. Generation of superoxide radicals and the fluidity of the membrane lipids of *Acholeplasma laidlawii* on aging of the cell culture. *Biophysics* **32**:99–104.
9. **Bevers, E. M., G. Leblanc, C. Le Grimellec, J. A. F. Op den Kamp, and L. L. M. van Deenen.** 1978. Disposition of phosphatidylglycerol in metabolizing cells of *Acholeplasma laidlawii*. *FEBS Lett.* **87**:49–51.
10. **Bevers, E. M., J. A. F. Op den Kamp, and L. L. M. van Deenen.** 1978. Physiochemical properties of phosphatidylglycerol in membranes of *Acholeplasma laidlawii*. A study with phospholipase A₂. *Eur. J. Biochem.* **84**:35–42.
11. **Bevers, E. M., J. A. F. Op den Kamp, and L. L. M. van Deenen.** 1978. The distribution of molecular classes of phosphatidylglycerol in the membrane of *Acholeplasma laidlawii*. *Biochim. Biophys. Acta* **511**:509–512.
12. **Bevers, E. M., S. A. Singal, J. A. F. Op den Kamp, and L. L. M. van Deenen.** 1977. Recognition of different pools of phosphatidylglycerol in intact cells and isolated membranes of *Acholeplasma laidlawii*. *Biochemistry* **16**:1290–1295.
13. **Bevers, E. M., H. H. Wang, J. A. F. Op den Kamp, and L. L. M. van Deenen.** 1979. On the interaction between intrinsic membrane proteins and phosphatidylglycerol in the membrane of *Acholeplasma laidlawii*. *Arch. Biochem. Biophys.* **193**:502–508.
14. **Bhakoo, M., R. N. A. H. Lewis, and R. N. McElhaney.** 1987. Isolation and characterization of a novel monoacylated glucopyranosyl neutral lipid from the plasma membrane of *Acholeplasma laidlawii* B. *Biochim. Biophys. Acta* **922**:34–45.
15. **Bhakoo, M., and R. N. McElhaney.** 1988. Regulation of membrane lipid composition in *Acholeplasma laidlawii* B in response to variations in temperature, fatty acid composition and cholesterol content. *Biochim. Biophys. Acta* **945**:307–314.
16. **Bittman, R., L. Blau, S. Clejan, and S. Rottem.** 1981. Determination of cholesterol asymmetry by rapid kinetics of filipin cholesterol association: effect of modifications of lipids and proteins. *Biochemistry* **20**:2425–2432.
17. **Bittman, R., S. Clejan, and S. W. Hui.** 1990. Increased rates of lipid exchange between *Mycoplasma capricolum* membranes and vesicles in relation to the propensity of forming nonbilayer lipid structures. *J. Biol. Chem.* **265**:15110–15117.
18. **Bittman, R., S. Clejan, B. P. Robinson, and N. M. Witzke.** 1985. Kinetics of cholesterol and phospholipid exchange from membranes containing cross-linked proteins or cross-linked phosphatidylethanolamines. *Biochemistry* **24**:1403–1409.
19. **Bittman, R. S. Clejan, and S. Rottem.** 1983. Transbilayer distribution of sterols in mycoplasma membranes: a review. *Yale J. Biol. Med.* **56**:397–403.
20. **Bittman, R., and S. Rottem.** 1976. Distribution of cholesterol between the outer and inner halves of the lipid bilayer of mycoplasma cell membranes. *Biochem. Biophys. Res. Commun.* **71**:318–324.
21. **Borochov, H., and M. Shinitzky.** 1976. Vertical displacement of membrane proteins mediated by changes in microviscosity. *Proc. Natl. Acad. Sci. USA* **73**:4526–4530.
22. **Bouvier, P., J. A. F. Op den Kamp, and L. L. M. van Deenen.** 1981. Studies on *Acholeplasma laidlawii* grown on branched-chain fatty acids. *Arch. Biochem. Biophys.* **208**:242–247.
23. **Burke, P. V., R. Kanki, and H. H. Wang.** 1985. Effect of positively charged local anesthetics on a membrane-bound phosphatase in *Acholeplasma laidlawii*. *Biochem. Pharmacol.* **34**:1917–1924.
24. **Butler, K. W., K. G. Johnson, and I. C. P. Smith.** 1978.

Acholeplasma laidlawii membranes: an electron spin resonance study of the influence on molecular order of fatty acid composition and cholesterol. *Arch. Biochem. Biophys.* **191:**289–297.

25. **Cameron, D. G., A. Martin, and H. H. Mantsch.** 1983. Membrane isolation alters the gel to liquid-crystalline transition of *Acholeplasma laidlawii. Science* **219:** 180–182.

26. **Cameron, D. G., A. Martin, D. J. Moffatt, and H. H. Mantsch.** 1985. Infrared spectroscopic study of the gel to liquid-crystal phase transition in live *Acholeplasma laidlawii* cells. *Biochemistry* **24:**4355–4359.

27. **Casal, H. L., D. G. Cameron, H. C. Jarrell, I. C. P. Smith, and H. H. Mantsch.** 1982. Lipid phase transitions in fatty acid-homogeneous membranes of *Acholeplasma laidlawii* B. *Chem. Phys. Lipids* **30:**17–26.

28. **Casal, H. L., D. G. Cameron, I. C. P. Smith, and H. H. Mantsch.** 1980. *Acholeplasma laidlawii* membranes: a Fourier transform infrared study of the influence of protein on lipid organization and dynamics. *Biochemistry* **19:**444–451.

29. **Casal, H. L., and H. H. Mantsch.** 1984. Polymorphic phase behavior of phospholipid membranes studied by infrared spectroscopy. *Biochim. Biophys. Acta* **779:** 381–401.

30. **Casal, H. L., and R. N. McElhaney.** 1990. Quantitative determination of hydrocarbon chain conformational order in bilayers of saturated phosphatidylcholines of various chain lengths by Fourier transform infrared spectroscopy. *Biochemistry* **29:**5423–5427.

31. **Casal, H. L., I. C. P. Smith, D. G. Cameron, and H. H. Mantsch.** 1979. Lipid reorganization in biological membranes: a study by Fourier transform infrared difference spectroscopy. *Biochim. Biophys. Acta* **550:**145–149.

32. **Chapman, D., and J. Urbina.** 1971. Phase transitions and bilayer structure of *Mycoplasma laidlawii* B. *FEBS Lett.* **12:**169–172.

33. **Christiansson, A., L. E. G. Eriksson, J. Westman, R. Demel, and Å. Wieslander.** 1985. Involvement of surface potential in regulation of polar membrane lipids in *Acholeplasma laidlawii. J. Biol. Chem.* **260:**3984–3990.

34. **Christiansson, A., H. Gutman, Å. Wieslander, and G. Lindblom.** 1981. Effects of anesthetics on water permeability and lipid metabolism in *Acholeplasma laidlawii* membranes. *Biochim. Biophys. Acta* **645:**24–32.

35. **Christiansson, A., and Å. Wieslander.** 1978. Membrane lipid metabolism in *Acholeplasma laidlawii* A EF22. Influence of cholesterol and temperature shift-down on the incorporation of fatty acids and synthesis of membrane lipid species. *Eur. J. Biochem.* **85:**65–76.

36. **Christiansson, A., and Å. Wieslander.** 1980. Control of membrane polar lipid composition in *Acholeplasma laidlawii* A by the extent of saturated fatty acid synthesis. *Biochim. Biophys. Acta* **595:**189–199.

37. **Church, S. E., D. J. Griffiths, R. N. A. H. Lewis, R. N. McElhaney, and H. H. Wickman.** 1986. X-ray structure study of thermotropic phases in isoacylphosphatidylcholine multibilayers. *Biophys. J.* **49:**597–605.

38. **Clejan, S., and R. Bittman.** 1984. Kinetics of cholesterol and phospholipid exchange between *Mycoplasma gallisepticum* cells and lipid vesicles. Alterations in membrane cholesterol and protein content. *J. Biol. Chem.* **259:**441–448.

39. **Clejan, S., and R. Bittman.** 1984. Distribution and movement of sterols with different side chain structures between the two leaflets of the membrane bilayer of mycoplasma cells. *J. Biol. Chem.* **259:**449–455.

40. **Clejan, S., and R. Bittman.** 1984. Decreases in rates of lipid exchange between *Mycoplasma gallisepticum* and unilamellar vesicles by incorporation of sphingomyelin. *J. Biol. Chem.* **259:**10823–10826.

41. **Clejan, S., R. Bittman, and S. Rottem.** 1978. Uptake, transbilayer distribution, and movement of cholesterol

42. **Clejan, S., R. Bittman, and S. Rottem.** 1981. Effects of sterol structure and exogenous lipids on the transbilayer distribution of sterols in the membrane of *Mycoplasma capricolum. Biochemistry* **20:**2200–2204.

43. **Clementz, T., A. Christiansson, and Å. Wieslander.** 1986. Transmembrane electrical potential affects the lipid composition of *Acholeplasma laidlawii. Biochemistry* **25:**823–830.

44. **Clementz, T., A. Christiansson, and Å. Wieslander.** 1987. Membrane potential, lipid regulation and adenylate energy charge in acyl chain modified *Acholeplasma laidlawii. Biochim. Biophys. Acta* **898:**299–307.

45. **Copps, T. P., W. S. Chelack, and A. Paetkau.** 1976. Variation in distribution of membrane particles in *Acholeplasma laidlawii* B with pH. *J. Ultrastruct. Res.* **55:**1–3.

46. **Dahl, C. E., J. S. Dahl, and K. Bloch.** 1980. Effect of alkyl-substituted precursors of cholesterol on artificial and natural membranes and on the viability of *Mycoplasma capricolum. Biochemistry* **19:**1462–1467.

47. **Dahl, C. E., J. S. Dahl, and K. Bloch.** 1983. Proteolipid formation in *Mycoplasma capricolum. J. Biol. Chem.* **258:**11814–11818.

48. **Dahl, J. S., and C. E. Dahl.** 1983. Coordinate regulation of unsaturated phospholipid, RNA, and protein synthesis in *Mycoplasma capricolum* by cholesterol. *Proc. Natl. Acad. Sci. USA* **80:**692–696.

49. **Dahl, J. S., and C. E. Dahl.** 1984. Effect of cholesterol on phospholipid, RNA, and protein synthesis in *Mycoplasma capricolum. Isr. J. Med. Sci.* **20:**807–811.

50. **Dahl, J. S., C. E. Dahl, and K. Bloch.** 1980. Sterols in membranes: growth characteristics and membrane properties of *Mycoplasma capricolum* cultured on cholesterol and lanosterol. *Biochemistry* **19:**1467–1472.

51. **Davis, J. A.** 1983. The description of membrane lipid conformation, order and dynamics by ^{2}H-NMR. *Biochim. Biophys. Acta* **737:**117–171.

52. **Davis, J. H., M. Bloom, K. W. Butler, and I. C. P. Smith.** 1980. The temperature dependence of molecular order and the influence of cholesterol in *Acholeplasma laidlawii* membranes. *Biochim. Biophys. Acta* **597:**477–491.

53. **Davis, P. J., H. Efrati, S. Razin, and S. Rottem.** 1984. Two cholesterol pools in *Acholeplasma laidlawii* membranes. *FEBS Lett.* **175:**51–54.

54. **de Kruijff, B., P. R. Cullis, G. K. Radda, and R. E. Richards.** 1976. Phosphorus nuclear magnetic resonance of *Acholeplasma laidlawii* cell membranes and derived liposomes. *Biochim. Biophys. Acta* **419:**411–424.

55. **de Kruijff, B., W. J. Gerritsen, A. Oerlemans, P. W. M. van Dijck, R. A. Demel, and L. L. M. van Deenen.** 1974. Polyene-antibiotic-sterol interactions in membranes of *Acholeplasma laidlawii* cells and lecithin liposomes. II. Temperature dependence of the polyene antibiotic-sterol complex formation. *Biochim. Biophys. Acta* **359:** 44–56.

56. **de Kruyff, B., R. A. Demel, and L. L. M. van Deenen.** 1972. The effect of cholesterol and epicholesterol incorporation on the permeability and on the phase transition of intact *Acholeplasma laidlawii* cell membranes and derived liposomes. *Biochim. Biophys. Acta* **255:** 331–347.

57. **de Kruyff, B., P. W. M. van Dijck, R. W. Goldback, R. A. Demel, and L. L. M. van Deenen.** 1973. Influence of fatty acid and sterol composition on the lipid phase transition and activity of membrane-bound enzymes in *Acholeplasma laidlawii. Biochim. Biophys. Acta* **330:** 269–282.

58. **Demel, R. A., and B. de Kruyff.** 1976. The function of sterols in membranes. *Biochim. Biophys. Acta* **457:** 109–132.

59. **Efrati, H., Y. Wax, and S. Rottem.** 1986. Cholesterol

uptake capacity of *Acholeplasma laidlawii* is affected by the composition and content of membrane glycolipids. *Arch. Biochem. Biophys.* **248**:282–288.

60. **Engelman, D. M.** 1970. X-ray diffraction studies of phase transitions in the membrane of *Mycoplasma laidlawii*. *J. Mol. Biol.* **47**:115–117.

61. **Engelman, D. M.** 1971. Lipid bilayer structure in the membrane of *Mycoplasma laidlawii*. *J. Mol. Biol.* **58**: 153–165.

62. **Eriksson, P.-O., L. Rilfors, Å. Wieslander, A. Lundberg, and G. Lindblom.** 1991. Order and dynamics in mixtures of membrane glucolipids from *Acholeplasma laidlawii* studied by ^{2}H NMR. *Biochemistry* **30**:4916–4924.

63. **Grant, C. W. M., and H. M. McConnell.** 1973. Fusion of phospholipid vesicles with viable *Acholeplasma laidlawii*. *Proc. Natl. Acad. Sci. USA* **70**:1238–1240.

64. **Green, F., and R. P. Hanson.** 1973. Ultrastructure and capsule of *Mycoplasma meleagridis*. *J. Bacteriol.* **116**:1011–1018.

65. **Gross, Z., and S. Rottem.** 1979. Lipid distribution in *Acholeplasma laidlawii* membrane. A study using lactoperoxidase. *Biochim. Biophys. Acta* **555**:547–552.

66. **Gruner, S. M., P. R. Cullis, M. J. Hope, and C. P. S. Tilcock.** 1985. Lipid polymorphism: the molecula basis of nonbilayer phases. *Annu. Rev. Biophys. Biophys. Chem.* **14**:211–238.

67. **Haberer, K., and D. Frosch.** 1982. Lateral mobility of membrane-bound antibodies on the surface of *Acholeplasma laidlawii*: evidence for virus-induced cell fusion in a procaryote. *J. Bacteriol.* **152**:471–478.

68. **Haberer, K., M. Pfisterer, and H.-J. Galla.** 1982. Virus capping on mycoplasma cells and its effect on membrane structure. *Biochim. Biophys. Acta* **688**:720–726.

69. **Huang, L., and A. Haug.** 1974. Regulation of membrane lipid fluidity in *Acholeplasma laidlawii*: effect of carotenoid pigment content. *Biochim. Biophys. Acta* **352**: 361–370.

70. **Huang, L., D. D. Jaquet, and A. Haug.** 1974. Effect of fatty acyl chain length on some structural and functional parameters of *Acholeplasma* membranes. *Can. J. Biochem.* **52**:483–490.

71. **Huang, L., S. K. Lorch, G. G. Smith, and A. Haug.** 1974. Control of membrane lipid fluidity in *Acholeplasma laidlawii*. *FEBS Lett.* **43**:1–5.

72. **Huang, T., A. J. DeSiervo, and Q.-X. Yang.** 1991. Effect of cholesterol and lanosterol on the structure and dynamics of the cell membrane of *Mycoplasma capricolum*. Deuterium magnetic resonance study. *Biophys. J.* **59**: 691–702.

73. **Hui, S.-W.** 1987. Non-bilayer-forming lipids: why are they necessary in biomembranes. *Comments Mol. Cell. Biophys.* **4**:233–248.

74. **Iwamoto, K., J. Sunamoto, K. Inoue, T. Endo, and S. Nojima.** 1982. Liposomal membranes. IV. Importance of surface structure in liposomal membranes of glyceroglycolipids. *Biochim Biophys. Acta* **691**:44–51.

75. **James, R., and D. Branton.** 1973. Lipid- and temperature-dependent structural changes in *Acholeplasma laidlawii* cell membranes. *Biochim. Biophys. Acta* **323**: 378–390.

76. **Jarrell, H. C., K. W. Butler, A. Byrd, R. Deslauriers, I. Ekiel, and I. C. P. Smith.** 1982. A ^{2}H-NMR study of *Acholeplasma laidlawii* membranes highly enriched in myristic acid. *Biochim. Biophys. Acta* **688**:622–636.

77. **Jarrell, H. C., A. P. Tulloch, and I. C. P. Smith.** 1983. Relative roles of cyclopropane-containing and *cis*-unsaturated fatty acids in determining membrane properties of *Acholeplasma laidlawii*: a deuterium nuclear magnetic resonance study. *Biochemistry* **22**:5611–5619.

78. **Johansson, K.-E., and S. Hjertén.** 1974. Localization of the Tween 20-soluble membrane proteins of *Acholeplasma laidlawii* by crossed immunoelectrophoresis. *J. Mol. Biol.* **86**:341–348.

79. **Johansson, K.-E., C. Jagersten, A. Christiansson, and Å. Wieslander.** 1981. Protein composition and extractibility of lipid-modified membranes from *Acholeplasma laidlawii*. *Biochemistry* **20**:6073–6079.

80. **Jost, P. C., O. H. Griffith, R. A. Capaldi, and G. Vanderkooi.** 1973. Evidence for boundary lipids in membranes. *Proc. Natl. Acad. Sci. USA* **70**:480–486.

81. **Kahane, I., Z. Ne'eman, and S. Razin.** 1973. Divalent cations in native and reaggregated mycoplasma membranes. *J. Bacteriol.* **113**:666–671.

82. **Kang, S.-Y., R. A. Kinsey, S. Rajan, H. S. Gutowsky, M. G. Gabridge, and E. Oldfield.** 1981. Protein-lipid interactions in biological and model membrane systems. Deuterium NMR of *Acholeplasma laidlawii* B, *Escherichia coli*, and cytochrome oxidase systems containing specifically deuterated lipids. *J. Biol. Chem.* **256**: 1155–1159.

83. **Kannenberg, E., A. Blume, R. N. McElhaney, and K. Poralla.** 1983. Monolayer and calorimetric studies of phosphatidylcholines containing branched-chain fatty acids and of their interactions with cholesterol and with a bacterial hopanoid in model membranes. *Biochim. Biophys. Acta* **733**:111–116.

84. **Khan, A., L. Rilfors, Å. Wieslander, and G. Lindblom.** 1981. The effect of cholesterol on the phase structure of glucolipids from *Acholeplasma laidlawii* membranes. *Eur. J. Biochem.* **116**:215–220.

85. **Kinsey, R. A., A. Kintanar, M.-D. Tsai, R. L. Smith, N. Janes, and E. Oldfield.** 1981. First observation of amino acid side chain dynamics in membrane proteins using high field deuterium nuclear magnetic resonance spectroscopy. *J. Biol. Chem.* **256**:4146–4149.

86. **Koblin, D. D., and H. H. Wang.** 1981. Chronic exposure to inhaled anesthetics increases cholesterol content in *Acholeplasma laidlawii*. *Biochim. Biophys. Acta* **649**: 717–725.

87. **Lala, A. K., T. M. Buttke, and K. Bloch.** 1979. On the role of the sterol hydroxyl group in membranes. *J. Biol. Chem.* **254**:10582–10585.

88. **Lange, Y., C. M. Cohen, and M. Poznansky.** 1977. Transmembrane movement of cholesterol in human erythrocytes. *Proc. Natl. Acad. Sci. USA* **74**:1538–1542.

89. **Langworthy, T. A.** 1979. Special features of thermoplasmas, p. 495–513. *In* M. F. Barile and S. Razin (ed.), *The Mycoplasmas*. Academic Press, New York.

90. **Le Grimellec, C., J. Cardinal, M.-C. Giocondi, and S. Carriere.** 1981. Control of membrane lipids in *Mycoplasma gallisepticum*: effect on lipid order. *J. Bacteriol.* **146**:155–162.

91. **Le Grimellec, C., D. Lajeunesse, and J.-L. Rigaud.** 1982. Effects of energization on membrane organization in mycoplasma. *Biochim. Biophys. Acta* **687**:281–290.

92. **Lelong, I., B. Luu, M. Mersel, and S. Rottem.** 1988. Effect of 7β-hydroxycholesterol on growth and membrane composition of *Mycoplasma capricolum*. *FEBS Lett.* **232**:354–358.

93. **Leon, O., and C. Panos.** 1981. Long-chain fatty acid perturbations in *Mycoplasma pneumoniae*. *J. Bacteriol.* **146**:1124–1134.

94. **Lewis, R. N. A. H., D. A. Mannock, and R. N. McElhaney.** 1990. Lamellar to nonlamellar phase transitions of phosphatidylethanolamines and monoglycosyl diacylglycerols. *Zentralbl. Bakteriol. Suppl.* **20**:643–645.

95. **Lewis, R. N. A. H., D. A. Mannock, R. N. McElhaney, D. C. Turner, and S. M. Gruner.** 1989. The effect of fatty acyl chain length and structure on the lamellar gel to liquid-crystalline and lamellar to reversed hexagonal phase transitions of aqueous phosphatidylethanolamine dispersions. *Biochemistry* **28**:541–547.

96. **Lewis, R. N. A. H., and R. N. McElhaney.** 1983. Purification and characterization of the membrane (Na[+] + Mg[2+])-ATPase from *Acholeplasma laidlawii*. *Biochim. Biophys. Acta* **735**:113–122.

97. **Lewis, R. N. A. H., A. W. B. Yue, R. N. McElhaney, D. C. Turner, and S. M. Gruner.** 1990. Thermotropic characterization of the 2-O-acyl, polyprenyl α-D-glucopyranoside isolated from palmitate-enriched *Acholeplasma laidlawii* B membranes. *Biochim. Biophys. Acta* **1026:**21–28.

98. **Lindblom, G., I. Brentel, M. Sjolund, G. Wikander, and Å. Wieslander.** 1986. Phase equilibria of membrane lipids from *Acholeplasma laidlawii*: importance of a single lipid forming nonlamellar phases. *Biochemistry* **25:**7502–7510.

99. **Macdonald, A. G., and A. R. Cossins.** 1983. Effects of pressure and pentanol on the phase transition in the membrane of *Acholeplasma laidlawii* B. *Biochim. Biophys. Acta* **730:**239–244.

100. **Macdonald, P. M., B. McDonough, B. D. Sykes, and R. N. McElhaney.** 1983. ^{19}F-nuclear magnetic resonance studies of lipid fatty acyl chain order and dynamics in *Acholeplasma laidlawii* B membranes. The effects of methyl-branch substitution and of *trans*-unsaturation upon membrane acyl chain orientational order. *Biochemistry* **22:**5103–5111.

101. **Macdonald, P. M., B. D. Sykes, and R. N. McElhaney.** 1984. ^{19}F-nuclear magnetic resonance studies of lipid fatty acyl chain order and dynamics in *Acholeplasma laidlawii* B membranes. ^{19}F NMR line shape and orientational order in the gel state. *Biochemistry* **23:** 4496–4502.

102. **Macdonald, P. M., B. D. Sykes, and R. N. McElhaney.** 1984. Fatty acyl chain structure, orientational order, and the lipid phase transition in *Acholeplasma laidlawii* B membranes. A review of recent ^{19}F nuclear magnetic resonance studies. *Can. J. Biochem. Cell Biol.* **62:** 1134–1150.

103. **Macdonald, P. M., B. D. Sykes, and R. N. McElhaney.** 1984. Calorimetric and spectroscopic studies of lipid hydrocarbon chain order in the *Acholeplasma laidlawii* membrane. *Isr. J. Med. Sci.* **20:**803–806.

104. **Macdonald, P. M., B. D. Sykes, and R. N. McElhaney.** 1985. ^{19}F nuclear magnetic resonance studies of lipid fatty acyl chain order and dynamics in *Acholeplasma laidlawii* B membranes. Orientational order in the presence of positional isomers of *trans*-octadecenoic acid. *Biochemistry* **24:**2237–2245.

105. **Macdonald, P. M., B. D. Sykes, and R. N. McElhaney.** 1985. Fluorine-19 nuclear magnetic resonance studies of lipid fatty acyl chain order and dynamics in *Acholeplasma laidlawii* B membranes. Gel-state disorder in the presence of methyl iso- and anteisobranched chain substituents. *Biochemistry* **24:**2412–2419.

106. **Macdonald, P. M., B. D. Sykes, and R. N. McElhaney.** 1985. Fluorine-19 nuclear magnetic resonance studies of lipid fatty acyl chain order and dynamics in *Acholeplasma laidlawii* B membranes. A direct comparison of the effects of *cis* and *trans* cyclopropane ring and double-bond substituents on orientational order. *Biochemistry* **24:**4651–4659.

107. **Macdonald, P. M., B. D. Sykes, R. N. McElhaney, and F. D. Gunstone.** 1985. ^{19}F nuclear magnetic resonance studies of lipid fatty acyl chain order and dynamics in *Acholeplasma laidlawii* B membranes. Orientational order in the presence of a series of positional isomers of *cis*-octadecenoic acid. *Biochemistry* **24:**177–184.

108. **Maniloff, J., and H. J. Morowitz.** 1972. Cell biology of the mycoplasmas. *Bacteriol. Rev.* **36:**263–290.

109. **Mannock, D. A., R. N. A. H. Lewis, and R. N. McElhaney.** 1990. The physical properties of glycosyl diacylglycerols. 1. Calorimetric studies of a homologous series of 1,2-di-O-acyl-3-O-(α-D-glucopyranosyl)-*sn*-glycerols. *Biochemistry* **29:**7790–7799.

110. **Mannock, D. A., R. N. A. H. Lewis, A. Sen, and R. N. McElhaney.** 1988. The physical properties of glycosyldiacylglycerols. Calorimetric studies of a homologous series of 1,2-di-O-acyl-3-O-(β-D-glucopyranosyl)-*sn*-glycerols. *Biochemistry* **27:**6852–6859.

111. **Mantsch, H. H., P. W. Yang, A. Martin, and D. G. Cameron.** 1988. Infrared spectroscopic studies of *Acholeplasma laidlawii* B membranes. Comparison of the gel to liquid-crystal phase transition in intact cells and isolated membranes. *Eur. J. Biochem.* **178:**335–341.

112. **Marsh, D.** 1985. ESR spin label studies of lipid-protein interactions, p. 143–172. *In* A. Watts and J. J. H. H. M. de Pont (ed.), *Progress in Protein-Lipid Interactions*, vol. 1. Elsevier, Amsterdam.

113. **McDonough, B., P. M. Macdonald, B. D. Sykes, and R. N. McElhaney.** 1983. Fluorine-19 nuclear magnetic resonance studies of lipid fatty acyl chain order and dynamics in *Acholeplasma laidlawii* B membranes. A physical, biochemical and biological evaluation of monofluoropalmitic acids as membrane probes. *Biochemistry* **22:**5097–5103.

114. **McElhaney, R. N.** 1974. The effect of membrane lipid phase transitions on membrane structure and on the growth of *Acholeplasma laidlawii* B. *J. Supramol. Struct.* **2:**617–628.

115. **McElhaney, R. N.** 1974. The effect of alterations in the physical state of the membrane lipids on the ability of *Acholeplasma laidlawii* B to grow at various temperatures. *J. Mol. Biol.* **84:**145–157.

116. **McElhaney, R. N.** 1982. The use of differential scanning calorimetry and differential thermal analysis in studies of model and biological membranes. *Chem. Phys. Lipids* **30:**229–259.

117. **McElhaney, R. N.** 1984. The relationship between membrane lipid fluidity and phase state and the ability of bacteria and mycoplasmas to grow and survive at various temperatures, p. 249–278. *In* M. Kates and L. Masen (ed.), *Biomembranes*, vol. 12. Academic Press, New York.

118. **McElhaney, R. N.** 1984. The structure and function of the *Acholeplasma laidlawii* plasma membrane. *Biochim. Biophys. Acta* **779:**1–42.

119. **McElhaney, R. N.** 1985. Membrane lipid fluidity, phase state and membrane function in prokaryotic microorgansims, p. 147–208. *In* R. A. Aloia and J. M. Boggs (ed.), *Membrane Fluidity in Biology*, vol. 4. Academic Press, New York.

120. **McElhaney, R. N.** 1989. The influence of membrane lipid composition and physical properties on membrane structure and function in *Acholeplasma laidlawii*. *Crit. Rev. Microbiol.* **17:**1–32.

120a. **McElhaney, R. N.** Unpublished data.

121. **McElhaney, R. N., J. de Gier, and L. L. M. van Deenen.** 1970. The effect of alterations in fatty acid composition and cholesterol content on the permeability of *Mycoplasma laidlawii* B cells and derived liposomes. *Biochim. Biophys. Acta* **219:**245–247.

122. **McElhaney, R. N., J. de Gier, and E. C. M. van der Neut-Kok.** 1973. The effect of alterations in fatty acid composition and cholesterol content on the nonelectrolyte permeability of *Acholeplasma laidlawii* B cells and derived liposomes. *Biochim. Biophys. Acta* **298:**500–512.

123. **Melchior, D. L., H. J. Morowitz, J. M. Sturtevant, and T. Y. Tsong.** 1970. Characterization of the plasma membrane of *Mycoplasma laidlawii*. VII. Phase transitions of membrane lipids. *Biochim. Biophys. Acta* **219:**114–122.

124. **Melchior, D. L., F. J. Scavitto, M. T. Walsh, and J. M. Steim.** 1977. Thermal techniques in biomembrane and lipoprotein research. *Thermochim. Acta* **18:**43–71.

125. **Melchior, D. L., and J. M. Steim.** 1977. Control of fatty acid composition of *Acholeplasma laidlawii* membranes. *Biochim. Biophys. Acta* **466:**148–159.

126. **Mendelsohn, R., M. A. Davies, J. W. Brauner, H. F. Schuster, and R. A. Dluhy.** 1989. Quantitative determination of conformational disorder in the acyl chains of

phospholipid bilayers by infrared spectroscopy. *Biochemistry* **28**:8934–8939.

127. **Mersel, M., A. Benenson, and F. Doljanski.** 1976. Lactoperoxidase-catalyzed iodination of surface membrane lipids. *Biochem. Biophys. Res. Commun.* **70**:1166–1171.

128. **Metcalfe, J. C., N. J. M. Birdsall, and A. G. Lee.** 1972. ¹³C NMR spectra of *Acholeplasma* membranes containing ¹³C labelled phospholipids. *FEBS Lett.* **21**:335–340.

129. **Metcalfe, J. C., S. M. Metcalfe, and D. M. Engelman.** 1971. Structural comparisons of native and reaggregated membranes from *Mycoplasma laidlawii* and erythrocytes by X-ray diffraction and nuclear magnetic resonance techniques. *Biochim. Biophys. Acta* **241**:412–421.

130. **Metcalfe, S. M., J. C. Metcalfe, and D. M. Engelman.** 1971. Structural comparisons of native and reaggregated membranes from *Mycoplasma laidlawii* and erythrocytes using a fluorescence probe. *Biochim. Biophys. Acta* **241**:422–430.

131. **Ne'eman, Z., I. Kahane, and S. Razin.** 1971. Characterization of the mycoplasma membrane proteins. II. Solubilization and enzyme activities of *Acholeplasma laidlawii* membrane proteins. *Biochim. Biophys. Acta* **249**:169–176.

132. **Nystrom, S., K.-E. Johansson, and Å. Wieslander.** 1986. Selective acylation of membrane proteins in *Acholeplasma laidlawii.* *Eur. J. Biochem.* **156**:85–94.

133. **Oldfield, E., D. Chapman, and W. Derbyshire.** 1972. Lipid mobility in *Acholeplasma* membranes using deuteron magnetic resonance. *Chem. Phys. Lipids.* **9**:69–81.

134. **Op den Kamp, J. A. F.** 1979. Lipid asymmetry in membranes. *Annu. Rev. Biochem.* **48**:47–71.

135. **Phillips, M. C., W. J. Johnson, and G. H. Rothblat.** 1987. Mechanisms and consequences of cellular cholesterol exchange and transfer. *Biochim. Biophys. Acta* **906**:223–276.

136. **Pink, D. A., and M. J. Zuckerman.** 1980. Lipid chain order in *Acholeplasma laidlawii* membranes. What does ²H-NMR tell us? *FEBS Lett.* **109**:5–8.

137. **Pisetsky, D., and T. M. Terry.** 1972. Are mycoplasma membrane proteins affected by membrane fatty acid composition? *Biochim. Biophys. Acta* **274**:95–104.

138. **Raetz, C. R. H.** 1982. Genetic control of phospholipid bilayer assembly, p. 435–477. *In* J. N. Hawthorne and G. B. Ansell (ed.), *Phospholipids.* Elsevier, Amsterdam.

139. **Rance, M., K. R. Jeffrey, A. P. Tulloch, K. W. Butler, and I. C. P. Smith.** 1980. Orientational order of unsaturated lipids in the membranes of *Acholeplasma laidlawii* as observed by ²H-NMR. *Biochim. Biophys. Acta* **600**:245–262.

140. **Rance, M., K. R. Jeffrey, A. P. Tulloch, K. W. Butler, and I. C. P. Smith.** 1982. Effects of cholesterol on the conformational order of unsaturated lipids in the membranes of *Acholeplasma laidlawii.* *Biochim. Biophys. Acta* **688**:191–200.

141. **Rance, M., I. C. P. Smith, and H. C. Jarrell.** 1983. The effect of headgroup class on the conformation of membrane lipids in *Acholeplasma laidlawii*: a ²H-NMR study. *Chem. Phys. Lipids.* **32**:57–71.

142. **Razin, S.** 1978. Cholesterol uptake is dependent on membrane fluidity in mycoplasmas. *Biochim. Biophys. Acta* **513**:401–404.

143. **Razin, S.** 1979. Membrane proteins, p. 289–322. *In* M. F. Barile and S. Razin (ed.), *The Mycoplasmas.* Academic Press, New York.

144. **Razin, S.** 1979. Isolation and characterization of mycoplasma membranes, p. 213–229. *In* M. F. Barile and S. Razin (ed.), *The Mycoplasmas.* Academic Press, New York.

145. **Razin, S.** 1982. The mycoplasma membrane, p. 165–250. *In* B. K. Ghosh (ed.), *Organization of Prokaryotic Cell Membranes.* CRC Press, Boca Raton, Fla.

146. **Razin, S., S. Kutner, H. Efrati, and S. Rottem.** 1980. Phospholipid and cholesterol uptake by mycoplasma

147. **Razin, S., and S. Rottem.** 1967. Role of carotenoids and cholesterol in the growth of *Mycoplasma laidlawii.* *J. Bacteriol.* **93**:1181–1182.

148. **Reinert, J. C., and J. M. Steim.** 1970. Calorimetric detection of a membrane-lipid phase transition in living cells. *Science* **168**:1580–1582.

149. **Rilfors, L.** 1985. Difference in packing properties between iso and anteiso methyl-branched fatty acids as revealed by incorporation into the membrane lipids of *Acholeplasma laidlawii* strain A. *Biochim. Biophys. Acta* **813**:151–160.

150. **Rilfors, L., G. Lindblom, Å. Wieslander, and A. Christiansson.** 1984. Lipid bilayer stability in biological membranes, p. 205–245. *In* M. Kates and L. A. Mason (ed.), *Membrane Fluidity,* vol. 12. *Biomembranes.* Plenum Press, New York.

151. **Rilfors, L., G. Wikander, and Å. Wieslander.** 1987. Lipid acyl chain-dependent effects of sterols in *Acholeplasma laidlawii* membranes. *J. Bacteriol.* **169**:830–838.

152. **Rodwell, A. W., and J. E. Peterson.** 1971. The effect of straight-chain saturated, monoenoic and branched-chain fatty acids on growth and fatty acid composition of *Mycoplasma* strain Y. *J. Gen. Microbiol.* **68**:173–186.

153. **Rothman, J. E., and J. Lenard.** 1977. Membrane asymmetry. *Science* **195**:743–753.

154. **Rottem, S.** 1975. Heterogeneity in the physical state of the exterior and interior regions of mycoplasma membrane lipids. *Biochem. Biophys. Res. Commun.* **64**:7–12.

155. **Rottem, S.** 1979. Molecular organization of membrane lipids, p. 259–288. *In* M. F. Barile and S. Razin (ed.), *The Mycoplasmas.* Academic Press, New York.

156. **Rottem, S.** 1981. Cholesterol is required to prevent crystallization of *Mycoplasma arginini* phospholipids at physiological temperatures. *FEBS Lett.* **133**:161–164.

157. **Rottem, S., V. P. Cirillo, B. de Kruyff, M. Shinitzky, and S. Razin.** 1973. Cholesterol in mycoplasma membranes. Correlation of enzymic and transport activities with physical state of lipids in membranes of *Mycoplasma mycoides* var. *capri* adapted to grow with low cholesterol concentrations. *Biochim. Biophys. Acta* **323**:509–519.

158. **Rottem, S., W. L. Hubbell, L. Hayflick, and H. M. McConnell.** 1970. Motion of fatty acid spins labels in the plasma membrane of mycoplasma. *Biochim. Biophys. Acta* **219**:104–113.

159. **Rottem, S., and O. Markowitz.** 1979. Carotenoids as reinforcers of the *Acholeplasma laidlawii* lipid bilayer. *J. Bacteriol.* **140**:944–948.

160. **Rottem, S., and S. Razin.** 1967. Uptake and utilization of acetate by mycoplasma. *J. Gen. Microbiol.* **48**:53–63.

161. **Rottem, S., and A. Samuni.** 1973. Effect of proteins on the motion of spin-labeled fatty acids in mycoplasma membranes. *Biochim. Biophys. Acta* **298**:32–38.

162. **Rottem, S., D. Shinar, and R. Bittman.** 1981. Symmetrical distribution and rapid transbilayer movement of cholesterol in *Mycoplasma gallisepticum* cell membranes. *Biochim. Biophys. Acta* **649**:572–580.

163. **Rottem, S., G. M. Slutzky, and R. Bittman.** 1978. Cholesterol distribution and movement in the *Mycoplasma gallisepticum* cell membrane. *Biochemistry* **17**:2723–2726.

164. **Rottem, S., and A. J. Verkleij.** 1982. Possible association of segregated lipid domains of *Mycoplasma gallisepticum* membranes with cell resistance to osmotic lysis. *J. Bacteriol.* **149**:338–345.

165. **Rottem, S., J. Yashouv, Z. Ne'eman, and S. Razin.** 1973. Composition, ultrastructure and biological properties of membranes from *Mycoplasma mycoides* var. *capri* cells adapted to grow with low cholesterol concentrations. *Biochim. Biophys. Acta* **323**:495–508.

166. **Saito, Y., and R. N. McElhaney.** 1977. Membrane lipid

Column 1 ending and column 2 continuation:

cells and membranes. *Biochim. Biophys. Acta* **598**:628–640.

biosynthesis in *Acholeplasma laidlawii* B: incorporation of exogenous fatty acids into membrane glyco- and phospholipids by growing cells. *J. Bacteriol.* **132**:485–496.

167. Saito, Y., J. R. Silvius, and R. N. McElhaney. 1977. Membrane lipid biosynthesis in *Acholeplasma laidlawii* B: de novo biosynthesis of saturated fatty acids by growing cells. *J. Bacteriol.* **132**:497–504.

168. Saito, Y., J. R. Silvius, and R. N. McElhaney. 1978. Membrane lipid biosynthesis in *Acholeplasma laidlawii* B: the chain elongation of medium- and long-chain exogenous fatty acids by growing cells. *J. Bacteriol.* **133**:66–74.

169. Schiefer, H.-G., H. Krauss, H. Brunner, and U. Gerhardt. 1976. Ultrastructural visualization of anionic sites on mycoplasma membranes by polycationic ferritin. *J. Bacteriol.* **127**:461–468.

170. Schindler, P. R. G., and M. Teuber. 1975. Differential fluorescence labelling with 5-dimethyl-aminonaphthalene-1-sulfonyl chloride of intact cells and isolated membranes in *Salmonella typhimurium* and *Acholeplasma laidlawii*. *Arch. Microbiol.* **102**:29–33.

171. Schreier, S., C. F. Polnaszek, and I. C. P. Smith. 1978. Spin labels in membranes. Problems in practice. *Biochim. Biophys. Acta* **515**:395–436.

172. Schuldiner, S., and H. R. Kaback. 1977. Fluorescent galactosides as probes for the *lac* carrier protein. *Biochim. Biophys. Acta* **472**:399–418.

173. Seddon, J. M., G. Cevc, and D. Marsh. 1983. Calorimetric studies of the gel-fluid (L_β-L_α) and lamellar-inverted hexogonal (L_α-H_{II}) phase transitions in dialkyl- and diacylphosphatidylethanolamines. *Biochemistry* **22**:1280–1289.

174. Seelig, J., and P. M. Macdonald. 1987. Phospholipids and proteins in biological membranes. ^{2}H NMR as a method to study structure, dynamics, and interactions. *Acc. Chem. Res.* **20**:221–228.

175. Seelig, J., and A. Seelig. 1980. Lipid conformation in model membranes and biological membranes. *Q. Rev. Biophys.* **13**:19–61.

176. Seguin, C., R. N. A. H. Lewis, H. H. Mantsch, and R. N. McElhaney. 1987. Calorimetric studies of the thermotropic phase behavior of cells, membranes and lipids from fatty acid-homogeneous *Acholeplasma laidlawii* B. *Isr. J. Med.* **23**:403–407.

177. Sen, A., and S.-W. Hui. 1989. Effects of lipid packing on polymorphic phase behavior and membrane proteins. *Proc. Natl. Acad. Sci. USA* **86**:5825–5829.

178. Sen, A., S.-W. Hui, D. A. Mannock, R. N. A. H. Lewis, and R. N. McElhaney. 1990. The physical properties of glycosyl diacylglycerols. 2. X-ray diffraction studies of a homologous series of 1,2-di-O-acyl-3-O-(α-D-glycopyranosyl)-sn-glycerols. *Biochemistry* **29**:7799–7804.

179. Shinitzky, M., and Y. Barenholz. 1978. Fluidity parameters determined by fluorescence polarization. *Biochim. Biophys. Acta* **515**:367–394.

180. Silvius, J. R., N. Mak, and R. N. McElhaney. 1980. Lipid and protein composition and thermotropic lipid phase transitions in fatty acid-homogeneous membranes of *Acholeplasma laidlawii* B. *Biochim. Biophys. Acta* **597**:199–215.

181. Silvius, J. R., N. Mak, and R. N. McElhaney. 1980. Why do prokaryotes regulate membrane fluidity?, p. 213–221. *In* M. Kates and A. Kuksis (ed.), *Control of Membrane Lipid Fluidity*. Humana Press, Clifton, N.J.

182. Silvius, J. R., and R. N. McElhaney. 1978. Growth and membrane lipid properties of *Acholeplasma laidlawii* B lacking fatty acid heterogeneity. *Nature* (London) **272**:645–646.

183. Silvius, J. R., and R. N. McElhaney. 1978. Lipid compositional manipulation in *Acholeplasma laidlawii* B. Effect of exogenous fatty acids on fatty acid composition

and cell growth when endogenous fatty acid production is inhibited. *Can. J. Biochem.* **56**:462–469.

184. Silvius, J. R., and R. N. McElhaney. 1980. Membrane lipid physical state and modulation of the (Na$^+$,Mg^{2+})-ATPase activity in *Acholeplasma laidlawii* B. *Proc. Natl. Acad. Sci. USA* **77**:1255–1259.

185. Sinensky, M. 1974. Homeoviscous adaptation—a homeostatic process that regulates the viscosity of membrane lipids in *Escherichia coli*. *Proc. Natl. Acad. Sci. USA* **71**:522–525.

186. Singer, S. J., and G. L. Nicolson. 1972. The fluid mosaic model of the structure of cell membranes. *Science* **175**:720–731.

187. Smith, I. C. P., K. W. Butler, A. P. Tulloch, J. H. Davis, and M. Bloom. 1979. The properties of gel state lipid in membranes of *Acholeplasma laidlawii* as observed by ^{2}H NMR. *FEBS Lett.* **100**:57–61.

188. Smith, I. C. P., and H. C. Jarrell. 1983. Deuterium and phosphorus NMR of microbial membranes. *Acc. Chem. Res.* **16**:266–272.

189. Steim, J. M., M. E. Tourtellotte, J. C. Reinert, R. N. McElhaney, and R. L. Rader. 1969. Calorimetric evidence for the liquid-crystalline state of lipids in a biomembrane. *Proc. Natl. Acad. Sci. USA* **63**:104–109.

190. Stockton, G. W., K. G. Johnson, K. W. Butler, C. F. Ponaszek, R. Cyr, and I. C. P. Smith. 1975. Molecular order in *Acholeplasma laidlawii* membranes as determined by deuterium magnetic resonance of biosynthetically-incorporated specifically-labelled lipids. *Biochim. Biophys. Acta* **401**:535–539.

191. Stockton, G. W., K. G. Johnson, K. W. Butler, A. P. Tulloch, Y. Boulanger, I. C. P. Smith, J. H. Davis, and M. Bloom. 1977. Deuterium NMR study of lipid organization in *Acholeplasma laidlawii* membranes. *Nature* (London) **269**:267–268.

192. Surewicz, W. K., and H. H. Mantsch. 1988. New insight into protein secondary structure from resolution-enhanced infrared spectra. *Biochim. Biophys. Acta* **952**:115–130.

193. Terry, T. M., and J. S. Zupnik. 1973. Weak association of glucosamine-containing polymer with the *Acholeplasma laidlawii* membrane. *Biochim. Biophys. Acta* **291**:144–148.

194. Tillack, T. W., R. Carter, and S. Razin. 1970. Native and reformed *Mycoplasma laidlawii* membranes compared by freeze-etching. *Biochim. Biophys. Acta* **219**:123–130.

195. Tourtellotte, M. E., D. Branton, and A. Keith. 1970. Membrane structure: spin labeling and freeze-etching of *Mycoplasma laidlawii*. *Proc. Natl. Acad. Sci. USA* **66**:909–916.

196. Tourtellotte, M. E., and J. S. Zupnick. 1973. Freeze-fractured *Acholeplasma laidlawii* membranes: nature of particles observed. *Science* **179**:84–86.

197. Verkleij, A. J., P. H. J. T. Ververgaert, L. L. M. van Deenen, and P. F. Elbers. 1972. Phase transitions of phospholipid bilayers and membranes of *Acholeplasma laidlawii* B visualized by freeze fracturing electron microscopy. *Biochim. Biophys. Acta* **288**:326–332.

198. Wallace, B. A., and D. M. Engelman. 1978. The planar distributions of surface proteins and intramembrane particles in *Acholeplasma laidlawii* are differently affected by the physical state of membrane lipids. *Biochim. Biophys. Acta* **508**:431–449.

199. Wallace, B. A., F. M. Richards, and D. M. Engelman. 1976. The influence of lipid state on the planar distribution of membrane proteins in *Acholeplasma laidlawii*. *J. Mol. Biol.* **107**:255–269.

200. Wieslander, Å., A. Christiansson, L. Rilfors, A. Khan, L. B.-A. Johansson, and G. Lindblom. 1980. Lipid bilayer stability in membranes. Regulation of lipid composition in *Acholeplasma laidlawii* as governed by molecular shape. *Biochemistry* **19**:3650–3655.

201. Wieslander, Å., A. Christiansson, L. Rilfors, A. Khan, L.

B.-A. Johansson, and G. Lindblom. 1981. Lipid phase structure governs the regulation of lipid composition in membranes from *Acholeplasma laidlawii*. *FEBS Lett.* **124**:273–278.

202. Wieslander, Å., and L. Rilfors. 1977. Qualitative and quantitative variations of membrane lipid species in *Acholeplasma laidlawii* A. *Biochim. Biophys. Acta* **466**:336–346.

203. Wieslander, Å., L. Rilfors, A. Dahlqvist, J. Jonsson, S. Hellberg, S. Rannar, M. Sjostrom, and G. Lindblom. In preparation.

204. Wieslander, Å., L. Rilfors, L. B.-A. Johansson, and G. Lindblom. 1981. Reversed cubic phase with membrane glucolipids from *Acholeplasma laidlawii*. ¹H, ²H, and diffusion nuclear magnetic resonance measurements. *Biochemistry* **20**:730–735.

205. Wieslander, Å., L. Rilfors, and G. Lindblom. 1986. Metabolic changes in membrane lipid composition in *Acholeplasma laidlawii* by hydrocarbons, alcohols, and detergents: arguments for effects on lipid packing. *Biochemistry* **25**:7511–7517.

206. Wieslander, Å., and E. Selstam. 1987. Acyl-chain-dependent incorporation of chlorophyll and cholesterol in membranes of *Acholeplasma laidlawii*. *Biochim. Biophys. Acta* **901**:250–254.

207. Wieslander, Å., J. Ulmius, G. Lindblom, and K. Fontell. 1978. Water binding and phase structures for different *Acholeplasma laidlawii* membrane lipids studied by deuteron nuclear magnetic resonance and X-ray diffraction. *Biochim. Biophys. Acta* **512**:241–253.

208. Wong, P. T. T., D. J. Siminovitch, and H. H. Mantsch. 1988. Structure and properties of model membranes: new knowledge from high-pressure vibrational spectroscopy. *Biochim. Biophys. Acta* **947**:139–171.

209. Yager, P., and E. L. Chang. 1983. Destabilization of a lipid non-bilayer phase by high pressure. *Biochim. Biophys. Acta* **731**:491–494.

210. Yue, A. W. B., R. N. A. H. Lewis, M. Monck, P. R. Cullis, and R. N. McElhaney. The effect of variations in fatty acyl chain length and structure on lipid polar headgroup composition in *Acholeplasma laidlawii* B membranes. *Biochim. Biophys. Acta*, submitted for publication.

9. Genome Structure and Organization

RICHARD HERRMANN

INTRODUCTION

In general, the essential genetic information of bacteria is contained in one circular double-stranded DNA molecule. So far, only a few exceptions have been reported. For instance, *Borrelia burgdorferi* seems to have a linear double-stranded genome (37), and *Rhodobacter spheroides* carries two different circular double-stranded chromosomes, both of which code for important information such as rRNA genes (98), but it has not been proven that both are indeed essential for survival.

The sizes of bacterial genomes vary considerably, ranging from 600 to 13,000 kbp (31, 43, 95). Until recently, the separation and size determination of DNA molecules larger than 50 kbp were laborious procedures. Development of the technique of pulsed-field gel electrophoresis (PFGE) (16, 87), which permits the separation of linear DNA molecules of up to several thousand kilobase pairs, initiated numerous new research activities in this area and led to the size determination of many bacterial genomes (Table 1) and to the construction of an increasing number of physical and genetic maps (89). In addition, refined cloning techniques and improvements in DNA sequencing technology will provide DNA sequences of complete bacterial genomes in the near future (4, 25, 40, 91, 94).

The mollicutes, possessing the smallest bacterial genomes known, are particularly suited for such analyses (Table 1). Members of this class have been divided into two genome size clusters, one composed of the genera *Mycoplasma* and *Ureaplasma*, with genomes of about 700 to 800 kbp, and the other composed of the genera *Acholeplasma*, *Spiroplasma*, and *Anaeroplasma*, with genomes about twice that size but displaying no genome with an intermediate size (60, 77).

In addition to their small genome size, the wide distribution of the mollicutes in nature, the parasitism of individual species with quite different hosts, and therefore their independent development under diverging conditions make these organisms ideal candidates for comparative studies. Besides answering the question of the minimal genetic constitution of a self-replicating cell (59), we expect to begin to understand evolutionary processes, such as the acquisition or loss of species-specific features during development, by analyzing different mollicutes species which live in similar habitats, such as *Mycoplasma pneumoniae* and *M. genitalium*, but differ in genome size by 200 kbp and also in G + C content (Table 2), and we also hope to determine the genetic differences between strains of the same species, such as *Ureaplasma urealyticum*, which differ considerably in genome size (80). Finally, by comparing genetic maps or partially sequenced genomes, we will have a much better basis for evaluating phylogeny, since we will not have to rely only on DNA sequences of a few selected conserved genes such as rRNA genes (102). Further, we can investigate an additional spectrum of parameters, such as gene placement on the chromosome, in correlation with a nonrandom G + C distribution which is suggested by a nonstatistical distribution of recognition sites for restriction endonucleases (27, 71) or the conservation of mechanisms regulating the organized expression of genes or operons, which have to function in a certain order.

This review of characterization of mollicutes genomes deals with the following topics: (i) base compositions, (ii) size and complexity, (iii) physical maps, (iv) genome stability, and (v) genetic maps. Extrachromosomal DNA elements such as plasmids and viral DNAs are discussed in chapter 3. As supplements to this review, the reader is referred to publications which also deal with the topic of mollicutes genome organization but with different emphases (12, 74, 75) and to the review by Krawiec and Riley, which summarizes present knowledge on the organization of bacterial chromosomes (52).

Richard Herrmann • Microbiology (ZMBH), University of Heidelberg, Im Neuenheimer Feld 282, 6900 Heidelberg, Germany.

Table 1. Examples of bacterial genome sizes determined by PFGE

Bacterial species	Size (10^6 bp)	Reference(s)
Mycoplasma genitalium G-37	0.6	31, 95
M. pneumoniae M129	0.8	51
Borrelia burgdorferi B31[a]	0.95	37
M. hyopneumoniae ATCC 25095	1.07	80
M. mycoides subsp. mycoides GC 1176-2	1.3	70, 80
Chlamydia trachomatis L2	1.45	39
Acholeplasma laidlawii A	1.6	62
Campylobacter jejuni 81116	1.7	63
Rickettsiella melolanthae	1.72	39
Haemophilus influenzae RdKW22	1.84	54
Methanococcus voltae PS	1.9	88
Rhodobacter sphaeroides 2.4.1[b]	3 / 0.9	98
Clostridium perfringens CPN50	3.58	15
Escherichia coli K-12	4.7	90
Bacillus cereus ATCC 10987	5.7	49
Pseudomonas aeruginosa PAO	5.94	81
Anabaena sp. strain PCC7120	6.37	8
Myxococcus xanthus DK 101	9.45	19

[a] Linear genome.
[b] Two genomes.

CHARACTERIZATION OF MOLLICUTES GENOMES

Base Composition

Besides their small size, mollicutes genomes are characterized by a low G+C content, which is below 30 mol% for most species. There are only a few species with a G+C content above 30 mol%, *M. pneumoniae* being the species with the highest value (41 mol%) (77) (Table 2). In the context of this review, the G+C content of individual species is of interest because of a suggestion that possible errors in molecular weight determination might be attributed to differences in G+C content (57).

Size and Complexity

Several techniques have been used to determine the sizes of mollicutes genomes. The former method of choice, DNA thermal renaturation kinetics (7, 41, 105), has now been replaced by PFGE (16, 87). Separation of DNA molecules by PFGE is achieved by subjecting the molecules to electric fields in alternating orientations. There are several modifications of the original PFGE technique. They all operate by the same principle but vary with respect to the way the alternating electric field is set up: field inversion gel electrophoresis (FIGE) (18), orthogonal-field-alternation gel electrophoresis, rotatory pulsed-field gel electrophoresis, and contour-clamped homogeneous electrical fields

(24) (for a summary, see reference 16). Among these modifications, the FIGE system must be used with caution for DNA size determination because it has been shown that in this system, DNA fragments do not always migrate according to size (18, 36).

The only precondition for DNA size analyses by PFGE is that the DNA must be linear in order to be separated according to size. Circular genomes can be linearized by partial digestion with infrequently cutting restriction endonucleases or by controlled gamma irradiation (67). Alternatively, genomes are digested to completion with a suitable restriction endonuclease, and the sizes of the individual fragments are determined by agarose gel electrophoresis and added up to obtain the total genome size.

The sizes of only a few mollicutes genomes have been calculated by methods other than DNA renaturation kinetics or PFGE. A rather elegant method of size determination is two-dimensional fingerprinting, whereby large DNAs are digested with a restriction endonuclease and the resulting fragments are separated by agarose gel electrophoresis. To generate a two-dimensional pattern, the agarose gel lane containing the separated DNA fragments is either placed on the top of an acrylamide gel containing a denaturant gradient or treated with a second endonuclease and placed on top of a second agarose gel. After electrophoresis perpendicular to the first dimension, a two-dimensional pattern of DNA fragments is generated, which can be used to calculate sizes of total bacterial genomes (68, 69, 109).

In a few instances, DNA size has been determined by electron microscopic contour length measurements (11, 33, 84, 100) or by conventional one-dimensional agarose gel electrophoresis of cloned (104) or native genomic (33) DNA. Neither method is very useful for routine genome analyses, either because of the expensive equipment and the tedious preparation of suitable samples of genomic DNA or because of the limited resolution of the one-dimensional gel electrophoresis, which requires that a genome be cleaved and separated in fragments smaller than 60 kbp. Recently, for the size determination of plant-pathogenic mycoplasmalike organisms, a method was applied (55) which compares fluorescence intensities of ethidium bromide-stained single-copy DNA restriction fragments of a genome with a known size with the intensities of an equivalent DNA fragment of a genome of an unknown size. The relative fluorescence intensities of these fragments should be inversely proportional to the relative genome size (108).

The sizes of mollicutes genomes determined by the aforementioned methods are summarized in Table 2. An evaluation of these results shows that with different methods, the same or similar apparent sizes were obtained for several strains (e.g., *M. hominis*, *M. orale*, *M. pneumoniae*, and *Acholeplasma laidlawii*), with an acceptable range of about 15%. On the other hand, there are values which are so far off that one has to question the method itself, whether the technique was properly executed in a particular case, or whether there are features of some of these genomes which make one of the methods preferable (see, for example, data for *M. bovirhinis*, *M. bovis*, *M. capricolum*, *M. fermentans*, and *M. gallisepticum* in Table 2). A priori, there is no obvious reason for the different results.

Table 2. Apparent sizes and G + C contents of mollicutes genomes

Organism	Genome size (kbp)[a]				Mol% G + C[b]
	PFGE	Renaturation kinetics	Electron microscopy	Other methods	
Mycoplasma					
agalactiae PG2		712 (5)			30.5–34.2
alkalescens PG51		742 (5)			25.9
arginini	735 (62)	606 (5)			27.6–28.6
arginini R16	685 (9)				
arthritidis PG6		667 (7)			30.0–32.6
bovigenitalium PG11		606 (5)			28.1–30.4
bovirhinis	955 (62)	666 (5)			24.5–27.3
bovis Donetta	1,080 (62)	666 (5)			27.8–32.9
capricolum California kid	1,120 (62)		1,020 (84)	724[c] (69)	24.1–25.5
	1,070 (107)				
dispar 462/2		803 (5)			28.5–29.3
edwardii PG24	980 (62)				29.2
ellychniae		585			
felis CO	1,055 (62)				25.2
fermentans GII	1,160 (62)				27.5–28.7
fermentans PG18		727 (7)			
fermentans	1,245 (9)				
flocculare ATCC 27716	890 (80)				
gallinarum		727 (5)			26.5–28.0
gallisepticum PG31	1,050 (70)	742 (7)			31.8–35.7
gallisepticum	1,170 (62)				
gallisepticum S6	1,435 (9)				
gallisepticum 5969	1,340 (9)				
gateae		667 (5)			28.5
genitalium G-37	600 (31)				32.5 (101)
	577–590 (95)				
hominis H39				773 (11)	27.3–33.7
hominis PG21	684 (62)	682 (7)			
hominis ATCC 14027	720 (80)				
hominis H34	745 (9)				
hominis K	635 (9)				
hyopneumoniae	1,070 (62)				
hyopneumoniae	1,140 (70)				
hyopneumoniae ATCC 25095	1,070 (80)				
hyorhinis ATCC 25021			818 (33)		27.3–27.8
			667 (100)		
hyorhinis BTS-7	610 (9)				
iowae 695	1,280 (70)				25
	1,315 (62)				
meleagridis 529		636 (1)			27.0–28.6
mobile ATCC 43663			780[d] (10)		
mustelae	895 (62)				
mycoides subsp. *capri* PG3		758 (5)			
mycoides subsp. *mycoides* PG1	1,280 (72)	760 (5)			26.2–27.1
mycoides subsp. *mycoides* KH₃	1,280 (72)				
mycoides subsp. *mycoides* Glysdale	1,260 (72)				
mycoides subsp. *mycoides* V5	1,230 (72)				
mycoides subsp. *mycoides* Y	1,240 (70)				
	1,180 (80)				
mycoides subsp. *mycoides* GC 1176-2	1,330 (70)				
	1,350 (80)				
neurolyticum A	1,075 (62)				22.8–26.2
orale	732 (62)				24.0–28.2
orale I (Patt)		712 (7)			
orale CH 19299	675 (9)				
Strain PG50	1,040 (72)	848 (5)			
pneumoniae MAC		727 (7)			
pneumoniae M129	785 (51)			840[e] (104)	
pneumoniae FH	840 (62)				
pullorum	995 (62)				29
pulmonis PG34	950 (62)				27.5–29.2
salivarium PG20		712 (7)			27.3–31.4
salivarium VV		636 (58)			
salivarium PG20	905 (9)				
synoviae WVU	900 (70)				34.2

(Continued)

Table 2. Apparent sizes and G + C contents of mollicutes genomes (*continued*)

Organism	Genome size (kbp)[a]				Mol% G + C[b]
	PFGE	Renaturation kinetics	Electron microscopy	Other methods	
Ureaplasma					
Human sources					
urealyticum T-960	910 (62)				26.9–28.0
T-strain no. 27 Ford		712 (7)			
T-strain no. 58 Ford		667 (7)			
urealyticum T-960 (ATCC 27618)	900 (70)				
urealyticum 7	760 (80)				
urealyticum 27	760 (80)				
urealyticum Pi	760 (80)				
urealyticum U26	760 (80)				
urealyticum 23	880 (80)				
urealyticum 58	910 (80)				
urealyticum 354 (NIH)	1,140 (80)				
urealyticum Co	880 (80)				
urealyticum T-960 (CX8)	890 (80)				
urealyticum Vancouver	950 (80)				
urealyticum S.F.	840 (80)				
urealyticum Western	890 (80)				
urealyticum U24	870 (80)				
urealyticum U38	900 (80)				
Animal sources					
diversum 2065-B	850 (79)				
diversum 1763	940 (79)				
diversum 95	940 (79)				
gallorale D6-1	730 (79)				
felinum FT2-B	1,140 (79)				
Strain CH3	850 (79)				
Strain PR-1	880 (79)				
Strain PR-2	860 (79)				
Strain 1625	850 (79)				
Strain 1202	850 (80)				
Strain 651	1,150 (80)				
Strain D6P	860 (80)				
Spiroplasma					24–30 (14)
apis B31	1,660 (14)				29–31
apis PPS1	1,568 (14)				
apis	1,700 (13)				
citri R8A2 (ATCC 27556)	1,379 (14)				25–27
	1,455–1,621 (85)				
citri ATCC 27665	1,379 (14)				
citri IB AS576	1,818 (53)				
citri IC I-747	1,363 (53)				
citri	1,400 (13)				
floricola 23-6	1,674 (14)				25
	2,575 (53)				
melliferum BC-3	1,342 (14)				27
Flower spiroplasma SR3	2,121 (53)				
Flower spiroplasma PPS1	1,530 (53)				
Leafhopper spiroplasma I-25	1,638 (14)				26
Acholeoplasma					
axanthum B 107 PA		1,621 (85)			31
		1,500 (5)			
granularum (Friend)		1,439 (7)			30.5–32.4
hippikon	1,540 (62)				
laidlawii A	1,600 (62)	1,682 (85)			31.7–35.7
laidlawii A (F1)		1,667 (7)			
laidlawii B	1,650 (80)				
laidlawii B (F8)		1,515 (7)			
laidlawii JA1				1,705[f] (68)	
				1,646[c] (69)	
laidlawii K2				1,483[f] (68)	
laidlawii PG8	1,580 (80)				
laidlawii FHM	1,525 (9)				
laidlawii A	1,640 (9)				
modicum PG49		1,500 (5)			29.3

(*Continued*)

Table 2. Apparent sizes and G+C contents of mollicutes genomes (*Continued*)

| Organism | Genome size (kbp)[a] | | | | Mol% G+C[b] |
	PFGE	Renaturation kinetics	Electron microscopy	Other methods	
MLOs[g]					
Oenothera MLO				1,050[h] (55)	
Beet leafhopper-transmitted virescence agent	660 (46)				
Severe western aster yellows agent	1,185 (46)				

[a] The average molecular weight of one base pair is 660. References are in parentheses.
[b] From reference 78 unless otherwise indicated by reference numbers in parentheses.
[c] Two-dimensional denaturing gradient gel electrophoresis.
[d] Two-dimensional FIGE.
[e] Combination of conventional agarose gel electrophoresis and FIGE, completely cloned genome.
[f] Two-dimensional fingerprinting.
[g] MLOs, mycoplasmalike organisms.
[h] Comparison of fluorescence intensities of restriction fragments.

However, it appears that in all but one case, the genome sizes derived from renaturation kinetics were smaller than those determined by PFGE. This difference is particularly pronounced for chromosomes with a PFGE-determined apparent size of between 900 and 1,200 kbp. Unfortunately, the publications on DNA renaturation kinetics-derived sizes of mollicutes genomes are often not detailed enough for a critical comparison. An exception is the genome size calculations for spiroplasmas by Bové et al. (12), which give much informative experimental data concerning reproducibility and margin of error. The authors demonstrate that the results obtained with the same strain fluctuate considerably from experiment to experiment. In contrast, PFGE-derived size determinations are reproducible and can be easily judged by the quality of the gel, which shows the widths of the DNA bands and the pattern of an appropriate DNA size marker, such as linear phage λ DNA polymers, showing the optimal resolution zone and therefore the limits of separation of a given gel.

The discrepancies between PFGE- and DNA renaturation kinetics-derived genome sizes caused some concern, and the validity of PFGE was questioned (57). It was argued that DNA migration in PFGE might be influenced (slowed down) by a low G+C content, simulating that of larger DNA fragment sizes. Further, it has been observed that for reasons not understood, some DNA fragments seem to migrate not according to their size or to migrate differently with respect to other fragments under various electrophoretic conditions (18, 36). The first argument could be refuted by experiments showing that there is no correlation between genome size and G+C content in mollicutes (62, 80). The latter argument is impossible to counter unless the real size of a fragment in question has been established by DNA sequencing, the only precise method. But this objection is valid for all of the other techniques as well. The good agreement between PFGE-based size calculations, derived either from linear full-length genomes or from adding up the sizes of individual restriction fragments, makes it unlikely that structural peculiarities like DNA bending (42) play a crucial role in the above-mentioned instances. There are, of course, a number of trivial explanations

for the observed differences, such as that the same strains of a species may have not been compared. The importance of this point is well documented by the results on genome size determination of ureaplasmas (80). Significant genome size differences exist within individual strains of the species *U. urealyticum*, ranging from 740 to 1,140 kbp, and the genome sizes of a given strain from different sources varied from 890 to 1,140 kbp (78a, 80). Another source of error might be that a genome contains repetitive DNA sequences, as shown for *M. flocculare*, *M. hyopneumoniae*, *M. hyorhinis* (38, 99), *M. pneumoniae* (30, 44, 83, 96, 103), and some *Spiroplasma* species (64). It has been calculated that about 6% of the *M. pneumoniae* genome is represented by multiple copies of four different repetitive DNA sequences (83). Similar results have been obtained for a repeated sequence in *M. hyorhinis* (38). Unfortunately, it is not known whether the strains showing large genome size differences contain repetitive DNA sequences. Therefore, it is still an open question whether the lower values of DNA renaturation kinetics-derived genome sizes can be attributed to repetitive DNA sequences.

It should also be mentioned that, depending on the methods, discrepancies in genome size determinations are quite common; for instance, DNA renaturation kinetics-derived data differ considerably from PFGE-derived sizes (Table 1) for *Myxococcus xanthus* (5.2×10^6 bp) (108), *Methanococcus voltae* (2.7×10^6 bp) (47), *Escherichia coli* (3.8×10^6 bp) (41), and *Chlamydia trachomatis* (0.6×10^6 to 0.85×10^6 bp) (45).

In conclusion, although the theory of PFGE has not been worked out, the many data on DNA size determination for many bacterial genomes from different laboratories leave no doubt that PFGE (if properly performed) is at least as reliable as DNA renaturation kinetics for calculating DNA fragment sizes. Therefore, the lesson from the PFGE-derived data is that mollicutes genomes do not fall into the two size clusters of 700 to 800 and 1,500 to 1,600 kbp as the early data indicated (60, 77); instead, any size between 600 and 1,700 kbp can be found in nature, as was first shown by Pyle et al. (70) and confirmed and extended by other investigators, mainly Robertson et al. (80) and Neimark and Lange (62). As a consequence of these results, genome size should not be considered a criterion for assigning a strain to any of the genera of the class *Mollicutes*.

Physical Maps

A physical map of a bacterial genome is presented in most cases as a map of restriction endonuclease cleavage sites or, in rare instances, as a collection of overlapping or adjacent clones in plasmids, cosmids, or λ phages, as is the map of *E. coli* (48). For the construction of a bacterial restriction map, one usually starts with a restriction endonuclease which cuts the genome 10 to 50 times. The resulting individual restriction fragments then have to be linked by standard techniques, such as multiple digestions with different enzymes, cloning of linking DNA fragments, or two-dimensional agarose electrophoresis as applied by Bautsch for constructing a map of *M. mobile* (10).

The advantage of this kind of restriction map is the ease of the procedure; the disadvantage is the relatively limited resolution. For instance, a mollicutes genome 1,000 kbp long with 20 restriction sites will give a mean resolution of about 50 kbp. Such maps might be improved by mapping sites of transposon insertions, which will give additional reference points on the genome (106).

A far better resolution can be achieved if a genome is represented by a complete ordered gene bank consisting of plasmids, cosmids, or λ phages (48, 104). Cloning of the genome in a cosmid provides better resolution, which can be improved further by subdividing the individual cosmid or λ phage DNA of a gene bank by restriction analysis. This approach is more time-consuming, requires cloning of a complete genome, and anticipates that the genome of choice can be cloned. Cloning could become a problem if the DNA of interest cannot be maintained in stable clones, as has been reported for *Spiroplasma* DNA (13). The reason for this instability is not known, but it might have to do with the difference in G + C content between the host DNA (*E. coli* DNA is 48 to 52 mol% G + C) and the mollicutes DNA (25 to 30 mol% G + C).

Table 3 summarizes the restriction maps of the mollicutes genomes that have been published. Discussion of this section and of the following sections on genome

stability and genome maps will be combined at the end of the latter section.

Genome Stability

Under the assumption that genomes of different strains of a species are derived from a common ancestor, the actual degree of sequence homology between them could be used as a measure of genome stability. It has been shown by immunological, physiological, and biochemical criteria (including DNA-DNA and DNA-RNA hybridization) that mollicute species display various degrees of intraspecies homogeneity (74, 75). Of course, the most meaningful criterion would be direct comparison between genomic DNA sequences, but we are not yet in a position to do this on a routine basis. Sequencing of a bacterial genome still requires an exceptional effort. A rather simple substitution for direct sequence analysis is comparison of restriction maps or of restriction endonuclease fragment patterns as they appear in an agarose gel after electrophoresis. Both serve as qualitative indicators of relatedness between strains of a species and of genome stability. The restriction pattern might be altered either because restriction sites were gained or lost by a single-base mutation or as a consequence of structural changes like inversion, deletion, insertion, gene amplification, or gene conversion.

All of these events may occur in mollicutes. The presence of numerous repetitive DNA sequences and the occurrence of two rRNA operons in some mollicute strains (2) indicate that these elements are still potential substrates for structural changes by recombinational processes.

It is obvious by this type of approach that only genomes with a high degree of homology and/or similar restriction patterns can be compared. Comparative restriction fragment analysis has been successfully applied to a number of mollicutes genomes (for a summary, see reference 75); for instance, spiroplasmas could be distinguished on the basis of DNA fragment profiles, which were specific and largely identical for strains of a given subgroup (*Spiroplasma citri*, *S. apis*, and *S. floricola*) but different for strains of different subgroups (12, 14). Darai et al. (33) studied several *M. hyorhinis* strains, and Razin (75) confirmed the data

Table 3. Physical and genetic maps of mollicutes genomes

Species	Genome size (10^6 bp)	No. of restriction sites mapped	No. of other mapped loci	Reference
Mycoplasma capricolum California kid	1.07	28	16	107
M. genitalium G37	0.6	18	4	31
M. mobile	0.78	19		10
Mycoplasma strain PG50	1.05	13	8	72
M. mycoides subsp. *mycoides* Y	1.2	32	11	71
M. mycoides subsp. *mycoides* PG1	1.28	16	9	72
M. mycoides subsp. *mycoides* KH₃	1.28	16	10	72
M. mycoides subsp. *mycoides* Glysdale	1.26	16	10	72
M. mycoides subsp. *mycoides* V5	1.24	16	9	72
M. pneumoniae M129	0.79	13	4	51
M. pneumoniae M129	0.8–0.85	25		104
Ureaplasma urealyticum T-960	0.9	29	2	27

derived from immunological and biochemical studies that ureaplasmas should be divided into two clusters and that *M. pneumoniae* seems to be a very homogeneous species (78). Similar studies on *M. hominis* also showed genome variation (23).

In the examples cited above, the restriction fragment patterns were compared after the individual DNA bands had been visualized by staining with ethidium bromide. This approach has only a limited sensitivity, because in order to recognize individual DNA bands in a stained agarose gel of a genomic DNA digest, the restriction endonuclease of choice should have only a limited number (20 to 50) of cleavage sites per genome. The sensitivity of this method increases with a larger number of restriction sites in the target genome, but 50 to 100 or more DNA fragments appear in an agarose gel after staining as a smear and not as a pattern of individual bands. This finding also depends, of course, on the size distribution of the generated fragments. It is now possible to identify and visualize individual DNA bands by Southern blotting of the genomic DNA digest and probing with defined cross-reacting labeled gene probes (93). The only prerequisite for such an analysis (also called genomic fingerprinting) is that the gene probe hybridizes with all of the DNAs to be tested. Therefore, conserved genes like the ones coding for rRNA, elongation factor EF-Tu, and ATPase were used initially (Table 4). By this technique, the heterogeneity of *A. laidlawii* (110) and *M. hominis* (21, 22, 110) strains, as well as the homogeneity of *M. pneumoniae* strains, was confirmed (110).

For *M. pneumoniae*, Dallo et al. (32) were able to demonstrate that, in contrast to the results with a conserved gene probe (rRNA), there is heterogeneity in this species. They found that because of a single cleavage site for endonuclease *Hin*dIII within the P1 gene coding for the major adhesin, restriction fragment length polymorphism (RFLP) could be exploited to divide individual isolates into one of two clusters. Similar experiments with repetitive DNA sequences as probes (83) confirmed these results. This analysis was further extended by using subsets of cosmids of a complete gene bank of the *M. pneumoniae* M129 genome (104), which allowed analysis of 145 individual *Eco*RI fragments of different independently isolated *M. pneumoniae* strains. Of the 145 *Eco*RI fragments in strains belonging to one of the proposed clusters, 130 were identical in length in all strains and 15 showed RFLP compared with strains of the other cluster (*M. pneu-*

moniae FH), but strains belonging to the same cluster showed RFLP in only one or two instances (43a). This finding indicates that despite minor changes, this species is very conserved and that the numerous repetitive DNA sequences do not destabilize the genome to an extent which can be detected readily by the applied methods. This genome stability stands in contradiction to the observation that an unusually high number of spontaneously arising mutants can be isolated (50). To understand these apparent or presumed differences in genetic homogeneity among mollicute species, more data need to be collected. For instance, are there favored regions for mutation in a genome? Has this anything to do with G+C content or genome size, assuming that a larger DNA codes for more nonessential genes? Or are there differences in fidelity of the DNA replication and repair processes and other processes?

Genetic Maps

The main reason for constructing physical maps is, of course, to have a basis for establishing a genetic map of an organism. This is specially true for bacteria like mollicutes (35), for which the classical tools for mapping genes are not as developed as are those for *E. coli* or *Bacillus subtilis*. The function of a genetic map is to have genes localized on the genome with respect to each other; therefore, the higher the resolution of the physical map, the better will be the genetic map. A restriction map with a mean resolution of 5 to 10 kbp will be a good basis with which to start. In the near future, we probably will have such high-resolution maps at least for some of the most extensively studied species.

There are several ways to convert a physical map into a genetic one. The simplest and most frequent approach takes advantage of cloned defined bacterial genes of the same or related species, using them as DNA probes to identify and localize the wanted gene by specific cross-hybridization. By this technique, several mollicute genome maps with up to 11 gene loci have been constructed (Fig. 1; Tables 3 and 4).

The most advanced genetic map study deals with strains within the *M. mycoides* subsp. *mycoides* cluster (72). Two large-colony strains, four small-colony strains, and one strain of a different serotype (*Mycoplasma* strain PG50) were compared with respect to genome size, restriction sites, and placement of 9 to 11

Table 4. Cloned mollicutes DNAs used as probes for identification and mapping of conserved genes in mollicutes

Gene	Symbol[a]	Source of cloned fragment	Reference
tRNA	*trn*	*Mycoplasma capricolum*	61
		M. mycoides	86
Ribosomal proteins (S10 operon)	*rpn*	*M. capricolum*	66
rRNA (5S, 16S, 23S)	*rrn*	*M. capricolum*	3
ATPase operon F1 sector subunit (δ, α, γ, β)	*uncH,A,GD*	*Mycoplasma* strain PG50	73
RNA polymerase (β'β subunit)	*rpoC,B*	*Mycoplasma* strain PG50	73
Serine hydroxymethyltransferase	*glyA*	*Mycoplasma* strain PG50	73
Deoxyribose phosphate aldolase	*deoC*	*M. pneumoniae*	56
Gyrase A/B subunit	*gyrA/B*	*M. pneumoniae*	29
EF-Tu	*tuf*	*M. pneumoniae*	111

[a] Gene symbols are the same as those proposed for the *E. coli* linkage map (6).

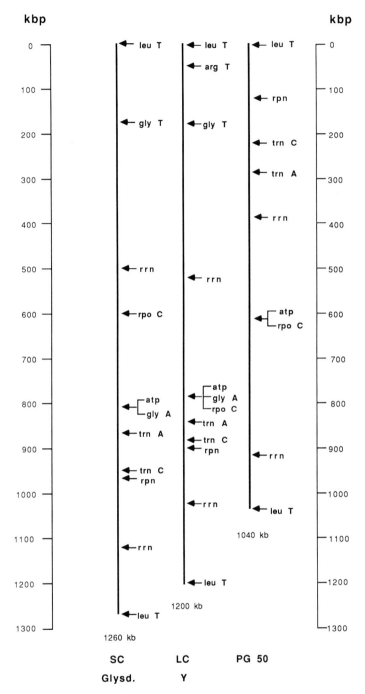

Figure 1. Comparison of genomic maps from two *M. mycoides* subsp. *mycoides* strains, Glysdale (Glysd.) and Y, and from strain PG50. SC, small-colony strain; LC, large-colony strain. Symbols identifying loci (see Table 4): *trnA,C*, cluster of several tRNAs; *argT*, tRNA^Arg; *glyT*, tRNA^Gly; *leuT*, tRNA^Leu. Arrows indicate approximate positions. These maps are simplified versions taken from Pyle et al. (72).

genes. The maps of the large- and small-colony strains were very similar with the exception of some restriction sites and the placement of the gene coding for the β subunit of the DNA-dependent RNA polymerase (*rpoC*). The *Mycoplasma* strain PG50 map differs from the other maps in size and placement of three gene loci. The modifications were such that all maps could be explained by inversion or translocation of distinct

regions of the chromosome (Fig. 1). Comparison with maps of other mollicutes genomes is presently not possible, since fewer and mostly different genes have been localized (Table 4).

The approach of using cloned defined genes as probes works well if the probe is derived from the same species or a closely related one, or if the gene desired is highly conserved, as are the rRNA and EF-Tu genes

(Fig. 1; Table 4). Otherwise, the method is not efficient enough for routinely identifying many genes, since the hybridization signals with the DNA probe are often not unambiguous and must be confirmed in all instances by DNA sequencing.

One also has to consider that most cloned and defined bacterial genes are from *E. coli* or *B. subtilis*, whose genomes have a significantly higher G + C content than do mollicutes genomes and therefore seem unlikely to give unambiguous signals. For constructing genomic maps, only a few useful mollicute-derived gene probes are now available (Table 4).

In my experience with *M. pneumoniae*, which has a genome with a relatively high (41 mol%) G + C content, probes derived from mollicutes genomes with a low (25 to 30 mol%) G + C content such as the genomes of *Mycoplasma* strain PG50 or *M. capricolum* do not give clear results. In such a case, it might be better to use probes from a distantly related bacterial species with a similar G + C content such as *B. subtilis*, as demonstrated by Colman et al. (29) in cloning the *M. pneumoniae* gyrase A and B genes with a *B. subtilis*-derived DNA probe.

In addition to those genes (and gene functions) which are shared by all mollicutes species, species-specific genes have to be individually identified by the appropriate techniques. Examples are the spiralin gene coding for the major membrane protein in spiroplasmas (20), the P1 gene coding for an adhesin in *M. pneumoniae* (44, 97), and the genes coding for membrane lipoproteins which are involved in generating surface diversity in *M. hyorhinis* (82). In the course of such studies, repetitive DNA sequences have been detected in several species (30, 38, 44, 64, 83, 96, 99, 103) (see also chapter 22).

From the viewpoint of constructing genetic maps, *M. pneumoniae* is noteworthy because four different repetitive elements, 150 to 2,200 bp long and with copy numbers between 8 and 10, have been localized on a cosmid-constructed *Eco*RI restriction map. These elements amount to 50 kbp, or 6% of the genome (83).

Adding up the bases of the different genes or DNA sequences that have been mapped so far on one or another genome (Table 4) yields about 100 kbp, or roughly 10% of an average mycoplasma genome (1,000 kbp). Of course, many more genes or gene products have been identified by immunological, physiological, or biochemical assays, but their gene loci have not yet been determined (26, 28, 34, 65).

CONCLUSION

Restriction fragment patterns and restriction maps are excellent tools for comparing different strains of a species, but they can be used only for related genomes. Both techniques are of practical value because they allow characterization of individual genomes, but they are not suitable for performing phylogenetic studies. An interesting approach to studying relatedness or phylogeny is to analyze gene placement on bacterial chromosomes to determine whether there is a conserved gene order. Because of their small size and wide distribution, mollicutes are excellent systems for these studies. Such analyses have been performed on the *M. mycoides* subsp. *mycoides* cluster. It is too early to draw any general conclusion because of the lack of sufficiently mapped gene loci. For future research, it would be beneficial to establish a stock of about 100 DNA probes for genes which are expected to occur in all mollicutes species and which could be used for such comparative analyses. It should be possible to find sets of probes for genomes similar in G + C content. Such probes must be gene specific and conserved, so that they cross-hybridize selectively with the corresponding gene, and DNA sequencing as further verification will be unnecessary. These gene probes probably could be generated by random sequencing, since one would expect that genes are closely spaced without extended noncoding regions particularly in the smaller mollicutes genomes.

The power of this approach has been demonstrated by Chevalier et al. (20), who reported that by sequencing a 5-kbp-long DNA fragment of the *S. citri* genome, five open reading frames, including the spiralin gene, were revealed, and four (encoding ribosomal protein S2, elongation factor EF-Ts, phosphofructokinase, and pyruvate kinase) were identified as genes by computer-aided homology search of the translated sequenced DNA. It will be interesting to test whether these genes can be successfully used as probes for detecting the corresponding genes in other mollicutes.

Independent of the outcome of this experiment, the direct approach, i.e., sequencing of the genome directly, seems to be the fastest way to identify many genes by a random approach. In this context, one must consider that identification of genes by cross-hybridization with cloned defined DNA probes from heterologous bacteria requires verification by DNA sequencing. Therefore, since only a small number of homologous DNA probes for individual mollicute species exist, a DNA fragment recognized by a heterologous DNA probe must be sequenced anyway.

At the moment, at least two mollicutes genomes, those of *M. capricolum* (40) and *M. pneumoniae* (104), are being sequenced. The two genomes differ considerably in G + C content and probably in size (Table 2). Therefore, besides laying the basis for defining the genetic makeup of a self-replicating cell (59), the sequence data will provide a large reservoir for many potential gene probes derived from bacteria with different codon usages, from which sets of 50 to 100 corresponding gene probes should be readily composed. The construction of genomic maps will be considerably facilitated by these probes. Although they might not cross-react in all instances, positive results among closely related species seem to be likely.

Development of the molecular cloning technique is compensating largely for the disadvantage of the mollicutes as a model for molecular biological studies—the lack of an efficient in vivo and in vitro gene transfer system. Therefore, mollicutes are now a very attractive model for investigating problems of molecular microbiology.

Acknowledgments. The experimental work from this laboratory was supported by the Bundesministerium für Forschung und Technologie (BCT 0318/5). I thank J. Maniloff for critically reading and S. Nazareth for preparing the manuscript.

REFERENCES

1. **Allen, T. C.** 1971. Base composition and genome size of *Mycoplasma meleagridis* deoxyribonucleic acid. *J. Gen. Microbiol.* **69:**285–286.

2. **Amikam, D., G. Glaser, and S. Razin.** 1984. Mycoplasmas (*Mollicutes*) have a low number of rRNA genes. *J. Bacteriol.* **158:**376–378.

3. **Amikam, D., S. Razin, and G. Glaser.** 1982. Ribosomal RNA genes in mycoplasma. *Nucleic Acids Res.* **10:**4215–4222.

4. **Ansorge, W., B. Sproat, J. Stegemann, C. Schwager, and M. Zenke.** 1987. Automated DNA sequencing: ultrasensitive detection of fluorescent bands during electrophoresis. *Nucleic Acids Res.* **15:**4593–4602.

5. **Askaa, G., C. Christiansen, and H. Erno.** 1973. Bovine mycoplasmas: genome size and base composition of DNA. *J. Gen. Microbiol.* **75:**283–286.

6. **Bachmann, B. J.** 1990. Linkage map of *Escherichia coli* K-12, edition 8. *Microbiol. Rev.* **54:**130–197.

7. **Bak, A. L., F. T. Black, C. Christiansen, and E. A. Freundt.** 1969. Genome size of mycoplasmal DNA. *Nature* (London) **224:**1209–1210.

8. **Bancroft, I., C. P. Wolk, and E. V. Oren.** 1989. Physical and genetic maps of the genome of the heterocyst-forming cyanobacterium *Anabaena* sp. strain PCC 7120. *J. Bacteriol.* **171:**5940–5948.

9. **Barlev, N. A., and S. N. Borchsenius.** 1990. Gradual distribution of mycoplasma genome sizes. *IOM Lett.* **1:**238–239.

10. **Bautsch, W.** 1988. Rapid physical mapping of the *Mycoplasma mobile* genome by two-dimensional field inversion gel electrophoresis techniques. *Nucleic Acids Res.* **16:**11461–11467.

11. **Bode, H. R., and H. J. Morowitz.** 1967. Size and structure of the *Mycoplasma hominis* H39 chromosome. *J. Mol. Biol.* **23:**191–199.

12. **Bové, J. M., P. Carle, M. Garnier, F. Laigret, J. Renaudin, and C. Saillard.** 1989. Molecular and cellular biology of spiroplasmas, p. 243–364. *In* R. F. Whitcomb and J. G. Tully (ed.), *The Mycoplasmas*, vol. 5. Academic Press, New York.

13. **Bové, J. M., F. Laigret, L. R. Finch, P. Carle, F. C. Ye, C. Citti, C. Saillard, O. Grau, J. Renaudin, C. Bové, J. Whitley, and D. Williamson.** 1990. Genome of spiroplasmas. *IOM Lett.* **1:**70–71.

14. **Bové, J. M., and C. Saillard.** 1979. Cell biology of spiroplasmas, p. 83–153. *In* R. F. Whitcomb and J. G. Tully (ed.), *The Mycoplasmas*, vol. 3. Academic Press, New York.

15. **Canard, B., and S. T. Cole.** 1989. Genome organization of the anaerobic pathogen *Clostridium perfringens*. *Proc. Natl. Acad. Sci. USA.* **86:**6676–6680.

16. **Cantor, C. R., C. L. Smith, and M. K. Mathew.** 1988. Pulsed-field gel electrophoresis of very large DNA molecules. *Annu. Rev. Biophys. Biophys. Chem.* **17:**287–304.

17. **Carle, G. F., M. Frank, and M. V. Olson.** 1986. Electrophoretic separations of large DNA molecules by periodic inversion of the electric field. *Science* **232:**65–68.

18. **Carle, G. F., and M. V. Olson.** 1985. An electrophoretic karotype for yeast. *Proc. Natl. Acad. Sci. USA* **82:**3756–3760.

19. **Chen, H., I. M. Keseler, and L. J. Shimkets.** 1990. Genome size of *Myxococcus xanthus* determined by pulsed-field gel electrophoresis. *J. Bacteriol.* **172:**4206–4213.

20. **Chevalier, C., C. Saillard, and J. M. Bové.** 1990. Organization and nucleotide sequences of the *Spiroplasma citri* genes for ribosomal protein S2, elongation factor Ts, spiralin, phosphofructokinase, pyruvate kinase, and an unidentified protein. *J. Bacteriol.* **172:**2693–2703.

21. **Christiansen, C., G. Christiansen, and O. F. Rasmussen.** 1987. Heterogeneity of *Mycoplasma hominis* as detected by a probe for *atp* genes. *Isr. J. Med. Sci.* **23:**591–594.

22. **Christiansen, G., and H. Andersen.** 1988. Hetrogeneity among *Mycoplasma hominis* strains as detected by probes containing parts of ribosomal ribonucleic acid genes. *Int. J. Syst. Bacteriol.* **38:**108–115.

23. **Christiansen, G., H. Andersen, S. Birkelund, and E. A. Freundt.** 1987. Genomic and gene variation in *Mycoplasma hominis* strains. *Isr. J. Med. Sci.* **23:**595–602.

24. **Chu, G., D. Vollrath, and R. W. Davis.** 1986. Separation of large DNA molecules by contour-clamped homogeneous electric fields. *Science* **234:**1582–1585.

25. **Church, G. M., and S. Kieffer-Higgins.** 1988. Multiplex DNA sequencing. *Science* **240:**185–188.

26. **Cocks, B. G., F. A. Brake, A. Mitchell, and L. R. Finch.** 1985. Enzymes of intermediary carbohydrate metabolism in *Ureaplasma urealyticum* and *Mycoplasma mycoides* subsp. *mycoides*. *J. Gen. Microbiol.* **131:** 2129–2135.

27. **Cocks, B. G., L. E. Pyle, and L. R. Finch.** 1989. A physical map of the genome of *Ureaplasma urealyticum* 960^T with ribosomal RNA loci. *Nucleic Acids Res.* **17:**6713–6719.

28. **Cocks, B. G., R. Youil, and L. R. Finch.** 1988. Comparison of enzymes of nucleotide metabolism in two members of the *Mycoplasmataceae* family. *Int. J. Syst. Bacteriol.* **38:**273–278.

29. **Colman, S. D., P.-C. Hu, and K. F. Bott.** 1990. *Mycoplasma pneumoniae* DNA gyrase genes. *Mol. Microbiol.* **4:**1129–1134.

30. **Colman, S. D., P.-C. Hu, and K. F. Bott.** 1990. Prevalence of novel repeat sequences in and around the *P1* operon in the genome of *Mycoplasma pneumoniae*. *Gene* **87:**91–96.

31. **Colman, S. D., P.-C. Hu, W. Litaker, and K. F. Bott.** 1990. A physical map of the *Mycoplasma genitalium* genome. *Mol. Microbiol.* **4:**683–687.

32. **Dallo, S. F., J. R. Horton, C. J. Su, and J. B. Baseman.** 1990. Restriction fragment length polymorphism in the cytadhesin P1 gene of human clinical isolate of *Mycoplasma pneumoniae*. *Infect. Immun.* **58:**2017–2020.

33. **Darai, G., L. Zöller, B. Matz, H. Delius, P. T. Speck, and R. M. Flügel.** 1982. Analysis of *Mycoplasma hyorhinis* genome by use of restriction endonucleases and by electron microscopy. *J. Bacteriol.* **150:**788–794.

34. **Desantis, D., V. V. Tryon, and J. D. Pollack.** 1989. Metabolism of Mollicutes: the Embden-Meyerhof-Parnas pathway and the hexose monophosphate shunt. *J. Gen. Microbiol.* **135:**683–691.

35. **Dybvig, K.** 1990. Mycoplasmal genetics. *Annu. Rev. Microbiol.* **44:**81–104.

36. **Ellis, T. H. N., W. G. Cleary, K. W. G. Burcham, and B. A. Bowen.** 1987. Ramped field inversion gel electrophoresis: a cautionary note. *Nucleic Acids Res.* **15:**5489.

37. **Ferdows, M. S., and A. G. Barbour.** 1989. Megabase-sized linear DNA in the bacterium *Borrelia burgdorferi*, the Lyme disease agent. *Proc. Natl. Acad. Sci. USA* **86:**5969–5973.

38. **Ferrell, R. V., M. B. Heidari, K. S. Wise, and M. A. McIntosh.** 1989. A *Mycoplasma* genetic element resembling prokaryotic insertion sequences. *Mol. Microbiol.* **3:** 957–967.

39. **Frutos, R., M. Pages, M. Bellis, G. Roizes, and M. Bergoin.** 1989. Pulsed-field gel electrophoresis determination of the genome size of obligate intracellular bacteria belonging to the genera *Chlamydia*, *Rickettsiella*, and *Porochlamydia*. *J. Bacteriol.* **171:**4511–4513.

40. **Gillevet, P. M.** 1990. Chemiluminescent multiplex DNA sequencing. *Nature* (London) **348:**657–658.

41. **Gillis, M., J. De Ley, and M. De Cleene.** 1970. The determination of molecular weight of bacterial genome DNA from renaturation rates. *Eur. J. Biochem.* **12:**143–153.

42. **Hagerman, P. J.** 1990. Sequence-directed curvature of DNA. *Annu. Rev. Biochem.* **59:**755–781.

43. **Herdman, M., M. Janvier, R. Rippka, and R. Y. Stanier.**

1979. Genome size of cyanobacteria. *J. Gen. Microbiol.* **111:**73–85.

43a. **Herrmann, R.** Unpublished data.

44. **Inamine, J. M., T. P. Denny, S. Loechel, U. Schaper, C.-H. Huang, K. F. Bott, and P.-C. Hu.** 1988. Nucleotide sequence of the P1 attachment-protein gene of *Mycoplasma pneumoniae. Gene* **64:**217–229.

45. **Kingsbury, D. T.** 1969. Estimate of the genome size of various microorganisms. *J. Bacteriol.* **98:**1400–1401.

46. **Kirkpatrick, B. C., and C. R. Kuske, P. O. Lim, and B. B. Sears.** 1990. Phylogeny of plant pathogenic mycoplasma-like organisms. *IOM Lett.* **1:**45–46.

47. **Klein, A., and M. Schnorr.** 1984. Genome complexity of methanogenic bacteria. *J. Bacteriol.* **158:**628–631.

48. **Kohara, Y., K. Akiyama, and K. Isono.** 1987. The physical map of the whole E. coli chromosome: application of a new strategy for rapid analysis and sorting of a large genomic library. *Cell* **50:**495–508.

49. **Kolsto, A. B., A. Gronstad, and H. Oppegaard.** 1990. Physical map of the *Bacillus cereus* chromosome. *J. Bacteriol.* **172:**3821–3825.

50. **Krause, D. C., D. K. Leith, R. M. Wilson, and J. B. Baseman.** 1982. Identification of *Mycoplasma pneumoniae* proteins associated with hemadsorption and virulence. *Infect. Immun.* **35:**809–817.

51. **Krause, D. C., and C. B. Mawn.** 1990. Physical analysis and mapping of the *Mycoplasma pneumoniae* chromosome. *J. Bacteriol.* **172:**4790–4797.

52. **Krawiec, S., and M. Riley.** 1990. Organization of the bacterial chromosome. *Microbiol. Rev.* **54:**502–539.

53. **Lee, I. M., and R. E. Davis.** 1980. DNA homology among diverse spiroplasma strains representing several serological groups. *Can. J. Microbiol.* **26:**1356–1363.

54. **Lee, J. J., and H. O. Smith.** 1988. Sizing of the *Haemophilus influenzae* Rd genome by pulsed-field agarose gel electrophoresis. *J. Bacteriol.* **170:**4402–4405.

55. **Lim, P. O., and B. B. Sears.** 1991. The genome size of a plant-pathogenic mycoplasmalike organism resembles those of animal mycoplasmas. *J. Bacteriol.* **173:**2128–2130.

56. **Loechel, S., J. M. Inamine, and P.-C. Hu.** 1989. Nucleotide sequence of the *deo*C gene of *Mycoplasma pneumoniae. Nucleic Acids Res.* **17:**801.

57. **Maniloff, J.** 1989. Anomalous values of Mycoplasma genome sizes determined by pulse-field gel electrophoresis. *Nucleic Acids Res.* **17:**1268.

58. **McGarrity, G. J., D. M. Phillips, and B. A. Vaidya.** 1980. Mycoplasmal infection of lymphocyte cell cultures: infection with M. salivarium. *In Vitro* **16:**346–356.

59. **Morowitz, H. J.** 1984. The completeness of molecular biology. *Isr. J. Med. Sci.* **20:**750–763.

60. **Morowitz, H. J., and D. C. Wallace.** 1973 Genome size and life cycle of the Mycoplasma. *Ann. N.Y. Acad. Sci.* **225:**62–73.

61. **Muto, A., Y. Andachi, H. Yuzawa, F. Yamao, and S. Osawa.** 1990. The organization and evolution of transfer RNA genes in *Mycoplasma capricolum. Nucleic Acids Res.* **18:**5037–5043.

62. **Neimark, H. C., and C. S. Lange.** 1990. Pulse-field electrophoresis indicates full-length mycoplasma chromosomes range widely in size. *Nucleic Acids Res.* **18:**5443–5448.

63. **Nuijten, P. J. M., C. Bartels, N. M. C. Bleumink-Pluym, W. Gaastra, and B. A. M. van der Zeijst.** 1990. Size and physical map of the *Campylobacter jejuni* chromosome. *Nucleic Acids Res.* **18:**6211–6214.

64. **Nur, I., D. J. LeBlanc, and J. G. Tully.** 1987. Short, interspersed, and repetitive DNA sequences in *Spiroplasma* species. *Plasmid* **17:**110–116.

65. **O'Brien, S. J., J. M. Simonson, M. W. Grabowski, and M. F. Barile.** 1981. Analysis of multiple isoenzyme expression among twenty-two species of *Mycoplasma* and *Acholeplasma. J. Bacteriol.* **146:**222–232.

66. **Ohkubo, S., A. Muto, Y. Kawauchi, F. Yamao, and S. Osawa.** 1987. The ribosomal protein gene cluster of *Mycoplasma capricolum. Mol. Gen. Genet.* **210:**314–322.

67. **Ostashevsky, J. Y., and C. S. Lange.** 1987. A model of the hydrodynamic behavior of irradiated DNA: dependence on molecular conformation. *Biopolymers* **26:**59–82.

68. **Poddar, S. K., and J. Maniloff.** 1986. Chromosome analysis by two-dimensional fingerprinting. *Gene* **49:**93–102.

69. **Poddar, S. K., and J. Maniloff.** 1989. Determination of microbial genome sizes by two-dimensional denaturing gradient gel electrophoresis. *Nucleic Acids Res.* **17:**2889–2895.

70. **Pyle, L. E., L. N. Corcoran, B. G. Cocks, A. D. Bergemann, J. C. Whitley, and L. R. Finch.** 1988. Pulsed-field electrophoresis indicates larger-than-expected sizes for mycoplasma genomes. *Nucleic Acids Res.* **16:**6015–6025.

71. **Pyle, L. E., and L. R. Finch.** 1988. A physical map of the genome of *Mycoplasma mycoides* subspecies *mycoides* Y with some functional loci. *Nucleic Acids Res.* **16:**6027–6039.

72. **Pyle, L. E., T. Taylor, and L. R. Finch.** 1990. Genomic maps of some strains within the *Mycoplasma mycoides* cluster. *J. Bacteriol.* **172:**7265–7268.

73. **Rasmussen, O. F., and C. Christiansen.** 1990. A 23 kb region of the Mycoplasma PG50 genome with three identified genetic structures. *Zentralbl. Bakteriol. Suppl.* **20:**315–323.

74. **Razin, S.** 1985. Molecular biology and genetics of mycoplasmas (*Mollicutes*). *Microbiol. Rev.* **49:**419–455.

75. **Razin, S.** 1989. Molecular approach to mycoplasma phylogeny, p. 33–69. *In* R. F. Whitcomb and J. G. Tully (ed.), *The Mycoplasmas*, vol. 5. Academic Press, New York.

76. **Razin, S., M. F. Barile, R. Harasawa, D. Amikam, and G. Glaser.** 1983. Characterization of the Mycoplasma genome. *Yale J. Biol. Med.* **56:**357–366.

77. **Razin, S., and E. A. Freundt.** 1984. The mycoplasmas, p. 740–793. *In* N. R. Krieg and J. G. Holt (ed.), *Bergey's Manual of Systematic Bacteriology*, vol. 1. The Williams & Wilkins Co., Baltimore.

78. **Razin, S., R. Harasawa, and M. F. Barile.** 1983. Cleavage patterns of the mycoplasma chromosome, obtained by using restriction endonucleases, as indicators of genetic relatedness among strains. *Int. J. Syst. Bacteriol.* **33:**201–206.

78a. **Robertson, J. A.** Personal communication.

79. **Robertson, J. A., L. Pyle, J. Kakulphimp, G. W. Stemke, and L. R. Finch.** 1990. The genomes of the genus Ureaplasma. *IOM Lett.* **1:**72–73.

80. **Robertson, J. A., L. E. Pyle, G. W. Stemke, and L. R. Finch.** 1990. Human ureaplasmas show diverse genome sizes by pulsed-field electrophoresis. *Nucleic Acids Res.* **18:**1451–1455.

81. **Römling, U., D. Grothues, W. Bautsch, and B. Tümmler.** 1989. A physical genome map of *Pseudomonas aeruginosa* PAO. *EMBO J.* **8:**4081–4089.

82. **Rosengarten, R., and K. S. Wise.** 1990. Phenotypic switching in mycoplasmas: phase variation of diverse surface lipoproteins. *Science* **247:**315–317.

83. **Ruland, K., R. Wenzel, and R. Herrmann.** 1990. Analysis of three different repeated DNA elements present in the P1 operon of *Mycoplasma pneumoniae*: size, number and distribution on the genome. *Nucleic Acids Res.* **18:**6311–6317.

84. **Ryan, J. F., and H. J. Morowitz.** 1969. Partial purification of native rRNA and tRNA cistrons from *Mycoplasma* sp. (kid). *Proc. Natl. Acad. Sci. USA* **63:**1282–1289.

85. **Saglio, P., M. L. Hospital, D. Laflèche, G. Dupont, J. M. Bové, J. G. Tully, and F. A. Freundt.** 1973. *Spiroplasma citri* gen. and sp.n.: a mycoplasma-like organism associ-

ated with "stubborn" disease of citrus. *Int. J. Syst. Bacteriol.* **23**:191–204.

86. **Samuelsson, T., P. Elias, F. Lustig, and Y. S. Guindy.** 1985. Cloning and nucleotide sequence analysis of transfer RNA genes from *Mycoplasma mycoides. Biochem. J.* **232**:223–228.

87. **Schwartz, D. C., and C. R. Cantor.** 1984. Separation of yeast chromosome-sized DNAs by pulsed field gradient gel electrophoresis. *Cell* **37**:67–75.

88. **Sitzmann, J., and A. Klein.** 1991. Physical and genetic map of the *Methanococcus voltae* chromosome. *Mol. Microbiol.* **5**:505–513.

89. **Smith, C. L., and G. Condemine.** 1990. New approaches for physical mapping of small genomes. *J. Bacteriol.* **172**:1167–1172.

90. **Smith, C. L., J. G. Econome, A. Schutt, S. Klco, and C. R. Cantor.** 1987. A physical map of the *Escherichia coli* K12 genome. *Science* **236**:1448–1453.

91. **Smith, L. M., J. Z. Sanders, R. J. Kaiser, P. Hughes, C. Dodd, C. R. Connell, C. Heiner, S. B. H. Kent, and L. E. Hood.** 1986. Fluorescence detection in automated DNA sequence analysis. *Nature* (London) **321**:674–679.

92. **Sorge, J. A., and L. A. Blinderman.** 1989. ExoMeth sequencing of DNA: eliminating the need for subcloning and oligonucleotide primers. *Proc. Natl. Acad. Sci. USA* **86**:9208–9212.

93. **Southern, E.** 1975. Detection of specific sequences among DNA fragments separated by gel electrophoresis. *J. Mol. Biol.* **98**:503–517.

94. **Studier, F. W.** 1989. A strategy for high-volume sequencing of cosmid DNAs: random and directed priming with a library of oligonucleotides. *Proc. Natl. Acad. Sci. USA* **86**:6917–6921.

95. **Su, C. J., and J. B. Baseman.** 1990. Genome size of *Mycoplasma genitalium. J. Bacteriol.* **172**:4705–4707.

96. **Su, C. J., A. Chavoya, and J. B. Baseman.** 1988. Regions of *Mycoplasma pneumoniae* cytadhesin P1 structural gene exist as multiple copies. *Infect. Immun.* **56**:3157–3161.

97. **Su, C. J., V. V. Tryon, and J. B. Baseman.** 1987. Cloning and sequence analysis of cytadhesin P1 gene from *Mycoplasma pneumoniae. Infect. Immun.* **55**:3023–3029.

98. **Suwanto, A., and S. Kaplan.** 1989. Physical and genetic mapping of the *Rhodobacter sphaeroides* 2.4.1 genome: presence of two unique circular chromosomes. *J. Bacteriol.* **171**:5840–5849.

99. **Taylor, M. A., R. V. Ferrel, K. S. Wise, and M. A. McIntosh.** 1987. Indentification of a repetitive genomic sequence that is distributed among a select group of mycoplasmas. *Isr. J. Med. Sci.* **23**:368–373.

100. **Teplitz, M.** 1977. Isolation of folded chromosome from *Mycoplasma hyorhinis. Nucleic Acids Res.* **4**:1505–1512.

101. **Tully, J. G., D. Taylor-Robinson, D. L. Rose, R. M. Cole, and J. M. Bové.** 1983. *Mycoplasma genitalium*, a new species from the human urogenital tract. *Int. J. Syst. Bacteriol.* **33**:387–396.

102. **Weisburg, W. G., J. G. Tully, D. L. Rose, J. P. Petzel, H. Oyaizu, D. Yang, L. Mandelco, J. Sechrest, T. G. Lawrence, J. van Etten, J. Maniloff, and C. R. Woese.** 1989. A phylogenetic analysis of the mycoplasmas: basis for their classification. *J. Bacteriol.* **171**:6455–6467.

103. **Wenzel, R., and R. Herrmann.** 1988. Repetitive DNA sequences in *Mycoplasma pneumoniae. Nucleic Acids Res.* **16**:8337–8350.

104. **Wenzel, R., and R. Herrmann.** 1989. Cloning of the complete *Mycoplasma pneumoniae* genome. *Nucleic Acids Res.* **17**:7029–7043.

105. **Wetmur, J. G., and N. Davidson.** 1968. Kinetics of renaturation of DNA. *J. Mol. Biol.* **31**:349–370.

106. **Whitley, J. C., and L. R. Finch.** 1989. Location of sites of transposon Tn*916* insertion in the *Mycoplasma mycoides* genome. *J. Bacteriol.* **171**:6870–6872.

107. **Whitley, J. C., A. Muto, and L. R. Finch.** 1991. A physical map for *Mycoplasma capricolum* Cal. kid with loci for all known tRNA species. *Nucleic Acids Res.* **19**:399–400.

108. **Yee, T., and M. Inouye.** 1981. Reexamination of the genome size of myxobacteria, including the use of a new method for genome size analysis. *J. Bacteriol.* **145**:1257–1265.

109. **Yee, T., and M. Inouye.** 1982. Two-dimensional DNA electrophoresis applied to the study of DNA methylation and the analysis of genome size in *Myxococcus xanthus. J. Mol. Biol.* **154**:181–196.

110. **Yogev, D., D. Halachmi, G. E. Kenny, and S. Razin.** 1988. Distinction of species and strains of mycoplasmas (Mollicutes) by genomic DNA fingerprints with an rRNA gene probe. *J. Clin. Microbiol.* **26**:1198–1201.

111. **Yogev, D., S. Sela, H. Bercovier, and S. Razin.** 1990. Nucleotide sequence and codon usage of the elongation factor Tu (EF-Tu) gene from *Mycoplasma pneumoniae. Mol. Microbiol.* **4**:1303–1310.

10. Ribosomes

GAD GLASER, HANA C. HYMAN, and SHMUEL RAZIN

INTRODUCTION

Apart from DNA, ribosomes are the only structures observed in the mycoplasma cytoplasm. Early reports (27, 30) had indicated the resemblance of mycoplasma ribosomes to those of *Escherichia coli* and other procaryotes in size and composition. Although no quantitative study has been done so far, the impression that one gets on observing sectioned logarithmically growing mycoplasma cells is that ribosome density (i.e., number of ribosomes per cytoplasmic unit) is lower in mycoplasmas than in logarithmically growing *E. coli* cells. If verified, this observation is in line with the slow growth rate of mycoplasmas. A peculiar corncoblike organization of ribosomes in *Mycoplasma gallisepticum* attracted attention in the 1960s. Maniloff (36) has shown these structures to consist of a helix repeat of 10 ribosomes in three turns. The failure to associate this peculiar ribosome organization in *M. gallisepticum* with function led to the conclusion that the helical ribosome structures do not represent polyribosomes active in polypeptide synthesis but rather are artifacts produced during preparation of the cells for sectioning.

In the absence of adequately sensitive methods for analysis, knowledge of mycoplasmal ribosomal proteins and rRNA showed little progress in the 1970s. With the introduction of molecular genetics methodology to mycoplasma research in the early 1980s, detailed information on ribosomal components has become available. In fact, much of the early work on the structure, organization, and control of mycoplasma genes has been carried out on rRNA and ribosomal protein genes, largely because the conserved nature of these genes among procaryotes facilitated their study.

RIBOSOMAL PROTEINS

Mycoplasmal ribosomes resemble typical eubacterial ribosomes in having a sedimentation coefficient of about 70S, three rRNA species (5S, 16S, and 23S), and about 50 protein species. Kawauchi et al. (28) detected 30 protein spots from the 50S subunits and 21 protein spots from the 30S subunits by two-dimensional polyacrylamide gel electrophoresis analysis of *M. capricolum* ribosomes. The *M. capricolum* ribosomal proteins resembled those of eubacteria in size and electrophoretic mobility. This resemblance was most pronounced to the ribosomal protein profiles of gram-positive bacilli (28). A significant portion of the *M. capricolum* genome encodes ribosome synthesis (about 55 genes of an estimated total of 400 to 600 genes). A recombinant plasmid carrying a cluster of genes for at least eight *M. capricolum* ribosomal proteins was constructed by Kawauchi et al. (29). The protein genes, organized apparently as an operon, were expressed in *E. coli* from their own promoter. A 1.3-kbp fragment of the recombinant plasmid DNA carrying the genes for ribosomal proteins S8 and L6 and a part of L18 was sequenced (40). The A + T content of the *M. capricolum* genes was much higher than that of corresponding *E. coli* genes. A more extensive study of the organization of the ribosomal protein gene cluster of *M. capricolum* was carried out by Ohkubo et al. (47). All 22 genes studied except *adk* corresponded to those found in the *E. coli* S10 and *spc* operons, and the gene order is essentially the same as that for *E. coli*. However, the genes for L30 and X protein in the *E. coli spc* operon are absent in *M. capricolum*. The 20 ribosomal protein genes and *secY* seem to consist of one operon in *M.*

Gad Glaser • Department of Cellular Biochemistry, The Hebrew University–Hadassah Medical School, Jerusalem 91010, Israel. **Hana C. Hyman and Shmuel Razin** • Department of Membrane and Ultrastructure Research, The Hebrew University–Hadassah Medical School, Jerusalem 91010, Israel.

capricolum. A promoterlike sequence is found 120 bp upstream of the S10 gene, and a terminatorlike sequence is found soon after *secY*. In *E. coli*, there are additional terminator and promoter sequences in the region between the genes for S17 and L14, so that the genes are in two operons. In *M. capricolum*, the spacer between S17 and L14 is 15 bp and does not include transcriptional signal sequences, so it appears that in *M. capricolum*, the two operons are fused into one operon.

It was demonstrated (47) that four of the intergenic regions, between the genes for L4 and L23, L16 and L29, L29 and S17, and L15 and *secY*, have overlapping translational stop/start codons, in which the third nucleotide of the stop codon TAA of the preceding gene overlaps the first nucleotide of the start codon ATG of the gene following. . . . TAATG. . . . This kind of overlapping was also reported in *E. coli* between the genes for L4 and L23, L16 and L29, and L29 and S17 (8, 81). All *M. capricolum* genes start with an ATG codon and a 3- to 8-bp stretch of a putative ribosome binding site (Shine-Dalgarno sequence) about 10 bp upstream from the start codon.

The amino acid sequences of 20 ribosomal proteins deduced from DNA sequences are similar to the corresponding *E. coli* sequences, although the average G + C content of the coding region of the *M. capricolum* gene cluster is 29%, which is much lower than the 51% G + C of the corresponding region of *E. coli*. The choice of synonymous codons in *M. capricolum* is clearly different from that in *E. coli* and is strongly biased to use A and U, as previously demonstrated by Muto et al. (40) (see chapter 19).

On the whole, the similarity in the arrangement of the ribosomal protein genes in *E. coli* and *M. capricolum* is remarkable, suggesting that the basic organization of the gene cluster was established before the phylogenetic separation of *M. capricolum* and *E. coli*.

rRNA

Number of Operons

The genes for rRNA and their products are highly conserved throughout procaryotic organisms, including the mollicutes. Thus, hybridization using defined segments of known procaryotic rRNA operons has been a primary tool to greatly facilitate the study of rRNA genes in mollicutes (6). Hybridization to restriction enzyme-digested mycoplasmal genomic DNA has enabled an estimation of rRNA gene copy number. All species of mollicutes tested so far carry only one or two sets of rRNA genes in their genomes (1, 17, 51–53, 59). Recently, it has been shown that the genomes of plant and insect noncultivable mycoplasmalike organisms (MLOs) also carry one or two copies of rRNA operons, supporting their inclusion in the class *Mollicutes* (30a, 32). This contrasts with the situation found in several eubacteria examined so far. The genome of *E. coli* carries seven independent rRNA transcription units for the 16S and 23S rRNAs (31, 45), *Bacillus subtilis* carries at least 10 copies of each of the three genes (33), and *Lactococcus cremoris* and *L. lactis* carry at least five or six sets of rRNA genes (42). Thus, the small size of the mycoplasma genome seems to be reflected in the small number of rRNA gene sets. However, there seems to be no strict correlation between genome size and number of rRNA genes. The genome of *Spiroplasma citri* is twice the size of the *M. arginini* genome, yet the former carries only one copy of rRNA genes and the latter carries two (51). Likewise, archaebacteria such as *Halobacterium halobium* contain only one set of rRNA genes, despite a genome size close to that of *E. coli* (22). The occurrence of few rRNA gene copies in the slowly growing mollicutes, archaebacteria, *Thermus thermophilus* (73), *Mycobacterium bovis* (63), *Mycobacterium lepraemurium* (62), and other mycobacteria (4) supports the idea proposed by Amikam et al. (1) that the copy number of rRNA genes may be related to growth rate. This view does not discount the possibility that the low number of rRNA genes in mollicutes is a result of extensive genetic deletions during their presumed evolution from gram-positive eubacterial ancestors (43, 77) (see chapter 33).

Order of Genes

Hybridization studies also led to the conclusion that in mycoplasmas, most rRNA gene sets are linked in the classical order found in procaryotes: 5'-16S-23S-5S-3' (14, 17, 58). The three genes were also found to be close to each other, occupying a chromosomal segment of about 5 kbp, suggesting an operon structure. As more mollicutes have been studied, several interesting exceptions have come to light. Organization of the single rRNA gene set of *M. hyopneumoniae* was determined by first cloning the rRNA genes and then hybridizing Southern blots of the cloned fragments and total genomic DNA by using the three rRNA species as probes (67). The 5S rRNA was found to be separated from the clustered 16S and 23S genes by more than 4 kb. Two *M. gallisepticum* strains, S6 and PG31, were analyzed by restriction of their DNAs followed by pulsed-field electrophoresis and Southern blotting (9). Selective hybridization of the resulting blots with fragments of an rRNA operon of *M. capricolum* led to the identification of three widely separated rRNA loci; one had a full set of rRNA genes, a second had a 23S gene and probably a 5S gene, and the third had only a 16S gene. Such unusual arrangements of procaryotic rRNA genes have been seen in some (but not all) archaebacteria, in which either all three rRNA genes are separated by spacers in the range of several kilobases or only the 5S rRNA is separated from the clustered 16S and 23S genes (44, 72). Similarly, the eucaryotic 5S rRNA gene is at a different locus from the 18S, 5.8S, and 28S genes (3).

Spacer Regions

Partial sequence information is available for the rRNA genes of four mycoplasma species (10–12, 13, 26, 48–50, 64, 67, 68): *M. capricolum*, *Mycoplasma* sp. strain PG50, *M. hyopneumoniae*, and *M. pneumoniae*. *M. capricolum* and *Mycoplasma* sp. strain PG50, two closely related species, each have two rRNA operons, *rrnA* and *rrnB*, with the usual eubacterial gene order. However, the spacer regions between the 16S and 23S rRNA genes of these mycoplasmas, as well as in *M. hyopneumoniae*, do not include tRNA genes. In contrast, tRNA genes have been found in the spacer regions of all seven *E. coli* rRNA operons, both *Anacystis nidulans* operons, and 8 of 10 *B. subtilis* operons (33). Recently, plant-pathogenic MLOs were shown to have a single tRNA^{Ile} gene in the spacer between the 16S and 23S rRNA genes (30a, 32). *Mycoplasma* sp. strain PG50 *rrnA* (48) and *M. pneumoniae* (21a) were also shown to have no tRNA sequences following their 5S rRNA genes as do most *B. subtilis* rRNA operons.

The sequences of the spacers in *M. capricolum rrnA* and *rrnB* (228 and 220 bp long, respectively) are highly conserved, showing 97% sequence identity. Furthermore, most of the differences are found in a limited part of the spacer, suggesting that the bulk of the spacer may play some functional role. Within *E. coli* and *B. subtilis*, spacer sequences are relatively conserved among the different rRNA operons of the same species, while little sequence homology has been found between the two species with the exception of the spacer tRNA gene regions. One suggestion is that the spacer sequence includes processing signals for rRNA maturation (5, 46, 58). Sequences flanking the 16S and 23S genes could generate large stem structures in *E. coli* and *B. subtilis* (60, 80). The stems may be the substrates for processing enzymes. These structures can also be generated in rRNA operons of *M. capricolum* and *Mycoplasma* sp. strain PG50 (see chapter 19). In *B. subtilis*, a stretch in the sequence preceding the 16S rRNA gene appears again in the spacer between the 23S and 5S rRNA genes. This feature also occurs in *M. capricolum* and *Mycoplasma* sp. strain PG50.

Furthermore, a great deal of homology was found between rRNA sequences from *M. capricolum*, *Mycoplasma* sp. strain PG50, and *B. subtilis* in the repeated stem regions. A sequence of 15 bp within this region is completely conserved, and a sequence of some 20 bp toward the 16S rRNA genes also shows significant homology (46). Ogasawara et al. (46) have proposed that these regions may be the target sites for processing enzymes such as RNase III. This would imply that the processing mechanisms in *M. capricolum* and *B. subtilis* are more highly conserved than between either of these organisms and *E. coli*. In several *B. subtilis* rRNA operons, a set of opposed G's is found in both stems, probably serving as RNase III cleavage sites. In *Mycoplasma* sp. strain PG50 (50), both sets of opposed G's have changed to a GC pair. If these ideas are correct, then the initial processing events in mycoplasmas have a strong resemblance to those in *B. subtilis* yet also show some distinct characteristics.

In *M. hyopneumoniae*, the 16S–23S spacer is 500 nucleotides long and the 5S rRNA gene is even further removed (67). In this mycoplasma, the transcription of the 16S–23S rRNA operon apparently terminates downstream from the putative 23S stem structure, where two alternative G + C-rich secondary structures are found. These structures may function as rho-independent terminators (56, 64).

Taschke and coworkers (64, 68) suggest that in both *M. hyopneumoniae* and *M. capricolum*, the primary transcript of 16S and 23S rRNAs is first cleaved to yield premature 16S and 23S rRNAs as in *E. coli* and *B. subtilis*. The cleavage sites fall within two putative stem structures surrounding the sequences of mature rRNAs. The inner parts of these recognition sequences in *M. hyopneumoniae* and in the *rrnB* operon of *M. capricolum* are homologous to the corresponding regions of the rRNA precursors of *B. subtilis* (34) but not to the corresponding *E. coli* rRNA operon sequences, in accord with the phylogenetic relationship between mycoplasmas and species of the *Bacillus-Clostridium* group deduced from comparisons of rRNA sequences. *M. pneumoniae* also has this conserved stem sequence of *B. subtilis* in its leader (25). However, a complementary sequence could not be found in its short (43-bp) 23S-5S spacer, indicating that the 23S rRNA of this mycoplasma may have a slightly different processing mechanism (our unpublished results).

The spacers and the 5′ and 3′ flanking sequences of the *M. capricolum* and *Mycoplasma* sp. strain PG50 rRNA operons are extremely low in G + C (20%), in contrast to a relatively high G + C content (48%) of the rRNA coding sequences (39). This value for the spacers is even lower than that of the total genomic *M. capricolum* DNA (25%). Mollicutes are known for their low G + C genomic content. Perhaps the combined restraints of a conserved rRNA gene sequence and a generally low G + C content led to the extremely low G + C spacer as a balance for the high G + C content in the conserved rRNA genes (41).

An unusual structural feature has been found in the *rrnA* operons of *M. capricolum* (13, 65) and *Mycoplasma* sp. strain PG50 (50). Upstream from the 16S rRNA are genes for two tRNA species, tRNA^{Lys} (−437 to −362) followed by tRNA^{Leu} (−360 to −277). The only other reports of genes coding for tRNA preceding rRNA operons have been for chloroplasts of higher plants, in which a tRNA^{Val} gene is located upstream of the 16S rRNA gene in all species examined (61).

TRANSCRIPTION CONTROL ELEMENTS OF rRNA OPERONS

Promoters

The accessibility of rRNA probes has facilitated the structural and functional analysis of the elements regulating mycoplasma rRNA synthesis. In the sequence analyses carried out by Rasmussen et al. (50) on *Mycoplasma* sp. strain PG50 and by Taschke and Herrmann (65) on *M. capricolum*, the two rRNA operons, *rrnA* and *rrnB*, of each organism were shown to have identical leader sequences of 114 bp. These sequences can participate in stem structures as described above.

The *rrnA* operon of *M. capricolum* has two promoters which have been identified functionally by primer extension and S1 nuclease mapping of the RNA species produced in vivo. The second promoter (P2) is associated with the transcription of the *rrnA* operon, whereas the first, P1, precedes the two tRNA genes located approximately 300 bp upstream from P2 (discussed above). Two promoters can also be identified in the corresponding locations of *rrnA* of *Mycoplasma* sp. strain PG50 (50). The two tRNA genes preceding the *rrnA* operon are succeeded by a stem and loop followed by T residues, a classical eubacterial transcription termination signal, suggesting that at least some of the transcripts initiated proximal to the tRNA genes terminate before transcription of the rRNA genes. Mapping methods could not definitively identify a read-through transcript produced by *M. capricolum*, although transcripts extending upstream from P2 were seen. In addition, when the cloned operon was expressed in *E. coli*, a read-through transcript could be detected both in vitro and in vivo (13). Primer extension studies (65), using oligonucleotide probes selective for *rrnA*, indicated that the putative precursor may be cleaved to yield tRNA and rRNA precursor molecules. The rRNA precursor is approximately 100 nucleotides longer than the precursor synthesized from P2. The second rRNA operon of *M. capricolum*, *rrnB*, also has two possible promoter structures. However, only the first, P1, could be shown to function in vivo in a study of *M. capricolum* (65). Results obtained in another study, based on primer extension analysis (13), suggested that a transcript initiated at P2 may be produced in vivo, but this result may be considered inconclusive because transcripts originating from the two different operons were not clearly distinguishable. Interestingly, extracts of *M. capricolum* cells transcribed from *rrnB* P2 more efficiently than from *rrnB* P1. Thus, Taschke and Herrmann (65) proposed that a growth control mechanism may be operating in vivo to inhibit transcription from P2 or that this transcript may have a short half-life in vivo.

The *rrnB* P1 promoter has one base change in the TTG −35 recognition sequence relative to TTA. This may explain why it is weaker than the *rrnA* promoters which have the exact consensus sequence. The other three promoter sequences in *M. capricolum* and the three corresponding promoter sequences of the rRNA operons of *Mycoplasma* sp. strain PG50 have the procaryotic consensus sequences. The two parts of the promoters are 17 bp apart, the optimal distance. Upstream from the promoters are A + T-rich regions (not surprising for an A + T-rich genome), especially in *rrnB*. This promoter resembles *B. subtilis* promoters which use the σ^{55} factor (37). These similar features suggest that these two mycoplasmas may have transcription systems very similar to those used during vegetative growth of *B. subtilis*. The mycoplasmal P2 promoters are located at approximately the same distance upstream of the repeated sequences as in the *B. subtilis rrnB* promoter. However, the *E. coli* and *B. subtilis* rRNA operons appear to be transcribed from two promoters. In *E. coli*, the upstream promoter, P1, is more active in cells during high growth rates and is the promoter that reacts during amino acid or carbon starvation, while P2 is a constitutive weak promoter, perhaps a maintenance promoter (16, 57). Only the second operon, *rrnB*, of *M. capricolum* may resemble the eubacterial promoter region, but the control mechanisms governing this mycoplasmal operon are not yet clear.

The single rRNA operon of *M. hyopneumoniae* studied by Taschke and Herrmann (64) has numerous unusual features. The 5S rRNA gene is separated from the 16S and 23S genes, and there is a 500-nucleotide spacer between the 16S and 23S genes, with no tRNAs present. The existence of a primary transcript including the 16S and 23S rRNAs is indicated by the observed promoter structure only upstream of the 16S rRNA as well as by the detection of premature rRNA species in mapping experiments. In addition, repeated processing signals occur before and after the 16S gene, and transcription termination was seen downstream from the 23S gene (56). Transcription of this operon occurs from two tandem promoters. Here, P2 seems to be used predominantly, possibly because of differential regulation or simply promoter strength. Both promoters have a consensus Pribnow box and start transcription with a purine as in other bacteria. It is striking that both promoters lack the −35 recognition region of eubacterial promoters. Instead, there are A + T-rich sequences which in *E. coli* influence promoter strength, but only together with a −35 region. In addition, two other promoters found in *M. hyopneumoniae* have the same structure (64, 66). Taschke and Herrmann (64) raise the question of whether the typical −35 consensus sequence can be replaced by an A + T-rich region or whether a recognition site is completely dispensable in *M. hyopneumoniae*.

Primer extension experiments on the single rRNA operon of *M. pneumoniae* identified one transcription start site 67 nucleotides upstream from the 16S rRNA gene (24, 25). This promoter also functioned in vitro with use of *E. coli* RNA polymerase. Its location is similar to that of the P2 promoter in *M. hyopneumoniae* (starting at position −87). In addition, the sequences of these two promoters are similar in that both have a −10 consensus sequence with an A + T-rich upstream region. The absence of a defined −35 recognition region may be responsible for our inability to detect transcripts in *E. coli* in vivo (25). This result differed from results of studies with the cloned *rrnA* operon of *M. capricolum* (13). The promoters of this operon were transcribed by *E. coli* RNA polymerase both in vivo and in vitro. This difference may be due to the presence of a −35 region resembling that of eubacterial promoters. It will be interesting to determine whether the novel promoter structure, described for *M. pneumoniae* and *M. hyopneumoniae*, occurs in these mycoplasmas only or also in other mycoplasma species.

Two main control mechanisms are known to affect stable RNA (rRNA and tRNA) synthesis in *E. coli*: growth rate control and stringent control (7). Stringent control in *E. coli* is related to the *relA* gene. Thus, wild-type *E. coli* cells respond to amino acid starvation by accumulation of the nucleotides guanosine 3′,5′-bis-diphosphate and guanosine 5′-triphosphate 3′-diphosphate (ppGpp and pppGpp) and by a concomitant inhibition of stable RNA synthesis. *relA* mutants of these bacteria have lost this control system (7). At least in the case of stringent control, the intracellular accumulation of ppGpp has been interpreted as the causative agent in the mechanism of inhibition of stable RNA synthesis.

M. capricolum, one of the least-exacting mycoplasmas, was selected (2, 13, 15) for studies on stringent control mechanisms in mollicutes because this mycoplasma can be grown in a partially defined medium. Stable RNA synthesis in *M. capricolum* was found to be markedly affected by omission of the amino acid supplement from the medium. The major conclusion from these experiments was that synthesis of stable RNA in *M. capricolum* is subject to a stringent control mechanism resembling that described in other procaryotes. However, in contrast to the findings with *E. coli*, the major nucleotide accumulated in the mycoplasma was pppGpp rather than ppGpp (15). Information is incomplete on cellular components involved in stringent control as well as on the mechanisms and factors controlling the synthesis and accumulation of ppGpp and pppGpp. A surprising observation was that the *M. capricolum* rRNA promoter that was expressed in vivo in *E. coli* was activated rather than repressed by ppGpp in *E. coli* (13). This result further emphasizes the need for additional studies to unravel the various elements that participate in the control of rRNA gene promoters in mycoplasmas. The fact that mollicute genomes carry only one or two copies of rRNA genes would seem to facilitate studies on the mode of control of rRNA promoters, since such studies become more complicated when the copy number of rRNA operons in a genome is high, as in *E. coli*.

Terminators

Several typical procaryotic transcription termination signals have been noted in mycoplasmal DNA sequences, but so far, only two have been proved functionally. The first was at the end of the *M. hyopneumoniae* rRNA operon (66), following the 23S gene, as described above. Hyman and Razin (25a) analyzed the 3' end of the *M. pneumoniae* rRNA operon by S1 nuclease mapping and DNA sequencing to determine the termination site. A putative stem-loop sequence followed by T's at the 3' end of the operon would be a potential terminator. A 3'-end-labeled DNA probe was prepared, starting within the 5S rRNA gene at an *Asu*II restriction site and extending 2,200 bp to a *Sma*I site, far beyond the 3' end of the operon. After hybridization to total RNA of *M. pneumoniae*, two DNA species were protected from S1 nuclease digestion. The results are shown in Fig. 1 next to a sequence ladder used as size markers. The protected DNA fragments (which end in a stutter due to either a technical artifact or termination stuttering) extended 67 and 110 bp from the *Asu*II site. These two bands map the 3' end of the 5S rRNA and the 3' end of the precursor RNA, respectively. The transcription termination site thus falls at the predicted site according to the stem-loop structure in the sequence. No additional site can be seen. Thus, in *M. pneumoniae* as in *M. hyopneumoniae*, the rRNA operon termination site resembles the structure of eubacterial factor-independent transcription terminators. Of course, these operons are evolutionarily conserved, and other mycoplasmal operons may have different terminator structures.

EVOLUTIONARY IMPLICATIONS OF STRUCTURE DIFFERENCES BETWEEN MYCOPLASMAL rRNAs

Comparison of the structural RNA sequences of organisms has contributed a great deal of information to the study of phylogenetic relationships, because these genes are present in all cells and thus evolved into their present form before the divergence of the precursors of any of the species now present (74). The 1,521-bp 16S *rrn*B rRNA gene of *M. capricolum* is 21 bp shorter than the corresponding *E. coli* sequence (38). Sequence similarities are 74% to *E. coli*, 82% to *B. subtilis*, and 75% to *A. nidulans*. The *M. hyopneumoniae* 16S gene shows 75% homology with *B. subtilis* and

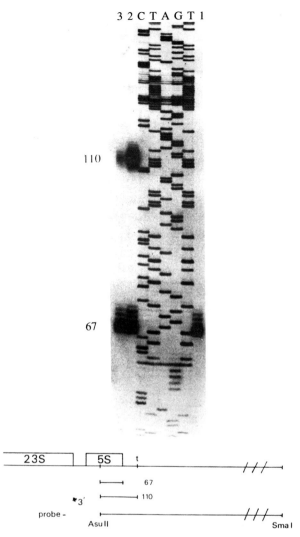

Figure 1. S1 nuclease mapping of the 3' end of the *M. pneumoniae* rRNA operon. S1 nuclease-protected DNA fragments were run on a 7% polyacrylamide–urea gel next to a known sequence (TGATC). Samples of 90 μg (lanes 1 and 2) and 30 μg (lane 3) were mixed with 150,000 cpm of *Asu*II-*Sma*I 3'-labeled DNA probe (shown in the diagram at the bottom) at 47°C (lanes 2 and 3) or 52°C (lane 1) as described previously (35). After 3 h of hybridization, 6 U of S1 nuclease (Bethesda Research Laboratories) was added, and incubation at 37°C was carried out for 30 min.

70% homology with *E. coli*. *Mycoplasma* sp. strain PG50 *rrn*B shares 99% identity with the corresponding *M. capricolum* gene. The 5S rRNA in *rrn*B is 109 bp, shorter than other bacterial 5S species, which fall into two groups, 116 bp (gram positive) and 120 bp (gram negative) (23).

The homologies to eubacterial 16S genes are often in the single-stranded loop regions. Often, the double-stranded stem regions contain compensatory base changes ensuring that the secondary structure is retained despite large differences in the primary sequence. In particular, a GC stem pair in *E. coli* may change to an AU pair in *Mycoplasma* sp. strain PG50 or *M. capricolum* sequences (12). Clearly, there is a very strong association between structure and function in these RNA species. Twelve guanine residues, which have all been implicated in the association of 30S and 50S subunits, are all conserved except for one in *Mycoplasma* sp. strain PG50. The 3' end, which is complementary to the Shine-Dalgarno sequence of mRNAs, is homologous in PG50 to the *B. brevis* sequence, whereas *E. coli* has a slightly shorter sequence. It is of interest that *B. subtilis* is known to be much stricter than *E. coli* regarding recognition of foreign transcription and translation signals. The ribosomes of *B. subtilis*, for example, fail to translate *E. coli* mRNAs. It has been proposed that differences at the 3' termini may be the cause (37). In general, variable regions in mycoplasma 16S rRNAs more closely resembled *B. brevis* sequences than *E. coli* sequences (76).

Extensive analyses have been carried out recently to compare a significant number of 16S (75) and 5S (55) rRNA sequences as a basis for constructing phylogenetic trees of organisms. The recent development of oligonucleotide technology enabled Weisburg et al. (75) to sequence 16S rRNAs of 40 mollicute species without cloning their genes. Because of the degree of similarity among all sequences, their alignment was not very difficult. Established secondary structural constraints and sequence conservation patterns enabled alignment of mollicute sequences and six of their walled relatives. The results obtained with the different types of rRNAs support the model (55, 77) that mycoplasmas form a coherent phylogenetic group that, with *Clostridium innocuum*, arose as a branch of the low-G + C gram-positive tree, near the lactobacilli and streptococci (see chapter 33). An additional study of plant-pathogenic MLOs using 16S rRNA comparisons led to the conclusion that MLOs have been appropriately placed in the class *Mollicutes*, but they are more closely related to the acholeplasmas than to the animal mycoplasmas (32). Thus, much of mycoplasma phylogeny is presently based on an analysis of structural RNA sequences.

rRNA GENE PROBES IN MYCOPLASMA TAXONOMY AND DIAGNOSIS

The finding that rRNA genes are conserved among mollicutes led to their use as probes in mycoplasma detection and identification. Southern blot hybridization of cloned *M. capricolum* rRNA genes with DNAs of various mycoplasmas digested by restriction endonucleases results in hybridization patterns specific for each of the tested mycoplasma strains (1, 51, 78, 79) (see also chapter 1). These patterns have been referred to as fingerprints and serve to reliably identify a given strain or isolate. This has been very useful as a method of detecting intraspecies genetic homogeneity or heterogeneity (78, 79), thereby aiding in studies of taxonomy and epidemiology of mycoplasma infections.

Laboratory diagnosis of mycoplasma infections generally suffers from the difficulty in cultivating the slowly growing mycoplasmas. In some cases, such as plant and insect infections by the uncultivable MLOs, diagnosis by conventional techniques is not possible. Serological techniques tend to be relatively nonspecific, as do indirect means such as DNA staining and enzymatic reactions. A more recent development in laboratory diagnosis is based on DNA probes. DNA sequences specific for a particular group or a single species of infectious agents are selected, cloned, and used as probes in hybridization tests with DNA of the infected tissue or clinical specimen (51).

DNA probes containing rRNA genes have been successfully applied to the detection and identification of mycoplasmas in contaminated cell cultures (53, 54). Eucaryotic rRNA genes show very little, if any, homology with the procaryotic genes. Fewer than 10^5 mycoplasmas per ml of culture could be detected, a level lower than that found in most contaminated animal cell cultures. This procedure, based on Southern blot hybridization of cloned *M. capricolum* rRNA genes with digested DNA of the tested culture, could also identify the contaminating mycoplasma. The more rapid dot blot technique can be used (69, 70) to detect mycoplasmas, but it is not specific to mycoplasmas and cannot identify a species.

Göbel and Stanbridge (20) used a cloned fragment of the *M. hyorhinis* 23S rRNA gene as a probe for the detection of mycoplasma contamination in cell cultures. Their probe had the advantage of being mycoplasma specific. Although it did not hybridize to *E. coli* DNA, it hybridized to all mycoplasma species tested and detected less than 0.5 pg of homologous DNA. The fact that this probe did not hybridize to *E. coli* does not ensure that it is mycoplasma specific, as mycoplasmal rRNA genes seem to be more homologous to those of gram-positive than gram-negative organisms. Göbel et al. (18, 19) refined the approach by using oligonucleotide probes. They carried out a computer-assisted sequence comparison of *M. pneumoniae* 16S rRNA sequences with sequences from various other mycoplasmal and bacterial species to construct mycoplasma group-specific oligonucleotide probes complementary to semiconserved regions of the *M. pneumoniae* 16S rRNA molecule. They also constructed *M. pneumoniae* species-specific oligonucleotide probes complementary to variable regions in the 16S rRNA molecule. Using a DNA-RNA dot blot hybridization procedure, they could detect fewer than 10^3 mycoplasmas as long as the cells were not frozen and thawed. A DNA-DNA hybridization procedure less sensitive to freezing easily detected 10^4 organisms applied to a filter. The presence of large amounts of rRNA in every cell makes rRNA an attractive target for diagnostic hybridization probes. In addition, the use of an oligonucleotide probe permits short hybridization and washing times.

The oligonucleotide probe method has been used by Gen-Probe (San Diego, Calif.) for the preparation of a kit for the detection of *M. pneumoniae*. Several reports of comparisons of the effectiveness of this kit with other diagnostic methods on clinical specimens have been published. In one such report (71), culture and probe tests were performed on respiratory specimens in transport media or on transport media in which colonies of suspected *M. pneumoniae* had been suspended. No respiratory specimen gave a positive culture test and a negative probe test, indicating 100% sensitivity. Only one specimen was negative in the culture test and positive in the probe test, indicating 98% specificity. Tilton et al. (71) conclude that the test is rapid (approximately 2 h), sensitive, and specific. Another report, by Harris et al. (21), compared the Gen-Probe method with the direct detection of specific antigens in respiratory exudates. They tested viable *M. pneumoniae* in negative nasopharyngeal aspirates. The Gen-Probe method proved to be more sensitive than the antigen capture indirect enzyme immunoassay (Ag-EIA), detecting 2×10^3 CFU/ml (10 to 100 times less sensitive than culture methods). They also tested 90 patients. All samples that were culture negative were also Gen-Probe negative. However, of 23 culture-positive or seropositive samples, 21 (91%) were detected by Ag-EIA and only 5 (22%) were detected by the Gen-Probe method. Thus, these authors found a close correspondence between positive cultures and Ag-EIA- and Gen-Probe-positive samples. The authors propose that protein antigen may remain intact in the respiratory tract much longer than rRNA. They also suggest that genomic DNA of *M. pneumoniae* would be more stable under conditions of natural infection; thus, the value of probes to genomic sequencing of *M. pneumoniae* merits investigation with clinical specimens.

REFERENCES

1. **Amikam, D., G. Glaser, and S. Razin.** 1984. Mycoplasmas (*Mollicutes*) have a low number of rRNA genes. *J. Bacteriol.* **158:**376–378.
2. **Amikam, D., S. Razin, and G. Glaser.** 1982. Ribosomal RNA genes in mycoplasma. *Nucleic Acids Res.* **10:**4215–4222.
3. **Bell, G. I., L. J. DeGennaro, D. H. Gelfand, R. J. Bishop, P. Valenzuela, and W. J. Rutter.** 1977. Ribosomal RNA genes of *Saccharomyces cerevisiae*. *J. Biol. Chem.* **252:**8118–8125.
4. **Bercovier, H., O. Kafri, and S. Sela.** 1986. Mycobacteria possess a surprisingly small number of ribosomal RNA genes in relation to the size of their genome. *Biochem. Biophys. Res. Commun.* **136:**1136–1141.
5. **Bram, R. J., R. J. Young, and J. A. Steitz.** 1980. The ribonuclease III site flanking 23S sequences in the 30S ribosomal precursor RNA of *E. coli*. *Cell* **19:**393–401.
6. **Brosius, J., T. J. Dull, D. D. Sleeter, and H. Noler.** 1981. Gene organization and primary structure of a ribosomal RNA operon from *Escherichia coli*. *J. Mol. Biol.* **148:**107–127.
7. **Cashel, M., and K. Rudd.** 1987. The stringent response, p. 1410–1438. *In* F. C. Neidhardt, J. L. Ingraham, K. B. Low, B. Magasanik, M. Schaechter, and H. E. Umbarger (ed.), *Escherichia coli and Salmonella typhimurium: Cellular and Molecular Biology*. American Society for Microbiology, Washington, D.C.
8. **Cerretti, D. P., D. Dean, G. R. Davis, D. M. Bedwell, and M. Nomura.** 1983. The *spc* ribosomal protein operon of *Escherichia coli*: sequence and cotranscription of the ribosomal protein genes and a protein export gene. *Nucleic Acids Res.* **11:**2599–2616.
9. **Chen, X., and L. R. Finch.** 1989. Novel arrangement of rRNA genes in *Mycoplasma gallisepticum*: separation of the 16S gene of one set from the 23S and 5S genes. *J. Bacteriol.* **171:**2876–2878.
10. **Christiansen, C.** 1987. The mycoplasma genome, part 1. *Microbiol. Sci.* **4:**168–172.
11. **Christiansen, C.** 1987. The mycoplasma genome, part 2. *Microbiol. Sci.* **4:**292–295.
12. **Frydenberg, J., and C. Christiansen.** 1985. The sequence of 16S rRNA from *Mycoplasma* strain PG50. *DNA* **4:**127–137.
13. **Gafny, R., H. C. Hyman, S. Razin, and G. Glaser.** 1988.

14. **Glaser, G., D. Amikam, and S. Razin.** 1984. Physical mapping of the ribosomal RNA genes of *Mycoplasma capricolum*. *Nucleic Acids Res.* **12:**2421–2426.
15. **Glaser, G., A. Razin, and S. Razin.** 1981. Stable RNA synthesis and its control in *Mycoplasma capricolum*. *Nucleic Acids Res.* **9:**3641–3646.
16. **Glaser, G., P. Sarmientos, and M. Cashel.** 1983. Functional inter-relationship between two tandem *E. coli* ribosomal RNA promoters. *Nature* (London) **302:**74–76.
17. **Göbel, U., G. H. Butler, and E. J. Stanbridge.** 1984. Comparative analysis of mycoplasma ribosomal RNA operons. *Isr. J. Med. Sci.* **20:**762–764.
18. **Göbel, U., R. Maas, G. Haun, C. Vinga-Martins, and E. J. Stanbridge.** 1987. Synthetic oligonucleotide probes complementary to rRNA for group- and species-specific detection of mycoplasmas. *Isr. J. Med. Sci.* **23:**742–846.
19. **Göbel, U. B., A. Geiser, and E. J. Stanbridge.** 1987. Oligonucleotide probes complementary to variable regions of ribosomal RNA discriminate between *Mycoplasma* species. *J. Gen. Microbiol.* **133:**1969–1974.
20. **Göbel, U. B., and E. J. Stanbridge.** 1984. Cloned mycoplasma rRNA genes for the detection of mycoplasma contamination in tissue cultures. *Science* **226:**1211–1213.
21. **Harris, R., B. P. Marmion, G. Varkanis, T. Kok, B. Lunn, and J. Martin.** 1988. Laboratory diagnosis of *M. pneumoniae* infection. II. Comparison of methods for the direct detection of specific antigen or nucleic acid sequences in respiratory exudates. *Epidemiol. Infect.* **101:**685–694.
21a. **Hayman, H., S. Razin, and G. Glaser.** Unpublished data.
22. **Hofman, J. D., R. H. Lan, and W. F. Doolittle.** 1979. The number, physical organization and transcription of ribosomal RNA cistrons in an archaebacterium: *Halobacterium halobium*. *Nucleic Acids Res.* **7:**1321–1333.
23. **Hori, H., and S. Osawa.** 1979. Evolutionary change in 5S RNA secondary structure and a phylogenetic tree of 54 5S RNA species. *Proc. Natl. Acad. Sci. USA* **76:**381–385.
24. **Hyman, H. C., R. Gafny, G. Glaser, and S. Razin.** 1987. Transcription control elements of the *Mycoplasma pneumoniae* rRNA operon. *Isr. J. Med. Sci.* **23:**585–590.
25. **Hyman, H. C., R. Gafny, G. Glaser, and S. Razin.** 1988. Promoter of the *Mycoplasma pneumoniae* rRNA operon. *J. Bacteriol.* **170:**3262–3268.
25a. **Hyman, H. C., and S. Razin.** Unpublished data.
26. **Iwami, M., A. Muto, F. Yamao, and S. Osawa.** 1984. Nucleotide sequence of the *rrn*B 16S ribosomal RNA gene from *Mycoplasma capricolum*. *Mol. Gen. Genet.* **196:**317–322.
27. **Johnson, J. D., and J. Horowitz.** 1971. Characterization of ribosomes and RNAs from *Mycoplasma hominis*. *Biochim. Biophys. Acta* **247:**262–279.
28. **Kawauchi, Y., A. Muto, and S. Osawa.** 1982. The protein composition of *Mycoplasma capricolum*. *Mol. Gen. Genet.* **188:**7–11.
29. **Kawauchi, Y., A. Muto, F. Yamao, and S. Osawa.** 1984. Molecular cloning of ribosomal protein genes from *Mycoplasma capricolum*. *Mol. Gen. Genet.* **196:**521–525.
30. **Kirk, R. G., and H. J. Morowitz.** 1969. Ribonucleic acids of *Mycoplasma gallisepticum* strain A5969. *Am. J. Vet. Res.* **30:**287–293.
30a. **Kirkpatrick, B. C., P. O. Lim, and B. B. Sears.** 1990. Phylogeny of plant-pathogenic mycoplasma-like organisms. *IOM Lett.* **1:**45–46.
31. **Kiss, A., B. Sain, and R. Venetianer.** 1977. The number of rRNA genes in *Escherichia coli*. *FEBS Lett.* **79:**7–78.
32. **Lim, P. O., and B. B. Sears.** 1989. 16S rRNA sequence indicates that plant-pathogenic mycoplasmalike organisms are evolutionarily distinct from animal mycoplasmas. *J. Bacteriol.* **171:**5901–5906.

33. **Loughney, K., E. Lund, and J. E. Dahlberg.** 1982. tRNA genes are found between the 16S and 23S rRNA genes in *Bacillus subtilis. Nucleic Acids Res.* **10**:1607–1623.

34. **Loughney, K., E. Lund, and J. E. Dahlberg.** 1983. Ribosomal RNA precursors of *Bacillus subtilis. Nucleic Acids Res.* **11**:6709–6721.

35. **Maniatis, T., E. F. Fritsch, and J. Sambrook.** 1982. *Molecular Cloning: A Laboratory Manual.* Cold Spring Harbor Laboratory, Cold Spring Harbor, N.Y.

36. **Maniloff, J.** 1971. Analysis of helical ribosome structures of *Mycoplasma gallisepticum. Proc. Natl. Acad. Sci. USA* **68**:43–47.

37. **Moran, C. P., Jr., N. Lang, S. F. J. LeGrice, G. Lee, M. Stephens, A. L. Sonenshein, J. Pero, and R. Losick.** 1982. Nucleotide sequences that signal the initiation of transcription and translation in *Bacillus subtilis. Mol. Gen. Genet.* **186**:339–346.

38. **Muto, A.** 1987. The genome structure of *Mycoplasma capricolum. Isr. J. Med. Sci.* **23**:334–341.

39. **Muto, A., H. Hori, M. Sawada, Y. Kawauchi, M. Iwami, F. Yamao, and S. Osawa.** 1983. The ribosomal RNA genes of *Mycoplasma capricolum. Yale J. Med. Sci.* **56**:373–376.

40. **Muto, A., Y. Kawauchi, F. Yamao, and S. Osawa.** 1984. Preferential use of A- and U-rich codons for *Mycoplasma capricolum* ribosomal proteins S8 and L6. *Nucleic Acids Res.* **12**:8209–8217.

41. **Muto, A., and S. Osawa.** 1987. The guanine and cytosine content of genomic DNA and bacterial evolution. *Proc. Natl. Acad. Sci. USA* **84**:166–169.

42. **Neimark, H.** 1983. Evolution of mycoplasmas and genome losses. *Yale J. Biol. Med.* **56**:377–383.

43. **Neimark, H.** 1984. Deletions, duplications and rearrangements in mycoplasma ribosomal RNA gene sequences. *Isr. J. Med. Sci.* **20**:765–767.

44. **Neumann, H., A. Gierl, J. Tu, J. Leibrock, D. Staiger, and W. Zillig.** 1983. Organization of the genes for ribosomal RNA in *Archaebacteria. Mol. Gen. Genet.* **192**:66–72.

45. **Noller, H. F., and M. Nomura.** 1987. Ribosomes, p. 104–125. *In* F. C. Neidhardt, J. L. Ingraham, K. B. Low, B. Magasanik, M. Schaechter, and H. E. Umbarger (ed.), *Escherichia coli and Salmonella typhimurium: Cellular and Molecular Biology.* American Society for Microbiology, Washington, D.C.

46. **Ogasawara, N., A. Moriya, and H. Yoshikawa.** 1983. Structure and organization of rRNA operons in the region of the replication origin of the *Bacillus subtilis* chromosome. *Nucleic Acids Res.* **11**:6301–6318.

47. **Ohkubo, S., A. Muto, Y. Kawauchi, F. Yamao, and S. Osawa.** 1987. The ribosomal protein gene cluster of *Mycoplasma capricolum. Mol. Gen. Genet.* **210**:314–322.

48. **Rasmussen, O. F., and C. Christiansen.** 1987. Nucleotide sequence of the 3′ end of the *Mycoplasma* strain PG50 *rrn*A operon. *Nucleic Acids Res.* **15**:1327.

49. **Rasmussen, O. F., and C. Christiansen.** 1987. Organization of the regions flanking the rRNA cistrons of *Mycoplasma* strain PG50. *Isr. J. Med. Sci.* **23**:342–346.

50. **Rasmussen, O. F., J. Frydenberg, and C. Christiansen.** 1987. Analysis of the leader and spacer regions of the two rRNA operons of *Mycoplasma* PG50: two tRNA genes are located upstream of *rrn*A. *Mol. Gen. Genet.* **208**:23–29.

51. **Razin, S.** 1985. Molecular biology and genetics of mycoplasmas (*Mollicutes*). *Microbiol. Rev.* **49**:419–455.

52. **Razin, S., M. F. Barile, R. Harasawa, D. Amikam, and G. Glaser.** 1983. Characterization of the mycoplasma genome. *Yale J. Biol. Med.* **56**:357–366.

53. **Razin, S., G. Glaser, and D. Amikam.** 1984. Molecular and biological features of *Mollicutes* (mycoplasmas). *Ann. Microbiol. (Inst. Pasteur)* **135A**:9–15.

54. **Razin, S., M. Gross, M. Wormser, Y. Pollack, and G. Glaser.** 1984. Detection of mycoplasmas infecting cell cultures by DNA hybridization. *In Vitro* **20**:404–408.

55. **Rogers, M. J., J. Simmons, R. T. Walker, W. G. Weisburg,** C. R. Woese, R. S. Tanner, I. M. Robinson, D. A. Stahl, G. Olsen, R. H. Leach, and J. Maniloff. 1985. Construction of the mycoplasma evolutionary tree from 5S rRNA sequence data. *Proc. Natl. Acad. Sci. USA* **82**:1160–1164.

56. **Rosenberg, M., and D. Court.** 1979. Regulatory sequences involved in the promotion and termination of RNA transcription. *Annu. Rev. Genet.* **13**:319–353.

57. **Sarmientos, P., and M. Cashel.** 1983. Carbon starvation and growth rate dependent regulation of the *Escherichia coli* ribosomal RNA promoters: differential control of dual promoters. *Proc. Natl. Acad. Sci. USA* **80**:7010–7013.

58. **Sawada, M., A. Muto, M. Iwami, F. Yamao, and S. Osawa.** 1984. Organization of ribosomal RNA genes in *Mycoplasma capricolum. Mol. Gen. Genet.* **196**:311–316.

59. **Sawada, M., S. Osawa, H. Kobayashi, H. Hori, and A. Muto.** 1981. The number of ribosomal RNA genes in *Mycoplasma capricolum. Mol. Gen. Genet.* **182**:502–504.

60. **Stewart, G. C., and K. F. Bott.** 1983. DNA sequence of the tandem ribosomal RNA promoter for *B. subtilis* operon *rrn*B. *Nucleic Acids Res.* **11**:6289–6300.

61. **Strittmatter, G., A. Gozkzicka-Jozefiak, and H. Kossel.** 1985. Identification of an rRNA operon promoter from *Zea mays* chloroplasts which excludes the proximal tRNA^{val} from the primary transcript. *EMBO J.* **4**:599–604.

62. **Suzuki, Y., T. Mori, Y. Miyata, and T. Yamada.** 1987. The number of ribosomal RNA genes in *Mycobacterium lepraemurium. FEMS Microbiol. Lett.* **44**:73–76.

63. **Suzuki, Y., K. Yoshinaga, Y. Ono, A. Nagata, and T. Yamada.** 1987. Organization of rRNA genes in *Mycobacterium bovis* BCG. *J. Bacteriol.* **169**:839–843.

64. **Taschke, C., and R. Herrmann.** 1986. Analysis of transcription and processing signals of the 16S/23S rRNA operon of *Mycoplasma hyopneumoniae. Mol. Gen. Genet.* **205**:434–441.

65. **Taschke, C., and R. Herrmann.** 1988. Analysis of transcription and processing signals in the 5′ regions of the two *Mycoplasma capricolum* rRNA operons. *Mol. Gen. Genet.* **212**:522–530.

66. **Taschke, C., M.-Q. Klinkert, E. Prikl, and R. Herrmann.** 1987. Gene expression signals in *Mycoplasma hyopneumoniae* and *Mycoplasma capricolum. Isr. J. Med. Sci.* **23**:347–351.

67. **Taschke, C., M.-Q. Klinkert, J. Wolters, and R. Herrmann.** 1986. Organization of the ribosomal RNA genes in *Mycoplasma hyopneumoniae*: the 5S rRNA is separated from the 16S and 23S rRNA genes. *Mol. Gen. Genet.* **205**:428–433.

68. **Taschke, C., K. Ruland, and R. Herrmann.** 1988. Nucleotide sequence of the 16S rRNA of *Mycoplasma hyopneumoniae. Nucleic Acids Res.* **15**:3918.

69. **Taylor, M. A., K. S. Wise, and M. A. McIntosh.** 1984. Species-specific detection of *Mycoplasma hyorhinis* using DNA probes. *Isr. J. Med. Sci.* **20**:778–780.

70. **Taylor, M. A., K. S. Wise, and M. A. McIntosh.** 1985. Selective detection of *Mycoplasma hyorhinis* using cloned genomic DNA fragments. *Infect. Immun.* **47**:827–830.

71. **Tilton, R. C., F. Dias, H. Kidd, and R. W. Ryan.** 1988. DNA probe versus culture for detection of *Mycoplasma pneumoniae* in clinical specimens. *Diagn. Microbiol. Infect. Dis.* **10**:109–112.

72. **Tu, J., and W. Zillig.** 1982. Organization of rRNA structural genes in the archaebacterium *Thermoplasma acidophilum. Nucleic Acids Res.* **10**:7231–7245.

73. **Ulbrich, N., I. Kumagai, and V. A. Erdmann.** 1984. The number of ribosomal RNA genes in *Thermus thermophilus* HB8. *Nucleic Acids Res.* **12**:2055–2060.

74. **Walker, R. T.** 1983. Mycoplasma evolution: a review of the use of ribosomal and transfer RNA nucleotide sequences in the determination of phylogenetic relationships. *Yale J. Biol. Med.* **56**:367–372.

75. **Weisburg, W. G., J. G. Tully, D. L. Rose, J. P. Petzel, H.**

Oyaizu, D. Yang, L. Mandelco, J. Sechrest, T. G. Lawrence, J. Van Etten, J. Maniloff, and C. R. Woese. 1989. A phylogenetic analysis of the mycoplasmas: basis for their classification. *J. Bacteriol.* **171**:6455–6467.

76. Woese, C. R., R. Gutell, R. Gupta, and H. F. Noller. 1983. Detailed analysis of the higher-order structure of the 16S-like ribosomal ribonucleic acids. *Microbiol. Rev.* **47**:621–669.

77. Woese, C. R., J. Maniloff, and L. B. Zablen. 1980. Phylogenetic analysis of the mycoplasmas. *Proc. Natl. Acad. Sci. USA* **77**:494–498.

78. Yogev, D., D. Halachmi, G. E. Keny, and S. Razin. 1988. Distinction of species and strains of mycoplasmas (*Molli-*

cutes) by genomic DNA fingerprints with an rRNA gene probe. *J. Clin. Microbiol.* **26**:1198–1201.

79. Yogev, D., S. Levisohn, S. H. Kleven, D. Halachmi, and S. Razin. 1988. Ribosomal RNA gene probes to detect intraspecies heterogeneity in *Mycoplasma gallisepticum* and *Mycoplasma synoviae*. *Avian Dis.* **32**:220–231.

80. Young, R. A., and J. A. Steitz. 1978. Complementary sequences 1700 nucleotides apart from a ribonuclease III cleavage site in *Escherichia coli* ribosomal precursor RNA. *Proc. Natl. Acad. Sci. USA* **75**:3593–3597.

81. Zurawski, G., and S. M. Zurawski. 1985. Structure of the *Escherichia coli* S10 ribosomal protein operon. *Nucleic Acids Res.* **13**:4521–4526.

III. METABOLISM AND ENERGY UTILIZATION

11. Carbohydrate Metabolism and Energy Conservation

J. DENNIS POLLACK

> Whenever we separate two things, we lose something which may have been the most essential feature.
> Albert Szent-Györgyi, 1963

INTRODUCTION

Perhaps 2,000 metabolic reactions occur during the synthesis of a bacterial cell like *Escherichia coli* (90). The reactions involve the formation of cellular structures such as envelopes, flagella, macromolecules, and their precursors. The 70 to 100 precursors in the form of nucleotides, sugars, amino acids, fatty acids, and coenzymes are all derived from only 12 central or core metabolites. The 12 core metabolites are glucose 6-phosphate (G6P), fructose 6-phosphate (F6P), triose phosphate, 3-phosphoglycerate, phosphoenolpyruvate (PEP), pyruvate, ribose 5-phosphate (R5P), erythrose 4-phosphate (E4P), 2-oxoglutarate, oxaloacetate, acetyl coenzyme A (acetyl-CoA), and succinyl-CoA (90).

The sequence of reactions, or pathways, by which 10 of these core metabolites are synthesized or utilized are known for mollicutes. Two major metabolic pathways are most involved. Eight core metabolites are synthesized by action of the Embden-Meyerhof-Parnas (EMP) pathway or its terminus. Two additional core metabolites are synthesized by action of the hexose monophosphate shunt (HMS).

The EMP pathway degrades G6P to pyruvate by reactions requiring ADP, NAD^+, and P_i. The products of this pathway are pyruvate, ATP, NADH, and H^+. During the conversion, G6P, F6P, triose phosphate, 3-phosphoglycerate, and PEP are also formed. Pyruvate at the terminus of the EMP pathway can be converted to lactate or alternatively to acetyl-CoA or oxaloacetate. The overall reaction of the EMP pathway in almost all procaryotic and eucaryotic cells is

$$\text{glucose} + 2\text{ ADP} + 2\text{ NAD}^+ + 2\text{ P}_i \longrightarrow$$

$$2\text{ pyruvate} + 2\text{ ATP} + 2\text{ NADH}$$

J. Dennis Pollack • Department of Medical Microbiology and Immunology, Ohio State University, 333 West 10th Avenue, Columbus, Ohio 43210.

The HMS produces two core metabolites: R5P and E4P. In most cells, the overall reaction for the HMS is

$$G6P + 12\ NADP^+ + 7\ H_2O \longrightarrow$$
$$6\ CO_2 + 12\ NADPH + 12\ H^+ + P_i$$

In the process of degradation of glucose or other carbohydrates by these two pathways, the coenzymes NAD^+ and $NADP^+$ are reduced to NADH and NADPH. For the pathways to continue to function, synthesis of NAD^+ or $NADP^+$ or reoxidation of NADH and NADPH becomes essential. Besides the reoxidation of NADH to NAD^+, protons are released from the cell and electrons are transported from one membrane component to another, each of higher (more positive) E_0' potential. In almost all cells other than mollicutes, the electrons are further processed by an electron transport chain composed of a variety of hydrogen carriers, including flavoproteins, lipoquinones, and cytochromes. In *E. coli*, a cytochrome finally transfers electrons to O_2, reducing it to water. During the passage of electrons to oxygen, part of the energy is removed and used to synthesize ATP from ADP and phosphate. The synthesis of ATP during this passage of protons and electrons involves a complex membrane integrated structure known as F_0F_1-ATPase.

Mollicutes differ strikingly from almost all procaryotes in possessing only a trace of lipoquinones (54), probably nonfunctional as significant electron carriers, and lacking cytochrome pigments. Mollicutes apparently directly pass electrons from NADH to molecular oxygen by way of a flavoprotein without lipoquinone or cytochrome intervention, mediated, at least in part, by an oxygen-dependent NADH oxidase (NOA). This reaction requires oxygen as the electron acceptor for all but the strictly anaerobic anaeroplasmas. The toxic superoxide radical (O_2^-) is formed as an intermediate. It is not known whether this oxidation of NADH in mollicutes is coupled to ATP synthesis. The role of a membrane-associated ATPase of mollicutes in the synthesis of ATP is discussed in chapter 15. This mollicute path is characterized as flavin-terminated respiration (FTR).

Alternate routes to the synthesis of ATP in mollicutes are less problematic. Substrate phosphorylation is a major mechanism. Substrate phosphorylation refers to the transfer of a phosphoryl group to ADP. The phosphorus-containing donor compounds are generally formed in the metabolism of carbohydrates. Two sites of substrate phosphorylation occur in the EMP pathway. They may be the major sites of substrate phosphorylation and ATP synthesis. The synthesis of ATP at these sites is mediated by 3-phosphoglycerate kinase and pyruvate kinase (PK). These activities have been found or indicated in all mollicutes.

In other procaryotes, a third site of substrate phosphorylation is located in the tricarboxylic acid (TCA) cycle, which is primarily fed by the products of the EMP pathway. Again, mollicutes differ strikingly from procaryotes since, except for the presence of malate dehydrogenase (MD) in all mollicutes and isocitrate dehydrogenase in the anaeroplasmas, an essentially complete functional TCA cycle has been reported in only one mollicute, and that single observation has not been confirmed.

GENERAL VIEW OF MOLLICUTES CARBOHYDRATE METABOLISM

In the apparent lactic fermentation that characterizes the glycolytic mollicutes, the continued need for NAD^+ and P_i is immediately apparent. Without NAD^+ and P_i, fermentation to lactate by the EMP pathway would not occur. An adequate supply of P_i is assumed in media used to cultivate mollicutes (13). It is not known whether mollicutes can synthesize the NAD nucleus, and except for semidefined and defined formulations, NAD derivatives are not routinely added to media (see chapter 2). A conceptual framework for discussing mollicutes metabolism might be built, in part, around the need for NAD^+.

Fermentation for mollicutes, in almost all cases, has been widely and loosely characterized as the process resulting in the production of acid in a supportive medium containing glucose as the major added carbohydrate. Those mollicutes that produce acid are described as fermentative, and those that do not are considered nonfermentative; in this discussion, the terms "glycolytic" and "nonglycolytic," respectively, will be substituted.

Glycolytic mollicutes grown anaerobically can convert glucose to lactate, in almost stoichiometric amounts; when grown aerobically, they produce lactate, acetate, and CO_2 (13, 14, 117–119, 150). Nonglycolytic mollicutes grown aerobically or anaerobically, although they possess portions of the EMP pathway, do not produce significant quantities of either lactate or acetate (39).

In one study (14), the nonglycolytic *Mycoplasma bovigenitalium* PG11, misrepresented as *M. bovis* PG45, showed no consumption of glucose and no change in the pH of the growth medium, while reaching a viable count of 5×10^9 CFU/ml, with a cellular adenylate energy charge of about 0.8. No lactate or pyruvate accumulated. This nonglycolytic strain, as noted below, apparently has the same enzymatic potential to synthesize lactate and acetate as do all glycolytic mollicutes (79, 98). Nonglycolytic mollicutes may gain energy and carbon by oxidizing short-chain fatty acids (78, 160) or by using amino acids such as glutamine (14) and arginine (14–17). Presumably, such amino acids are the major sources of carbon for *M. bovigenitalium* PG11 (14).

The strictly anaerobic mollicutes, members of the family *Anaeroplasmataceae*, are killed by oxygen. The end products of their metabolism have not been identified, but they possess the EMP pathway as do aerotolerant fermentative mollicutes (98).

Fermentations that occur in the presence of air often result in the production of toxic products like O_2^- and H_2O_2. Microorganisms, especially (and perhaps all) aerobes, produce superoxide dismutase (SOD) and catalase to convert these toxic agents to water and oxygen (47). All mollicutes tested produce SOD (83), and many produce catalase (77, 83, 94).

In the production of lactate by the EMP pathway, glycolytic mollicutes process hexoses through a series of reactions generally common to most cells. But there is a significant difference. The glycolytic *Acholeplasma* spp. use PP_i rather than ATP as the phosphoryl donor in the phosphofructokinase (PFK) reaction (109), as does *Anaeroplasma intermedium* (98). All other glycolytic mollicutes use ATP in the PFK reaction (39, 106).

The few nonglycolytic mollicutes that have been analyzed (*M. bovigenitalium* PG11 is an example) all lack PFK and fructose 1,6-phosphate aldolase activities yet possess all of the enzymes of the triose (C_3) arm of the EMP pathway (39). They express all of the enzymes necessary to produce lactate from trioses but apparently cannot synthesize trioses from hexoses, like glucose, or obtain trioses by other mechanisms in sufficient quantity to synthesize detectable levels of lactate. The nonglycolytic *Acholeplasma parvum* has not been tested (4).

The C_3 arm is where all substrate phosphorylation of the EMP pathway occurs. Two enzymes are involved: phosphoglycerate kinase and PK. These enzyme activities have been detected in both glycolytic and nonglycolytic *Mycoplasma* spp. (39, 79), *Ureaplasma urealyticum* (34), *Spiroplasma* spp. (106), and *Anaeroplasma intermedium* (98). *Asteroleplasma anaerobium* does not have PK activity (98).

As described more fully in later sections, an additional pathway that may carry significant metabolic traffic in the mollicutes is the HMS. *Acholeplasma* spp. are the only mollicutes that can generate NADPH by this pathway. Acholeplasmas presumably use NADPH to synthesize fatty acids from acetate. All other mollicutes lack the initiating dehydrogenases of the classical HMS and are presumably unable to reduce $NADP^+$ to NADPH, are unable to convert acetate to lipids, and need exogenous lipid for survival.

The HMS also interconverts sugars, feeds the EMP pathway at the level of F6P and glyceraldehyde 3-phosphate (G3P) and acts as a source of precursors for nucleic acid and aromatic amino acid synthesis. It is an important linker path and has been found in all mollicutes except the nonglycolytic *Mycoplasma* spp. The nonglycolytic *Mycoplasma* spp. examined, therefore, lack both a functional HMS and the enzymatic points of attachment in the hexose arm of the EMP pathway, where the HMS would connect (i.e., feed) glycolysis.

Although mollicutes can oxidize pyruvate in a series of reactions with CoA to acetyl-CoA, they cannot degrade the acetate moiety to CO_2 because they lack a functional TCA cycle (79). In *Acholeplasma* spp., acetyl-CoA is probably used in the synthesis of lipids; in other mollicutes, it may be converted to malate and then oxaloacetate. All mollicutes can also carboxylate pyruvate with CO_2 directly to oxaloacetate. Oxaloacetate can be transaminated. Many of these reactions are known to be reversible. The interplay of mollicutes reactions at the pyruvate locus is complex. In addition to pyruvate, PEP, lactate, acetyl-CoA, malate, and oxaloacetate are involved. The major differences are that (i) *Acholeplasma* spp. can carboxylate PEP to oxaloacetate, whereas *Mycoplasma* spp. cannot, and (ii) *Mycoplasma* spp. can synthesize malate from acetyl-CoA and glyoxylate, whereas *Acholeplasma* spp. cannot (79). The levels of ATP and ADP and of NAD^+ and NADH may modulate the interactions.

Mollicutes are aerotolerant. They produce SOD, some produce catalase, and they can grow at a reduced pO_2. Except for the strictly anaerobic family *Anaeroplasmataceae*, oxygen, when available, may be the major electron acceptor for all mollicutes. In this role, mediated by NOA, oxygen is reduced by nutrient-derived electrons carried by an intermediate, NADH. Emphasis cannot be placed entirely on oxygen as the terminal electron acceptor, since NADH participating in reductions of organic molecules would be reoxidized to NAD^+ without oxygen such as in the reduction of pyruvate to lactate.

Lactate may have a more important role in mollicutes metabolism than has been appreciated. The lactococci, in many metabolic respects, are similar to mollicutes; for example, they lack cytochromes (62, 67). Konings et al. (68) have shown that lactococci generate metabolic energy not only by substrate phosphorylation or arginine metabolism but also by proton motive force generation linked to lactate efflux. The process involving lactate is electrogenic and carrier mediated. The concept and data indicate that lactate efflux occurs by symport with protons. The model is called the energy recycling model (23, 68) and was first described by Michels et al. (84).

CARBOHYDRATE METABOLISM IN MOLLICUTES

The doctoral thesis in medicine of Edouard Dujardin-Beaumetz to the Faculté de Médicine de Paris, entitled "Le Microbe de la Péripneumonie et sa Culture," was presented on 5 April 1900 (40). His collaborator was Edmond Isidore Étienne Nocard of Alfort, who with Pierre Paul Émil Roux discovered the mollicutes. Dujardin-Beaumetz was the first investigator to study the pattern of carbohydrate utilization, i.e., metabolism, in mollicutes. He found that the péripneumonie agent, presumably *M. mycoides* subsp. *mycoides*, grown in the presence of 5% glucose or maltose produced one volatile acid, acetic acid. There was no acid when lactose, sucrose, or galactose was substituted. There was no report of lactic acid recovery. In 1932, Holmes and Pirie (55) made a detailed study of the glucose metabolism of the "bovine pleuropneumonia virus." They found that the organism could produce acid from glucose and reduce methylene blue in the presence of lactate. They indicated that growth could be estimated by monitoring the increase in lactic dehydrogenase (LDH) activity. Warren (161) studied eight pleuropneumonia strains and found that they all produced acid from glucose and contained LDH. Edward (41) studied 18 strains of pleuropneumonia(like) organisms in fermentation tests with eight carbohydrates. Only eight strains produced acid from the sugars, without gas. Miles and Wadher (85) have studied substrate utilization in *Mycoplasma* spp. as evidenced by O_2 consumption by a sensitive polarographic technique.

Rodwell and Rodwell's landmark studies in 1954 with *Asterococcus* (now known as *Mycoplasma*) *mycoides* V5 described the pathway by which this organism processed glucose (117–119). Under anaerobic conditions, lactate was the major end product, whereas aerobically acetate and CO_2 accumulated. No evidence was found for a cytochrome system, peroxidase, or metabolism of TCA cycle intermediates. The data suggested that under anaerobic conditions, pyruvate acted as the major electron acceptor and was reduced by NADH and LDH to form lactate which accumulated in the culture. Aerobically, NADH was oxidized by other systems such as NOA, and less lactate and acetate were formed. This model is apparently the pattern followed by most and perhaps all glycolytic mollicutes except *Ureaplasma* spp. and the anaerobic mollicutes, whose methods for disposing of electrons are least known. The pattern that the Rodwells described is similar in most respects to the homofermentative or homolactic pathway (122). By this route, comprising the EMP pathway, each mole of glucose is converted to 2 mol of lactate and 2 mol of ATP. The path is characteristic of many lactic acid bacteria, e.g., *Lactococcus*, *Lactobacillus*, *Streptococcus*, and *Leuconostoc* spp. Lactate with lesser amounts of pyruvate and acetate has been reported to accumulate in the culture fluids of various mollicutes (13, 14, 24, 55, 93, 150).

The second major path by which mollicutes metabolize glucose was first revealed by the work of Castrejon-Diez et al. (24). Using *A. laidlawii* Adler, a strain related to the more generally studied strain B, they found that the complete HMS system was functional. They detected NADP-dependent G6P dehydrogenase (G6Pde), transketolase (TK), and phosphoribose isomerase. Under some experimental conditions, heptose and fructose accumulated. The presence of the HMS has been generally associated with *Acholeplasma* spp. (29, 70, 94, 95, 130). Recently, a truncated form lacking the two initiating NADP-dependent dehydrogenase reactions has been found to be widespread in mollicutes genera (29, 34, 39, 98, 106). In these studies, the two dehydrogenases of the HMS (G6Pde and 6-phosphogluconate dehydrogenase [6PGde]) were found only in the *Acholeplasma* spp. and have not been reported in any other mollicutes genus.

The carbohydrate metabolism of mollicutes is apparently centered upon the interaction of glycolysis, the EMP pathway, and the HMS. ATP may also be synthesized by proton translocation coupled to oxidation of reduced pyridines such as NADH or to the synthesis and transport of lactate. The relative paucity of metabolic opportunity is reflected by the absence of cytochromes and the TCA cycle in all mollicutes examined.

GLYCOLYSIS

Entry to Glycolysis

Mollicutes can utilize a variety of sugars. A compilation of the sugars utilized by different species with the production of acid was first published in 1954 (41). More recent analyses (53, 116) and very comprehensive surveys (154, 155) are available.

The transport of sugars into mollicutes cells is reported to proceed either by a carrier-mediated active transport process in some *Acholeplasma* spp. or by a group translocation process involving PEP in *Mycoplasma* and *Spiroplasma* spp. (27, 125, 156, 158). In the former case, glucose is finally phosphorylated in the cytoplasm, presumably by hexokinase or glucokinase, to G6P and enters the EMP pathway. In the group translocation process, glucose is phosphorylated to G6P without the apparent intervention of hexokinase. The topic of the transport of sugars into mollicutes

cells has been presented elsewhere (125) and is discussed in chapter 15.

EMP Pathway

The priming steps and the hexose arm

The EMP pathway (Fig. 1) is virtually ubiquitous and is considered to be the most ancient type of energy metabolism (96). It is composed of 15 enzymes, if hexokinase and alcohol dehydrogenase are included. The structural cores of the glycolytic enzymes are similar: they are eight mostly parallel β strands surrounded by eight α helices in a cylindrical barrel structure, and their amino acid sequences are strongly conserved (45).

Glycolytic enzymes mutate slowly, about $\frac{1}{3}$ to $\frac{1}{10}$ the rate of trypsin or RNase (37). Their use of ATP or NAD$^+$, in seven cases, has suggested that they evolved from a common ancestor. Fothergill-Gilmore believes that the glycolytic path has not evolved from a common ancestor but resulted from the random assembly of independently evolving enzymes (45). In this model, the similarities in the glycolytic enzymes and their barrel structures are the result of evolutionary convergence toward stable protein structures that bind negatively charged moieties, such as hexose and triose phosphates.

Hexokinase is the first priming step of glycolysis. A neutral D-sugar is phosphorylated by ATP to form, in the case of D-glucose, G6P. The reaction requires a divalent cation, e.g., Mg^{2+}. The actual substrate of the reaction is Mg-ATP. There are two types of enzymes: hexokinase (EC 2.7.1.1), which catalyzes the phosphorylation of glucose and other hexoses, and glucokinase (EC 2.7.1.2), which phosphorylates only glucose. This distinction has not been generally made in the mollicutes literature. Hexokinase activity has been reported in *Acholeplasma* spp. (39, 70) and in *Anaeroplasma intermedium* (98) but not in *Spiroplasma* spp. (39), *Mycoplasma* spp. (39), *U. urealyticum* (17, 29) or *Asteroleplasma anaerobium* (98).

G6P is converted by the EMP pathway to F6P. The reaction is mediated by G6P isomerase (EC 5.3.1.9). G6P can take another path, of great import in mollicutes metabolism: the HMS (see below). The G6P isomerase reaction is reversible and has been found in *Acholeplasma* spp. (39, 94, 95), *Mycoplasma* spp. (29, 39, 94), *Spiroplasma* spp. (106), *Anaeroplasma intermedium* (98), and *Asteroleplasma anaerobium* (98) but not in *U. urealyticum* (29). The presence of G6P isomerase in two nonglycolytic species, *M. bovigenitalium* and *M. hominis*, is noteworthy, because both of these mycoplasmas lack detectable levels of the next two enzyme activities of the EMP pathway (39). This enzyme activity was also not found in other nonglycolytic *Mycoplasma* spp. (94).

The next step of the EMP pathway is the second priming reaction of glycolysis and requires energy in the form of a high-energy phosphate bond. In mollicutes, the high-energy phosphate bond can be supplied by either ATP or, in some cases, PP$_i$. The reaction is mediated by PFK (EC 2.7.1.11 when ATP is used; EC 1.7.1.90 when PP$_i$ is used). The reaction is irreversible when ATP is required. The phosphorylation of F6P by

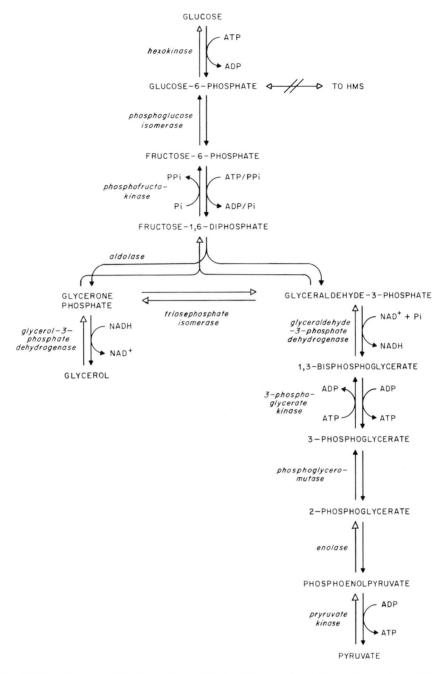

Figure 1. The EMP pathway as it is known in mollicutes. The nonglycolytic mollicutes lack PFK and aldolase activities (see text). Filled arrowheads indicate that the reactions are reported in mollicutes; unfilled arrowheads indicate that the reactions are presumed to be present.

PFK is recognized as the rate-limiting reaction of the entire glycolytic pathway (49, 73). PFK is allosteric in some cells, being inhibited by high concentrations of ATP and other compounds and stimulated by ADP or AMP. Therefore, when ATP levels are high, glycolysis can be shut off by the inhibition of a functional PFK. The ATP-dependent PFK reaction in mollicutes was first described in *M. gallisepticum* by Tourtellotte (149a).

Egan et al. (42) found, in ^{31}P nuclear magnetic reso-

nance studies of growing cells of *M. gallisepticum*, that under glycolytic conditions, high levels of fructose 1,6-diphosphate (F1,6P$_2$) were produced. Under the same conditions, PEP levels were low.

In 1984, it was discovered that ATP could not serve as the donor for the PFK activity of *A. laidlawii* B-PG9 and that PP$_i$ was required (109). PP$_i$ (not ATP)-dependent PFK has been found in *A. laidlawii* B-PG9 (109), *A. florum* L1 (109), *A. axanthum* (39), and *A. equifetale* (39). Petzel et al. (98, 99) have reported that *Anaer-*

oplasma intermedium and *Anaeroplasma bactoclasticum* also use PP_i in this reaction. However, these workers reported that ATP could also serve as the donor, although PP_i was clearly the preferred form (98, 99).

Only ATP (not PP_i)-dependent PFK has been reported in six glycolytic *Mycoplasma* spp. (39) and *M. mycoides* subsp. *mycoides* (29), eight *Spiroplasma* spp. (109), *U. urealyticum* (29), and *Asteroleplasma anaerobium* (98). No ATP- or PP_i-dependent PFK has been found in seven strains of *M. hominis* and *M. bovigenitalium* PG11 (39). Are the *Anaeroplasma* spp., which can use both ATP and PP_i for their PFK reactions, metabolic intermediates between the PP_i-dependent PFK-requiring *Acholeplasma* spp. and the ATP-dependent PFK-requiring *Mycoplasma*, *Spiroplasma*, and *Ureaplasma* spp. or their metabolic progenitors? The question is unanswerable at present.

Phylogenetic analyses of the mollicutes by Weisburg et al. (165) have indicated that *Anaeroplasma intermedium* and *Acholeplasma* spp. comprise a distinct clade, as determined by small-subunit rRNA sequence analyses. The overall phylogenetic unit included six related walled bacteria. Three of the walled relatives were found to have PP_i-dependent PFK activity (99). The data, also involving pyruvate-P_i dikinase activity, were interpreted as phenotypic evidence supporting the phylogenetic relationship between mollicutes and their walled relatives (99).

The PP_i-dependent PFK (EC 2.7.1.90) of *A. laidlawii* B-PG9 has been purified (109). ATP, CTP, GTP, and UTP, or their deoxy forms, and ITP, TTP, ADP, or P_i could not substitute for PP_i. The activity was not altered by $(NH_4)_2SO_4$, fructose 2,6-diphosphate, AMP, citrate, GDP, or PEP. The enzyme had an approximate molecular mass of 74 kDa, representing a dimeric form, and had a sedimentation coefficient of 6.7S.

PP_i is strongly favored as Earth's first biological energy-rich compound (8, 69, 76, 112, 170). In 1957, M. Calvin (quoted by Baltscheffsky [7]) postulated a model for primitive energy conversion, assuming coupling between electron transport involving the Fe^{2+}-Fe^{3+} redox system and the phosphorylation of P_i to PP_i. Iron storage has been reported in *M. capricolum* (12). Lipman indicated the importance of PP_i in primitive biological transformations and suggested that what he termed "metabolic fossils" may exist today (75). Many consider *Rhodospirillum rubrum* a metabolic fossil. I also suggest acholeplasmas or the anaeroplasmas as possible metabolic fossils.

The cellular source of PP_i is unknown, but there are many possibilities (171). In mollicutes, these include the synthetic activities of dUTPase (168, 169) and phosphoribosyltransferases (82, 152) (both discussed in chapter 13), DNA polymerase (see chapter 17), and RNA polymerase and aminoacyl-tRNA synthetases (chapter 19). The medium may also be a source of PP_i. Jones and Pollack found 0.7 μg of PP_i per ml in modified Edward's medium (13) containing 3% (vol/vol) horse serum and 2.2 μg of PP_i per ml with 9% (vol/vol) horse serum (58a). No evidence indicating that phosphatase or pyrophosphatase activities reported in mollicutes modulate the ATP- or PP_i-dependent PFK system has been presented (18, 21, 35, 94).

Acholeplasmas and *Anaeroplasma* spp. require PP_i not only for their PFK activities but also for their unique PP_i-dependent nucleoside kinase activities (82,

153) (see chapter 13). These PP_i requirements emphasize the importance of PP_i metabolism in mollicutes. It has been suggested that the use of PP_i by acholeplasmas represents a conserved remnant of ancient cellular development processes, as PP_i may be an evolutionary precursor of ATP (109).

The protein encoded by an open reading frame (ORF) identified on the *S. citri* insert of a plasmid (pES3') had 45.8% homology with the ATP-dependent PFK sequence from *Bacillus stearothermophilus* (26). The authors indicated that this sequence (ORF IV) may be the PFK gene of *S. citri*.

The product of PFK activity is $F1,6P_2$. In the next reaction of the EMP pathway, $F1,6P_2$ is cleaved by fructose bisphosphate aldolase (EC 4.1.2.13) or aldolase. The products of this reversible aldol condensation are glycerone (dihydroxyacetone) phosphate and G3P. The two C_3 products are in equilibrium in the presence of triose phosphate isomerase (EC 5.3.1.1).

Synthesis of G3P has been detected in *Acholeplasma* spp. (24, 39), *Mycoplasma* spp. (29, 39), *U. urealyticum* (29), *Spiroplasma* spp. (106), *Anaeroplasma intermedium* (98), and *Asteroleplasma anaerobium* (98). Aldolases of *Acholeplasma* spp. were critically examined by Neimark (91). His studies suggested a phylogenetic relationship between acholeplasmas and two other bacteria, *Streptococcus faecalis* and the pneumococcus.

Aldolase activity has not been found in two nonglycolytic *Mycoplasma* spp. that also lack PFK activity: *M. bovigenitalium* PG11 and *M. hominis* (39). This finding indicates that these isolates cannot metabolize hexoses that are presented as G6P or F6P. Parenthetically, these two species also lack a functional HMS. The energy source of these mollicutes is presumably arginine added to the growth medium or medium-derived amino acids. An untested premise is that whether glucose is available or not, the presence of arginine suppresses expression of the enzymes of the EMP pathway and the HMS.

The triose arm and substrate phosphorylation

The triose, or C_3, arm of the EMP pathway has five reaction steps leading to the synthesis of pyruvate (Fig. 1). The reactions (Fig. 1) are mediated by G3P dehydrogenase (G3Pde) (EC 1.2.1.12), phosphoglycerate kinase (EC 2.7.2.3), phosphoglyceromutase (EC 5.4.2.1), enolase (EC 4.2.1.11), and PK (EC 2.7.1.40), respectively. The C_3 reaction sequence is of undoubted major importance in mollicutes metabolism, because the C_3 arm may be where most ATP of mollicutes is synthesized. The synthesis of ATP occurs at the two kinase sites: 3-phosphoglycerate kinase and PK. Alternate possibilities for ATP synthesis outside the C_3 arm of glycolysis, such as acetate kinase, the arginine dihydrolase pathway, and the reoxidation of NADH, will be discussed later.

By spectrophotometric techniques, most of the multistep C_3 arm of the EMP pathway has been found in all species of mollicutes tested (29, 39, 79, 98, 106). The exceptions are *Asteroleplasma anaerobium*, which was reported to lack PK activity (98). It has a substitute, pyruvate-P_i dikinase, which will be discussed later. Also, there is some uncertainty as to whether *M. bovigenitalium* PG11 (39) and *U. urealyticum* (29) have phosphoglycerate kinase activity. The operating hypothesis is that the latter two organisms have this activity. Therefore, the C_3 arm of the EMP pathway is reported or considered to be in glycolytic and nonglycolytic, arginine-utilizing mollicutes as well as in strictly anaerobic mollicutes. It follows that, if functional, the C_3 path when supplied G3P or perhaps another triose can give rise to 2 equivalents of ATP, one ATP at the beginning of the C_3 path by 3-phosphoglycerate kinase and another ATP at the end of the path by PK. O'Brien et al., in starch gel electrophoresis studies of 22 mollicutes, reported G3Pde and triose phosphate isomerase activities in glycolytic *Mycoplasma* and *Acholeplasma* spp. (94).

Grossato et al. (50) studied purified enolases from several mollicutes. The enolases had a molecular mass of about 100 kDa, were inhibited by fluoride and phosphate, and had reaction optima at pH 7.7 and 1 mM Mg^{2+}. The authors indicated that the enolases were similar to those reported from *E. coli*. Lanham et al., by starch gel electrophoresis, has found enolase in four strains of *A. laidlawii* (70).

The last or next to last enzyme in the EMP (some authorities include LDH) is PK (EC 2.7.1.40). PK converts PEP and ADP to pyruvate and ATP. It is the second site of substrate phosphorylation in glycolysis, 3-phosphoglycerate kinase in the C_3 arm of the EMP pathway being the other. In other systems, this irreversible reaction requires Mg^{2+} or Mn^{2+} and other cations. PK is an allosteric enzyme: it turns off when cellular ATP concentrations are high or when fatty acids or acetyl-CoA are available (73). PK turns on when PEP or $F1,6P_2$ levels build up (22). PK has been reported in eight *Spiroplasma* spp. (106), *Anaeroplasma intermedium* (98), two *Acholeplasma* spp. (70), seven *Mycoplasma* spp. (79), *M. mycoides* subsp. *mycoides* (29), and *U. urealyticum* (29) but not in *Asteroleplasma anaerobium* (98).

A number of investigators have studied a side reaction of the C_3 arm involving glycerol 3-phosphate dehydrogenase (EC 1.1.1.8) in *U. urealyticum* and *M. mycoides* subsp. *mycoides* (29, 120, 133). This enzyme reduces glycerone (dihydroxyacetone) phosphate to glycerol 3-phosphate, which may be used in the synthesis of lipids and nucleotides. This step, analogous to the NADH shuttle seen in eucaryotic cells (73), has been largely ignored by other investigators and deserves scrutiny, because it serves as another reaction whereby NADH is reoxidized to NAD^+.

Since LDH is almost always present, lactate may accumulate even in cultures of nonglycolytic mollicutes. In these cases, the amount of lactate will be dependent on the concentrations of ADP and NADH and the degree of aeration. In the nonglycolytic mollicutes tested, the source of G3P is unknown, since these mollicutes lack the HMS. Control or modulation of the C_3 arm may occur by modification of the G3Pde activity of nonglycolytic as well as glycolytic mollicutes (110).

The obligate use of PP_i by *Acholeplasma* spp. alters their glycolytic balance sheet. For mycoplasmas, spiroplasmas, and ureaplasmas, the sum reaction for glycolysis probably is, as already noted,

$$\text{glucose} + 2 \text{ ADP} + 2 \text{ NAD}^+ + 2 \text{ P}_i \longrightarrow$$
$$2 \text{ pyruvate} + 2 \text{ ATP} + 2 \text{ NADH}$$

The balance sheet for the PP_i-requiring acholeplasmas and anaeroplasmas when PP_i is used may be

$$\text{glucose} + 3 \text{ ADP} + 2 \text{ NAD}^+ + \text{PP}_i + \text{P}_i \longrightarrow$$
$$2 \text{ pyruvate} + 3 \text{ ATP} + 2 \text{ NADH}$$

HMS

Mollicutes, like many other cells, can participate in the metabolism of glucose by the HMS, also called the Warburg-Dickens, phosphogluconate, or pentose phosphate pathway. The HMS is a multifunctional pathway. In photosynthetic organisms, its activity results in the fixation of CO_2 to form carbohydrate. In nonphotosynthetic organisms, it serves four functions: production of NADPH; synthesis of pentoses as precursors for nucleic acid intermediates; interconversion of three-, four-, five-, six- and seven-carbon sugars; and linkage of these reactions to the EMP pathway through F6P and G3P (172).

The pathway as it is known in mollicutes is shown in Fig. 2.

Castrejon-Diez et al. (24) gave [1-^{14}C]glucose to *A. laidlawii* cells and found a high specific activity in CO_2, suggesting for the first time that the HMS was present in mollicutes. They also found G6Pde, ribose 5-isomerase, TK activities and an accumulation of fructose in cell-free reaction systems.

The first step of the HMS, as generally presented, involves dehydrogenation of the G6P of the EMP pathway in the presence of $NADP^+$ to a hydrated form of 6-phosphogluconate (6PG) and NADPH. The enzyme G6Pde, or Zwischenferment (EC 1.1.1.49), catalyzes the reaction. After dehydration, the next enzyme dehydrogenates and decarboxylates 6PG in the presence of $NADP^+$ to ribulose 5-phosphate (R5P), NADPH, and CO_2. The enzyme 6PGde (EC 1.1.1.44) catalyzes this reaction.

These G6Pde and 6PGde activities have been found in all *Acholeplasma* spp. studied: *A. laidlawii* (39, 70, 108), *A. granularum* (39, 94), *A. axanthum* (39, 94), *A. oculi* (94), *A. modicum* (94), and *A. equifetale* (39, 70). The activities have not been found in any *Mycoplasma* (29, 39, 108), *Ureaplasma* (29), *Spiroplasma* (106), *Anaeroplasma* (98), or *Asteroleplasma* (98) spp. The action of these two dehydrogenases is considered to be the principal source of a cell's NADPH. The major cellular requirement for NADPH is for lipid synthesis. As noted before, *Acholeplasma* spp., which in almost all cases can synthesize lipids from acetate (105), can also synthesize NADPH by these reactions. Other mollicutes, such as *Mycoplasma*, *Ureaplasma*, and *Spiroplasma* spp., require exogenous lipid for growth, cannot synthesize lipids from acetate (105), and lack these two dehydrogenases.

The remaining enzymes of the HMS, ribulose phosphate 3-epimerase (EC 5.1.3.1), R5P isomerase (EC 5.3.1.6), TK (EC 2.2.1.1), and transaldolase (TA) (EC 2.2.1.2), were detected in *M. mycoides* subsp. *mycoides* (29). The enzyme activities were also detected, except for a probably weak reaction for TA in *U. ureaplasma* (29). The same enzymes were detected in eight other glycolytic *Mycoplasma* spp. (39), in eight *Spiroplasma* spp. (106), and in *Anaeroplasma intermedium* and *Aster-*

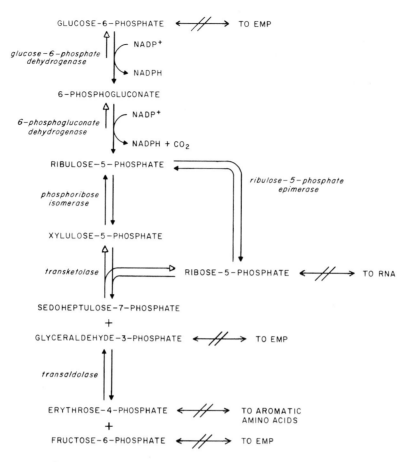

Figure 2. The HMP as it is known in mollicutes. The G6P and 6PGde activities have been found only in *Acholeplasma* spp. Nonglycolytic mollicutes have only ribulose phosphate epimerase activity (see text). Filled arrowheads indicate that the reactions are reported in mollicutes; unfilled arrowheads indicate that the reactions are presumed to be present.

oleplasma anaerobium (98). The reactions have been detected in both directions, using extracts of acholeplasmas and mycoplasmas (39).

DeSantis et al. (39) also studied five strains of the nonglycolytic *M. hominis* and *M. bovigenitalium* PG11. They found that these two species lacked not only G6Pde and 6PGde activities, as already noted, but also R5P isomerase, TK, and TA activities. Both had only the ribulose phosphate epimerase activity. The authors had no explanation for this anomaly and suggested that it might be an unrecognized nonspecific enzyme activity in nonglycolytic strains.

Workers have had difficulty in detecting TA activity in some strains (29, 39). TA mediates the interconversion of sedoheptulose 7-phosphate and G3P to E4P and F6P. Since TK activity was found and TK requires E4P, a product of TA, our working presumption is that TA activity is present. Technical factors probably account for the inability to detect TA in all strains. E4P is a reactant in the committed step of the aromatic amino acid pathway reported in acholeplasmas (16) (see chapter 12).

Cocks et al. (29), studying *M. mycoides* subsp. *mycoides* and *U. urealyticum*, were able to link the HMS and two important intermediates of nucleic acid metabolism: deoxyribose 1-phosphate and ribose 1-phos-

phate. The key enzyme was phosphopentomutase (EC 5.4.2.7). This enzyme converts ribose 1-phosphate or deoxyribose 1-phosphate to R5P or dR5P. R5P directly enters the HMS; dR5P is converted to G3P by dR5P aldolase (EC 4.1.2.4) (89). By the action of this system, the sugars derived from RNA and DNA can be salvaged and may reenter the HMS and the EMP pathway. The dR5P aldolase has been found in three *Acholeplasma* spp. (39), in six *Mycoplasma* spp. (39), in six *Spiroplasma* spp. (106), and in *Anaeroplasma intermedium* and *Asteroleplasma anaerobium* (98). The activity was not detected in *Spiroplasma citri*, *S. kunkelii*, *M. lactucae*, or *M. gallisepticum* (39, 106).

In mollicutes, it appears that the HMS and the EMP pathway may interact. Acholeplasmas apparently possess the activities of both pathways and therefore may be more capable of balancing their needs for R5P and NADPH. All other mollicutes must either be supplied, scavenge, or synthesize $NADP^+$ by routes not yet described. Acholeplasmas and all other mollicutes may be able to utilize a variety of C_{3-7} sugars, exogenously supplied or derived from DNA or RNA, after conversion by the HMS to EMP pathway intermediates F6P and G3P. This suggests that metabolic thrust is toward the ubiquitous C_3 arm of the EMP pathway and its two sites of substrate phosphorylation.

In acholeplasmas, and presumably anaeroplasmas, the reactions of the hexose arm of the EMP pathway are reversible. Therefore, in these organisms, the synthesis of G6P, or gluconeogenesis, from F6P or G3P is theoretically possible. G6P synthesized from EMP pathway intermediates by this "backward-moving" EMP pathway may continuously recycle through the HMS. At each revolution, 1 equivalent of CO_2 is lost, 2 equivalents of NADPH are formed, and new intermediates become available for both nucleic acid and aromatic amino acid synthesis. In acholeplasmas, the EMP pathway–HMS cyclic system differs from that of most cells in requiring P_i. Also, PP_i is synthesized by the reverse-acting PP_i-dependent PFK. The synthesis of PP_i during gluconeogenesis could be energetically favorable, because upon hydrolysis PP_i yields a $\Delta G^{0'}$ of -4.6 kcal (1 cal = 4.184 J) mol^{-1}. Alternatively, the PP_i might be used by the PP_i-dependent nucleoside kinase (see chapter 13).

On the other hand, mycoplasmas, ureaplasmas, and spiroplasmas, like most other cells, only have an irreversible-acting, unidirectional, lactate-directed ATP-dependent PFK. Most other organisms with this ATP-dependent PFK also possess a fructose 1,6-phosphatase activity. During gluconeogenesis, this phosphatase hydrolytically removes a phosphate from $F1,6P_2$ to form F6P. It is not known whether mollicutes have this gluconeogenic activity. $M.$ $capricolum$ 14 apparently does not (104a). In the absence of this phosphatase activity, mycoplasmas, ureaplasmas, and spiroplasmas may be unable to convert G3P from the HMS to G6P. This is because the G3P would be "trapped" below the unidirectional (lactate-directed) ATP-dependent PFK locus. There is no other bypass reaction known.

However, F6P entering the same hexose arm of the EMP pathway, above the "missing" gluconeogenic reaction at the PFK locus, could be converted to G6P. Presently, this reaction does not make metabolic sense, since all of the organisms in question (mycoplasmas, ureaplasmas, and spiroplasmas) lack both of the two initial dehydrogenases of the HMS. In effect, they cannot process G6P further, i.e., by way of the HMS. Therefore, except for the acholeplasmas and possibly the anaeroplasmas, the glycolytic mollicutes can synthesize G6P from HMS-derived F6P but not from HMS-derived G3P. Further, in the absence of G6Pde and 6PGde, they cannot process G6P through the balance of the HMS, which they do possess.

In the three groups of sterol-requiring glycolytic mollicutes, carbon processed through the truncated HMS may be diverted to other systems through R5P or E4P or to lactate by G3P. Since recycling through the HMS is apparently impossible, the source of G6P may need to be continuous in order to synthesize F6P, which presumably enters the truncated HMS, but may pass through that system only once.

Nonglycolytic $Mycoplasma$ spp. apparently lack a functional HMS and also lack the two access points from the HMS to the EMP pathway; i.e., they have no PFK or aldolase activities. The metabolic needs of these nonglycolytic strains, therefore, require direct entry to the C_3 arm of the EMP pathway at the triose level, or alternate modes of ATP synthesis (22), such as utilization of amino acids like arginine. Proof of the former concept requires, among other points, the necessity of showing that G3P carbon derived from hexose, via the HMS, can supply the carbon for pyruvate.

THE PYRUVATE ROUNDHOUSE

In mollicutes, there are a number of alternative paths that PEP and pyruvate may take (Fig. 3). These alternate paths are separated for this discussion into those leading from PEP to oxaloacetate, pyruvate to lactate, pyruvate to acetyl-CoA, pyruvate to oxaloacetate via acetyl-CoA and malate, and pyruvate to oxaloacetate. It is not certain whether all of these paths can operate simultaneously, nor is it known under what growth conditions they are stimulated. Since lactate and acetate accumulate in cultures, it is understood that more than one path is operative during the growth cycle. Aerobically, and with adequate cofactors, the routes to acetate apparently predominate. As the culture ages, or is maintained anaerobically, and with adequate grow factors, lactate will accumulate (117–119, 150).

PEP to Oxaloacetate and an Uncommon Route to Pyruvate

The EMP pathway precursor to pyruvate is PEP. Beaman and Pollack (15) indicated that $A.$ $laidlawii$ could fix CO_2 by carboxylation of PEP to oxaloacetate (79). The PEP carboxylase (PEP-C) (EC 4.1.1.31) activity was found in $Acholeplasma$ spp. and $Anaeroplasma$ $intermedium$ (98) but not in $Mycoplasma$ spp. (79), $U.$ $urealyticum$ (34), or $Asteroleplasma$ $anaerobium$ (98). It is uncertain whether the enzyme is present in $Spiroplasma$ spp. (104a).

This enzyme belongs to a class of enzymes known as anaplerotic or C_4-acid replenishing enzymes that are usually associated with the TCA cycle (49). In mollicutes, PEP-C is found in the absence of a TCA cycle (79). PEP-C has been purified from $A.$ $laidlawii$ B-PG9 (80) and reported to have a molecular mass of between 353 and 384 kDa. At low bicarbonate concentrations, the enzyme activity was stimulated by $F1,6P_2$. Aspartate was a noncompetitive inhibitor. It has been suggested that the enzyme is involved in the interdependent regulation of protein, lipid, and nucleic acid metabolism.

Petzel et al. (98) reported that $Asteroleplasma$ $anaerobium$ lacks PK and that PEP in this organism is converted to pyruvate by the action of pyruvate P_i dikinase (EC 2.7.9.1). The latter activity was not found in $Anaeroplasma$ $intermedium$ (98) or in $Mycoplasma$ or $Acholeplasma$ spp. (79). This interesting reaction requires PP_i and synthesizes not only pyruvate but also ATP. This reaction, together with the PP_i-dependent PFK (98) and PP_i-dependent nucleoside kinases (82), also reported in $Anaeroplasma$ $intermedium$ (98), accentuates the role of PP_i in mollicutes metabolism. The metabolic similarities of $Anaeroplasma$ and $Acholeplasma$ spp. and their relatively close phylogenetic relationship have been emphasized (98, 99). PEP carboxykinase (EC 4.1.1.49) activity has been reported in $Anaeroplasma$ $intermedium$ (98) but not in $Mycoplasma$ or $Acholeplasma$ spp. (79).

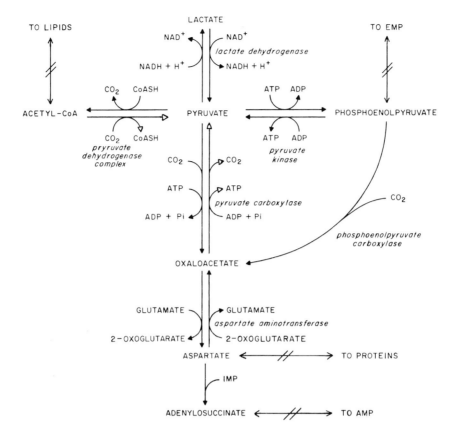

Figure 3. The pyruvate roundhouse as it is known in *Acholeplasma* spp. Filled arrowheads indicate that the reactions are reported in mollicutes (see text).

Pyruvate to Lactate

Lactate production is a characteristic of mollicutes metabolism. Its production is mediated by LDH (EC 1.1.1.27), and its presence is reported in all mollicutes, including nonglycolytic species (2, 24, 48, 55, 73, 79, 93, 98, 106, 117–119, 150), but not in *Ureaplasma* spp. (29). Neimark and Lemcke (92) studied the LDHs of six *Mycoplasma* and two *Acholeplasma* spp. and reported three patterns of LDH activity: an NAD$^+$-dependent L-(+)-LDH, or an NAD$^+$-dependent L-(−)-LDH in *Mycoplasma* spp., and both an F1,6P$_2$-activated NAD$^+$-dependent L-(+)-LDH and an NAD$^+$-dependent L-(−)-LDH in *Acholeplasma* spp. The F1,6P$_2$-activated LDH shared specific characteristics with the F1,6P$_2$-activated LDHs from streptococci (91).

The LDH content of *M. mycoides* T1 (vaccine strain) has been used as an indicator of viable count during log-phase growth (170). From these data, it was calculated that each CFU contained a mean of 4.1×10^{-10} U of LDH.

Pyruvate to Acetyl-CoA

Another pathway from pyruvate leads to the synthesis of acetyl-CoA via the pyruvate dehydrogenase complex. The complex is composed of three enzymes, with three polypeptide chains catalyzing the oxidative decarboxylation of pyruvate. The reaction requires NAD$^+$ and CoASH. Flavin adenine denucleotide (FAD) is a tightly bound reducible prosthetic group of one of the enzymes and is involved in the final transfer of electrons to the NAD$^+$ acceptor. The reaction requires the cofactors thiamine PP$_i$, hydroxyethylthiamine PP$_i$, and lipoic acid (73). The overall reaction is

pyruvate + NAD$^+$ +

CoASH → acetyl-CoA + NADH + H$^+$ + CO$_2$

The complex is regulated by ATP and, in some systems, by Ca^{2+}. Therefore, when ATP levels are high, the formation of acetyl-CoA is down-regulated, and when the levels of ADP and pyruvate are high, acetyl-CoA may be synthesized in greater yield, depending on competing reactions for pyruvate.

The presence of the pyruvate dehydrogenase complex in mollicutes, as indicated by pyruvate oxidation, was reported by a number of investigators. The activity was found in *Mycoplasma* spp. (28, 31, 79, 117–119, 150), *Acholeplasma* spp. (31, 79), *Spiroplasma* spp. (106), and *U. urealyticum* (34) but not in *Anaeroplasma* or *Asteroleplasma* spp. (98).

Constantopoulos and McGarrity (31) studied the pyruvate dehydrogenase complex in three glycolytic and two nonglycolytic mollicutes, grown aerobically or anaerobically. The presence of air modulated the activity. Activity was higher in an aerobic environment, perhaps because NADH is an inhibitor of pyruvate dehydrogenase. In air, NADH is probably more rapidly oxidized to NAD^+ by the action of NOA; in this circumstance, the NADH levels decrease.

Pyruvate to Oxaloacetate via Acetyl-CoA and Malate

Acetyl-CoA formed by the pyruvate dehydrogenase complex is generally considered to play a major role in lipid synthesis in *Acholeplasma* spp. The function of acetyl-CoA in *Mycoplasma* spp., which cannot synthesize lipids from acetate, is less appreciated.

Manolukas et al. (79) have detected malate synthase (EC 4.1.3.2) in eight *Mycoplasma* spp., glycolytic and nonglycolytic, but not in the two *Acholeplasma* spp. tested. Petzel et al. (98) did not detect the activity in either *Anaeroplasma intermedium* or *Asteroleplasma anaerobium*, and it was not found in any of nine *Spiroplasma* spp. (106). Davis et al. (34) have detected malate synthase in *U. urealyticum*, *U. diversum*, and two ovine ureaplasmas. The reaction requires glyoxalate; the source of glyoxalate in mollicutes is unknown. Since the TCA cycle is absent (see below), glyoxalate probably does not arise from isocitrate.

In this route to oxaloacetate, malate, the product of malate synthase action, is converted to oxaloacetate by MDH (EC 1.1.1.37). The reaction in mollicutes is reversible (79, 98). MDH activity was reported in *Mycoplasma* spp. (29, 79), in *Spiroplasma* spp. (106), in *U. urealyticum* (29, 38), and in *Anaeroplasma intermedium* and *Asteroleplasma anaerobium* (98). MDH was not detected in two *Acholeplasma* spp. tested, the same two (*A. laidlawii* and *A. morum*) that lacked malate synthase. However, Salih et al. (130) reported weak MDH activity in *A. laidlawii*. The function of MDH in mollicutes presumably involves modulation of NAD^+ and NADH levels. Malic enzyme (EC 1.1.1.38; EC 1.1.1.39) has not been detected in mollicutes (79).

Therefore, *Mycoplasma* and *Ureaplasma* spp. can synthesize malate from acetyl-CoA. They can convert malate to oxaloacetate with NAD^+, possibly produced from NADH by NADH oxidase or by other reactions. This path to oxaloacetate has not been detected in other mollicutes. Mollicutes can transaminate oxaloacetate to aspartate (79) (see chapter 12). In eucaryotic cells, these latter enzyme activities comprise a system known as the malate-aspartate shuttle, which is involved in the transfer of reducing equivalents from the cytosol to the mitochondria (73).

Pyruvate to Oxaloacetate

A more direct route to oxaloacetate from pyruvate is the final reaction in the pyruvate roundhouse. In this step, CO_2 is fixed in the carboxylation of pyruvate directly to oxaloacetate. The enzyme that mediates the reaction is pyruvate carboxylase (EC 6.4.1.1). ATP is required. Pyruvate carboxylase activity has been reported in *Acholeplasma* and *Mycoplasma* spp. (79), *Anaeroplasma intermedium* (98), and *U. urealyticum* (34). The activity was not detected in *Asteroleplasma anaerobium* (98). Unfortunately, the studies with *Spiroplasma* spp. for pyruvate carboxylase were preliminary (106).

The Two Major Patterns at the Pyruvate Roundhouse

PEP-C, PK, pyruvate-P_i dikinase, pyruvate dehydrogenase complex, pyruvate carboxylase, malate synthase, and MDH make up the pyruvate roundhouse. Two major patterns emerge (79).

The acholeplasma pattern (Fig. 3) is characterized by the carboxylation (CO_2 fixation) of PEP to oxaloacetate and by the absence of malate synthase and MDH activities. The mycoplasma-ureaplasma pattern (Fig. 4) is the converse, possessing malate synthase and MDH activities but lacking PEP-C activity. Less well characterized patterns for the anaerobic mollicutes suggest that acetyl-CoA requirements must be met by a route other than glycolysis (EMP pathway)-derived pyruvate. The spiroplasma pattern, if a distinctive one exists, at present does not link oxaloacetate to pyruvate or, more certainly, to PEP. Further, the source of malate in the spiroplasmas is unknown, but it might be amino acids if not pyruvate. More study is obviously required.

The two major patterns reveal an energy-related aspect deserving comment. The acholeplasma pattern (Fig. 3) does not yield a gain of ATP, whereas the mycoplasma-ureaplasma pattern (Fig. 4) does. As Manolukas et al. (79) indicated, the acholeplasmas do not have a malate bypass option to oxaloacetate. Acholeplasmas can reach oxaloacetate from PEP by two routes: by direct carboxylation with no involvement of ATP and through pyruvate by action of PK and then pyruvate carboxylase. In the second case, ATP is involved in both steps but the net gain or loss of ATP is zero, since at PK 1 equivalent is gained and at pyruvate carboxylase 1 equivalent is consumed.

The mycoplasma-ureaplasma pattern lacks PEP-C, but they also have two routes from PEP to oxaloacetate. One is identical to the second alternative of the acholeplasmas, i.e., from PEP to pyruvate to oxaloacetate with no net gain or loss of ATP. The other alternative route, absent from acholeplasmas, is from PEP to pyruvate to acetyl-CoA and malate and then to oxaloacetate. By this pathway, the pyruvate carboxylase step that requires ATP is avoided. NADH is also formed, which may be involved in some energy-conserving mechanism perhaps associated with NOA activity. This malate bypass found in all of the few *Mycoplasma* and *Ureaplasma* spp. studied permits these mollicutes to synthesize oxaloacetate when ATP is limiting. The role of oxaloacetate as a source of amino acids is discussed elsewhere (see chapter 12).

THE TCA CYCLE

Except for studies with *M. hominis* 07, now called *M. arthritidis* 07, there is essentially no evidence for the existence of a complete TCA cycle in any mollicutes (159). Only MDH has been reported in some mollicutes (see above), and Petzel et al. (98) have reported the somewhat anomalous presence of isocitrate dehydrogenase (EC 1.1.1.41) activity in *Anaeroplasma intermedium*.

Manolukas et al. (79) studied 10 mollicutes, including two strains of *M. hominis*, and did not detect cit-

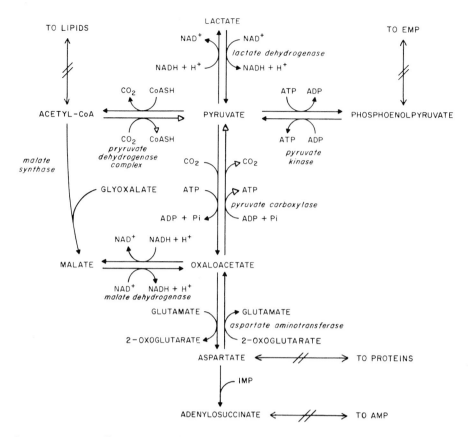

Figure 4. The pyruvate roundhouse as it is known in *Mycoplasma* spp. and *U. urealyticum*. Filled arrowheads indicate that the reactions are reported in mollicutes (see text).

rate synthase, aconitase, isocitrate dehydrogenase, 2-oxoglutarate dehydrogenase, succinic synthase, succinic dehydrogenase, or fumarase. Data indicating the absence of the TCA cycle had been found earlier (117–119, 150). Rodwell and Rodwell found that *M. mycoides* subsp. *mycoides* could not utilize citrate, 2-oxoglutarate, succinate, or fumarate (117–119).

In procaryotes with a TCA cycle, this cycle plays a major catabolic role. Aerobic heterotrophs use the TCA cycle to provide cellular precursors, such as oxaloacetate for biosynthesis and NADH for oxidative phosphorylation. All parts of the TCA cycle are not always expressed. Many aerobes lack part of the cycle. Methylotrophs growing on C_1 compounds lack 2-oxoglutarate dehydrogenase, and some acetic acid bacteria lack succinate thiokinase but have the remaining components of the cycle (49). Mollicutes do not express much of the TCA cycle whether grown aerobically or anaerobically. The parts that are expressed in mollicutes are the "stand-alone" MDH found in all strains studied and isocitrate dehydrogenase activity found only in *Anaeroplasma intermedium*, as noted above.

It may be that the conditions of growth suppress the formation of TCA enzymes. If so, since mollicutes grow in relatively rich media, different investigations are likely to lead to the same impression. This possibility can be explored when mollicutes are grown in defined media or in two or more media of sufficiently variable composition. The studies of Rodwell with *M. mycoides* subsp. *mycoides* (121) and of Hackett et al. (51) and

Chang and Chen (25) with *Spiroplasma* spp. suggest that a completely defined medium for mollicutes is possible (see chapter 2). It is also possible that gene networks encoding the TCA enzymes are controlled by gene regulators, such as the *arcA* and *arcB* genes effecting aerobic respiration control (57). The action of gene network regulators in the mollicutes, if they exist, may result in repression of the translation of TCA enzymes. Further, it has been suggested that mollicutes are metabolically limited by virtue of their relatively small genome size and cell volume (86). It is estimated that *M. capricolum* expresses about 400 gene products (63). Such genome limitations may result in the absence of sequences coding for enzymes or even entire enzymatic networks, such as the TCA cycle. Many of the same arguments can be used to critique the reported absence of lipoquinone-cytochrome components of an electron transport system in mollicutes (107).

THE FATE OF ELECTRONS

The respiratory pathways and energy-yielding mechanisms of mollicutes were reviewed in 1979 (102). At that time, glycolytic mollicutes were considered to lack oxidative phosphorylation involving quinones (54) and cytochromes (102–104, 117). Flavins were associated with the final transfer of electrons, presumably to oxygen. It was suggested that an NADH-ferricyanide oxidoreductase activity might be involved in ATP synthesis (58, 102). In nonglycolytic mollicutes, a quinone-cytochrome-containing system and oxidative phosphorylation, coupled to a TCA cycle, oxidation of fatty acids, and the metabolism of amino acids, were reported to be present. At that time, there was no description of energy-conserving pathways in *Ureaplasma*, *Spiroplasma*, or *Anaeroplasma* spp. (102).

VanDemark first described FTR in mollicutes (157). He associated the pathway with glycolytic mollicutes. The data now suggest that this pathway is common to all aerobic mollicutes. The mollicutes FTR pathway may include a copper- or iron-flavin-containing NOA that, upon reduction by NADH, transfers an electron to oxygen, initially forming O_2^-. This toxic radical is dismutated to oxygen and hydrogen peroxide by the action of SOD. In some mollicutes, the peroxide is converted to oxygen and water by the action of catalase. Although the overall reaction sequence has not been determined in mollicutes, O_2^- may be protonated to the reactive hydroperoxyl radical, which may react with reduced copper or iron to form the reactive hydroxyl radical or iron-oxygen complexes or may decompose to singlet oxygen. The reactive hydroxyl radical may be capable of oxidizing anything but ozone and hence is one of the most reactive moieties known.

The Flavin NOA and NADH Dehydrogenase

Major components of the mollicutes FTR chain are NADH dehydrogenase and NOA. These activities may both be mediated by the same protein. The NOA of mollicutes is localized in the membrane or cytoplasmic fraction of the cell (87, 101, 102, 106). In *Mycoplasma* and *Spiroplasma* spp., NOA is localized in the cytoplasmic fraction; in *Acholeplasma* spp., the activity is localized in the membrane. There are exceptions; for example, the localization of NOA in *A. florum* L1 is apparently cytoplasmic (104a). *A. florum* is a metabolically interesting, perhaps unique, acholeplasma. Like other *Acholeplasma* spp. studied, it has a PP$_i$-dependent PFK. Unlike other acholeplasmas, besides the apparent localization of NOA in the cytoplasmic fraction as in the sterol-requiring mollicutes, *A. florum* L1 cannot synthesize lipids from acetate (105).

NOA has generally not been detected in *Ureaplasma* spp. (81, 103, 138). Davis and Villanueva (36) have reported an NADH diaphorase in *U. urealyticum*, *U. diversum*, and ovine *Ureaplasma* strains. The presence or absence of NOA in anaeroplasmas has not been reported.

Arora and Sinha (3) purified mycoplasmalike organisms from aster yellows-infected plants. They localized NOA in the membrane fraction and NADPH oxidase and G6Pde activities in the cytoplasmic fraction. This distribution pattern is the same as found in all *Acholeplasma* spp. but in no other mollicutes genera studied.

Jinks and Matz (58) first purified an NADH dehydrogenase (EC 1.6.99.3) from *A. laidlawii* membranes. Reinards et al. (114) extracted NOA from the membranes of *A. laidlawii* and purified the activity to apparent homogeneity. In their extensive studies, the enzyme was found to be a copper-containing iron-sulfur flavin mononucleotide (FMN) flavoprotein (FMN:Cu:-

Fe:labile S::1:1:6:6). It was composed of three subunits of molecular masses 65, 40, and 19 kDa, contained a high fraction of hydrophobic amino acids, and had a strong fluorescence at $\lambda_{max} = 526$ nm. Oxygen used as an electron acceptor catalyzed the formation of H_2O_2 in stoichiometric amounts. NADH, but not NADPH, could serve as a substrate. Ferricyanide, dichlorophenolindophenol (DCPIP), and cytochrome c could serve as electron acceptors. The authors obtained evidence that the flavin shuttles between the fully reduced and the semiquinone state during oxidation of NADH. SOD inhibited the oxidation of NADH with O_2, indicating that O_2^- was an intermediate. The involvement of an Fe-S center(s) was indicated. The purified enzyme had properties that corresponded to those observed in whole membranes.

Klomkes et al. (65) studied the cytoplasmic NOA from *M. capricolum*. They purified the enzyme to apparent homogeneity and determined its molecular mass to be 71.5 kDa. No subunits were detected. The enzyme contained FAD with a fluorescence at $\lambda_{max} = 526$ nm, but no copper, zinc, or molybdenum, and had traces of iron and manganese. The enzyme catalyzed the transfer of electrons from NADH to oxygen, and weakly to ferricyanide, but not to DCPIP, cytochrome c, or methylene blue. The transfer to O_2 was not inhibited by SOD, and Fe-S clusters were presumed to be absent.

The studies of Reinards et al. (114) and Klomkes et al. (65) are significant, as they describe the enzymes that may be at the terminus of *Mycoplasma* and *Acholeplasma* energy metabolism. The enzymes, perhaps representative of each genera, are different; both accept NADH or ferricyanide as electron donors and both mediate the reduction of oxygen. Whether these processes are linked to the synthesis of ATP is not known.

Sjostrom and Kenny (138) compared the NADH dehydrogenases of 14 strains of mollicutes by quantitative electrophoresis. They were able to identify five serologically distinct NADH dehydrogenases in 10 species and suggested the use of such specificities as taxonomic criteria.

SOD

SOD (EC 1.15.1.1) eliminates the highly toxic O_2^- that may be generated by the action of NOA. SOD is considered to be indispensable for aerobic organisms (47). SOD was first reported in mollicutes by Petkau and Chelack (97). Lee and Kenny (72) have indicated that the SODs of five *Acholeplasma* spp. are immunologically heterogeneous and have suggested that their findings indicate evolutionary diversity of SODs.

Some *Acholeplasma* and *Mycoplasma* spp. and *U. urealyticum* were reported to lack SOD (64, 65, 77, 94). Meier and Habermehl (83) found SOD in extracts from 21 strains of mollicutes, including *Mycoplasma*, *Acholeplasma*, and *Ureaplasma* strains previously reported to lack SOD. Their ability to detect SOD was related to their dialysis of the fresh cell lysates and the subsequent heating of the dialyzed extract. Heating presumably destroyed labile interfering enzymatic activities. The data are convincing and suggest that aerobic mollicutes, like other aerobes, produce SOD, which protects against oxygen toxicity. The toxic component,

O_2^-, is generated during the one electron transfer from NOA to oxygen.

Reinards et al. (113) have purified and characterized the SOD from *A. laidlawii*. The apparently homogeneous SOD had a molecular mass of 41.5 kDa and was composed of two apparently identical subunits of 21.6 kDa. Mn^{2+} was detected by electron paramagnetic resonance at 0.5 atom per subunit; the iron content was less than 0.02 atom. The activity was resistant to H_2O_2 and potassium cyanide. The data are compatible with those obtained from other procaryotic Mn^{2+}-dependent SODs.

Catalase

Catalase (EC 1.11.1.5) was first described in mollicutes by Lecce and Morton (71). Some workers have reported catalase in mollicutes (30, 117); others did not detect catalase in some mollicutes (46, 61, 100, 162). Meier and Habermehl (83) studied catalase activity polarographically and found none in any mollicutes strains. They commented that induction of catalase is more dependent on cultural conditions than is induction of SOD.

The presence of catalase is correlated with the presence of SOD. According to the model of Reinards et al. (113, 114), the action of SOD produces H_2O_2, which is converted to O_2 and water by catalase. Peroxidases are apparently not present in mollicutes.

The Absence of Cytochromes from Mollicutes

Excluding the report of cytochromes in *M. hominis* (*M. arthritidis*) 07 (157), already discussed in relationship to the TCA cycle, all attempts to find cytochromes in *Mycoplasma*, *Acholeplasma*, or *Ureaplasma* spp. have been unsuccessful (48, 103, 117, 144, 148). No cytochrome pigments were found upon examination of four *Spiroplasma* spp. and *Anaeroplasma intermedium* (104). Asteroleplasmas have not been studied.

The opinion that cytochrome pigments are absent from mollicutes can be criticized by using the same arguments presented for the absence of the TCA cycle. The expression of cytochromes may be mediated by components of the growth medium or the presence of oxygen (90, 104, 115, 166, 167). Their absence may be the result of genomic repression; perhaps they are not coded for in mollicutes. Proof may require conclusive identification of the genomic sequences coding for these proteins and certainty that such sequences are absent from mollicutes DNA.

Oxygen-Dependent Mollicutes Respiration

To recapitulate, as a working hypothesis, by using the glycolytic *A. laidlawii* and *M. capricolum* as models, the terminal electron chain of aerobic mollicutes appears to be a flavin-terminated respiration (157). NADH is the apparent electron donor and is a terminal reduction product of mollicutes metabolism. The role of transhydrogenase is uncertain. In *Acholeplasma* spp., NADH reduces a Fe-Cu FAD flavoprotein, and in *Mycoplasma* spp. it reduces an FMN flavo-protein. In a one-electron transfer from reduced flavoprotein to oxygen, an O_2^- intermediate is formed. The radical is dismutated to H_2O_2 and O_2 by an Mn-dependent SOD. In some aerobic mollicutes, catalase converts H_2O_2 to water and O_2. The generation of ATP may somehow be coupled or related to these reactions.

Spiroplasmas may have a pattern resembling the mycoplasma scheme but have been much less extensively studied. The system may also be similar in the anaeroplasmas, but the final electron acceptor is not oxygen. O_2^-, therefore, may not be formed. The identity of the final electron acceptor in these anaerobes is unknown. In ureaplasmas, the system may be different, since no FAD or FMN flavoprotein or NOA has been detected. However, as indicated before, Davis and Villanueva (36) reported an NADH diaphorase activity in ureaplasmas.

OTHER SOURCES OF ENERGY

Fatty Acids

VanDemark and Smith (160) showed that cell extracts of butyrate-grown *M. hominis* (*M. arthritidis*) 07 possessed a β-oxidative pathway for the oxidation of fatty acids. It was suggested that this cyclic path was operative in nonglycolytic species and that the process was linked to the TCA cycle, which was at that time believed to be present. There is suggestive evidence that supports the concept of energy conservation linked to fatty acid oxidation. Lynn (78) reported that nonglycolytic species were capable of oxidizing short-chain fatty acids. Acetyl-CoA synthase (EC 6.2.1.1) (160), phosphotransacetylase (EC 2.3.1.8) (60, 143), and acetate kinase (EC 2.7.2.1) (24, 60, 88, 126) have been reported in *M. arthritidis* and *M. gallisepticum*. These enzyme activities may effect the oxidation of pyruvate and may be involved in energy-conserving reactions. Kahane et al. (60), however, suggested that the action of acetate kinase did not result in a significant synthesis of ATP.

The role of fatty acid transport in mollicutes has been studied by Dahl (33), who found that *M. capricolum* fatty acid transport is tightly coupled to the esterification of phospholipid. There was little accumulation of free fatty acid. The process was energy linked and protein mediated. The activity was not dependent on CoA but was stimulated by ATP.

Amino Acids

Smith (140–142) studied the production of ATP by mollicutes from glutamine. The phosphorolytic deamidation of glutamine yields ATP. Smith, however, considered that the reaction was not a significant contributor to the energy requirements of the cell.

Arginine serves as an energy source for nonglycolytic mollicutes, but there is some difference of opinion as to the magnitude of its role (9, 11, 17, 44, 52, 56, 131, 132, 137, 164). The sequence of reactions by which ATP is generated is called the arginine dihydrolase (ADI) pathway (32). The reaction sequence is as follows:

arginine + H_2O $\longrightarrow$ citrulline + NH_4^+

citrulline + P_i $\longleftrightarrow$ ornithine + carbamyl phosphate

carbamyl phosphate + ADP $\longleftrightarrow$

$$ATP + HCO_3^- + NH_4^+$$

The first step is irreversible and considered to be unique to the ADI path. It is mediated by arginine deiminase (EC 3.5.3.6). In the second step, ornithine is synthesized by the action of ornithine carbamoyltransferase (EC 2.1.2.2). Ornithine is also the product of the hydrolytic action of arginase (EC 3.5.3.1) (1). Therefore, ornithine must be used warily as an indicator of the complete ADI path. In the last step of the ADI pathway, carbamate kinase (EC 2.7.2.2) catalyzes the phosphorylation of ADP to produce ATP.

Arginine deiminase was purified to apparent homogeneity from *M. arginini* and *M. arthritidis* (66, 164). The enzyme has a molecular mass of 87.3 kDa, contains two subunits, requires no cofactors or metal ions for activity, and distinctively contains 36 half-cysteine residues (164). Neither citrulline nor ornithine inhibits arginine deiminase activity. Arginine deiminase constitutes about 10% of the cytoplasmic protein of *M. arthritidis* (132, 164) and perhaps *M. hominis* (74). The enzyme has been cloned and sequenced from *M. arginini* (66). The ORF for the enzyme encoded a 385-amino-acid polypeptide of molecular mass 43.9 kDa.

Nonglycolytic mollicutes may not use arginine as a sole or perhaps even primary energy source. Beaman and Pollack (14) showed that the nonglycolytic *M. arginini* G230^T consumes glucose during growth in the presence of arginine. The pH, as expected, rose slightly, and no accumulation of lactate or pyruvate was observed. Other *Mycoplasma* spp. (e.g., *M. fermentans* [10] and *M. iowae* [59]) can also use glucose and arginine.

Sjostrom et al. (137) have shown that species generally regarded as glycolytic and unable to utilize arginine, as indicated by a trivial alkaline shift of the medium, can produce end products which are indicators of arginine metabolism. They found that the glycolytic, apparently non-arginine-utilizing species (*M. putrefaciens*, *M. capricolum*, a bovine *Mycoplasma* sp., and two strains of *M. gallisepticum*) all produced citrulline from arginine. The first three also produced ornithine.

The widespread occurrence of the ADI pathway is also suggested by studies of *S. citri* and *S. kunkelii* (56, 147, 151). The ADI path was reported to be present in both of these spiroplasmas. As these spiroplasmas can be characterized as glycolytic (104, 106), they are additional examples of the ability of a growing number of mollicutes known to use both glucose and arginine.

The activities of ornithine carbamoyltransferase and carbamate kinase are less frequently reported. They have been purified from *M. hominis* 07 (132). The importance of carbamate kinase is related to its mediation of ATP synthesis. This enzyme may be lacking in some arginolytic strains (137). In this case, the ADI path would be characterized as truncated (137) and represented by those strains producing citrulline and ornithine but no ATP. This feature suggests that a measure of the presence of the ADI pathway and its usefulness requires an estimation of the presence and quantity of ATP synthesized from arginine.

Carbamate kinase may be in competition with aspartate transcarbamylase (EC 2.1.3.2) for carbamyl phosphate. Carbamyl phosphate is not only an intermediate in the ADI pathway but also an initial intermediate in the synthesis of the pyrimidine UMP. Both carbamate kinase of the ADI pathway and aspartate transcarbamylase, leading to UMP, require carbamyl phosphate. This sequence of reactions leading to the synthesis of UMP has not been reported in mollicutes.

The question of whether arginine or glucose is the preferred substrate is difficult to answer (32). Hahn and Kenny (52) reported that not all arginine-utilizing species of mollicutes showed an arginine requirement for the initiation of growth and that the function of the pathway may not be entirely associated with energy production. Fenske and Kenny (44) reported that arginine deiminase was first detected late in the log phase of *M. hominis* cultures and concluded that the ADI pathway is not the major energy-generating system in this mollicutes. Igwegbe and Thomas (56) concluded that the pathway was inducible in *S. citri*.

Cunin et al. (32) suggested that energy depletion is an essential signal for inducing the ADI pathway in most bacteria studied so far. Beaman and Pollack (13, 14) indicated that mollicutes, apart from *A. laidlawii* B-PG9, are in a relative energy deficit during mid-exponential-phase growth. These authors suggested that the low levels of ATP or the low cellular adenylate energy charge levels in nonglycolytic species may be a stimulus to activate alternate metabolic pathways.

Saglio et al. (129) determined the ATP content in growing *S. citri* cells. From their data, it was calculated that growing *S. citri* contained 1.9×10^{-17} mol of ATP per CFU (14). They also concluded that during mid-exponential-phase growth of *A. laidlawii* B-PG9, the value was 2.3×10^{-17} mol of ATP per CFU; in *M. arginini*, it was 0.08×10^{-17} mol of ATP per CFU (14). Stemler et al. (146) found 47.0×10^{-17} mol of ATP per cell of *U. urealyticum*. In studying the ADI path of mollicutes as a source of energy, more attention might be paid to the production of ATP and the preferential use of sensitive biochemical techniques (137) rather than pH changes. Such studies may be affected by medium induction (139), the possible presence of a variety of arginine-active enzymes (5, 6, 129, 134–136), the possible role of arginine in amino acid transport (74, 111), and the presence of two forms of the deiminase (163). It is probable that arginine does not serve as a sole energy source for *Mycoplasma* spp. (32). Speculatively, the ADI path may provide nitrogen in the form of NH_4^+ when other nitrogen sources are depleted.

Using preparations of *S. melliferum*, Rottem and Shirazi (127) have described an arginine-ornithine exchange system in mollicutes. The data were characterized as the first report of an exchange system for cationic metabolites in bacteria.

Urea

Urease, the enzyme activity that characterizes the genus *Ureaplasma*, may have a significant role in ATP synthesis. It has been proposed that urea hydrolysis generates ATP through a chemiosomotic process (123,

124). A number of investigators have purified urease from *U. urealyticum* (19, 20, 38, 43, 128, 145, 149). Urease mediates the hydrolysis of urea to ammonia and carbon dioxide. Thirkell et al. (149) found that urease was composed of three subunits: 72, 14, and 11 kDa. The native enzyme had a molecular mass of 190 kDa, was a hexamer, and contained, like the 72-kDa subunit, nickel ion. Blanchard (19) carried out nucleotide sequence analysis of a *U. urealyticum* DNA fragment which was homologous to cloned urease genes from other procaryotes and found three ORFs. The molecular masses calculated for the proteins encoded by these three ORFs were 66.6, 13.6, and 11.2 kDa, values very close to those found by Thirkell et al. (149). Sequences of genomic DNA from *U. urealyticum* in hybridization studies were shown to be homologous to urease genes from *Campylobacter pylori*, *E. coli*, and *Providencia stuartii* (20). These findings indicate that phylogenetically distant procaryotes have urease genes with conserved sequences.

REFERENCES

1. **Abdelel, A. T.** 1979. Arginine catabolism by microorganisms. *Annu. Rev. Microbiol.* **33:**139–168.
2. **Allsopp, B. A., and K. P. Matthews.** 1975. Studies of lactate dehydrogenase of *Mycoplasma mycoides* var. *mycoides. J. Gen. Microbiol.* **88:**58–64.
3. **Arora, Y. K., and R. C. Sinha.** 1985. Enzymatic activities in cell fractions of mycoplasmalike organisms purified from aster yellows-infected plants. *J. Bacteriol.* **164:**811–815.
4. **Atobe, H., J. Watabe, and M. Ogata.** 1983. *Acholeplasma parvum*, a new species from horses. *Int. J. Syst. Bacteriol.* **33:**344–349.
5. **Ball, H. J., S. D. Neill, and L. R. Reid.** 1982. Use of arginine aminopeptidase activity in characterization of arginine-utilizing mycoplasmas. *J. Clin. Microbiol.* **15:**28–34.
6. **Ball, H. J., S. D. Neill, and R. L. Reid.** 1985. Aminopeptidase activity in arginine-utilizing *Mycoplasma* spp. *J. Clin. Microbiol.* **21:**859–860.
7. **Baltscheffsky, H.** 1971. Inorganic pyrophosphate and the origin and evolution of biological energy transformation, p. 466–474. *In* R. Buvet and C. Ponnamperuma (ed.), *Chemical Evolution and the Origin of Life*. North Holland Publishing Co., Amsterdam.
8. **Baltscheffsky, H., M. Lundin, C. Luxemburg, P. Nyrén, and M. Baltscheffsky.** 1986. Inorganic pyrophosphate and the molecular evolution of biological energy coupling. *Chem. Scr.* **26B:**259–262.
9. **Barile, M. F.** 1983. Arginine hydrolysis, p. 345–349. *In* S. Razin and J. G. Tully (ed.), *Methods in Mycoplasmology*, vol. 1. Academic Press, Inc., New York.
10. **Barile, M. F., R. A. Del Giudice, T. R. Carski, C. J. Gibbs, and J. A. Morris.** 1968. Isolation and characterization of *Mycoplasma arginini* spec. nov. *Proc. Soc. Exp. Biol. Med.* **129:**489–494.
11. **Barile, M. F., R. T. Schimke, and D. B. Riggs.** 1966. Presence of the arginine dihydrolase pathway in *Mycoplasma. J. Bacteriol.* **91:**189–192.
12. **Bauminger, E. R., S. G. Cohen, F. Labenski de Kanter, A. Levy, S. Ofer, M. Kessel, and S. Rottem.** 1980. Iron storage in *Mycoplasma capricolum. J. Bacteriol.* **141:**378–381.
13. **Beaman, K. D., and J. D. Pollack.** 1981. Adenylate energy charge in *Acholeplasma laidlawii* B-PG9. *J. Bacteriol.* **146:**1055–1058.
14. **Beaman, K. D., and J. D. Pollack.** 1983. Synthesis of

15. **Beaman, K. D., and J. D. Pollack.** 1984. Enzymatic assimilation of ^{14}C from $NaH^{14}CO_3$ by extracts of *Acholeplasma laidlawii* B-PG9. *Yale J. Biol. Med.* **57:**897.
16. **Berry, A., S. Ahmad, A. Liss, and R. A. Jenson.** 1987. Enzymological features of aromatic amino acid biosynthesis reflect the phylogeny of mycoplasmas. *J. Gen. Microbiol.* **133:**2147–2154.
17. **Black, F. T.** 1973. Biological and physical properties of human T-mycoplasmas. *Ann. N.Y. Acad. Sci.* **225:**131–143.
18. **Black, F. T.** 1973. Phosphatase activity in T-mycoplasmas. *Int. J. Syst. Bacteriol.* **23:**65–66.
19. **Blanchard, A.** 1990. *Ureaplasma urealyticum* urease genes; use of a UGA tryptophan codon. *Mol. Microbiol.* **4:**669–676.
20. **Blanchard, A., and M. F. Barile.** 1989. Cloning of *Ureaplasma urealyticum* DNA sequences showing genetic homology with urease genes from Gram negative bacteria. *Res. Microbiol.* **140:**281–290.
21. **Bradbury, J.** 1977. Rapid biochemical tests for characterization of the *Mycoplasmatales. J. Clin. Microbiol.* **5:**531–534.
22. **Bridger, W. A., and J. F. Henderson.** 1983. *Cell ATP*. John Wiley & Sons, New York.
23. **Brink, B. T., R. Otto, U.-P. Hansen, and W. N. Konings.** 1985. Energy recycling by lactate efflux in growing and nongrowing cells of *Streptococcus cremoris. J. Bacteriol.* **162:**383–390.
24. **Castrejon-Diez, J., T. N. Fisher, and E. Fisher, Jr.** 1963. Glucose metabolism in two strains of *Mycoplasma laidlawii. J. Bacteriol.* **86:**627–636.
25. **Chang, C.-J., and T. A. Chen.** 1981. Spiroplasmas: cultivation in chemically defined medium. *Science* **215:**1121–1122.
26. **Chevalier, C., C. Saillard, and J. M. Bové.** 1990. Organization and nucleotide sequences of the *Spiroplasma citri* genes for ribosomal protein S2, elongation factors Ts, spiralin, phosphofructokinase, pyruvate kinase, and an unidentified protein. *J. Bacteriol.* **172:**2693–2703.
27. **Cirillo, V. P., and S. Razin.** 1973. Distribution of a phosphoenolpyruvate-dependent sugar phosphotransferase system in mycoplasmas. *J. Bacteriol.* **113:**212–217.
28. **Clark, A. F., D. F. Farrell, W. Burke, and C. R. Scott.** 1978. The effect of mycoplasma contamination on the *in vitro* assay of pyruvate dehydrogenase activity in cultured fibroblasts. *Clin. Chim. Acta* **82:**119–124.
29. **Cocks, B. J., F. A. Brake, A. Mitchell, and L. R. Finch.** 1985. Enzymes of intermediary carbohydrate metabolism in *Ureaplasma urealyticum* and *Mycoplasma mycoides* subsp. *mycoides. J. Gen. Microbiol.* **131:**2129–2135.
30. **Cole, B. C., J. R. Ward, and C. H. Martin.** 1968. Hemolysin and peroxide activity of *Mycoplasma* species. *J. Bacteriol.* **95:**2022–2030.
31. **Constantopoulos, G., and G. J. McGarrity.** 1987. Activities of oxidative enzymes in mycoplasmas. *J. Bacteriol.* **169:**2012–2016.
32. **Cunin, R., N. Glansdorff, A. Piérard, and V. Stalon.** 1986. Biosynthesis and metabolism of arginine in bacteria. *Microbiol. Rev.* **50:**314–352.
33. **Dahl, J.** 1988. Uptake of fatty acids by *Mycoplasma capricolum. J. Bacteriol.* **170:**2022–2026.
34. **Davis, J. W., Jr., J. T. Manolukas, B. E. Capo, and J. D. Pollack.** 1990. Pyruvate metabolism and the absence of a tricarboxylic acid cycle in *Ureaplasma urealyticum. Zentralbl. Bakteriol. Suppl.* **20:**666–669.
35. **Davis, J. W., Jr., I. S. Moses, C. Ndubuka, and R. Ortiz.** 1987. Inorganic pyrophosphatase activity in cell-free extracts of *Ureaplasma urealyticum. J. Gen. Microbiol.* **133:**1453–1459.
36. **Davis, J. W., Jr., and I. Villanueva.** 1990. Enzyme differ-

ences in serovar clusters of *Ureaplasma urealyticum, U. diversum,* and ovine ureaplasmas. *Zentralbl. Bakteriol. Suppl.* **20:**661–665.

37. **Dayhoff, M. O.** 1971. Evolution of proteins, p. 392–419. *In* R. Buvet and C. Ponnamperuma (ed.), *Chemical Evolution and the Origin of Life.* North Holland Publishing Co., Amsterdam.

38. **Delisle, G. J.** 1977. Multiple forms of urease in cytoplasmic fractions of *Ureaplasma urealyticum. J. Bacteriol.* **130:**1390–1392.

39. **DeSantis, D., V. V. Tryon, and J. D. Pollack.** 1989. Metabolism of Mollicutes: the Embden-Meyerhof-Parnas pathway and the hexose monophosphate shunt. *J. Gen. Microbiol.* **135:**683–691.

40. **Dujardin-Beaumetz, E.** 1900. Le Microbe de la péripneumonie et sa culture. Etude bacteriologique d'un microorganisme à la limite de la visibilité. Thèse, Faculté de Médecine de Paris. Octave Doin, Paris.

41. **Edward, D. G. ff.** 1954. The pleuropneumonia group of organisms: a review together with some new observations. *J. Gen. Microbiol.* **10:**27–64.

42. **Egan, W., M. Barile, and S. Rottem.** 1986. ^{31}P-NMR studies of *Mycoplasma gallisepticum* cells using a continuous perfusion technique. *FEBS Lett.* **204:**373–376.

43. **Eng, H., J. A. Robertson, and G. W. Stemke.** 1986. Properties of urease from *Ureaplasma urealyticum:* kinetics, molecular weight, and demonstration of multiple enzyme isoelectric point forms. *Can. J. Microbiol.* **32:**487–493.

44. **Fenske, J. D., and G. E. Kenny.** 1976. Role of arginine deiminase in growth of *Mycoplasma hominis. J. Bacteriol.* **126:**501–510.

45. **Fothergill-Gilmore, L. A.** 1986. Domains of glycolytic enzymes, p. 85–174. *In* D. G. Hardie and J. R. Coggins (ed.), *Multidomain Proteins—Structure and Evolution.* Elsevier, Amsterdam.

46. **Freundt, E. A.** 1958. *The Mycoplasmataceae.* Munksgaard, Copenhagen.

47. **Fridovich, I.** 1981. Superoxide radical and superoxide dismutases, p. 250–272. *In* D. L. Gilbert (ed.), *Oxygen and Living Processes.* Springer-Verlag, New York.

48. **Gill, J. W.** 1960. Culture and metabolism of *Mycoplasma gallisepticum. J. Bacteriol.* **83:**213–218.

49. **Gottschalk, G.** 1986. *Bacterial Metabolism,* 2nd ed. Springer-Verlag, New York.

50. **Grossato, A., E. Boccu, and F. M. Veronese.** 1976. Ricerche sugli enzimi dei micoplasmi: enolasi del *Mycoplasma hominis. Boll. Ist. Sieroter. Milan.* **55:**104–109.

51. **Hackett, K. J., A. S. Ginsberg, S. Rottem, R. B. Henegar, and R. F. Whitcomb.** 1987. A defined medium for a fastidious spiroplasma. *Science* **237:**525–527.

52. **Hahn, R., and G. E. Kenny.** 1974. Differences in arginine requirement for growth among arginine-utilizing *Mycoplasma* species. *J. Bacteriol.* **117:**611–618.

53. **Henrikson, C. V., M. Kunze, and H. Flamm.** 1971. Biochemische Untersuchungen an 10 Stammen von *Mykoplasma laidlawii. Zentralbl. Bakteriol. Abt. 1 Orig.* **216:**333–338.

54. **Höllander, R.** 1977. Lipoquinones of some bacteria and mycoplasmas, with considerations of their functional significance. *Antonie van Leeuwenhoek J. Microbiol. Serol.* **43:**177–185.

55. **Holmes, B. E., and A. Pirie.** 1932. Growth and metabolism of the bovine pleuropneumonia virus. *Br. J. Exp. Pathol.* **13:**364–370.

56. **Igwegbe, E. C. K., and C. Thomas.** 1978. Occurrence of enzymes of arginine dihydrolase pathway in *Spiroplasma citri. J. Gen. Appl. Microbiol.* **24:**261–269.

57. **Iuchi, S., D. C. Cameron, and E. C. C. Lin.** 1989. A second global regulator gene (*arcB*) mediating repression of enzymes in aerobic pathways of *Escherichia coli. J. Bacteriol.* **171:**868–873.

58. **Jinks, D. C., and L. L. Matz.** 1976. Reduced nicotinamide adenine dinucleotide oxidase of *Acholeplasma laidlawii* membranes. *Biochim. Biophys. Acta* **430:**71–82.

58a.**Jones, M., and J. D. Pollack.** Unpublished data.

59. **Jordan, F. T. W., G. Erno, G. S. Cottew, K. H. Hinz, and L. Stipkovits.** 1982. Characterization and taxonomic description of five mycoplasma serovars (serotypes) of avian origin and their elevation to species rank and further evaluation of the taxonomic status of *Mycoplasma synoviae. Int. J. Syst. Bacteriol.* **32:**108–115.

60. **Kahane, I., A. Muhlrad, and S. Razin.** 1978. Possible role of acetate kinase in ATP generation in *Mycoplasma hominis* and *Acholeplasma laidlawii. FEMS Microbiol. Lett.* **3:**143–145.

61. **Kandler, G., and O. Kandler.** 1955. Ernahrungs und stoff-wechselphysiologische Untersuchungen an pleuropneumonie-ahnlichen Organismen under der L-Phase der Bakterien. *Zentralbl. Bakteriol. Abt. 2* **108:**383.

62. **Kandler, O.** 1983. Carbohydrate metabolism in lactic acid bacteria. *Antonie van Leeuwenhoek J. Microbiol. Serol.* **49:**209–224.

63. **Kawauchi, Y., A. Muto, and S. Osawa.** 1982. The protein composition of *Mycoplasma capricolum. Mol. Gen. Genet.* **188:**7–11.

64. **Kirby, T., J. Blum, I. Kahane, and I. Fridovich.** 1980. Distinguishing between manganese-containing and iron-containing superoxide dismutases in crude extracts of cells. *Arch. Biochem. Biophys.* **201:**551–555.

65. **Klomkes, M., R. Altdorf, and H.-D. Ohlenbusch.** 1985. Purification and properties of an FAD-containing NADH-oxidase from *Mycoplasma capricolum. Biol. Chem. Hoppe-Seyler* **366:**963–969.

66. **Kondo, K., H. Sone, H. Yoshida, T. Toida, K. Kanatani, Y.-M. Hong, N. Nishino, and J. Tanaka.** 1990. Cloning and sequence analysis of the arginine deiminase gene from *Mycoplasma arginini. Mol. Gen. Genet.* **221:**81–86.

67. **Konings, W. N.** 1985. Generation of metabolic energy by end-product efflux. *Trends Biochem. Sci.* **10:**317–319.

68. **Konings, W. N., B. Poolman, and A. J. M. Driessen.** 1989. Bioenergetics and solute transport in lactococci. *Crit. Rev. Microbiol.* **16:**419–476.

69. **Kulaev, I. S., and V. M. Vagabov.** 1983. Polyphosphate metabolism in micro-organisms. *Adv. Microbiol. Physiol.* **24:**83–171.

70. **Lanham, S. M., R. M. Lemcke, C. M. Scott, and J. M. Grendon.** 1980. Isoenzymes in two species of *Acholeplasma. J. Gen. Microbiol.* **117:**19–31.

71. **Lecce, J. G., and H. E. Morton.** 1953. Metabolic studies on the three strains of pleuropneumonia-like organisms isolated from man. *J. Bacteriol.* **67:**62–68.

72. **Lee, G. Y., and G. E. Kenny.** 1984. Immunological heterogeneity of superoxide dismutases in the *Acholeplasmataceae. Int. J. Syst. Bacteriol.* **34:**74–76.

73. **Lehninger, A. L.** 1982. *Principles of Biochemistry.* Worth Publishers, New York.

74. **Lin, J.-S. L.** 1986. Arginine deiminase of *Mycoplasma hominis:* cytoplasmic and membrane-associated forms. *J. Gen. Microbiol.* **132:**1467–1474.

75. **Lipman, F.** 1965. Projecting backward from the present stage of evolution of biosynthesis, p. 259–280. *In* S. W. Fox (ed.), *The Origins of Prebiological Systems.* Academic Press, New York.

76. **Liu, C.-L., and H. D. Peck, Jr.** 1981. Comparative bioenergetics of sulfate reduction in *Desulfovibrio* and *Desulfotomaculum* spp. *J. Bacteriol.* **145:**966–973.

77. **Lynch, R. E., and B. C. Cole.** 1980. *Mycoplasma pneumoniae:* a prokaryote which consumes oxygen and generates superoxide but which lacks superoxide dismutase. *Biochem. Biophys. Res. Commun.* **96:**98–105.

78. **Lynn, R.** 1960. Oxidative metabolism of pleuropneumonia-like organisms. *Ann. N.Y. Acad. Sci.* **79:**538–542.

79. **Manolukas, J., M. F. Barile, D. K. F. Chandler, and J. D. Pollack.** 1988. Presence of anaplerotic reactions and

transamination, and the absence of the tricarboxylic acid cycle in Mollicutes. *J. Gen. Microbiol.* **134:**791–800.

80. **Manolukas, J. T., M. V. Williams, and J. D. Pollack.** 1989. The anaplerotic phosphoenolpyruvate carboxylase of the tricarboxylic acid cycle deficient *Acholeplasma laidlawii* B-PG9. *J. Gen. Microbiol.* **135:** 251–256.

81. **Masover, G. K., S. Razin, and L. Hayflick.** 1977. Localization of enzymes in *Ureaplasma urealyticum* (T-strain mycoplasma). *J. Bacteriol.* **130:**297–302.

82. **McElwain, M. C., D. K. F. Chandler, M. F. Barile, T. F. Young, V. V. Tryon, J. W. Davis, Jr., J. P. Petzel, C.-J. Chang, M. V. Williams, and J. D. Pollack.** 1988. Purine and pyrimidine metabolism in *Mollicutes* species. *Int. J. Syst. Bacteriol.* **38:**417–423.

83. **Meier, B., and G. G. Habermehl.** 1990. Evidence for superoxide dismutase and catalase in Mollicutes and release of reactive oxygen species. *Arch. Biochem. Biophys.* **277:**74–79.

84. **Michels, P. A. M., J. P. J. Michels, J. Boonstra, and W. N. Konings.** 1979. Generation of electrochemical proton gradient in bacteria by excretion of metabolic end products. *FEMS Microbiol. Lett.* **5:**357–364.

85. **Miles, R. J., and B. J. Wadher.** 1990. Kinetics and patterns of substrate utilization by *Mycoplasma* spp. *Zentralbl. Bakteriol. Suppl.* **20:**675–677.

86. **Morowitz, H. J.** 1984. The completeness of molecular biology. *Isr. J. Med. Sci.* **20:**750–753.

87. **Mudd, J. B., M. Ittig, B. Roy, J. Latrille, and J. M. Bové.** 1977. Composition and enzyme activities of *Spiroplasma citri* membranes. *J. Bacteriol.* **129:**1250–1256.

88. **Muhlrad, A., I. Peleg, J. A. Robertson, I. M. Robinson, and I. Kahane.** 1981. Acetate kinase activity in mycoplasmas. *J. Bacteriol.* **147:**271–273.

89. **Neale, G. A. M., A. Mitchell, and L. R. Finch.** 1983. Pathways of pyrimidine deoxyribonucleotide biosynthesis in *Mycoplasma mycoides* subsp. *mycoides. J. Bacteriol.* **154:**17–22.

90. **Neidhardt, F. C., J. L. Ingraham, and M. Schaechter.** 1990. *Physiology of the Bacterial Cell. A Molecular Approach.* Sinauer Associates, Inc., Sunderland, Mass.

91. **Neimark, H.** 1979. Phylogenetic relationships between mycoplasmas and other prokaryotes, p. 43–61. *In* M. F. Barile and S. Razin (ed.), *The Mycoplasmas,* vol. 1. *Cell Biology.* Academic Press, New York.

92. **Neimark, H., and R. M. Lemcke.** 1972. Occurrence and properties of lactic dehydrogenases of fermentative mycoplasmas. *J. Bacteriol.* **111:**633–640.

93. **Neimark, H., and M. J. Pickett.** 1960. Products of glucose metabolism of pleuropneumonia-like organisms. *Ann. N.Y. Acad. Sci.* **79:**531–537.

94. **O'Brien, S. J., J. M. Simonson, M. W. Grabowski, and M. F. Barile.** 1981. Analysis of multiple isoenzyme expression among twenty-two species of *Mycoplasma* and *Acholeplasma. J. Bacteriol.* **146:**222–232.

95. **O'Brien, S. J., J. M. Simonson, S. Razin, and M. F. Barile.** 1983. On the distribution and characteristics of isozyme expression in *Mycoplasma, Acholeplasma* and *Ureaplasma* species. *Yale J. Biol. Med.* **56:**701–708.

96. **Pantskhava, E.** 1971. Some information on the possibility of preglycolytic ways in evolution, p. 475–479. *In* R. Buvet and C. Ponnamperuma (ed.), *Chemical Evolution and the Origin of Life.* North Holland Publishing Co., Amsterdam.

97. **Petkau, A., and W. S. Chelack.** 1974. Radioprotection of *Acholeplasma laidlawii* B by cysteine. *Int. J. Radiat. Biol.* **26:**421–426.

98. **Petzel, J., M. C. McElwain, D. DeSantis, J. Manolukas, M. V. Williams, P. A. Hartman, M. J. Allison, and J. D. Pollack.** 1989. Enzymic activities of carbohydrate, purine, and pyrimidine metabolism in the *Anaeroplasmataceae* (class Mollicutes). *Arch. Microbiol.* **152:** 309–316.

99. **Petzel, J. P., P. A. Hartman, and M. J. Allison.** 1989. Pyrophosphate-dependent enzymes in walled bacteria phylogenetically related to the wall-less bacteria of the class *Mollicutes. Int. J. Syst. Bacteriol.* **39:**413–419.

100. **Pirie, A.** 1938. The effect of catalase on the respiration of a filterable organism from sewage. *Br. J. Exp. Pathol.* **19:**9.

101. **Pollack, J. D.** 1975. Localization of reduced nicotinamide adenine dinucleotide oxidase activity in *Acholeplasma* and *Mycoplasma* species. *Int. J. Syst. Bacteriol.* **25:**108–113.

102. **Pollack, J. D.** 1979. Respiratory pathways and energy yielding mechanisms, p. 187–211. *In* M. F. Barile and S. Razin (ed.), *The Mycoplasmas,* vol. 1. Academic Press, Inc., New York.

103. **Pollack, J. D.** 1986. Metabolic distinctiveness of ureaplasmas. *Pediatr. Infect. Dis.* **5:**S305–S307.

104. **Pollack, J. D.** 1990. Metabolism of the *Spiroplasmataceae. IOM Lett.* **1:**199–200.

104a. **Pollack, J. D.** Unpublished data.

105. **Pollack, J. D., K. D. Beaman, and J. A. Robertson.** 1984. Synthesis of lipids from acetate is not characteristic of *Acholeplasma* or *Ureaplasma* species. *Int. J. Syst. Bacteriol.* **34:**124–126.

106. **Pollack, J. D., M. C. McElwain, D. DeSantis, J. T. Manolukas, J. G. Tully, C.-J. Chang, R. F. Whitcomb, K. J. Hackett, and M. V. Williams.** 1989. Metabolism of members of the *Spiroplasmataceae. Int. J. Bacteriol.* **39:**406–412.

107. **Pollack, J. D., A. J. Merola, M. Platz, and R. L. Booth, Jr.** 1981. Respiration-associated components of Mollicutes. *J. Bacteriol.* **146:**907–913.

108. **Pollack, J. D., S. Razin, and R. C. Cleverdon.** 1965. Localization of enzymes in mycoplasma. *J. Bacteriol.* **90:**617–622.

109. **Pollack, J. D., and M. V. Williams.** 1986. PPi-dependent phosphotransferase (phosphofructokinase) activity in the mollicutes (mycoplasma) *Acholeplasma laidlawii. J. Bacteriol.* **165:**53–60.

110. **Poolman, B., B. Bosman, J. Kiers, and W. N. Konings.** 1987. Control of glycolysis by glyceraldehyde-3-phosphate dehydrogenase in *Streptococcus cremoris* and *Streptococcus lactis. J. Bacteriol.* **169:**5887–5890.

111. **Razin, S., L. Gottfried, and S. Rottem.** 1968. Amino acid transport in mycoplasma. *J. Bacteriol.* **95:**1685–1691.

112. **Reeves, R. E.** 1987. Metabolic energy supplied by PPi, p. 255–259. *In* F. G. Rothman, S. Silver, A. Wright, and E. Yagil (ed.), *Phosphate Metabolism and Cellular Regulation in Microorganisms.* American Society for Microbiology, Washington, D.C.

113. **Reinards, R., R. Altdorf, and H.-D. Ohlenbusch.** 1984. Purification and properties of a manganese-containing superoxide dismutase from *Acholeplasma laidlawii. Hoppe-Seyler's Z. Physiol. Chem.* **365:**577–585.

114. **Reinards, R., J. Kubicki, and H.-D. Ohlenbusch.** 1981. Purification and characterization of NADH oxidase from membranes of *Acholeplasma laidlawii,* a copper-containing iron-sulfur flavoprotein. *Eur. J. Biochem.* **120:**329–337.

115. **Ritchie, T. W., and H. W. Seeley, Jr.** 1976. Distribution of cytochrome-like respiration in streptococci. *J. Gen. Microbiol.* **93:**195–203.

116. **Robertson, J. A., and L. A. Howard.** 1987. Effect of carbohydrates on growth of *Ureaplasma urealyticum* and *Mycoplasma hominis. J. Clin. Microbiol.* **25:**160–161.

117. **Rodwell, A., and E. S. Rodwell.** 1954. The breakdown of carbohydrates by *Asterococcus mycoides,* the organism of bovine pleuropneumonia. *Aust. J. Biol. Sci.* **7:**18–30.

118. **Rodwell, A., and E. S. Rodwell.** 1954. The breakdown of pyruvate by *Asterococcus mycoides,* the organism of bovine pleuropneumonia. *Aust. J. Biol. Sci.* **7:**31–36.

119. **Rodwell, A., and E. S. Rodwell.** 1954. The pathway for glucose oxidation by *Asterococcus mycoides,* the organ-

ism of bovine pleuropneumonia. *Aust. J. Biol. Sci.* **7:**37–46.

120. **Rodwell, A. W.** 1960. Nutrition and metabolism of *Mycoplasma mycoides* var. *mycoides. Ann. N.Y. Acad. Sci.* **79:**499–507.

121. **Rodwell, A. W.** 1968. Fatty acid composition of mycoplasma lipids: biomembrane with only one fatty acid. *Science* **160:**1350–1351.

122. **Rodwell, A. W.** 1969. Nutrition and metabolism of the mycoplasmas, p. 413–449. *In* L. Hayflick (ed.), *The Mycoplasmatales and the L-Phase of Bacteria.* Appleton-Century-Crofts, New York.

123. **Romano, N., R. LaLicata, and D. R. Alesi.** 1986. Energy production in *Ureaplasma urealyticum. Pediatr. Infect. Dis.* **5:**S308–S312.

124. **Romano, N., G. Tolone, F. Ajello, and R. LaLicata.** 1980. Adenosine 5′-triphosphate synthesis induced by urea hydrolysis in *Ureaplasma urealyticum. J. Bacteriol.* **144:**830–832.

125. **Rottem, S., and V. P. Cirillo.** 1986. Transport in mycoplasmas. *Methods Enzymol.* **125:**259–264.

126. **Rottem, S., and S. Razin.** 1967. Uptake and utilization of acetate by mycoplasma. *J. Gen. Microbiol.* **48:**53–63.

127. **Rottem, S., and I. Shirazi.** 1990. An arginine-ornithine exchange system in spiroplasmas. *IOM Lett.* **1:**102–103.

128. **Saada, A. B., and I. Kahane.** 1988. Purification and characterization of urease from *Ureaplasma urealyticum. Zentralbl. Bakteriol. Mikrobiol. Hyg. Abt. A* **269:**160–167.

129. **Saglio, P. H. M., M. I. Daniels, and A. Pradet.** 1979. ATP and energy charge as criteria of growth and metabolic activity of Mollicutes: application to *Spiroplasma citri. J. Gen. Microbiol.* **110:**13–20.

130. **Salih, M. M., V. Simonsen, and H. Erno.** 1983. Electrophoretic analysis of isoenzymes of *Acholeplasma* species. *Int. J. Syst. Bacteriol.* **33:**166–172.

131. **Schimke, R. T., and M. F. Barile.** 1963. Arginine metabolism in pleuropneumonia-like organisms isolated from mammalian cell cultures. *J. Bacteriol.* **86:**195–206.

132. **Schimke, R. T., C. M. Berlin, E. W. Sweeney, and W. R. Carroll.** 1966. The generation of energy by the arginine dihydrolase pathway in *Mycoplasma hominis* 07. *J. Biol. Chem.* **241:**2228–2236.

133. **Shepard, M. C., and G. K. Masover.** 1979. Special features of ureaplasmas, p. 452–494. *In* M. F. Barile and S. Razin (ed.), *The Mycoplasmas,* vol. 1. Academic Press, New York.

134. **Shibata, K.-I., and T. Watanabe.** 1986. Carboxypeptidase activity in human mycoplasmas. *J. Bacteriol.* **168:**1045–1047.

135. **Shibata, K.-I., and T. Watanabe.** 1987. Purification and characterization of an aminopeptidase from *Mycoplasma salivarium. J. Bacteriol.* **169:**3409–3413.

136. **Shibata, K.-I., and T. Watanabe.** 1988. Purification and characterization of an arginine-specific carboxypeptidase from *Mycoplasma salivarium. J. Bacteriol.* **170:**1795–1799.

137. **Sjostrom, K. E., K. C. S. Chen, and G. E. Kenny.** 1986. Detection of end products of the arginine dihydrolase pathway in both fermentative and nonfermentative *Mycoplasma* species by thin-layer chromatography. *Int. J. Syst. Bacteriol.* **36:**60–65.

138. **Sjostrom, K. E., and G. E. Kenny.** 1983. Distinctive antigenic specificities of adenosine triphosphates and reduced nicotinamide, adenine dinucleotide dehydrogenases as means for classification of the order *Mycoplasmatales. Int. J. Syst. Bacteriol.* **33:**218–228.

139. **Smith, D. W., R. L. Ganaway, and D. E. Fahrney.** 1978. Arginine deiminase from *Mycoplasma arthritidis.* Structure-activity relationships among substrates and competitive inhibitors. *J. Biol. Chem.* **253:**6016–6025.

140. **Smith, P.** 1960. Amino acid metabolism of PPLO. *Ann. N.Y. Acad. Sci.* **79:**543–550.

141. **Smith, P. F.** 1955. Amino acid metabolism by pleuropneumonia-like organisms. I. General catabolism. *J. Bacteriol.* **70:**552–556.

142. **Smith, P. F.** 1957. Conversion of citrulline to ornithine by pleuropneumonia-like organisms. *J. Bacteriol.* **74:**801–806.

143. **Smith, P. F., and C. V. Henrikson.** 1965. Comparative biosynthesis of mevalonic acid by mycoplasma. *J. Bacteriol.* **89:**146–153.

144. **Smith, S. L., P. J. VanDemark, and J. Fabricant.** 1963. Respiratory pathways in the mycoplasma. I. Lactate oxidation by *Mycoplasma gallisepticum. J. Bacteriol.* **86:**893–897.

145. **Stemke, G. W., J. A. Robertson, and M. Nhan.** 1987. Purification of urease from *Ureaplasma urealyticum. Can. J. Microbiol.* **33:**857–862.

146. **Stemler, M. E., G. W. Stemke, and J. A. Robertson.** 1987. ATP measurements obtained by luminometry provide rapid estimation of *Ureaplasma urealyticum* growth. *J. Clin. Microbiol.* **25:**427–429.

147. **Stevens, C., R. M. Cody, and R. T. Gudauskas.** 1980. Arginine metabolism by the corn stunt spiroplasma. *Curr. Microbiol.* **4:**139–142.

148. **Tarshis, M. A., A. G. Bekkouzjin, and V. G. Ladygina.** 1976. On the possible role of respiratory activity of *Acholeplasma laidlawii* cells in sugar transport. *Arch. Microbiol.* **109:**295–299.

149. **Thirkell, D., A. D. Mils, B. L. Precious, J. S. Frost, J. C. Woodall, M. G. Burdon, and W. C. Russell.** 1989. The urease of *Ureaplasma urealyticum. J. Gen. Microbiol.* **135:**315–323.

149a.**Tourtellotte, M. E.** 1960. Ph.D. thesis. University of Connecticut, Storrs.

150. **Tourtellotte, M. E., and R. E. Jacobs.** 1960. Physiological and serological comparison of PPLO from various sources. *Ann. N.Y. Acad. Sci.* **79:**521–530.

151. **Townsend, R.** 1976. Arginine metabolism by *Spiroplasma citri. J. Gen. Microbiol.* **94:**417–420.

152. **Tryon, V. V., and J. D. Pollack.** 1984. Purine metabolism in *Acholeplasma laidlawii* B: a novel PP$_i$-dependent nucleoside kinase activity. *J. Bacteriol.* **159:**265–270.

153. **Tryon, V. V., and J. D. Pollack.** 1985. Distinctions in *Mollicutes* purine metabolism: pyrophosphate-dependent nucleoside kinase and dependence on guanylate salvage. *Int. J. Syst. Bacteriol.* **35:**497–501.

154. **Tully, J. G., and S. Razin.** 1977. The Mollicutes: mycoplasmas and ureaplasmas, p. 417–443. *In* A. I. Laskin and H. Lechevalier (ed.), *Handbook of Microbiology,* vol. 1. CRC Press, Cleveland.

155. **Tully, J. G., and S. Razin.** 1977. The Mollicutes: acholeplasmas, spiroplasmas, thermoplasmas, and anaeroplasmas, p. 445–459. *In* A. I. Laskin and H. Lechevalier (ed.), *Handbook of Microbiology,* vol. 1. CRC Press, Cleveland.

156. **Ullah, A. H. J., and V. Cirillo.** 1976. *Mycoplasma* phosphoenolpyruvate-dependent sugar phosphotransferase system: purification and characterization of the phosphocarrier protein. *J. Bacteriol.* **127:**1298–1306.

157. **VanDemark, P. J.** 1969. Respiratory pathways in the mycoplasmas, p. 491–501. *In* L. Hayflick (ed.), *The Mycoplasmatales and the L-Phase of Bacteria.* Appleton-Century Crofts, New York.

158. **VanDemark, P. J., and P. Plackett.** 1972. Evidence for a phosphoenolpyruvate-dependent sugar phosphotransferase in mycoplasma strain Y. *J. Bacteriol.* **111:**454–458.

159. **VanDemark, P. J., and P. F. Smith.** 1964. Evidence for a tricarboxylic acid cycle in *Mycoplasma hominis. J. Bacteriol.* **88:**1602–1607.

160. **VanDemark, P. J., and P. F. Smith.** 1965. Nature of butyrate oxidation by *Mycoplasma hominis. J. Bacteriol.* **89:**373–377.

161. **Warren, J.** 1942. Observations on some biological char-

acteristics of organisms of the pleuropneumonia group. *J. Bacteriol.* **43:**211–227.

162. **Weibull, C., and K. Hammarberg.** 1962. Occurrence of catalase in pleuropneumonia-like organism and bacterial L-forms. *J. Bacteriol.* **84:**520–525.

163. **Weickmann, J. L., and D. E. Fahrney.** 1977. Arginine deiminase from *Mycoplasma arthritidis.* Evidence for multiple forms. *J. Biol. Chem.* **252:**2615–2620.

164. **Weickmann, J. L., M. E. Himmel, P. G. Squire, and D. E. Fahrney.** 1978. Arginine deiminase from *Mycoplasma arthritidis.* Properties of the enzyme from log phase cultures. *J. Biol. Chem.* **253:**6010–6015.

165. **Weisburg, W. G., J. G. Tully, D. L. Rose, J. P. Petzel, H. Oyaizu, D. Yang, L. Mandelco, J. Sechrest, T. G. Lawrence, J. Van Etten, J. Maniloff, and C. R. Woese.** 1989. A phylogenetic analysis of the mycoplasmas: basis for their classification. *J. Bacteriol.* **171:**6455–6467.

166. **White, D. C., and P. R. Sinclair.** 1971. Branched electron-transport systems in bacteria. *Adv. Microb. Physiol.* **5:**173–211.

167. **Whittenbury, R.** 1960. Two types of catalase-like activity in lactic acid bacteria. *Nature* (London) **187:**433–434.

168. **Williams, M. V., and J. D. Pollack.** 1984. Purification and characterization of a dUTPase from *Acholeplasma laidlawii* B-PG9. *J. Bacteriol.* **159:**278–282.

169. **Williams, M. V., and J. D. Pollack.** 1990. The importance of differences in the pyrimidine metabolism of the Mollicutes. *Zentralbl. Bakteriol. Suppl.* **20:**163–171.

170. **Windsor, R. S., and C. D. H. Boarer.** 1972. A method for the rapid enumeration of *Mycoplasma* species growing in broth culture. *J. Appl. Bacteriol.* **35:**37–42.

171. **Wood, H. G.** 1985. Inorganic pyrophosphate and polyphosphates as sources of energy. *Curr. Top. Cell. Regul.* **26:**355–369.

172. **Wood, T.** 1985. *The Pentose Phosphate Pathway.* Academic Press, Inc., Orlando, Fla.

12. Sources of Amino Acids

RANDY S. FISCHER, BRENDA E. FISCHER, and ROY A. JENSEN

INTRODUCTION

The investigation of amino acid metabolism in the mycoplasmas has been complicated because of the complex nutritional requirements of these organisms. For some *Mycoplasma* species, contemporary pessimism about prospects for elucidation of amino acid metabolism is probably unwarranted because the amino acid requirements have not always been systematically defined. The application of new molecular genetic techniques is also a basis for optimism. Because of the limited progress in delineating amino acid pathways, there has been a tendency to assume that all mycoplasmas are deficient in amino acid biosynthesis. However, direct enzymological analyses have generated scattered reports indicating that some mycoplasmas may possess intact or partial pathways of amino acid metabolism. The extent to which mycoplasmas may harbor additional enzymes or unique arrangements of amino acid metabolism is an emerging focal point of research that merits additional attention.

Various nutritional, physiological, and, less often, enzymological approaches have been used to assess the biochemical capabilities of the mycoplasmas (6, 37, 42). Recent studies by Berry et al. (4) and Petzel and Hartman (27) in *Acholeplasma laidlawii* and *Anaeroplasma* species, respectively, have demonstrated the presence of several enzymes central to aromatic amino acid biosynthesis. *Thermoplasma acidophilum*, which is generally believed to have considerable biosynthetic capacity because of its ability to grow in an inorganic salt medium containing glucose and a polypeptide fraction of yeast extract (43), has now been excluded from the class *Mollicutes* and assigned to a branch of the archaebacteria, even though it lacks a cell wall (30).

In this chapter, we present an overview of existing nutritional, biochemical, and enzymological information pertaining to amino acid metabolism in the mollicutes. When enzyme activities have been characterized, distinctive enzymological features (e.g., character states such as cofactor specificity) will be related to phylogenetically near microorganisms so that future analyses may be oriented to the potential character states shared by organismal clusters.

AMINO ACID REQUIREMENTS FOR GROWTH

The amino acid requirements of the various mycoplasma species have been difficult to define because many media formulations have contained basal components of beef heart infusion and peptone, to which supplements of yeast extract and horse serum have been added. Bovine serum albumin, lipoproteins, or tryptic digests of casein are often added to defined media to serve as a carrier and detoxifier of free fatty acids. As a result, the complex growth requirements of these microorganisms have generally hindered identification of essential amino acids. Nevertheless, considerable progress has been made with a few mycoplasmas.

Among mycoplasmas able to grow in at least partially defined media, those listed in Table 1 exemplify the distinctions in amino acid requirements among species, ranging from 3 amino acids for *Spiroplasma melliferum* (an insect pathogen) to 17 for *Mycoplasma mycoides* (isolated from goats). Only *A. laidlawii* B and *M. mycoides* Y are capable of growing in a fully defined medium (i.e., a medium lacking any supplement of peptides or protein). *M. mycoides* Y (36, 37) required all amino acids except cystine, aspartic acid, and glutamic acid. These nonessential amino acids appear, however, to be derived from the essential amino acids—cysteine, asparagine, and glutamine. Alanine was required only in the absence of pyridoxal. *A. laidlawii* B (44) is able to grow without a supplement of

Randy S. Fischer, Brenda E. Fischer, and Roy A. Jensen • Department of Microbiology and Cell Science, University of Florida, Gainesville, Florida 32611-0100.

Table 1. Amino acid requirements for growth of diverse mycoplasmas

Amino acid	Requirement for amino acid					
	S. melliferum[a] AS576 (6)[b]	M. arthritidis[c] 07 (41)	M. gallinarum[d] J (23)	A. laidlawii[a] A (31)	A. laidlawii B (44)	M. mycoides Y (36, 37)
Alanine	−	−	+	+	+	−
Arginine	−	+	+	+	+	+
Asparagine	+	−	+	+	−	+
Aspartic acid	−	+	−	−	+	−
Cysteine	+	+	−	−	−	+
Cystine	−	−	+	+	+	−
Glutamine	+	+	−	+	+	+
Glutamic acid	−	+	+	−	+	−
Glycine	−	−	+	+	+	+
Histidine	−	−	+	+	+	+
Isoleucine	−	+	+	+	+	+
Leucine	−	−	+	+	+	+
Lysine	−	−	−	−	+	+
Methionine	−	+	+	+	+	+
Phenylalanine	−	+	+	+	−	+
Proline	−	−	−	−	+	+
Serine	−	−	−	−	+	+
Threonine	−	−	+	+	+	+
Tryptophan	−	+	−	−	+	+
Tyrosine	−	−	+	+	−	+
Valine	−	−	−	−	+	+

[a] Medium contains bovine serum albumin.
[b] Reference numbers are given in parentheses.
[c] Medium contains serum lipoprotein fraction.
[d] Medium contains tryptic digest of casein.

phenylalanine and tyrosine if alanine is included in the medium. Asparagine and cysteine are not essential if aspartic acid and cystine are medium components. A. laidlawii A requires at least 13 amino acids (31), while M. arthritidis 07 needs 9 (41). M. gallinarum J grows in a medium supplied with 13 amino acids (23). However, dialyzed protein included in the latter three media could potentially supply some of the amino acid requirements.

The spiroplasmas include several species which have minimal requirements for amino acids. Rapid advances in the in vitro cultivation of spiroplasmas have occurred since the first isolate was cultivated in 1971. This progress was recently reviewed by Chang (6). The first defined medium (CC-494), formulated in 1982, allowed growth of three spiroplasmas (S. melliferum AS576, S. floricola 23-6, and S. apis SR3) when supplemented with the 20 common amino acids. This medium also contained bovine serum albumin as a carrier and detoxifier of free fatty acids. S. floricola and S. apis appeared to exhibit minimal requirements for amino acids, showing the ability to grow in CC-494 supplemented with each of 10 groups of combinations of the 20 amino acids. S. melliferum, in contrast, was able to grow in only 4 of the 10 combinations. Following systematic investigation, the essential amino acids were recognized as asparagine, cysteine, and glutamine, whereas the remaining 17 amino acids were nonessential. Whether S. melliferum can grow in medium devoid of bovine serum albumin or whether bovine serum albumin can serve as a source of nitrogen in this bacterium is not known. Success in ongoing searches for compounds to replace bovine serum

albumin as a carrier and detoxifier would be most helpful.

Anaeroplasma intermedium 5LA, placed in the same phylogenetic group as A. laidlawii (45), shows potential for development of a defined medium for assessing amino acid requirements, since it was demonstrated to grow, albeit slowly, in S-2 broth (28) which had been modified by substituting amino acids (exclusive of phenylalanine, tryptophan, and tyrosine) for peptones and reducing the concentrations of yeast extract and malt extract.

TRANSPORT OF AMINO ACIDS

In view of the limited capacity for amino acid biosynthesis in the mycoplasmas studied to date, one would predict a well-developed and efficient capability for amino acid transport. This expectation, however, has yet to be realized because of lack of data. Only two amino acid transport systems, L-histidine transport in M. fermentans and L-methionine transport in M. hominis, have been characterized to date (32). Both transport processes appear to meet the criteria for active transport. The transport of L-methionine by M. hominis was highly specific, not being affected by a number of amino acids. L-Histidine transport in M. fermentans is mediated by a transport system recognizing basic amino acids, since histidine transport was competitively inhibited by L-arginine and L-lysine. These results reveal properties that generally resemble those of the permease systems of other microorganisms.

Since free amino acids are generally required in the presence of peptides, proteolytic capability or transport of peptides may be minimal in mycoplasmas.

METABOLISM OF AMINO ACIDS

Catabolism

Microorganisms exhibit a variety of capabilities for conversion of one amino acid to another. Information on the role of catabolism in supplying amino acids for biosynthesis in mycoplasmas is minimal at present. *M. arthritidis* is able to catabolize a variety of amino acids, including arginine, glutamine, glutamic acid, aspartic acid, histidine, leucine, and threonine under aerobic conditions and tyrosine and tryptophan under anaerobic conditions (42). *M. mycoides* is able to degrade serine and threonine by dehydrases to yield the corresponding 2-keto acids (35). Whether the majority of these amino acids can be transformed via catabolic reaction sequences to other amino acids remains to be determined.

Two amino acids, glutamine and arginine, undergo catabolic reactions related to energy generation, and both generate amino acid products. Glutamine at pH 6 was demonstrated to undergo a phosphorolytic deamidation (requiring ADP, Mg^{2+}, and P_i) which forms glutamic acid, ATP, and NH_3 (42). By the arginine dehydrolase pathway, arginine is degraded by quantitative hydrolytic deimidation to citrulline (3, 40, 42) in a reaction catalyzed by arginine deiminase (EC 3.5.3.6). Citrulline then may undergo phosphorolysis by ornithine transcarbamylase to give ornithine and carbamyl phosphate. Cleavage of the carbamyl phosphate by carbamate kinase then yields ATP. Among the species screened (3), most of the nonfermentative organisms contained arginine deiminase activity, whereas only one fermentative species (*M. fermentans*) possessed the enzyme activity. The full significance of the production of ATP from glutamine or arginine is unclear. Whether the resultant amino acid product (glutamate or ornithine, respectively) has additional metabolic significance is unknown.

Ornithine can also be generated by degradation of arginine by arginase (EC 3.5.3.1), an enzyme activity found in 24 mycoplasma strains of veterinary interest (39). Glutamate may also be degraded to 2-ketoglutarate by oxidative deamination in *A. laidlawii* A (48) by glutamate dehydrogenase (EC 1.4.1.3), although the apparent absence of a tricarboxylic acid cycle in this organism (24, 37) raises questions about the fate of the 2-ketoglutarate product.

Biosynthesis

Transamination

Transaminations are ubiquitous in nature, essential to amino acid metabolism, and of importance in many other metabolic pathways. Although more than 60 aminotransferases are known (8), their presence in the mollicutes has sometimes been questioned. Electrophoretic analyses were used to provide evidence for aspartate aminotransferase (EC 2.6.1.1) in *A. laidlawii*

(22) and for both aspartate aminotransferase and alanine aminotransferase (EC 2.6.1.2) in mycoplasmas of veterinary interest (39). Another study, however, failed to detect an electrophoretic band for aspartate aminotransferase in 22 *Mycoplasma* and *Acholeplasma* species (26). Recently, enzyme activities identified as aspartate aminotransferase or alanine aminotransferase have been demonstrated in cell extracts of *Acholeplasma* (7, 24), *Mycoplasma* (7, 24), *Anaeroplasma* (28), and *Asteroleplasma* (28) species (Table 2). Aspartate aminotransferase appears to be more widely distributed among the mycoplasmas studied to date. However, this finding may simply reflect the relative activities of these enzymes, since alanine aminotransferase is generally present at low specific activity.

Aminotransferase functions in vivo are not easily identified solely from in vitro data because of broad substrate specificity; furthermore, aminotransferases seem to be highly variable from organism to organism in nature. Genetic data to establish gene-enzyme relationships are usually necessary to assign in vivo function. Apparently dissimilar conclusions in the identity of a particular aminotransferase can sometimes be due to pitfalls arising from overlapping activities of unknown aminotransferases in crude extracts or to the fact that only a limited number of arbitrarily selected substrates were examined. The intracellular roles of microbial aminotransferases and the overlap of these enzymes across different biochemical pathways have been reviewed elsewhere (15).

Table 2. Distribution of aspartate and alanine aminotransferase activities in mycoplasmas

Mycoplasma (reference)	Enzyme	
	Aspartate amino-transferase	Alanine amino-transferase
Acholeplasma laidlawii B-PG9 (24)	+	ND[a]
Acholeplasma laidlawii MG (7)	+	+
Acholeplasma morum S2 (24)	+	ND
Anaeroplasma intermedium 5LA (28)	+	ND
Asteroleplasma anaerobium 161[T] (28)	+	ND
Mycoplasma bovigenitalium PG11 (24)	+	ND
Mycoplasma capricolum 14 (24)	+	ND
Mycoplasma genitalium G-37 (24)	+	ND
Mycoplasma hominis PG21 (24)	+	ND
Mycoplasma hominis 1620 (24)	+	ND
Mycoplasma hyopneumoniae J (24)	+	ND
Mycoplasma pneumoniae FH (7, 24)	+	+
Mycoplasma salivarium VV (7)	+	+

[a] ND, not determined.

Do the aspartate and alanine aminotransferases present in the mollicutes function in vivo? All information to date is based on assumptions implied by nutritional studies. *A. laidlawii*, interestingly, is able to grow without supplementation of L-phenylalanine and L-tyrosine if L-alanine is included in the medium. No allosteric link of alanine and the aromatic amino acid pathway enzymes was detected by in vitro assay (4). Aminotransferases able to transaminate phenylpyruvate or 4-hydroxyphenylpyruvate were not studied; perhaps L-alanine is specifically required as the amino donor for aromatic aminotransferase function. Since two molecules of phosphoenolpyruvate (PEP) are needed for synthesis of each phenylalanine or tyrosine molecule, another possibility is that alanine boosts PEP production via transamination of alanine to pyruvate.

Anaeroplasma intermedium 5LA is also able to grow slowly in defined medium without aromatic amino acids (27). It is of considerable interest that *A. laidlawii* and *Anaeroplasma intermedium* have aspartate aminotransferase activity, since both of these mycoplasmas possess the key enzymes for tyrosine and phenylalanine biosynthesis. This aminotransferase could potentially function for aromatic amino acid biosynthesis in mycoplasmas, since aspartate aminotransferase and aromatic aminotransferase have been demonstrated to have overlapping substrate specificities in *Escherichia coli* (12) and *Pseudomonas aeruginosa* (46). Any one of three aminotransferases in *E. coli* (coded by *ilvE*, *tyrB*, or *aspC*) is able to transaminate phenylpyruvate to L-phenylalanine in vivo (12). In *P. aeruginosa*, any one of five aminotransferases that can transaminate aspartate is capable of transamination in vitro with any of the three keto acid intermediates of the aromatic amino acid pathway (46).

The generation of an alanine requirement by withholding pyridoxal, the interrelationship of alanine with tyrosine and phenylalanine requirements, and the potential linkage to glycolysis via pyruvate are suggestive of important in vivo functions for alanine aminotransferase. Aspartate aminotransferase may have an interpathway function if it plays a role in aromatic amino acid biosynthesis in *A. laidlawii* and *Anaeroplasma intermedium*. However, the existence of a separate aromatic aminotransferase cannot be ruled out, since to our knowledge no attempt to assay this enzyme activity in these species has been reported. Another possibility is that the apparent aspartate aminotransferase is in fact the aromatic aminotransferase in these mycoplasmas. The lack of evidence for a tricarboxylic acid cycle in *A. laidlawii* (24, 37) raises additional questions pertaining to in vivo capabilities of these aminotransferases.

Glutamate: glutamate dehydrogenase (EC 1.4.1.3)

Glutamate dehydrogenases catalyze the reductive amination of 2-ketoglutarate to glutamate and the oxidative deamination of glutamate. This enzyme, therefore, can function in either ammonia assimilation or glutamate catabolism. *A. laidlawii* A possesses a glutamate dehydrogenase with dual coenzyme specificity for NAD(H) and NADP(H) (48). The characteristic of dual coenzyme specificity may reflect phylogenetic relationships, since *Bacillus subtilis* (20, 21) possesses a glutamate dehydrogenase showing preference for NAD(H) but retaining some ability to use NADP(H). Interestingly, a number of dehydrogenases from the thermoacidophilic archaebacteria are noted for accepting both NAD⁺ and NADP⁺ (13). Otherwise, the *A. laidlawii* enzyme was typical of glutamate dehydrogenases from other microorganisms in that it was not inhibited by purine nucleotides (AMP, ADP, or ATP).

Fourteen mycoplasmas of animal origin contained activities that were identified as glutamate dehydrogenase following isoenzyme electrophoresis (39). The possibility of widespread distribution of glutamate dehydrogenase among the mycoplasmas is important because the enzyme in other microorganisms is pivotal in cellular metabolism by linking carbohydrate and nitrogen metabolism. Although the *A. laidlawii* enzyme has been known for several years, little information is available concerning its ability to synthesize or catabolize glutamate in vivo. The ability of the glutamate dehydrogenase to function biosynthetically seems unlikely because of the reputed absence of a tricarboxylic acid cycle in *A. laidlawii* (24, 37).

Tyrosine and phenylalanine

The enzymes. Prior to the report by Berry et al. (4) in 1987, demonstrating the aromatic amino acid biosynthetic pathway in *A. laidlawii*, no biosynthetic pathway for amino acids had been confirmed for the mycoplasmas. Nutritional studies (37, 42) had previously revealed that *A. laidlawii*, perhaps the least fastidious mycoplasma species, did not require L-phenylalanine and L-tyrosine for growth (provided that L-alanine was supplied), and ¹⁴C-labeled shikimic acid was incorporated into protein. A recent investigation of *Anaeroplasma* species (27) reports the activities of four aromatic amino acid pathway enzymes, augmenting the results for *A. laidlawii*. Enzymological analyses of cell extracts demonstrated that *A. laidlawii* Jgct, *Anaeroplasma intermedium* 5LA, and *Anaeroplasma varium* A-2T, which are all on the same phylogenetic branch (45), possess the key metabolic sequences necessary to synthesize L-phenylalanine and L-tyrosine from the initial precursors, erythrose 4-phosphate and PEP (Fig. 1). The activities of 3-deoxy-D-*arabino*-heptulosonate 7-phosphate (DAHP) synthase (EC 4.1.2.15) (the first enzyme of the pathway), dehydroshikimate reductase (EC 1.1.1.25) of the common trunk, and two postprephenate enzymes, prephenate dehydratase (EC 4.2.1.51) and prephenate dehydrogenase (EC 1.3.1.12), were present in all three mycoplasmas. The activities of 5-enolpyruvylshikimate 3-phosphate (EPSP) synthase (EC 2.5.1.19), chorismate mutase (EC 5.4.99.5), and arogenate dehydrogenase were also found in extracts of *A. laidlawii* but were not assayed in the *Anaeroplasma* species (27a).

With species outside the anaeroplasma group, Berry et al. (4) were unable to detect any of the aforementioned enzyme activities in extracts of either *M. iowae* or *M. gallinarum* assayed in parallel with those of *A. laidlawii*. Of interest in this context is the fact that *M. iowae* and *M. gallinarum* are small-genome mycoplasmas, in contrast to *A. laidlawii*, *Anaeroplasma intermedium*, and *Anaeroplasma varium*.

The pathway for biosynthesis of aromatic amino acids shown in Fig. 1 exhibits considerable diversity

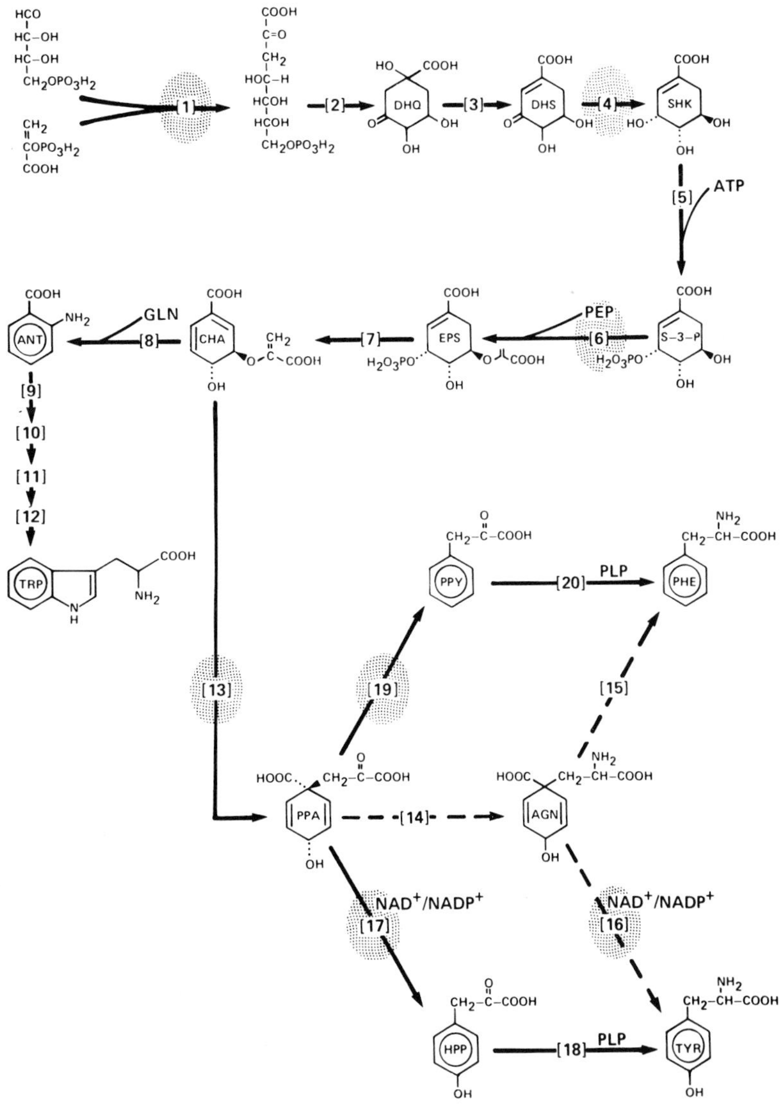

Figure 1. Outline of the divergent, multibranched pathway of aromatic amino acid biosynthesis identified in mycoplasmas. Shading highlights the enzyme activities found in *Acholeplasma* and *Anaeroplasma* species. Enzymes [1] to [7] catalyze steps within the common shikimate branch; enzyme [13] catalyzes the single reaction of the midbranch; enzymes [8] to [12] and [14] to [20] catalyze terminal branchlet reactions culminating with L-tryptophan (TRP), L-phenylalanine (PHE), or L-tyrosine (TYR) synthesis. Only some organisms possess the entire array of dual branches to phenylalanine and tyrosine, i.e., enzymes [14] to [20]. The dotted arrows show the arogenate branches for phenylalanine and tyrosine biosynthesis. Enzymes [16] and [17] may be NAD linked, NADP linked, or both, depending on the organism. The pathway begins (upper left) with the condensation of erythrose 4-phosphate and PEP to form DAHP. Other abbreviations: DHQ, dehydroquinate; DHS, dehydroshikimate; SHK, shikimate; S-3-P, shikimate 3-phosphate; EPS, 5-enolpyruvylshikimate 3-phosphate; CHA, chorismate; GLN, glutamine; ANT, anthranilate; PPA, prephenate; AGN, L-arogenate; PPY, phenylpyruvate; HPP, 4-hydroxyphenylpyruvate; PLP, pyridoxal 5'-phosphate. Enzymes: [1], DAHP synthase; [2], dehydroquinate synthase; [3], dehydroquinase; [4], dehydroshikimate reductase; [5], shikimate kinase; [6], EPSP synthase; [7], chorismate synthase; [8], anthranilate synthase; [9], anthranilate phosphoribosylpyrophosphate transferase; [10], phosphoribosyl-anthranilate isomerase; [11], indoleglycerol phosphate synthase; [12], tryptophan synthase; [13], chorismate mutase; [14], prephenate aminotransferase; [15], arogenate dehydratase; [16], arogenate dehydrogenase; [17], prephenate dehydrogenase; [18], 4-hydroxyphenylpyruvate aminotransferase; [19], prephenate dehydratase; and [20], phenylpyruvate aminotransferase.

in nature with respect to the following character state features: alternative enzymatic steps which may be used for L-phenylalanine or L-tyrosine synthesis, specificity of tyrosine pathway dehydrogenases for NAD[+] or NADP[+], allosteric specificities, presence or absence of regulatory isozymes, presence or absence of multi-

functional proteins, and genetic organization of pathway genes (1, 5, 17). The data emerging from just two studies of aromatic amino acid pathway enzymes in the mycoplasmas promise to enrich the documentation of microbial diversity for aromatic biosynthesis.

Pathway arrangement and substrate specificity. Although the existence of DAHP synthase activity was substantiated in *A. laidlawii* and *Anaeroplasma* species, neither study attempted to determine the existence of DAHP synthase isozymes, commonly found in gram-negative bacteria. The dehydroshikimate reductase (shikimate dehydrogenase) and EPSP synthase of *A. laidlawii* exhibited some typical properties of eubacterial enzymes. Thus, dehydroshikimate reductase accepted only NADPH as a coenzyme substrate, and the EPSP synthase was sensitive to inhibition by the broad-spectrum herbicide glyphosate. In *Anaeroplasma intermedium* and *Anaeroplasma varium*, however, the dehydroshikimate reductase exhibited a unique character state by utilizing NADH but not NADPH. To our knowledge, these are the only examples in the literature of NADH-specific dehydroshikimate reductases.

Prephenate dehydratase, but not arogenate dehydratase, was found in *A. laidlawii*, indicating that phenylalanine synthesis occurs solely via the phenylpyruvate route (i.e., through the actions of prephenate dehydratase and phenylpyruvate aminotransferase).

The prephenate dehydrogenase activity present in *A. laidlawii* accepted both NADH and NADPH as coenzyme substrates, although NADH was preferred. This enzyme is probably a cyclohexadienyl-type dehydrogenase that is able to recognize L-arogenate as an alternative, less-preferred substrate when NADH is present. The abilities of the NADH-specific prephenate dehydrogenases of *Anaeroplasma intermedium* and *Anaeroplasma varium* to use arogenate as a substrate were not tested (27a).

Allosteric control. The allosteric control of enzymes of aromatic biosynthesis in *A. laidlawii* and *Anaeroplasma intermedium* is shown in Table 3.

(i) DAHP synthase. DAHP synthase enzymes in nature are feedback inhibited by aromatic amino acids or by the mid-pathway intermediate chorismate or prephenate. The diversity of allosteric control patterns makes this enzyme an important reference for delineation of evolutionary relationships within a defined genealogy. The DAHP synthase activity of *A. laidlawii* was inhibited by L-tyrosine and activated by L-tryptophan. Neither combinations of aromatic amino acids

(to detect synergistic effects) nor chorismate and prephenate were effective inhibitors. This pattern of allosteric control has no precedent in the literature. In *Anaeroplasma intermedium*, DAHP synthase was also activated by L-tryptophan but was not inhibited by L-tyrosine. The potential allostery of prephenate, chorismate, and L-phenylalanine was not determined with the *Anaeroplasma intermedium* enzyme (27a). Two isozymes may exist, one activated by tryptophan and the other inhibited by tyrosine. In *Anaeroplasma intermedium*, the tyrosine-sensitive isozyme may have been lost (or may be labile). However, because the extent of inhibition of enzyme activity by L-tyrosine was either incomplete or absent in extracts of *A. laidlawii* or *Anaeroplasma intermedium*, the residual uninhibited activity could be due to the presence of a second, allosterically insensitive isozyme similar to the DS-O isozyme in superfamily B of the purple bacteria (2).

(ii) Chorismate mutase. Chorismate mutase from *A. laidlawii* was not subject to allosteric control by any of the aromatic amino acids or by L-arogenate. The enzyme was, however, subject to partial product inhibition by prephenate.

(iii) Prephenate and arogenate dehydrogenase. The activities of the tyrosine biosynthetic dehydrogenases from *A. laidlawii* and *Anaeroplasma intermedium* were subject to feedback inhibition by L-tyrosine. The NADH-linked prephenate dehydrogenase of *A. laidlawii* was inhibited by 85% by L-tyrosine. The NADH-linked arogenate dehydrogenase in this strain was completely inhibited by L-tyrosine. This finding probably reflects the existence of a single cyclohexadienyl dehydrogenase, competitively inhibited by tyrosine and exhibiting a lower K_m for prephenate than for L-arogenate. The prephenate dehydrogenase (NADH) from *Anaeroplasma intermedium* was completely inhibited by L-tyrosine.

(iv) Prephenate dehydratase. L-Phenylalanine was a strong feedback inhibitor of prephenate dehydratase activities in both *A. laidlawii* and *Anaeroplasma intermedium*. With the *A. laidlawii* enzyme, other aromatic end products and the group of nonaromatic metabolites known to affect prephenate dehydratase in *B. subtilis* (33) also proved to be effective modulators

Table 3. Allosteric control of aromatic pathway enzyme activities demonstrated in extracts of *A. laidlawii* Jgct and *Anaeroplasma intermedium* 5LA

Acholeplasma laidlawii Jgct		Anaeroplasma intermedium 5LA	
Enzyme[a]	Effector[b]	Enzyme	Effector
[1] DAHP synthase	Tyr (−), Trp (+)	[1] DAHP synthase	Trp (+)
[4] Dehydroshikimate reductase (NADP+)	ND[c]	[2] Dehydroshikimate reductase (NAD+)	ND
[6] EPSP synthase	ND		
[13] Chorismate mutase	PPA (−)		
[16] Arogenate dehydrogenase (NAD+)	Tyr (−)		
[17] Prephenate dehydrogenase (NAD+/NADP+)	Tyr (−)	[17] Prephenate dehydrogenase (NAD+)	Tyr (−)
[19] Prephenate dehydratase	Phe (−), Tyr (+), Trp (+), Val (+), Ile (+), Met (+)	[19] Prephenate dehydratase	Phe (−)

[a] Enzyme numbers correspond to those depicted in Fig. 1. Coenzyme substrates are given in parentheses.
[b] Abbreviations: Tyr, L-tyrosine; Trp, L-tryptophan; PPA, prephenate; Phe, L-phenylalanine; Val, L-valine; Ile, L-isoleucine; Met, L-methionine.
[c] ND, none determined.

of enzyme activity. Both L-tyrosine and L-tryptophan stimulated enzyme activity and appeared to antagonize the inhibitory effect of L-phenylalanine. The nonaromatic hydrophobic amino acids, L-valine and L-isoleucine, stimulated prephenate dehydratase activity, while L-leucine had no effect. L-Methionine activated the *A. laidlawii* prephenate dehydratase the most, reaching a peak of 62% at an L-methionine concentration of 1.0 mM. With the prephenate dehydratase from *Anaeroplasma intermedium*, however, L-methionine showed no ability to stimulate enzyme activity. Whether the latter enzyme is preferentially modulated by one of the other known effectors, a frequent finding, is not known, since potential allostery of L-tyrosine, L-tryptophan, L-leucine, L-isoleucine, and L-valine was not investigated (27a).

Evolutionary relationships. Mycoplasmas are part of an evolutionary branch of the low-G+C gram-positive eubacterial (*Bacillus-Lactobacillus-Clostridium-Streptococcus*) line of descent, as determined by oligonucleotide cataloging of 16S rRNA (11, 47), 5S rRNA sequencing (38), and comparative enzyme-immunological studies (25). The *Acholeplasma* and *Anaeroplasma* species are reported to be close phylogenetic relatives belonging to one of five primary groups within the class *Mollicutes* (45). The apparent ability to synthesize aromatic amino acids and the presence of several key metabolic activities in common distinguish acholeplasmas and anaeroplasmas from other mollicutes.

The character state of the prephenate dehydratase of *A. laidlawii* is potentially significant, since it exhibits the allosteric properties termed metabolic interlock, which was originally described in *B. subtilis* (14) as one of several examples of interpathway regulation. Prephenate dehydratase activity from *A. laidlawii* was feedback inhibited by L-phenylalanine and either positively or negatively modulated by remote effectors (L-tryptophan, L-tyrosine, L-valine, L-isoleucine, and L-methionine), as is the enzyme of *B. subtilis* (14, 29, 33, 34). Since the mycoplasmas are believed to have branched off from the gram-positive eubacterial lineage at a deep phylogenetic position, regulation of prephenate dehydratase is probably characteristic of the ancestral enzyme of the entire gram-positive lineage. This conclusion is supported by the discovery that the gram-positive coryneforms (10) represent another major assemblage that has interlock-type prephenate dehydratases. An extreme halophile (16), interestingly, also possesses an interlock type of prephenate dehydratase.

Although the regulation of prephenate dehydratase by remote effectors seems to be a character state that is conserved at a very deep hierarchical level in the gram-positive lineage of eubacteria, the pattern of allosteric control for DAHP synthase in this phylogenetic group is conserved at much shallower hierarchical levels. Thus, in DAHP synthase regulatory mechanisms, (i) feedback inhibition of the *B. subtilis* enzyme by chorismate and prephenate operates through a mechanism of sequential feedback inhibition (18), (ii) feedback inhibition of the enzyme of clostridial species is mediated solely by L-phenylalanine (19), and (iii) synergistic control of the enzyme from coryneform bacteria is accomplished by the combination of L-tyrosine and L-phenylalanine (9). It remains to be determined

whether *A. laidlawii* and *Anaeroplasma intermedium* share two isozymes (as discussed earlier) or whether evolutionary divergence has occurred at this level with respect to DAHP synthase.

SUMMARY AND OUTLOOK

Enzyme activities of the aromatic amino acid biosynthetic pathway have been found and characterized in *Acholeplasma* and *Anaeroplasma* species, demonstrating the likelihood that L-tyrosine and L-phenylalanine are synthesized in these mycoplasmas. These findings correlate with nutritional studies which have shown that these mycoplasmas are able to grow in defined media not requiring supplementation by these aromatic amino acids. Among other mycoplasmas for which defined media have been developed, certain species of *Spiroplasma* (e.g., *S. melliferum*) reveal substantial potential for biosynthesis of amino acids. The contributions of amino acid transport, catabolic sequences, and transaminative conversions to the supply of amino acids for general metabolism are largely unknown at present. Rigorous investigation, employing enzymological and molecular biological techniques, may reveal additional genes of amino acid metabolism which are cryptic or otherwise poorly expressed because of genetic or physiological constraints. Techniques such as the polymerase chain reaction (PCR) offer great potential for further elucidation of amino acid pathways in the mycoplasmas. With PCR, the ability to amplify genomic DNA for sequencing (by using degenerate primers derived from known sequences of amino acid pathway genes from phylogenetically related organisms) will circumvent many of the pitfalls inherent to the microbiology of mycoplasmas.

The ability to analyze genes without primary selection for function will be less complicated than the molecular biological approaches of a few years ago. For example, aromatic amino acid pathway genes of *A. laidlawii*, cloned and characterized following PCR amplification, may be used to probe DNA libraries of small-genome mycoplasmas to answer questions concerning genome reduction in the mycoplasmas. The fact that the *A. laidlawii* genome is roughly twice the size of the smallest mycoplasma genomes (30) suggests that the inability to detect activities of the aromatic biosynthetic pathway in *M. iowae* and *M. gallinarum* may reflect the loss of a portion of the original ancestral mycoplasma genome.

Acknowledgment. This chapter is Florida Agricultural Experiment Station Journal Series no. N-00613.

REFERENCES

1. **Ahmad, S., and R. A. Jensen.** 1988. New prospects for deducing the evolutionary history of metabolic pathways in prokaryotes: aromatic biosynthesis as a case-in-point. *Origins Life* **18**:41–57.
2. **Ahmad, S., B. Rightmire, and R. A. Jensen.** 1986. Evolution of the regulatory isozymes of 3-deoxy-D-*arabino*-heptulosonate 7-phosphate synthase present in the *Escherichia coli* genealogy. *J. Bacteriol.* **165**:146–154.

3. **Barile, M. F., R. T. Schimke, and D. B. Biggs.** 1966. Presence of the arginine dihydrolase pathway in *Mycoplasma. J. Bacteriol.* **91:**189–192.

4. **Berry, A., S. Ahmad, A. Liss, and R. A. Jensen.** 1987. Enzymological features of aromatic amino acid biosynthesis reflect the phylogeny of mycoplasmas. *J. Gen. Microbiol.* **133:**2147–2154.

5. **Byng, G. S., J. F. Kane, and R. A. Jensen.** 1982. Diversity in the routing and regulation of complex biochemical pathways as indicators of microbial relatedness. *Crit. Rev. Microbiol.* **9:**227–252.

6. **Chang, C. J.** 1989. Nutrition and cultivation of spiroplasmas, p. 201–241. *In* R. F. Whitcomb and J. G. Tully (ed.), *The Mycoplasmas,* vol. 5. *Spiroplasmas, Acholeplasmas, and Mycoplasmas of Plants and Arthropods.* Academic Press, Inc., San Diego, Calif.

7. **Constantopoulos, G., and G. J. McGarrity.** 1989. Activities of aspartate and alanine aminotransferases in the Mollicutes *A. laidlawii* MG, *M. pneumoniae* FH, and *M. salivarium* VV. *Curr. Microbiol.* **19:**213–216.

8. **Cooper, A. J. L., and A. Meister.** 1985. Metabolic significance of transamination, p. 534–563. *In* P. Christen and D. E. Metzler (ed.), *Transaminases.* John Wiley & Sons, New York.

9. **Fazel, A. M., J. R. Bowen, and R. A. Jensen.** 1980. Arogenate (pretyrosine) is an obligatory intermediate of L-tyrosine biosynthesis: confirmation in a microbial mutant. *Proc. Natl. Acad. Sci. USA* **77:**1270–1273.

10. **Fazel, A. M., and R. A. Jensen.** 1980. Regulation of prephenate dehydratase in coryneform species of bacteria by L-phenylalanine and by remote effectors. *Arch. Biochem. Biophys.* **200:**165–176.

11. **Fox, G. E., E. Stackebrandt, R. B. Hespell, J. Gibson, J. Maniloff, T. A. Dyer, R. S. Wolfe, W. E. Balch, R. S. Tanner, L. J. Magrum, L. B. Zablen, R. Blakemore, R. Gupta, L. Bonen, B. J. Lewis, D. A. Stahl, K. R. Luehrsen, K. N. Chen, and C. R. Woese.** 1980. The phylogeny of prokaryotes. *Science* **209:**457–463.

12. **Gelfand, D. H., and R. A. Steinberg.** 1977. *Escherichia coli* mutants deficient in the aspartate and aromatic amino acid aminotransferases. *J. Bacteriol.* **130:**429–440.

13. **Hough, D. W., and M. J. Danson.** 1989. Archaebacteria: ancient organisms with commercial potential. *Lett. Appl. Microbiol.* **9:**33–39.

14. **Jensen, R. A.** 1969. Metabolic interlock. Regulatory interactions exerted between biochemical pathways. *J. Biol. Chem.* **244:**2816–2823.

15. **Jensen, R. A., and D. H. Calhoun.** 1981. Intracellular roles of microbial aminotransferases: overlap enzymes across different biochemical pathways. *Crit. Rev. Microbiol.* **8:**229–261.

16. **Jensen, R. A., T. A. d'Amato, and L. I. Hochstein.** 1988. An extreme-halophile archaebacterium possesses the interlock type of prephenate dehydratase characteristic of the Gram-positive eubacteria. *Arch. Microbiol.* **148:**365–371.

17. **Jensen, R. A., and R. S. Fischer.** 1987. The post-prephenate biochemical pathways to phenylalanine and tyrosine. *Methods Enzymol.* **142:**472–478.

18. **Jensen, R. A., and E. W. Nester.** 1965. The regulatory significance of intermediary metabolites: control of aromatic acid biosynthesis by feedback inhibition in *Bacillus subtilis. J. Mol. Biol.* **12:**468–481.

19. **Jensen, R. A., and R. Twarog.** 1972. Allostery of 3-deoxy-D-*arabino*-heptulosonate 7-phosphate synthetase in *Clostridium:* another conserved generic characteristic. *J. Bacteriol.* **111:**641–648.

20. **Kane, J. F., J. Wakim, and R. S. Fischer.** 1981. Regulation of glutamate dehydrogenase in *Bacillus subtilis. J. Bacteriol.* **148:**1002–1005.

21. **Kimura, K., A. Miyakawa, T. Imai, and T. Sasakawa.** 1977. Glutamate dehydrogenase from *Bacillus subtilis* PCI219. I. Purification and properties. *J. Biochem.* **81:**467–476.

22. **Lanham, S. M., R. M. Lemcke, C. M. Scott, and J. M. Grendon.** 1980. Isoenzymes in two species of *Acholeplasma. J. Gen. Microbiol.* **117:**19–31.

23. **Lund, P. G., and M. S. Shorb.** 1966. Growth of *Mycoplasma gallinarum* strain J without serum. *Proc. Soc. Exp. Biol. Med.* **121:**1070–1075.

24. **Manolukas, J. T., M. F. Barile, D. K. F. Chandler, and J. D. Pollack.** 1988. Presence of anaplerotic reactions and transamination, and the absence of the tricarboxylic acid cycle in mollicutes. *J. Gen. Microbiol.* **134:**791–800.

25. **Neimark, H., and J. London.** 1982. Origins of the mycoplasmas: sterol-nonrequiring mycoplasmas evolved from streptococci. *J. Bacteriol.* **150:**1259–1265.

26. **O'Brien, S. J., J. M. Simpson, M. W. Grabowski, and M. F. Barile.** 1981. Analysis of multiple isoenzyme expression among twenty-two species of *Mycoplasma* and *Acholeplasma. J. Bacteriol.* **146:**222–232.

27. **Petzel, J. P., and P. A. Hartman.** 1991. Aromatic amino acid biosynthesis and carbohydrate catabolism in strictly anaerobic mollicutes (*Anaeroplasma* spp.). *Syst. Appl. Microbiol.* **13:**240–247.

27a.**Petzel, J. P., and P. A. Hartman.** Personal communication.

28. **Petzel, J. P., M. C. McElwain, D. DeSantis, J. Manolukas, M. V. Williams, P. A. Hartman, M. J. Allison, and J. D. Pollack.** 1989. Enzymic activities of carbohydrate, purine, and pyrimidine metabolism in the *Anaeroplasmataceae* (class *Mollicutes*). *Arch. Microbiol.* **152:**309–316.

29. **Pierson, D. L., and R. A. Jensen.** 1974. Metabolic interlock: control of an interconvertible prephenate dehydratase by hydrophobic amino acids in *Bacillus subtilis. J. Mol. Biol.* **90:**563–579.

30. **Razin, S.** 1989. Molecular approach to mycoplasma phylogeny, p. 33–69. *In* R. F. Whitcomb and J. G. Tully (ed.), *The Mycoplasmas,* vol. 5. *Spiroplasmas, Acholeplasmas, and Mycoplasmas of Plants and Arthropods.* Academic Press, Inc., San Diego, Calif.

31. **Razin, S., and A. Cohen.** 1963. Nutritional requirements and metabolism of *Mycoplasma laidlawii. J. Gen. Microbiol.* **30:**141–154.

32. **Razin, S., L. Gottfried, and S. Rottem.** 1968. Amino acid transport in *Mycoplasma. J. Bacteriol.* **95:**1685–1691.

33. **Rebello, J. L., and R. A. Jensen.** 1970. Metabolic interlock. The multi-metabolite control of prephenate dehydratase activity in *Bacillus subtilis. J. Biol. Chem.* **245:**3738–3744.

34. **Riepl, R. G., and G. I. Glover.** 1979. Regulation and state of aggregation of *Bacillus subtilis* prephenate dehydratase in the presence of allosteric effectors. *J. Biol. Chem.* **254:**10321–10328.

35. **Rodwell, A. W.** 1960. Nutrition and metabolism of *Mycoplasma mycoides* var. *mycoides. Ann. N.Y. Acad. Sci.* **79:**499–507.

36. **Rodwell, A. W.** 1969. A defined medium for mycoplasma strain Y. *J. Gen. Microbiol.* **58:**39–47.

37. **Rodwell, A. W., and A. Mitchell.** 1979. Nutrition, growth, and reproduction, p. 103–139. *In* M. F. Barile and S. Razin (ed.), *The Mycoplasmas,* vol. 1. *Cell Biology.* Academic Press, Inc., New York.

38. **Rogers, M. J., J. Simmons, R. T. Walker, W. G. Weisburg, C. R. Woese, R. S. Tanner, I. M. Robinson, D. A. Stahl, G. Olsen, R. H. Leach, and J. Maniloff.** 1985. Construction of the mycoplasma evolutionary tree from 5S rRNA sequence data. *Proc. Natl. Acad. Sci. USA* **82:**1160–1164.

39. **Salih, M. M., H. Erno, and V. Simonsen.** 1983. Electrophoretic analysis of isoenzymes of mycoplasma species. *Acta Vet. Scand.* **24:**14–33.

40. **Schimke, R. T., and M. F. Barile.** 1963. Arginine metabolism in pleuropneumonia-like organisms isolated from mammalian cell culture. *J. Bacteriol.* **86:**195–206.

41. **Smith, P. F.** 1955. Synthetic media for pleuropneumonia-like organisms. *Proc. Soc. Exp. Biol. Med.* **88:**628–631.

42. **Smith, P. F.** 1971. Dynamics of reproduction and growth, p. 99–161. *In* P. F. Smith (ed.), *The Biology of Mycoplasmas.* Academic Press, Inc., New York.

43. **Smith, P. F., T. A. Langworthy, and M. R. Smith.** 1975. Polypeptide nature of growth requirement in yeast extract for *Thermoplasma acidophilum. J. Bacteriol.* **124:**884–892.

44. **Tourtellotte, M. E., H. J. Morowitz, and P. Kasimer.** 1964. Defined medium for *Mycoplasma laidlawii. J. Bacteriol.* **88:**11–15.

45. **Weisburg, W. G., J. G. Tully, D. L. Rose, J. P. Petzel, H. Oyaizu, D. Yang, L. Mandelco, J. Sechrest, T. G. Lawrence, J. Van Etten, J. Maniloff, and C. R. Woese.** 1989. A phylogenetic analysis of the mycoplasmas: basis for their classification. *J. Bacteriol.* **171:**6455–6467.

46. **Whitaker, R. J., C. G. Gaines, and R. A. Jensen.** 1982. A multispecific quintet of aromatic aminotransferases that overlap different biochemical pathways in *Pseudomonas aeruginosa. J. Biol. Chem.* **257:**13550–13556.

47. **Woese, C. R., J. Maniloff, and L. B. Zablen.** 1980. Phylogenetic analysis of the mycoplasmas. *Proc. Natl. Acad. Sci. USA* **77:**494–498.

48. **Yarrison, G., D. W. Young, and G. L. Choules.** 1972. Glutamate dehydrogenase from *Mycoplasma laidlawii. J. Bacteriol.* **110:**494–503.

13. Sources of Nucleotides

LLOYD R. FINCH and ALANA MITCHELL

OVERVIEW

Chemical Forms of Purines and Pyrimidines in the Cell

Normally, purines and pyrimidines are present intracellularly almost entirely as nucleotides, i.e., linked through an N-glycosylic bond to phosphorylated derivatives of either ribose or deoxyribose. Most of this nucleotide material is present in acid-precipitable polymeric form as RNA or DNA. Razin et al. (59) have

reported contents of RNA ranging from 8 to 17%, of DNA ranging from 4 to 7%, and of protein ranging from 54 to 63% (dry weight) for eight mollicute strains. In general, these values do not vary much from those for most bacteria. Very approximately for mollicutes, they imply total net requirements of 280, 220, 170, 170, and 120 μmol per g of protein per generation for the bases adenine, guanine, cytosine, uracil, and thymine, respectively. Even for the most rapidly growing mollicutes, these values correspond to rates not much above 1 to 3 μmol/min per g of protein.

Among the acid-soluble components are the nucleo-

Lloyd R. Finch • Department of Biochemistry, University of Melbourne, Parkville, Victoria, Australia, 3052. **Alana Mitchell** • Baker Institute of Medical Research, Prahran, Australia, 3181.

side 5'-monophosphates, 5'-diphosphates, and 5'-triphosphates (NMP, NDP, and NTP, respectively), coenzymes with nucleotide moieties (e.g., NDP sugars and pyridine nucleotides), and regulatory nucleotides. Table 1 presents some data on concentrations, or evidence for the existence, of these nucleotides in *Mycoplasma mycoides*.

Functions and Turnover of NTP

NTPs are the immediate precursors of nucleic acids and the nucleotide coenzymes. Synthesis of stable nucleic acids, i.e., DNA, rRNA, and tRNA, as major components of the cell generates the greatest net demand for nucleotides. However, high turnovers resulting from the use of nucleotides for incorporation into mRNA and as coenzymes or substrates in other reactions also create a strong demand for the regeneration of NTPs. The latter uses include involvement as NDP sugars and pyridine nucleotides, and particularly the use of ATP and GTP as free energy sources for many reactions. NMPs and NDPs are the major products from these reactions leading to NTP turnover.

Phosphorylation of Nucleotides

As well as arising from NTP turnover, NMPs are the immediate products of nucleotide synthesis by salvage pathways and in many cases de novo pathways. Formation of the metabolically important NTPs, the major components of the free nucleotide pool, requires successive phosphorylations from NMP to NDP to NTP. These reactions are catalyzed by nucleotide kinases. NMP kinase activity has been detected for AMP,

GMP, CMP, UMP, and dTMP in mollicutes. In other organisms, e.g., enterobacteria (44), the specificity of the kinases for the first three of these nucleotides includes the corresponding dNMP, whereas UMP and dTMP have separate kinases. The preferred phosphate donor for all of these kinases is Mg-ATP.

AMP kinase has been reported as ubiquitous in members of the order *Mycoplasmatales* (47). It has been assayed in *M. mycoides* subsp. *mycoides* and *Ureaplasma urealyticum* (6) and partly fractionated from extracts of the latter (7). There are no reports of dAMP kinase in mollicutes, although its presence may be inferred in *M. mycoides* from the observed in vivo phosphorylation of [^{32}P]dAMP to labeled dADP and dATP (42). GMP kinase has also been studied in *M. mycoides* (32), but no data on its activity with dGMP are available. With respect to CMP kinase, competition studies on extracts of *M. mycoides* (41) indicate that the enzyme from this organism also has dCMP kinase activity. Neale (38) (see Table 4) has reported that the V_{max} value is higher (30 versus 15 µmol/min per g of protein) and the K_m value is lower (70 versus 94 µM) for dCMP than for CMP, suggesting greater specificity for the former nucleotide as a substrate. No evidence was found for competition from UMP despite the observation that extracts of *M. mycoides* show UMP kinase activity ($K_m = 60 \pm 10$ µM) with a V_{max} approximately 13-fold greater (31) than that for the CMP/dCMP kinase. Among the other mollicutes tested for dCMP kinase, *Acholeplasma laidlawii* (76) clearly showed activity, whereas levels were low or not detected in extracts of several *Spiroplasma* strains (50) and *Asteroleplasma anaerobium* (48).

Thymidylate (dTMP) kinase is the most broadly studied of the NMP kinases. The activity in 100,000 × g supernatants from *M. mycoides* was 13 µmol/min per

Table 1. Intracellular amounts of some nucleotides and PRPP in *M. mycoides* subsp. *mycoides*[a]

Compound	Amt (µmol/g of protein)[d] in cells grown in medium[e]:			RNA composition[b]		DNA composition[c]	
	A	B	C	Nucleotide	Amt (mol%)	Nucleotide	Amt (mol%)
ATP	4.3	5.2		AMP	27.6	dAMP	38
GTP	2.7	2.4		GMP	26.8	dGMP	12
UTP	3.8	2.6		UMP	26.1	dTMP	38
CTP	1.2	1.2		CMP	19.3	dCMP	12
ADP	1.6	1.2					
GDP	0.7	0.4					
dATP	0.105						
dGTP	0.04						
dTTP	0.125						
dCTP	0.07						
cAMP[f]			0.005–0.015				
PRPP[g]			0.5–1.0				

[a] From references 29, 38, and 40.
[b] From reference 29.
[c] From reference 38.
[d] Protein content in *M. mycoides* cells is approximately 60% (dry weight) (29).
[e] Log-phase cultures in minimal medium with guanine as purine (A), minimal medium with guanine plus adenine as purines (B) or PPLO broth (C).
[f] Early to mid-log phase to late log phase (9a).
[g] From reference 29.

g of protein, with a K_m of 12 μM for dTMP (38, 41) and inhibition by dTTP. Activity in 250,000 × g supernatants from extracts of several other mollicutes (24, 48, 76) was somewhat lower (<1 μmol/min per g of protein) and very low (0.01 μmol/min per g of protein) in some *Spiroplasma* strains (50). Current knowledge of metabolism indicates that dTMP kinase may be essential for an organism containing thymidine in its DNA. Therefore, we presume that the low values observed for spiroplasmas are indicative of possession of the enzyme. On this basis, the similar values observed for dCMP kinase activity in spiroplasma extracts would probably also indicate possession of that enzyme. No dUMP kinase activity was detectable (41) from *M. mycoides* or from *A. laidlawii* B-PG8 (76), the only other mollicutes tested.

The products of kinase activity on the NMPs are the corresponding NDPs. Conversion of these to NTPs is catalyzed by an NDP kinase able to transfer the γ-phosphate from any NTP to any NDP. The activity of NDP kinase in cells is generally observed to be higher than that of the NMP kinases, so there is rapid equilibration of the NDP/NTP ratios determined by the ADP/ATP ratio within the cell. When assayed, NDP kinase has been observed at significant levels in mollicutes (7, 31, 41, 76).

Nutritional Sources of Nucleotides or Nucleotide Precursors

Mycoplasmas are usually found living parasitically in host tissues, where presumably they can scavenge a steady supply of preformed precursors. A variety of media have been found to support the growth of several species of mollicutes, though only rarely has the minimal requirement for precursors of nucleotides been determined. It has been suggested that the growth-promoting activity of yeast extract may in part be ascribed to its high content of nucleic acids and nucleic acid precursors (26).

DNA is also added to some media, since early studies suggested that it served as a complete source of nucleotide requirements for *A. laidlawii*. Optimum provision of nucleic acid precursors for *A. laidlawii* B and A and *M. mycoides* subsp. *capri* came from a balanced supply of RNA and DNA (55, 60) rather than from their component bases or nucleosides. Oligonucleotides were also effective. Later study showed that the requirement for DNA precursors was met by thymidine, but RNA remained the best source of the other requirements. The simplest requirements defined for nucleic acid precursors are guanine, uracil, and thymine for *M. mycoides* subsp. *mycoides* (62). For the closely related *M. capricolum*, adenine is also required (62). A partly defined medium for *A. laidlawii* PG8 and PG9 includes adenosine, guanosine, and cytidine but no uridine or thymidine (62). The latter, however, was required if folinic acid (N^5-formyltetrahydrofolate) was omitted from the medium (63). As precursors of the pyridine nucleotides, the defined media noted above contain nicotinic acid. However, a medium for *M. synoviae* requires NADH (11).

The nutritional requirements of the mollicutes indicate that they lack most capacities for de novo synthesis of nucleotides from the simplest precursors but must possess a range of enzyme activities and transport functions to facilitate the use of the more complex derivatives required.

PRPP

Physiological Function

The capability of mycoplasmas to use bases for efficient synthesis of ribonucleotides by salvage pathways is predicated on their possession of phosphoribosyltransferase activities and hence 5-phosphoribosyl-1-diphosphate (abbreviated PRPP from its former name, 5-phosphoribosyl-1-pyrophosphate). Depending on the organism, PRPP has various functions in the biosynthesis of histidine, tryptophan, and nicotinamide coenzymes in addition to purine and pyrimidine nucleotides. Synthesis of the first two of these products is probably unlikely in mollicutes, but provision of the others nonetheless imposes a major demand for PRPP.

Biosynthesis and Pools

The enzyme PRPP synthetase catalyzes the formation of PRPP from ATP and ribose 5-phosphate, yielding AMP as the second product. In the direction of PRPP synthesis, the equilibrium constant is 29 (44). The synthetases from *Escherichia coli* and *Salmonella typhimurium* have been purified to homogeneity and studied in detail. The two enzymes are similar in amino acid composition and subunit molecular mass (of 31 kDa). Free magnesium ion is required for activity in addition to that required to chelate ATP as substrate, and P_i also plays an activating role. Only ADP of many nucleotides tested seems to be a candidate for a physiological inhibitor of PRPP synthetase. It is an allosteric inhibitor, the effectiveness of which is influenced by the concentration of ribose 5-phosphate. The presence of a similar PRPP synthetase in mollicutes has not been established by enzymatic studies. However, Chen and Finch (5a) have identified a sequence in DNA from *M. gallisepticum* containing an open reading frame showing similarity in amino acid sequence to a region of the PRPP synthetases of the rat, *E. coli*, and *Bacillus subtilis* (46).

Intracellular contents of PRPP have been determined in bacteria and to a limited extent in *M. mycoides* subsp. *mycoides* (10, 29). In *E. coli*, there is a close correlation between the PRPP concentration and growth rate (1). Starvation for carbon, nitrogen, or phosphate resulted in rapid depletion of the pool. Rapid and marked changes are to be expected in a pool of small size (Table 1), which is subject to the very high rates of influx and efflux necessary to support the requirements of a major pathway such as nucleotide and nucleic acid synthesis. Changes in media and incubation conditions were observed to lead to rapid changes in the PRPP pool of *M. mycoides* (29). The most marked of these was an almost total depletion (98%) of the pool upon addition of adenine to cultures growing with guanine as the sole purine source (10).

PURINES

The existence of a defined growth medium for *M. mycoides* subsp. *mycoides* (62) has caused it to be the mollicute strain with the most-studied and best-characterized systems for nucleotide biosynthesis. Considering nucleotide metabolism, the medium has glucose as a potential source of nucleotide pentose plus a purine base (guanine) and two pyrimidine bases (uracil and thymine) as the minimal requirements. Folate, or folinic acid, is not required for growth and does not remove the guanine requirement if provided. This characteristic makes it unlikely that the organisms can effect purine biosynthesis de novo.

This conclusion has been substantiated in experiments to determine the fractions of the individual RNA ribonucleotides (30) or DNA deoxyribonucleotides (40) derived from an added ^{14}C-labeled precursor. Labeling with ^{32}P$_i$ was used to quantitate the amount of nucleotide isolated from the nucleic acid; thus, the ^{14}C/^{32}P ratio defined the fraction of isolated nucleotide derived from the ^{14}C-labeled precursor. The effect of competition from unlabeled precursors was also examined. Results showed that *M. mycoides* (30) derives all of its purine ribonucleotides in RNA from guanine when this is the only purine present and derives its guanine nucleotide from guanine and adenine nucleotide from adenine when both purine precursors are present. Hypoxanthine could provide about 50% of the adenine nucleotide in competition with guanine but none in competition with adenine. Purine nucleosides added to overnight cultures were equivalent to their corresponding bases, suggesting that they were rapidly broken down by *M. mycoides*. This rapid breakdown to free base was observed with early-log-phase cultures (30). From these studies, together with the assay and kinetic examination of enzymatic activities in extracts (32, 41) (Table 2), it has been possible to outline pathways of purine nucleotide biosynthesis for

M. mycoides (Fig. 1) which are similar to those proposed by Pollack et al. (51, 70, 71) for *A. laidlawii*. The extensive studies of Pollack and coworkers suggest these pathways apply, with variations, to mollicutes generally.

Purine Ribonucleotide Biosynthesis from Bases

Purine ribonucleotide biosynthesis from bases would in most circumstances be dependent on the activity of phosphoribosyltransferases utilizing PRPP as the phosphoribosyl donor. These activities for the bases adenine, guanine, and hypoxanthine (23, 32, 48, 50, 70, 71) have been detected generally in mollicutes. An absence of hypoxanthine or guanine phosphoribosyltransferase activity from extracts of *U. urealyticum* has been reported (24). However, activity with hypoxanthine (guanine was not tested) has been observed in fresh extracts but not in fractionated extracts of this organism (7). Since the phosphoribosyltransferase activities observed are usually high, they will probably continue to meet rates of cellular nucleic acid synthesis even when substrate concentrations are less than saturating. This ability also gives them a capacity and a requirement to be effectively regulated. The use of bases to synthesize ribonucleotides via the initial formation of nucleosides seems unlikely in most mollicutes, as discussed below.

Guanine, hypoxanthine, and xanthine

Some organisms, e.g., *E. coli* and *S. typhimurium* (44), have two phosphoribosyltransferases, each able to utilize 6-oxopurine substrates. One has greater efficiency for hypoxanthine; the other has greater efficiency for guanine. Whether mollicutes also possess two such enzymes has not been established. For *M. mycoides*, the two activities cofractionated in ammo-

Table 2. Enzymes of purine nucleotide biosynthesis in *M. mycoides*[a]

Enzyme	Substrate	K_m (μM[b])	V_{max}[c] (μmol/min/g of protein)	Negative effectors
Guanine phosphoribosyltransferase	Guanine	1.3	200	GMP, GTP, IMP
	PRPP	11		
GMP kinase	GMP	30	150	
	ATP	5 mM		
GMP reductase	GMP	10	3	IMP, AMP, (ATP)[d]
	NADPH	<10		
Adenylosuccinate synthetase	IMP	45	1.5	
	GTP	30		
Hypoxanthine phosphoribosyltransferase	Hypoxanthine	80	250	GMP, GTP, IMP
	PRPP	66		
Adenine phosphoribosyltransferase	Adenine	<0.5	200	GMP, AMP, ATP
	PRPP	~5		
Purine nucleoside phosphorylase	Adenosine	ND[e]	730	ND
	Inosine	ND	415	ND
Purine nucleoside kinase	Deoxyadenosine	ND	4	ND
	Adenosine	ND	3	ND

[a] From reference 10.
[b] Except as noted.
[c] From cultures grown on PPLO broth.
[d] Inhibition by MgATP only observed with GMP below 10 μM.
[e] ND, not determined.

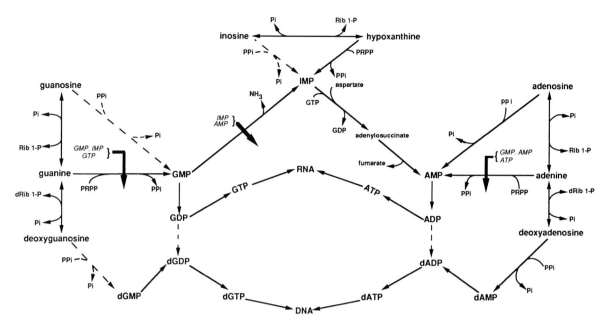

Figure 1. Pathways of purine salvage and interconversion. Reactions indicated by broken arrows have not been detected in *M. mycoides* subsp. *mycoides*, but some have been observed in other mollicutes. Heavy arrows parallel to the reaction pathway indicate activation by the effector(s) shown in italics, and those across the reaction pathway indicate inhibition. Rib 1-P, ribose 1-phosphate; dRib 1-P, deoxyribose 1-phosphate.

nium sulfate precipitation and eluted in a single peak in Sephadex G-100 chromatography, consistent with, but not proving, the existence of both activities in a single protein. The extracts for these studies were obtained from cells grown on PPLO broth; however, the ratio of activity with hypoxanthine to activity with guanine varied with growth in different media over a range from 1.3 for PPLO broth to 4.0 for minimal medium with adenine and guanine as defined purine sources (32). As shown in Table 2, the K_m for guanine is much lower than that for hypoxanthine and the K_m for PRPP is significantly lower with guanine as the base. Strong inhibitory effects, increasing at lower PRPP concentrations, were observed with GMP, IMP, and GTP but not adenine or pyrimidine nucleotides. These observations were made for activities in extracts from cells grown in PPLO broth. A possibility remains that a phosphoribosyltransferase with preference for hypoxanthine is coded for by *M. mycoides* but is not strongly expressed during growth in PPLO broth.

Adenine

The adenine phosphoribosyltransferase of *M. mycoides* shows complex kinetics by comparison with the *E. coli* enzyme, which shows simple Michaelis-Menten kinetics (67). The *M. mycoides* enzyme has a sigmoidal response to PRPP concentration, accentuated with an increase in concentrations of adenine and the nucleotide inhibitors. At high concentrations of PRPP (>40 μM), the enzyme shows Michaelis-Menten kinetics for adenine, with a K_m (Table 2) of 300 nM (K_m for the *E. coli* enzyme is 1.3 μM, and it has weaker responses to inhibitors), but adenine becomes inhibitory at concentrations in the nanomolar range when PRPP is low (67). An effect of inhibitory nucleotides in promoting

an increased sigmoidality in response to PRPP concentration is accentuated when the adenine concentration increases. The most effective inhibitor is GMP, followed by AMP and ATP. GTP inhibits at pH 7.8 and above but activates at pH 7.1. The pyrimidine nucleotides all activate strongly at pH 7.1, and CMP and UMP also activate at pH 7.8.

Interconversions of Purine Ribonucleotides

The use of guanine as a sole source of purines, as in *M. mycoides*, would involve an initial step to form GMP by the action of guanine (hypoxanthine) phosphoribosyltransferase. GMP kinase and NDP kinase would then provide GDP (for reduction to the deoxyribonucleotide) and GTP (for metabolic reactions and an energy source in protein synthesis and for RNA synthesis). Production of the adenine nucleotides can occur through the reduction of GMP to IMP for conversion to AMP via the action of adenylosuccinate synthetase and adenylosuccinate lyase. AMP kinase and NDP kinase would then provide the necessary ADP and ATP. Similarly, IMP produced from hypoxanthine by the action of hypoxanthine (guanine) phosphoribosyltransferase could be converted to AMP. Pathways for the formation of guanine nucleotide from other purine ribonucleotides have not been demonstrated in mollicutes. Assays for IMP dehydrogenase, GMP synthetase, AMP deaminase, and adenosine deaminase (70, 71) have failed to detect any significant levels of activity, implying a generalized requirement of mollicutes for a source of preformed guanine.

GMP reductase

GMP reductase has been observed in *M. mycoides* (32), all *Acholeplasma* species tested, and *Spiroplasma floricola* but not in *M. gallisepticum* or *M. arginini* (70, 71). Lack of reductase implies that guanine cannot act as a sole purine source for the latter two strains. GMP reductase of *M. mycoides* (Table 2) is inhibited by IMP and AMP and has low V_{max}, or specific activity, and low K_m values for both GMP and NADPH. Inhibition by IMP and AMP is stronger at lower concentrations of GMP, and ATP may also inhibit strongly at low GMP concentrations. These properties will tend to ensure that an adequate, but not excessive, production of intermediates for ATP synthesis can be maintained with only low GMP concentrations and that the production can be turned off if the levels of intermediates build up. Compared with GMP reductase, GMP kinase (Table 2) has a very high V_{max} and a somewhat high (30 μM) K_m for GMP and very high K_m (5 mM) for ATP. It will always be less saturated by GMP than is the reductase but will readily respond to increases in ATP concentration to divert GMP away from reduction when ATP is high. Degradation to guanosine and P_i is another possible pathway (32), but this route is strongly inhibited by P_i.

Adenylosuccinase synthetase and adenylosuccinate lyase

Adenylosuccinase synthetase and adenylosuccinate lyase activities have been observed in extracts from *M. mycoides*, *M. gallisepticum*, *M. arginini*, *A. laidlawii*, *A. axanthum*, and *A. granulosum* but not *A. florum* or *S. floricola* (32, 70, 71). The absence of these activities implies that the latter two species are unable to use hypoxanthine or guanine as a source of adenine nucleotides. The adenylosuccinate synthetase of *M. mycoides* has a quite low K_m for GTP but a rather high K_m for IMP (Table 2). Its V_{max} in extracts from cultures grown on PPLO broth is low, which may suggest regulation of the enzyme level in response to the availability of preformed adenine precursors in this medium.

Purine Nucleotide Biosynthesis from Nucleosides

The studies of Mitchell and Finch (30) noted above showed purine ribonucleosides to be equivalent to bases in their incorporation into RNA in overnight cultures of *M. mycoides*. This finding was accounted for by rapid purine nucleoside phosphorylase activity to convert the nucleoside to the free base for use by the appropriate phosphoribosyltransferase. However, direct synthesis of purine nucleotides from purine nucleosides is made possible in some mollicutes by a novel PP_i-dependent purine nucleoside kinase activity discovered by Tryon and Pollack (70). The only ATP-dependent purine nucleoside kinase activity found in any mollicute is a strong ATP-dependent phosphorylation of deoxyguanosine observed for all spiroplasmas tested (50) except *S. floricola*.

Purine nucleoside phosphorylase

Phosphorolysis of adenosine, guanosine, inosine, deoxyadenosine, deoxyguanosine, and deoxyinosine and the reverse reaction to form the nucleosides have been observed in extracts from most mollicutes that have been studied (14, 23, 24, 32, 48, 50, 70, 71). In an earlier report (14), adenosine phosphorylase was reported as common but probably not universal to members of the *Mycoplasmatales*, and its detection in mammalian cell cultures was suggested as the basis for a test for mycoplasmal contamination in such cultures. In enterobacteria, these activities are usually properties of a single purine nucleoside phosphorylase (44). Competition studies indicated that a single purine nucleoside phosphorylase was involved for catalysis of the reaction with the three purine ribonucleosides by extracts of *M. mycoides* (32). With the general occurrence of adenine or hypoxanthine-guanine phosphoribosyltransferases in mollicutes, the phosphorolysis activities will make bases from the nucleosides available for synthesis of the corresponding ribonucleotides. The other product is ribose 1-phosphate (or deoxyribose 1-phosphate), which could react with other bases to form the corresponding nucleosides or more generally be catabolized via isomerization to the 5-phosphate (6).

The reverse reaction to form the nucleoside from the base and ribose 1-phosphate or deoxyribose 1-phosphate could provide a pathway to the corresponding NMPs (23). This would be possible only in mollicutes that possess the appropriate nucleoside kinase activity and a ready source of pentose phosphate. Such a pathway seems unlikely to be a significant contributor of purine ribonucleotides or a sole pathway to purine deoxyribonucleotides. The limitation in both cases appears to be the effective maintenance of an adequate source of pentose phosphate. Its provision through phosphorolysis of other nucleosides from the medium could be of limited duration, since phosphorylase activities are usually orders of magnitude greater than rates of cellular nucleic acid synthesis. This is the situation noted earlier with respect to purine nucleosides in overnight cultures of *M. mycoides*. Phosphorolysis of nucleosides produced continuously in vivo would provide a more sustained source of pentose phosphate. Such effects could account for the capacity of exogenous [U-^{14}C]cytidine to contribute a small amount of deoxyribose to the dAMP and dGMP in DNA of *M. mycoides* (40).

Nucleoside kinases

PP_i-dependent purine nucleoside kinase activities have been observed with adenosine, guanosine, inosine, deoxyadenosine, and guanosine in extracts from *A. laidlawii* (70), all spiroplasmas tested except possibly *S. floricola* (50), *Anaeroplasma intermedium*, and some strains of *M. hominis* (24). Activity with some of these nucleosides was found with *A. axanthum* and *A. granulosum* (71), *A. morum* (23), *Asteroleplasma anaerobium* (48), and *M. mycoides* (10, 38). *U. urealyticum* and seven other mycoplasma strains tested lacked activity (23, 24, 71). As noted above, the ATP-dependent deoxyguanosine kinase appears to be unique to the spiroplasmas among the mollicutes.

Regulation of Purine Ribonucleotide Biosynthesis

The regulation of purine ribonucleotide biosynthesis in mollicutes has been addressed only in relation to *M. mycoides* (10). Measurement was made of the intracellular concentrations of ribonucleotides and their changes in *M. mycoides* growing in defined media under various conditions. These results were used with the data on kinetic properties and allosteric effectors of the participating enzymes to suggest mechanisms for regulation of the pathways. The measurements followed the time course for the variation in intracellular contents of ATP, GTP, CTP, UTP, ADP, and GDP from the period 10 min before and up to 30 min after the addition of further purine precursors to cultures growing with guanine or guanine plus adenine as the defined purine source(s). The effect of addition of hypoxanthine or inosine to cultures growing on guanine as the sole purine source was to increase the level of all of the nucleotides at least temporarily. The increases appeared more rapid with inosine than with hypoxanthine. An explanation of these effects was that the formation of IMP from hypoxanthine or inosine provided an alternative source of this substrate for AMP synthesis and also served to spare some GMP from reduction and allow increased ATP and GTP content. Increased GTP would activate uracil phosphoribosyltransferase (31) (Table 3), leading to increased UTP content. The increase in UTP and ATP as substrates and GTP as an activator of CTP synthetase (31) (Table 3) would lead to some increase in CTP content.

With the addition of adenine or adenosine to a culture with guanine as the sole purine source, the levels of ATP and GTP rose much more than when hypoxanthine or inosine was added. With the addition of adenine, UTP initially dropped by about 60% and then rose to about 80% of its original level, the rise being coincident with the increase in GTP, the activator of uracil phosphoribosyltransferase. UTP did not change greatly with addition of adenosine, and CTP was not strongly affected by either addition. Again, the rises in nucleotides appeared to be achieved more quickly with addition of the nucleoside rather than the corresponding base. Cultures grown overnight with both guanine and adenine as purine sources were very similar in nucleotide contents to those grown with guanine only. Addition of adenosine to these cultures caused an immediate rise in ATP and UTP but not GTP.

Another aspect investigated was the effect of the additions on PRPP content. Hypoxanthine, inosine, and adenosine caused only small changes to the PRPP content in cultures grown with guanine as the sole purine source, with decreases of up to 20% over the first 5 to

10 min. Adenine, however, caused a decrease of 98 to 99% (to below 4 μM) within 2 min, with only a slight rise to about 8 μM over the subsequent 18 min.

The results were discussed in relation to the kinetic and regulatory parameters (listed in Table 2) for the enzymes involved. The guanine phosphoribosyltransferase activity with low K_m values for guanine and PRPP has a high specific activity by comparison with a total required rate of 1.5 to 3 μmol/min per g of protein for incorporation of purines to produce nucleic acids for growth of cells in the guanine-only defined medium. The strong feedback inhibition from guanine nucleotides and IMP should effectively regulate this activity, particularly when PRPP levels decrease upon addition of adenine. Once GMP is formed, its utilization would be balanced between reduction for adenine nucleotide synthesis and phosphorylation for GTP synthesis by the characteristics of GMP reductase and GMP kinase as noted above. With hypoxanthine added to the medium, the need for GMP reduction to IMP for adenylate nucleotide synthesis would be spared by the IMP produced from 5-phosphoribosylation of hypoxanthine. If both guanine and hypoxanthine are acted on by the one phosphoribosyltransferase, this phosphoribosylation of hypoxanthine could well be restricted by competition from guanine when both bases are present at similar concentrations, a suggestion which could account for the observation that hypoxanthine provided only about 50% of the adenine nucleotide in competition with guanine.

Competition at the 5-phosphoribosyltransferase step would not occur with the addition of adenine to the guanine-only medium, and so the levels of ATP and GTP would both rise more strongly. These rises would be limited by feedback inhibition and by the great decrease in PRPP concentration down to 2 to 4 μM, the range within which higher adenine concentrations become strongly inhibitory to adenine phosphoribosyltransferase. It is also well below the K_m values for PRPP of 11, 66, and 50 μM for the guanine, hypoxanthine, and uracil phosphoribosyltransferases, respectively. The lower degree of saturation of the uracil phosphoribosyltransferase would account for the immediate drop in UTP content, while the increased activation of the enzyme by higher levels of GTP would contribute to the subsequent partial restoration of the original level.

Table 3. Enzymes of pyrimidine nucleotide biosynthesis in *M. mycoides*[a]

Enzyme	Substrate	K_m (μM)	V_{max} (μmol/min/g of protein)	Effectors
Uracil phosphoribosyltransferase[b]	Uracil	2.6	120	UMP(−), UDP(−)
	PRPP	51		UTP(−), GTP(+)
Uridine phosphorylase	Uridine	2,160	860	
	P_i	2,000		
Uridine/cytidine kinase	Uridine	ND[c]	12.5	CTP(−), UTP(−)
	Cytidine	ND	6.5	CTP(−), UTP(−)
UMP kinase	UMP	60	200	
	ATP	530		
CTP synthetase	UTP	ND	2.5	CTP(−), GTP(+)
CMP kinase	CMP	94 ± 27	15 ± 1.6	
	ATP	ND		

[a] From reference 31.
[b] Assayed in the presence of 1 mM GTP.
[c] ND, not determined.

As well as decreasing the saturation of these phosphoribosyltransferases, the decrease in PRPP concentration would increase their sensitivity to feedback inhibitors. These effects, together with the high K_m of adenylosuccinate synthetase for IMP, would act toward the complete exclusion of hypoxanthine from adenine nucleotide formation when adenine is available. Similarly, GMP synthesis would be partially restricted, but the greater saturation of the GMP kinase by ATP would allow flowthrough to GTP to be maintained at lower GMP concentrations, affording some relaxation of feedback inhibition on the guanine phosphoribosyltransferase. GMP reduction would be inhibited by the stronger action of feedback inhibition at low GMP concentrations. For AMP synthesis, feedback inhibition from increased concentrations of the adenine and guanine nucleotides would be potentiated by sensitization of adenine phosphoribosyltransferase to them by high adenine as well as low PRPP levels. In the studies of nucleotide levels in *M. mycoides* cultures, the addition of nucleosides had effects slightly different from those of the corresponding bases. Some of these differences could have been related to an elevation or a maintenance of the initial PRPP level, but most are best interpreted as resulting from the action of PP$_i$-dependent purine nucleoside kinase in *M. mycoides*. Longer-term effects of purine nucleosides, such as those observed with overnight cultures, probably result from their conversion to the corresponding bases by purine nucleoside phosphorylase.

Experiments measuring nucleotide levels in cells immediately before and after supply of additional purine precursors to the cultures showed immediate changes interpreted in terms of the properties of the enzymes concerned and the levels of related metabolites. After overnight growth, however, the nucleotide contents in cells from a culture in guanine-plus-adenine minimal medium were similar to those in a guanine-only culture. Longer-term regulation of enzyme activity was suggested by the specific activities for GMP kinase and GMP reductase measured under the different growth conditions. These values were 145 and 3.7 μmol/min per g of protein, respectively, from cells grown in a medium with guanine plus adenine, whereas they were 90 and 7.6 μmol/min per g of protein from cells grown with guanine as the sole purine source (32).

PYRIMIDINES

Among mollicutes, the simplest requirement for precursors to supply all pyrimidine ribonucleotides appears to be that defined for *M. mycoides* subsp. *mycoides*, namely, uracil alone. This conclusion is based on the minimal growth requirements of the organism (62) and was substantiated by determination of the specific activities of pyrimidine nucleotides isolated from the RNA of cultures labeled with [^{14}C]uracil and ^{32}P$_i$ (30) as described above. Uracil provided all of the cytidine and uridine nucleotides, confirming the absence of any contribution from de novo synthesis of pyrimidine nucleotides. The utilization of uracil involves conversion to UMP by action of uracil phosphoribosyltransferase as the first step. The next steps are phosphorylations catalyzed by UMP kinase and NDP

kinase to give UDP and UTP, respectively, followed by amination of UTP to CTP catalyzed by CTP synthetase. Cytidine, but not cytosine, can also serve as a source of pyrimidine ribonucleotides in *M. mycoides*. This utilization involves phosphorylation (by uridine-cytidine kinase) to produce cytidine ribonucleotides and limited deamination in some form to produce precursors for uridine ribonucleotides. For *A. laidlawii*, cytosine is effective as a pyrimidine source (19, 55), presumably through initial action of cytosine deaminase, since cytosine can be metabolized only through deamination to uracil (44). The overall data for *M. mycoides* (30) suggested pathways as outlined in Fig. 2. Observations of enzymatic activities in *M. mycoides* (31), summarized in Table 3, support these suggestions.

Pyrimidine Ribonucleotide Biosynthesis from Uracil

Utilization of uracil in *E. coli* under normal conditions depends on uracil phosphoribosyltransferase (43). The enzyme from *E. coli* is activated by GTP and inhibited by uridine nucleotides (35) and ppGpp (44). This activity was first reported for a number of mollicutes by Long et al. (20) and subsequently found in all mollicutes tested (7, 20, 27, 31). It has been the subject of more detailed studies in *M. mycoides* (31). The enzyme was activated three- to sixfold by saturating concentrations (>0.5 mM) of GTP, depending on the PRPP concentration, and was inhibited by uridine nucleotides (Table 3), most strongly by UMP.

With 1 mM GTP, the reaction rate followed Michaelis-Menten kinetics with respect to PRPP concentration (K_m = 51 μM) but sigmoidal kinetics in the absence of GTP. Inhibition by uridine nucleotides appeared to be competitive with respect to PRPP. The high potential level of activity allows for strong down-regulation (Table 3) while still adequately meeting the pyrimidine ribonucleotide requirements of the cell. Some evidence for the action of these regulatory effects was noted above in the discussion of purine nucleotide biosynthesis. The enzyme from *A. laidlawii* has also been studied in detail (27), showing K_m values (66 μM for PRPP and 4.2 μM for uracil) similar to those of the enzyme from *M. mycoides*. The effect of GTP on the *A. laidlawii* enzyme was not reported.

A second possible route for incorporation of uracil into nucleotides is via the sequential actions of uridine phosphorylase and uridine kinase. As discussed later, this pathway may be of minor significance in *M. mycoides* as it is in enterobacteria, in which it is operative only if uracil and ribose 1-phosphate are available in high concentrations (44). The sequential phosphorylations catalyzed by UMP kinase and NDP kinase would complete the formation of UTP. The ability of uracil to serve as the precursor of cytidine nucleotides depends on the CTP synthetase catalysis of the amination of UTP with the amido group from glutamine in a reaction energized by ATP (44). The enzyme, which requires GTP as a positive effector, has been demonstrated in cell extracts of *M. mycoides* (31). The formation of cytidine nucleotides by the extracts required UTP, glutamine, magnesium ions, ATP, and GTP.

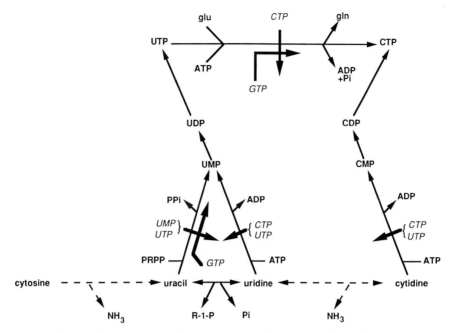

Figure 2. Pathways of pyrimidine salvage and interconversion. Reactions indicated by broken arrows have not been detected in *M. mycoides* subsp. *mycoides*, but some have been observed in other mollicutes. Heavy arrows parallel to the reaction pathway indicate activation by the effector(s) shown in italics, and those across the reaction pathway indicate inhibition. R-1-P, ribose 1-phosphate.

Pyrimidine Ribonucleotide Biosynthesis from Nucleosides

Mollicutes have a capacity for incorporation of pyrimidine nucleosides provided in the growth medium, although this is not a universal characteristic. Of eight *Mycoplasmatales* species tested (26), all but the arginine-utilizing species, *M. hominis* and *M. arginini*, were able to incorporate both cytidine and uridine. For *M. mycoides*, a study of the fraction of individual RNA nucleotides derived from ^{14}C-labeled nucleosides in the presence of uracil revealed that the relative levels of incorporation of uracil and uridine by overnight cultures are proportional to the relative concentrations in the medium (30). Competition between cytidine and uracil is more complex, with cytidine virtually excluding uracil from cytidine nucleotide while supplying approximately 20% of the uridine nucleotide. In cultures of *M. mycoides*, some of the radioactivity lost from [^{14}C]cytidine appears as uridine and uracil in the growth medium and the remainder accumulates intracellularly in nucleic acids. Cytidine will substitute for uracil to support the growth of *M. mycoides* (79) in C4 minimal medium (62).

Two possible routes exist for the conversion of uridine to UMP. One is via phosphoribosyl transfer after uracil has been released by the action of uridine phosphorylase. The second is via direct phosphorylation by uridine kinase. The data on relative uptake of uracil and uridine in overnight cultures suggested that the nucleoside is incorporated as uracil, and studies of uridine metabolism in early- to mid-log-phase cultures showed that 90 µM uridine was 80 to 90% degraded to uracil within 60 min. This degradation was catalyzed by a very active uridine phosphorylase (V_{max} = 860

µmol/min per g of protein) of high K_m (2 mM). Uridine phosphorylase prepared from *A. laidlawii* (28) had lower K_m values (uridine, 170 µM; P_i, 120 µM). For the reverse, potentially anabolic reaction, K_m values were 110 µM for uracil and 17 µM for ribose 1-phosphate. The K_m of the uridine kinase for uridine was 3.2 µM. Taking account of the relative activities and kinetic constants of the enzymes involved, and the intracellular concentrations of the relevant substrates, the authors concluded that uridine phosphorylase would have only a catabolic role and that the utilization of uracil would occur via uracil phosphoribosyltransferase (28).

Uridine phosphorylase appears to be present in all mollicutes (13, 23, 25, 27, 31) except spiroplasmas (23, 25, 50). It could play a role in making ribose 1-phosphate available for other purposes, e.g., catabolism or reaction with other bases, as noted for purine nucleoside phosphorylase. Decreased incorporation of [^{3}H]uridine into RNA in cultured mammalian cells contaminated with mycoplasmas has been attributed to the uridine phosphorylase activity of the mycoplasmas. Uncontaminated cell lines do not incorporate [^{3}H]uracil appreciably, but it is rapidly incorporated with contaminated cells, presumably because of the uracil phosphoribosyltransferase activity of the mycoplasma cells. From these observations (65), measurement of the ratio of uracil incorporation to uridine incorporation was developed as a measure of mycoplasmal contamination of cultured cells. Such methods have been reviewed elsewhere (64).

Uridine-cytidine kinase, which phosphorylates uridine and cytidine, has been detected in dialyzed cell extracts of *M. mycoides* (31) and *A. laidlawii* (28). Both reports comment on the instability of the kinase and the difficulties of its assay in the presence of high levels of uridine phosphorylase activity. It is perhaps not surprising that there appear to be no other reports of this activity in mycoplasmas, although its presence may be anticipated from the effective use of pyrimidine nucleosides and bases by many of these organisms. In *M. mycoides*, the specific activity with uridine was twice that with cytidine as a substrate (Table 3). Whereas in *E. coli* the preferred phosphate donor is GTP with either nucleoside, cytidine kinase of *M. mycoides* used only ATP, and uridine kinase showed a marked preference for ATP over GTP.

Analogy with other procaryotes suggests two potential routes for incorporation of cytidine in mollicutes. As for uridine, cytidine may be directly phosphorylated to NMP by uridine-cytidine kinase. Alternatively, activity of cytidine deaminase may enable cytidine to be made available as uridine or ultimately uracil. It is probable that both alternatives exist within the mollicutes. Cytidine deaminase, which in other procaryotes also catalyzes deamination of deoxycytidine (43, 44), has been detected in a number of mycoplasmas, *U. urealyticum*, and *Anaeroplasma intermedium* (77). Extracts from only three of nine members of the family *Spiroplasmataceae* catalyzed deamination of cytidine to uridine (50). *Asteroleplasma anaerobium* was also deficient in this enzyme (48). Surprisingly, no deamination of cytidine was detectable in extracts of *M. mycoides* (31), despite strong evidence for its occurrence from the pattern of labeling of RNA when cells were grown on medium containing [^{14}C]cytidine and from the capacity of cytidine to act as a sole source of pyrimidines (79).

Regulation of Pyrimidine Nucleotide Biosynthesis

The kinetic parameters, K_m and V_{max}, and regulatory effectors have been determined for several enzymes of pyrimidine metabolism in *M. mycoides* (31). These data (Table 3), although subject to some limitations because assays were on dialyzed unfractionated cell extracts and therefore competing reactions may have influenced the substrate concentrations of the enzymes under investigation, provide insight into possible mechanisms for regulation of the supply of pyrimidine nucleotides. The effectiveness of the postulated mechanisms was tested by measurement of the changes occurring to the intracellular contents of the major ribonucleotides in response to the addition to cultures of potential precursors of pyrimidine nucleotides (31).

Steady-state cultures growing on uracil with guanine or guanine plus adenine presumably meet their pyrimidine nucleotide requirements at balanced rates determined by the combination of effects of PRPP, GTP, and uridine nucleotides acting on uracil phosphoribosyltransferase and of UTP, ATP, GTP, and CTP acting on CTP synthetase. When such cultures were supplemented with uridine or cytidine, the ribonucleotide contents of the cells were altered rapidly and markedly. Uridine caused an immediate, though transitory, doubling in the level of UTP, presumably due to the provision of a second pathway via uridine kinase, since there was no change in the PRPP level (29). GTP also increased briefly. The rapid rise in UTP

would impose feedback inhibition on both uridine kinase and uracil phosphoribosyltransferase, whereas the elevation in GTP would activate the latter enzyme, tending to augment the rise in UTP concentration. The subsequent fall in GTP and decreased availability of uridine would then tend to limit the rate of UMP production, requiring that there be a lower concentration of the feedback inhibitor, UTP, to allow the supply of uridine nucleotides to be maintained at an adequate rate. In this uridine-supplemented growth condition, the CTP concentration also increases as a predictable consequence of elevation in the concentrations of both the NTP substrates (UTP and ATP) and the activator (GTP) of CTP synthetase. Regulation of CTP back to the original level would occur through inhibition of the enzyme by its product, CTP.

Cytidine caused dramatic increases in the concentrations of both CTP and UTP, but to various extents in the presence or absence of adenine. In the former situation, the large sustained increase in both pyrimidine NTPs, particularly CTP, may reflect the greater capacity of these cultures to support additional phosphorylations. With the addition of cytidine, a pathway for direct synthesis of cytidine nucleotides independently of UTP is enlisted via cytidine kinase. Feedback inhibition by CTP of its synthesis from UTP and activation of uracil phosphoribosyltransferase by GTP would both contribute to the rise in UTP concentration. Any conversion of cytidine to uridine would make available an additional pathway for UTP synthesis via uridine kinase. Since the concentrations of both CTP and UTP rise markedly, it is likely that the concentration of CTP required to inhibit CTP synthetase is appreciably less than that needed to inhibit cytidine kinase.

The rate of pyrimidine ribonucleotide biosynthesis from uracil, or uracil plus uridine, appears to be determined by the activities of uracil phosphoribosyltransferase and CTP synthetase. With cytidine supplementing uracil, regulation of cytidine kinase may also be important.

DEOXYRIBONUCLEOTIDES

Various components have been included in growth media for mycoplasmas as precursors of deoxyribonucleotides and therefore DNA. However, as noted above, it is not always clear whether the requirements described are minimal or merely effective in supporting growth. Such components include DNA itself, oligonucleotides, thymidine, and thymine. Whereas thymine is a sufficient requirement for *M. mycoides*, not replaceable by folinic acid, *A. laidlawii* has been reported to require thymidine in addition to adenosine, guanosine, and cytidine unless folinic acid is also present, in which case thymidine is unnecessary (55). For *A. laidlawii* B, both uridine and thymidine were reported to be absolute requirements for growth, with thymine failing to support growth when substituted for thymidine (68). In a third strain of *A. laidlawii*, LA-1, guanine, thymine, and either uracil or cytosine were sufficient as precursors of nucleic acids (19). In the latter two publications, there was no report of the effect of folinic acid, which appears to enable the folate-dependent conversion of dUMP to dTMP by dTMP synthase in *A. laidlawii*. McIvor and Kenny reported that addition of other deoxyribonucleosides greatly increased incorporation of [³H]thymine into the DNA of *A. laidlawii* (26). This increase would be consistent with the need for a source of deoxyribose for the utilization of thymine.

Such a source might be endogenous, allowing thymine to be used without deoxyribonucleosides in the medium, or exogenous from added deoxyribonucleosides. In general, the base or nucleoside component of thymidylate must be provided intact, indicating a probable lack of dTMP synthase for the conversion of dUMP to thymidylate among the mollicutes. An exception is *A. laidlawii*, which was shown to be extremely sensitive to the drugs methotrexate and trimethoprim in comparison with *M. gallisepticum*, despite the similarity in properties of the dihydrofolate reductases from the two organisms (22). A suggested explanation for the different sensitivities was that *M. gallisepticum* might be impaired in transport of the drugs. Another possibility is that *A. laidlawii* generates dihydrofolate to a greater extent through dTMP synthase activity and therefore requires greater dihydrofolate reductase activity to maintain tetrahydrofolate for growth.

Formation of Deoxyribonucleotides and Deoxyribose 1-Phosphate

Formation of deoxyribonucleotides can occur most simply by phosphorylation of the corresponding deoxyribonucleosides when these deoxyribonucleosides are available. If not present in the medium, the necessary deoxyribonucleosides might be formed by the action of phosphorylases on the corresponding bases and deoxyribose 1-phosphate, provided that a source of the latter is available. An alternative to the direct phosphorylation pathway is provided by reduction of ribonucleotides.

Phosphorylation of Deoxyribonucleosides

The direct phosphorylation of deoxyribonucleosides potentially provides one avenue for the generation of deoxyribonucleotides by mycoplasmas. Deoxyribonucleoside kinases have been detected in several members of the mollicutes. Kinetic properties of the enzymes from *M. mycoides* (38) are listed in Table 4. All organisms tested had thymidine kinase activity (24, 48, 50, 77), and most had deoxycytidine kinase activity. Only the anaerobic organisms *Anaeroplasma intermedium* and *Asteroleplasma anaerobium* are reported to lack the latter kinase activity (48).

For the phosphorylation of purine deoxyribonucleosides, the novel PP$_i$-dependent purine nucleoside kinase (70) noted above is active with deoxyribonucleosides as well as ribonucleosides. An ATP-dependent deoxyguanosine kinase has been observed for most spiroplasmas examined (50). Except for thymidine kinase, the deoxyribonucleoside kinases would probably function as the major agent for nucleotide synthesis only if deoxyribonucleosides were available in the medium. For thymidine and the purine nucleosides, but not for deoxycytidine, the competing reactions catalyzed by the corresponding nucleoside phosphorylase

Table 4. Enzymes for proposed pathways of pyrimidine deoxyribonucleotide biosynthesis in *M. mycoides*[a]

Enzyme	K_m + SE (μM)	V_{max} ± SE (μmol/min/g of protein)	Effector
CMP kinase	94 ± 27	15.0 ± 1.6	
dCMP kinase	70 ± 23	29.7 ± 4.0	
dCTPase	ND[b]	1.5[c], 1.3[d]	
Deoxycytidine kinase	88 ± 18	5.2 ± 0.2	dTTP(−)
dCMP deaminase	46 ± 16[e]	285 ± 37	dCTP(+) dTTP(−)
dUTPase	5[f]	50.2[g]	
dUMP phosphatase	1,570 ± 220	72.0 ± 5.3	
dTMP phosphatase	3,720 ± 530	29.4 ± 2.2	
Thymidine/deoxyuridine phosphorylase with substrate:			
Deoxyuridine at 0.2 mM P$_i$	2,090 ± 540	1,120	
Thymidine at 0.2 mM P$_i$	617 ± 72	1,240	
P$_i$ at 10 mM deoxyuridine	114 ± 22	1,570 ± 173	
P$_i$ at 2.5 mM thymidine	106 ± 23	1,350 ± 135	
Uracil at 0.2 mM dRib 1-P[h]	138 ± 36	891 ± 72	
Thymine at 0.2 mM dRib 1-P	51 ± 14	1,170 ± 68	
dRib 1-P at 2 mM uracil	157 ± 73	2,100 ± 560	
dRib 1-P at 2 mM thymine	98 ± 33	1,700 ± 280	
Thymidine kinase	129 ± 41	26.3 ± 2.4	dTTP(−)
Deoxyuridine kinase	559 ± 161	40.5 ± 4.6	dTTP(−)
dTMP kinase	9 ± 3	11.8 ± 0.6	dTTP(−)

[a] From reference 38.
[b] ND, not determined.
[c] Rate of dCMP production at 20 μM dCTP.
[d] Rate of dCDP production at 20 μM dCTP.
[e] In the presence of 150 μM dCTP.
[f] From reference 7.
[g] Rate of dUMP production at 10 μM dUTP.
[h] dRib 1-P, deoxyribose 1-phosphate.

should lead to rapid depletion of the exogenous deoxyribonucleosides. However, these reactions would also metabolize a given deoxyribonucleoside to yield deoxyribose 1-phosphate, which could then be used with the appropriate base to generate another deoxyribonucleoside for phosphorylation to the corresponding dNMP. The lack of an exogenous source of deoxyribonucleosides would require that the deoxyribose moieties be generated endogenously by reduction of ribonucleotides.

Endogenous Generation of Deoxyribose 1-Phosphate

The major means for the synthesis of deoxyribonucleotides in eucaryotes and most procaryotes is reduction of substrate rNDPs by the enzyme rNDP reductase. Whereas ADP, GDP, and CDP undergo reduction and a single phosphorylation to give rise to dATP, dGTP, and dCTP respectively, the synthesis of dTTP from UDP proceeds via a series of reactions. The dUTP formed from the reduction and phosphorylation is acted on by dUTPase to form dUMP, which is then methylated by thymidylate synthase to dTMP. An alternative and probably major source of dUMP is reduction of CDP to dCDP, followed by deamination of deoxycytidine nucleotide in the form of dCTP in enterobacteria or of dCMP in eucaryotes and gram-positive bacteria (34). rNDP reductase has much higher activity toward CDP than toward UDP (9, 16, 17), a characteristic which would make deoxycytidine nucleotide available in excess.

rNDP reductase activity was not detected in extracts of *M. mycoides* (41), possibly because of the complex nature of both the enzyme and the assay system. However, indirect evidence was strongly suggestive of its presence in this organism. Thus, labeling of the deoxyribose moiety of dCMP and dTMP in DNA from [U-14C]cytidine (40) could have arisen only from reduction of the ribosyl group. Furthermore, the effects of hydroxyurea in causing inhibition of growth and a marked decrease in the intracellular contents of dATP were consistent with the properties of rNDP reductase from other organisms (9, 16, 17). This study of Neale et al. (40) on *M. mycoides* sought to define the source of deoxyribose 1-phosphate necessary for synthesis of thymidine, and hence dTMP, from preformed thymine. By measuring the specific activity of deoxyribonucleotides isolated from DNA after the incorporation of 14C-labeled precursors with and without competition from other nucleotide precursors, it was found that cytidine competed effectively with uracil to provide all of the deoxycytidine nucleotide as well as most of the deoxyribose 1-phosphate for synthesis of dTMP. Competition studies with other pyrimidine nucleosides showed that deoxyuridine was most effective in excluding the cytidine label from dTMP, whereas deoxycytidine excluded a small amount of cytidine label from dCMP and a considerable amount from dTMP. Although growth studies have shown that thymidine can fully meet the requirement of *M. mycoides* for thymine, thymidine was unable to compete with cytidine for the provision of deoxyribose in thymidylate. This apparent inability of thymidine to serve as a precursor of dTTP may have arisen through its failure to compete with the thymine present as a normal constituent of the growth medium to which the cells were adapted. The data (40) were consistent with *M. mycoides*, growing on guanine, uracil, thymine, and cytidine, having a pathway for the derivation of deoxyribose 1-phosphate from cytidine for synthesis of dTMP, as outlined in Fig. 3. Some kinetic properties for most of the enzymes involved in the pathway are shown in Table 4.

Incorporation of dNMPs

In assessing the contribution of cytidine ribose to thymidylate deoxyribose, Neale et al. (40) found that dUMP, dCMP, and dTMP each excluded the contribution to some extent. Apparently, appreciable incorporation of exogenous dNMP into DNA took place without prior dephosphorylation. A later, more detailed examination of this phenomenon (42) showed the dNMPs to be rapidly phosphorylated to the triphosphate level inside the cell and incorporated into DNA. This uptake and utilization of dNMPs by *M. mycoides* is considered in more detail below.

Biosynthesis of Thymidylate and dTTP

Two different pathways exist in microorganisms for the synthesis of dTTP. The first of these is the endogenous pathway, in which dUMP undergoes tetrahydrofolate-dependent methylation to dTMP. Thymidylate synthase, which catalyzes this reaction, has been identified in all microorganisms examined except some of the mollicutes (34). Although assay data have not been reported, this enzyme is indicated in *A. laidlawii* by the lack of a thymidine requirement in the presence of folinic acid (62). The second, or exogenous, pathway involves the supply of thymidine or thymine in the medium. Use of thymine requires a source of deoxyribose 1-phosphate to form thymidine and then sequential phosphorylations to dTMP and ultimately dTTP. The substrate for synthesis of thymidine nucleotides by methylation in the former pathway, dUMP, can also serve as the source of deoxyribose 1-phosphate in the latter. This ability depends on the processes of dephosphorylation and phosphorolysis as outlined in Fig. 3 for *M. mycoides* subsp. *mycoides*. The enzymatic activities for these processes have been defined in *M. mycoides* (40, 41) and *A. laidlawii* B-PG9 (76) and a number of other mollicutes (77).

As noted above, the deoxyribose for thymidine biosynthesis in *M. mycoides* was found to derive from the ribose of cytidine (40). In enteric bacteria, 75% of the dUMP required for synthesis of thymidine nucleotide is derived from a cytidine nucleotide via reduction of CDP (44), followed by a reaction sequence involving phosphorylation to dCTP, deamination to dUTP, and finally hydrolysis of dUTP to dUMP. Thus, an important link in this pathway is the deamination of deoxycytidine nucleotide at the level of the triphosphate. Both *M. mycoides* (41) and *A. laidlawii* (76) were found to lack dCTP deaminase. Instead, they had a highly active dCMP deaminase to effect the formation of dUMP, a property that they share with *B. subtilis* (33), *Lactobacillus acidophilus* (66), and *Staphylococcus aureus* (8). Since these early reports, several other mem-

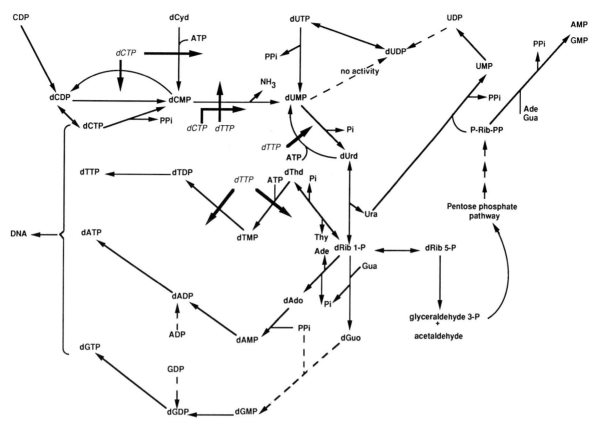

Figure 3. Pathways of deoxyribonucleotide biosynthesis and interconversion. Reactions indicated by broken arrows have not been detected in *M. mycoides* subsp. *mycoides*, but some have been observed in other mollicutes. Heavy arrows parallel to the reaction pathway indicate activation by the effector(s) shown in italics, and those across the reaction pathway indicate inhibition. P-Rib-PP, 5-phosphoribosyl 1-pyrophosphate; dRib 1-P, deoxyribose 1-phosphate; dRib 5-P, deoxyribose 5-phosphate.

bers of the mollicutes have also been shown to possess dCMP deaminase. It has been observed in *Anaeroplasma intermedium* (24), all *Mycoplasma* strains tested (24, 77), several other *Acholeplasma* species (77), several *Spiroplasma* species (50), and *U. urealyticum* (7).

M. mycoides and *A. laidlawii* displayed a close similarity with regard to the enzymatic activities associated with dTMP (and dTTP) synthesis. They both possessed kinases for thymidine, deoxycytidine, deoxyuridine, dTMP, (d)CMP, and NDPs as well as thymidine (deoxyuridine) phosphorylase. Neither organism was capable of phosphorylating dUMP. The major difference in activities of enzymes for deoxyribonucleotide synthesis was the absence from *A. laidlawii* of activities to generate dCMP from dCTP or dCDP. It was proposed (76) that this absence may account for the inability of *A. laidlawii* to use exogenous thymine for the formation of thymidine. Thus, *A. laidlawii* would generate insufficient dCMP from CDP, via dCDP and dCTP, to support the supply of dUMP as a source of deoxyribose 1-phosphate needed for thymidine and dTMP synthesis. The effect of other deoxyribonucleosides in stimulating the incorporation of thymine into DNA in *A. laidlawii* (26) is consistent with this proposal. Nonetheless, *A. laidlawii* would require a supply of dUMP for a pathway to dTMP via thymidylate syn-

thase. Bearing in mind the properties of ribonucleotide reductase, which include a very much lower activity toward UDP than toward CDP, it is likely that dCMP deaminase would make some contribution to such a supply.

Regulation of Deoxyribonucleotide and dTTP Synthesis

Figure 3 outlines proposed pathways for deoxyribonucleotide biosynthesis in *M. mycoides* modified from that of Neale et al. (41) to include data on possible regulatory effectors of enzymes (38, 41) and potential pathways for the purine nucleotides. The outline indicates that provision of the four dNTPs for DNA synthesis would depend on reduction of CDP, GDP, ADP, and possibly UDP in the absence of deoxyribonucleosides or dNMPs in the medium. The only measurements of dNTP concentrations in *M. mycoides* (41) gave results consistent with the reduction occurring via an rNDP reductase with properties similar to those of the enzyme in most other organisms, including *E. coli*. The overall activity of the *E. coli* enzyme is determined by the positive effector ATP and the negative effector dATP, and the affinity (specificity) of the enzyme toward different substrates is determined by ATP, dTTP, and dGTP (44). The specificities promoted are CDP or UDP reduction by ATP, GDP reduction by dTTP, and ADP reduction by dGTP, with dATP inhibiting all reactions. This pattern of regulation predicts that a decrease in total enzyme capacity would be compensated for by a decrease in negative feedback through a decreased dATP concentration. Such an effect of decreased dATP level was observed with *M. mycoides* cultures when hydroxyurea was added to give partial inhibition of the reductase (40).

The high activity of dCMP deaminase suggests that this enzyme provides the major means of dUMP formation in *M. mycoides*. This suggestion receives support from some of the kinetic properties of the enzyme which shows a sigmoidal curve for the response of rate to dCMP concentration and to the activating and inhibitory effects of dCTP and dTTP, respectively. These properties could serve to regulate the use of deoxycytidine nucleotide in the production of deoxyribose for thymidine nucleotide synthesis. Similar regulatory effects have been observed for the dCMP deaminase from other procaryotes (8, 33, 66). Comparison of the kinetic data for dCMP deaminase and dCMP kinase (Table 4) suggests that the former would provide the major avenue for dCMP metabolism, a suggestion which receives support from the observation that deoxycytidine and dCMP compete with [U-^{14}C]cytidine more effectively in the provision of deoxyribose for DNA thymidylate than in the synthesis of DNA cytidylate.

With dUMP available, its utilization as a precursor of deoxyribose in DNA thymidylate is favored by the properties (Table 4) of the enzymes dUMP (dTMP) phosphatase, thymidine (deoxyuridine) phosphorylase, thymidine (deoxyuridine) kinase, and dTMP kinase, together with uracil phosphoribosyltransferase (31). The preference (higher V_{max} and lower K_m) of the phosphatase for dUMP would result in the formation of deoxyuridine without appreciable breakdown of dTMP. The phosphorylase would rapidly convert deoxyuridine to deoxyribose 1-phosphate and uracil, and removal of the latter product by the highly active uracil phosphoribosyltransferase (V_{max} = 120 µmol/min per g of protein; K_m for uracil = 2.6 µM) (31) would greatly limit the reverse reaction. With thymine present, the deoxyribose 1-phosphate produced from dUMP would rapidly and reversibly be used by the phosphorylase for the formation of thymidine. The kinetic characteristics of thymidine kinase would then ensure that thymidine was phosphorylated with little corresponding phosphorylation of deoxyuridine. The resulting dTMP would be further phosphorylated to dTDP by dTMP kinase and to dTTP by NDP kinase. Similar steps could not occur for dUMP because of the absence of dUMP kinase activity. Thus, the kinetic and thermodynamic considerations are well suited to ensuring that the direction of flow through the pathway is from dUMP to dTMP. Feedback effects on the thymidine and dTMP kinases by dTTP would modulate the production of dTTP in relation to its use. However, the formation of dUMP is not tightly regulated by the level of dTTP when dCMP and dCTP concentrations are high (41). Under these conditions, the production of thymidine or deoxyribose 1-phosphate may exceed the cell's requirement for thymidine nucleotide. Further metabolism of either excess thymidine or its equivalent as deoxyribose 1-phosphate may account in part for the

observed incorporation of deoxyribose from carbon atoms of [U-^{14}C]cytidine into other deoxyribonucleotides (40).

The activity of the PP$_i$-dependent purine nucleoside kinase would enable phosphorylation of purine deoxyribonucleosides which may arise from purine bases and deoxyribose 1-phosphate through the action of purine nucleoside phosphorylase (32). Cytidine ribose appearing in rNMPs (40) may arise either through a pathway from deoxyribose 1-phosphate to PRPP via glyceraldehyde 3-phosphate (6) or through deamination of cytidine. Uridine from the latter reaction could form uridine nucleotides or, by phosphorolysis, provide ribose 1-phosphate for synthesis of purine nucleotides through purine nucleoside phosphorylase and purine nucleoside kinase or through PRPP synthetase and purine phosphoribosyltransferases.

Another enzyme worthy of comment is the NMP phosphohydrolase which is unusual in its high activity for dUMP, namely, dUMPase. This property has obvious advantages for the function of the enzyme in the pathway to thymidine nucleotides proposed in Fig. 3. The lack of activity toward dCMP suggests that the observed in vivo release of phosphate from dCMP (40, 42) depends on prior conversion of dCMP to dUMP. A dUMPase has been found both in *E. coli* (72) and *S. typhimurium* (34). The only nucleotides which were cleaved by the enzymes were dUMP, dTMP, and UMP. No activity was observed with purine NMPs. These organisms and *A. laidlawii*, in which somewhat similar activity was also observed (76), are usually incapable of providing an endogenous source of deoxyribose 1-phosphate for utilization of thymine. Thus, it appears the enzyme may serve another function, namely, to assist in limiting the presence of deoxyuridine nucleotides in the cell.

Mechanisms To Limit dUTP Concentrations

Although uracil residues may arise in DNA through incorporation of dUTP by DNA polymerase or by deamination of deoxycytidine in DNA, there is usually no significant appearance of uracil in DNA. Several enzyme activities could assist to limit the accumulation of dUMP in DNA. One of these, dUTPase, prevents the initial incorporation by hydrolyzing dUTP to dUMP plus PP$_i$. As noted above, the dUMP could then be degraded by dUMPase and thymidine phosphorylase. A further enzyme, uracil-DNA glycosylase, breaks the bond between uracil and the 3',5'-phosphodiester-linked deoxyribose in the DNA to remove the base. The apyrimidinic site left behind in the DNA is replaced by repair processes which enable the incoming deoxyribonucleotide residue to be matched to the corresponding residue on the complementary strand of the DNA helix. As noted by Williams and Pollack (78), both dUTPase and uracil-DNA glycosylase have been found in all procaryote and eucaryote organisms examined with the possible exception of some mollicutes. These authors examined the distribution of the two enzymes among the mollicutes (78) and noted that *M. mycoides* is the only member of the *Mycoplasmataceae* in which dUTPase has been observed (7, 41). Three members of the *Mycoplasmataceae* tested also lacked uracil-DNA glycosylase. Williams and Pollack (78) have suggested that the lack of these enzymes could correlate with a rapid rate of evolution and an AT-biased mutation pressure. For *M. mycoides*, the reasonably high activity of dUTPase (50 μmol/min per g of protein) and its low K_m (5 μM) (Table 4) coupled with the presence of dUMP phosphatase activity and absence of dUMP kinase should be effective in limiting availability of dUTP for incorporation into DNA.

FOLIC ACID METABOLISM

In the context of the basic cellular functions of gene expression and replication, folic acid is important through the role of tetrahydrofolic acid derivatives in the synthesis of purine nucleotides and dTMP, in the formylation of methionyl-tRNA$_f^{Met}$, and in the provision of methyl groups, via *S*-adenosylmethionine, for the methylation of nucleic acids. The derivatives and the processes in which they participate are N^{10}-formyltetrahydrofolic acid in formylation of methionyl-tRNA$_f^{Met}$ and purine biosynthesis; N^5,N^{10}-methenyltetrahydrofolic acid in purine biosynthesis; N^5,N^{10}-methylenetetrahydrofolic acid in dTMP synthesis and provision of N^5-methyltetrahydrofolic acid; and N^5-methyltetrahydrofolic acid in methionine formation from homocysteine. The methylation reactions depend on activation of the methyl group of methionine by the formation of *S*-adenosylmethionine. Transfer of the methyl group generates *S*-adenosylhomocysteine, from which homocysteine can be regenerated.

Synthesis of folic acid from simple precursors involves a complex pathway which is the site of action of the sulfonamides (4). This complexity and the insensitivity of the mollicutes to sulfonamides make it unlikely that these organisms possess such a pathway. Formation of tetrahydrofolic acid from folic acid is achieved by two reductive steps. The second of these, catalyzed by dihydrofolate reductase, also functions in regeneration of tetrahydrofolic acid from dihydrofolic acid when the latter is produced in the synthesis of dTMP from N^5,N^{10}-methylenetetrahydrofolic acid and dUMP.

No form of folic acid is included in the defined growth media for *M. mycoides* subsp. *mycoides* (C4 medium) and *M. capricolum* (C5 medium), whereas folinic acid (N^5-formyltetrahydrofolic acid) is a component of the partly defined medium for *A. laidlawii* (62). The latter medium does not include thymidine, which is required in media without folinic acid (55). Thus, at least some strains of *A. laidlawii* have the capacity to synthesize dTMP when folinic acid is available. This finding suggests that they must at least possess thymidylate synthase to catalyze the methylation of dUMP to dTMP, with concurrent conversion of N^5,N^{10}-methylenetetrahydrofolic acid to dihydrofolic acid. Regeneration of tetrahydrofolic acid for further use as a coenzyme requires the activity of dihydrofolate reductase. This enzyme has been demonstrated and investigated in *A. laidlawii* and *M. gallisepticum* (22). The enzymes show similar specific activities in crude extracts from both sources, similar K_m values for dihydrofolic acid, and similar inhibition constants for methotrexate, a specific inhibitor of the mammalian and bacterial enzyme. In contrast, studies of growth inhibition by methotrexate showed that *A. laidlawii* was about 3,300-fold more susceptible than *M. gallisepticum* (22). The affinity of another inhibitor, trimethoprim, was 130-fold lower for the *M. gallisepticum* enzyme than for that of *A. laidlawii*, but the susceptibility of *M. gallisepticum* to the drug was 3,300-fold lower. The authors concluded that these differences in the relative effects of inhibitors on the enzyme in comparison with whole cells are apparently due to impaired drug entrance into *M. gallisepticum* cells. An alternative explanation could be that *M. gallisepticum* lacks thymidylate synthase and therefore does not generate the same demand for dihydrofolic acid reduction as does *A. laidlawii*.

Further evidence of a capacity for tetrahydrofolic acid metabolism in mollicutes comes from *M. mycoides* subsp. *mycoides*, in which it was observed that either N^{10}-formyltetrahydrofolic acid or N^5,N^{10}-methenyltetrahydrofolic acid could support formylation of methionyl-tRNA$_f^{Met}$ to formylmethionyl-tRNA^{Met} (39) when added to cultures in C4 minimal defined medium. Formylation of methionyl-tRNA$_f^{Met}$ is apparently not essential for initiation of protein synthesis in *M. mycoides*, possibly because the tRNA lacks ribothymidine in the pseudouridine loop (74). It is interesting that there is a complete lack of ribothymidine, for 23S rRNA as well as for tRNA, in the closely related *M. capricolum* but not in *A. laidlawii* (15). These observations demonstrated a capacity for *M. mycoides* to take up and utilize these preformed tetrahydrofolic acid derivatives. Folic acid itself had no effect. Experiments with N^5,N^{10}-methylenetetrahydrofolic acid, both labeled and unlabeled, gave no evidence that it was able to replace the thymine requirement of *M. mycoides*, supporting the conclusion that *M. mycoides* lacks thymidylate synthase (38).

Since methylation is generally observed in the nucleic acids of mollicutes (58), a methyl donor, presumably *S*-adenosylmethionine, must be available in the cells. Bergemann et al. (2) have observed the derivation of methyl groups in *M. mycoides* DNA from [*methyl*-^{14}C]methionine in the medium. The demand for methionine for methylation reactions has the potential to raise the nutritional requirement for the amino acid above that needed for protein synthesis.

If, as suggested above, *M. mycoides* does lack thymidylate synthase, it may seem a little surprising that it contains a gene, *glyA*, coding for serine-tetrahydrofolic acid hydroxymethyltransferase, which catalyzes the synthesis of N^5,N^{10}-methylenetetrahydrofolic acid. This gene, cloned and sequenced from PG50 (54) in the closely related bovine serogroup 7, is also found in other members of the *M. mycoides* cluster (53) as well as in *M. pneumoniae* (75). The significance of retention of the gene in these mollicutes may lie in use of the one-carbon group from N^5,N^{10}-methylenetetrahydrofolate to maintain the supply of methyl groups, via N^5-methyltetrahydrofolate and remethylation of homocysteine, in circumstances in which the supply of methionine may be limiting. This limitation could occur readily, since methionine is a relatively minor component in proteins and thus in the mixtures of amino acids or peptides derived from them as nutritional sources.

TRANSPORT OF NUCLEOTIDES AND NUCLEOTIDE PRECURSORS

The use of nucleosides and bases as precursors for nucleotide synthesis by mollicutes implies that they have transport systems for the penetration of these hydrophilic solutes through the hydrophobic phase of the cell membrane. Such transport processes are widely known in other organisms, including procaryotes (37, 44). For mycoplasmas, detailed study of these processes is mostly confined to *M. mycoides* subsp. *mycoides*. For this organism, there is also evidence of an unusual process for transport of intact NMP into the cell for use in DNA synthesis without prior dephosphorylation (40, 42, 79).

Nucleotides

Early evidence from nutritional studies on mollicutes suggested that nucleic acids and in some cases NMPs supported the nucleotide requirements of these organisms very effectively (55, 60). There has been some study of the possibility that nucleases of mollicutes degrade environmental nucleic acids to more assimilable precursors necessary for growth (49, 56, 57, 61). In most other procaryotes, the use of exogenous nucleotides in this fashion has been explicable by uptake of the nucleosides derived from prior dephosphorylation of the NMPs by periplasmic phosphatases (43–45). With *M. mycoides*, however, it was observed that the NMP phosphoryl group can remain attached to the nucleoside when it has been incorporated into DNA (40, 42). Kinetic investigations involving competition studies indicated that there was a single system mediating the uptake of the usual four dNMPs and rNMPs (42). The system showed twofold higher affinity for dNMPs than rNMPs and was capable of half-saturating the nucleotide requirement for DNA synthesis at concentrations down to 27 nM (for dGMP) in competition with the corresponding bases at 80 μM. The comparative rates of uptake at 500 nM were 1.3, 1.0, 1.1, 0.8, and 3.6 μmol/min per g of protein for dTMP, dCMP, dAMP, dGMP, and CMP, respectively. The intact rNMP was used more for DNA synthesis than for RNA synthesis. This finding was interpreted as indicating that the exogenous rNMP might contribute more readily to the pool of rNDP for ribonucleotide reduction and subsequent incorporation into DNA, via the dNTP, than to the pool of rNTP for incorporation into RNA.

There was also rapid degradation of much (about 50% with 500 nM added NMP) of the nucleotide taken up, yielding P_i, free base, some nucleoside, and presumably the corresponding pentose 1-phosphate and its metabolic products (40, 42, 79). (An erratum to the report of Neale et al. [42] indicated that Fig. 2 should read "10 μg atoms of $^{14}C \cdot g^{-1}$" instead of "μmole·g^{-1}" on the ordinate and have "thymine" instead of "thymidine" in line 6 of the legend.) The base and nucleoside products are found almost totally released into the extracellular medium, whereas much of the P_i is retained intracellularly as a preferential source of phosphate. The existence of this NMP transport system has been substantiated by the isolation and characterization of

mutants defective in the transport (79). To select mutants, log-phase cells were incubated with high-specific-activity [^{32}P]dAMP and then stored at $-20°C$ for several weeks to allow ^{32}P decay before plating. Colonies were then screened for lack of labeling by tracer amounts of [^{32}P]dAMP. The wild type was able to grow well with dUMP, UMP, CMP, or cytidine substituting for uracil in modified C4 medium, whereas only cytidine served as a replacement with the two mutants tested. Similarly, dGMP or GMP substituted for guanine in the wild type but not in the mutants. However, substitution of dTMP for thymine supported good growth of both the mutants and the wild type. Further studies on the metabolism of dTMP indicated that the mutants retained less capacity to dephosphorylate dTMP than did the wild type and less capacity to use ^{32}P released from NMPs in preference to medium P_i. The data were consistent with the mutants and the wild type being able to effect extracellular dephosphorylation of dTMP at a rate sufficient to meet the thymine and thymidine requirements but still much slower than the rate of intracellular dephosphorylation of dTMP after uptake by wild-type cells. Mutants incorporated very little label from [^3H]dTMP in competition with thymine in the medium, whereas the wild type incorporated it very strongly.

Demonstration of a transport system for NMPs has been reported for a few other organisms but not for other mollicutes. Such a system appears to be absent from *U. urealyticum* 960 (80). However, its effectiveness in allowing economical labeling of DNA for cells growing in complex media (see below) should provide an incentive to test for its occurrence in other mollicutes if DNA labeling is required.

For mollicutes lacking the NMP transport system, utilization of NMPs as nucleic acid precursors might depend on their prior degradation by extracytoplasmic phosphatases, as noted for some other procaryotes (43–45), or as found for the use of dTMP by the NMP transport-deficient mutants of *M. mycoides*. Phosphatase (or nucleotidase) activities against NMPs have been observed generally in mollicutes (7, 23, 24, 48, 50). A comparison of these activities in *U. urealyticum* and *M. mycoides* showed them to be very much higher and mostly membrane associated in *U. urealyticum*, whereas about half of the activity was cytoplasmic in *M. mycoides* (7). It is not known whether *U. urealyticum* can use NMPs as nucleic acid precursors.

Nucleosides

Two high-affinity nucleoside transport systems energized by proton motive force have been identified in *E. coli* (44). One transports all nucleosides, and the other transports only pyrimidine and adenine nucleosides. The exogenous nucleosides are rapidly metabolized after their entry into cells. Neale (38), using the techniques reported for uptake of NMP (42), examined uptake of nucleosides by *M. mycoides* subsp. *mycoides*. He observed half-saturating concentrations of 0.13, 0.85, and 15 μM for the uptake of thymidine, deoxycytidine, and cytidine, respectively. Tests were made of the competitive effects of nucleosides and NMPs on the uptake of these three nucleosides. All of the deoxyribonucleoside competitors at 5 μM completely inhibited the uptake of cytidine, whereas cytidine was ineffective as a competitor for uptake of the deoxyribonucleosides. There was competition from other deoxyribonucleosides, most effectively from deoxythymidine and deoxyuridine, and the ribonucleosides uridine, adenosine and guanosine also caused some inhibition of the uptake of the three nucleosides. Nucleotides had less effect. The results suggested that *M. mycoides* possessed a nucleoside transport system for both ribo- and deoxyribonucleosides, distinct from that for NMP uptake and having a much lower affinity for cytidine than for the other nucleosides.

Bases

Several studies suggest that uptake of the purine bases uracil and cytosine into *E. coli* involves specific transport systems energized by proton motive force (37, 44). There is no information on such systems in mollicutes. Their existence might be expected from the need for a mechanism to allow the polar bases through the cell membrane and from a need for efficient scavenging mechanisms for bases in these organisms that are dependent on exogenous sources of nucleic acid precursors. It has been suggested that processes for active uptake of bases by proton symport could be used for generation of a proton gradient if driven in reverse by efflux of the bases generated by phosphorolysis of nucleosides (10).

LABELING OF NUCLEIC ACIDS

Use of C4 defined medium (62) for the growth of *M. mycoides* subsp. *mycoides* has allowed ready use of ^{14}C- or ^{3}H-labeled bases, nucleosides, or NMPs as well as ^{32}P$_i$ or ^{32}P-labeled dNMPs for labeling nucleic acids (31, 40, 42). Similar labeling should be readily possible in other mollicutes for which defined or partly defined media are available. Complex media did not allow significant incorporation of nucleosides and bases into acid-insoluble material for *A. laidlawii* and seven *Mycoplasma* species, possibly because of competition from nucleic acid breakdown products of the yeast extract component in the medium (26). It was also observed that incorporation was unsatisfactory in cells suspended in saline. However, modest growth and DNA labeling were obtained in Eagle's basal medium. With *M. mycoides*, incorporation of dNMPs was quite effective from complex media (52, 79) and should be similarly effective for other mollicutes if they possess the NMP transport system.

PYRIDINE NUCLEOTIDES

NAD and its phosphorylated derivative (NADP) are ubiquitous in their participation in cellular oxidation-reduction reactions. In addition, NAD can be degraded at either of two high-energy bonds to drive DNA ligations or to effect ADP ribosylation of proteins (69). The DNA ligation reaction, as it occurs in *E. coli* and *S. typhimurium*, involves hydrolysis of NAD to nicotinamide mononucleotide (NMN) and AMP and is a major contributor to NAD turnover. ADP ribosylation occurs but is probably a minor contributor to turnover. Synthesis of NAD from exogenous preformed precursors can occur from nicotinic acid, nicotinamide, NMN, or NAD. NAD is not transported into the cell but is degraded by extracellular enzymes to produce nicotinamide. A variety of pathways are known for NAD synthesis or recycling in different organisms, but the reactions in *E. coli* and *S. typhimurium* appear to go through the intermediate formation of nicotinate mononucleotide (NaMN) to deamido-NAD (NaAD) to NAD. NaMN can derive from deamination of NMN or from the reaction with PRPP catalyzed by nicotinate phosphoribosyltransferase. This enzyme reacts with ATP, catalyzed by NaMN adenylyltransferase, to give NaAD.

There appear to have been no studies on the synthesis of pyridine nucleotides in mollicutes or on the possible use of NAD for DNA ligations or ADP ribosylation. The defined and partially defined media for growth of *M. mycoides* and *A. laidlawii* contain nicotinic acid (62), whereas Frey's medium, which supports the growth of *M. synoviae*, contains NADH (11). Considering other examples showing that mollicutes require intact coenzymes, e.g., coenzyme A in C4 medium for *M. mycoides* (62), rather than vitamins as nutrients, the addition of NAD or NADH to media might be tested more widely.

REGULATORY NUCLEOTIDES

Regulatory nucleotides observed in *E. coli* include cyclic AMP (cAMP), ppGpp, ppGppp, and AppppA. There is only limited information on these nucleotides in mollicutes.

cAMP

The role of cAMP in the regulation of carbon metabolism in enteric bacteria has been reviewed recently (21). cAMP is synthesized from ATP by adenylate cyclase and binds to a protein factor known as the catabolite activator protein (CAP), also called the cAMP receptor protein. The cAMP-CAP complex binds to a consensus sequence at or near promoters for several gene systems concerned with carbon catabolism, enabling them to be available for initiation of transcription when derepressed by the presence of the appropriate inducer. Lowering of cAMP levels through modulation of adenylate cyclase activity by the presence of glucose, or some other substrates for carbon catabolism, diminishes formation of the cAMP-CAP complex, thereby preventing transcription from the cAMP-dependent promoters. Various observations suggest that the functions of cAMP and CAP may be more complex than outlined here (21, 73). Mugharbil and Cirillo (36) observed cAMP in *M. capricolum* and reported that its level was low while free glucose or fructose was in the culture medium but rose when the sugar was exhausted. With a mutant defective in the phosphoenolpyruvate-dependent sugar phosphotransferase system for glucose, the level remained high in the presence of glucose but was depressed by fructose. Assay of cAMP and adenylate cyclase has also been performed with *M. mycoides* (9a) (Table 1).

ppGpp

The nucleotide ppGpp is considered to be the major regulatory signal during the stringent response, a cellular response to amino acid starvation that entails regulation of numerous cellular activities, including inhibition of synthesis of stable RNAs (5). Mutants lacking this response have been termed relaxed (*rel* mutants), and the product of the *relA* gene has been identified as (p)ppGpp synthetase. The enzyme catalyzes ATP-dependent pyrophosphorylation of GDP or GTP. For activity, it needs to be associated with ribosomes having bound mRNA and codon-specified uncharged tRNA at the tRNA acceptor (A) site. Another mechanism of synthesis, associated with carbon starvation, may also exist. Glaser et al. (12) demonstrated that amino acid starvation of *M. capricolum* caused an inhibition of stable RNA synthesis and was accompanied by an increase in pppGpp and ppGpp, indicating that this mycoplasma employs a stringent control mechanism resembling that in *E. coli* (see chapters 10 and 19).

ApppppA

ApppppA and related dinucleotides are products of reactions catalyzed by aminoacyl-tRNA synthetases, which result when nucleotides such as ATP are adenylated in place of PP$_i$ in the back-reaction of aminoacyl-tRNA synthetases (81). They are found in a wide variety of procaryotic and eucaryotic cells (81) and accumulate in *S. typhimurium* and *E. coli* during heat shock and oxidative stress, leading to the suggestion that they serve as signals to generate responses to these stresses (3, 18). Neither their role nor their occurrence in mollicutes has been investigated.

REFERENCES

1. **Bagnara, A. S., and L. R. Finch.** 1973. The effects of bases and nucleosides on the intracellular contents of nucleotides and 5-phosphoribosyl-1-pyrophosphate in *Escherichia coli. Eur. J. Biochem.* **41:**421–430.
2. **Bergemann, A. D., J. C. Whitley, and L. R. Finch.** 1990. Taxonomic significance of differences in DNA methylation within the 'Mycoplasma mycoides cluster' detected with restriction endonucleases MboI and DpnI. *Lett. Appl. Microbiol.* **11:**48–51.
3. **Bochner, B. R., P. C. Lee, S. W. Wilson, C. W. Cutler, and B. N. Ames.** 1984. ApppppA and related adenylated nucleotides are synthesized as a consequence of oxidative stress. *Cell* **37:**225–232.
4. **Brown, G. M., and J. M. Williamson.** 1987. Biosynthesis of folic acid, riboflavin, thiamine, and pantothenic acid, p. 521–538. *In* F. C. Neidhardt, J. L. Ingraham, K. B. Low, B. Magasanik, M. Schaechter, and H. E. Umbarger (ed.), *Escherichia coli and Salmonella typhimurium: Cellular and Molecular Biology.* American Society for Microbiology, Washington, D.C.
5. **Cashel, M., and K. E. Rudd.** 1987. The stringent response, p. 1410–1438. *In* F. C. Neidhardt, J. L. Ingraham, K. B. Low, B. Magasanik, M. Schaechter, and H. E. Umbarger (ed.), *Escherichia coli and Salmonella typhimurium: Cellular and Molecular Biology.* American Society for Microbiology, Washington, D.C.
5a.**Chen, X., and L. R. Finch.** Unpublished data.

6. **Cocks, B. G., F. A. Brake, A. Mitchell, and L. R. Finch.** 1985. Enzymes of intermediary carbohydrate metabolism in *Ureaplasma urealyticum* and *Mycoplasma mycoides* subsp. *mycoides. J. Gen. Microbiol.* **131:**2129–2135.
7. **Cocks, B. G., R. Youil, and L. R. Finch.** 1988. Comparison of enzymes of nucleotide metabolism for two members of the *Mycoplasmataceae* family. *Int. J. Syst. Bacteriol.* **38:**273–278.
8. **Duncan, B. K., G. R. Diamond, and M. J. Bessman.** 1972. Regulation of enzyme activity through subunit interaction. *J. Biol. Chem.* **247:**8136–8138.
9. **Eriksson, S., L. Thelander, and M. Akerman.** 1979. Allosteric regulation of calf thymus ribonucleoside diphosphate reductase. *Biochemistry* **18:**2948–2952.
9a.**Favaloro, J. M., and L. R. Finch.** Unpublished data.
10. **Finch, L. R., and A. Mitchell.** 1990. Purine nucleotide metabolism and its regulation in the mollicutes. *Zentralbl. Bakteriol. Suppl.* **20:**172–180.
11. **Freundt, E. A.** 1983. Culture media for classic mycoplasmas, p. 127–135. *In* S. Razin and J. G. Tully (ed.), *Methods in Mycoplasmology,* vol. 1. *Mycoplasma Characterization.* Academic Press, Inc., New York.
12. **Glaser, G., A. Razin, and S. Razin.** 1981. Stable RNA synthesis and its control in *Mycoplasma capricolum. Nucleic Acids Res.* **9:**3641–3646.
13. **Hamet, M., C. Bonissol, and P. Carter.** 1980. Enzymatic activity of purine and pyrimidine metabolism in nine *Mycoplasma* species contaminating cell cultures. *Clin. Chim. Acta* **103:**15–22.
14. **Hatanaka, M., R. Del Giudice, and C. Long.** 1975. Adenine formation from adenosine by mycoplasmas: adenosine phosphorylase activity. *Proc. Natl. Acad. Sci. USA* **72:**1401–1405.
15. **Hsuchen, C.-C., and C. T. Dubin.** 1988. Methylation patterns of mycoplasma transfer and ribosomal ribonucleic acid. *J. Bacteriol.* **144:**991–998.
16. **Larsson, A., and P. Reichard.** 1966. Allosteric effects in the reduction of pyrimidine nucleotides by the ribonucleoside diphosphate reductase system of *Escherichia coli. J. Biol. Chem.* **241:**2533–2539.
17. **Larsson, A., and P. Reichard.** 1966. Reduction of purine ribonucleotides: allosteric behaviour and substrate specificity of the enzyme from *Escherichia coli. J. Biol. Chem.* **241:**2540–2549.
18. **Lee, P. C., B. R. Bochner, and B. N. Ames.** 1983. ApppppA, heat-shock, stress and cell oxidation. *Proc. Natl. Acad. Sci. USA* **80:**7496–7500.
19. **Liska, B., and P. F. Smith.** 1974. Requirements of *Acholeplasma laidlawii* A, strain LA 1, for nucleic acid precursors. *Folia Microbiol.* **19:**107–117.
20. **Long, C. W., R. Del Giudice, R. S. Gardella, and M. Hatanaka.** 1977. Uracil phosphoribosyltransferase activity of mycoplasma and infected cell cultures. *In Vitro* **13:**429–433.
21. **Magasanik, B., and F. C. Neidhardt.** 1987. Regulation of carbon and nitrogen utilization, p. 1318–1325. *In* F. C. Neidhardt, J. L. Ingraham, K. B. Low, B. Magasanik, M. Schaechter, and H. E. Umbarger (ed.), *Escherichia coli and Salmonella typhimurium: Cellular and Molecular Biology.* American Society for Microbiology, Washington, D.C.
22. **Mandelbaum-Shavit, F., and I. Kahane.** 1988. Activity of dihydrofolate reductase in the Mollicutes *Acholeplasma laidlawii* and *Mycoplasma gallisepticum* and their susceptibility to antifolates. *Curr. Microbiol.* **17:**351–354.
23. **McElwain, M. C., D. K. Chandler, M. F. Barile, T. F. Young, V. V. Tryon, J. W. Davis, Jr., T. P. Petzel, C.-J. Chang, M. V. Williams, and J. D. Pollack.** 1988. Purine and pyrimidine metabolism in *Mollicutes* species. *Int. J. Syst. Bacteriol.* **38:**417–423.
24. **McElwain, M. C., and J. D. Pollack.** 1987. Synthesis of deoxyribomononucleotides in *Mollicutes:* dependence

and deoxyribose-1-phosphate and PP$_i$. *J. Bacteriol.* **169:** 3647–3653.

25. **McGarrity, G. J., L. Gamon, T. Steiner, J. Tully, and H. Kotani.** 1985. Uridine phosphorylase activity among the class *Mollicutes. Curr. Microbiol.* **12:**107–112.

26. **McIvor, R. S., and G. E. Kenny.** 1978. Differences in incorporation of nucleic acid bases by various *Mycoplasma* and *Acholeplasma laidlawii. J. Bacteriol.* **135:**483–489.

27. **McIvor, R. S., R. M. Wohlhueter, and P. G. W. Plageman.** 1983. Uracil phosphoribosyltransferase from *Acholeplasma laidlawii:* partial purification and kinetic properties. *J. Bacteriol.* **156:**192–197.

28. **McIvor, R. S., R. M. Wohlhueter, and P. G. W. Plageman.** 1983. Uridine phosphorylase from *Acholeplasma laidlawii:* purification and kinetic properties. *J. Bacteriol.* **156:**198–204.

29. **Mitchell, A.** 1976. The ribonucleotides of *Mycoplasma mycoides.* Ph.D. thesis. University of Melbourne, Parkville, Victoria, Australia.

30. **Mitchell, A., and L. R. Finch.** 1977. Pathways of nucleotide biosynthesis in *Mycoplasma mycoides* subsp. *mycoides. J. Bacteriol.* **130:**1047–1054.

31. **Mitchell, A., and L. R. Finch.** 1979. Enzymes of pyrimidine metabolism in *Mycoplasma mycoides* subsp. *mycoides. J. Bacteriol.* **137:**1073–1080.

32. **Mitchell, A., I. L. Sin, and L. R. Finch.** 1977. Enzymes of purine metabolism in *Mycoplasma mycoides* subsp. *mycoides. J. Bacteriol.* **137:**706–712.

33. **Mollgaard, H., and J. Neuhard.** 1978. Deoxycytidylate deaminase from *Bacillus subtilis.* Purification, characterization and physiological function. *J. Biol. Chem.* **253:** 3536–3542.

34. **Mollgaard, H., and J. Neuhard.** 1983. Biosynthesis of deoxythymidine triphosphate, p. 149–201. *In* A. Munch-Peterson (ed.), *Metabolism of Nucleotides, Nucleosides and Nucleobases in Microorganisms.* Academic Press, Inc. (London), Ltd., London.

35. **Molloy, A., and L. R. Finch.** 1969. Uridine 5′-monophosphate pyrophosphorylase activity from *Escherichia coli. FEBS Letts.* **5:**211–213.

36. **Mugharbil, U., and V. P. Cirillo.** 1978. Mycoplasma phosphoenolpyruvate-dependent sugar phosphotransferase system: glucose-negative mutant and regulation of intracellular cyclic AMP. *J. Bacteriol.* **133:**203–209.

37. **Munch-Petersen, A., and B. Mygind.** 1983. Transport of nucleic acid precursors, p. 259–305. *In* A. Munch-Peterson (ed.), *Metabolism of Nucleotides, Nucleosides and Nucleobases in Microorganisms.* Academic Press, Inc. (London), Ltd., London.

38. **Neale, G. A. M.** 1984. Deoxyribonucleotide and one-carbon metabolism in *Mycoplasma mycoides* subsp. *mycoides.* Ph.D. thesis. University of Melbourne, Parkville, Victoria, Australia.

39. **Neale, G. A. M., A. Mitchell, and L. R. Finch.** 1981. Formylation of methionyl-transfer ribonucleic acid in *Mycoplasma mycoides* subsp. *mycoides. J. Bacteriol.* **146:** 816–818.

40. **Neale, G. A. M., A. Mitchell, and L. R. Finch.** 1983. Pathways of pyrimidine deoxynucleotide biosynthesis in *Mycoplasma mycoides* subsp. *mycoides. J. Bacteriol.* **154:** 17–22.

41. **Neale, G. A. M., A. Mitchell, and L. R. Finch.** 1983. Enzymes of pyrimidine deoxynucleotide metabolism in *Mycoplasma mycoides* subsp. *mycoides. J. Bacteriol.* **156:** 1001–1005.

42. **Neale, G. A. M., A. Mitchell, and L. R. Finch.** 1984. Uptake and utilization of deoxynucleoside 5′-monophosphates by *Mycoplasma mycoides* subsp. *mycoides. J. Bacteriol.* **158:**943–947. (Erratum, **160:**1207.)

43. **Neuhard, J.** 1983. Utilization of preformed pyrimidine bases and nucleosides, p. 95–148. *In* A. Munch-Peterson (ed.), *Metabolism of Nucleotides, Nucleosides and Nucleo-*

44. **Neuhard, J., and P. Nygaard.** 1983. Purines and pyrimidines, p. 445–473. *In* F. C. Neidhardt, J. L. Ingraham, K. B. Low, B. Magasanik, M. Schaechter, and H. E. Umbarger (ed.), *Escherichia coli and Salmonella typhimurium: Cellular and Molecular Biology.* American Society for Microbiology, Washington, D.C.

45. **Nygaard, P.** 1983. Utilization of preformed purine bases and nucleosides, p. 27–93. *In* A. Munch-Peterson (ed.), *Metabolism of nucleotides, Nucleosides and Nucleobases in Microorganisms.* Academic Press, Inc. (London), Ltd., London.

46. **Nilsson, D., B. Hove-Jensen, and K. Arnvig.** 1989. Primary structure of the *tms* and *prs* genes of *Bacillus subtilis. Mol. Gen. Genet.* **218:**565–571.

47. **O'Brien, S. J., J. M. Simonsen, M. W. Grabowski, and M. F. Barile.** 1981. Analysis of multiple isozyme expression among twenty-two species of *Mycoplasma* and *Acholeplasma. J. Bacteriol.* **158:**222–232.

48. **Petzel, J. P., M. C. McElwain, D. DeSantis, J. Manolukas, M. V. Williams, P. A. Hartmann, M. J. Allison, and J. D. Pollack.** 1988. Enzymic activities of carbohydrate, purine, and pyrimidine metabolism in the *Anaeroplasmataceae* (class *Mollicutes*). *Arch. Microbiol.* **152:**309–316.

49. **Pollack, J. D., and P. J. Hoffman.** 1982. Properties of the nucleases of Mollicutes. *J. Bacteriol.* **152:**538–541.

50. **Pollack, J. D., M. C. McElwain, D. DeSantis, T. J. Manolukas, J. G. Tully, C.-J. Chang, R. F. Whitcomb, K. J. Hackett, and M. V. Williams.** 1989. Metabolism of members of the *Spiroplasmataceae. Int. J. Syst. Bacteriol.* **39:**406–412.

51. **Pyle, L. E., V. V. Tryon, and K. D. Beaman.** 1983. The metabolic pathways of *Acholeplasma* and *Mycoplasma:* an overview. *Yale J. Biol. Med.* **56:**709–716.

52. **Pyle, L. E., and L. R. Finch.** 1988. A physical map of the genome of *Mycoplasma mycoides* subsp. *mycoides* Y with some functional loci. *Nucleic Acids Res.* **16:**6027–6039.

53. **Pyle, L. E., T. Taylor, and L. R. Finch.** 1990. Genomic maps of some strains within the *Mycoplasma mycoides* cluster. *J. Bacteriol.* **172:**7265–7268.

54. **Rasmussen, O. F., and C. Christiansen.** 1990. A 23 kb region of the *Mycoplasma* PG50 genome with three identified genetic structures. *Zentralbl. Bakteriol. Suppl.* **20:** 315–323.

55. **Razin, S.** 1962. Nucleic acid precursor requirements of *Mycoplasma laidlawii. J. Gen. Microbiol.* **28:**243–250.

56. **Razin, S.** 1969. Structure and function in mycoplasma. *Annu. Rev. Microbiol.* **23:**317–356.

57. **Razin, S.** 1973. Physiology of mycoplasmas. *Adv. Microb. Physiol.* **10:**1–80.

58. **Razin, S.** 1985. Molecular biology and genetics of mycoplasmas (*Mollicutes*). *Microbiol. Rev.* **49:**419–455.

59. **Razin, S., M. Argaman, and J. Avigan.** 1963. Chemical composition of mycoplasma cells and membranes. *J. Gen. Microbiol.* **33:**477–487.

60. **Razin, S., and B. C. J. G. Knight.** 1960. The effects of ribonucleic acid and deoxyribonucleic acid on the growth of *Mycoplasma. J. Gen. Microbiol.* **22:**504–519.

61. **Razin, S., A. Knyszynski, and Y. Lifshitz.** 1964. Nucleases of *Mycoplasma. J. Gen. Microbiol.* **36:**323–350.

62. **Rodwell, A. W.** 1983. Defined and partly defined media, p. 163–172. *In* S. Razin and J. G. Tully (ed.), *Methods in Mycoplasmology,* vol. 1. *Mycoplasma Characterization.* Academic Press, Inc., New York.

63. **Rodwell, A. W., and A. Mitchell.** 1979. Nutrition, growth and reproduction, p. 163–172. *In* M. R. Barile and S. Razin (ed.), *The Mycoplasmas,* vol. 1. Academic Press, Inc., New York.

64. **Schneider, E. L., and E. J. Stanbridge.** 1975. Comparison of methods for the detection of mycoplasma contamination of cell cultures: a review. *In Vitro* **11:**20–34.

65. **Schneider, E. L., E. J. Stanbridge, and C. J. Epstein.** 1974.

Incorporation of ^{3}H-uridine and ^{3}H-uracil into RNA. A simple technique for the detection of mycoplasma contamination of cultured cells. *Exp. Cell Res.* **84**:311–318.

66. **Sergott, R. C., L. J. Debeer, and M. J. Bessman.** 1971. On the regulation of a bacterial deoxycytidylate deaminase. *J. Biol. Chem.* **246**:7755–7758.

67. **Sin, I. L., and L. R. Finch.** 1972. Adenine phosphoribosyltransferase in *Mycoplasma mycoides* and *Escherichia coli.* *J. Bacteriol.* **112**:439–444.

68. **Smith, D. W., and P. C. Hanawalt.** 1968. Macromolecular synthesis and thymineless death in *Mycoplasma laidlawii* B. *J. Bacteriol.* **96**:2066–2076.

69. **Tritz, G. J.** 1987. NAD biosynthesis and recycling, p. 557–563. *In* F. C. Neidhardt, J. L. Ingraham, K. B. Low, B. Magasanik, M. Schaechter, and H. E. Umbarger (ed.), *Escherichia coli and Salmonella typhimurium: Cellular and Molecular Biology.* American Society for Microbiology, Washington, D.C.

70. **Tryon, V. V., and J. D. Pollack.** 1984. Purine metabolism in *Acholeplasma laidlawii* B-PG 9: novel PPi-dependent nucleoside kinase activity. *J. Bacteriol.* **159**:265–270.

71. **Tryon, V. V., and J. D. Pollack.** 1985. Distinctions in *Mollicutes* purine metabolism: pyrophosphate-dependent nucleoside kinase and dependence on guanylate salvage. *Int. J. Syst. Bacteriol.* **35**:497–501.

72. **Uerkwitz, W., O. Karlstrom, and A. Munch-Petersen.** 1973. A deoxyuridine monophosphate phosphatase de-

tected in mutants of *Escherichia coli* lacking alkaline phosphatase and 5′-nucleotidase. *Mol. Gen. Genet.* **121**: 337–346.

73. **Ullman, A., and A. Danchin.** 1983. Role of cyclic AMP in bacteria. *Adv. Cyclic Nucleotide Res.* **15**:1–15.

74. **Walker, R. T., and U. L. RajBhandary.** 1978. The nucleotide sequence of formylmethionine tRNA from *Mycoplasma mycoides* subsp. *capri. Nucleic Acids Res.* **5**:57–70.

75. **Wenzel, R., and R. Herrmann.** 1990. From a physical to a genetic map of *Mycoplasma pneumoniae. IOM Lett.* **1**:76.

76. **Williams, M. V., and J. D. Pollack.** 1985. Pyrimidine deoxyribonucleotide metabolism in *Acholeplasma laidlawii* B-PG9. *J. Bacteriol.* **161**:1029–1033.

77. **Williams, M. V., and J. D. Pollack.** 1985. Pyrimidine deoxyribonucleotide metabolism in members of the class *Mollicutes. Int. J. Syst. Bacteriol.* **35**:227–230.

78. **Williams, M. V., and J. D. Pollack.** 1990. The importance of differences in pyrimidine metabolism of the mollicutes. *Zentralbl. Bakteriol. Suppl.* **20**:163–171.

79. **Youil, R., and L. R. Finch.** 1988. Isolation and characterization of mutants of *Mycoplasma mycoides* subsp. *mycoides* deficient in nucleoside monophosphate transport. *J. Bacteriol.* **170**:5922–5925.

80. **Youil, R., and L. R. Finch.** Unpublished data.

81. **Zamecnik, P.** 1983. Diadenosine 5′,5‴-P[1,2]-tetraphosphate (Ap$_4$A): its role in cellular metabolism. *Anal. Biochem.* **134**:1–10.

14. Lipid Incorporation, Biosynthesis, and Metabolism

RONALD N. McELHANEY

INTRODUCTION

As documented in chapter 6, the mycoplasmas as a group contain a large number of membrane lipid structures. However, the biochemical pathways by which these various lipids or their precursors are incorporated from the growth medium or are biosynthesized and metabolized are known for only a small proportion of these compounds. In this chapter, I summarize what is currently known about the incorporation, biosynthesis, and metabolism of the mycoplasma membrane lipids. The important roles of membrane lipids in the structure and function of mycoplasma cell membranes are discussed in chapters 8 and 15, respectively. Since the biophysical aspects of membrane lipid compositional variations and their possible regulation are also discussed in chapter 8, I will concentrate here on the biochemical aspects, which are less well understood. For previous summaries of mycoplasma membrane lipid biochemistry, the reader is referred to reviews by Razin (84) and by Smith (148, 150).

INCORPORATION OF EXOGENOUS LIPIDS AND THEIR PRECURSORS

Fatty Acids

The fatty acid requirements of the sterol-nonrequiring *Acholeplasma laidlawii* strains A and B have been the most extensively studied to date among the various mycoplasma species and will be discussed first. As discussed later in this chapter, *A. laidlawii* A and B are capable of the de novo biosynthesis of saturated fatty acids, and this fact should be borne in mind when one considers their exogenous fatty acid requirements.

Razin and Rottem (90) were the first to study the specific fatty acid requirements for the growth of *A. laidlawii* A and B in a semidefined growth medium. These workers found that of the exogenous fatty acids tested, oleic acid is the most effective in promoting cell growth, followed by linolenic, linoleic, and lauric acids in that order, with palmitic and stearic acids being completely inactive. Moreover, the addition of saturated fatty acids to growth medium containing

Ronald N. McElhaney • Department of Biochemistry, University of Alberta, Edmonton, Alberta, Canada T6G 2H7.

oleic acid does not further improve cell growth. Growth promotion by oleic acid occurs only within a certain concentration range, with growth inhibition being observed at higher concentrations. The toxic effect of higher concentrations of oleic acid can be decreased by increasing the concentration of bovine serum albumin in the growth medium, by substituting methyl oleate for oleate, or by utilizing Tween 80 as a source of oleic acid. These results confirm those of earlier studies indicating that high concentrations of surface-active agents such as uncomplexed fatty acids inhibit growth by causing the lysis of these lytic-sensitive, cell wall-less microorganisms.

Tourtellotte et al. (162) subsequently studied the fatty acid requirements of *A. laidlawii* B in a completely defined (but not necessarily minimal) growth medium. These workers reported optimal growth with an equimolar mixture of myristic, palmitic, oleic, linoleic, and linolenic acids. Although these fatty acids were apparently not tested individually, Tourtellotte and coworkers reported that oleic acid alone supports only about half-optimal growth, suggesting some synergy between these different species of exogenous fatty acids. These workers also found that these exogenous fatty acids support growth only within a limited concentration range and that exogenous acetate cannot replace the exogenous fatty acid requirement. Furthermore, they demonstrated that radiolabeled oleic and linoleic acids are incorporated almost exclusively into the polar glycerolipid fraction of the total membrane lipids, indicating that these exogenous fatty acids serve as precursors in the biosynthesis of the glyco- and phospholipids of the cell membrane of this organism.

Although the results of Razin and Rottem (90) and of Tourtellotte et al. (162) indicate that an exogenous unsaturated fatty acid is required for the growth of *A. laidlawii* B, Henrikson and Panos (41) later reported that this organism and *Acholeplasma* sp. strain KHS, another sterol-nonrequiring mycoplasma, both grow well in a complex but exhaustively delipidated growth medium. Moreover, the membrane lipids from these organisms contain only very small amounts of unsaturated fatty acids derived from residual levels in the lipid-depleted growth medium. They concluded either that *A. laidlawii* B may have lost its original requirements for unsaturated fatty acids over many years of laboratory culture or that such a requirement is manifest only in more minimal growth medium. The absence of an unsaturated fatty acid growth requirement was also reported by McElhaney (58) and by McElhaney and Tourtellotte (63) for *A. laidlawii* B cells capable of de novo saturated fatty acid biosynthesis and by Silvius and McElhaney (134) for cells whose capability for fatty acid biosynthesis had been inhibited.

Razin et al. (87, 95) later confirmed that the fatty acid composition of the *A. laidlawii* B membrane polar lipids can be significantly altered by variations in the exogenous fatty acids added to the growth medium and that these variations in fatty acid composition can affect the growth, morphology, and osmotic fragility of this organism. These workers reported that exogenous oleic, linoleic, or linolenic acid supports the highest levels of growth, with lauric and arachidonic acids being less effective in this regard. Myristic acid is without effect relative to control cells grown without exogenous fatty acids, while palmitic and stearic acids actually inhibit growth. Cells enriched in unsaturated fatty acids consist of long, thin, branched filaments which are relatively resistant to osmotic lysis, whereas those enriched in saturated fatty acids exist primarily as single spheres or short, swollen filaments which are more sensitive to osmotic lysis. Although the ratio of saturated to unsaturated fatty acids in the membrane polar lipids can be varied considerably by varying the relative amounts of palmitic or oleic acid added to the growth medium, cells grown without exogenous fatty acids contain polar lipids consisting primarily of palmitate (55% [dry weight]), myristate (20%), and smaller amounts of laurate and stearate (3 to 4%), with very little oleate (<2%). In contrast, the residual fatty acids present in the tryptose growth medium are primarily palmitic, stearic, and oleic acids. Thus, although the fatty acid composition of the *A. laidlawii* membrane lipids reflects to some extent that of the medium in which it is grown, as also observed by Smith et al. (155), the great preponderance of saturated fatty acids in the lipids of cells grown without exogenous fatty acid supplementation suggests that *A. laidlawii* is capable of synthesizing saturated but not unsaturated fatty acids. This conclusion follows from the fact that exogenous radiolabeled palmitic and oleic acids are biosynthetically incorporated into the membrane glycerolipids of this organism at comparable rates; thus, the preponderance of saturated fatty acids in unsupplemented cells must arise primarily from endogenous sources. This suggestion was later confirmed by other studies (discussed below).

McElhaney and Tourtellotte (63), using a lipid-poor growth medium, later showed that not only exogenous saturated and unsaturated fatty acids but also elaidic, isopalmitic, and dihydrosterculic acids can be incorporated into the *A. laidlawii* B membrane lipids. Moreover, under growth conditions designed to maximize exogenous fatty acid incorporation, the levels of exogenous fatty acid in the membrane can reach 60 to 80 mol%. Since these rather drastic alterations in fatty acid composition in most cases do not adversely affect the viability of this organism, these workers concluded that membrane structure and function are not critically dependent on the specific chemical structure of the lipid hydrocarbon chains, a conclusion later supported by a variety of other studies (see chapters 8 and 15). The increased ability to alter membrane lipid fatty acid composition in a predictable fashion by incorporation of large amounts of a wide range of fatty acid types further enhanced the suitability of *A. laidlawii* B for studies of the roles of membrane lipids in biological membranes (see references 60 and 61).

Romijn et al. (110) subsequently studied the fatty acid composition of the total membrane lipids and of the phosphatidylglycerol (PG) from *A. laidlawii* B and their relationship to the permeability of intact cells of this organism. In these experiments, cells were grown in the presence of equimolar mixtures of palmitic or stearic acid and either elaidic, oleic, linoleic, or arachidonic acid. Although the fatty acid composition of both the total membrane lipids and PG reflects the exogenous fatty acid composition and varies roughly in parallel, the PG was generally found to be more highly enriched in the two exogenous fatty acids and to contain fewer endogenous saturated fatty acids than did the total lipid fraction. This finding suggests that the neutral glycolipids, monoglucosyl diglyceride (MGDG) and diglucosyl diglyceride (DGDG), the other major membrane lipids in this organism, must be enriched in endogenous saturated fatty acids, particularly of shorter chain length, compared with PG, a suggestion later confirmed experimentally (see below). In both fractions, decreasing amounts of exogenous unsaturated fatty acids are incorporated in the order elaidic > oleic > linoleic > linolenic > arachidonic acid, and this decrease is counterbalanced primarily by an increased uptake of exogenous saturated fatty acid. Since the order of decrease in the uptake of the exogenous unsaturated fatty acids parallels their increasing degree of unsaturation and thus their decreasing melting temperatures, the increase in the saturated/unsaturated fatty acid ratio observed with the decreasing melting points of the unsaturated fatty acids appears to be compensatory. However, this compensatory regulation of membrane fluidity is not complete, since the passive permeability of intact cells still increases with the degree of unsaturation of the exogenous fatty acid, although to a lesser extent than when equal amounts of saturated and unsaturated fatty acids are incorporated (62). Moreover, subsequent calorimetric studies demonstrated that the gel-to-liquid-crystalline phase transition temperature also continues to decrease as the degree of unsaturation of the exogenous fatty acid increases (58). Thus, this organism can only poorly regulate the phase state and fluidity of its membrane lipids by alterations in the degree of incorporation of exogenous fatty acids.

Saito and McElhaney (128) later studied the incorporation of homologous series of exogenous saturated, methyl iso- and anteiso-branched, and cis- and trans-monounsaturated fatty acids, as well as selected cis- and trans-cyclopropane and cis-polyunsaturated fatty acids, into the total membrane lipid fraction and into the individual polar lipids of A. laidlawii B cells. Within each homologous series of fatty acids, the extent of incorporation increases markedly with increasing chain length, reaches a maximum, and then declines progressively but less sharply with further increases in chain length. The chain length giving optimal incorporation is 15 for the linear saturated, 16 for the methyl iso-branched, 17 for the methyl anteiso-branched and trans-monounsaturated, and 18 for the cis-monounsaturated fatty acids, so that the optimal chain length for incorporation increases as the melting point of the exogenous fatty acid decreases. Again, this can be viewed as a potential compensatory regulatory mechanism, although not a very effective one, since the phase transition temperature of the membrane lipid varies markedly with changes in fatty acid composition (see chapter 8). In terms of the effect of fatty acid structure on the maximum extent of incorporation, the highest levels of enrichment (>80 mol%) are obtained with the methyl iso- and anteiso-branched and trans-unsaturated fatty acids, with levels of enrichment somewhat lower for the linear saturated and lower still for the cis-monounsaturated fatty acids. As reported earlier by Romijn et al. (110), the maximum levels of incorporation progressively decline with the number of double bonds in the unsaturated fatty acids. With the exception of the cis- and trans-cyclopropane fatty acids tested, which are incorporated to a smaller extent than are their corresponding lower melting cis- and trans-monounsaturated analogs, the degree of incorporation appears to be maximal with intermediate-melting-point fatty acids and to decline as the melting point increases or decreases.

Saito and McElhaney (128) also observed that the fatty acid compositions of the individual polar lipid fractions differ to some extent from one another. When cells are grown without exogenous fatty acid supplementation so that >90 mol% of the fatty acids are endogenous saturated fatty acids, the phosphatides PG and O-amino acid esters of PG (O-PG) are relatively enriched in palmitate and stearate, while the neutral glycolipids MGDG and DGDG are enriched in myristate and lauric acid. Moreover, the phosphorylated glycolipid, glycerylphosphoryldiglucosyl diglyceride (GPDGDG), is even more enriched in short-chain saturates, with the level of lauric acid being markedly elevated and the level of stearic acid markedly repressed. Interestingly, since the gel-to-liquid-crystalline phase transition temperatures of MGDG and DGDG are greater than that of PG when their fatty acid compositions are similar (133), these characteristic differences in fatty acid composition can be viewed as compensatory in that they minimize intrinsic differences in phase transition temperatures, thus producing a more physicochemically homogeneous mixture of membrane lipids than would result from a nonspecific incorporation of fatty acids into the various polar lipid fractions. Moreover, these characteristic differences in fatty acid composition between the GPDGDG, the MGDG-DGDG, and the PG–O-PG fractions are usually maintained when various exogenous fatty acids are added to the growth medium. The unique fatty composition of the GPDGDG, with its markedly elevated levels of short-chain saturated fatty acids and markedly depressed levels of exogenous fatty acid, has also been observed by de Kruyff et al. (27) for elaidic acid-enriched A. laidlawii B membranes. As well, Panos and Henrikson (69) have reported that when cultured in palmitelaidic acid, the MGDG of Acholeplasma sp. strain KHS is also relatively enriched in endogenous saturated fatty acids, particularly of shorter chain lengths, and depleted in palmitelaidic acid compared with the phospholipid fraction.

Silvius and McElhaney (134) and Silvius et al. (133) subsequently studied the fatty acid requirements for the growth of A. laidlawii B rendered totally fatty acid auxotropic by the addition of avidin to a complex but lipid-extracted growth medium. Avidin functions by irreversibly binding all of the biotin present in the growth medium. Since biotin is required as a prosthetic group for the enzyme acetyl coenzyme A (acetyl-CoA) carboxylase, which catalyzes the first committed step in de novo fatty acid biosynthesis, cells grown in the presence of avidin are unable to synthesize their normal spectrum of linear saturated fatty acids or to carry out the chain elongation of certain exogenous fatty acids. Cells cultured with avidin grow only when one or more exogenous medium- or long-chain fatty acids are added to the growth medium, and the membrane lipids produced by these cells contain essentially (usually >97 mol%) only the fatty acid or acids added. These workers found that of the single exogenous fatty acids tested, a variety of different fatty acid classes produce normal growth, including certain linear saturated, methyl iso- and anteiso-branched, and *trans*-monounsaturated and *trans*-cyclopropane fatty acids. Subsequent unpublished work has shown that certain dimethyl iso-branched (ω-tertiary butyl) and ω-cyclohexyl fatty acids, as well as the all-*trans* form of linoleic acid, also support good growth. In contrast, naturally occurring *cis*-monounsaturated or *cis*-cyclopropane fatty acids, as well as all of the *cis*-polyunsaturated fatty acids tested, support markedly reduced or no growth. As well, although very short (<14-carbon) or very long (>19-carbon) fatty acids do not support growth, the range of chain lengths supporting normal growth varies markedly within the various fatty acid classes. For example, in the linear saturated fatty acid series, only pentadecanoic acid supports good growth; growth-supporting ability decreases progressively but markedly with decreasing chain length, with lauric acid being totally ineffective. Increasing the chain length only slightly results in a complete loss of growth-supporting ability, so that palmitic acid is completely ineffective. Interestingly, the range of growth-supporting chain lengths for the *trans*-monounsaturated and *trans*-cyclopropane fatty acids is wider (about three carbon atoms) and is wider still for the branched-chain and ω-cyclohexyl fatty acids (four or five members of these homologous series can support good growth). All of these growth data can be explained by the finding that high-melting-point fatty acids, which produce predominantly gel-state membrane lipids at the growth temperature, and low-melting-point fatty acids, which produce hyperfluid liquid-crystalline bilayers, do not support growth and that the hydrocarbon core of the membrane lipid bilayer of this organism must be neither too thin nor too thick (see chapter 15 for a more detailed discussion). This interpretation is supported by the finding that equimolar binary mixtures of a high-melting-point and a low-melting-point fatty acid, such as palmitate and oleate, will support good growth, whereas mixtures of two high-melting-point or two low-melting-point fatty acids will not. A similar result is seen when binary mixtures of short-chain and long-chain fatty acids are tested. Of course, the ability to produce fatty acid-homogeneous membranes, exhibiting a wide range of membrane lipid phase transition temperatures and cooperativities as well as a range of bilayer thicknesses, further enhances the suitability of this organism for membrane lipid structural and functional studies (see chapters 8 and 15, respectively).

A particularly striking illustration of the relationship between the melting properties of a series of fatty acids and their growth-promoting abilities in *A. laidlawii* B is provided by Silvius and McElhaney's study of a series of *cis*-octadecanoic acids in which the position of the double bond within the hydrocarbon chain is systematically varied (134). These workers found that *cis*-octadecanoates with double bonds at positions 4 and 15 support the best growth, whereas moving the double bond toward either end or toward the middle of the hydrocarbon chain results in a progressive loss of growth-promoting ability. These results can be explained readily if one assumes that only *cis*-octadecanoates with intermediate melting points support good growth. Since a plot of the melting points of these *cis*-octadecanoates versus the position of the double is U shaped, it is precisely those *cis*-octadeca-

noates with double bonds about halfway between the carbonyl group or the methyl terminus and the chain center that fulfill this criterion. Octadecanoates with the *cis*-double bond near either end of the hydrocarbon chain behave essentially as saturated fatty acids and would produce membranes whose lipids would be predominantly in the gel state at the growth temperature, whereas a fatty acid with the *cis*-double bond near the center of the chain, like oleic acid, has a very low melting point and would produce a hyperfluid lipid bilayer. Again, support for this conclusion is provided by the results of the appropriate mixing experiments, which show that binary mixtures of high- and low-melting-point *cis*-octadecanoates will generally support good growth. These studies also demonstrate not only that this organism has no intrinsic unsaturated fatty acid requirement but also that in the absence of a capacity for saturated fatty acid biosynthesis, many unsaturated fatty acids alone cannot support cell growth.

The fatty acid growth requirements of *A. laidlawii* A have been studied by Panos and Rottem (71, 119) and by Panos and Leon (70). These workers found that strain A, unlike strain B, requires an exogenous long-chain unsaturated fatty acid when cultured in a complex but lipid-extracted growth medium, as previously reported by Razin and Rottem (90). However, elaidic and *trans*-vaccenic acids were found to support greater growth than did either oleic acid or its positional isomer, *cis*-vaccenic acid. The cyclopropane ring-containing fatty acids dihydrosterculic acid and lactobacillic acid also promote growth but exhibit a greater toxicity at higher concentrations in the medium and a lower growth response. Interestingly, shorter-chain *cis*-monounsaturated fatty acids cannot replace the growth requirement for octadecenoic acid, despite the fact that they are biosynthetically incorporated into the membrane glycerolipids after some degree of chain elongation. However, the shorter-chain cyclopropane fatty acid *cis*-9,10-methylene hexadecanoate is as effective as its longer-chain homologs. In contrast to strain B, the phospho- and glycolipid fractions exhibit virtually identical fatty acid compositions. However, since the phospholipid fraction also contains GPDGDG, it is possible that the fatty acid compositions of the individual phospho- and glycolipids are not the same. Interestingly, these results generally parallel those reported by Silvius and McElhaney (134) for *A. laidlawii* B, since only *trans*-unsaturated fatty acids support growth in the absence of saturated fatty acid synthesis, and when paired with equimolar amounts of a saturated fatty acid, *cis*-monounsaturated fatty acids support better growth than do the analogous *cis*-cyclopropane fatty acids.

Wieslander and Selstam (168) have recently studied the growth of *A. laidlawii* A cells supplemented with palmitic acid or with various unsaturated fatty acids in the presence and absence of cholesterol. In the absence of exogenous cholesterol, growth yields decrease in the order palmitic > oleic > linoleic acid and no growth occurs in the linolenic acid-supplemented medium. However, the addition of cholesterol increases growth yields in linoleic acid-supplemented cells and permits some growth to occur in the linolenic acid-supplemented medium. Thus, in the highly unsaturated linoleic or linolenic acid-enriched growth medium, *A. laidlawii* A becomes dependent on cholesterol for optimal growth or for any growth at all, respectively. These workers attribute the growth-promoting effects of cholesterol molecules in these highly unsaturated membranes to their well-known ability to increase the orientational order and closeness of packing of the lipid hydrocarbon chains in model membranes and in *A. laidlawii* B membranes (see chapter 8). Whether or not the level of cholesterol incorporation affects the fatty acid growth requirements of the sterol-requiring mycoplasmas has not been rigorously determined but is a distinct possibility that should be investigated.

Leaver et al. (52) have shown that *A. laidlawii* A can be grown on media containing synthetic conjugated diacetylenic fatty acids instead of the conventional unsaturated fatty acids. Although growth is poor on the C_{23} diacetylenic acid tested, growth is good on its C_{20} analog, and as much as 90% of the fatty acyl groups of the membrane lipid consist of the exogenous shorter-chain diacetylenic fatty acid. Because these diacetylenic fatty acids form chemical cross-links with one another when irradiated with UV light, the lipid bilayer of the membrane of this organism can be converted to a conjugated polymeric structure in which essentially all of the fatty acyl chain-containing lipids are covalently associated with one another. Since the physical properties of the lipid bilayer will obviously be altered by such polymerization, this technique can be used to study lipid-protein interactions in the membrane. In fact, these workers reported that the activity of NADH oxidase, an intrinsic membrane-bound enzyme in this organism, decreases upon lipid bilayer polymerization, whereas the activity of RNase, an extrinsic membrane-bound enzyme, is not affected.

Liss et al. (56) have studied the cytotoxic and cytolytic activities of nonadecafluoro-*n*-decanoic acid (NDFDA) on *A. laidlawii* JA1 grown with different serum supplements. When grown in medium supplemented with PPLO serum fraction, this organism is rapidly killed by low concentrations (<1.0 mM) of NDFDA, but higher concentrations (>10 mM) are required to lyse cells. When grown in medium supplemented with horse serum, however, cells are killed and lysed at the same high NDFDA concentration (>10 mM). These workers concluded that this perfluorinated fatty acid can be cytotoxic and cytolytic to mycoplasmas just as to eucaryotic cells and suggested that NDFDA probably interacts primarily with the membrane of these cells. Although much more work will be required to confirm this latter suggestion and to determine whether NDFDA is incorporated into the membrane lipids, this use of *A. laidlawii* as a model system for evaluating the potential cytotoxic or cytolytic effects of suspected animal or plant toxicants which may act on cell membranes is novel and interesting.

The fatty acid growth requirements of the sterol-requiring mycoplasmas have generally been studied in much less detail than have those of the sterol-nonrequiring *Acholeplasma* species, with the exception of the rigorous studies of Rodwell and coworkers on *Mycoplasma* strain Y (closely related in *Mycoplasma mycoides*) described below. With only one reported exception, none of the *Mycoplasma*, *Ureaplasma*, or *Spiroplasma* species studied are able to synthesize sat-

urated or unsaturated fatty acids or to elongate or otherwise modify exogenous fatty acids (see later discussion). These organisms are thus fatty acid auxotrophic and are typically grown in a mixture of saturated and unsaturated fatty acids, usually palmitate and oleate.

The initial studies of Rodwell (99) of the fatty acid requirements of *Mycoplasma* strain Y in a complex medium suggested that only oleic acid is required for growth. However, a subsequent study by Rodwell and Abbott (106), using a partially defined medium, clearly showed that both a saturated and an unsaturated fatty acid are required for optimal growth. The requirement for a saturated fatty acid can be met equally well with palmitic, margaric, or stearic acid; myristic acid produces a similar yield of cells but the growth rate is slower, while lauric acid is considerably less effective in supporting growth. When grown in the presence of palmitate, oleic acid is most effective in promoting growth, followed by linolenic and linoleic acids. Organisms incubated in a medium deficient in exogenous fatty acids die rapidly, and death is accompanied by cell lysis. These workers postulated that exogenous long-chain fatty acids are required for the synthesis of an undetermined cell component (presumably membrane phospholipids) necessary for the structural integrity of the cell, a suggestion later confirmed by other studies.

In further studies using a partly defined medium, Rodwell (101, 102, 104) showed that the chain length and the position and geometrical configuration of the double bond in the exogenous monounsaturated fatty acid all influence the range of saturated fatty acids supporting good growth of *Mycoplasma* strain Y. Elaidic acid is unique among the saturated and unsaturated acids tested in that good growth is obtained in the absence of other exogenous fatty acids. Moreover, under these conditions, membranes whose lipids are essentially homogeneous in elaidic acid can be obtained. However, when elaidic acid is paired with saturated fatty acids of intermediate chain length or with oleic acid, both fatty acids are incorporated in equal proportions throughout the growth cycle. On the other hand, when grown with elaidic acid plus either a short-chain or long-chain saturated fatty acid, elaidate is incorporated preferentially during the early stages of growth and the saturated fatty acids are incorporated during the later stages of growth. This finding was attributed to a competition between the two fatty acids for binding to the bovine serum albumin required to detoxify the exogenous fatty acids rather than to an intrinsic change in the specificity of the enzymes involved in the biosynthetic incorporation of exogenous fatty acids into the membrane lipids with age.

Rodwell and Peterson (107) later showed that elaidic acid is not the only single exogenous fatty acid that can support the growth of *Mycoplasma* strain Y. When cultured at 37°C in a lipid-poor growth medium containing exogenous cholesterol plus one of a large number of exogenous fatty acids, this organism grows well in the presence of several different classes of fatty acids. Specifically, two *trans*-monounsaturated fatty acids (elaidate and *trans*-vaccenate), two methyl iso-branched fatty acids (isopalmitate and isostearate), a methyl anteiso-branched fatty acid of moderate chain length (anteisoheptadecanoate), and a few positional isomers of oleic acid support growth. Straight-chain saturated fatty acids or naturally occurring cis-unsaturated fatty acids do not support growth alone, nor do short-chain or long-chain trans-unsaturated or branched-chain fatty acids. However, binary combinations of a high-melting-point fatty acid (such as palmitate) with a low-melting-point fatty acid (such as oleate), or of a long-chain saturated fatty acid with a short-chain saturated fatty acid, do support good growth. The correspondence between these results and those of studies of the growth of fatty acid-auxotrophic A. laidlawii by Silvius and McElhaney (134) discussed earlier is striking. Almost all of the results of Rodwell and Peterson can be explained by postulating that even in the presence of cholesterol, Mycoplasma strain Y, like A. laidlawii B, requires fatty acids which will produce a liquid-crystalline bilayer of moderate fluidity and thickness for proper membrane function and normal cell growth to occur.

Le Grimellec et al. (53) studied both the exogenous fatty acid growth requirements of and the degree of incorporation of various exogenous fatty acids into M. gallisepticum grown with both high and low amounts of exogenous cholesterol. In cholesterol-enriched cells, supplementation with myristic, palmitic, or stearic acid alone results in good growth, with palmitate being most effective. In fact, palmitic acid-supplemented cells were reported to support a higher degree of cell growth than was observed for cells grown on an equimolar mixture of palmitate and oleate! Palmitelaidic and oleic acids are comparable but less effective in promoting the growth of this organism, with palmitoleic acid being least effective (elaidic acid was not tested). In cholesterol-depleted cells, growth yields are generally lower, but similar results were obtained with the narrower range of exogenous fatty acids tested, except that in this case elaidic acid supports a higher level of growth than does oleic acid. Although these results appear to be somewhat at variance with those obtained with strain Y in that a wider range of single exogenous fatty acids support good growth, it should be noted that the growth medium used by Le Grimellec and coworkers was not lipid extracted and therefore contained appreciable exogenous palmitic, stearate, oleic, and linoleic acids. Thus, the maximum incorporation of the various single exogenous fatty acids tested ranged between only 50 and 70 mol%, as opposed to the >95 mol% observed in Mycoplasma strain Y. The fact that cells enriched in a single exogenous saturated fatty acid still contain appreciable amounts of exogenous unsaturated fatty acids and vice versa would clearly result in less stringent fatty acid growth requirements. Although an estimate of the relative extents of incorporation of the single exogenous fatty acids added to the growth medium is complicated by the relatively high levels of residual exogenous fatty acid in the growth medium, it appears that the efficiency of incorporation into the membrane polar lipids decreases in the order elaidic > palmitic > stearic > oleic acids. Interestingly, a very similar order is generally observed for the magnitude of incorporation of single exogenous fatty acids into the A. laidlawii B membrane lipids in cells capable of de novo saturated fatty acid biosynthesis, except that oleic

acid is usually incorporated more efficiently than is stearic acid (58, 63, 128).

There have been several attempts to study the fatty acid growth requirements of some of the more nutritionally fastidious Mycoplasma species, such as that by Gadir et al. (35) on three strains of bovine mycoplasma and that of Leon and Panos (55) on M. pneumoniae. However, in these and similar studies, growth media containing residual sources of fatty acids were used and the exogenous fatty acids were added without bovine serum albumin or detergents to detoxify them. Under these conditions, the addition of at least some exogenous fatty acids actually inhibited cell growth and even caused the lysis of cells in the inoculum. Under these conditions, a definitive determination of the intrinsic fatty acid growth requirements of these organisms is not possible, and the results of these studies will not be discussed further.

Although Rottem and Razin (124) did not study the fatty acid growth requirements of M. hominis, they did observe that this organism exhibits a marked preference for the incorporation of exogenous palmitic (and apparently also stearic) acid over oleic acid and a marked discrimination against the incorporation of exogenous linoleic acid in the membrane polar lipids. This observation contrasts with the results usually obtained with A. laidlawii, M. capricolum, and M. gallisepticum, in which roughly equal amounts of palmitic and oleic acids are incorporated. Rottem and Greenberg (115) later presented evidence that the enzymatic basis of this unusual preference for saturated fatty acids may reside in the slight and marked preferences, respectively, of the M. hominis acyl-CoA synthetase and acyl-CoA:α-glycerophosphate transacylase for palmitic acid and palmitoyl-CoA over oleic acid and oleoyl-CoA. Interestingly, in A. laidlawii, this latter enzyme actually has a slight preference for oleoyl-CoA over palmitoyl-CoA, adding support to this suggestion.

Freeman et al. (34) and Mudd et al. (67) have published some preliminary studies of the fatty acid growth requirements of Spiroplasma citri and of the biosynthetic incorporation of various exogenous fatty acids into the membrane lipids of this organism. Unfortunately, their use of the detergent Tween 80, which can liberate free fatty acids (primarily oleate) upon hydrolysis by extracellular lipases, prevented a rigorous determination of the fatty acid requirements of this organism. However, the fact that exogenous palmitic acid increases growth in the presence of Tween 80, and that oleic, linoleic, or linolenic acid cannot fully substitute for palmitate, suggests that both an exogenous saturated and an unsaturated fatty acid are required for optimal growth. When grown in the presence of sera, S. citri preferentially incorporates palmitic, and to a lesser extent oleic, acid and discriminates against linoleic acid, while stearic acid is present in the membrane lipids in about the same relative proportion as in the growth medium.

More recently, Chang and Chen (12) and Chang (11) used a chemically defined medium to investigate the fatty acid growth requirements of two flower spiroplasmas, including S. floricola, and a honey bee spiroplasma. Initial studies indicated that exogenous oleic acid is essential for the growth of all three spiroplasma species and that exogenous palmitic acid markedly increases growth. Subsequently, the abilities of other saturated and unsaturated fatty acids to replace palmitic and oleic acid, respectively, were studied. In the two flower spiroplasmas, lauric, myristic, or stearic acid can, to some extent, replace palmitic acid, although the best growth continued to be observed in the palmitate-oleate combination. In one of these species the myristate-oleate, and in another the stearate-oleate, combination is the next-most-effective combination. However, in the honey bee spiroplasma, the laurate-oleate and myristate-oleate combinations are slightly more effective than the palmitate-oleate combination. Similarly, in the two flower spiroplasmas, palmitoleic, linoleic, or linolenic acid can replace oleic acid, but again the palmitate-oleate combination produces the best growth. In both of these flower spiroplasmas, the palmitic acid-linoleate combination is the next most effective in promoting growth and the palmitate-linolenate combination is least effective. In contrast, the palmitate-palmitoleate combination is clearly the most effective in promoting the growth of the honey bee spiroplasma and the palmitate-oleate and palmitate-linoleate combinations are next, with the palmitate-linolenate combination again being least effective. Thus, although in general combinations of saturated fatty acids of medium chain length and unsaturated fatty acids containing one or two double bonds are most effective, the fatty acid requirements for optimal growth seem to vary somewhat among these three spiroplasma species.

Dahl and coworkers (21, 22, 24) have studied the mechanism of exogenous fatty acid uptake in *M. capricolum* and its relationship to the growth and sterol content of the cell membrane of this organism. They found that in *M. capricolum*, lipid, protein, and RNA are synthesed essentially synchronously during growth and that optimal growth depends on the presence of at least small amounts of exogenous cholesterol. However, increasing the exogenous fatty acid concentration in the growth medium can at least partially restore growth even in the absence of small amounts of exogenous cholesterol. Studies of the kinetics of exogenous fatty acid incorporation into the membrane phospholipids revealed that this process is protein mediated, since it exhibits saturation, is energy dependent, and can be blocked by certain sulfhydryl group inhibitors. Moreover, fatty acid transport and activation appear to be tightly coupled to phospholipid synthesis, since there is little accumulation of free fatty acids or acyl-CoA, and since fatty acid uptake requires the presence of glycerol, a precursor for phospholipid biosynthesis in this organism. Interestingly, the presence of small amounts of cholesterol necessary for optimal growth decreases the K_m and increases the V_{max} for oleic or elaidic acid incorporation but has no effect on the K_m or V_{max} for palmitic acid uptake. However, the incorporation of exogenous egg phosphatidylcholine (PC) in place of cholesterol can restore growth as well as RNA and protein synthesis without stimulating endogenous phospholipid biosynthesis. These workers therefore concluded that small amounts of cholesterol are required by *M. capricolum* to stimulate the uptake of the exogenous unsaturated fatty acids required for the synthesis of the unsaturated phospholipids, which are in turn necessary to support protein and RNA synthesis and optimal cell growth. The question of whether small amounts of cholesterol stimulate the transport of unsaturated fatty acid across the membrane, their biochemical activation in the cytoplasm, or the biosynthetic incorporation of the activated fatty acids into phospholipids remains to be answered. However, this very interesting work illustrates well the complexities of fatty acid incorporation and its sometimes subtle relationships to growth and overall cellular metabolism.

Acetate, Glycerol, Glucose, and P_i

It is well established that acetate is utilized by *A. laidlawii* for the biosynthesis of saturated fatty acids, for the chain elongation of exogenous fatty acids, and for the biosynthesis of carotenoids (see below). Thus, the provision of radioactive acetate in the growth medium is a convenient, albeit less specific, way of radiolabeling these compounds in growing cells of this organism (112). Of course, radioactive acetate will not be incorporated into the membrane lipid fraction of the sterol-requiring *Mycoplasma* species, since they are incapable of synthesizing fatty acids or carotenoids (112).

In principle, the acetate required by *A. laidlawii* for fatty acid and carotenoid synthesis can be supplied exogenously or can be derived from the glycolysis of sugars such as glucose. In fact, the work of McElhaney and Tourtellotte (65) strongly suggests that radioactivity derived from exogenous radiolabeled glucose can be found in both the glycerol and fatty acid moieties of the phospho- and glycolipids of the *A. laidlawii* B membrane. However, Tourtellotte et al. (162) reported that in their defined medium, optimal growth of this organism requires either a mixture of five exogenous fatty acids or exogenous acetate plus Tween 80 as a source of oleic acid (41), implying that exogenous acetate is required for optimal rates of endogenous fatty acid biosynthesis to be maintained. However, Razin and Cohen (86) reported that the addition of exogenous acetate to their minimal defined medium for *A. laidlawii* strains does not improve cell growth. Therefore, the question of whether exogenous acetate is an actual growth requirement for *A. laidlawii* and related organisms, at least in the absence of exogenous fatty acids, seems to be an open one, despite the fact that the rate of production of acetate from glucose would seem to be more than sufficient to furnish the acetate required for fatty acid and carotenoid biosynthesis.

Glycerol has been shown by Rodwell and Abbott (106) to be a specific growth requirement for *M. mycoides* Y and for *M. capricolum* and is expected to be required by all nonfermentative mycoplasma species or by fermentative strains that may lack NAD-linked glycerol phosphate dehydrogenase activity. This enzyme is required for the synthesis of glycerol 3-phosphate from the dehydroxyacetone phosphate produced during glycolysis, the former compound being the initial precursor for the biosynthesis of all the glycerophospho- and glyceroglycolipids found in the mycoplasma membrane (see below). Thus radioactive glycerol added to the growth medium has been shown to be biosynthetically incorporated not only into the neutral and polar lipid fractions of *M. mycoides* (73) and *Mycoplasma* strain Y (75) but also into the membrane lipids of other sterol-requiring species such as

M. pneumoniae (74, 79) and a *Ureaplasma* species (109) and of the sterol-nonrequiring *Anaeroplasma axanthum* (76). Moreover, Dahl (21) has shown that glycerol is specifically required for fatty acid uptake and phospholipid biosynthesis in *M. capricolum*. Presumably, all of the above-named mycoplasma species must possess an active glycerol kinase in order to convert exogenous glycerol to glycerol 3-phosphate. In contrast, the fermentative, sterol-nonrequiring *A. laidlawii* strains and the nonfermentative, sterol-requiring *M. hominis* do not incorporate exogenous radiolabeled glycerol into their membrane lipids (112), presumably because they lack an active glycerol kinase.

Although glucose is usually considered an essential growth requirement for fermentative mycoplasmas because of its central role in energy metabolism, it seems certain that this and possibly other sugars also function as essential precursors in the biosynthesis of the glycolipids found in most mycoplasma species. The fact that the glycolipids of *A. laidlawii* (65), *M. mycoides* (73), and *M. pneumoniae* (74) are more heavily radiolabeled than are the phospholipids when these organisms are cultured in radioactive glucose indicates that this sugar has been directly incorporated into the polar headgroups of the glycolipids. However, since some radioactivity is also present in the phospholipid fractions, glucose must label the glycerol moieties of all of the glycerolipids as well, through its conversion via glycolysis to glycerol 3-phosphate. In addition, in *A. laidlawii*, some of the glucose-derived radioactivity is found in the endogenous saturated fatty acyl groups of both the glyco- and phospholipids, since glucose gives rise to the acetate utilized in de novo fatty acid biosynthesis (see below). Thus, radiolabeled sugars, while often useful in lipid analytical and metabolic studies, are not specific labels of the glycolipid polar headgroups, at least in fermentative mycoplasma species. In contrast, radioactive P_i salts are useful and specific radiolabeling agents for the phosphate portions of the polar headgroups of the phosphatides and phosphoglycolipids of all mycoplasma species studied to date (see below).

Sterols

Cholesterol and related sterols are generally found only in eucaryotes, in which they appear to play an essential structural role in the plasma membrane and may serve other specific metabolic and regulatory functions (see Yeagle [169] and Dahl and Dahl [19], respectively, for comprehensive reviews). Although some eubacteria and their derived L forms can incorporate exogenous cholesterol into their inner membranes, these organisms neither synthesize sterols nor require them for growth (29, 82, 94). In contrast, many mycoplasma species are unique among the procaryotes in having an absolute growth requirement for cholesterol, just as found in the eucaryotes. Specifically, members of the genera *Mycoplasma* (28, 29, 35, 96, 100, 106, 158), *Ureaplasma* (121), and *Spiroplasma* (11, 12, 26, 34, 67) require exogenous cholesterol for growth and incorporate substantial quantities of this or a closely related sterol into their plasma membranes (see chapter 6). The sterol-nonrequiring *Acholeplasma* species (86, 88, 111) are also capable of incorporating

exogenous cholesterol into their plasma membranes, although generally in smaller amounts. Not only is cholesterol not required by *A. laidlawii* A or B, but exogenous cholesterol normally does not stimulate growth (88, 95, 168; but see reference 9). None of the mycoplasmas studied to date, including the sterol-nonrequiring species, is capable of cholesterol synthesis, and the cholesterol incorporated from the growth medium is usually not esterified or otherwise chemically modified (see below). Certain *Mycoplasma* species also incorporate exogenous cholesterol esters into their plasma membranes, but the *Acholeplasma* species do not (see 92).

The specificity of the sterol requirement of mycoplasmas (3, 30, 35, 100, 101, 140, 142, 158), ureaplasmas (121), and spiroplasmas (11, 12, 34, 67) has been investigated in considerable detail by a number of workers. Although some variation among species is observed, in general most structural alterations in the cholesterol molecule result in a decrease in its ability to support cell growth. Specifically, changing the configuration of the hydroxyl group at C-3 of ring A from β to α, converting the β-hydroxyl group to an ester, or replacing the β-hydroxyl group with a keto group results in loss of the ability of the sterol to support growth. Although the degree of unsaturation of the ring system is of secondary importance, cholesterol is more effective at supporting growth than are its fully saturated or multiply unsaturated analogs. Moreover, sterols with nonplanar ring systems are ineffective as growth promoters, as are sterols which lack an aliphatic side chain. Although in none of the studies just summarized were the effects of these structural variations on membrane lipid fluidity and phase state determined, it is significant to note that the structural features required for cell growth, namely, a planar sterol nucleus with a free hydroxyl at the 3β position and a hydrocarbon side chain, are precisely those required for the sterol to exert its maximum effect on ordering the lipid hydrocarbon chains and on reducing the permeability of liquid-crystalline model and biological membranes (169). This good correlation provides strong support for the idea that one of the major roles of sterols in biological membranes is to regulate the fluidity and phase state of the lipid bilayer. The effects of cholesterol and other sterols on the structure and function of mycoplasma membranes are reviewed in chapters 8 and 15, respectively.

It appears that *M. capricolum* is much less specific in its sterol requirements than are the other sterol-requiring mycoplasmas studied to date. For example, Odriozola et al. (68) and Lala et al. (51) report that the sterol requirements of this organism can be met by a variety of sterols and sterol esters or ethers, all of which lack one or more of the structural attributes which seem necessary to support the growth of the other sterol-requiring mycoplasma species. Moreover, Kannenberg and Poralla (49) found that even a hopanoid, a member of the group of bacterial pentacyclic triterpenoids which appear to function similarly to cholesterol, can support the moderate growth of this organism. In contrast, Archer (3) has shown that a free β-hydroxyl group at C-3 of ring A is a strict structural requirement for sterols to support significant growth of the closely related *M. mycoides* subsp. *capri*. It has been suggested that the broad sterol specificity of *M.*

capricolum may be associated with its ability to grow with low concentrations of exogenous cholesterol (89). However, *M. mycoides* (3, 127) and *M. gallisepticum* (53) can also be adapted to grow with relatively low cholesterol levels in the growth medium, yet these organisms appear to have much more stringent sterol structural requirements for growth. A possible resolution to this apparent discrepancy in results may be found in the work of Dahl et al. (23) and Lelong et al. (54), who demonstrated that very small amounts of cholesterol can support reasonably good growth of *M. capricolum* in the presence of larger amounts of lanosterol or 7β-hydroxycholesterol, sterols which when present alone either do not support growth or can even inhibit growth when present at high concentrations. These workers suggest that small amounts of cholesterol, or of a closely related sterol, are required for specific metabolic and regulatory processes in this organism, whereas other less structurally related sterols can fulfill at least some of the physiochemical roles played by cholesterol in the lipid bilayer (for a further discussion, see chapter 8). Thus, the unrecognized presence of trace amounts of cholesterol in the growth medium, insufficient on its own to support normal growth, could explain the surprisingly broad sterol specificity observed by Odriozola et al. (68) and Lala et al. (51), since small amounts of cholesterol and larger amounts of other sterols can act synergistically to support the growth of this organism.

Although it seems clear that *A. laidlawii* strains do not require cholesterol for optimal growth under most conditions, there may be special circumstances under which these normally sterol-nonrequiring organisms do require exogenous cholesterol or other sterols. As discussed earlier, Wieslander and Selstam (168) have reported that in growth medium enriched in the highly unsaturated linoleic or linolenic acid, *A. laidlawii* A requires exogenous cholesterol for optimal growth, whereas this is not true when this organism is grown in the presence of palmitic or oleic acid. Moreover, Rilfors et al. (98) have found that epicoprostanol, cholest-4-en-3-one, and cholest-5-en-3-one stimulate the growth of this same organism when cells are enriched in saturated fatty acids but actually cause the lysis of cells enriched in unsaturated fatty acids. In these cases, the sterol seems to optimize growth by reducing the fluidity of the highly fluid polyunsaturated fatty acid-enriched membranes or by increasing the fluidity of the rather rigid saturated fatty acid-enriched membranes (see chapter 15). In addition, Smith and Henrikson (153) have reported that exogenous cholesterol can at least partially reverse the inhibition of the growth of *A. laidlawii* B caused by inhibitors of carotenoid biosynthesis. Finally, Butler and Knight (9) found that exogenous cholesterol is required for the growth of *A. laidlawii* A and B in certain growth media but not in others, and these workers suggested that cholesterol might promote growth indirectly by detoxifying fatty acids or other compounds present in some of their undefined growth media, rather than by serving directly as an intrinsic growth requirement. These studies illustrate well the complex interactions that can occur between an organism and its chemical and physical environment and the resulting difficulty in unambiguously establishing the growth requirements of microorganisms which require a complex medium for growth.

Serum lipoproteins presumably serve not only as the natural source of cholesterol for the sterol-requiring mycoplasma species found in animals but also as the major cholesterol donors for all mycoplasma species grown in complex, serum-containing media. Slutzky et al. (136–138) have studied the uptake of cholesterol from purified human serum lipoproteins and cholesterol-PC vesicles by the sterol-requiring *M. hominis* and the sterol-nonrequiring *A. laidlawii*. Under similar growth conditions, *M. hominis* incorporates about three times more free cholesterol into its plasma membrane than does *A. laidlawii*. The low-density lipoprotein (LDL) serves as a better cholesterol donor than does the high-density lipoprotein (HDL) in both organisms, in that considerably more cholesterol is incorporated into growing cells and isolated membranes, although in *A. laidlawii*, the rate of cholesterol uptake is the same for both LDL and HDL. Interestingly, the very low density lipoprotein actually inhibits the growth of both organisms (but not the growth of *M. capricolum*) despite the fact that the lipoproteins serve as effective cholesterol donors. These workers suggested that the higher molar ratio of cholesterol to phospholipid in LDL than in HDL might be responsible, at least in part, for the greater effectiveness of the former as a cholesterol donor, although clearly the results for very low density lipoprotein indicate that this is not the only important variable. This suggestion was supported by the study of Kahane and Razin (48), who showed that the ability of cholesterol-PC vesicles to donate cholesterol to both organisms and to stimulate the growth of *M. hominis* increases with the increasing cholesterol/phospholipid molar ratio of the vesicles. Interestingly, although cholesterol uptake by *A. laidlawii* from LDL and HDL is actually slower than uptake from vesicles, a larger total cholesterol incorporation is obtained with the serum lipoproteins than with the vesicles.

These workers also studied the mechanism of cholesterol transfer between the lipoprotein particles or the cholesterol-PC vesicles and the membrane. They found that in *A. laidlawii*, only free cholesterol is incorporated into the membrane, with no concomitant uptake of cholesterol esters, phospholipid, or radiolabeled protein. Moreover, the lipoprotein particles or vesicles do not appear to be degraded or altered in any way by this organism, except for the depletion of free cholesterol. These results were interpreted to suggest that cholesterol is transferred from the donor to the *A. laidlawii* membrane only by transient contact, rather than by fusion (although the diffusion of cholesterol through the aqueous phase without direct contact was not ruled out). In contrast, *M. hominis* incorporates some cholesterol esters from the serum lipoproteins and some phospholipid from both the lipoprotein and vesicle donors, suggesting that some particle adherence or even fusion may take place. However, subsequent work by Rottem et al. (125) with *M. gallisepticum* and by Efrati et al. (31) with *M. capricolum* suggested that in these organisms, LDL adhesion and fusion would represent only a minor portion of the total uptake of free and esterified cholesterol. Whether this is true for the other sterol-requiring mycoplasma species requires further study.

The serum lipoproteins used in conventional, undefined growth media can be most effectively replaced by phospholipid-cholesterol vesicles (15, 16, 48, 89), egg yolk lipid dispersions (30), Tween 80-cholesterol micelles (96), certain serum lipoprotein-cholesterol complexes (103, 157), or ethanolic solutions of cholesterol-fatty acid mixtures (59, 62, 95, 96). In fact, as shown by Smith and Boughton (151), a variety of amphiphilic compounds can function to provide cholesterol in a form that can be assimilated by mycoplasmas. These workers also demonstrated that as long as the amphiphilic agents themselves are not toxic, the ability of these compounds to support the growth of sterol-requiring mycoplasmas correlates only with their ability to solubilize cholesterol. Cluss and Somerson (16) have shown that cholesterol-phospholipid vesicles made from mixtures of phospholipids are more effective than are those made from a single phospholipid in promoting the growth of a number of sterol-requiring *Mycoplasma* species and that the sources of the phospholipids utilized are also important. Although cholesterol alone is sometimes added to complex growth media after dissolution in ethanol (30, 46, 96), this is often not an effective means of providing this sterol in a usable form, since most of the cholesterol added crystallizes out of the growth medium and may cosediment with cells or membranes upon harvesting by centrifugation. It has also been suggested that exogenous cholesterol can function to detoxify surface-active agents such as fatty acids when these agents are not otherwise rendered nonlytic by complexation with bovine serum albumin or other agents (148).

Smith and Rothblat (159) and Smith (142) studied the mechanism of the incorporation of cholesterol and other steroids by several other sterol-requiring and sterol-nonrequiring mycoplasmas. They found that cholesterol uptake occurs at comparable rates and to comparable extents in both resting and growing cells and that cholesterol incorporation follows a typical absorption isotherm. The rate of incorporation is not particularly rapid, and some uptake continues to occur even after 8 h of incubation. Cholesterol uptake rates increase with temperature, and competition between cholesterol and other sterols is not observed. Interestingly, sterols with nonplanar ring systems are incorporated almost as well as is cholesterol, despite the fact that these sterols do not support cell growth. However, sterols without an aliphatic side chain like that of cholesterol are not incorporated. Pretreatment of these organisms with heat, various protein-modifying agents, or metabolic inhibitors does not affect cholesterol incorporation. In contrast, growth in excess cholesterol or extraction with ethanol-ether reduces cholesterol uptake, while chloroform-methanol extraction abolishes it. These authors concluded that cholesterol incorporation occurs primarily by a passive partitioning of sterol molecules into the hydrophobic core of the membrane lipid bilayer of these organisms.

Gershfeld et al. (37) and Razin et al. (93, 97) studied the mechanism of cholesterol uptake by isolated membranes of the sterol-nonrequiring *A. laidlawii*. Cholesterol incorporation was found to obey simple first-order kinetics and to exhibit a low activation energy (about 6 kcal/mol [1 cal = 4.184 J]). Cholesterol uptake was also found to be unaffected by the removal of some of the membrane lipid by an aqueous acetone extraction. The activation energy for cholesterol incorporation and the amount of cholesterol taken up are the same for membranes enriched in palmitic or oleic acid, but the rate constant for incorporation is significantly higher for the oleate-enriched membranes. Thus, the mechanism of cholesterol uptake by *A. laidlawii* membranes also seems to occur by a simple passive, nonsaturable, lipid bilayer-mediated process, as reported earlier for intact cells of *M. arthritidis* and for other sterol-requiring and sterol-nonrequiring mycoplasmas. However, these workers report that isolated membranes take up about twice as much cholesterol at equilibrium as do nongrowing cells, which in turn take up about three times more cholesterol than do growing cells. It was therefore proposed that although the processes of cholesterol incorporation are similar in all three systems, growing cells possess a mechanism for limiting or even excluding cholesterol from their membranes.

Razin (83) later studied cholesterol uptake into growing cells of *A. laidlawii*, the membrane lipid fluidity and phase state of which were varied by changing the fatty acid composition of the membrane lipids. He reported that in elaidate-enriched cells, the rate and extent of cholesterol incorporation are markedly lower at 4°C than at 37°C, whereas in oleate-enriched cells, the rate and extent of cholesterol uptake are only moderately lower at 4°C than at 37°C. Moreover, at 37°C, the rate and extent of cholesterol incorporation are significantly greater into oleate-enriched cells than into elaidate-enriched cells. Razin therefore suggested that cholesterol incorporation is slower and that the amount of cholesterol incorporated is smaller when the lipid bilayer is in the gel state than when it is in the liquid-crystalline state. Moreover, the higher rate and extent of cholesterol incorporation by oleate-enriched cells than by elaidate-enriched cells at 37°C also suggest that the efficiency of cholesterol uptake increases with increases in membrane lipid fluidity in the liquid-crystalline state. Support for this suggestion comes from studies on the steady-state level of cholesterol incorporation in *A. laidlawii* A (168) and B (6) cells grown at 37°C; in both cases, the amount of cholesterol found in the membrane increases as the degree of unsaturation of the membrane lipid fatty acyl chains increases. One important difference in results between this study on growing cells and the earlier studies on isolated membranes was the finding that the maximum amount of cholesterol that can be incorporated appears to be fatty acid dependent in growing cells but not in isolated membranes. The apparent lack of a dependence of the extent of cholesterol uptake on the fluidity and phase state of the lipid bilayer in isolated membranes is puzzling and may be related to the use of the detergent Tween 80 in these studies.

Razin (81) provided further support for the crucial role of the lipid bilayer in controlling the amount of cholesterol incorporated into the cell membrane by investigating cholesterol uptake into growing *A. laidlawii*, *M. hominis*, and *M. mycoides* subsp. *capri* cells whose membrane lipid/protein ratios were decreased markedly by aging or increased markedly by growth in the presence of the protein synthesis inhibitor chloramphenicol. In all three species, alterations in the protein content of the membrane have little influence on the amount of cholesterol incorporated, whereas the molar ratio of cholesterol to membrane glycerolipid is maintained almost constant, although his characteristic ratio varied markedly among the three mycoplasma species studied. Moreover, Efrati and coworkers (32) showed that the phospholipase A_2-catalyzed hydrolysis of about 30 and 70% of the total polar lipids of membranes of *A. laidlawii* and *M. capricolum*, respectively, resulted in proportional decreases in the amount of cholesterol incorporated. However, although extensive trypsin digestion of the proteins of isolated membranes or growing cells of *A. laidlawii* has no effect on cholesterol uptake, a similar treatment of *M. capricolum* membranes and cells reduces cholesterol uptake by about one-half. Efrati et al. therefore proposed that the ability of *Mycoplasma* species to incorporate larger quantities of cholesterol (and also to incorporate cholesterol ester and phospholipids) may depend on the presence of protein receptors for cholesterol donors, whereas such receptors are absent in *Acholeplasma* species. Such a suggestion was also made earlier by Razin et al. (89) on the basis of the observations that (i) cells of *Mycoplasma* but not *Acholeplasma* species incorporate exogenous cholesterol esters, phospholipids, and sphingomyelin (SM) as well as higher levels of cholesterol; (ii) isolated membranes of *M. capricolum* and *A. laidlawii* incorporate lower amounts of cholesterol (and no phospholipid) compared with growing cells (but see below); and (iii) the inhibition of the growth of *M. capricolum* decreases cholesterol uptake. However, since a subsequent study by Efrati et al. (31) concluded that LDL particles do not bind tightly to or fuse with the *M. capricolum* membrane, it was proposed that cholesterol (and cholesterol esters and phospholipids) exchange between donor and membranes by a simple exchange process. However, one could argue that these later results with isolated membranes are not definitive, since the results of Razin et al. (89) suggest a significantly greater capacity for cholesterol (and cholesterol ester and phospholipid) uptake by growing cells than by membranes. Thus, the question of the existence and role of receptors for lipoprotein particles or other cholesterol donors in *Mycoplasma* species is presently unresolved, as is the related question regarding the location of incorporated cholesterol, cholesterol esters, and phospholipid in the cell membrane. Although there is a considerable body of evidence that at least some of the incorporated cholesterol is present in the lipid bilayer (see chapters 8 and 15), the existence of multiple pools of cholesterol in some *Mycoplasma* species and in *A. laidlawii* suggests that some cholesterol may exist in another form, possibly simply absorbed in hydrophobic sites on some of the membrane proteins. This may also be true of the phospholipid and especially of the cholesterol esters associated with the membranes of *Mycoplasma* species, since studies with model phospholipid bilayer membranes indicate that they can incorporate only very small amounts of esterified cholesterol. Clearly, considerable additional experimental work will be required to resolve these questions.

Efrati et al. (33) have proposed that the difference in the cholesterol uptake capacities of *Acholeplasma* and *Mycoplasma* species may be due to the much higher glycolipid content of the former and to a reduced affinity of glycolipids for cholesterol. This proposal was based essentially on a statistical analysis of a large number of *Acholeplasma* strains which revealed a negative correlation between glycolipid content and the level of cholesterol incorporation by growing cells. Also given as evidence for this hypothesis was (i) the observation that cholesterol uptake capacity increases in aging cells in conjunction with a decreased glycolipid level and (ii) the existence of two pools of cholesterol in *A. laidlawii* membranes (25), one suggested to consist of phospholipid binding cholesterol relatively strongly and another suggested to consist of glycolipid binding cholesterol relatively weakly. However, Razin (81) reported earlier that the incorporation of cholesterol into cells of *A. laidlawii* (and into cells of *M. hominis* and *M. mycoides*) decreases upon aging, and as discussed in chapter 8, the roughly equal sizes of the slowly and rapidly exchanging pools in *A. laidlawii* and *M. gallisepticum* membranes are not compatible with their markedly different relative proportions of glycolipids. Moreover, the retention of a considerable cholesterol-binding capability by *A. laidlawii* cells whose membrane lipids have been essentially depleted of phospholipids by phospholipase A_2 treatment (32) and the ability of isolated *A. laidlawii* membranes to take up much larger amounts of cholesterol than do growing cells (37, 97) are observations which seem incompatible with this proposal, as is the reported ability of glycolipid dispersions from the membrane of this organism to incorporate cholesterol as efficiently as do total membrane lipid dispersions (84).

Although most studies of cholesterol uptake by growing cells do support the notion that *Mycoplasma* species incorporate higher levels of cholesterol into their cell membranes than do *Acholeplasma* species, it should be noted that in some studies, nearly comparable amounts of cholesterol are found when uptake is expressed as the amount of cholesterol incorporated per unit weight of membrane or total cell protein or per mole of total lipid rather than as per mole of phospholipids (see, for example, references 81 and 89). Moreover, the levels of cholesterol incorporated by different sterol-requiring *Mycoplasma* species can vary significantly, and several species can be adapted to grow with rather low levels of cholesterol. In addition, several groups have claimed to have obtained *A. laidlawii* membranes containing much more than the 10 to 20 mol% of cholesterol usually reported (see chapter 8). Therefore, the question of whether a difference in the extent of cholesterol uptake is an important and fundamental difference between the sterol-requiring and sterol-nonrequiring mycoplasmas remains to some extent an open one.

Carotenoids

Henrikson and Smith (43) have shown that exogenous C_{40} all-*trans*-3,3′-dihydroxycarotenes can replace the sterol growth requirement for both *M. arthritidis* and *M. gallinarum*, whereas other carotenoids with only a single hydroxyl group at C-3,3′, or with hydroxyl groups elsewhere in the molecule, are ineffective. Interestingly, the carotenoids from the *A. laidlawii* membrane, now known to be C_{30} apocarotenoids rather than C_{40} carotenoids (see chapter 6), can also support the growth of these organisms, presumably due to the presence of 3,3'-dihydroxy-aponeurosporene or a closely related compound. Since the sterol-requiring mycoplasma species are incapable of synthesizing carotenoids (see below), Smith (148) has suggested that this fact accounts for their dependence on exogenous cholesterol for growth and has proposed that carotenoids and sterols fulfill similar functions in the sterol-nonrequiring and sterol-requiring strains, respectively. Evidence for and against this proposal is discussed later in this chapter. The role of carotenoids in the structure and function of mycoplasma membranes is discussed in chapters 8 and 15, respectively.

Phospholipids and Sphingolipids

Although PC and SM are not synthesized by any mycoplasma species studied to date, significant quantities of these and other exogenous phospholipids are incorporated into membranes of sterol-requiring *Mycoplasma* and *Spiroplasma* species when the organisms are grown in the presence of serum or of phospholipid-cholesterol or SM-cholesterol dispersions (5, 7, 8, 14, 31, 32, 34, 38, 73, 74, 88, 89, 113, 117). Although some *Mycoplasma* species preferentially incorporate more exogenous PC than SM, others resemble the *Spiroplasma* species in preferentially incorporating exogenous SM. As mentioned earlier, *Acholeplasma* species do not take up exogenous phospholipids or sphingolipids when cultured under identical conditions. Although the exogenous PC and SM are normally incorporated unchanged from the growth medium by most *Mycoplasma* and *Spiroplasma* species, certain *Mycoplasma* species modify the PC molecules by replacing the unsaturated fatty acid at glycerol position 2 with a saturated fatty acid (39, 117). There is some evidence that the exogenous phospholipids taken up are incorporated into the membrane lipid bilayer, since exogenous and endogenous phospholipids resemble each other in ether extractability and susceptibility to phospholipase A_2 hydrolysis (32). As well, the incorporation of exogenous phospholipids by *M. gallisepticum* inhibits endogenous PG synthesis (84) and alters the PG/diphosphatidylglycerol (DPG) ratio in *M. capricolum* (35, 39). It would be desirable, however, to confirm the localization of these exogenous phospholipids exclusively to the membrane lipid bilayer by the use of selectively labeled exogenous phospholipids and suitable physical techniques. Rodwell (105) has shown that exogenous PC or SM is required for the growth of *M. gallisepticum* in a defined medium, and Hackett et al. (40) have shown that exogenous SM is required for the growth of *S. mirum*.

MEMBRANE LIPID BIOSYNTHESIS

Fatty Acids

The first direct evidence for the ability of certain mycoplasma species to synthesize fatty acids was provided by Pollack and Tourtellotte (80), who demonstrated that *A. laidlawii* A and B and another sterol-nonrequiring *Acholeplasma* species are capable of biosynthetically incorporating radioactive acetate into lauric, myristic, palmitic, and stearic acids but not into oleic or linoleic acid, indicating that only saturated fatty acids can be synthesized by these organisms. Rottem and Razin (123) later reported that *A. laidlawii* incorporates radioactive acetate mainly into the polar lipids and that most of that radioactivity is located in the esterified fatty acids. Exogenous palmitic and stearic acids markedly inhibit acetate incorporation, whereas oleic acid does not, again suggesting that acetate is utilized primarily for the synthesis of saturated fatty acids. Acetate uptake by washed *A. laidlawii* cells requires glucose, CoA, and Mg^{2+}, is temperature and pH dependent, and is inhibited by several metabolic inhibitors, especially iodoacetate. Although pyruvate enhances acetate incorporation into the membrane lipids in the presence of glucose, it cannot replace glucose as an energy source for acetate uptake. Propionate and butyrate markedly decrease acetate uptake. This was suggested to be due to the inhibition of the acetokinase activity of this organism, although the preferential utilization of these short-chain fatty acids as primers in de novo fatty acid biosynthesis may have contributed to the decreased acetate uptake observed (see below). The probable biochemical pathway for fatty acid biosynthesis in *A. laidlawii* is presented in Fig. 1.

Pollack and coworkers (45, 77, 78) later demonstrated that the ability to synthesize saturated fatty acids (or indeed any lipid) from acetate is shared by most but not all of the sterol-nonrequiring *Acholeplasma* species, whereas all of the many sterol-requiring *Mycoplasma* and *Ureaplasma* species tested lack this ability. This later finding contrasts with the original report of Rottem and Razin (123) that radiolabeled acetate is incorporated into the polar or neutral lipid fractions of several *Mycoplasma* species. However, Rottem (112) later presented data showing insignificant acetate incorporation into the total lipids of these same species. Miura et al. (66) have also found that *A. laidlawii* A, but not any of several *Mycoplasma* species, is capable of the incorporation of acetate into fatty acids; however, these workers reported that radiolabeled acetate is found in oleic acid as well as in even-chain saturated fatty acids, a finding not supported by previous or subsequent work (see below).

Figure 1. Biochemical pathway for the de novo synthesis of linear, even-chain saturated fatty acids in *A. laidlawii*. Only reaction 1 has been demonstrated in vitro; reactions 2 to 7 are presumed to occur but have not been directly demonstrated. Propionyl-CoA, isobutryl-CoA, or anteisovaleryl-CoA can apparently be formed from the corresponding short-chain fatty acids and can largely replace acetyl-CoA as the primer. Under these conditions, linear odd-chain saturated, methyl iso-branched, or methyl anteiso-branched fatty acids are the primary products. The metabolic sources of acetyl-CoA are discussed in chapter 11. The enzymes catalyzing the various individual reactions are indicated.

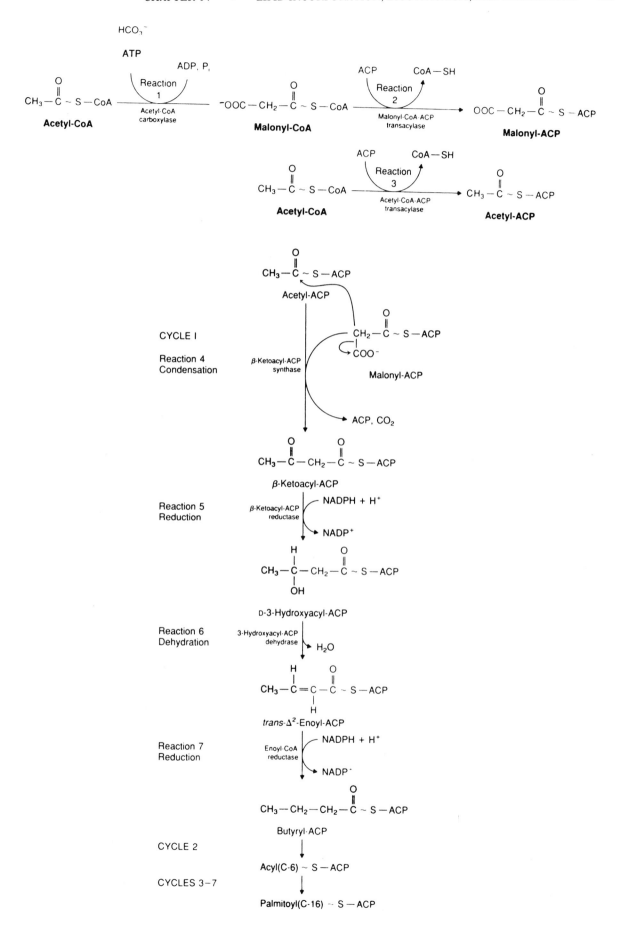

Finally, Romano et al. (108) have reported that *U. urealyticum* can synthesize both saturated and unsaturated fatty acids from exogenous radiolabeled acetate, a surprising finding not confirmed by Pollack et al. (78). Since Freeman et al. (34) have found that *S. citri* also does not synthesize fatty acids (or other lipids) from acetate, it appears most likely that none of the sterol-requiring mycoplasma species have de novo fatty acid biosynthetic ability.

Rottem et al. (118) have shown that the fatty acid biosynthetic activities of three *Acholeplasma* species correlates positively with their acyl carrier protein (ACP) content and that ACP levels in the five *Mycoplasma* species tested are all very low or possibly absent. Although it is also possible that these *Mycoplasma* species lack one or more of the requisite enzymes for fatty acid biosynthesis, the virtual absence of ACP in these organisms may be at least a contributing factor to their inability to carry out de novo fatty acid biosynthesis or even the chain elongation of exogenous fatty acids. Since the *Mycoplasma* species tested all incorporate exogenous fatty acids into their membrane lipids, these results suggest that acyl-CoA rather than acyl-ACP serves as the activated fatty acyl group donor in glycerolipid biosynthesis in these organisms. However, as these workers estimated ACP levels by the activity of the malonyl-CoA–CO_2 exchange reaction, it is not clear whether this activity reflects the levels of ACP or simply the activity of the enzymes responsible for fixing CO_2. However, these workers also reported that the addition of pantetheine or, to a lesser degree, CoA to *A. laidlawii* B cultures results in a significantly increased malonyl-CoA–CO_2 exchange activity and carotenoid biosynthetic output, suggesting that ACP levels may be rate limiting for lipid synthesis in this organism. Moreover, Christiansson and Wieslander (13) later found that the low level of endogenous saturated fatty acid and carotenoid biosynthesis in *A. laidlawii* A can be stimulated markedly by the addition of pantetheine and that exogenous palmitic acid can partially inhibit saturated fatty acid biosynthesis.

Rottem et al. (126) have detected a thioesterase acting specifically on long-chain fatty acyl-CoAs in the membranes of several mycoplasma species. Since its activity was found to be much higher in the *Acholeplasma* than in the *Mycoplasma* species tested, it was suggested that this enzyme may have a regulatory role in fatty acid biosynthesis. However, what this role might be is presently unclear.

Rottem and Panos (120) demonstrated that a soluble system derived from *A. laidlawii* A cells can synthesize long-chain saturated fatty acids from radiolabeled acetate. The addition of malonyl-CoA is absolutely required for fatty acid synthesis to occur, and the addition of ATP, $MgCl_2$, and reduced NADP stimulates synthesis. The requirement for malonyl-CoA and the low levels of acetyl-CoA carboxylase activity present indicate that in this cell-free system, almost all of the radiolabeled acetate is incorporated as acetyl-ACP rather than as malonyl-ACP (i.e., that the radiolabeled acetate is functioning only as the "primer" in this fatty acid-synthesizing system). In this system, the ACP content does not appear to be rate limiting for fatty acid synthesis, in apparent contrast to the later findings of Rottem and Markowitz (116) for whole cells of *A.*

laidlawii B. However, appreciable acetyl-CoA carboxylase activity may have been lost during the preparation of this soluble system, which may account for the difference in results. Only saturated fatty acids can be synthesized by this cell-free system, but the addition of β-hydroxy thioester dehydrase from *E. coli* results in the formation of both saturated and monounsaturated fatty acids, indicating that the lack of this enzyme in *A. laidlawii* A is responsible for its inability to synthesize unsaturated fatty acids. Interestingly, the primary product of this cell-free synthetase system is stearic acid, with smaller amounts of palmitic and arachidic acids also being formed, whereas intact cells of this organism produce primarily myristic and palmitic acids. Although the factors controlling the termination of fatty acid synthesis and thus the chain length of the final product have not been elucidated completely in any organism, evidence will be discussed below that the longer chain lengths produced by the soluble system than by the in vivo system may be due, at least in part, to the absence of the membrane-associated glycerolipid-synthesizing enzymes in the former, which may compete for the medium-chain fatty acyl-ACP being synthesized. Also interesting is the observed lack of any inhibition of the soluble system by exogenous saturated or unsaturated fatty acids, which do appear to inhibit acetate incorporation into endogenous saturated fatty acids in vivo.

Saito and McElhaney (128), in their studies of the incorporation of exogenous fatty acids by growing *A. laidlawii* B cells, found a "biphasic maximum" when the amount of incorporation of members of a homologous series of linear saturated, methyl iso-, or methyl anteiso-branched fatty acids is plotted against the chain length of the exogenous fatty acid. That is, very short chain fatty acids (containing three to five carbon atoms) are incorporated reasonably well, with the degree of uptake and biosynthetic utilization falling to low values at intermediate chain lengths before rising and peaking again at longer chain lengths. This result indicated that short-chain fatty acids other than acetate can serve as primers in the de novo fatty acid biosynthetic system of this organism. This conclusion was confirmed by Saito et al. (131), who demonstrated that although endogenous acetate and propionate are the predominant primers for the biosynthesis of even- and odd-chain saturated fatty acids, respectively, exogenous isobutyric and anteisovaleric acids are also efficiently utilized, giving rise to the synthesis of up to 80% endogenous methyl iso- and anteiso-branched fatty acids, respectively. These results demonstrated that the primer specificity, and thus the type of fatty acid synthesized, is quite broad in this organism. However, as more highly branched short-chain fatty acids or those possessing halogen substituents or double bonds are not utilized, the enzymes responsible for the production of the primer do have some substrate specificity. In contrast to the results of Rottem and Panos (120) for the soluble fatty acid-synthesizing system of *A. laidlawii* A, Saito and coworkers found that radiolabeled acetate served in vivo as a precursor of both the primer and chain-elongating unit, since the amount of radioactivity incorporated into the endogenous fatty acids increases linearly as a function of chain length. As well, this study showed clearly that radiolabeled acetate is not incorporated into unsaturated fatty acids, thus supporting most of the earlier findings. Interestingly, the output spectrum of the de novo fatty acid biosynthetic pathway in *A. laidlawii* B was found to be essentially independent of temperature or of the amount of cholesterol present in the cell membrane, indicating that this pathway is not regulated by the fluidity of the membrane lipid bilayer, confirming the earlier findings of McElhaney (58) for this organism and of Rottem and Panos (119) for *A. laidlawii* A.

Silvius et al. (135) later investigated the regulation of the quantity and chain length of the endogenous saturated fatty acids synthesized by growing *A. laidlawii* B cells by the presence of various kinds of exogenous long-chain fatty acids. These workers found that exogenous fatty acids significantly reduce the amount of de novo-synthesized fatty acids in the cell by two different mechanisms. The major mechanism is an actual inhibition of the total output of the de novo fatty acid biosynthetic pathway, and exogenous even-chain saturated and unsaturated fatty acids are both effective in this regard. A minor mechanism is the excretion of endogenous free fatty acids into the growth medium, which is most marked with exogenous medium-chain saturated fatty acids. These two mechanisms do not suffice to maintain total membrane lipid levels constant but do moderate the effect of the incorporation of exogenous fatty acids on increasing the lipid/protein ratio of the membrane. As well, exogenous long-chain saturated or other high-melting-point fatty acids were found to decrease the average chain length of the endogenous fatty acids, whereas exogenous unsaturated or other low-melting-point fatty acids were found to increase the average chain length of the saturated fatty acids synthesized by this organism. Since the direction and magnitude of the shifts in the average chain length of the de novo-synthesized fatty acids correlates very well with the specificity of the exogenous fatty acid for esterification to the 1 or 2 position of the glycerol moiety of the membrane glycerolipids (see below), these workers proposed that the competition of endogenous and exogenous fatty acids for esterification to a particular position can selectively repress the synthesis of endogenous fatty acids of similar specificity. For example, exogenous oleic acid, which is highly specific for esterification at the 2 position during glycerolipid biosynthesis in this organism, would successfully compete with the shorter-chain endogenous lauric and myristic acids normally also occupying this position, thereby reducing the relative amounts of these fatty acids incorporated into the membrane glycerolipids, while having little effect on the incorporation of the longer-chain endogenous palmitic and stearic acids, which are specific for the 1 position. The net effect of this particular competition would be both to reduce the total amount of endogenous esterified fatty acids in the membrane lipids and to increase their average chain length, as observed. However, further experimental work in cell-free systems will clearly be required to confirm this hypothesis.

The effect of cerulenin, a potent inhibitor of fatty acid biosynthesis in bacteria, on the growth and lipid biosynthesis of several *Acholeplasma* and *Mycoplasma* species was examined by Rottem and Barile (114). Cerulenin was found to markedly inhibit the growth of all species tested, but the *Acholeplasma* species (especially *A. laidlawii*) are inhibited at much lower cerulenin concentrations. Although cerulenin markedly inhibits the incorporation of radiolabeled acetate into endogenous saturated fatty acids in *A. laidlawii*, it actually stimulates the incorporation of acetate into the carotenoid fraction; cerulenin also inhibits the chain elongation of exogenous medium-chain fatty acids. The growth inhibition of *A. laidlawii* is not, however, reversed by the addition of exogenous fatty acids to the growth medium, indicating that cerulenin inhibits the growth of this organism by effects other than the inhibition of fatty acid biosynthesis. Although low levels of cerulenin can be used to increase the incorporation of exogenous fatty acids into the membrane lipids of *A. laidlawii*, the nonspecific toxicity of this compound prevents its use in concentrations high enough to completely inhibit endogenous fatty acid biosynthesis. Thus, the membrane lipids from cells grown with low levels of cerulenin still contain 20 to 40% endogenous saturated fatty acids. Generally similar results for the cerulenin treatment of *A. laidlawii* B were later reported by Saito et al. (131), except that in this strain, exogenous elaidic acid relieves the growth inhibition even at relatively high cerulenin concentrations. However, the complete inhibition of fatty acid biosynthesis cannot be achieved at nontoxic cerulenin concentrations. These workers also found that low concentrations of cerulenin decrease the average chain length of the endogenous fatty acids without affecting total biosynthetic output, whereas higher concentrations also markedly decrease the amount of endogenous fatty acid synthesized by the organism. Saito and coworkers thus suggested that low concentrations of cerulenin preferentially inhibit a β-ketoacyl thioester synthetase which is specific for medium-chain (C_{10} to C_{13}) fatty acids, and which is largely responsible for the chain elongation of exogenous fatty acids (130), and that the analogous enzyme(s) specific for the shorter-chain fatty acyl-ACPs is inhibited only at higher cerulenin concentrations.

Silvius and McElhaney (134) later studied a variety of other potential inhibitors of de novo fatty acid biosynthesis in *A. laidlawii* B. Although CM-55, an antimicrobial fatty acid amide, was found to more strongly inhibit endogenous fatty acid synthesis than did cerulenin, this compound is also unable to completely inhibit endogenous fatty acid production at nontoxic levels. However, the addition of the biotin-binding protein avidin to the complex growth medium completely inhibits growth, fatty acid biosynthesis, and the elongation of exogenous medium-chain fatty acids. Moreover, this growth inhibition can be completely relieved by the addition of appropriate exogenous long-chain fatty acids to the growth medium. Apparently, the avidin tightly binds all of the biotin available in the growth medium, denying this vitamin to the cell and thus preventing the synthesis of functional acetyl-CoA carboxylase, which requires biotin as a prosthetic group. By using avidin, it is possible to produce exogenous fatty acid-homogeneous *A. laidlawii* B membranes whose lipids are essentially free of endogenous saturated fatty acids, thus permitting a much greater control over the thickness and the fluidity and phase state of the membrane lipid bilayer of this organism (see chapters 8 and 15).

Sterols

No mycoplasma species examined to date, including the sterol-nonrequiring species, is capable of the biosynthesis of cholesterol or related sterols (148, 150). Moreover, exogenous cholesterol or other steroids incorporated from the growth medium do not appear to be structurally altered in any way by these organisms (4, 32, 100, 111, 140). The cholesterol esters containing long-chain fatty acyl groups found in the membranes of some sterol-requiring species appear to arise exclusively from exogenous esterified cholesterol present in the serum or serum lipoproteins present in the growth medium (31, 117, 124), although it has been reported that a few mycoplasma species are capable of esterifying exogenously incorporated cholesterol with very short chain fatty acids (148, 150). However, most mycoplasma species do not form cholesterol esters from exogenous cholesterol (84). Smith (140, 147) has reported that a cholesteryl-β-D-glucopyranose is formed by both *A. laidlawii* and *M. gallinarum* from exogenous cholesterol.

Carotenoids

Most but apparently not all (78) of the sterol-nonrequiring *Acholeplasma* species examined to date are capable of the synthesis of carotenoids, as evidenced by the incorporation by radiolabeled acetate or mevalonate into polyterpenes found in the neutral lipid fraction of the cell membrane (1, 111, 141, 156). It should be noted, however, that in *Escherichia coli* and some other bacteria, exogenous radiolabeled acetate is not utilized in polyterpene biosynthesis (170), so the lack of acetate incorporation into the neutral lipid fraction of some *Acholeplasma* species (78) is not definitive evidence for the absence of carotenoid synthesis. Although the carotenoids of most *Acholeplasma* species contain a series of conjugated double bonds which impart an intense yellow color to them, *A. axanthum* appears to synthesize carotenoids which are almost colorless, presumably as a result of the at least partial absence of oxidation of the polyterpenes produced (156). In contrast to most of the *Acholeplasma* species, none of the sterol-requiring *Mycoplasma*, *Spiroplasma*, or *Ureaplasma* species thus far examined appears capable of carotenoid pigment biosynthesis (34, 45, 78, 112, 160).

Smith and coworkers (44, 144, 152, 166) and Castrejon-Diez et al. (10) have examined the enzymes in the pathway from acetate to the polyprenols in the sterol-requiring *A. laidlawii* and in the sterol-nonrequiring *M. arthritidis* and *M. gallinarum*. These workers found that although all three organisms are capable of the formation of acetyl-CoA, only *A. laidlawii* possesses all of the appropriate enzymes for carotenoid biosynthesis (Fig. 2). *M. gallinarum* was found to lack only the three enzymes responsible for the conversion of mevalonic acid to isopentenyl pyrophosphate but to possess the enzymes beyond this stage in the polyterpene biosynthetic pathway. In contrast, *M. arthritidis* is completely deficient in the requisite enzymes beyond the formation of acetoacetyl-CoA. Interestingly, the biosynthesis of carotenoids by *A. laidlawii* has been reported to be partially inhibited by cholesterol (141), although inhibition is not complete, since other polyterpenoid compounds probably play important metabolic roles in this organism, such as in the formation of isopentenyl adenosine and lipopolysaccharides (148, 150). The site of cholesterol inhibition of carotenoid biosynthesis in *A. laidlawii* B has been reported to be the conversion of isopentenyl pyrophosphate to dimethylallyl pyrophosphate (161), an enzymatic step not usually sensitive to cholesterol inhibition in organisms normally synthesizing sterols. As mentioned earlier, the addition of pantetheine, a CoA precursor, stimulates carotenoid biosynthesis in *A. laidlawii* A (13) and B (118), suggesting that CoA may be limiting in some growth media. Moreover, cerulenin, an inhibitor of fatty acid biosynthesis in *A. laidlawii*, also stimulates carotenoid biosynthesis (119), presumably by increasing available acetyl-CoA levels.

Smith (141) has proposed that the carotenoids of the sterol-nonrequiring *Acholeplasma* species fulfill functions analogous to those of cholesterol in the sterol-requiring mycoplasmas. Evidence in support of this hypothesis includes the observations that exogenous cholesterol spares carotenoid biosynthesis in *A. laidlawii* (141) and that inhibition of the early steps of polyterpene biosynthesis completely inhibits the growth of this organism, an inhibition reversed by exogenous cholesterol (153). On the other hand, inhibitors of carotenoid synthesis in *A. laidlawii* also inhibit the growth of *M. arthritidis*, which lacks almost all of the enzymes for polyterpene synthesis, and the reversal of the growth inhibition of *A. laidlawii* by cholesterol is only partial. Moreover, when exogenous isopentenyl pyrophosphate is supplied to *M. gallinarum* in lieu of cholesterol, this normally cholesterol-requiring species is supposedly capable of growth (43) and of the synthesis of polyterpenols (144). However, the growth observed is less than with cholesterol supplementation, and a significant growth response is observed only at high isopentenyl pyrophosphate concentrations. Finally, the observation that certain exogenous polyterpenes can substitute for the cholesterol growth requirement of *M. arthritidis* and *M. gallinarum* (43) lends further support to this hypothesis. On the other hand, Razin and Rottem (91, 123) have reported that

Figure 2. Biochemical pathway for the synthesis of the 30-carbon apocarotenoids in *A. laidlawii*. The enzymes catalyzing the various reactions are as follows: 1, acetoacetyl-CoA thiolase; 2, hydroxymethylglutaryl-CoA synthetase; 3, hydroxymethylglutaryl-CoA reductase; 4, mevalonate kinase; 5, phosphomevalonate kinase; 6, pyrophosphomevalonate kinase; 7, pyrophosphomevalonate decarboxylase; 8, isopentenyl pyrophosphate isomerase; 9, geranyltransferase; and 10, squalene synthetase. The biochemical reactions catalyzed by enzymes 1 through 8 have been demonstrated to occur in this organism (148), as has the biosynthetic incorporation of radiolabeled acetate and mevalonate into the apocarotenoids (see text); the remaining biochemical reactions are presumed to occur but have not been directly demonstrated.

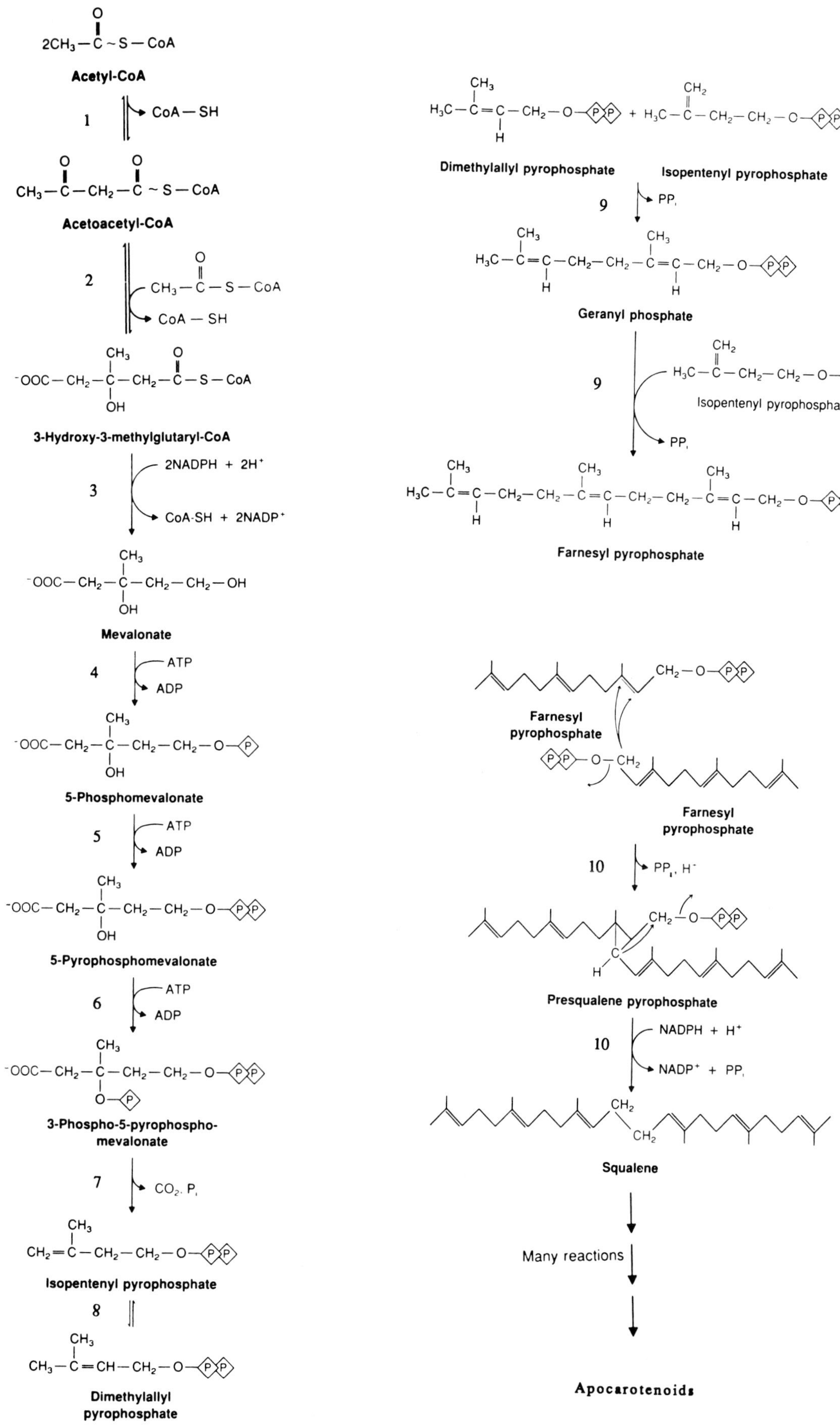

O
‖
2CH₃—C ∼ S—CoA

Acetyl-CoA

1   CoA—SH

O   O
‖   ‖
CH₃—C—CH₂—C ∼ S—CoA

Acetoacetyl-CoA

O
‖
2   CH₃—C—S—CoA

CoA—SH

CH₃   O
| ‖
⁻OOC—CH₂—C—CH₂—C—S—CoA
|
OH

3-Hydroxy-3-methylglutaryl-CoA

3   2NADPH + 2H⁺

CoA·SH + 2NADP⁺

CH₃
|
⁻OOC—CH₂—C—CH₂—CH₂—OH
|
OH

Mevalonate

4   ATP
ADP

CH₃
|
⁻OOC—CH₂—C—CH₂—CH₂—O—Ⓟ
|
OH

5-Phosphomevalonate

5   ATP
ADP

CH₃
|
⁻OOC—CH₂—C—CH₂—CH₂—O—ⓅⓅ
|
OH

5-Pyrophosphomevalonate

6   ATP
ADP

CH₃
|
⁻OOC—CH₂—C—CH₂—CH₂—O—ⓅⓅ
|
O—Ⓟ

**3-Phospho-5-pyrophospho-
mevalonate**

7   CO₂, Pᵢ

CH₃
|
CH₂=C—CH₂—CH₂—O—ⓅⓅ

Isopentenyl pyrophosphate

8

CH₃
|
CH₃—C=CH—CH₂—O—ⓅⓅ

**Dimethylallyl
pyrophosphate**

CH₃   CH₂
| ‖
H₃C—C=C—CH₂—O—ⓅⓅ + H₃C—C—CH₂—CH₂—O—ⓅⓅ
     |
     H

Dimethylallyl pyrophosphate   **Isopentenyl pyrophosphate**

9   PPᵢ

CH₃   CH₃
| |
H₃C—C=C—CH₂—CH₂—C=C—CH₂—O—ⓅⓅ
     | |
     H   H

Geranyl phosphate

9   CH₂
‖
H₃C—C—CH₂—CH₂—O—ⓅⓅ

Isopentenyl pyrophosphate

PPᵢ

CH₃   CH₃   CH₃
| | |
H₃C—C—C—CH₂—CH₂—C=C—CH₂—CH₂—C=C—CH₂—O—ⓅⓅ
     | | |
     H   H   H

Farnesyl pyrophosphate

CH₂—O—ⓅⓅ

**Farnesyl
pyrophosphate**

ⓅⓅ—O—CH₂

**Farnesyl
pyrophosphate**

10   PPᵢ, H⁺

CH₂—O—ⓅⓅ
|
C
|
H

Presqualene pyrophosphate

10   NADPH + H⁺

NADP⁺ + PPᵢ

CH₂
|
CH₂

Squalene

Many reactions

Apocarotenoids

247

A. laidlawii can grow normally in the absence of cholesterol when carotenoid biosynthesis is inhibited by the absence of CoA in the growth medium or by the presence of exogenous propionate. However, in the first study, the inhibition of radiolabeled acetate into the neutral lipid fraction may not have reflected actual carotenoid levels in the membrane, since unlabeled acetate derived from glucose metabolism may have supported some carotenoid synthesis, and in the second study, the authors measured carotenoids only by their absorption in the visible region, thereby possibly overlooking the presence of colorless carotenoids, which apparently function as well as those with extensive conjugated double bonds (153). (This controversy could be readily resolved by experiments using any of a number of specific inhibitors of hydroxymethylglutaryl-CoA reductase now available and by a direct chemical assay for polyterpenes.) Moreover, Razin and Cleverdon (85) showed that inhibition of the synthesis of at least the colored carotenoids by thallium acetate or diphenylamine, or stimulation of their synthesis by acetate, does not affect the uptake of exogenous cholesterol, nor do changes in the levels of cholesterol incorporation affect carotenoid synthesis in *A. laidlawii*. Similarly, Tully and Razin (164) and Pollack et al. (78) have reported that several *Acholeplasma* species do not synthesize carotenoids, as measured either by their characteristic absorbance spectra or by the uptake of radiolabeled acetate into the neutral lipid fraction. As well, the levels of carotenoids in the membranes of most *Acholeplasma* species are small, often of the order of a few moles percent. Therefore, although the bulk of the available evidence seems to support the hypothesis that carotenoids can at least partially fulfill the function of cholesterol in at least some of the sterol-requiring *Mycoplasma* species, the hypothesis that carotenoids fulfill an essential cholesterol-like role in the membranes of *Acholeplasma* species remains controversial. As discussed in chapters 8 and 15, although carotenoids and cholesterol do have generally similar effects on the organization and dynamics of the membrane lipid bilayer of this organism, carotenoids, like cholesterol, are probably not required by *A. laidlawii*, at least not in order to regulate the fluidity and phase state of its membrane lipids.

Smith (141) has reported that carotenyl acetate and carotenyl glucosides can be synthesized by various *Acholeplasma* species, but the mechanism of their biosynthesis is largely unknown. Smith (146) has also postulated a role for these lipids in the active transport of glucose and acetate in *A. laidlawii*. This postulate is discussed in detail in a later section of this chapter.

Phospholipids

The acidic phospholipids PG and DPG, which appear to be found in all mycoplasma species, can be synthesized de novo, as shown by their appearance in mycoplasmas grown in defined or lipid-free medium (see chapter 6) and by the incorporation of radiolabeled P_i, fatty acids, and in some cases glycerol or glycerol-3-phosphate into these compounds (26, 46, 65, 72, 73, 75, 76, 112, 115, 128, 143, 146). However, the actual biochemical pathway by which these compounds are formed has not been definitively determined, although

it is presumed to be the same as in *E. coli* and other eubacteria (Fig. 3). Observations compatible with this suggestion include the finding of small amounts of lysophosphatidic and phosphatidic acids in *Acholeplasma* (65, 110), *Mycoplasma* (124, 150), and *Ureaplasma* (109) species, the synthesis of cytidine diphosphate diglyceride from CTP and phosphatidic acid by *A. laidlawii* B (148), the synthesis of PG from CTP and glycerol-3-phosphate by *Mycoplasma* strain Y (75), and the presence of PG phosphate in *M. gallinarum* (154). However, the virtual absence of this latter compound in most mycoplasma species suggests the presence of an active PG phosphate phosphatase. The slow metabolic turnover of PG observed in some mycoplasmas (73, 75, 146) and the reciprocal relationship between decreasing levels of this compound and increasing levels of DPG in aging cells (38, 115, 146) suggests a precursor-product relationship between these two acidic phosphatides. Indeed, Gross and Rottem (38) have shown that exogenous PG can be converted to DPG by *M. capricolum*. However, an actual determination of the biochemical mechanism of this interconversion is currently lacking. The biosynthesis of these phospholipids in cell-free systems has been only preliminarily studied (115), and thus we know little of the biochemical regulation of this pathway or of the characteristics of the enzymes involved in it.

As discussed earlier, free glycerol is utilized for phospholipid biosynthesis by some *Mycoplasma* species (presumably those with an active glycerol kinase) but not by many others, suggesting that glycerol-3-phosphate and not free glycerol is the actual substrate for acylation. Support for this suggestion comes from the observation that the glycerol moiety of the phospholipids of the fermentative *A. laidlawii* (65) and *Mycoplasma* strain Y (75) can be labeled by radioactive glucose and from the fact that glycerol-3-phosphate rather than glycerol is utilized for PG synthesis by isolated membranes of *M. hominis* (115). Moreover, although the dihydroxyacetone phosphate derived from glucose is probably an intermediate in the formation of glycerol-3-phosphate in *Mycoplasma* strain Y, there is no evidence for its acylation (75). In *M. hominis*, the presence of a soluble acyl-CoA synthetase and a membrane-bound acyl-CoA:glycerol-3-phosphate transacylase activity (115), plus the apparently low levels of ACP present in all of the sterol-requiring mycoplasmas tested (118), suggests that the exogenous fatty acids utilized by these organisms are biosynthetically incorporated into the membrane phospholipids as CoA thiol esters. However, in the *Acholeplasma* species, which are capable of de novo fatty acid biosynthesis and which appear to contain high levels of ACP, fatty acyl-ACP may function in the acylation of glycerol 3-phosphate, at least for the endogenous fatty acids. The question of whether exogenous fatty acids are activated by conversion into CoA or ACP derivatives in the *Acholeplasma* species has not been definitively determined.

The distribution of a number of fatty acids between the 1 and 2 positions of the PG from *A. laidlawii* B has been studied by McElhaney and Tourtellotte (64). The positional distribution of any particular fatty acid was found to be independent of the amount of that acid biosynthetically incorporated into the PG, provided that the fatty acid in question was not present in suffi-

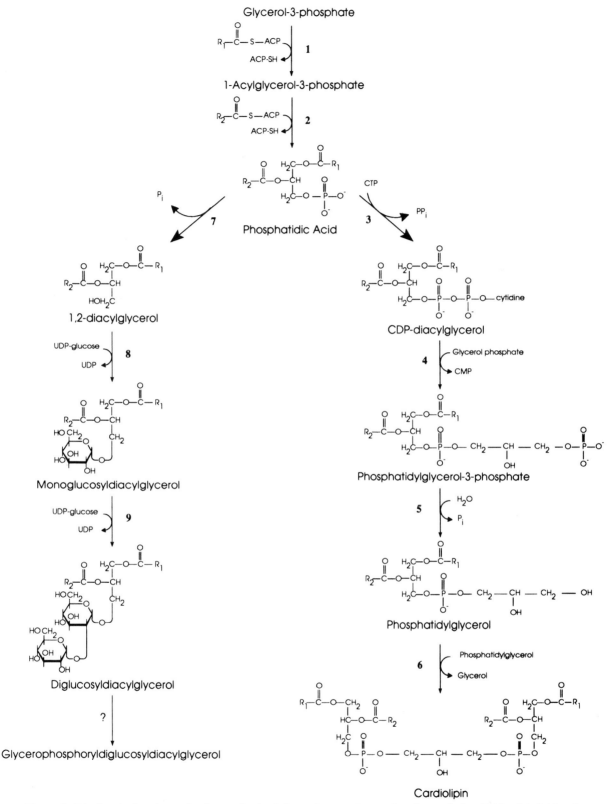

Figure 3. Biochemical pathway for the synthesis of the major membrane phospho- and glycolipids of *A. laidlawii*. The enzymes catalyzing the various reactions are as follows: 1, glycerol-3-phosphate acyltransferase; 2, 1-acylglycerol-3-phosphate acyltransferase; 3, phosphatidic acid cytidylyltransferase; 4, glycerophosphate phosphatidyltransferase; 5, phosphatidylglycerol phosphate phosphatase; 6, cardiolipin synthetase; 7, phosphatidic acid phosphatase; 8, diacylglycerol UDP-glucosyltransferase; and 9, monoglucosyldiacylglycerol UDP-glucosyltransferase. Reactions 3, 8, and 9 have been demonstrated to occur in this organism, and there is indirect evidence for reactions 1, 2, 6, and 7; reaction 6 has been demonstrated in *M. capricolum*, and evidence for reactions 4 and 5 has been found in several *Mycoplasma* species (see text).

cient quantity to saturate the preferred position. Within any single class of fatty acid, the positional specificity is markedly dependent on chain length, with the affinity for the 1 position decreasing (and that for the 2 position increasing) as a function of decreasing chain length. At comparable chain lengths, the affinities of different classes of fatty acids for the 1 position decrease (and those for the 2 position increase) in the order straight-chain saturated > methyl iso-branched > *trans*-monounsaturated > *cis*-monounsaturated > *cis*-diunsaturated fatty acids. These results were confirmed by Romijn et al. (110), who showed in addition that the asymmetric positional distribution of saturated and unsaturated fatty acyl chains in the PG of this organism is introduced exclusively during the first steps in its de novo biosynthesis, namely, during the formation of phosphatidic acid. Saito et al. (130) later demonstrated that the positional distribution of a number of different fatty acids in the neutral glycolipids of *A. laidlawii* B, the MGDG and DGDG, is essentially identical to that found in the anionic phospholipid PG, suggesting that these two classes of lipids share a common biosynthetic pathway (Fig. 3). Interestingly, in all of the studies cited above and in a study of the positional distribution of a series of positional isomers of *cis*-octadecenoic acid in the PG of this organism (129), an excellent correlation was observed between the relative positional specificity and the physicochemical rather than the chemical properties of a given fatty acid, with the highest-melting-point fatty acids exhibiting the greatest affinity for position 1 and the lowest-melting-point fatty acids showing the greatest affinity for position 2. Thus, the fatty acid specificity of the enzymes catalyzing the sequential esterification of glycerol 3-phosphate must be markedly different and will function to produce primarily mixed-acid membrane glycerolipids having a much higher degree of physicochemical homogeneity than would be the case if fatty acids were esterified randomly at each position of the glycerol backbone.

Although the positional distribution of fatty acids seen in *A. laidlawii* is typical of that observed in most eubacteria and in all eucaryotes, this does not seem to be the case with the sterol-requiring *Mycoplasma* species tested. Rottem and Markowitz (116, 117) have shown that in *M. gallisepticum* and in five other *Mycoplasma* species, longer-chain saturated fatty acids such as palmitate are found chiefly at the 2 position and oleic acid is found chiefly at the 1 position of the PG synthesized by these organisms, and Davis et al. (26) report a similar finding for *S. floricola*. Interestingly, this unusual reversed fatty acid positional distribution is also found in a few other eubacterial groups, among them the clostridia, which have been suggested to be closely related to the mycoplasmas (see chapter 33). However, since the *Acholeplasma* and *Mycoplasma* species are also purported to be closely related, the "typical" fatty acid positional distribution observed in the two *Acholeplasma* species thus far studied becomes difficult to explain if indeed a clostridial subline also gave rise to this group of mycoplasmas.

Koostra and Smith (50) have characterized the mechanism of the biosynthesis of the principal O-amino acid esters of PG which are synthesized by *A. laidlawii* B in acidic growth medium. The biosynthesis of L-alanylphosphatidylglycerol was found to involve a membrane-associated, enzyme-catalyzed transesterification of the amino acid from L-alanyl-tRNA and requires exogenous PG. Biosynthesis of the D-alanyl-phosphatidylglycerol does not involve tRNA but does require PG and a complex of D-alanine with ATP and an amino acid-activating enzyme. The biosynthesis of each of these isomeric O-amino acid esters of PG is stereospecific and is not inhibited by the opposite stereoisomer, and the conformation of the alanine-containing substrate is maintained in the product.

As discussed earlier, Dahl and coworkers (22, 24) have shown that small amounts of cholesterol are specifically required to stimulate phospholipid synthesis in *M. capricolum*, possibly by enhancing the rates of the uptake and/or esterification of exogenous oleic acid (21), and that the rate of unsaturated phospholipid synthesis in turn coordinately controls the rate of RNA and protein synthesis in this organism. This finding may explain, in part at least, the observation of Archer (3) that large changes in the amount of cholesterol incorporated into the membrane of the closely related *M. mycoides* subsp. *capri* produce only small changes in the cholesterol/phospholipid ratio, a result supporting a coordinate regulation of cholesterol uptake and phospholipid biosynthesis. On the other hand, Rottem et al. (125) and Le Grimellec et al. (53) have reported that *M. mycoides* subsp. *capri* and *M. gallisepticum*, respectively, adapted to grow on low levels of exogenous cholesterol, also exhibit markedly reduced cholesterol/phospholipid ratios. Moreover, the lipid/protein ratio in the membranes of *A. laidlawii* B (163) and of several *Mycoplasma* species (2, 47, 81) can be substantially altered by inhibiting either lipid or protein biosynthesis, suggesting that these two processes are not tightly coupled in these organisms. Clearly, a great deal more experimental work on the regulation of phospholipid biosynthesis in mycoplasmas is required to achieve even a rudimentary understanding of the mechanisms of such regulation.

Glycolipids

Smith (145) has studied the biosynthesis of MGDG and DGDG in *A. laidlawii* B in considerable detail. The MGDG was found to be synthesized by a membrane-bound enzyme from 1,2-diglyceride and UDP-glucose. The 1,2-diglycerides derived from the phospholipids of this organism were reported to be by far the best substrate, although mixed-acid 1,2-diglycerides from egg yolk exhibit some activity. Interestingly, 1,2-diglycerides containing either two identical saturated or two identical unsaturated fatty acids are not utilized (although they obviously can be utilized in vivo), nor are 1,3-diglycerides. A medium of high ionic strength containing some sodium dodecyl sulfate is required for optimal MGDG synthesis. The DGDG was also found to be synthesized by a membrane-bound enzyme from MGDG and UDP-glucose. A monogalactosyl diglyceride could not substitute for MGDG. Both reactions are specific for both the nucleotide and the sugar portion of the UDP-glucose substrate, and both require Mg^{2+} and exhibit an optimal pH of 8.0. The optimal rate of MGDG formation was found to be about 10-fold greater than the optimal rate of DGDG formation, qualitatively consistent with the usual predominance of the former lipid under most growth conditions. In view of the many similarities between these two reactions and because both are membrane associated, it is not clear whether both reactions are catalyzed by a single enzyme or whether two distinct enzymes are involved. The details of neutral glycolipid synthesis in the sterol-requiring mycoplasmas which contain these lipids have not been studied.

In contrast to the neutral glycolipids of *A. laidlawii*, practically nothing is known about the mechanisms of biosynthesis of the different phosphoglycolipids that have been found to occur in several *Acholeplasma* species (149). However, the previously discussed similarity in the fatty acid compositions of the neutral glycolipids and GPDGDG (27, 128) suggests that DGDG may be the biosynthetic precursor to this phosphoglycolipid in these organisms.

Sphingolipids

Plackett et al. (76) have shown that *A. axanthum* is unique among the mycoplasmas thus far studied in having the capacity to synthesize sphingosine-type bases from various exogenous fatty acids (and presumably serine) and to convert these bases into the corresponding *O*-acyl ceramide 1-phosphoglycerol and their deacylated derivatives. However, the mechanism of the synthesis of these compounds by this organism has not been studied. The SM found associated with the membranes of a number of sterol-requiring *Mycoplasma* and *Spiroplasma* species grown in complex, serum-containing medium is not synthesized but represents exogenous lipid incorporated unchanged from the growth medium (see previous section).

MEMBRANE LIPID METABOLISM

Fatty Acids

The fermentative mycoplasmas, including both the sterol-nonrequiring *Acholeplasma* species and the sterol-requiring *Mycoplasma* species, are not capable of oxidizing fatty acids (see chapter 11). However, Lynn (57) has shown that some nonfermentative *Mycoplasma* species, such as *M. arthritidis*, are able to oxidize short-chain fatty acids and to derive a considerable portion of their metabolism energy via this process. This organism was found to oxidize saturated fatty acids containing 2 to 10 carbon atoms, although the rate of oxidation decreased with increasing chain length. VanDemark and Smith (166) have demonstrated that in *M. hominis*, butyrate oxidation proceeds by the typical fatty acid β-oxidation pathway described for *E. coli* and other bacteria and that the acetyl-CoA produced is further metabolized via the tricarboxylic acid cycle (165). Apparently, the longer-chain saturated and unsaturated exogenous fatty acids that are required for the biosynthesis of the membrane glycerolipids by these organisms are not substrates for β oxidation. One should note, however, that subsequent work has failed to confirm the existence of the tricarboxylic cycle in *M. hominis* or in any other *Mycoplasma* species and has suggested that the *M. hominis*

strain used by VanDemark and Smith may have been contaminated by a bacterial species (see chapter 11). Therefore, the question of the existence of a fatty acid β-oxidation pathway in this or other *Mycoplasma* species should probably be regarded as an open one at this point.

None of the mycoplasmas studied to date are capable of modifying the chemical structure of exogenous long-chain fatty acids by, for example, introducing a double bond into the hydrocarbon chain, altering the geometrical configuration of a double bond already present, or shortening or lengthening the hydrocarbon chains (84, 148, 150; see also earlier sections in this chapter). The only exceptions to this rule described to date are *A. laidlawii* A and B, which are capable of the chain elongation of a variety of exogenous medium- and long-chain fatty acids. For example, Panos and coworkers have shown that *A. laidlawii* A can elongate both *cis*- and *trans*-monounsaturated tetra- or hexadecenoic acids (71) or *cis*-9,10-methylene hexadecanoic acid (69), a cyclopropane ring-containing fatty acid, and that *Acholeplasma* sp. strain KHS can elongate palmitoleic acid but not palmitelaidic acid, its geometrical isomer (69). In the case of *A. laidlawii* A, the degree of elongation of the *cis*-monounsaturated fatty acids was found to be greater than that of the *trans*-monounsaturated fatty acids. Romijn et al. (110) also reported that *A. laidlawii* B is capable of elongating palmitoleic acid to *cis*-vaccenic acid.

Saito and McElhaney (128) and Saito et al. (132) subsequently studied the chain elongation process in *A. laidlawii* B in more detail, using a wide variety of exogenous fatty acids of different chain lengths. Within each chemical class of fatty acids examined, the extent of chain elongation increases with increases in chain length, reaches a maximum value, and then declines to zero with further increases in chain length. Depending on chemical structure, exogenous fatty acids containing fewer than 6 to 9 carbon atoms or more than 15 to 18 carbon atoms are not substrates for the chain elongation system. The substrate specificity of this fatty acid elongation system is strikingly broad, and certain straight-chain, methyl iso-branched, and methyl anteiso-branched saturated fatty acids, as well as *cis*- and *trans*-monounsaturated, *cis*-cyclopropane, and *cis*-polyunsaturated fatty acids, undergo chain elongation in vivo. The extent of chain elongation and the average chain length of the primary elongation products correlate well with the physical properties (melting temperatures) of the exogenous fatty acid substrates. That is, the lower the melting point of a particular exogenous fatty acid, the higher is the proportion of that fatty acid elongated and the greater is the number of two-carbon units added to it. The specificity of fatty acid chain elongation in *A. laidlawii* B thus maintains the fluidity and physical state of the membrane lipids within a rather wide but definitely limited range.

Saito et al. (132) also found that the fatty acid chain elongation system of this organism could be markedly influenced by the presence of a second exogenous fatty acid that is not itself a substrate for the chain elongation system but which is incorporated directly into the membrane lipids. The presence of a relatively low-melting-point exogenous fatty acid increases both the extent of chain elongation and the average chain length of the elongation products generated, whereas the presence of a relatively high-melting-point fatty acid has the opposite effect. The extent of chain elongation and nature of the elongation products formed are not, however, dependent on the fluidity and physical state of the membrane lipids per se. The second exogenous fatty acid appears instead to exert its characteristic effect by competing with the chain elongation substrate and elongation products for the stereospecific acylation of positions 1 and 2 of sn-glycerol-3-phosphate. The similar effects of alterations in environmental temperature, cholesterol content, and exposure to the antibiotic cerulenin on the fatty acid chain elongation and de novo biosynthetic activities suggest that the chain elongation system of this organism may be a component of the de novo biosynthetic system. Support for this suggestion was provided by Saito et al. (131), who presented evidence that the low concentrations of cerulenin which decrease the average chain length of endogenous saturated fatty acids (by preferentially inhibiting the β-ketoacyl thioesterase component of the de novo fatty acid biosynthetic pathway that is specific for medium-chain fatty acids) also preferentially inhibit the elongation of exogenous medium-chain fatty acids.

Sterols and Their Derivatives

Cholesterol or other sterols incorporated into the membranes of all mycoplasma species studied to date remain chemically unmodified and therefore do not exhibit metabolic turnover in growing cells (4, 34, 100, 111, 140). The same appears to be true for the exogenous cholesterol esters which are apparently incorporated into the membranes of certain *Mycoplasma* and *Spiroplasma* species (26, 31, 117, 124). Moreover, in most cases, metabolic interconversions between cholesterol and cholesterol esters are not observed once these compounds have been taken up and incorporated into the membrane. However, Smith (139) has reported the presence of a membrane-associated sterol esterase in *A. laidlawii*, *M. gallinarum*, and *M. arthritidis* and characterized this enzyme in the latter organism in some detail. This esterase is capable of the hydrolytic or thiolytic cleavage of steryl esters and carotenyl esters and requires that the substrate be in micellar form with an amphiphilic lipid for maximal activity. Although not highly specific with regard to the fatty acyl moiety, esters formed from short-chain fatty acids are attacked most readily, and the enzyme exhibits considerable specificity for the sterol portion of the molecule. Apparently, the function of this esterase in mycoplasma cells is to hydrolyze exogenous cholesterol esters into cholesterol and free fatty acids, so that each may be incorporated into the membrane most readily.

Henrikson and Smith (42) have demonstrated the presence of membrane-associated α- and β-glucosidases in the fermentative *A. laidlawii* and *M. gallisepticum*, respectively, but not in the nonfermentative *M. hominis*, and have suggested that these enzymes may be involved in the synthesis and hydrolysis of carotenyl glucoside and cholesteryl glucoside, respectively, by these organisms. The metabolic turnover of the glucose moiety of these glucosides led Smith (146)

to postulate a role for carotenyl glucosides in the transport of glucose into *A. laidlawii* cells. However, in view of the well-established and sufficient role of membrane proteins in all active transport processes studied in detail to date (see chapter 15), this postulate now appears unlikely.

Carotenoids and Their Derivatives

Carotenoids, once synthesized by the appropriate *Acholeplasma* species, also appear not to undergo degradation or chemical modification in growing cells (146). However, Smith (146) has reported that the acetyl moiety of the carotenyl ester found in *A. laidlawii* undergoes a rapid turnover during the metabolism of glucose and has suggested that the turnover of this compound may be involved in transporting acetate out of glucose-metabolizing cells. The idea is that the acetate formed intracellularly would be utilized to form carotenoyl acetate on the inner surface of the membrane lipid bilayer, and that after flipping across the bilayer, the acetate would be liberated to the medium by the action of the carotenyl (or sterol) esterase discussed above. Again, however, the passive or protein-mediated diffusion of acetate across the lipid bilayer down its concentration gradient would appear to be a simpler, more efficient, and less energetically costly route of acetate translocation out of the cell.

Phospholipids

Smith (143, 146) has studied the metabolic turnover of the glycerophosphatides of *A. laidlawii*, using radioactive P_i to pulse-radiolabel these compounds. He found that no metabolic turnover of PG or DPG occurs, indicating that at least the phosphate portions of the polar headgroups of these phosphatides are metabolically stable. McElhaney and Tourtellotte (65) carried out similar studies of this organism by using growth in radioactive fatty acids, glucose, and P_i to label the fatty acyl groups, the glycerol backbone, and the polar headgroups, respectively, of these phospholipid molecules. These workers also found that no loss of radioactivity from any of the phospholipids present in the membrane occurs upon subsequent growth, indicating that all portions of these phospholipid molecules are metabolically stable in growing cells. A similar result was earlier reported by Kahane and Razin (47), who used radioactive oleate to label the total membrane polar lipid fraction of *A. laidlawii*. However, these workers did detect a small amount of lipid turnover after several hours of growth of washed cells originally harvested in the mid-log phase of growth and an immediate and more pronounced lipid turnover in cells from stationary-phase cultures. Since McElhaney and Tourtellotte (65) did not detect any metabolic turnover in any of the membrane lipids of this organism even after 4 h of growth, the lipid turnover observed by Kahane and Razin may have resulted from the heavy suspension of cells used in their experiments. This may have resulted in a depletion of essential nutrients from the growth medium over time, which in turn induced cell lysis.

Smith (143) and Smith and Koostra (154) have also

carried out studies of phospholipid turnover in two sterol-requiring mycoplasmas, *M. hominis* and *M. gallisepticum*, using radioactive P_i to label the phospholipid polar headgroups. Again, no metabolic turnover was observed in any of the phospholipids, indicating that these lipids play only a structural role in the membranes of these organisms. However, Dahl and co-workers (18, 20) have reported that in *M. capricolum*, endogenous or exogenous phospholipids containing radiolabeled palmitate, oleate, or glycerol moieties can serve as acyl donors (and possibly also as diglyceride donors) to a number of membrane proteins, implying that at least a small amount of phospholipid turnover should occur in this organism. Interestingly, the palmitate and oleate moieties radiolabel a different set of membrane proteins, and the addition of exogenous cholesterol stimulates the acylation of certain proteolipids by oleate but not by palmitate. As well, the radiolabeled glycerol moiety is incorporated primarily into the same membrane proteins labeled by oleate, suggesting the involvement of a bound diglyceride moiety.

The general lack of phospholipid turnover in mycoplasmas is compatible with the failure thus far to demonstrate active phospholipase A, C, or D in most of the organisms studied (36, 84, 148, 150, 167). However, the presence of a very active, membrane-associated lysophospholipase has been demonstrated by van Golde et al. (167) in *A. laidlawii* B and by Gatt et al. (36) in *M. gallisepticum*. The *A. laidlawii* enzyme exhibits a much higher activity for exogenous lysophosphatidylglycerol than for the analogous lysophosphatidylcholine and hydrolyzes 1-acyl lysophospholipids at slightly greater rates than it hydrolyzes their 2-acyl homologs, and the *M. gallisepticum* enzyme was shown to be capable of degrading pancreatic phospholipase A_2-generated lysophospholipids in the same or adjacent membranes. In both organisms, the lysophospholipase appears to be located on the external surface of the membrane of whole cells. It has been suggested that the function of these enzymes may be to hydrolyze and thus detoxify any highly lytic lysophospholipids encountered in the environment.

Rottem and Markowitz (117) have reported that exogenous PCs taken up by *M. gallisepticum* are modified by replacing the largely unsaturated fatty acid found at position 2 with a saturated fatty acid, thus producing primarily disaturated molecular species. This reaction apparently occurs by a phospholipase A_2-catalyzed deacylation followed by a reacylation of position 2 with a saturated fatty acid; although an active phospholipase A_2 could not be demonstrated in this first study, the acylation of exogenous 1-lysophosphatidylcholine could be. However, Rottem et al. (113) later demonstrated a very low endogenous phospholipase A_2 activity in isolated membranes of this organism but one that could be markedly stimulated by detergents. As well, these workers showed that exogenous diunsaturated and saturated-unsaturated PCs are modified to various extents by *M. gallisepticum* but disaturated PCs, although incorporated into the membrane, are not. Moreover, Rottem and coworkers found that *M. pulmonis* and *M. pneumoniae* were also capable of modification of exogenous PCs but that most of the other *Mycoplasma* and all of the *Spiroplasma* species tested were not. The placement of a saturated rather

than an unsaturated fatty acid at position 2 of exogenous PCs by these three *Mycoplasma* species is probably related to the unusual positional distribution of fatty acids in the endogenous PG of these organisms. As discussed earlier, the predominant PGs synthesized by many *Mycoplasma* species contain unsaturated fatty acids at position 1 and saturated fatty acids at position 2 (116, 117).

Glycolipids

Smith (143) and Smith and Koostra (154) have also studied the turnover of the glycolipids of the *A. laidlawii* membrane by using a pulse-chase sequence with highly radioactive glucose. These workers found no metabolic turnover of the neutral glycolipids MGDG and DGDG but did find rapid metabolic turnover of the phosphorylated glycolipid GPDGDG, which was also manifest by radioactive P_i labeling. However, McElhaney and Tourtellotte (65), who radiolabeled these lipids by growth with exogenous palmitate and oleate as well as with glucose and P_i, reported no dilution of any of these labels upon subsequent growth in complete growth medium containing the same unlabeled lipid precursors. The reason for this discrepancy in results is unclear but may be related to differences in the conditions under which radiolabeling and subsequent incubation of the cells were carried out and to the use of different time scales in the two experiments. Plackett (73) has also reported an absence of monogalactosyl diglyceride turnover in *M. mycoides*.

Sphingolipids

As discussed earlier, none of the sterol-requiring mycoplasma species studied to date which have been shown to incorporate exogenous SM into their cell membranes appear to modify it in any way after incorporation. The metabolic turnover of the phosphosphingolipids synthesized by *A. axanthum* has not been investigated (76).

Glycerides

Although the metabolic turnover of the small quantities of di- and triglycerides apparently synthesized by many mycoplasma species (see chapter 6) has not been studied, a nonspecific lipase has been reported in a number of mycoplasma species (17, 122, 139). This enzyme attacks synthetic triglycerides, natural fats, and fatty acid esters and is distinct from the sterol esterase discussed earlier. The nonspecific lipase is not membrane associated, has no inorganic ion requirement, and exhibits an alkaline pH optimum. Since cultures of many mycoplasma species exhibit lipolytic activity (see reference 17 and references therein), this or a similar enzyme is presumably secreted by cells growing either on solid or in liquid culture. The function of this lipase is probably to liberate the free fatty acids required for the optimal growth of most mycoplasma species.

CONCLUSIONS AND OUTLOOK

We currently know a considerable amount about the general aspects of mycoplasma membrane lipid incorporation, biosynthesis, and metabolism at the descriptive or whole-cell level, particularly for *A. laidlawii*. However, the detailed biochemical pathways for the biosynthesis and metabolism of only a few membrane lipid classes are definitively established at present. Although some progress has been made in understanding the qualitative aspects of the regulation of mycoplasma lipid biosynthesis and metabolism, the biochemical mechanisms by which such regulation is accomplished are virtually unknown. As well, the isolation, characterization, and functional reconstitution of even a single enzyme involved in any aspect of lipid biochemistry has yet to be accomplished. Clearly, the lack of mutants defective in the various steps of membrane lipid biosynthesis and metabolism has impeded progress in these areas. Despite the fact that much remains to be done, and although these organisms offer many intrinsic advantages in studies of lipid biochemistry, the small number of researchers currently working in this area does not bode well for future progress.

REFERENCES

1. **Al-Shammari, A. J. N., and P. F. Smith.** 1979. Lipid and lipopolysaccharide composition of *Acholeplasma oculi*. *J. Bacteriol.* **139:**356–361.
2. **Amar, A., S. Rottem, and S. Razin.** 1979. Is the vertical disposition of mycoplasma membrane proteins affected by membrane fluidity? *Biochim. Biophys. Acta* **552:** 457–467.
3. **Archer, D. B.** 1975. Modification of the membrane composition of *Mycoplasma mycoides* subsp. *capri* by the growth medium. *J. Gen. Microbiol.* **88:**329–338.
4. **Argamon, M., and S. Razin.** 1965. Cholesterol and cholesterol esters in mycoplasma. *J. Gen. Microbiol.* **38:** 153–168.
5. **Beckman, B. L., and G. E. Kenny.** 1968. Immunochemical analysis of serologically active lipids of *Mycoplasma pneumoniae*. *J. Bacteriol.* **96:**1171–1180.
6. **Bhakoo, M., and R. N. McElhaney.** 1988. The effect of variations in growth temperature, fatty acid composition and cholesterol content on the lipid polar headgroup composition of *Acholeplasma laidlawii* B membranes. *Biochim. Biophys. Acta* **945:**307–314.
7. **Bittman, R., S. Clejan, and S. W. Hui.** 1990. Increased rates of lipid exchange between *Mycoplasma capricolum* membranes and vesicles in relation to the propensity of forming nonbilayer lipid structures. *J. Biol. Chem.* **265:**15110–15117.
8. **Bittman, R., S. Clejan, B. P. Robinson, and N. M. Witzke.** 1985. Kinetics of cholesterol and phospholipid exchange from membranes containing cross-linked proteins or cross-linked phosphatidylethanolamine. *Biochemistry* **24:**1403–1409.
9. **Butler, M., and B. C. J. G. Knight.** 1960. Steroid growth requirements and steroid growth inhibitors of mycoplasma. *J. Gen. Microbiol.* **22:**483–491.
10. **Castrejon-Diez, J., J. N. Fisher, and E. Fisher.** 1962. Acetokinase reaction in several pleuropneumonia-like organisms. *Biochem. Biophys. Res. Commun.* **9:**416–420.
11. **Chang, C. J.** 1985. Lipid utilization of two flower spiroplasmas and honeybee spiroplasma. *Can. J. Microbiol.* **31:**173–176.
12. **Chang, C. J., and T. A. Chen.** 1983. Nutritional require-
ments of two flower spiroplasmas and honey bee spiroplasma. *J. Bacteriol.* **153:**452–457.
13. **Christiansson, A., and Å. Wieslander.** 1980. Control of membrane polar lipid composition in *Acholeplasma laidlawii* A by the extent of saturated fatty acid synthesis. *Biochim. Biophys. Acta* **595:**189–199.
14. **Clejan, S., and R. Bittman.** 1984. Decreases in rates of lipid exchange between *Mycoplasma gallisepticum* and unilamellar vesicles by incorporation of sphingomyelin. *J. Biol. Chem.* **259:**10823–10826.
15. **Cluss, R. G., J. K. Johnson, and N. L. Somerson.** 1983. Liposomes replace serum for cultivation of fermenting mycoplasmas. *Appl. Environ. Microbiol.* **46:**370–374.
16. **Cluss, R. G., and N. L. Somerson.** 1986. Interaction of albumin phospholipid:cholesterol liposomes in growth of *Mycoplasma* spp. *Appl. Environ. Microbiol.* **51:** 281–287.
17. **Cole, B. C., and P. Pease.** 1967. Lipolytic activity by oral pleuropneumonia-like (mycoplasma) organisms.*J. Gen. Microbiol.* **47:**171–174.
18. **Dahl, C. E., and J. S. Dahl.** 1984. Phospholipids as acyl donors to membrane proteins of *Mycoplasma capricolum*. *J. Biol. Chem.* **259:**10771–10776.
19. **Dahl, C. E., and J. S. Dahl.** 1988. Cholesterol and cell function, p. 148–171. *In* P. L. Yeagle (ed.), *Biology of Cholesterol*. CRC Press, Boca Raton, Fla.
20. **Dahl, C. E., J. S. Dahl, and K. Bloch.** 1983. Proteolipid formation in *Mycoplasma capricolum*. Influence of cholesterol on unsaturated fatty acid acylation of membrane proteins. *J. Biol. Chem.* **258:**11814–11818.
21. **Dahl, J.** 1988. Uptake of fatty acids by *Mycoplasma capricolum*. *J. Bacteriol.* **170:**2022–2026.
22. **Dahl, J. S., and C. E. Dahl.** 1983. Coordinate regulation of unsaturated phospholipid, RNA, and protein synthesis in *Mycoplasma capricolum* by cholesterol. *Proc. Natl. Acad. Sci. USA* **80:**692–696.
23. **Dahl, J. S., C. E. Dahl, and K. Bloch.** 1980. Sterols in membranes: growth characteristics and membrane properties of *Mycoplasma capricolum* cultured on cholesterol and lanosterol. *Biochemistry* **19:**1467–1472.
24. **Dahl, J. S., C. E. Dahl, and K. Bloch.** 1981. Effect of cholesterol on macromolecular synthesis and fatty acid uptake by *Mycoplasma capricolum*. *J. Biol. Chem.* **256:**87–91.
25. **Davis, P. J., H. Efrati, S. Razin, and S. Rottem.** 1984. Two cholesterol pools in *Acholeplasma laidlawii* membranes. *FEBS Lett.* **175:**51–54.
26. **Davis, P. J., A. Katznel, S. Razin, and S. Rottem.** 1985. Spiroplasma membrane lipids. *J. Bacteriol.* **161:** 118–122.
27. **de Kruyff, B., R. A. Demel, A. J. Slotboom, L. L. M. van Deenen, and A. F. Rosenthal.** 1973. The effect of the polar headgroup on the lipid-cholesterol interaction: a monolayer and differential scanning calorimetry study. *Biochim. Biophys. Acta* **307:**1–19.
28. **Edward, D. G. A.** 1971. Determination of sterol requirement for mycoplasmatales. *J. Gen. Microbiol.* **69:** 205–210.
29. **Edward, D. G. ff.** 1953. A difference in growth requirements between bacteria in the L-phase and organisms of the pleuropneumonia group. *J. Gen. Microbiol.* **8:** 256–262.
30. **Edward, D. G. ff., and W. A. Fitzgerald.** 1951. Cholesterol in the growth of organisms of the pleuropneumonia group. *J. Gen. Microbiol.* **5:**576–586.
31. **Efrati, H., Y. Oschry, S. Eisenberg, and S. Razin.** 1982. Preferential uptake of lipids by mycoplasma membranes from human plasma low-density lipoproteins. *Biochemistry* **21:**6477–6482.
32. **Efrati, H., S. Rottem, and S. Razin.** 1981. Lipid and protein membrane components associated with cholesterol uptake by mycoplasmas. *Biochim. Biophys. Acta* **641:**386–394.

33. **Efrati, H., Y. Wax, and S. Rottem.** 1986. Cholesterol uptake capacity of *Acholeplasma laidlawii* is affected by the composition and content of membrane glycolipids. *Arch. Biochem. Biophys.* **248:**282–288.

34. **Freeman, B. A., R. Sissenstein, T. T. McManus, J. E. Woodward, I. M. Lee, and J. B. Mudd.** 1976. Lipid composition and lipid metabolism of *Spiroplasma citri. J. Bacteriol.* **125:**946–954.

35. **Gadir, F. A., R. J. Hidalgo, and L. C. Grumbles.** 1973. Lipid nutrition of mycoplasma of bovine origin. *Am. J. Vet. Res.* **34:**335–339.

36. **Gatt, S., B. Morag, and S. Rottem.** 1982. Lysophospholipase-catalyzed hydrolysis of lysophospholipids in *Mycoplasma gallisepticum* membranes. *J. Bacteriol.* **151:**1095–1101.

37. **Gershfeld, N. L., M. Wormser, and S. Razin.** 1974. Cholesterol in mycoplasma membranes. I. Kinetics and equilibrium studies of cholesterol uptake by the cell membrane of *Acholeplasma laidlawii. Biochim. Biophys. Acta* **352:**371–384.

38. **Gross, Z., and S. Rottem.** 1986. Lipid interconversions in aging *Mycoplasma capricolum* cultures. *J. Bacteriol.* **167:**986–991.

39. **Gross, Z., S. Rottem, and R. Bittman.** 1982. Phospholipid interconversions in *Mycoplasma capricolum. Eur. J. Biochem.* **122:**169–174.

40. **Hackett, K. J., A. S. Ginsberg, S. Rottem, R. B. Henegar, and R. F. Whitcomb.** A defined medium for a fastidious Spiroplasma. *Science* **237:**525–527.

41. **Henrikson, C. V., and C. Panos.** 1969. Fatty acid composition, distribution, and requirements of two nonsterol-requiring mycoplasmas from complex but defatted growth media. *Biochemistry* **8:**646–651.

42. **Henrikson, C. V., and P. F. Smith.** 1964. β-Glucosidase activity in mycoplasma. *J. Gen. Microbiol.* **37:**78–80.

43. **Henrikson, C. V., and P. F. Smith.** 1966. Growth response of mycoplasma to carotenoid pigments and carotenoid intermediates. *J. Gen. Microbiol.* **45:**73–82.

44. **Henrikson, C. V., and P. F. Smith.** 1966. Conversion of mevalonic acid to γ,γ-dimethylallyl pyrophosphate by *Mycoplasma. J. Bacteriol.* **92:**701–706.

45. **Herring, P. K., and J. D. Pollack.** 1974. Utilization of [1-^13C]acetate in the synthesis of lipids by *Acholeplasmas. Int. J. Syst. Bacteriol.* **24:**73–78.

46. **Johnson, J. K., and N. L. Somerson.** 1980. Cholesterol as a limiting factor in the growth of *Mycoplasma pneumoniae. Appl. Environ. Microbiol.* **40:**391–399.

47. **Kahane, I., and S. Razin.** 1969. Synthesis and turnover of membrane protein and lipid in *Mycoplasma laidlawii. Biochim. Biophys. Acta* **183:**79–89.

48. **Kahane, I., and S. Razin.** 1977. Cholesterol-phosphatidylcholine dispersions as donors of cholesterol to mycoplasma membranes. *Biochim. Biophys. Acta* **471:**32–38.

49. **Kannenberg, E., and K. Poralla.** 1982. The influence of hopanoids on growth of *Mycoplasma mycoides. Arch. Microbiol.* **133:**100–102.

50. **Koostra, W. L., and P. F. Smith.** 1969. D- and L-alanylphosphatidylglycerols from *Mycoplasma laidlawii,* strain B. *Biochemistry* **12:**4794–4806.

51. **Lala, A. K., T. M. Buttke, and K. Bloch.** 1979. On the role of the sterol hydroxyl group in membranes. *J. Biol. Chem.* **254:**10582–10585.

52. **Leaver, J., A. Alonso, A. A. Durranic, and D. Chapman.** 1983. The biosynthetic incorporation of diacetylenic fatty acids into the biomembranes of *Acholeplasma laidlawii* A cells and polymerization of the biomembranes by irradiation with ultraviolet light. *Biochim. Biophys. Acta* **727:**327–335.

53. **Le Grimellec, C., J. Cardinal, M.-C. Giocondi, and S. Carriere.** 1981. Control of membrane lipids in *Mycoplasma gallisepticum:* effect on lipid order. *J. Bacteriol.* **146:**155–162.

54. **Lelong, I., B. Luu, M. Mersel, and S. Rottem.** 1988. Effect of 7β-hydroxylcholesterol on growth and membrane composition of *Mycoplasma capricolum. FEBS Lett.* **232:**354–358.

55. **Leon, O., and C. Panos.** 1981. Long-chain fatty acid perturbations in *Mycoplasma pneumoniae. J. Bacteriol.* **146:**1124–1134.

56. **Liss, A., J. C. Pfeil, and D. Levitt.** 1987. Cytotoxic and cytolytic activity of nonadecafluoro-*n*-decanoic acid on *Acholeplasma laidlawii. Appl. Environ. Microbiol.* **53:**1236–1240.

57. **Lynn, R. J.** 1960. Oxidative metabolism of pleuropneumonia-like organisms. *Ann. N.Y. Acad. Sci.* **79:**538–542.

58. **McElhaney, R. N.** 1974. The effect of alterations in the physical state of the membrane lipids on the ability of *Acholeplasma laidlawii* B to grow at various temperatures. *J. Mol. Biol.* **84:**145–157.

59. **McElhaney, R. N.** 1983. Manipulation of membrane lipid composition, p. 235–239. *In* S. Razin and J. G. Tully (ed.), *Methods in Mycoplasmology,* vol. 1. Academic Press, New York.

60. **McElhaney, R. N.** 1984. The structure and function of the *Acholeplasma laidlawii* membrane. *Biochim. Biophys. Acta* **779:**1–42.

61. **McElhaney, R. N.** 1989. The influence of membrane lipid composition and physical properties on membrane structure and function in *Acholeplasma laidlawii. Crit. Rev. Microbiol.* **17:**1–32.

62. **McElhaney, R. N., J. de Gier, and E. C. M. van der Neut-Kok.** 1973. The effect of alterations in fatty acid composition and cholesterol content on the nonelectrolyte permeability of *Acholeplasma laidlawii* cells and derived liposomes. *Biochim. Biophys. Acta* **298:**500–512.

63. **McElhaney, R. N., and M. E. Tourtellotte.** 1969. Mycoplasma membrane lipids: variations in fatty acid composition. *Science* **164:**433–434.

64. **McElhaney, R. N., and M. E. Tourtellotte.** 1970. The relationship between fatty acid structure and the positional distribution of esterified fatty acids in the phosphatidylglycerol from *Mycoplasma laidlawii. Biochim. Biophys. Acta* **202:**120–128.

65. **McElhaney, R. N., and M. E. Tourtellotte.** 1970. Metabolic turnover of the polar lipids of *Mycoplasma laidlawii* strain B. *J. Bacteriol.* **101:**72–76.

66. **Miura, Y., N. Imaeda, M. Shinoda, H. Tamura, and N. Ueta.** 1978. An analysis of the fatty acid composition of total lipids from mycoplasma. *Jpn. J. Exp. Med.* **48:**525–531.

67. **Mudd, J. B., M. Ittig, B. Roy, J. Latrille, and J.-M. Bové.** 1977. Composition and enzyme activities of *Spiroplasma citri* membranes. *J. Bacteriol.* **129:**1250–1256.

68. **Odriozola, J. M., E. Waitzkin, T. L. Smith, and K. Bloch.** 1978. Sterol requirement of *Mycoplasma capricolum. Proc. Natl. Acad. Sci. USA* **75:**4107–4109.

69. **Panos, C., and C. V. Henrikson.** 1969. Fatty acid interconversions in *Mycoplasma* sp. KHS. *Biochemistry* **8:**652–658.

70. **Panos, C., and O. Leon.** 1974. Replacement of the octadecenoic acid growth-requirement for *Acholeplasma laidlawii* A by *cis*-9,10-methylene-hexadecanoic acid, a cyclopropane fatty acid. *J. Gen. Microbiol.* **80:**93–100.

71. **Panos, C., and S. Rottem.** 1970. Incorporation and elongation of fatty acid isomers by *Mycoplasma laidlawii* A. *Biochemistry* **9:**407–412.

72. **Plackett, P.** 1967. The glycolipids of *Mycoplasma mycoides. Biochemistry* **6:**2746–2754.

73. **Plackett, P.** 1967. The synthesis of polar lipids by mycoplasma. *Ann. N.Y. Acad. Sci.* **143:**158–164.

74. **Plackett, P., B. P. Marmion, E. J. Shaw, and R. M. Lemcke.** 1969. Immunochemical analysis of *Mycoplasma pneumoniae.* 3. Separation and chemical identification of serologically active lipids. *Aust. J. Exp. Biol. Med. Sci.* **47:**171–195.

75. **Plackett, P., and A. W. Rodwell.** 1970. Glycerolipid bio-

synthesis by *Mycoplasma* strain Y. *Biochim. Biophys. Acta* **210**:230–240.

76. **Plackett, P., P. F. Smith, and W. R. Mayberry.** 1970. Lipids of a sterol-nonrequiring mycoplasma. *J. Bacteriol.* **104**:798–807.

77. **Pollack, J. D.** 1978. Differentiation of *Mycoplasma* and *Acholeplasma*. *Int. J. Syst. Bacteriol.* **28**:425–426.

78. **Pollack, J. D., K. D. Beaman, and J. A. Robertson.** 1984. Synthesis of lipids from acetate is not characteristic of *Acholeplasma* or *Ureaplasma* species. *Int. J. Syst. Bacteriol.* **34**:124–126.

79. **Pollack, J. D., N. L. Somerson, and L. B. Senterfit.** 1970. Isolation, characterization, and immunogenicity of *Mycoplasma pneumoniae* membranes. *Infect. Immun.* **2**:326–339.

80. **Pollack, J. D., and M. E. Tourtellotte.** 1967. Synthesis of saturated long chain fatty acids from sodium acetate-1-^{14}C by *Mycoplasma*. *J. Bacteriol.* **93**:636–641.

81. **Razin, S.** 1974. Correlation of cholesterol to phospholipid content in membranes of growing mycoplasmas. *FEBS Lett.* **47**:81–85.

82. **Razin, S.** 1975. Cholesterol incorporation into bacterial membranes. *J. Bacteriol.* **124**:570–572.

83. **Razin, S.** 1978. Cholesterol uptake is dependent on membrane fluidity in mycoplasmas. *Biochim. Biophys. Acta* **513**:401–404.

84. **Razin, S.** 1982. The mycoplasma membrane, p. 165–250. *In* B. K. Ghosh (ed.), *Organization of Prokaryotic Cell Membranes*. CRC Press, Boca Raton, Fla.

85. **Razin, S., and R. C. Cleverdon.** 1965. Carotenoids and cholesterol in membranes of *Mycoplasma laidlawii*. *J. Gen. Microbiol.* **41**:409–415.

86. **Razin, S., and A. Cohen.** 1963. Nutritional requirements and metabolism of *Mycoplasma laidlawii*. *J. Gen. Microbiol.* **30**:141–154.

87. **Razin, S., B. J. Cosenza, and M. E. Tourtellotte.** 1966. Variations in mycoplasma morphology induced by long-chain fatty acids. *J. Gen. Microbiol.* **42**:139–145.

88. **Razin, S., and B. C. J. G. Knight.** 1960. A partially defined medium for the growth of Mycoplasma. *J. Gen. Microbiol.* **22**:492–503.

89. **Razin, S., S. Kutner, H. Efrati, and S. Rottem.** 1980. Phospholipid and cholesterol uptake by mycoplasma cells and membranes. *Biochim. Biophys. Acta* **598**:628–640.

90. **Razin, S., and S. Rottem.** 1963. Fatty acid requirements of *Mycoplasma laidlawii*. *J. Gen. Microbiol.* **33**:459–470.

91. **Razin, S., and S. Rottem.** 1967. Role of carotenoids and cholesterol in the growth of *Mycoplasma laidlawii*. *J. Bacteriol.* **93**:1181–1182.

92. **Razin, S., and S. Rottem.** 1978. Cholesterol in membranes: studies with mycoplasmas. *Trends Biochem. Sci.* **3**:51–55.

93. **Razin, S., S. Rottem, M. Hasin, and N. L. Gershfeld.** 1973. Binding of exogenous proteins and lipids to mycoplasma membranes. *Ann. N.Y. Acad. Sci.* **225**:28–37.

94. **Razin, S., and Z. Shafer.** 1969. Incorporation of cholesterol by membranes of bacterial L-phase variants. *J. Gen. Microbiol.* **58**:327–339.

95. **Razin, S., M. E. Tourtellotte, R. N. McElhaney, and J. D. Pollack.** 1966. Influence of lipid components of *Mycoplasma laidlawii* membranes on osmotic fragility of cells. *J. Bacteriol.* **91**:609–616.

96. **Razin, S., and J. S. Tully.** 1970. Cholesterol requirement for mycoplasmas. *J. Bacteriol.* **102**:306–310.

97. **Razin, S., M. Wormser, and N. L. Gershfeld.** 1974. Cholesterol in mycoplasma membranes. II. Components of *Acholeplasma laidlawii* cell membranes responsible for cholesterol binding. *Biochim. Biophys. Acta* **352**:385–396.

98. **Rilfors, L., G. Wikander, and Å Wieslander.** 1987. Lipid acyl chain-dependent effects on sterols in *Acholeplasma laidlawii* membranes. *J. Bacteriol.* **169**:830–838.

99. **Rodwell, A. W.** 1956. The role of serum in the nutrition of *Asterococcus mycoides*. *Aust. J. Biol. Sci.* **9**:105–116.

100. **Rodwell, A. W.** 1963. The steroid growth-requirement of *Mycoplasma mycoides*. *J. Gen. Microbiol.* **32**:91–101.

101. **Rodwell, A. W.** 1967. The nutrition and metabolism of mycoplasma: progress and problems. *Ann. N.Y. Acad. Sci.* **143**:88–109.

102. **Rodwell, A. W.** 1968. Fatty-acid composition of mycoplasma lipids: biomembrane with only one fatty acid. *Science* **160**:1350–1351.

103. **Rodwell, A. W.** 1969. The supply of cholesterol and fatty acids for the growth of mycoplasmas. *J. Gen. Microbiol.* **58**:29–37.

104. **Rodwell, A. W.** 1971. The incorporation of elaidate, oleate and straight-chain saturated fatty acids by *Mycoplasma* strain Y. *J. Gen. Microbiol.* **68**:167–172.

105. **Rodwell, A. W.** 1983. *Mycoplasma gallisepticum* requires exogenous phospholipid for growth. *FEMS Microbiol. Lett.* **17**:265–268.

106. **Rodwell, A. W., and A. Abbott.** 1961. The function of glycerol, cholesterol and long-chain fatty acids in the nutrition of *Mycoplasma mycoides*. *J. Gen. Microbiol.* **25**:210–214.

107. **Rodwell, A. W., and J. E. Peterson.** 1971. The effect of straight-chain saturated, monoenoic and branched-chain fatty acids on growth and fatty acid composition of *Mycoplasma* strain Y. *J. Gen. Microbiol.* **68**:173–186.

108. **Romano, N., S. Rottem, and S. Razin.** 1976. Biosynthesis of saturated and unsaturated fatty acids by a T-strain mycoplasma (ureaplasma). *J. Bacteriol.* **128**:170–173.

109. **Romano, N., P. F. Smith, and W. R. Mayberry.** 1972. Lipids of a T strain of *Mycoplasma*. *J. Bacteriol.* **109**:565–569.

110. **Romijn, J. C., L. M. G. van Golde, R. N. McElhaney, and L. L. M. van Deenen.** 1972. Some studies on the fatty acid composition of total lipids and phosphatidylglycerol from *Acholeplasma laidlawii* B and their relation to the permeability of intact cells of this organism. *Biochim. Biophys. Acta* **280**:22–32.

111. **Rothblat, G. H., and P. F. Smith.** 1961. Nonsaponifiable lipids of representative pleuropneumonia-like organisms. *J. Bacteriol.* **82**:479–491.

112. **Rottem, S.** 1983. Labeling of cellular components during growth, p. 179–184. *In* S. Razin and J. G. Tully (ed.), *Methods in Mycoplasmology*, vol. 1. Academic Press, New York.

113. **Rottem, S., L. Adar, Z. Gross, Z. Ne'eman, and P. J. Davis.** 1986. Incorporation and modification of exogenous phosphatidylcholines by mycoplasmas. *J. Bacteriol.* **167**:299–304.

114. **Rottem, S., and M. F. Barile.** 1976. Effect of cerulenin on growth and lipid metabolism of mycoplasmas. *Antimicrob. Agents Chemother.* **9**:301–307.

115. **Rottem, S., and A. S. Greenberg.** 1975. Changes in composition, biosynthesis, and physical state of membrane lipids occurring upon aging of *Mycoplasma hominis* cultures. *J. Bacteriol.* **121**:631–639.

116. **Rottem, S., and O. Markowitz.** 1979. Unusual positional distribution of fatty acids in phosphatidylglycerol of sterol-requiring mycoplasmas. *FEBS Lett.* **107**:379–382.

117. **Rottem, S., and O. Markowitz.** 1979. Membrane lipids of *Mycoplasma gallisepticum*: a disaturated phosphatidylcholine and a phosphatidylglycerol with an unusual positional distribution of fatty acids. *Biochemistry* **18**:2930–2935.

118. **Rottem, S., O. Muhsam-Peled, and S. Razin.** 1973. Acyl carrier protein in mycoplasmas. *J. Bacteriol.* **113**:586–591.

119. **Rottem, S., and C. Panos.** 1969. The effect of long chain fatty acid isomers on growth, fatty acid composition and osmotic fragility of *Mycoplasma laidlawii* A. *J. Gen. Microbiol.* **59**:317–328.

120. **Rottem, S., and C. Panos.** 1970. The synthesis of long-chain fatty acids by a cell-free system from *Mycoplasma laidlawii* A. *Biochemistry* **9:**57–63.

121. **Rottem, S., E. A. Pfendt, and L. Hayflick.** 1971. Sterol requirements of T-strain mycoplasmas. *J. Bacteriol.* **105:**323–330.

122. **Rottem, S., and S. Razin.** 1964. Lipase activity of mycoplasma. *J. Gen. Microbiol.* **37:**123–134.

123. **Rottem, S., and S. Razin.** 1967. Uptake and utilization of acetate by mycoplasma. *J. Gen. Microbiol.* **48:**53–63.

124. **Rottem, S., and S. Razin.** 1973. Membrane lipids of *Mycoplasma hominis.* *J. Bacteriol.* **113:**565–571.

125. **Rottem, S., G. M. Slutzky, and R. Bittman.** 1978. Cholesterol distribution and movement in the *Mycoplasma gallisepticum* cell membrane. *Biochemistry* **17:**2723–2726.

126. **Rottem, S., S. L. Trotter, and M. F. Barile.** 1977. Membrane-bound thioesterase activity in mycoplasmas. *J. Bacteriol.* **129:**707–713.

127. **Rottem, S., J. Yashouv, Z. Ne'eman, and S. Razin.** 1973. Composition, ultrastructure and biological properties of membranes from *Mycoplasma mycoides* var. *capri* cells adapted to grow with low cholesterol concentrations. *Biochim. Biophys. Acta* **323:**495–508.

128. **Saito, Y., and R. N. McElhaney.** 1977. Membrane lipid biosynthesis in *Acholeplasma laidlawii* B: incorporation of exogenous fatty acids into membrane glyco- and phospholipids by growing cells. *J. Bacteriol.* **132:**485–496.

129. **Saito, Y., and R. N. McElhaney.** 1978. The positional distribution of a series of positional isomers of *cis*-octadecanoic acid in phosphatidylglycerol from *Acholeplasma laidlawii.* B. *Biochim. Biophys. Acta* **529:**224–229.

130. **Saito, Y., J. R. Silvius, and R. N. McElhaney.** 1977. Membrane lipid biosynthesis in *Acholeplasma laidlawii* B. Relationship between fatty acid structure and the positional distribution of esterified fatty acids in phospho- and glycolipids from growing cells. *Arch. Biochem. Biophys.* **182:**443–454.

131. **Saito, Y., J. R. Silvius, and R. N. McElhaney.** 1977. Membrane lipid biosynthesis in *Acholeplasma laidlawii* B: de novo biosynthesis of saturated fatty acids by growing cells. *J. Bacteriol.* **132:**497–504.

132. **Saito, Y., J. R. Silvius, and R. N. McElhaney.** 1978. Membrane lipid biosynthesis in *Acholeplasma laidlawii* B: elongation of medium- and long-chain exogenous fatty acids by growing cells. *J. Bacteriol.* **133:**66–74.

133. **Silvius, J. R., N. Mak, and R. N. McElhaney.** 1980. Lipid and protein composition and thermotropic lipid phase transition in fatty acid-homogeneous membranes of *Acholeplasma laidlawii* B. *Biochim. Biophys. Acta* **597:**199–215.

134. **Silvius, J. R., and R. N. McElhaney.** 1978. Lipid compositional manipulation in *Acholeplasma laidlawii* B. Effect of exogenous fatty acids on fatty acid composition and cell growth when endogenous fatty acid production is inhibited. *Can. J. Biochem.* **56:**462–469.

135. **Silvius, J. R., Y. Saito, and R. N. McElhaney.** 1977. Membrane lipid biosynthesis in *Acholeplasma laidlawii* B. Investigations into the *in vivo* regulation of the quantity and hydrocarbon chain lengths of *de novo* biosynthesized fatty acids in response to exogenously supplied fatty acids. *Arch. Biochem. Biophys.* **182:**455–464.

136. **Slutzky, G. M., S. Razin, and I. Kahane.** 1976. Serum lipoproteins as cholesterol donors to mycoplasma membranes. *Biochem. Biophys. Res. Commun.* **68:**592–536.

137. **Slutzky, G. M., S. Razin, I. Kahane, and S. Eisenberg.** 1977. Inhibition of mycoplasma growth by human very low-density lipoproteins. *FEMS Microbiol. Lett.* **2:**185–188.

138. **Slutzky, G. M., S. Razin, I. Kahane, and S. Eisenberg.**

139. **Smith, P. F.** 1959. Cholesterol esterase activity of pleuropneumonia-like organisms. *J. Bacteriol.* **77:**682–689.

140. **Smith, P. F.** 1962. Fate of ergosterol and cholesterol in pleuropneumonia-like organisms. *J. Bacteriol.* **84:**534–538.

141. **Smith, P. F.** 1963. The carotenoid pigments of mycoplasma. *J. Gen. Microbiol.* **32:**307–319.

142. **Smith, P. F.** 1964. Relation of sterol structure to utilization in pleuropneumonia-like organisms. *J. Lipid Res.* **5:**121–125.

143. **Smith, P. F.** 1967. Comparative lipid biochemistry of mycoplasma. *Ann. N.Y. Acad. Sci.* **143:**139–151.

144. **Smith, P. F.** 1968. Nature of unsaponifiable lipids of a *Mycoplasma* strain growth with isopentenyl pyrophosphate as a substitute for sterol. *J. Bacteriol.* **95:**1718–1720.

145. **Smith, P. F.** 1969. Biosynthesis of glucosyl diglycerides by *Mycoplasma laidlawii* strain B. *J. Bacteriol.* **99:**480–486.

146. **Smith, P. F.** 1969. The role of lipids in membrane transport in *Mycoplasma laidlawii. Lipids* **4:**331–336.

147. **Smith, P. F.** 1971. Biosynthesis of cholestryl glucoside by *Mycoplasma gallinarum. J. Bacteriol.* **108:**986–991.

148. **Smith, P. F.** 1971. *The Biology of the Mycoplasmas,* p. 107–109, 114–124, 133–143. Academic Press, New York.

149. **Smith, P. F.** 1972. A phosphatidyl diglucosyl diglyceride from *Acholeplasma laidlawii* B. *Biochim. Biophys. Acta* **280:**375–382.

150. **Smith, P. F.** 1979. The composition of membrane lipids and lipopolysaccharides, p. 231–257. *In* S. Razin and J. G. Tully (ed.), *The Mycoplasmas,* vol. 1. Academic Press, New York.

151. **Smith, P. F., and J. E. Boughton.** 1960. Role of protein and phospholipid in the growth of pleuropneumonia-like organisms. *J. Bacteriol.* **80:**851–860.

152. **Smith, P. F., and C. V. Henrikson.** 1965. Comparative biosynthesis of mevalonic acid by *Mycoplasma. J. Bacteriol.* **89:**146–153.

153. **Smith, P. F., and C. V. Henrikson.** 1966. Growth inhibition of *Mycoplasma* by inhibitors of polyterpene biosynthesis and its reversal by cholesterol. *J. Bacteriol.* **91:**1854–1858.

154. **Smith, P. F., and W. L. Koostra.** 1967. Phospholipids and glycolipids of sterol-requiring *Mycoplasma. J. Bacteriol.* **93:**1853–1862.

155. **Smith, P. F., W. L. Koostra, and C. V. Henrikson.** 1965. Diphosphatidyl glycerol in *Mycoplasma laidlawii. J. Bacteriol.* **90:**282–283.

156. **Smith, P. F., and T. A. Langworthy.** 1979. Existence of carotenoids in *Acholeplasma axanthum. J. Bacteriol.* **137:**185–188.

157. **Smith, P. F., J. G. Lecce, and R. J. Lynn.** 1954. A lipoprotein as a growth factor for certain pleuropneumonialike organisms. *J. Bacteriol.* **68:**627–633.

158. **Smith, P. F., and R. J. Lynn.** 1958. Lipid requirements for the growth of pleuropneumonialike organisms. *J. Bacteriol.* **76:**264–269.

159. **Smith, P. F., and G. H. Rothblat.** 1960. Incorporation of cholesterol by pleuropneumonia-like organisms. *J. Bacteriol.* **80:**842–850.

160. **Smith, P. F., and G. H. Rothblat.** 1962. Comparison of lipid composition of pleuropneumonia-like and L-type organisms. *J. Bacteriol.* **83:**500–506.

161. **Smith, P. F., and M. R. Smith.** 1970. Cholesterol inhibition of isopentenyl pyrophosphate Δ^3,Δ^2-isomerase in *Mycoplasma laidlawii. J. Bacteriol.* **103:**27–31.

162. **Tourtellotte, M. E., H. J. Morowitz, and P. Kasimer.** 1964. Defined medium for *Mycoplasma laidlawii. J. Bacteriol.* **88:**11–15.

163. **Tourtellotte, M. E., and J. S. Zupnick.** 1973. Freeze-frac-

1977. Cholesterol transfer from serum lipoproteins to mycoplasma membranes. *Biochemistry* **16:**5158–5163.

tured Acholeplasma laidlawii membranes: nature of particles observed. *Science* **179**:84–86.

164. **Tully, J. G., and S. Razin.** 1969. Characteristics of a new sterol-requiring *Mycoplasma. J. Bacteriol.* **98**:970–978.

165. **VanDemark, P. J., and P. F. Smith.** 1964. Evidence for a tricarboxylic acid cycle in *Mycoplasma hominis. J. Bacteriol.* **88**:1602–1607.

166. **VanDemark, P. J., and P. F. Smith.** 1965. Nature of butyrate oxidation by *Mycoplasma hominis. J. Bacteriol.* **89**:373–377.

167. **van Golde, L. M. G., R. N. McElhaney, and L. L. M. van Deenen.** 1971. A membrane-bound lysophospholipase from *Mycoplasma laidlawii* strain B. *Biochim. Biophys. Acta* **321**:245–249.

168. **Wieslander, Å., and E. Selstam.** 1987. Acyl-chain-dependent incorporation of chlorophyll and cholesterol in membranes of *Acholeplasma laidlawii. Biochim. Biophys. Acta* **901**:250–254.

169. **Yeagle, P. L.** 1988. Cholesterol and the cell membrane, p. 121–145. *In* P. L. Yeagle (ed.), *Biology of Cholesterol.* CRC Press, Boca Raton, Fla.

170. **Zhou, D., and R. W. White.** 1991. Early steps of isoprenoid biosynthesis in *Escherichia coli. Biochem. J.* **273**:627–634.

15. Membrane Function

RONALD N. McELHANEY

INTRODUCTION

The development of our knowledge of membrane function in the mycoplasmas has proceeded rather unevenly and in general is not as far advanced as our knowledge of membrane structure (see chapter 8). Probably because of our ability to induce marked variations in membrane lipid fatty acid composition and cholesterol content in *Acholeplasma laidlawii* and several *Mycoplasma* species, we know a great deal about the dependence of cell growth, passive permeability, and activity of a few membranous enzymes and active transport systems on membrane lipid fluidity and phase state and, in a few instances, even on the thickness and surface charge density of the lipid bilayer. In contrast, only a relatively small number of mycoplasma active transport systems have been studied in detail in vivo, and only a handful of membrane enzymes or transport proteins have been isolated, purified, and characterized in their active state. Moreover, not a single mycoplasma membrane protein has been sequenced and its detailed topology in the native membrane firmly established (see chapter 7). Therefore, much of what follows is somewhat descriptive and preliminary, reflecting the current state of the art in this area of research, although sugar and ion transport are fairly well characterized in some mycoplasma species.

The interested reader is referred to previous general reviews on mycoplasma membrane function and on permeability and active transport by Rottem (100) and Razin (86, 87) and by Cirillo (11), respectively. For later reviews focusing exclusively on membrane function in *A. laidlawii*, see references 71 and 72.

CELL GROWTH

Perhaps the most fundamental and comprehensive indicator of cellular function in general, and of cell membrane function in particular, is cell growth, a process which can usually be conveniently and accurately monitored with a minimum of perturbation to the microorganism under study. Although in principle growth can be (and sometimes is) limited by processes occurring in the cytoplasm rather than in the membrane, the fact that alterations in membrane lipid phase state and fluidity can markedly affect cell

---

Ronald N. McElhaney • Department of Biochemistry, University of Alberta, Edmonton, Alberta, Canada T6G 2H7.

growth in mycoplasmas and bacteria indicates that lipid-influenced membrane processes can limit both the range of temperatures over which an organism can grow and the rate and efficiency of growth within that range. Studies of the effects of alterations in membrane lipid fatty acid composition and cholesterol content on the growth of *A. laidlawii* and of several *Mycoplasma* species are summarized below. A more comprehensive discussion of the relationship of lipid physical properties and the ability of bacteria and mycoplasmas to grow and survive at various temperatures is presented in reference 70.

Dependence on Membrane Lipid Fatty Acid Composition

The first study of the relationship between the physical state of lipids in a biological membrane and the ability of cells to grow was that of Steim et al. (138), who used differential scanning calorimetry (DSC) to monitor the phase state of the lipids of the *A. laidlawii* B membrane. These investigators found that *A. laidlawii* B is capable of normal growth at 37°C so long as cells are supplemented with exogenous fatty acids giving rise to membrane lipids with phase transitions centered from just below 0°C to near the growth temperature of 37°C. However, cells grown in the presence of exogenous stearic acid exhibit a decreased rate of growth and eventual cell lysis as the biosynthetic incorporation of this high-melting-point fatty acid raises the phase transition temperature above 37°C. This study was thus the first to demonstrate that cells can grow normally when their membrane lipids exist entirely or predominantly in the liquid-crystalline state but not when gel-state lipid predominates.

McElhaney (67, 68) later carried out more detailed studies of the relationship between membrane lipid fluidity and phase state, using a wide variety of fatty acid supplements to alter the phase transition temperature and differential thermal analysis to monitor the proportion of gel and liquid-crystalline lipid in the membrane at the growth temperature. In these studies, both the temperature range over which *A. laidlawii* B cells could grow and the rate of growth within the permissible temperature range were measured. McElhaney found that the minimum growth temperature of these cells could be varied from 8 to 30°C, depending on the fatty acid supplement used. The lower temperature limit of growth of 8°C appeared to be an intrinsic feature of these cells, since it cannot be reduced further, even when fatty acids giving rise to phase transitions well below 0°C are used. However, the minimum growth temperatures of 10 to 30°C, observed when cells were supplemented with various medium- or high-melting-point fatty acids, are clearly correlated with the lower boundaries of the gel-to-liquid-crystalline phase transition of the membrane lipids. Although the optimum and maximum growth temperatures observed are not determined directly by the lipid phase transition midpoint or upper boundary, these temperatures can be significantly influenced by the fatty acid composition of the membrane lipids. In particular, cells having lipid phase transition temperatures occurring near or below 0°C exhibit progressively reduced optimum and maximum growth temperatures,

suggesting that an upper limit on membrane lipid fluidity compatible with membrane function must exist. Within the growth temperature range characteristic of each fatty acid supplement, both the absolute rates and temperature coefficients of growth are similar for all fatty acid compositions tested, provided that the membrane lipids exist entirely or predominantly in the liquid-crystalline state. Below the midpoint temperature of the lipid transition, however, growth rates decline rapidly with decreasing temperature, and the temperature coefficient of growth increases markedly within this temperature range, irrespective of the particular fatty acid supplement used. Cell growth ceases entirely when more than about 90% of the membrane lipid is converted to the solid state. Qualitatively similar results were obtained in a number of similar studies of *Escherichia coli* unsaturated fatty acid auxotrophs (70). Thus, the fluidity and phase state of the membrane lipids can have a profound effect on the ability of *A. laidlawii* B and other bacteria to grow effectively over a variety of environmental temperatures.

It is interesting to note that of all the many exogenous fatty acids tested by McElhaney (67, 68), no single exogenous fatty acid supplement permits *A. laidlawii* B to grow at its maximum potential rate over its maximum potential growth temperature range of 8 to 44°C. Also, cells grown without fatty acid supplementation grow poorly below about 25°C and not at all below about 18°C. Two conclusions can be drawn from these observations. First, *A. laidlawii* B does not possess an effective homeostatic mechanism for regulating either the fluidity or the physical state of its membranes; otherwise, it would be able to exploit more fully its growth potential. Second, if this organism did possess such a mechanism, as many other procaryotic microorganisms do, this property would certainly significantly extend the range of environmental temperatures over which effective growth can occur, and thus have great survival value, at least in the free-living state.

Silvius and McElhaney (130) have studied the effect of exogenous fatty acid incorporation on the growth of *A. laidlawii* B rendered totally auxotrophic for fatty acids by selective inhibition of de novo fatty acid biosynthesis and chain elongation, and this study also provides support for the existence of an upper limit for membrane lipid fluidity. These investigators demonstrated that *A. laidlawii* B can grow relatively normally when various single exogenous *n*-saturated, methyl iso- and anteiso-branched, or *trans*-monounsaturated or *trans*-cyclopropane fatty acids make up 95 to 99 mol% of the total membrane lipid fatty acyl groups. As expected, high-melting-point exogenous fatty acids such as long-chain *n*-saturated fatty acids do not support growth at 37°C, since these fatty acids produce membrane lipids which exist entirely in the gel state at this temperature. Interestingly, however, the low-melting-point, short-chain *n*-saturated and branched-chain fatty acids, as well as all *cis*-cyclopropane and *cis*-polyunsaturated fatty acids tested, also do not support significant growth. Silvius et al. (129) subsequently showed by differential thermal analysis that the gel-to-liquid-crystalline lipid phase transition midpoint temperatures of these normally growing, fatty acid-homogeneous cells range from −14.9 to

36.7°C. Since the relative fluidities of the lipids from these various membranes must be appreciably different at 37°C, these results also indicate that a broad range of lipid fluidities are compatible with at least relatively normal membrane function in this organism. Although a minimum chain length of 14 carbon atoms also appeared to be a requirement for exogenous fatty acid growth-supporting ability, even for fatty acids which produce lipids having moderate phase transition temperatures (i.e., tridecanoic acid), the inability of cis-cyclopropane and cis-polyunsaturated fatty acids to support growth could be explained by postulating that exogenous fatty acids giving rise to membrane lipids having phase transitions centered below about −15 to −20°C produce a hyperfluid state at 37°C.

Direct evidence for this hypothesis was provided by Silvius and McElhaney (130) in a study of the ability of a series of cis-octadecenoic acid positional isomers to support the growth of totally fatty acid auxotrophic A. laidlawii B. cis-Octadecanoates with the double bond located near the center of the hydrocarbon chain, which produce membrane lipids with the lowest phase transition temperatures, are unable to support growth, as are cis-octadecanoates with the double bond very near the carbonyl group or methyl terminus, which produce lipids with very high melting points. On the other hand, positional isomers having the double bond at intermediate positions in either half of the hydrocarbon chain, which produce lipids having moderate phase transition temperatures (about −10 to 30°C), support fair to good growth. In this regard, it may be significant that in A. laidlawii B cells that retain the ability to biosynthesize endogenous saturated fatty acids (67, 68) and in a totally fatty acid auxotrophic mutant of E. coli (1), the minimum phase transition midpoint temperatures which can be achieved by decreasing the saturated/unsaturated fatty acid ratio of the membrane lipids are about −19 and −13°C, respectively. Although these studies and an investigation of a Bacillus stearothermophilus mutant unable to regulate its fatty acid composition with temperature (75) strongly suggest that an upper limit for membrane lipid fluidity does exist, no quantitative physical measurements of this maximum fluidity limit are available. Rigorous studies utilizing several nonperturbing spectroscopic techniques, which are sensitive to lipid orientational order and motional rates over a range of time scales, are a clear priority in this regard.

The effects of pressure and of pressure antagonists on the growth of A. laidlawii were studied by Mac-Naughton and Macdonald (64). These workers found that at 37°C cell growth is progressively inhibited by increases in hydrostatic pressure over the range of 200 to 600 atm (1 atm = 101.29 kPa). However, this inhibition of growth is greater in magnitude than expected if increases in hydrostatic pressure act solely to increase the gel-to-liquid-crystalline phase transition of the lipid bilayer or to decrease membrane lipid fluidity (63). However, the observed partial reversal of pressure-induced growth inhibition by helium and hydrogen may be caused by a partial reversal of the ordering effect of hydrostatic pressure on the A. laidlawii membrane lipid bilayer, since these lipid-soluble gases partially antagonize the effects of high hydrostatic pres-

sure in lipid bilayer model membranes (63). Pentanol, which is also known to decrease the lipid phase transition temperature and to increase the fluidity of the lipid bilayer in model and A. laidlawii membranes, not only failed to offset the inhibitory effects of high pressure but further inhibited growth. This finding suggests that pentanol acts predominantly by binding directly to enzymes and other cellular components involved in growth and inhibiting their function rather than by stimulating their activity by antagonizing the effect of pressure on the membrane lipid bilayer. These results are probably best rationalized by postulating the hydrostatic pressure inhibits the growth of this organism both by direct effects on membrane proteins and other cellular constituents and by indirect effects mediated through the lipid bilayer, with the former being the more important.

The relationship between membrane lipid fatty acid composition and cell growth has also been studied, albeit less extensively, in Mycoplasma strain Y (serologically and biochemically related to Mycoplasma mycoides subsp. mycoides) by Rodwell and Peterson (96). In contrast to A. laidlawii, Mycoplasma species require both exogenous cholesterol (or other sterol) and an appropriate long-chain fatty acid (or acids) for growth. When cultured at 37°C in a lipid-poor growth medium containing exogenous cholesterol plus one of a large number of exogenous fatty acids, Mycoplasma strain Y will grow only in the presence of a limited number of fatty acids. Specifically, two trans-monounsaturated fatty acids (elaidate and trans-vaccenate), two methyl iso-branched fatty acids (isopalmitate and isosterate), a methyl anteiso-branched fatty acid of moderate chain length (anteisoheptadecanoate), and a few positional isomers of oleic acid are the only exogenous fatty acids that support growth. Straight-chain saturated fatty acids or naturally occurring cis-unsaturated fatty acids do not support growth alone, nor do short-chain or long-chain trans-unsaturated or branched-chain fatty acids. However, binary combinations of a high-melting-point fatty acid (such as palmitate) with a low-melting-point fatty acid (such as oleate) do support good growth. Although the fluidity and physical state of membrane lipids were not determined in this study, the correspondence between these results and the studies of the growth of fatty acid auxotrophic A. laidlawii by Silvius and McElhaney (130) discussed above are striking. The results of Rodwell and Peterson can all be explained by postulating that even in the presence of cholesterol, Mycoplasma strain Y, like A. laidlawii B, requires fatty acids which will produce a liquid-crystalline bilayer of moderate fluidity and thickness in order to support proper membrane function and thus normal cell growth.

Dependence on Membrane Sterol Composition

Wieslander and Selstam (150) recently studied the relative abilities of chlorophyll and cholesterol to affect cell growth and membrane lipid polar headgroup composition in A. laidlawii A cells supplemented with palmitic acid or with various unsaturated fatty acids. In the absence of chlorophyll or cholesterol, growth yields decrease in the order palmitic > oleic > linoleic acid-enriched cells, and no growth occurs in the linolenic acid-supplemented medium. However, the addition of either chlorophyll or cholesterol increases growth yields in linoleic acid-supplemented cells and permits some growth to occur in the linolenic acid-supplemented medium. Thus, in the highly unsaturated linoleic and linolenic acid-enriched growth media, A. laidlawii A is dependent on these additives for optimal growth and survival, respectively. Moreover, the amount of chlorophyll, and to a lesser extent cholesterol, incorporated into the membrane increases markedly with an increase in the degree of unsaturation of the lipid hydrocarbon chains. These authors attribute the growth-promoting effects of incorporated cholesterol molecules in highly unsaturated membranes to their well-known ability to increase the orientation order and the closeness of packing of lipid hydrocarbon chains in model membranes and A. laidlawii membranes. Whether or not chlorophyll also promotes cell growth in cells enriched in highly unsaturated fatty acids by a similar mechanism remains to be determined.

Rilfors and coworkers (94) recently carried out a very detailed study of the effects of the incorporation of various sterols on A. laidlawii A membranes highly enriched in a variety of fatty acids. The following two effects were observed with respect to cell growth: (i) with a given acyl chain composition of the membrane lipids, growth was stimulated, unaffected, reduced, or completely inhibited (lysis), depending on the sterol structure, and (ii) the effect of a certain sterol depended on the acyl chain composition (most striking for epicorostanol, cholest-4-en-3-one, and cholest-5-en-3-one, which stimulated growth with saturated acyl chains but caused lysis with unsaturated chains). Generally, the observed effects could be explained by an influence of the various sterols either on the fluidity and phase state of the membrane lipid bilayer or on the bilayer/nonbilayer phase preference of the membrane lipids (see chapter 8).

Several studies of sterol-requiring mycoplasmas provide support for the conclusion that the lower boundary of the gel-to-liquid-crystalline membrane lipid phase transition may limit the minimal growth temperature under certain conditions. Rottem et al. (102, 110) have shown that the native strain of M. mycoides subsp. capri, which efficiently incorporates both saturated and unsaturated exogenous fatty acids and contains relatively large amounts of cholesterol in its cell membrane, grows well over the temperature range of 25 to 37°C, as measured by cell yield. In contrast, a strain adapted to grow with a much reduced level of membrane cholesterol grows relatively well at 37°C but quite poorly at 25°C. Several physical techniques all show the absence of a discrete phase transition in the cholesterol-rich native strain membranes, whereas a phase transition occurring over the temperature range of 20 to 30°C is detected in membranes of the cholesterol-poor adapted strain. The adapted strain also exhibits an increased osmotic fragility in comparison with the native strain, particularly at temperatures below 20°C. Similar results have been reported by Le Grimellec et al. (52) for cholesterol-rich and cholesterol-poor strains of M. gallisepticum. Rottem et al. (102, 110) suggested that solidification of the membrane lipids around 25°C, which occurs only in the adapted strain, is responsible for the inability to grow

at lower temperatures. Using similar physical techniques, Rottem (101) has also demonstrated that the membrane lipids of M. arginini would exist predominantly in the gel state, even at its optimal growth temperature of 37°C, in the absence of large amounts of membrane cholesterol. He suggested that the strict cholesterol requirement for the growth of this and several other mycoplasma species which are unable to efficiently incorporate exogenous unsaturated fatty acids into their membrane lipids results from the need to fluidize their highly saturated membrane lipids in order to permit cell growth and membrane function at physiological temperatures. This situation is in contrast to that existing in eucaryotic membranes, whose polyunsaturated fatty acid-containing lipids are well above their phase temperatures at physiological temperatures, where cholesterol is thought to act as a rigidifier rather than as a fluidizer of membrane lipids (25).

Dahl and coworkers (16, 20) have studied the effects of structural modifications of the cholesterol molecule on growth and membrane lipid organization in M. capricolum. They found that the effectiveness of a series of alkyl-substituted sterols in promoting the growth of this sterol auxotrophic organism increases in the order lanosterol < 4,4-dimethyl cholestanol < 4β-methyl cholestanol < 4α-methyl cholestanol < cholestanol < cholesterol. Interestingly, this is also the order of increasing effectiveness of these sterols in ordering the hydrocarbon chains of the membrane lipid bilayer at 37°C (in the liquid-crystalline state) and the order in which these compounds are formed in the cholesterol biosynthetic pathway. These workers concluded that the sequential biosynthetic removal of the three methyl groups from the lanosterol ring nucleus and the introduction of a double bond into ring B improve the membrane function of the sterol molecule by increasing the planarity and decreasing the bulk of the sterol ring system, thus permitting a closer interaction with and a higher degree of ordering of the hydrocarbon chains of the membrane lipids. In contrast, Lala et al. (48) showed that cholesterol methyl ether and cholesterol acetate are almost as effective as cholesterol itself in promoting cell growth and membrane ordering, indicating that the free hydroxyl group at C-3 of ring A is not strictly required for cholesterol function. This finding, however, is at odds with earlier work with other mycoplasmas (see below).

Dahl et al. (20) also found that the provision of exogenous cholesterol allowed M. capricolum cells to grow on media containing a wider variety of exogenous fatty acids than did provision of lanosterol, a finding compatible with the greater effectiveness of cholesterol in regulating membrane lipid fluidity. An unexpected finding, however, was that low levels of cholesterol, which on their own are unable to support cell growth, are able to support good growth when high levels of lanosterol are also present, despite the fact that the microviscosity values of the membrane lipid remain low in these circumstances. These workers suggested that lanosterol may fulfill one of the more primitive functions of sterols in membranes, namely, to separate polar lipid headgroups and decrease surface density (15, 25), even though it cannot effectively regulate the fluidity of the lipid hydrocarbon chains. Alternatively, small amounts of cholesterol were suggested to serve other, more specialized cellular functions, a suggestion confirmed by subsequent studies from this laboratory (17–19). In particular, the addition of a small amount of cholesterol to *M. capricolum* cells growing slowly on a large amount of lanosterol first stimulates the biosynthesis of phospholipid molecules containing unsaturated fatty acids, which in turn is followed by a stimulation of RNA and protein synthesis. As well, the phospholipid molecules synthesized were shown to serve as acyl donors for the large number of fatty acylated membrane proteins found in this organism. In particular, cholesterol addition causes a marked increase in the phospholipid-derived oleate found in two specific membrane proteins as well as a general increase in phospholipid-derived palmitate. Interestingly, the cholesterol stimulation of growth, and of phospholipid, RNA, and protein synthesis, can be reversed by the addition of epicoprostanol, a sterol known to specifically inhibit the growth of cholesterol-requiring mycoplasmas (16, 19). These results strongly suggest that exogenous cholesterol plays a specific role (or roles) as a signal for membrane biogenesis and, in turn, for macromolecular synthesis and cell growth, as well as a general role in regulating the fluidity and phase state of the membrane lipid bylayer. Considerable evidence for multiple roles for ergosterol in membrane biogenesis and function, and in the promotion of cell growth in general, has also been gathered for the yeast *Saccharomyces cerevisiae* (15).

Lelong et al. (55) studied the effect on 7β-hydroxycholesterol on the growth of *M. capricolum* adapted to grow on low levels of cholesterol. When sufficient exogenous cholesterol is not provided, cells are unable to grow even in the presence of high levels of the hydroxy sterol. However, in the presence of very low levels of cholesterol, which alone would not support significant cell growth, the addition of moderate to high levels of hydroxycholesterol produces reasonably good growth. The growth response to combinations of cholesterol and hydroxycholesterol is synergistic rather than additive, just as observed previously by Dahl et al. (20) for combinations of cholesterol and lanosterol. These workers therefore suggested that 7β-hydroxycholesterol probably fulfills the normal bulk roles of cholesterol in the membrane. However, since the introduction of a hydroxyl group into ring B of the cholesterol molecule, which is normally situated in a hydrophobic environment within the hydrocarbon core of the lipid bilayer, would be expected to disrupt sterol-lipid interactions, it is unlikely that 7β-hydroxycholesterol can produce the characteristic ordering of the liquid-crystalline lipid hydrocarbon chains produced by cholesterol. It seems more likely that hydroxycholesterol performs only the primitive role of sterols in the *M. capricolum* membrane, namely, to reduce the negative surface charge density of the lipid bilayer surface, as appears to be the case also for lanosterol (20).

The studies on the relationship between sterol structure, sterol-lipid interactions, and cell growth described above are generally in accord with earlier studies of the ability of various sterols to support the growth of various *Mycoplasma*, *Ureaplasma*, and *Spiroplasma* species (28, 95, 105, 135). Although some variation among species was observed, in general most structural alterations in the cholesterol molecule were found to result in a decrease in its ability to support cell growth. Specifically, changing the configuration of the hydroxyl group at C-3 of ring A from β to α, converting the β-hydroxyl group to an ester, or replacing the β-hydroxyl group with a keto group results in loss of the ability of the sterol to support growth (87). Although the degree of unsaturation of the ring system is of secondary importance, cholesterol is more effective at supporting growth than are its fully saturated or multiply unsaturated analogs. Moreover, sterols with nonplanar ring systems are ineffective as growth promoters. Although the actual structure and size of the alkyl side chain at C-17 are relatively unimportant, the removal of this alkyl chain results in a loss of the ability to support cell growth. Although in none of the studies just summarized were the effects of these structural variations on membrane lipid fluidity and phase state determined, it is significant that the structural features required for cell growth, namely, a planar sterol nucleus with a free hydroxyl at the 3β position and a hydrocarbon side chain, are precisely those required for the sterol to exert its maximum effect on ordering the lipid hydrocarbon chains and reducing the permeability of liquid-crystalline model (25) and biological (22, 25) membranes. This good correlation provides strong support for the idea that one of the major roles of sterols in biological membranes is to regulate the fluidity and phase state of the lipid bilayer.

Dependence on Membrane Carotenoid Composition

The presence of carotenoids only in the sterol-nonrequiring *Acholeplasma* species led Smith (134) to propose that these polyterpenoid compounds fulfill functions analogous to those of cholesterol in the sterol-requiring mycoplasmas (136). In support of this proposal, Smith and Henrikson (137) showed that several inhibitors of carotenoid biosynthesis can inhibit the growth of *A. laidlawii* and that this inhibition can be reversed by the addition of cholesterol to the growth medium. Indeed, as discussed in chapter 8, carotenoid pigments do have a cholesterol-like effect on the *A. laidlawii* membrane lipid bilayer, increasing the degree of orientational order and restricting the rates of motion of the lipid hydrocarbon chains in the liquid-crystalline state. However, since the amount of carotenoid pigment normally found in the *A. laidlawii* membrane is quite low (less than 1 wt% of the total lipid fraction), it is doubtful that these compounds play a major or a crucial role in regulating the physical properties of the lipid bilayer of the *A. laidlawii* membrane. Indeed, Razin and Rottem (90, 100, 107) report that this organism grows well on a sterol-free medium in the complete absence of carotenoid synthesis.

The reader is referred to chapter 14 for additional discussion of the incorporation and possible biochemical functions of sterols and carotenoids in *Acholeplasma* and *Mycoplasma* species.

PASSIVE PERMEABILITY

Although a great deal of indirect experimental evidence had long suggested that one of the major functions of lipids in biological membranes was to provide a selective permeability barrier (59), studies of *A. laidlawii* B cells provided the first direct and compelling evidence for this hypothesis. McElhaney et al. (73) investigated the relationship between the rates of glycerol passive diffusion into intact cells whose membrane lipid fatty acid composition and cholesterol content were systematically varied. These workers found that the rate of glycerol permeation is dependent on the geometrical configuration and number of double bonds present in the membrane lipid hydrocarbon chains. The rate of glycerol permeation at a given temperature was observed to increase in the order elaidic acid- < oleic acid- < linoleic acid-enriched cells, in agreement with trends noted in previous studies with model membranes generated from synthetic phosphatidylcholines. Also, the incorporation of cholesterol into the cell membrane decreases the rate of glycerol passive entry, also as previously observed for model membranes in the fluid state. In all respects, the permeability properties of intact cells mirror those of liposomes prepared from the *A. laidlawii* B total membrane lipids.

Romijn et al. (99), McElhaney et al. (74), and de Kruyff et al. (22, 23) extended the study just described. Romijn and coworkers showed that the glycerol and erythritol permeability of intact *A. laidlawii* B cells increases with the number of *cis*-double bonds in the membrane lipid fatty acyl chains, even for polyunsaturated fatty acids containing as many as four double bonds in the membrane lipid fatty acyl chains. These investigators also demonstrated that the non-electrolyte passive permeability rates increase as the chain length of the fatty acyl group decreases. These observations were confirmed and extended by McElhaney et al. (74), who also studied the temperature dependence of ethylene glycol, glycerol, and erythritol passive diffusion into intact cells and derived liposomes. The mean activation energies calculated for the permeation of ethylene glycol, glycerol, and erythritol into both cells and liposomes are about 14, 18, and 21 kcal (1 cal = 4.184 J)/mol, respectively. In contrast to permeation rates, which are markedly dependent on membrane lipid fatty acid composition and cholesterol content as well as permeant structure, activation energies for permeation are not affected by lipid composition changes and are dependent only on permeant structure. As discussed by de Gier et al. (21), the activation energies for nonelectrolyte passive diffusion correlate well with the net number of hydrogen bonds which must be broken in removing these compounds from water, suggesting that these nonelectrolyte molecules permeate both biological and model membranes in their fully dehydrated state. These results also imply that lipid compositional variations influence permeation rates by altering the entropy rather than the enthalpy of permeation. Since the permeability of cells and liposomes was found to be inversely proportional to their gel-to-liquid-crystalline phase transition temperatures (74), these differences in permeation entropies presumably reflect either the increased ease of insertion of the dehydrated nonelectrolyte molecules into the hydrophobic core of the more fluid and disordered lipid bilayers or an increased rate of diffusion within these bilayers (21).

In addition to studying the fatty acid compositional dependence of erythritol efflux from *A. laidlawii* B

cells, de Kruyff and coworkers (22, 23) investigated the effects of the structures of various steroids incorporated into the plasma membrane on its erythritol permeability. These investigators found that in order to produce the significant reduction in the erythritol permeability of liquid-crystalline *A. laidlawii* membranes characteristic of cholesterol itself, a 3β-hydroxy sterol with a flat (all-*trans*) steroid nucleus is required. The replacement of the 3β-hydroxyl group with a 3-keto function, a change in the configuration of the 3-hydroxy group from β to α, or the introduction of a *cis*-structured ring system resulted in a loss of the ability to reduce erythritol efflux, just as observed for liposomes prepared from egg phosphatidylcholine.

McElhaney et al. (73, 74) demonstrated that the nonelectrolyte permeability of *A. laidlawii* cells and derived liposomes is not affected by the conversion of most of the membrane lipids from the liquid-crystalline to the gel state. Since de Kruyff et al. (22, 23) presented evidence that glycerol permeation occurs at significant rates only through fluid lipid domains, this observation suggests that those lipid domains remaining in the liquid-crystalline state have an enhanced nonelectrolyte permeability, possibly due to the presence of disordered boundary regions at the interfaces of the solid and fluid lipid domains. This suggestion was later supported by the work of Silvius et al. (128) on the glycerol and Na$^+$ permeability of fatty acid-homogeneous *A. laidlawii* B cells. However, both groups presented evidence that *A. laidlawii* cells and derived liposomes, whose membrane lipids exist predominantly in the gel state, readily lyse if subjected to mechanical or osmotic stress, and this finding was later confirmed by the work of van Zoelen et al. (149). Cells and liposomes do remain intact and essentially impermeable to nonelectrolytes at temperatures below the phase transition lower boundary, however, if not subjected to stress. De Kruyff and coworkers (22, 23) also showed that the incorporation of cholesterol reduces the temperature of onset of mechanical osmotic fragility in intact cells, as expected from its fluidizing effect on the membrane lipids below their characteristic gel-to-liquid-crystalline phase transition temperatures.

The valinomycin-mediated K$^+$ and Rb$^+$ permeability of *A. laidlawii* B cells differing in membrane lipid fatty acid composition and cholesterol content were studied by van der Neut-Kok et al. (147). The rate at which the lipid-soluble valinomycin molecules carry ions across the membrane was found to increase in the order elaidic acid- < oleic acid- < linoleic acid-enriched cells and to decrease slightly when cholesterol was present, just as observed for nonelectrolyte permeation in earlier studies. The valinomycin-mediated ion flux rates were found to be only weakly temperature dependent when the membrane lipids exist entirely in the liquid-crystalline state, but flux rates decrease markedly as the proportion of gel-state lipid increases, becoming essentially zero at temperatures below the lipid phase transition lower boundary. This observation provided additional evidence that valinomycin functions as a mobile carrier rather than as an ion channel in a biological membrane, just as in model membrane systems.

Huang and Haug (36) have reported that an elevation in the carotenoid content of the membrane of *A.*

laidlawii results in a slightly lower glycerol permeability of intact cells, a finding compatible with the observation of these and other workers that carotenoids tend to rigidify the hydrocarbon chains of the membrane lipid bilayer in its liquid-crystalline state (see chapter 8). However, since the levels of carotenoid pigments in the *A. laidlawii* membrane are normally quite low, this reduction in permeability, if real, is not likely to be biologically significant.

All of the permeability studies reviewed above provide strong support for the concept that a continuous lipid bilayer is a central structural feature of the *A. laidlawii* membrane and that one of the major functions of this lipid bilayer is to provide a selective, semipermeable barrier at the surface of the cell (for a review, see reference 69).

ACTIVE TRANSPORT

Sugar Transport in *A. laidlawii*

Tarshis and coworkers (81, 143–145) were the first to study the uptake and utilization of sugars in *A. laidlawii* cells. They were able to show that glucose transport and metabolism by this organism do not occur via the phosphoenolpyruvate (PEP):sugar phosphotransferase system (PTS) present in some bacteria, since α-methyl-D-glucoside, the normal glucose analog for this transport system, is not taken up by *A. laidlawii* and because cell extracts lack the ability to catalyze the transfer of the phosphate group from PEP to glucose. However, free glucose is taken up by this organism by a saturable process which is relatively specific for this particular hexose (although maltose has some ability to compete for uptake), and glucose is phosphorylated by ATP in cell extracts. The uptake of glucose was reported to be inhibited by inhibitors of glycolysis, by various sulfhydryl group reagents, and by several inhibitors of mitochondrial and bacterial oxidative phosphorylation. Glucose uptake was also reported to be temperature and pH dependent, with maximal rates of uptake being observed near 47°C and pH 7.0. These workers concluded that glucose is actively transported into *A. laidlawii*. However, since glucose is actively metabolized by this organism upon entering the cell, one cannot distinguish between facilitated diffusion and active transport processes on the basis of the data presented. In fact, the similarity between the K_ms calculated for glucose uptake in whole cells and glucose phosphorylation in cell extracts suggests that the kinetics of glucose metabolism rather than glucose transport may have been measured in these experiments. The very slow time course of glucose uptake, with a steady state not being reached until 60 min, lends support to this suggestion, as does the fact that the apparent K_m for the transport of 3-*O*-methylglucoside (3-*O*-MG), a nonmetabolizable analog of glucose, is less than 1/100 that of glucose itself (see below), whereas the opposite is true for most of the other glucose transport systems studied to date.

Read and McElhaney (91) also studied glucose uptake and metabolism in *A. laidlawii*, using both a swelling rate assay for measuring the rate of glucose entry into cells when high concentrations of glucose are present extracellularly as well as the standard radiolabeled glucose uptake assay to monitor the uptake of low levels of sugar. The swelling rate assay revealed that glucose enters *A. laidlawii* cells by a saturable process at a rate at least 100 times greater than by simple passive diffusion and with a considerably reduced apparent activation energy compared with passive permeation. Moreover, glucose entry is inhibited by low concentrations of phloretin and phlorizin, fairly specific inhibitors of glucose transport in other organisms, and by exposure of cells to temperatures above 45°C. These results clearly establish that glucose entry under these conditions is via a protein-mediated, facilitated-diffusion process.

These workers found that the metabolism of radiolabeled glucose by this organism once the sugar enters the cell is quite rapid, and when low levels of glucose are used, the total intracellular radioactivity is a reflection of the net effect of glucose transport, glucose metabolism, and loss from the cells of radiolabeled metabolic products. In fact, under the assay conditions used by Tarshis et al. (81, 143–145), most of the intracellular radioactivity present even at the earliest time point resides in glucose metabolic products rather than in free sugar. These authors have found the addition of iodoacetate markedly inhibits overall glucose uptake. However, this compound also markedly inhibits the metabolism of glucose, so it is not clear whether iodoacetate inhibits net glucose uptake exclusively by inhibiting glucose metabolism or whether glucose transport itself is inhibited as well. Interestingly, the addition of small amounts of unlabeled glucose was found to increase the rate of radiolabeled glucose uptake by intact cells, presumably by stimulating of glycolysis and the production of ATP, suggesting that glucose uptake is energy limited under these conditions. The rapid, energy-limited metabolism of intracellular glucose observed under these conditions precluded the determination of whether the accumulation of glucose against a concentration gradient occurs and prevented a meaningful determination of the K_m and V_{max} values of the glucose transport system itself.

Read and McElhaney (91) studied the dependence of the initial rates of glucose uptake on the membrane lipid fatty acid composition and cholesterol content of *A. laidlawii* cells under conditions in which the effect of glucose metabolism on these rates are minimal. They found that the rates of glucose transport increase with the degree of unsaturation of the membrane lipids and decrease upon the incorporation of cholesterol, suggesting that the rate of transmembrane movement of the glucose carrier increases with an increase in the fluidity of the lipid bilayer. In contrast to initial rates, the apparent activation energy for glucose transport does not depend on the fatty acid composition or cholesterol content of the membrane, suggesting that entropic factors must account for the observed differences in rates, just as has been observed for the passive diffusion of nonelectrolytes into this organism (see above). Glucose uptake could not be detected at temperatures below the membrane lipid gel-to-liquid-crystalline phase transition temperatures because cells become leaky and mechanically fragile, which may explain in part why Tarshis and coworkers could not detect glucose or 3-*O*-MG uptake at temperatures below 10 to 20°C.

Tarshis and coworkers subsequently carried out several more definitive studies of glucose transport in *A. laidlawii* in both cells (139, 140) and membrane vesicles (26, 27, 80) by using 3-*O*-MG. The transport of 3-*O*-MG was shown to be a saturable process with a K_m of 4.6 µM (as opposed to a K_m of 480 µM for glucose uptake reported in their earlier studies). The pH and temperature optima for 3-*O*-MG transport were reported to be 7.2 and 40°C, respectively, (as opposed to 7.0 and 47°C for the uptake of glucose). Glucose itself and 6-deoxyglucose were found to be competitive inhibitors of 3-*O*-MG transport, whereas maltose was a noncompetitive inhibitor. However, a variety of other hexoses and pentoses did not inhibit 3-*O*-MG uptake. The efflux of preloaded 3-*O*-MG was also shown to be a carrier-mediated process, and "entrance counterflow" (accelerated exchange) of extra- and intracellular substrate could be demonstrated. The transport of 3-*O*-MG was reported to be concentrative, with a ratio of internal to external concentration of a saturating external concentration of substrate of about 10:1. A mutant supposedly defective in glucose and 3-*O*-MG transport but normal in glycolytic ability was also isolated and biochemically characterized (47).

The energetics of 3-*O*-MG transport were also studied by Tarshis and coworkers (139, 141). Anaerobic conditions did not appear to reduce 3-*O*-MG uptake rates significantly, nor did incubation of cells or vesicles in glucose-free buffer for up to 4 h. A variety of sulfhydryl reagents, however, markedly inhibit 3-*O*-MG uptake, as do a number of uncoupling agents and several agents which inhibit glycolysis. Some electron transport inhibitors are without effect, while others produce moderate inhibition. It could be shown that respiration and 3-*O*-MG transport are not necessarily coupled in *A. laidlawii* cells.

Tarshis and Kapitanov (142) subsequently provided evidence for H⁺/3-*O*-MG symport in *A. laidlawii* cells. The addition of 3-*O*-MG to a lightly buffered cell suspension was reported to result in a decrease in the pH. Such a 3-*O*-MG-induced alkalinization of the incubation buffer does not occur with glucose analogs which are not transported and can be prevented by sulfhydryl reagents or by uncouplers. The stoichiometry of symport was estimated to be one H⁺ per 3-*O*-MG molecule taken up. Moreover, these workers provided evidence that 3-*O*-MG transport can be driven either by an electrical potential (due to a depletion of intracellular K⁺ by valinomycin) or by a pH gradient (due to the addition of acid to the incubation buffer), even when inhibitors of energy-transducing ATPases are present. In addition, evidence was presented that artificially imposed K⁺ or H⁺ gradients can result in ATP synthesis in intact cells. These authors therefore suggested that the hydrolysis of glycolytically formed ATP by a membrane-bound ATPase causes the extrusion of H⁺ from cells, resulting in an electochemical potential gradient of proteins across the membrane. The entry of 3-*O*-MG is in turn suggested to be directly coupled to H⁺ entry via the sugar carrier protein, with the movement of H⁺ down its electrochemical gradient providing the energy for the accumulation of 3-*O*-MG against its concentration gradient within the cell.

Although it is clear that metabolizing *A. laidlawii* cells do indeed maintain a transmembrane electrochemical potential (see below), which can drive active transport, the manner in which this potential is established remains in doubt. The proposal by Tarshis and coworkers, that the transmembrane electrochemical potential arises exclusively from the action of an energy-transducing, F_1F_0-type (H⁺ + Mg²⁺)-ATPase, is a reasonable one. However, the major Mg²⁺-ATPase of the *A. laidlawii* membrane is not stimulated by H⁺ or Ca²⁺, as is generally the case with bacterial energy-transducing ATPases, but is stimulated by Na⁺. In fact, the (Na⁺ + Mg²⁺)-ATPase clearly functions as an Na⁺ pump when reconstituted in lipid vesicles (see below). Although indirect evidence for an F_1F_0-type (H⁺ + Mg²⁺)-ATPase in this organism has been presented, this evidence is weak (see below). Therefore, whether such an ATPase exists in the *A. laidlawii* membrane, and whether it functions as proposed, remains to be definitely established.

There are several other potential sources for the generation of a transmembrane electrochemical potential in metabolizing *A. laidlawii* cells. Although it is clear that mycoplasmas in general contain a truncated electron transport chain in comparison with those of most bacteria and mitochondria, Tarshis and coworkers have themselves presented evidence for an inhibition of sugar transport by inhibitors of mitochondrial site I (but not site II and III) respiration (139, 141), suggesting that a transmembrane electrochemical potential capable of driving transport can be produced by respiration as well as by ATP hydrolysis. Moreover, the NADH oxidase of the *A. laidlawii* membrane has been shown to be a multisubunit, copper-containing, iron-sulfur flavoprotein which, at least in principle, is the type of enzyme capable of carrying out the vectorial separation of protons and electrons and thus of establishing a transmembrane electrochemical potential (92). As well, it has been proposed that in certain groups of bacteria which are dependent primarily on glycolysis for energy, an electrochemical potential can be generated by coupling the efflux of lactate to the efflux of protons (45). Additional work will clearly be necessary to identify the source (or sources) and the transmembrane electrochemical potential in *A. laidlawii*.

There are a number of apparent inconsistencies in the work of Tarshis and colleagues which require resolution. In their early papers, Tarshis et al. (81, 143–145) claim that 2-deoxyglucose is not a competitor for the glucose transport system in *A. laidlawii* and is not phosphorylated in cell extracts. However, Read and McElhaney (91) report that 2-deoxyglucose competes with glucose for transport and is partially metabolized in intact cells. Tarshis et al. (139, 141) also claim that succinate, malate, and ethanol stimulate respiration and glucose uptake (but not 3-*O*-MG transport), but several workers report that these substrates are not utilized for respiration by growing cells of this organism (see chapter 11). Equally puzzling is the finding that the addition of NADH or ADP to cell suspensions stimulates respiration and glucose uptake (139, 141), since these substrates are impermeable to intact cells and, unlike in mitochondria, carrier-mediated NADH-NAD⁺ and ADP-ATP exchange systems do not exist in free-living procaryotes (indeed, their presence would be lethal since scarce intracellular coenzymes and nucleotides would be lost to the external medium). Another puzzling aspect of the work of Tarshis and colleagues is the reported ability of *A. laidlawii* cells and vesicles to transport 3-*O*-MG for long periods of time in the absence of an energy source, even if they are incubated in buffer for long periods of time before transport is assayed. Read and McElhaney (91) have shown that an energy source is required for maximal rates of glucose (and 2-deoxyglucose and 3-*O*-MG) transport, and several other workers have shown that the ability to support Na^+ extrusion and K^+ uptake, or to maintain an electrochemical potential across the membrane, is progressively lost when cells are incubated in buffer in the absence of glucose or another energy source (see below). Finally, the observation that glucose transport in resealed membrane vesicles appears to be driven by respiration and not ATP hydrolysis (27), whereas the reverse is true in intact cells (139, 141), is a finding hard to rationalize.

K^+ Transport in *A. laidlawii*

The active transport of K^+ into *A. laidlawii* cells was first demonstrated by Rottem and Razin (106), who showed that cells previously incubated in K^+-poor growth medium can accumulate about 7 mg of K^+ per g of cell protein within 30 min when incubated at 37°C with growth media containing glucose and 2.6 mM K^+. The presence of glucose is essential for K^+ accumulation, and iodoacetate inhibits K^+ transport, apparently by inhibiting glucose metabolism. Ouabain, an inhibitor of $(Na^+ + K^+)$-ATPases and thus of Na^+ and K^+ transport in eucaryotic cells, does not inhibit K^+ uptake in *A. laidlawii*. Variations in the Na^+ content of the incubation medium do not affect the rate or extent of K^+ uptake, and K^+ accumulation does not seem to be associated with changes in intracellular Na^+ content.

Cho and Morowitz (8) subsequently studied both the monovalent cation requirements for growth and K^+ transport in *A. laidlawii*. They demonstrated that K^+ is an absolute requirement for the growth of this organism and that K^+ is growth limiting for unadapted cells below a concentration of 5.37 mM, although cultures can be adapted to grow with K^+ concentrations as low as 0.034 mM. Rb^+ can partially substitute for K^+, but Na^+, Li^+, or Cs^+ cannot. Interestingly, normal growth is obtained in the virtual absence of Na^+ provided that the osmotic strength of the growth medium is maintained above a certain limit. Unadapted growing cells were shown to maintain an intracellular K^+ concentration of about 70 mM over a range of external K^+ concentrations of 1.35 to 5.37 mM, but the intracellular K^+ concentration is reduced at lower external potassium concentrations. In contrast, cells adapted to grow on low external K^+ concentrations can maintain an intracellular K^+ concentration of about 110 mM even at an external K^+ concentration of only 0.537 mM. It should be noted that Schummer and Schiefer (116) and Clementz et al. (13) have reported that growing *A. laidlawii* cells can maintain intracellular K^+ concentrations of 150 and 190 mM, respectively, when the external K^+ concentration is <5 mM.

Cho and Morowitz (8) also studied the kinetics of K^+ uptake (actually exchange) at 37°C by adding $^{42}K^+$ to exponentially growing *A. laidlawii* cells and monitoring the accumulation of intracellular radioactivity. In unadapted cells growing in the presence of 5.37 mM K^+, intracellular $^{42}K^+$ reaches its maximum level in about 40 min but half of the intracellular K^+ is exchanged in about 5 min. As observed by Rottem and Razin (106), iodoacetate strongly inhibits K^+ exchange and ouabain is without effect. K^+ exchange is also inhibited by several sulfhydryl group reagents and by NaF. On the other hand, uncouplers of oxidative phosphorylation, such as sodium arsenite, sodium azide, and dinitrophenol, have little effect. These two studies indicate that K^+ is actively transported by this organism by a saturable, protein-mediated process and that the energy required to drive K^+ accumulation derives ultimately from glycolysis rather than respiration.

Cho and Morowitz (9) also investigated the effects of variations in both growth and assay temperatures on the rates and steady-state levels of both K^+ influx and K^+ efflux in *A. laidlawii*. The initial rates of K^+ uptake and K^+ efflux were found to be slightly higher for 37°C-grown than for 25°C-grown cells. However, the steady-state level of intracellular K^+ is independent of growth temperature. On the other hand, the initial rates of K^+ influx and efflux are moderately dependent on the assay temperature, as expected, but somewhat surprisingly so are the steady-state levels of K^+. In particular, steady-state levels of intracellular K^+ decrease fairly markedly with temperature. Interestingly, the efflux of K^+ was shown to be markedly reduced by the absence of K^+ in the external medium and by the presence of sulfhydryl group reagents and the metabolic inhibitor iodoacetate, indicating that K^+ efflux is primarily an active, protein-mediated process in growing cells rather than a passive leakage across the lipid bilayer. The fact that the apparent activation energy for K^+ efflux is about 18 kcal/mol also supports this finding, since the activation energy for K^+ passive permeation of lipid bilayers is much higher.

The earlier observation of Cho and Morowitz (8), that treatment of *A. laidlawii* cells with phospholipase A (but not phospholipase C) inhibited K^+ uptake, suggests that intact, diacyl phospholipids are required to maintain the integrity of the membrane lipid bilayer or to support the activity of the K^+ transport protein itself, or both. However, the fact that Arrhenius plots of the initial rates of K^+ efflux are linear over the temperature range of 15 to 37°C, whereas a gel-to-liquid-crystalline phase transition of the membrane lipids occurs over this same temperature range, indicates that the rates of K^+ transport are not sensitive to the physical state of the membrane lipids. Moreover, the fact that initial uptake rates for K^+ at 25°C are actually slightly higher for 37°C-grown than for 25°C-grown cells, even though the former might be expected to contain lipids with a slightly higher gel-to-liquid-crystalline phase transition temperature, suggests that membrane lipid fluidity is not a major factor in determining the kinetics of K^+ transport in this organism. However, experiments in which larger and more controlled variations in membrane lipid fatty acid composition and cholesterol content are obtained are required to confirm this point.

Na^+ Transport in *A. laidlawii*

Mahajan et al. (65) have studied Na^+ transport in live *A. laidlawii* cells by using $^{23}Na^+$ nuclear magnetic resonance spectroscopy and a nonpermeable shift reagent to permit the differentiation of intra- and extracellular Na$^+$ pools. When energy-depleted, sodium-loaded cells are provided with glucose, a time-dependent extrusion of Na$^+$ from cells is observed, with about half of the intracellular Na$^+$ removed in 5 min and a steady-state level reached in about 20 min. In the presence of excess glucose, intracellular Na$^+$ concentrations of roughly 15 mM are obtained in isotonic buffer containing 156 mM Na$^+$. Moreover, nonmetabolizable glucose analogs cannot substitute for glucose, and the presence of glucose metabolic poisons such as sodium fluoride and Merthiolate inhibit Na$^+$ extrusion. These results clearly show that Na$^+$ efflux in this organism is an active transport process ultimately driven by glycolysis.

Mahajan et al. (65) also investigated the influx of ^{22}Na$^+$ into *A. laidlawii* cells which had depleted the glucose initially present in the isotonic assay buffer. At 37°C, Na$^+$ enters the cell down its concentration gradient at a rate much slower than the rate at which it was pumped out, with about half of the maximum intracellular Na$^+$ entering at 30 to 40 min. This rate of Na$^+$ entry is nevertheless much faster than that expected for the passive diffusion of Na$^+$ across the lipid bilayer. However, the rate of Na$^+$ entry is markedly temperature dependent and at temperatures below about 20°C becomes too slow to measure. Using ^{31}P nuclear magnetic resonance spectroscopy, these workers were able to show that in glucose-deprived cells maintained at 37°C, the entry of Na$^+$ ions is accompanied initially only by the loss of intracellular sugar phosphates and then by a loss of nucleoside triphosphates. If glucose is added before the nucleoside triphosphate level falls, Na$^+$ efflux is again observed. However, the addition of glucose to nucleoside triphosphate-depleted cells (1 h more of glucose starvation) does not result in Na$^+$ efflux or an increase in intracellular sugar phosphate or nucleoside triphosphate levels.

Mahajan et al. (65) also studied the temperature and lipid phase state dependence of Na$^+$ extrusion. Cells enriched in oleic acid, whose membrane lipids are exclusively in the liquid-crystalline state throughout the physiological temperature range, exhibit increasing rates of Na$^+$ extrusion with temperatures from 20 to 37°C. However, no decrease in intracellular Na$^+$ levels with time is detected at 15°C or below. In contrast, cells enriched in palmitic acid, which exhibit a gel-to-liquid-crystalline membrane lipid phase transition over the temperature range of 15 to 37°C, exhibit glucose-dependent Na$^+$ efflux at 37°C but not at 20°C. The lack of Na$^+$ efflux in palmitate-enriched cells at 20°C is not due to a disruption in energy metabolism, since normal levels of sugar phosphates and nucleotide triphosphates are present. The absence of net Na$^+$ efflux at 20°C in palmitate-enriched cells could be due either to an inhibition of the function of the glucose transporter by gel-state lipid or to a leakage of Na$^+$ ions at the boundaries of gel and liquid-crystalline lipid domains, or both. However, the latter suggestion is unlikely, since palmitate-enriched, glucose-depleted cells maintained in Na$^+$-containing buffer at 20°C do not exhibit a detectable inward movement of Na$^+$. In fact, extensive evidence for inhibition of the function of the (Na$^+$ + Mg^{2+})-ATPase sodium transporter in

this organism by gel-state lipid is available and will be discussed in a subsequent section.

Lelong et al. (56) have provided evidence for a monovalent cation/proton antiport activity in *A. laidlawii*. They showed that an artificially created ΔpH (inside acid) in intact cells can be dissipated more rapidly when Na$^+$ is added and that the addition of K$^+$ after Na$^+$ further stimulates the collapse of the pH gradient, although the reverse is not true. However, the addition of K$^+$ is without effect in resealed membrane vesicles, as is the addition of HCl. The addition of nigericin, a K$^+$/H$^+$ antiporter, collapses the imposed ΔpH when added along with KCl, but the addition of large amounts of tetraphenylphosphonium, which is known to collapse the transmembrane electrical potential, has no effect in intact cells. These workers suggest that a K$^+$-dependent Na$^+$/H$^+$ exchange may exist in intact cells of *A. laidlawii* and that this exchange may function both in pH homeostasis in the alkaline pH range and in the extrusion of excess intracellular Na$^+$. They further suggest that the osmotic balance may be maintained by the activity of an H$^+$-ATPase and a secondary Na$^+$/H$^+$ exchanger rather than by the (Na$^+$ + Mg^{2+})-ATPase. However, as the existence and function of an H$^+$-ATPase have not been conclusively demonstrated in this organism whereas the existence of an Na$^+$-transporting ATPase has, it is possible that the (Na$^+$ + Mg^{2+})-ATPase is the primary system for osmoregulation, with the Na$^+$/H$^+$ exchanger playing a secondary role in maintaining cell volume and intracellular pH.

Energization of Active Transport in *A. laidlawii*

Schummer and coworkers have studied the electrical potential across the membrane of *A. laidlawii* cells by using both a potential-sensitive fluorescence dye (120) and a null point concentration technique based on the valinomycin-mediated flow of K$^+$ from cells (115, 122). These techniques were both applied to freshly harvested cells that had been incubated in Tris buffer containing NaCl and KCl but no energy source for 10 min. These two techniques yielded almost comparable values for the membrane potential of this organism, namely, -27 and -28 mV, respectively. Similar values of -23 to -26 mV were reported by Lelong et al. (56), who used a technique based on the partitioning of a lipophilic cation between cells and buffer as well as cells suspended in a Tris-morpholinepropanesulfonic (MOPS) buffer containing high levels of NaCl and 10 mM glucose. Lelong and coworkers also report the absence of a ΔpH in cells of this organism below pH 7.5 but an increasing though still small ΔpH of 0.2 to 0.3 at higher external pHs. This is a very unusual result, since in most bacteria and in other mycoplasmas, ΔpH values decrease with increasing external pH. In fact, Schummer et al. (123) report that in glucose-metabolizing *A. laidlawii*, ΔpH values decrease from nearly 0.5 at an external pH of 6.0 to near zero at an external pH of 8.5; at an external pH of 7.0, a ΔpH of about 0.3 was observed.

Clementz et al. (13, 14) also determined both the membrane electrical potential and the ΔpH in *A. laidlawii* cells, using the partitioning of a lipophilic cation and a weak organic acid, respectively. In contrast to the previous studies, however, these determinations were made with cells growing in complete growth medium rather than in monovalent cation-containing buffers. Interestingly, membrane electrical potential values of -52 to -62 mV were recorded in these studies, and no ΔpH was present. Although these higher electrical potential values might in principle be ascribed to the use of growth media rather than buffer to suspend cells, these workers report similar results for centrifuged cells resuspended in Tris-HCl buffer containing 130 mM NaCl, 2 mM MgCl$_2$, 5 mM CaCl$_2$, and 1.2 mM Na$_2$HPO$_4$ plus 20 mM glucose. Perhaps the presence of divalent cations in this buffer stabilized the cell membrane, thus accounting for the difference in results. Since in the absence of a ΔpH, an electrical potential of about -60 mV would be necessary to effect a 10-fold concentration difference of transport substrates, and since variations in the extracellular to intracellular concentrations of 3-O-MG, Na$^+$, and K$^+$ of 10-fold (or more) have been observed in *A. laidlawii*, the higher values for the transmembrane electrical reported by Clementz and coworkers seem the more reasonable, particularly considering that the earlier studies of bacteria often underestimated the electrochemical potential since a portion of the intracellular contents was lost during centrifugation. In this regard, it is noteworthy that only in the studies of Clementz et al. (13, 14) was the loss of intracellular material during processing carefully monitored and shown to be negligible.

Clementz and coworkers also studied the effects of variations in the degree of unsaturation of the lipid fatty acyl chains on the membrane potential and adenylate energy charge in *A. laidlawii* A. Despite the fact that variations in the degree of unsaturation are known to affect the passive membrane permeability of a number of ions and nonelectrolytes, no significant correlation between membrane lipid fatty acid composition and the magnitude of the electrical potential maintained by this organism is apparent. However, the adenylate energy charge of these cells does exhibit a modest dependence on membrane lipid fatty acid composition. Specifically, the adenylate energy charge increases steadily as the oleic acid/palmitic acid ratio in the membrane lipids increases but is substantially lower in cells supplemented with linoleic acid. Thus, an intermediate degree of lipid acyl chain unsaturation seems to be optimal for maintaining a highly energized state in this organism. Interestingly, however, Wieslander and Selstam (150) reported that cell growth yields were highest in palmitic acid-enriched cells and declined with the increasing degree of unsaturation of the membrane lipids. Taken together, these results imply that the adenylate energy charge maintained by *A. laidlawii* is not a major determinant of the growth efficiency of this organism, a somewhat surprising but not unprecedented finding.

Sugar Transport in *Mycoplasma* and *Spiroplasma* Species

In contrast to the classical active transport of glucose observed in acholeplasmas, sugar transport by the glucose-utilizing species of the genera *Mycoplasma* (12, 37, 38, 108, 146) and *Spiroplasma* (37, 38) occurs

via the PEP:PTS, first described by Kundig and coworkers for *E. coli* (46) and later found to occur in a number of anaerobic and facultative anaerobic bacteria (85, 111). In this vectorial phosphorylation system, transport of the sugar molecule across the cell membrane occurs in concert with its phosphorylation, such that the sugar phosphate rather than the free sugar appears in the cytoplasm. The ultimate phosphoryl donor for sugar phosphorylation is PEP, which is formed by glycolysis. In *E. coli*, the phosphoryl group from PEP is transferred by enzyme I to a histidine-containing phosphocarrier protein (HPr), which in turn serves as the phosphate donor for two sugar-specific classes of proteins (enzymes II and III), which are involved in the actual phosphorylation of sugars and their transport across the membrane. Enzyme I and HPr are constitutive, cytoplasmic proteins, whereas enzymes II and III are usually membrane bound and may be inducible by the presence of the specific sugars upon which they act. The PTS seems to be unique to procaryotes. For recent reviews of this complex and fascinating transport system, see references 85 and 111.

Jaffor Ullah and Cirillo (37, 38) have characterized the PTS in several *Mycoplasma* and *Spiroplasma* species, using the nonmetabolizable analog α-methylglucoside (α-MG), which seems to be a reasonably specific substrate for this particular sugar transport system. The uptake of α-MG occurs by a saturable, carrier-mediated process dependent on a source of metabolic energy. Specifically, iodoacetate and fluoride, which inhibit glycolysis, also inhibit α-MG transport, presumably by depleting cells of the phosphoryl donor PEP. The uptake of α-MG however, is not sensitive to uncouplers of oxidative phosphorylation which do inhibit the active transport of glucose in *A. laidlawii*. Mutants of *M. capricolum* defective in PTS enzyme activity are also unable to transport α-MG (76), demonstrating the obligatory link between phosphorylation and transport in this system.

Rottem et al. (102) compared the rate and temperature dependence of α-MG transport in cells of *M. mycoides* subsp. *capri* adapted to grow with low levels of exogenous cholesterol with those of native cells in which the normal high level of cholesterol was present in the membrane. In the native strain, rates of α-MG uptake are higher than in the adapted strain except at the highest temperature studied. In fact, the adapted strain cannot transport α-MG at temperatures below 25°C. Since a cooperative membrane lipid gel-to-liquid-crystalline phase transition is observed only in the adapted strain, it would appear that α-MG uptake cannot occur in the presence of predominantly gel-state lipid, although whether the absence of transport at low temperatures is due to the inhibition of cell growth and energy metabolism, to a leaky membrane, or to an actual inhibition of a portion of the PTS is not clear. Interestingly, a break in the Arrhenius plot of α-MG at 30°C was observed in the native but not in the adapted strain, which is opposite to the result expected if such a break is due to a lipid phase transition. However, since alterations in the fatty acid composition of the membrane lipids do not alter the temperature of this break, the authors concluded that it was not induced by a lipid phase transition. Surprisingly, however, Arrhenius plots of α-MG efflux show a break at 23°C in the adapted but not in the native strain, and the temperature of this break can be shifted by changing the membrane lipid fatty acid composition. In contrast, the rates and temperature dependences of α-MG phosphorylation by isolated membranes of the adapted and native strains of this organism are identical. Although the molecular basis for the cholesterol and membrane lipid fatty acid compositional dependence of α-MG uptake and efflux remains unclear, these results imply that the PTS is sensitive to the fluidity and phase state of the membrane lipids in *M. mycoides* subsp. *capri*. These results contrast with those of Shechter et al. (124), who found that the rate-temperature profiles of PTS-mediated glucose transport in an *E. coli* unsaturated fatty acid auxotroph are independent of the fatty acid composition and thus of the fluidity and phase state of the membrane lipids.

Jaffor Ullah and Cirillo (37, 38) have also purified and characterized two components of the PTS from *M. capricolum*, HPr and enzyme I. The *M. capricolum* HPr, like that of *E. coli* and *Staphylococcus aureus*, is a heat-stable protein of molecular weight about 9,000 having a single histidine residue. However, the mycoplasma HPr has two cysteine residues rather than one. Interestingly, despite the apparent structural similarity of the HPr proteins in the three organisms and the fact that the phosphorylated mycoplasma HPr functions well with *E. coli* membranes, the *M. capricolum* HPr does not cross-react with antibodies to the *E. coli* HPr, indicating that immunochemical techniques do not always provide reliable information on structural relatedness (see below). Enzyme I from *M. capricolum* was reported to have a molecular weight of about 220,000 and to consist of four subunits, two of 44,500 and one each of 62,000 and 64,000, whereas the enzymes I from *E. coli* and *S. aureus* consist of a single polypeptide chain having a molecular weight of between 70,000 and 90,000. Despite the apparent significant differences between the structures of the mycoplasmal and eubacterial enzymes I, the *M. capricolum* enzyme phosphorylates *E. coli* HPr at a respectable rate. As expected, HPr proteins and enzymes I from several *Mycoplasma* and *Spiroplasma* species complement each other very well in in vitro reconstitution experiments.

In eubacteria, the PTS is involved in a variety of regulatory functions as well as in sugar transport, one of the most important of these functions being the regulation of intracellular levels of cyclic AMP (cAMP). Mugharbil and Cirillo (76) have shown that sugars such as glucose and fructose, which are substrates for the PTS, can alter cAMP levels in wild-type *M. capricolum*. However, in a mutant of this organism unable to take up glucose by the PTS, this sugar does not alter cAMP levels. In eubacteria possessing the PTS, the presence of sugar substrates inhibits the induction of enzymes and transport systems required for the uptake and utilization of alternate energy sources. This inhibitory effect is mediated in part by a reduction in intracellular cAMP levels. The data of Mugharbil and Cirillo suggest that the PTS may play a similar regulatory role in this organism, although additional work will be required to establish this fact.

Although characterization of the PTS in mycoplasmas is incomplete, one is struck by the fact that the components of this system studied thus far seem as structurally complex as, or more complex than, those in many eubacteria, despite the restricted genome size of the former. Also striking is the fact that acholeplasmas, mycoplasmas, and spiroplasmas, although apparently evolutionarily closely related (see chapters 1 and 33), contain two completely different types of transport systems for the uptake of glucose and related sugars.

Amino Acid Transport in *Mycoplasma* Species

Razin et al. (88) studied L-histidine uptake in *M. fermentans* and L-methionine uptake in *M. hominis*, using incubation media containing chloramphenicol to inhibit protein synthesis. The rates of uptake of both amino acids are maximal in mid-log-phase cells. The uptake of L-histidine by *M. fermentans* exhibits a sharp pH optimum at 5.4, whereas L-methionine uptake by *M. hominis* shows a broad pH optimum between 6.8 and 8.0. The optimal temperature for L-histidine uptake by *M. fermentans* is 37°C, and that for L-methionine uptake by *M. hominis* is 42°C. Both uptake systems exhibit large Q_{10} values (near 3.0) over the physiological temperature range, and there is no measurable uptake of either amino acid below 10°C. Steady-state levels of L-histidine and L-methionine are obtained in about 20 and 30 min, respectively.

The amino acid uptake systems of both organisms exhibited Michaelis-Menten kinetics. The K_m and V_{max} values for L-histidine uptake in *M. fermentans* are 8 × 10^{-5} M and 17 μmol per mg of cell protein per min, respectively, whereas those for L-methionine uptake in *M. hominis* are 3 × 10^{-5} M and 0.04 μmol per mg of cell protein per min. The intracellular concentration of L-histidine in *M. fermentans* was estimated to be about 200 times the external concentration, while the intracellular concentration of L-methionine in *M. hominis* is only about three times the external concentration. The transport of L-histidine by *M. fermentans* is inhibited by the basic amino acids L-arginine, L-lysine, and L-ornithine but only to a small extent by D-histidine. In contrast, the transport system of L-methionine exhibits a high degree of specificity, with none of the other amino acids tested, including D-methionine, inhibiting uptake even at 1,000-fold-higher concentrations. The efflux of radiolabeled L-histidine from preloaded *M. fermentans* cells can be stimulated by about fivefold by the addition of unlabeled L-histidine to the reaction mixture.

Razin et al. (88) also studied the energy dependence and inhibitor spectra of these two amino acid transport systems. Incubation of *M. fermentans* cells in buffer progressively decreases their ability to take up L-histidine. Surprisingly, however, the addition of glucose to the incubation buffer does not restore L-histidine uptake, despite the fact that this organism appears to utilize glucose as an energy source. In contrast, L-methionine uptake in *M. hominis* is substantially reduced when L-arginine is omitted or modestly reduced when acetate and butyrate, the normal energy sources for this organism, are absent. The uptake of both amino acids can be inhibited strongly by sulfhydryl reagents and modestly by inhibitors of glycolysis (iodoacetate and fluoride) and respiration (cyanide and azide) but not by dinitrophenol, a proton uncoupler. Additional work will be required to determine the molecular mechanisms of these transport systems and the nature of their coupling to the energy metabolism of these organisms.

Sodium Transport and Cell Volume Regulation in *Mycoplasma* Species

Rottem et al. (104) studied the relationship between the proton motive force, sodium movement, and cell volume regulation in *M. gallisepticum*. When cells are incubated at 37°C in NaCl-containing buffer at pH 7.1 in the presence of glucose, a proton motive force of -70 mV is observed, intracellular ATP levels near 4 mM are measured, and cells maintain their normal volumes. When glucose is not added, both the proton motive force and the intracellular levels of ATP progressively decline with time, and cells swell and eventually lyse. The tendency of cells to swell and lyse under these conditions increases with the age of the culture. Interestingly, incubation of cells with glucose and N,N'-dicyclohexylcarbodiimide (DCCD), an ATPase inhibitor, results in a low transmembrane electrochemical potential and a more rapid swelling and lysis, despite the fact that high levels of intracellular ATP are maintained. The substitution of NaCl by KCl does not prevent cell swelling in the absence of glucose at 37°C, but cells do not swell significantly when incubated in sucrose-containing buffer, indicating that the observed increase in cell volume is due to the entry of ions (and water) into the cells. These authors concluded that an energy source and a functional ATPase are required for the regulation of cell volume in this organism, as demonstrated earlier for *A. laidlawii* (42, 127).

These results were confirmed and extended by Linker and Wilson (60, 61), who demonstrated that *M. gallisepticum* cells incubated in NaCl-containing buffer began to swell when intracellular ATP levels fell below about 40 μM; such swelling was not observed in the presence of several impermeable solutes. Interestingly, cell swelling in NaCl-containing buffers without glucose is not observed at 20°C or below, presumably because cells are relatively impermeable to sodium ions at low temperatures. The addition of nigericin alone or valinomycin alone, which in the presence of extracellular KCl collapses the transmembrane pH or electrical potential gradients, respectively, does not induce cell swelling in the presence of NaCl and glucose, but these agents do induce swelling and lysis when added together. Similarly, other selective inhibitors of either the transmembrane pH or electrical potential gradients do not induce swelling under similar conditions, but the addition of gramicidin, which forms a nonspecific cation channel, does. Again, the addition of DCCD alone induces cell swelling in NaCl even in the presence of glucose. It thus appears that either a transmembrane pH or electrical potential gradient can provide the energy required for the membrane ATPase to maintain cell volume.

Linker and Wilson (60, 61) also showed that when washed cells of *M. gallisepticum* are incubated at 37°C in 250 mM ^{22}NaCl, intracellular Na$^+$ increases and K$^+$ decreases. The addition of glucose to these Na$^+$-loaded cells causes Na$^+$ efflux and K$^+$ uptake, with both ions

moving against their concentration gradients. This effect of glucose is blocked by the ATPase inhibitor DCCD, which prevents the generation of a proton motive force in these cells. In additional experiments, Na$^+$ extrusion was studied by diluting the ^{22}Na$^+$-loaded cells into Na$^+$-free medium and monitoring the loss of ^{22}Na$^+$ from the cells. Glucose stimulates ^{22}Na$^+$ extrusion in such cells by a DCCD-sensitive mechanism. As well, proton movement was studied by measuring the pH gradient across the cell membrane with the 9-aminoacridine fluorescence technique. Glucose addition to cells preincubated with cations other than Na$^+$ results in cell alkalinization, which is prevented by DCCD. This observation is consistent with the operation of a proton-extruding ATPase. When glucose is added to Na$^+$-loaded cells and diluted into Na$^+$-free medium, intracellular acidification is observed, followed several minutes later by a DCCD-sensitive alkalinization process. The initial acidification was ascribed to the operation of an Na$^+$/H$^+$ antiport, since Na$^+$ exit was occurring simultaneously with H$^+$ entry. When Na$^+$-loaded cells are diluted into Na$^+$-containing medium, the subsequent addition of glucose results in a weak acidification, presumably due to H$^+$ entry in exchange for Na$^+$ (driven by the ATPase) plus a continuous passive influx of Na$^+$. These workers explain their data by postulating the combined operation of an ATP-driven proton pump and an Na$^+$/H$^+$ exchange reaction in this organism.

This interpretation was subsequently challenged by Shirvan et al. (125, 126), who studied the role of Na$^+$ extrusion in the volume regulation of *M. gallisepticum* in more detail. Na$^+$ efflux from cells was studied by diluting ^{22}Na$^+$-loaded cells into an iso-osmotic NaCl solution and measuring the residual ^{22}Na$^+$ in the cells. Uphill ^{22}Na$^+$ efflux was found to be glucose dependent and linear with time over a 60-s period and to exhibit almost the same rate in the pH range of 6.5 to 8.0. ^{22}Na$^+$ efflux was markedly inhibited by DCCD but not by proton-conducting ionophores over the entire pH range tested. An ammonium diffusion potential and a pH gradient were created by diluting intact cells or sealed membrane vesicles of *M. gallisepticum* loaded with NH$_4$Cl into a choline chloride solution. The imposed H$^+$ gradient (inside acid) is not affected by the addition of either NaCl or KCl to the medium. Dissipation of the proton motive force has no effect on the growth of *M. gallisepticum* in the pH range of 7.2 to 7.8 in an Na$^+$-rich medium. Additionally, energized cells are stable in an iso-osmotic NaCl solution, even in the presence of proton conductors, whereas nonenergized cells tend to swell and lyse. These results show that in *M. gallisepticum*, Na$^+$ movement is neither driven nor inhibited by the collapse of the electrochemical gradient of H$^+$, suggesting that in this organism, Na$^+$ is extruded by an electrogenic, primary Na$^+$ pump rather than by an Na$^+$/H$^+$ exchange system energized by the proton motive force.

Shirvan et al. (125, 126) provided additional evidence that Na$^+$ is extruded via a primary ion pump rather than by an Na$^+$/H$^+$ exchange process in this organism. The primary extrusion of Na$^+$ from *M. gallisepticum* cells was demonstrated by showing that when Na$^+$-loaded cells are incubated with both glucose and an uncoupler, rapid acidification of the cell interior occurs, resulting in the quenching of acridine orange fluorescence. No acidification is obtained with Na^+-depleted cells or with cells loaded with either KCl, RbCl, LiCl, or CsCl. Acidification is inhibited by DCCD and diethylstilbestrol but not by vanadate. By collapsing the transmembrane electrical potential with tetraphenylphosphonium or KCl, the fluorescence can be dequenched. These results are consistent with an electrical potential-driven, uncoupler-dependent proton gradient generated by an electrogenic ion pump specific for Na^+.

Shirvan and coworkers (125, 126) also report that the ATPase activity of *M. gallisepticum* membranes is Mg^{2+} dependent over the entire pH range tested (5.5 to 9.5). Na^+ (>10 mM) causes a threefold increase in the ATPase activity at pH 8.5 but has only a small effect at pH 5.5. In Na^+-free medium, the enzyme exhibits a pH optimum of 7.0 to 7.5, with a specific activity of 30 ± 5 μmol of phosphate released per h per mg of membrane protein. In the presence of Na^+, the optimum pH is between 8.5 and 9.0, with a specific activity of 52 ± 6 μmol. The Na^+-stimulated ATPase activity at pH 8.5 is much more stable to prolonged storage than is the Na^+-independent activity. Further evidence that two distinct ATPases exist was obtained by showing that *M. gallisepticum* membranes possess a protein of molecular weight 52,000 that reacts with antibodies raised against the β subunit of *E. coli* F_0F_1-ATPase as well as a protein of molecular weight 68,000 that reacts with the anti-yeast plasma membrane ATPase antibodies. These workers postulated that the Na^+-stimulated ATPase functions as the electrogenic Na^+ pump.

Romano et al. (97) have shown that the age of the culture and the membrane lipid composition of *M. capricolum* can affect its cell volume. In cells grown in the presence of exogenous palmitic and oleic acids plus high levels of cholesterol, the cellular water volumes are constant throughout the exponential phase of growth. However, the cell water volume of stationary-phase cells is considerably higher than in exponentially growing cells, possibly as a result either of changes in the membrane lipid composition and physical properties or of a decrease in the activities of active transport systems and membrane-bound ATPases which are known to accompany culture aging in mycoplasmas. Cell water volumes are dramatically reduced in late-stationary-phase cells, presumably because of cell lysis. An increase in the cholesterol/phospholipid molar ratio in the membranes also produces an increase in cell water volume and a decrease in membrane fluidity, as measured by electron spin resonance (ESR) spectroscopy. When *M. capricolum* cells are grown with exogenous egg phosphatidylcholine, a 50% increase in membrane phospholipid composition occurs without a change in the cholesterol/phospholipid molar ratio. This increase in the phospholipid content of the cell membrane also produces an increase in cell volume but in this case an increased membrane lipid fluidity. It is therefore probable that the increases in cell volume observed upon increasing both the cholesterol and the phospholipid contents of the cell membrane of this organism are due primarily to an increase in the surface area of the membrane caused by an increase in lipid content rather than to a change in membrane lipid physical properties.

K^+ and Na^+ Transport in *M. mycoides* subsp. *capri*

Leblanc and Le Grimellec (50) have studied K^+ and Na^+ transport in *M. mycoides* subsp. *capri* in great detail. These workers found that in growing cells, a high intracellular K^+ concentration (200 to 300 mM) and a low Na^+ concentration (20 mM) are maintained. Since the K^+ and Na^+ concentrations in the growth medium were 9 and 100 mM, respectively, active transport systems for these two monovalent cations clearly are operative. The intracellular K^+ concentration decreases with the age of the culture, but the intracellular Na^+ concentration remains constant.

The uptake of K^+ in washed organisms resuspended in buffered saline exhibits saturation kinetics. In cells depleted of intracellular K^+, the K_m and V_{max} for K^+ uptake are 0.3 mM and 80 neq/mg of cell protein per min, respectively, while in cells containing their normal intracellular K^+ levels, these values are 1.5 mM and 20 neq/mg of cell protein per min, suggesting that two different transport mechanisms for K^+ may exist. In fact a further kinetic analysis shows that both a net K^+ uptake and an autologous K^+/K^+ system are operative, the former predominating when intracellular K^+ is low and the latter predominating when intracellular K^+ is high. Both systems are energy dependent, being energized ultimately by glycolysis. Interestingly, pyruvate is almost as effective as glucose in maintaining high intracellular K^+ concentrations, and lactate can also support appreciable K^+ uptake activity.

In energy-starved cells, intracellular K^+ steadily decreases with time and K^+ loss is partially compensated for by a gain of Na^+. However, since cell volume does not increase under these conditions, entry of another cation, presumably H^+, must occur. The readdition of glucose essentially completely reverses these effects. Ouabain and anoxia have no effect on K^+ transport, nor do a number of respiratory inhibitors, but both processes are inhibited by DCCD, presumably by inhibiting the Mg^{2+}-ATPase activity present in the membrane of this organism.

Leblanc and Le Grimellec (51) also studied the relationship between K^+ transport, transmembrane electrical potential, and ATPase activity in *M. mycoides* subsp. *capri*. The addition of DCCD was found to result in a progressive loss of intracellular K^+ from metabolizing cells, despite the fact that it does not inhibit glucose metabolism. This loss is due to an inhibition of K^+ entry, since K^+ efflux is not affected by DCCD. The influx of K^+ can be totally blocked by DCCD. Addition of the K^+ ionophore valinomycin to metabolizing cells has little effect on K^+ distribution but causes a complete loss of K^+ in starved cells. Interestingly, various uncoupling agents alone, although they can be shown to dissipate the transmembrane pH difference, do not interfere with the maintenance of higher intracellular K^+ levels, although the K^+ concentration gradient can be dissipated when these agents are combined with valinomycin.

A transmembrane electrical potential of about 125 mV could be measured in glucose-metabolizing cells. This potential progressively decays when glucose is exhausted and can also be dissipated by a mixture of valinomycin with an uncoupler but not by either alone. As well, the addition of DCCD prevents the regeneration of a transmembrane electrical potential when glucose is added to starved cells. Interestingly, however, DCCD inhibits Mg^{2+}-ATPase activity by 30 to 40%, possibly suggesting the presence of two different ATPases. These authors interpreted their results as indicating that K^+ transport is driven by an electrochemical potential gradient generated by a membrane-bound ATPase activity, which in turn depends on the ATP generated at least primarily by glycolysis.

Benyoucef et al. (4, 5) have investigated some additional features of K^+ accumulation by glycolyzing *M. mycoides* cells. They found that when Na^+ is absent from the external medium, K^+ accumulates up to the level predicted by the amplitude of the transmembrane electrical potential, as measured by Rb^+ and methyltriphenylphosphonium cation distribution. Therefore, under these experimental conditions, the coupling mechanism of K^+ uptake consists of a potential-driven uniport. However, when Na^+ is present in the external medium, the level of K^+ accumulation by glycolyzing cells is too high to be in equilibrium with the transmembrane electrical potential. These results clearly indicate the presence of an active K^+ transport system specifically stimulated by Na^+. Furthermore, by controlling the amplitude of the energy-dependent electrical potential, evidence was obtained that this specific Na^+-stimulated K^+ transport is also modulated by the transmembrane electrical potential. Finally, these workers showed that ATP is consumed by both the K^+ uniport and the Na^+-dependent K^+ uptake systems.

Benyoucef et al. (4, 5) have also studied the relationship between the movements of Na^+, K^+, and H^+ in glycolyzing *M. mycoides* cells. In the light of previous work implicating the membrane-bound ATPase in these movements, its ionic requirements and sensitivity to specific inhibitors were investigated. Although Na^+ stimulates ATPase activity, K^+ does not affect it, and DCCD and 7-chloro-4-nitrobenzo-2-oxa-1,3-diazole are potent inhibitors of the basal ATPase activity, which is unaffected by vanadate and ouabain. It was also found that when Na^+-loaded cells previously equilibrated with $^{22}Na^+$ are diluted in sodium-free medium, addition of glucose induces a rapid efflux of $^{22}Na^+$. This energy-dependent efflux is independent of the presence of KCl in the medium. Studies of the changes in internal pH by 9-aminoacridine fluorescence or [^{14}C]methylamine distribution indicate that the movement of Na^+ is coupled to that of protons moving in the opposite direction, a finding that supports the presence of an Na^+/H^+ antiport system. When Na^+-loaded cells are diluted into Na^+-rich medium, Na^+/H^+ antiport is still active but cannot decrease the intracellular Na^+ concentration. Under such conditions, net $^{22}Na^+$ extrusion is specifically dependent on the presence of K^+ in the medium. These results and those derived from the previous studies of K^+ accumulation can be rationalized by assuming that this organism contains two transport systems for Na^+ extrusion, an Na^+/H^+ antiport and an ATP-consuming Na^+/K^+-exchange system.

Le Grimellec and Leblanc (53) investigated the relationship of membrane lipid fatty acid composition and cholesterol content to potassium transport rates and levels of accumulation in *M. mycoides* subsp. *capri*. These workers studied the growth characteristics, intracellular K^+ content, and ability to extrude protons of native *M. mycoides* cells grown on medium supplemented with cholesterol and either palmitic and oleic acids or with elaidic acid and of a strain adapted to grow on low levels of cholesterol in the presence of elaidic acid; cholesterol accounts for 20 to 25% of the total membrane lipid in the native strain and less than 2% in the adapted strain. Native organisms grown on cholesterol-rich medium exhibit identical growth characteristics, intracellular K^+ contents, and medium acidification properties, irrespective of fatty acid supplementation. In contrast, cholesterol-deficient organisms are unable to grow below pH 6.5 (instead of pH 5.2 as in the native strain), and they exhibit lower intracellular K^+ levels and a reduced ability to extrude protons. Moreover, K^+ passive permeability is drastically increased in the adapted strain, although K^+ remains in equilibrium with the (reduced) transmembrane potential, and the intracellular Na^+ content increases. Replenishment of cholesterol in membranes of cholesterol-deficient cells results in a recovery of native growth characteristics, intracellular K^+ level, and acidification potential. These authors suggested that cholesterol depletion produces its characteristic effects by inducing an increase in proton permeability, which, in turn, reduces the transmembrane electrochemical proton gradient that can be generated by this organism, thereby reducing intracellular K^+ accumulation and limiting growth at lower pH values. The changes observed in K^+ passive permeability do not appear to be involved in determining intracellular K^+ levels. This study is an important one in that it demonstrates that lipid-dependent changes in the energy state of a cell can affect transport processes.

Using the same organism, Le Grimellec and Leblanc (54) subsequently investigated the temperature-activity relationship of active K^+ influx, Mg^{2+}-ATPase activity, transmembrane potential, and membrane lipid composition. Arrhenius plots of the initial rates of K^+ exchange influx in the native strain enriched in palmitic and oleic acids give a linear relationship. On the other hand, the native strain enriched with elaidic acid produces a biphasic linear Arrhenius plot with a discontinuity at about 28 to 30°C. Finally, the adapted strain grown in the presence of elaidic acid exhibits a biphasic linear Arrhenius plot with a break at about 23°C. A broad endothermic lipid phase transition, occurring between 20 and 48°C, is observed by DSC for membranes from the cholesterol-deficient strain, whereas no phase transitions can be detected by this technique in membranes of the native strain, irrespective of fatty acid composition. However, diphenyl hexatriene fluorescence polarization results suggest the presence of a phase separation between 29 and 31°C both in palmitic-plus-oleic acid-containing and in elaidic acid-containing native strain membranes. Thus, the rates of active K^+ influx appear to be sensitive in a complex manner to the phase state, and possibly to the fluidity, of the membrane lipids. However, at temperatures above the Arrhenius inflection points, the relative rates of K^+ influx do not correlate with the relative membrane lipid fluidities. In contrast, Arrhenius plots of Mg^{2+}-ATPase activity and of transmembrane potential do not exhibit discontinuities or breaks, and the activity-temperature profiles of the native and adapted strains are not significantly different.

These workers thus concluded that the absolute Mg^{2+}-ATPase activity and its temperature dependence, as well as the temperature dependence of the transmembrane potential difference, are not affected by the order-disorder phase transition of the membrane lipids. Therefore, the observed alterations in the K^+ influx rates with membrane lipid composition must reflect the dependence of the K^+ carrier itself on the phase state of the membrane lipids.

Energization of Active Transport in *Mycoplasma* and *Spiroplasma* Species

Schummer and coworkers have applied several techniques to determine the transmembrane electrochemical potentials across the membranes of several *Mycoplasma* and *Spiroplasma* species and the contributions of various transmembrane ion fluxes to these potentials. Utilizing potential-sensitive fluorescent dyes, Schummer et al. (117, 120, 121) estimated the transmembrane potentials of *M. gallisepticum* and *M. mycoides* subsp. *capri* cells, suspended in NaCl- or KCl-containing buffer in the absence of glucose or other endogenous energy source, to be about -48 mV (inside negative), although another publication by this group reported a lower value of about -30 mV for *M. mycoides* with use of a similar technique. Schummer et al. (120) later estimated the transmembrane electrical potentials of *M. gallisepticum* and *M. mycoides* to be -35 and -53 mV, respectively, using a technique based on the distribution of K^+ ions in the presence and absence of valinomycin (115) in cells incubated in NaCl-plus-KCl buffers containing various extracellular K^+ ion concentrations. In subsequent work, Schiefer and Schummer (112, 116) demonstrated that both K^+ and Na^+ diffusion potentials contribute significantly to the membrane potential of *M. mycoides* but that Cl^- is freely permeable to the membrane and does not contribute to the membrane potential. Under normal growth conditions and in the presence of an energy source, the *M. mycoides* membrane potential was estimated to be -68 to -80 mV, somewhat higher than the -48 to -53 mV reported for cells suspended in buffer in the absence of an energy source.

Schummer et al. (123) and Schiefer and Schummer (112) also studied the proton gradient across the membranes of *M. mycoides* subsp. *capri* and *M. gallisepticum*, using several different membrane-permeable probes which distribute between the extra- and intracellular space according to their relative pH values. For both species, the intracellular pH is higher than the extracellular pH when cells are incubated in the presence of an energy source, with the difference between the two pH values decreasing as the external pH increases. At an extracellular pH of 7.0, the intracellular pH is 7.4, so the ΔpH is 0.4. Without an energy source, no ΔpH is observed, and the addition of DCCD, an inhibitor of membrane-bound ATPases, also reduces the ΔpH, as does the addition of carbonyl cyanide *m*-chlorophenylhydrazone (CCCP), a proton conductor, and gramicidin, a cation-conducting antibiotic. These results imply that the proton gradient maintained across mycoplasma membranes is generated by an electrogenic, proton-translocating ATPase which uses the ATP formed by glycolysis to

effect proton extrusion. Since a ΔpH value of 0.4 at an external pH of 7.0 contributes about another -24 mV to the total transmembrane electrochemical potential, the total electrical and chemical potential across the membranes of these organisms was calculated to be about -72 mV, assuming an electrochemical potential value of -48 mV due to the K^+ and Na^+ diffusion potentials. If the later estimates of the electrical potential of metabolizing cells in their normal growth medium of -68 to -80 mV are used, then the total transmembrane electrochemical potential of these two organisms would be -92 to -104 mV.

Schiefer et al. (113) also studied the effects of various membrane-active antimicrobial agents on the membrane electrical potential and the viability of *M. mycoides* subsp. *capri*. Valinomycin, an ionophore with extreme potassium selectivity, induces a membrane hyperpolarization. Valinomycin is not cidal but is static to this mycoplasma. Obviously, the potassium drain induced by valinomycin can be compensated for by this organism. Gramicidin is an antibiotic forming cation conduction channels across membranes. It induces a rapid depolarization of mycoplasma membranes. At low concentrations, gramicidin has a static effect, whereas at high concentrations, it is cidal to *M. mycoides*. The rapid permeation of cations through the stationary ion channels formed by gramicidin obviously exerts an inhibitory or even lethal effect on mycoplasma metabolism and growth. Polymyxin B induces a depolarization of mycoplasma membranes only when the cells have been pretreated and hyperpolarized with valinomycin. After treatment with both valinomycin and polymyxin B, a slight inhibition of growth is observed. Clotrimazole, a synthetic imidazole antimycotic agent, also hyperpolarized mycoplasma membranes, being cidal at high concentrations but static at low concentrations. Although the depolarization of *M. mycoides* membranes by clotrimazole is less than that induced by valinomycin, its greater cidal and static effects on growth and metabolism are probably due to its greater general damage to the membrane permeability barrier, since this antibiotic can induce the leakage of amino acids, phosphates, and nucleotides as well as K^+ from cells.

The transmembrane electrochemical potential of *M. gallisepticum* cells under various conditions was also investigated by Rottem et al. (104). The electrical potential of cells suspended in glucose-containing buffer was found to vary from about -45 to -65 mV, depending on the extracellular pH, with maximum values being observed at about pH 6.5. In contrast, the ΔpH increases from a value of 0.2 to 0.3 at an extracellular pH of 8.0 to a value of about 1.3 at pH 5.5. At an external pH of 7.0, then, the total transmembrane electrochemical potential was calculated to be about -100 mV. This value is somewhat higher than the values of -59 to -72 mV reported by Schummer and coworkers, but these latter values are for cells suspended in buffer without an energy source. In the absence of glucose, the ΔpH decreases to zero within 15 min; intracellular ATP concentrations also decrease markedly, but the electrical potential is maintained. Longer periods (up to 4 h) of glucose starvation result in a further decrease in intracellular ATP and a progressive decline in the electrical potential to a constant value of -15 mV, which may represent the Donnan potential. Cells incubated with glucose plus DCCD maintain high intracellular ATP levels but only a small electrical potential and no detectable transmembrane pH gradient, confirming the roles of glycolysis and of a functional membrane-bound ATPase in maintaining a substantial electrochemical potential across the membrane of this organism.

Benyoucef et al. (2) investigated the transmembrane electrochemical potential of *M. mycoides* subsp. *capri* cells under a variety of conditions, using the preferred flow dialysis technique. In the presence of glucose only, cells maintain a ΔpH (inside alkaline) which varies from almost 1.0 pH unit at an external pH of 5.7 to 0.2 pH unit at an external pH of 7.7; at neutral pH, the ΔpH was determined to be about 0.5, corresponding to an electrical potential of about −30 mV. In contrast, the electrical potential increases almost linearly with increasing pH, rising from −58 mV at pH 5.7 to −90 mV at pH 7.7. As a result of the opposite variations in ΔpH and electrical potential with external pH, the total electrochemical potential across the membrane of this organism remains constant at about −115 mV. The addition of DCCD to glucose-metabolizing cells abolishes both the transmembrane ΔpH and the electrical potential generated by this organism. A proton uncoupler and nigericin also prevent the generation of a ΔpH in cells incubated with glucose. These results, which agree fairly well with those of Schummer and coworkers, again indicate that the membrane-bound ATPase is involved in generating both the electrical potential gradient and the proton chemical gradient across the membrane of glycolyzing *M. mycoides* subsp. *capri* cells.

Benyoucef et al. (3) also demonstrated that α-MG, a nonmetabolizable glucose analog, can be used to regulate the amount of glucose uptake and consequently the level of intracellular ATP in *M. mycoides* subsp. *capri* cells. The level of intracellular ATP, in turn, determines the rate of proton extrusion catalyzed by the membrane-bound Mg^{2+}-ATPase and thus the magnitude of both the electrical potential and the proton chemical gradient across the membrane. When the amount of intracellular ATP is limiting, no transmembrane ΔpH is formed and only an electrical potential exists. In fact, only when sufficient ATP is present to generate about 75% of the maximal total transmembrane electrochemical potential does a ΔpH begin to be established. These results indicate that the ΔpH is not generated at the expense of the electrical potential and imply that compensatory movements of cations and/or anions (most likely K^+ and Na^+) primarily generate the electrochemical potential. Thus, the primary form of energy stored in the transmembrane electrochemical potential gradient generated by this organism is the electrical potential. Because of the low electrical capacity of the *M. mycoides* subsp. *capri* membrane, the extrusion of only a small number of protons can apparently develop a relatively high membrane potential, while much higher rates of proton flow are required to generate a significant chemical potential of protons (a ΔpH). The ability to produce a gradation in the magnitude of the transmembrane electrochemical gradient in this organism was used to good effect in the studies of the energization of K^+ and Na^+ movements by this group discussed above (4, 5).

Schummer and Schiefer (118) have also recently studied the transmembrane electrochemical potential gradient of *Spiroplasma floricola* in a glucose-containing buffer over a range of external pH values. The electrical potential was found to increase with pH from −55 mV at pH 5.5 to −100 mV at pH 8.5. The ΔpH was found to also depend on pH but in the opposite direction, with ΔpH equal to 1.8 at pH 5 and to 0.5 at pH 8.0. Thus, the total electrochemical potential across the membrane of this organism varies from a minimum of −103 mV at pH 6.5 to −130 to −140 mV at pH 5.5 or 8.0. At an external pH of 7.0 and above, DCCD, an ATPase inhibitor, and CCCP, a proton carrier, both dissipate the ΔpH, and the presence of glucose is required to generate and to maintain both the electrical and chemical components of the total transmembrane electrochemical potential in this organism. These results are generally similar to those obtained for *M. gallisepticum* and *M. mycoides* subsp. *capri* except that the maximal electrochemical potentials obtained are somewhat lower with these organisms than with *S. floricola* and are obtained at near-neutral pH values.

The membrane surface potentials (the electrical potential difference located at the boundary between the membrane surface and the external medium) have been measured in *M. mycoides* subsp. *capri* by Rigaud et al. (93) and in *S. floricola* by Schummer and Schiefer (119). In the former organism, the addition of glucose to resting cells results in the outer surface of the membrane becoming more negatively charged. The glucose-induced increase in the negative membrane surface potential can be largely abolished by the prior addition of DCCD or CCCP, suggesting that this change in surface potential is dependent on an Mg^{2+}-ATPase-generated ΔpH across the membrane. In the latter organism, the membrane surface potential was calculated to be −118 mV in Ca^{2+}-free buffer, but this value can be progressively reduced to zero by the addition of up to 100 mM Ca^{2+}. Cytochemical evidence suggests the anionic lipid phosphate groups are largely responsible for the negative surface potential of *S. floricola* membranes, and variations in the cholesterol content or treatment of cells with pronase do not change the membrane surface potential. The increase in membrane surface charge observed upon the energization of *M. mycoides* subsp. *capri* membranes was suggested to be due to changes in membrane protein conformation induced by local pH changes, such that the ionizable carboxyl groups of membrane proteins become exposed at the outer surface.

ENZYME ACTIVITIES

Electron Transport Enzymes

The components of the aerobic and anaerobic electron transport systems are membrane associated in almost all eubacteria studied to date. However, the electron transport activity of *Mycoplasma* and *Spiroplasma* species, measured as the transfer of electrons from NADH to oxygen, is located in their cytoplasmic rather than membrane fractions (49, 87). The truncated, flavin-terminated respiratory systems of these organisms, which lack quinones and cytochromes and which apparently do not catalyze a vectorial transport of protons and electrons, may explain their lack of a dependence on the plasma membrane for their organization and function (see chapter 11). However, the NADH oxidase activities of *Acholeplasma* species are membrane bound (49, 83, 84), despite the fact that these organisms also appear to contain a truncated electron transport system.

Jinks and Matz (39, 40) studied a number of properties of the NADH oxidase of *A. laidlawii* both in isolated membranes and in a partially purified form. They reported that this dehydrogenase contains only trace amounts of iron, has a flavin ratio of flavin adenine nucleotide to flavin mononucleotide (FMN) of 2:1, and consists of one major and two minor bands on sodium dodecyl sulfate-polyacrylamide gel electrophoresis (molecular weights were not reported). The K_m for NADH was found to be 0.5 mM, and the V_{max} was found to be 0.24 μmol/min. The purified enzyme efficiently utilizes a number of electron acceptors, including ferricyanide, menadione, and dichloroindophenol, but not O_2, ubiquinone Q_{10}, or cytochrome *c*, and is susceptible to inhibition by a number of heavy-metal cations but less so to Mg^{2+} or Ca^{2+}. The *A. laidlawii* NADH oxidase is not stimulated by the addition of ADP, flavin adenine dinucleotide, FMN, or cysteine and is relatively insensitive to several respiratory inhibitors and to oligomycin. These workers also reported that this enzyme does not require lipid for activity, nor are the K_m and V_{max} values changed by alterations in the membrane lipid fatty acid composition. This finding is in accord with those of earlier studies reporting no influence of lipid phase state or fluidity on the NADH oxidase activity of isolated *A. laidlawii* membranes (24) and the presence of this enzyme activity in a solubilized membrane fraction devoid of lipid (77). Moreover, the NADH oxidase activity of isolated *A. laidlawii* membranes has been shown to be unaffected by the phospholipase-catalyzed hydrolysis of the membrane phosphatidylglycerol (PG), which does inhibit the activity of the lipid-requiring Mg^{2+}-ATPase (6). Nevertheless, this enzyme appears to be an integral membrane protein, since it cannot be released from the membrane by EDTA and low-ionic-strength buffers (78).

Reinards et al. (92) also purified and characterized the NADH oxidase from *A. laidlawii* membranes, and in some respects their findings do not entirely agree with those of Jinks and Matz (39, 40). The NADH oxidase was extracted with 3% Triton X-100 and subsequently purified by several chromatographic steps. The final preparation is essentially homogeneous, as judged by gel electrophoresis under nondenaturing conditions. The enzyme appears to be a copper-containing iron-sulfur flavoprotein (FMN:Cu:Fe:labile S = 1:1:6:6). It contains a high fraction of hydrophobic amino acids and is composed of three subunits of molecular weights 65,000, 40,000, and 19,000. When oxygen is used as an electron acceptor, the purified enzyme has a specific activity of 58.0 IU/mg of protein and catalyzes the formation of H_2O_2 in nearly stoichiometric amounts. The apparent K_m value for NADH was estimated to be 0.4 mM (pH 7.4). NADPH cannot serve as a substrate for the enzyme. In addition to the NADH oxidase activity, the enzyme is able to catalyze electron transfer from NADH to various other electron acceptors (ferricyanide, dichloroindophenol, and cytochrome *c*). Metal-chelating and mercurial agents were shown to inhibit the activity of the enzyme. From electron paramagnetic resonance and optical absorption measurements, evidence was obtained that the flavin semiquinone radical in the NADH oxidase has a high air stability and that the flavin shuttles between the fully reduced and semiquinone states upon electron transport from NADH to the electron acceptors. Inhibition of the NADH oxidoreductase activities by superoxide dismutase indicates that O_2 serves as an intermediate in the electron transfer from NADH to all electron acceptors used in this work. In addition to electron transfer via the superoxide radical O_2, an alternative pathway probably involving Fe-S centers is operative. An NADH oxidase of this complexity and one tightly associated with the *A. laidlawii* membrane could in principle carry out the vectorial transfer of protons and electrons and thus have a direct role in the generation of the transmembrane electrochemical gradient in this organism. Future studies directed to this question are in order.

ATPases

An Mg^{2+}-ATPase activity has been detected in the membrane of every mycoplasma species studied so far (87), but the *A. laidlawii* enzyme is by far the best characterized. The *A. laidlawii* Mg^{2+}-ATPase cannot be released by the techniques usually used to detach peripheral membrane proteins (78) and is firmly bound to the membrane (77, 84), indicating that it is an integral membrane protein. Since no Mg^{2+}-ATPase activity can be detected in intact cells, the ATP hydrolytic site is presumed to be located on the cytoplasmic side of the membrane (84, 106). Because the Mg^{2+}-ATPase of this organism is inactivated by detergents and organic solvents, early attempts to isolate and characterize it failed (77). However, it was reported that in its native, membrane-associated form, the *A. laidlawii* ATPase is not activated by Na^+ or K^+ and that it is insensitive to ouabain, a specific inhibitor of eucaryotic $(Na^+ + K^+)$-ATPases (106). However, the activity of this enzyme in isolated membranes is sensitive to the fluidity and phase state of the membrane lipids (see below), indicating that it is probably an integral, transmembrane, lipid-requiring enzyme.

The first investigation of the lipid and temperature dependence of the major ATPase of the *A. laidlawii* B membrane was that of de Kruyff et al. (24), who studied the temperature dependence of three membrane-bound enzymes in cells whose fatty acid and sterol compositions were widely varied. For NADH oxidase and *p*-nitrophenylphosphatase activities, Arrhenius plots are linear over the temperature range of 5 to 35°C, and no breaks or slope changes are observed. Moreover, the absolute activity of these enzymes in isolated membranes does not vary with membrane lipid fatty acid or sterol composition. De Kruyff and coworkers thus concluded that NADH oxidase and *p*-nitrophenylphosphatase, despite being integral membrane proteins, are unaffected by the fluidity and phase state of the membrane lipids. In contrast, the Mg^{2+}-ATPase activity seems to exhibit biphasic linear Arrhenius plots in membranes enriched in relatively high-melting-point fatty acids. The Arrhenius plot break temperatures always fall a few degrees above the lower boundary of the gel-to-liquid-crystalline lipid phase transition as measured by DSC. When grown in the presence of cholesterol, the Arrhenius break temperatures are reduced by 6 to 7°C, as is the lower boundary of the lipid phase transition. Treatment of cholesterol-enriched membranes with the polyene antibiotic filipin, which specifically complexes cholesterol and withdraws it from interaction with the membrane glycerolipids, reverses the effect of cholesterol incorporation on both ATPase activity and the lipid phase transition. Finally, the incorporation of epicholesterol instead of cholesterol has no effect on either the ATPase activity-temperature profile or the membrane lipid phase transition. De Kruyff et al. concluded that the activity of the *A. laidlawii* B Mg^{2+}-ATPase is markedly influenced by the phase state of the membrane lipids and that, within the phase transition temperature range at least, this enzyme preferentially associates with the lipid molecular species having the lowest phase transition temperatures. Qualitatively similar results were subsequently presented by Hsung et al. (35), who used ESR spectroscopy to monitor membrane lipid phase behavior.

Bevers et al. (6) investigated the phospholipid requirement of the three membrane-bound enzymes studied earlier by de Kruyff et al., using various phospholipases to selectively degrade the PG in *A. laidlawii* B membranes. These workers found that the complete hydrolysis of PG, the only phosphatide present in this *A. laidlawii* strain, by phospholipase A_2, C, or D had no effect on the activity of NADH oxidase or of *p*-nitrophenylphosphatase. Similarly, phospholipase A_2 and C hydrolysis of about 90% of the membrane PG could occur without effect on Mg^{2+}-ATPase activity, but hydrolysis of the final 10% of this phospholipid, which proceeded at a slower rate, resulted in a marked and progressive loss of activity. The complete conversion of PG to phosphatidic acid by phospholipase D treatment did not affect Mg^{2+}-ATPase activity, indicating that the glycerol portion of the PG headgroup is not required for activity. The inactivated Mg^{2+}-ATPase in PG-depleted membranes could be reactivated by adding PG, phosphatidic acid, or phosphatidylserine but not phosphatidylcholine, phosphatidylethanolamine, or any of the *A. laidlawii* glycolipids. These results indicate that this enzyme requires small amounts of a diacyl phosphatide bearing a net negative charge for optimal activity. Phospholipid reconstitution experiments demonstrated that the fatty acid compositions both of the residual PG present in the membrane and of the added phospholipid determine the activation energy of the Mg^{2+}-ATPase and the Arrhenius plot break temperature. In these reconstitution experiments, a preferential association of this enzyme with the more fluid phospholipid species does not seem to occur, in contrast to the suggestion made earlier by de Kruyff et al. It is noteworthy that the ability to restore Mg^{2+}-ATPase activity by adding exogenous phospholipid to membranes containing less than 2% of their original PG is gradually lost with time. This result probably means that a certain minimal amount of phospholipid is required for stabilization of this enzyme in an active

conformation in the native membrane, such as appears to be the case for the isolated enzyme (58).

The dependence of the kinetic parameters of the *A. laidlawii* ATPase on the fluidity and phase state of the membrane lipids has been investigated in more detail by McElhaney and coworkers. These investigators showed that the K_m of this enzyme for ATP is markedly temperature dependent, increasing roughly 10-fold as the temperature is increased from 5 to 40°C (42). This temperature dependence of substrate-binding affinity appears to be an intrinsic property of the enzyme molecule, since it is not affected by the fatty acid composition, cholesterol content, or phase state of the membrane lipids. Moreover, Silvius et al. (132) demonstrated that this and other enzymes with a temperature-dependent K_m can yield a variety of Arrhenius plot artifacts, most notably erroneous breaks, if enzyme activity is assayed at a fixed substrate concentration; in fact, the positions of the Arrhenius plot breaks previously reported by de Kruyff et al. (24) were actually significantly underestimated (by 7 to 10°C) because ATPase activity was becoming substrate limited at the higher assay temperatures. These investigators also demonstrated that the Mg^{2+}-ATPase of *A. laidlawii* B is strongly and specifically stimulated by Na^+ and therefore that this enzyme is actually an $(Na^+ + Mg^{2+})$-ATPase.

The results of initial studies of the activity-temperature profile of the *A. laidlawii* $(Na^+ + Mg^{2+})$-ATPase, under conditions in which the true maximum velocity of the enzyme was being measured, appeared to produce the classic biphasic linear Arrhenius plots for membranes enriched with fatty acid giving a lipid phase transition in the physiological temperature range, except that the break temperatures now occur slightly below but generally near the phase transition midpoint temperature instead of at the lower boundary of the transition (42, 127). Interestingly, the Arrhenius plots of ATPase activity in membranes enriched in low-melting-point fatty acids appear to be curved downward instead of being linear as previously reported (42, 127). Subsequent studies by Silvius and McElhaney (131) and by Silvius et al. (128), in which more accurate ATPase activity values at additional temperature points were determined, confirmed that in membranes containing exclusively liquid-crystalline lipid in the physiological temperature range, Arrhenius plots of $(Na^+ + Mg^{2+})$-ATPase activity are clearly nonlinear (slope gently downward). The temperature dependence of the ATPase activity is not dependent on membrane lipid fatty acid composition as long as the lipids exist in the fluid state. The absolute activity of this enzyme, however, does vary significantly with fatty acid composition, but there is no discernible relationship between enzyme activity and lipid fluidity per se. If a gel-to-liquid-crystalline phase transition occurs within the physiological range, however, a gently curving biphasic or triphasic Arrhenius plot is observed, in which the $(Na^+ + Mg^{2+})$-ATPase activity falls off more steeply with decreasing temperature than would otherwise be the case. No effect of the lipid phase transition on the ATPase activity is noted until about half of the membrane lipid is converted to the solid state, and some ATPase activity remains at temperatures considerably below the lower boundary of the lipid phase transition, although eventually all ATPase seems to be lost. These results suggest that the *A. laidlawii* ($Na^+ + Mg^{2+}$)-ATPase is active only in association with liquidlike boundary lipids and that the ATPase hydrolytic reaction exhibits a significant heat capacity of activation in this case. This enzyme appears to become progressively inactivated when its boundary lipids undergo a liquidlike-to-solidlike phase transition that is driven by the liquid-crystalline-to-gel phase transition of the bulk membrane lipid phase but that is less cooperative and takes place over a lower temperature range than does the bulk lipid transition. The lateral aggregation of intramembranous protein particles normally observed as the bulk lipid enters the gel state is apparently not responsible for the loss of ATPase activity, since membranes enriched in methyl iso-branched fatty acids give Arrhenius plots indistinguishable from those described above, despite the fact that no significant clustering of intramembranous particles occurs in iso-branched acid-enriched membranes. These results suggest that the familiar biphasic linear Arrhenius plots commonly reported for many membrane enzymes and transport systems may in fact have a more complex shape, the analysis of which can furnish useful information regarding the behavior of the enzyme molecule in its membrane environment.

The effects of pressure and of pentanol on the activity and temperature dependence of the ATPase of the *A. laidlawii* plasma membrane were studied by MacNaughton and Macdonald (64). Increases in hydrostatic pressure increase the temperature at which the break in the Arrhenius plot of ATPase activity versus temperature is observed. Since this Arrhenius plot break is known to be induced by a gel-to-liquid-crystalline phase transition of the membrane lipids, this finding implies that the effect of hydrostatic pressure is mediated predominantly through its action on the membrane lipid bilayer. Moreover, the increases in the Arrhenius plot slopes (apparent activation energies) observed at temperatures above the break temperature with increases in hydrostatic pressure can also be explained by changes in the physical properties of the lipid bilayer, since hydrostatic pressure increases the order of liquid-crystalline lipid bilayers (63). Pentanol, however, which is known to decrease the lipid phase transition temperature and to increase the fluidity of liquid-crystalline bilayers of this organism (63), inhibits ATPase activity without affecting the Arrhenius break temperature at 37°C and atmospheric pressure, suggesting that it can act directly on the enzyme to inhibit its function. However, pentanol can partially offset the inhibitory effects of high hydrostatic pressure, which is consistent with a bilayer-fluidizing effect of this alcohol. It thus appears that pentanol can exert two opposite effects on the activity of this ATPase, with the net effect being determined by the temperature and pressure and by the alcohol concentration used.

Lewis and McElhaney (58) have succeeded in isolating the ($Na^+ + Mg^{2+}$)-ATPase from the *A. laidlawii* B membrane in a relatively pure and enzymatically active form. This enzyme has been shown to consist of five subunits (α, β, γ, δ, and ϵ) ranging in apparent molecular weight from 68,000 to 16,000; the probable subunit stoichiometry is $\alpha_3\beta\gamma\delta_2\epsilon_3$. All of the subunits of the purified, phospholipid-reconstituted ATPase can

be labeled by water-soluble, group-specific reagents, suggesting that at least a portion of each of these subunits is exposed to the aqueous phase (34, 57). On the other hand, the α (and possibly the ϵ) subunit can be photolabeled by phospholipids containing a photosensitive fatty acyl group, indicating that portions of at least this subunit(s) penetrate into or traverse the hydrophobic core of the phospholipid bilayer (30). Studies with a variety of reagents that specifically modify various amino acid residues indicate that the modification of one reactive lysine, one reactive arginine, or two reactive tyrosine residues completely inactivates this enzyme. A partial inactivation of enzyme activity by certain sulfhydryl and carboxyl group reagents also occurs, suggesting that these groups may also be involved in catalysis, although nonspecific effects such as subunit cross-linking may be responsible for these effects (57). The ($Na^+ + Mg^{2+}$)-ATPase can also be labeled by the 2′,3′-dialdehyde derivative of ATP; however, since all subunits except the ϵ subunit are labeled, localization of the ATP-binding subunit is not achieved (34). However, a nucleotide analog that reacts with phenolic or sulfhydryl groups, or both, specifically labels the α subunit, suggesting that it contains the active site (57).

With the development of a successful reconstitution procedure for the purified *A. laidlawii* B ($Na^+ + Mg^{2+}$)-ATPase (31, 41), George and coworkers have recently investigated in more detail than is possible in vivo the lipid and temperature dependence of the ATP hydrolytic activity of this enzyme (29, 32). To investigate the influence of lipid fluidity and phase state on the temperature dependence of the purified *A. laidlawii* ($Na^+ + Mg^{2+}$)-ATPase, this enzyme was reconstituted with phosphatidylcholines containing saturated, branched-chain, or unsaturated fatty acids having a wide range of chain lengths, and Arrhenius plots of ATPase activity versus assay temperature were constructed. In proteoliposomes made from phospholipids having gel-to-liquid-crystalline phase transition temperatures below 0°C, so that they exist entirely in the fluid state over the physiological temperature range, almost identical, smoothly curving Arrhenius plots are observed, indicating that the nature of the fatty acid has little or no effect on the absolute activity or temperature dependence of this enzyme. These Arrhenius plots are essentially identical to those observed in isolated *A. laidlawii* B membranes whose lipids have been highly enriched in various low-melting-point fatty acids (128, 131).

Arrhenius plots of ($Na^+ + Mg^{2+}$)-ATPase activity in vesicles composed of phosphatidylcholines containing saturated or unsaturated fatty acids and that exhibit gel-to-liquid-crystalline phase transitions in the physiological temperature range were also constructed. In all cases, these Arrhenius plots are clearly biphasic. The high-temperature portion of each plot exhibits a gentle downward slope, as observed for vesicles whose lipids exist entirely in the liquid-crystalline state above 0°C. The low-temperature portions of the plots are more nearly linear and exhibit much greater slopes. The temperature at which the change in slope occurs correlates well with the midpoint of the gel-to-liquid-crystalline lipid phase transition temperature of the ATPase-containing vesicle as determined by DSC. These results indicate that this enzyme is fully active only when most of the phospholipid is in the liquid-crystalline state. However, at temperatures above the phospholipid phase transition temperature, the absolute activities obtained for the ATPase are fairly similar. This result indicates again that moderate alterations in phospholipid fatty acid structure and chain length, and thus membrane lipid fluidity, have only a small effect on enzyme activity. These Arrhenius plots are also essentially identical to those observed in isolated membranes whose lipids have been highly enriched in various higher-melting-point fatty acids (128, 131). These results also indicate that the wide variations in ATPase activity observed in *A. laidlawii* B membranes differing in fatty acid composition are due primarily to variations in the number, rather than to the specific activity, of the ATPase molecules present (29, 32).

To investigate the effect of cholesterol on the activity and temperature dependence of the $(Na^+ + Mg^{2+})$-ATPase, this enzyme was reconstituted into dimyristoylphosphatidylcholine vesicles containing various amounts of cholesterol, and Arrhenius plots of enzyme activity versus temperature were constructed (32). The presence of relatively small amounts of cholesterol (13 to 24 mol%) reduces ATPase activity slightly at higher temperatures but does not change the temperature at which the change in slope of the Arrhenius plot occurs. However, these low levels of cholesterol decrease the slope of the lower-temperature portions of these plots. At higher cholesterol concentrations (33 and 45 mol%), ATPase activity markedly and progressively decreases, and the temperature at which the change in slope of the Arrhenius plot occurs is reduced. Calorimetric analyses of the ATPase-containing vesicles reveal that at the two lower cholesterol concentrations, the phospholipid phase transition is broadened compared with that of cholesterol-free vesicles, while at the higher cholesterol levels, no cooperative lipid phase transition can be detected. These results can probably be rationalized by considering the well-known effect of cholesterol on phospholipid bilayer membranes. Cholesterol is known to produce an intermediate phase state by fluidizing gel-state lipids and rigidifying liquid-crystalline lipids. Since this ATPase is active in the presence of fluid lipid but comparatively inactive in the presence of gel-state lipid, one would predict that the incorporation of increasing quantities of cholesterol into a phospholipid model membrane would decrease the ATPase activity observed at higher temperatures and increase that observed at lower temperatures. This is essentially what is observed.

To investigate the effect of the nature of the phospholipid polar headgroup on ATPase activity, this enzyme was reconstituted into vesicles composed of one of four different phospholipids and its activity was assayed at 37°C, a temperature at which all of these phospholipids exist in the liquid-crystalline state (29, 32). The two zwitterionic phospholipids tested, phosphatidylcholine and phosphatidylethanolamine, both support high levels of activity, while the anionic phosphatidylserine is much less effective; PG, an anionic lipid that is the major phosphatide of the *A. laidlawii* B membrane, alone does not support any ATPase activity. Moreover, when reconstituted with mixtures of zwitterionic and anionic phospholipids, enzyme activity is progressively diminished when the anionic phospholipid constitutes more than 20 mol% of the binary

mixture. Interestingly, however, when increasing quantities of PG are combined with equimolar amounts of the major glycolipids of the *A. laidlawii* B membrane, the added phospholipid actually stimulates ATPase activity up to 15 to 20 mol% and does not begin to inhibit ATP hydrolysis until levels of 35 to 40 mol% are reached. It is noteworthy, however, that even in the complete absence of anionic phospholipids, these neutral glycolipids support a relatively high enzyme activity. This latter finding is surprising in view of the study of Bevers et al. (6) discussed earlier, which seemed to show an absolute requirement for small amounts (about 10 mol%) of PG for optimal Mg^{2+}-ATPase activity in *A. laidlawii* B membranes.

George et al. (33) reconstituted the purified $(Na^+ + Mg^{2+})$-ATPase from *A. laidlawii* B plasma membranes with synthetic phospholipids and used DSC to examine the lipid thermotropic phase behavior of the proteoliposomes formed. The effect of this ATPase on the host lipid phase transition is markedly dependent on the amount of protein incorporated. At low protein/lipid ratios, the presence of increasing quantities of ATPase in the proteoliposomes increases the temperature and enthalpy while decreasing the cooperativity of the phospholipid gel-to-liquid-crystalline phase transition. At higher protein/lipid ratios, the incorporation of increasing amounts of this enzyme does not further alter the temperature and cooperativity of the phospholipid chain-melting transition but progressively and markedly decreases the transition enthalpy. Plots of lipid phase transition enthalpy versus protein concentration suggest that at the higher lipid/protein ratios, each ATPase molecule removes approximately 1,000 dimyristoylphosphatidylcholine molecules from participation in the cooperative gel-to-liquid-crystalline phase transition of the bulk lipid phase. These results indicate that this integral transmembrane protein interacts in a complex, concentration-dependent manner with its host phospholipid and that such interactions involve both hydrophobic interactions with the lipid bilayer core and electrostatic interactions with the lipid polar headgroups at the bilayer surface.

Jinks et al. (42) reported that whole cells of *A. laidlawii* incubated in NaCl- or KCl-containing buffer swell and lyse if deprived of glucose or if treated with several $(Na^+ + Mg^{2+})$-ATPase inhibitors in the presence of glucose. In contrast, cells incubated in $MgSO_4$ buffer or sucrose do not swell or lyse under these same conditions. These and other results led these workers to postulate that this enzyme is intimately involved in regulation of the intracellular osmolarity and cellular volume of this organism, probably by functioning as an ion pump which actively extrudes monovalent cations (probably Na^+) from cells. This hypothesis has recently been confirmed by Mahajan et al. (65, 66), who showed that the purified $(Na^+ + Mg^{2+})$-ATPase catalyzes the ATP-dependent translocation of Na^+ when reconstituted into liposomes. Moreover, the amount of Na^+ transported increases with the concentration of ATP added, and both Na^+ transport and ATPase activity are inhibited to comparable extents by inhibitors of the *A. laidlawii* $(Na^+ + Mg^{2+})$-ATPase such as vanadate and leucinostatin. Although some Na^+/Na^+ exchange is observed in the reconstituted proteoliposomes studied, a net accumulation of Na^+ is observed with a stoichiometry (corrected for leakage and exchange) of about 1 mol of Na$^+$ per mol of ATP hydrolyzed.

Kapitanov et al. (44) claim to have isolated an F$_1$F$_0$-type H$^+$-ATPase from the *A. laidlawii* membrane by extensive sonication followed by chromatography. This "water-soluble" ATPase binds ATP with a K_m of 7.4×10^{-4} M, and ADP acts as a competitive inhibitor. The enzyme was reported to be cold labile but could be stabilized by lecithin, a rather unusual result for a supposedly water-soluble enzyme. In contrast to bacterial F$_1$F$_0$-ATPases, this enzyme was initially reported to be insensitive to inhibition by DCCD up to a concentration of 10^{-4} M. This enzyme was also reported to be inhibited by Na$^+$ and K$^+$, although only relatively high concentrations were tested. No evidence for stimulation by H$^+$ or Ca^{2+} was presented, and no characterization of the nature or assessment of the purity of the isolated enzyme was attempted. Since Rottem and Razin (106) had shown previously that sonication of *A. laidlawii* membranes results in the production of small, nonsedimentable membrane fragments to which the Mg^{2+}-ATPase remains firmly bound, it is unlikely that the enzyme responsible for the ATP hydrolytic activity observed by Kapitanov et al. (44) was actually solubilized. Moreover, since the kinetic, inhibitor, and storage properties of this enzyme are rather similar to those of the (Na$^+$ + Mg^{2+})-ATPase as reported by McElhaney and coworkers (42, 58) and by Chen et al. (7), it seems likely that the activity actually being monitored was due to this enzyme rather than to the F$_1$ portion of an F$_1$F$_0$-type H$^+$-ATPase.

Kapitanov et al. (43) subsequently used a detergent solubilization procedure to supposedly isolate the entire "F$_1$F$_0$-ATPase complex" from *A. laidlawii* membranes. The kinetic constants and inhibitor spectrum of this enzyme were reported to be similar to those of the "water-soluble" ATPase isolated previously. Interestingly, the activity of the purified ATPase could be markedly stimulated by lecithin. Moreover, the F$_1$ portion of this enzyme was reported to consist of five subunits ranging from 64,500 to 17,000 in molecular weight, whereas the F$_0$ portion supposedly consisted of six subunits of higher molecular weight. Again, the addition of Ca^{2+} resulted in a marked inhibition of ATPase activity, and the enzyme was relatively insensitive to DCCD.

It is quite clear from the properties reported that these workers have not isolated an F$_1$F$_0$-type H$^+$-ATPase, for a number of reasons. First, the F$_1$ portion of bacterial H$^+$-ATPases can invariably be removed as a truly water-soluble complex by procedures which liberate peripheral membrane proteins, but this is not true of the *A. laidlawii* ATPase. Second, bacterial F$_1$F$_0$-type H$^+$-ATPases are stimulated by H$^+$ and Ca^{2+} and are completely inhibited by very low concentrations of DCCD, in contrast to the behavior reported for the mycoplasmal enzyme. Third, the F$_1$ portion of bacterial F$_1$F$_0$-ATPases does not require lipid for activity, as the *A. laidlawii* ATPase does. Fourth, the F$_0$ portion of bacterial F$_1$F$_0$-ATPases typically consists of three (or fewer) subunits of relatively low molecular weight, whereas six polypeptides of high molecular weight were assigned to the F$_0$ portion of the *A. laidlawii* ATPase by Kapitanov and coworkers (see Schneider and Altendorf [114] for a review of bacterial F$_1$F$_0$-ATPases). In contrast to the poor correspondence between the

properties of the *A. laidlawii* ATPase and bacterial F$_1$F$_0$-type H$^+$-ATPases, the properties of the former correspond closely to those of the (Na$^+$ + Mg^{2+})-ATPase as reported by McElhaney and coworkers (42, 58) and by Chen et al. (7). Thus, it follows that Kapitanov et al. (43, 44) have actually isolated a slightly impure form of the (Na$^+$ + Mg^{2+})-ATPase and not an F$_1$F$_0$-type H$^+$-ATPase.

The only other evidence for the presence of an F$_1$F$_0$-type H$^+$-ATPase in the *A. laidlawii* membrane is that of Zilberstein et al. (151), who have reported that polyclonal antibodies to the β subunit of the F$_1$ portion of the *E. coli* F$_1$F$_0$-type H$^+$-ATPase cross-react with proteins in isolated membranes from *A. laidlawii* (and a number of other mycoplasma species) having ATP hydrolytic activity. However, immunological cross-reactivity is a weak and unreliable criterion for typing bacterial ATPases. For example, antibodies to the *E. coli* β subunit also react with the β subunit of the (Na$^+$ + Mg^{2+})-ATPase, despite the fact that the amino acid sequences at the N-terminal regions of these two subunits indicate that they are not closely related (149a). This does not mean that an F$_1$F$_0$-type H$^+$-ATPase might not exist in the membrane of *A. laidlawii* and fulfill a key role in cellular bioenergetics and transport, only that there is presently no creditable evidence for its existence.

As mentioned earlier, an Mg^{2+}-dependent ATPase activity has been detected in the membrane of every *Acholeplasma*, *Mycoplasma*, *Spiroplasma*, and *Ureaplasma* species studied to date (85), and in several species it has been established that this ATPase plays a key role in cell volume regulation (see preceding sections). Although it has often been postulated that these Mg^{2+}-ATPases function as electrogenic proton pumps, a direct demonstration that any mycoplasma Mg^{2+}-ATPase can catalyze the vectorial translocation of protons requires that the ATPase in question be purified to homogeneity and reconstituted into lipid vesicles. The only mycoplasmal ATPase for which this has been accomplished thus far is the (Na$^+$ + Mg^{2+})-ATPase of *A. laidlawii*, which functions in vitro and probably also in vivo as an ATP-requiring Na$^+$ pump rather than as a proton-translocating ATPase (see above). Although the generation of a transmembrane electrochemical potential can often be inhibited in vivo in several mycoplasma species by inhibitors of the Mg^{2+}-ATPases such as sulfhydryl reagents and DCCD, it should be noted that these reagents are not specific for proton-translocating ATPases at the concentrations used and that inhibition of ATPases which translocate other ions can lead indirectly to a dissipation of the transmembrane electrochemical gradient in any case. Therefore, although there is circumstantial evidence for the presence of H$^+$-ATPases in a few mycoplasma species, an unequivocal demonstration of their existence remains for future work.

It is clear, however, that the mycoplasma Mg^{2+}-ATPases studied to date are generally different both structurally and functionally from most bacterial H$^+$-ATPases (14). Eubacterial ATPases typically consist of two portions, the BF$_1$ portion containing the ATP hydrolytic site and the BF$_0$ portion containing the proton channel. The BF$_1$ portion, which is usually made up of five subunits, can be readily detached from the bacterial membrane by washing in low-ionic-strength buffers and does not usually require lipid for activity. In contrast, the BF_0 portion, which also consists of three or more subunits, behaves as an integral membrane protein. Another characteristic of BF_1F_0-type H^+-ATPases is their stimulation by Ca^{2+} but relative insensitivity to Na^+ and K^+ and their inhibition by very low levels of DCCD. The mycoplasma Mg^{2+}-ATPases, on the other hand, cannot be dissociated into two portions, and the entire ATPase complex behaves like an integral membrane protein. As well, most mycoplasma Mg^{2+}-ATPases are not stimulated by Ca^{2+} but may be stimulated by Na^+ or K^+ and are inhibited by DCCD only at relatively high concentrations. Moreover, several of the mycoplasma Mg^{2+}-ATPases are sensitive to the fluidity and phase state of their membrane lipid environment, in contrast to most of the BF_1F_0-ATPases studied to date. Until the amino acid sequences and detailed topological arrangement of the mycoplasma Mg^{2+}-ATPases in their native membranes are determined, the molecular basis for these structural and functional differences between the mycoplasmal and bacterial ATPase will remain obscure.

The purification and characterization of the membranous $Na^+ + Mg^{2+}$-ATPase from *A. laidlawii*, and its dependence on the physical properties of its lipid environment, have been discussed in detail earlier. Here I briefly summarize the properties of some other mycoplasma Mg^{2+}-ATPases in their native membranes and speculate on their functions in the mycoplasma species in which they are found.

Benyoucef et al. (5) have studied the properties of the Mg^{2+}-ATPase from *M. mycoides* subsp. *capri* membranes and attempted to relate them to the H^+, K^+, and Na^+ transport systems operating in this organism. This ATPase was found to be stimulated up to two-fold by Na^+, but only at relatively high concentrations; the maximal Na^+ stimulation of ATP hydrolytic activity is observed at about 100 mM and the K_m for Na^+ stimulation is about 30 mM. Other monovalent cations, such as K^+, Li^+, and Rb^+, are without effect even at a concentration of 100 mM, and K^+ does not affect Na^+ stimulation. Ouabain and vanadate, potent inhibitors of eucaryotic $(Na^+ + K^+)$-ATPases, do not affect ATPase activity, either in the presence or in the absence of Na^+. On the other hand, DCCD and nitrobenzoxadiazole, which are inhibitors of H^+-ATPases in bacteria, do significantly inhibit ATP hydrolytic activity, but inhibition is only partial even at relatively high concentrations of inhibitor; both the basal and Na^+-stimulated activities are inhibited to comparable extents by these compounds. Since these results are quite similar to those reported earlier for the $(Na^+ + Mg^{2+})$-ATPase of *A. laidlawii* (42, 58), except for the greater stimulation observed at a much lower concentration of Na^+ in the latter enzyme, these workers tentatively concluded that the *M. mycoides* enzyme was most likely an Na^+-transporting ATPase. However, Benyoucef et al. (5) were unable to rationalize this conclusion with their studies of cation movements in *M. mycoides* subsp. *capri*, which suggested the presence of both an ATP-consuming Na^+/K^+ exchange and an Na^+/H^+ antiport system in this organism. One possible explanation for this apparent discrepancy might be that during cell lysis and the preparation of membranes, a protein component of this enzyme responsible for the Na^+/K^+ exchange activity was lost or that

the relative affinities of this enzyme for monovalent cations were altered. However, since monovalent cations at relatively high concentrations can stimulate some bacterial H^+-ATPases by 20 to 100%, it is also possible that these workers were in fact observing primarily the ATP hydrolytic activity of the proton-extruding ATPase, which they also postulated to be present in the membrane of this organism. Additional experimental work is clearly required to resolve this uncertainty.

There have been two studies of the membrane-bound ATPase activity of *M. gallisepticum* which have reached somewhat dissimilar conclusions. Linker and Wilson (62) found that the major ATPase of isolated membranes exhibits a pH optimum of 7.0 to 7.5 and requires Mg^{2+} for maximal activity, Ca^{2+} being rather ineffective. All monovalent cations tested show a slight stimulation of activity at lower concentrations only, which was ascribed to nonspecific salt effects. Ouabain, an inhibitor of eucaryotic $(Na^+ + K^+)$-ATPases, is without effect, while vanadate, an inhibitor of ATPases that involve a phosphorylated intermediate but not of bacterial H^+-ATPases, inhibits about 60% of the ATPase activity. On the other hand, DCCD, the classical inhibitor of bacterial H^+-ATPases, inhibits the *M. gallisepticum* membrane ATPase in a biphasic fashion, producing 50% inhibition at a concentration of about 20 μM and 90% inhibition at a concentration of 100 μM. It was also found that the DCCD-insensitive ATPase activity is not stimulated by Na^+ or K^+. This enzyme is also markedly inhibited by mercurial compounds and by diethylstilbestrol but is relatively insensitive to azide, CCCP, oligomycin, and efrapeptin. Although the properties of this enzyme are not completely consistent with those of any other known class of ATPases, these authors postulated that this enzyme most likely functions in vivo as an ATP-requiring electrogenic proton pump.

Shirvan et al. (126) subsequently reported that the ATPase activity of *M. gallisepticum* membranes is Mg^{2+} dependent over the entire pH range tested (5.5 to 9.5). Na^+ (>10 mM) causes a threefold increase in the ATPase activity at pH 8.5 but has only a small effect at pH 5.5. In an Na^+-free medium, the enzyme exhibits a pH optimum of 7.0 to 7.5, with a specific activity of 30 ± 5 μmol of phosphate released per h per mg of membrane protein. In the presence of Na^+, the optimum pH is between 8.5 and 9.0, with a specific activity of 52 ± 6 μmol. The Na^+-stimulated ATPase activity at pH 8.5 is much more stable to prolonged storage than is the Na^+-independent activity. At pH 7.5, ATP hydrolysis is strongly inhibited by DCCD, diethylstilbestrol, and quercetin, moderately inhibited by azide and vanadate, but not inhibited by oligomycin, ouabain, or N-ethylmaleimide. The pH profile and the inhibition pattern suggest the presence of two distinct ATPases. Further evidence that two distinct ATPases exist was obtained by showing that *M. gallisepticum* membranes possess a protein of molecular weight 52,000 that reacts with antibodies raised against the β subunit of *E. coli* F_1F_0-ATPase as well as a protein of molecular weight 68,000 that reacts with the anti-yeast plasma membrane ATPase antibodies. Shirvan et al. postulated that the Na^+-stimulated ATPase functions as the electrogenic Na^+ pump and that the Na^+-nonstimulated ATPase is an H^+-ATPase. This is a reasonable suggestion but one that must be confirmed by additional experiments.

Romano et al. (98) investigated the properties of the membrane-bound ATPase of *Ureaplasma urealyticum*. Like the other mycoplasmal ATPases, this enzyme behaves as an integral membrane protein which cannot be detached from the membrane by EDTA-containing, low-ionic-strength buffers. The ATP hydrolytic activity of this enzyme in its native membrane exhibits a progressive increase with increases of temperature up to at least 40°C and a broad pH optimum ranging from 6.8 to 8.4. This ATPase requires Mg^{2+} for optimal activity, with the amount of Mg^{2+} required being dependent on the ATP concentrations used; the highest enzyme activity is observed at an Mg^{2+}/ATP ratio of 1. Mn^{2+} and Co^{2+} can replace Mg^{2+} to some extent, but Ca^{2+} is rather ineffective in this regard. Interestingly, the *U. urealyticum* ATPase is stimulated 3- to 4-fold by Na^{2+} and 2.5- to 3.0-fold by Li^+ but not by H^+, K^+, and NH_4^+. Although activity is highest with ATP, other nucleotide triphosphates exhibit substantial activity, and even ADP is hydrolyzed at 40% of the rate for ATP. Among the various inhibitors tested, DCCD inhibits ATP hydrolytic activity by 50% at 10^{-4} M and 90% at 10^{-3} M, concentrations much higher than those required to inhibit most bacterial H^+-ATPases, and several sulfhydryl-blocking reagents also were found to be potent inhibitors. In contrast, ouabain and oligomycin do not inhibit this enzyme, but quercetin and nitrobenzoxadiazole, inhibitors of F_1F_0-ATPases in bacteria, are potent inhibitors. Although these authors did not speculate on the function of this ATPase in vivo, it is noteworthy that its properties are generally rather similar to those of the $(Na^+ + Mg^{2+})$-ATPases of *A. laidlawii* and *M. gallisepticum*, which appear to function as electrogenic Na^+ pumps.

Most mycoplasma membranes also contain a firmly bound *p*-nitrophenylphosphatase activity (87). The weight of evidence now strongly suggests that the ATPase and *p*-nitrophenylphosphatase activities reside on two different proteins, at least in *A. laidlawii*, since these two activities differ in their sensitivities to detergents, organic solvents, and pronase treatment (78, 79) and in their sensitivities to DCCD (42). Moreover, the *p*-nitrophenylphosphatase activity does not depend on the physical state of the membrane lipids (24) or on the presence of intact PG in the membrane (6), in contrast to the behavior of the $(Na^+ + Mg^{2+})$-ATPase of this organism. Finally, the purified $(Na^+ + Mg^{2+})$-ATPase of *A. laidlawii* does not exhibit *p*-nitrophenylphosphatase activity (58). The insensitivity of the *p*-nitrophenylphosphatase of *U. urealyticum* to DCCD concentrations which almost completely inhibit ATPase activity also suggests that these two enzyme activities arise from two different proteins in this organism (96).

Other Hydrolytic Enzymes

The membranes of *A. laidlawii* and some other mycoplasma species contain a number of hydrolytic enzymes. These include phosphatases acting on nucleotides other than ATP (106), RNase and DNase (79, 84), peptidases (10, 82), a sterol esterase (133), and a lysophospholipase (146, 148). The function of these enzymes, most of which are expressed on the outer surface of the plasma membrane, is probably to degrade macromolecules present in the growth medium or host organism into smaller components which can then be taken up, either actively or passively, and utilized in various biosynthetic pathways. For example, the action of the nucleases present on the surface of *A. laidlawii* allows these cells to utilize RNA and DNA as the source of the purine and pyrimidine bases that it requires for nucleic acid biosynthesis and growth (89). However, since these hydrolytic enzymes have not been isolated and purified and are generally poorly characterized, they will not be discussed further.

Lipid Biosynthetic Enzymes

The enzymes responsible for de novo fatty acid biosynthesis in *A. laidlawii* (87, 136) and for the activation of endogenous free fatty acids by their conversion to their coenzyme A (CoA) derivatives in *A. laidlawii* and *M. hominis* (103) are localized in the cytoplasmic fraction of these organisms. However, the enzymes responsible for the biosynthesis of the phospholipids and glucolipids, and of the carotenoids pigments of *Acholeplasma* species, are membrane associated (87, 136). A thioesterase acting specifically on long-chain fatty acyl-CoA thiol esters has been detected in the membranes of several mycoplasmas (109). Since its activity is much higher in *Acholeplasma* than in *Mycoplasma* species, the enzyme has been postulated to have a regulatory role in fatty acid biosynthesis.

Rottem et al. (109) studied the temperature dependence of this membrane-associated long-chain fatty acyl-CoA thioesterase activity in *A. laidlawii* PG8 that had been grown in the presence of palmitic, elaidic, or oleic acid. The absolute activity of this enzyme was found to be quite similar in all isolated membranes studied, regardless of their membrane lipid fatty acid compositions. However, Arrhenius plots of thioesterase activity in elaidic acid- and palmitic acid-enriched membranes exhibit slight breaks in slope at temperatures of about 12 and 18°C, respectively, while in oleic acid-enriched membranes, the Arrhenius plot is linear over the entire temperature range of 5 to 40°C. The lipid phase transition temperatures of these membranes were reported to be 26 and 35°C for elaidate- and palmitate-enriched membranes, respectively, as determined by ESR spectroscopy using an intercalated 12-nitroxide stearic acid, and no phase transition could be detected in oleate-enriched membranes. These ESR spectroscopy-determined phase transition temperatures are reasonably close to the phase transition midpoint temperatures determined by DSC, differential thermal analysis, and X-ray techniques in studies reviewed in chapter 8. These workers concluded that either this enzyme is preferentially associated with the lowest-melting-point lipid species or the low-temperature-induced conversion of the membrane lipid from the liquid-crystalline to the gel state reduces the solubility of the palmitoyl-CoA substrate in the lipid bilayer, thereby reducing enzyme activity. Since the thioesterase activity break temperatures, as determined from the Arrhenius plots, lie near the lower boundary of the lipid phase transition as determined by other techniques, these suggestions seem reasonable. Unlike the *A. laidlawii* (Na$^+$ + Mg^{2+})-ATPase, however, the thioesterase retains a fairly high level of activity even at temperatures well below the lower boundary of the membrane lipid phase transition.

CONCLUSION

As discussed in the introduction, our understanding of the relationship between membrane lipid fluidity and phase state and cell growth, passive permeability, and activity of the (Na$^+$ + Mg^{2+})-ATPase of *A. laidlawii* is well advanced. Nevertheless, even in these areas, important questions remain. For example, the molecular basis (or bases) for the inhibition of growth and ATPase activity by both gel and hyperfluid lipid remains to be determined, as does the apparent dependence of this ATPase on the lipid polar headgroup and surface charge of the lipid bilayer. The question of whether nonbilayer-forming lipids play important roles in the function of this and other membrane proteins is also an open one. The mechanisms by which ions are transported in *A. laidlawii* and in many *Mycoplasma* species remain to be completely elucidated. As well, the exact mechanism (or mechanisms) by which the transmembrane electrochemical potential is established and coupled to active transport systems is not firmly established for any mycoplasma species, and in most cases the actual physiological role of the various membranous ATPases present remains unclear. Finally, many more membrane-bound enzymes and transport proteins need to be isolated, purified, characterized, and sequenced so that their function, disposition in the membrane, and evolutionary relationship to other bacterial membrane proteins can be established. In principle, the genetic and morphological simplicity of mycoplasmas, and the ease of isolation of their plasma membranes, should make these organisms excellent candidates for studies of the structure and function of membrane proteins. The factor currently limiting our progress appears to be the relatively small number of investigators working in this important research area.

Acknowledgments. The work described in this review that emanated from my laboratory was supported by operating and major equipment grants from the Medical Research Council of Canada and by major equipment and personnel support grants from the Alberta Heritage Foundation for Medical Research.

REFERENCES

1. **Baldassare, J. J., K. B. Rhinehart, and D. F. Silbert.** 1976. Modification of membrane lipid: physical properties in relation to fatty acid structure. *Biochemistry* **15:**2986–2994.
2. **Benyoucef, M., J.-L. Rigaud, and G. Leblanc.** 1981. The electrochemical proton gradient in *Mycoplasma* cells. *Eur. J. Biochem.* **113:**491–498.
3. **Benyoucef, M., J.-L. Rigaud, and G. Leblanc.** 1981. Gradation of the magnitude of the electrochemical proton gradient in *Mycoplasma* cells. *Eur. J. Biochem.* **113:**499–506.
4. **Benyoucef, M., J.-L. Rigaud, and G. Leblanc.** 1982. Cation transport mechanisms in *Mycoplasma mycoides* var. *capri* cells. Na$^+$-dependent K$^+$ accumulation. *Biochem. J.* **208:**529–538.
5. **Benyoucef, M., J.-L. Rigaud, and G. Leblanc.** 1982. Cation transport mechanisms in *Mycoplasma mycoides* var. *capri* cells. The nature of the link between K$^+$ and Na$^+$ transport. *Biochem. J.* **208:**539–547.
6. **Bevers, E. M., G. T. Snoek, J. A. F. Op den Kamp, and L. L. M. van Deenen.** 1977. Phospholipid requirement of the membrane-bound Mg^{2+}-dependent adenosine triphosphatase in *Acholeplasma laidlawii. Biochim. Biophys. Acta* **467:**346–356.
7. **Chen, J.-W., Q. Sun, and F. Hwang.** 1984. Properties of the membrane-bound Mg^{2+}-ATPase isolated from *Acholeplasma laidlawii. Biochim. Biophys. Acta* **777:**151–154.
8. **Cho, H. W., and H. J. Morowitz.** 1969. Characterization of the plasma membrane of *Mycoplasma laidlawii.* VI. Potassium transport. *Biochim. Biophys. Acta* **183:**295–303.
9. **Cho, H. W., and H. J. Morowitz.** 1972. Characterization of the plasma membrane of *Mycoplasma laidlawii.* VIII. Effect of temperature shift and antimetabolites on K$^+$ transport. *Biochim. Biophys. Acta* **274:**105–110.
10. **Choules, G. L., and W. R. Gray.** 1971. Peptidase activity in the membranes of *Mycoplasma laidlawii. Biochem. Biophys. Res. Commun.* **45:**849–855.
11. **Cirillo, V. P.** 1979. Transport systems, p. 323–349. *In* M. F. Barile and S. Razin (ed.), *The Mycoplasmas*, vol. 1. Academic Press, New York.
12. **Cirillo, V. P., and S. Razin.** 1973. Distribution of a phosphoenolpyruvate-dependent sugar phosphotransferase system in mycoplasmas. *J. Bacteriol.* **113:**212–217.
13. **Clementz, T., A. Christiansson, and Å. Wieslander.** 1986. Transmembrane electrical potential affects the lipid composition of *Acholeplasma laidlawii. Biochemistry* **25:**823–830.
14. **Clementz, T., A. Christiansson, and Å. Wieslander.** 1987. Membrane potential, lipid regulation and adenylate energy charge in acyl chain modified *Acholeplasma laidlawii. Biochim. Biophys. Acta* **898:**299–307.
15. **Dahl, C., and J. S. Dahl.** 1988. Cholesterol and cell function, p. 147–171. *In* P. L. Yeagle (ed.), *Biology of Cholesterol.* CRC Press, Boca Raton, Fla.
16. **Dahl, C. E., J. S. Dahl, and K. Bloch.** 1980. Effect of alkyl-substituted precursors of cholesterol on artificial and natural membranes and on the viability of *Mycoplasma capricolum. Biochemistry* **19:**1462–1467.
17. **Dahl, C. E., J. S. Dahl, and K. Bloch.** 1983. Proteolipid formation in *Mycoplasma capricolum. J. Biol. Chem.* **258:**11814–11818.
18. **Dahl, J. S., and C. E. Dahl.** 1983. Coordinate regulation of unsaturated phospholipid, RNA, and protein synthesis in *Mycoplasma capricolum* by cholesterol. *Proc. Natl. Acad. Sci. USA* **80:**692–696.
19. **Dahl, J. S., and C. E. Dahl.** 1984. Effect of cholesterol on phospholipid, RNA, and protein synthesis in *Mycoplasma capricolum. Isr. J. Med. Sci.* **20:**807–811.
20. **Dahl, J. S., C. E. Dahl, and K. Bloch.** 1980. Sterols in membranes: growth characteristics and membrane properties of *Mycoplasma capricolum* cultured on cholesterol and lanosterol. *Biochemistry* **19:**1467–1472.
21. **de Gier, J., J. G. Mandersloot, J. V. Hupkes, R. N. McElhaney, and W. P. van Beck.** 1971. On the mechanism of non-electrolyte permeation through lipid bilayers and through biomembranes. *Biochim. Biophys. Acta* **233:**610–618.
22. **de Kruyff, B., W. J. de Greef, R. V. W. van Eyk, R. A. Demel, and L. L. M. van Deenen.** 1973. The effect of different fatty acid and sterol composition on the erythritol flux through the cell membrane of *Acholeplasma laidlawii. Biochim. Biophys. Acta* **298:**479–499.
23. **de Kruyff, B., R. A. Demel, and L. L. M. van Deenen.** 1972. The effect of cholesterol and epicholesterol incor-

poration on the permeability and on the phase transition of intact *Acholeplasma laidlawii* cell membranes and derived liposomes. *Biochim. Biophys. Acta* **255**:331–347.

24. **de Kruyff, B., P. W. M. van Dijck, R. W. Goldback, R. A. Demel, and L. L. M. van Deenen.** 1973. Influence of fatty acid and sterol composition on the lipid phase transition and activity of membrane-bound enzymes in *Acholeplasma laidlawii. Biochim. Biophys. Acta* **330**:269–282.

25. **Demel, R. A., and B. de Kruyff.** 1976. The function of sterols in membranes. *Biochim. Biophys. Acta* **457**:109–132.

26. **Fedotov, N. S., L. F. Panchenko, A. P. Logachev, A. G. Bekkouzhin, and M. A. Tarshis.** 1975. Transport properties of membrane vesicles from *Acholeplasma laidlawii.* I. Isolation and general characteristics. *Folia Microbiol.* (Prague) **20**:470–479.

27. **Fedotov, N. S., L. F. Panchenko, and M. A. Tarshis.** 1975. Transport properties of membrane vesicles from *Acholeplasma laidlawii.* III. Evidence of active nature of glucose transport. *Folia Microbiol.* (Prague) **20**:488–495.

28. **Freeman, B. A., R. Sissenstein, T. T. McManus, J. E. Woodward, I. M. Lee, and J. B. Mudd.** 1976. Lipid composition and lipid metabolism of *Spiroplasma citri. J. Bacteriol.* **125**:946–954.

29. **George, R., R. N. A. H. Lewis, S. Mahajan, and R. N. McElhaney.** 1989. Studies on the purified, lipid-reconstituted (Na$^+$ + Mg^{2+})-ATPase from *Acholeplasma laidlawii* B membranes: dependence of enzyme activity on lipid headgroup and hydrocarbon chain structure. *J. Biol. Chem.* **264**:11598–11604.

30. **George, R., R. N. A. H. Lewis, and R. N. McElhaney.** 1985. Reconstitution and photolabeling of the purified (Na$^+$ + Mg^{2+})-ATPase from the plasma membrane of *Acholeplasma laidlawii* B with phospholipids containing a photosensitive fatty acyl group. *Biochim. Biophys. Acta* **821**:253–258.

31. **George, R., R. N. A. H. Lewis, and R. N. McElhaney.** 1987. Reconstitution of the purified (Na$^+$ + Mg^{2+})-ATPase from *Acholeplasma laidlawii* B membranes into lipid vesicles and a characterization of the resulting proteoliposomes. *Biochim. Biophys. Acta* **903**:282–291.

32. **George, R., R. N. A. H. Lewis, and R. N. McElhaney.** 1987. Lipid modulation of the activity and temperature dependence of the purified (Na$^+$ + Mg^{2+})-ATPase from *Acholeplasma laidlawii* B membranes. *Isr. J. Med. Sci.* **23**:374–379.

33. **George, R., R. N. A. H. Lewis, and R. N. McElhaney.** 1990. Studies on the purified (Na$^+$ + Mg^{2+})-ATPase from *Acholeplasma laidlawii* B membranes. A differential scanning calorimetric study of the ATPase-dimyristoylphosphatidylcholine interactions. *Biochem. Cell Biol.* **68**:161–168.

34. **George, R., and R. N. McElhaney.** 1985. Affinity labeling of the (Na$^+$ + Mg^{2+})-ATPase from *Acholeplasma laidlawii* B membranes by the 2',3'-dialdehyde derivative of adenosine 5'-triphosphate. *Biochim. Biophys. Acta* **813**:161–166.

35. **Hsung, J.-C., L. Huang, D. J. Hoy, and A. Haug.** 1974. Lipid and temperature dependence of membrane-bound ATPase activity of *Acholeplasma laidlawii. Can. J. Biochem.* **52**:974–980.

36. **Huang, L., and A. Haug.** 1974. Regulation of membrane fluidity in *Acholeplasma laidlawii*: effect of carotenoid pigment content. *Biochim. Biophys. Acta* **352**:361–370.

37. **Jaffor Ullah, A. H., and V. P. Cirillo.** 1976. Mycoplasma phosphoenolpyruvate-dependent sugar phosphotransferase system: purification and characterization of the phosphocarrier protein. *J. Bacteriol.* **127**:1298–1306.

38. **Jaffor Ullah, A. H., and V. P. Cirillo.** 1977. Mycoplasma phosphoenolpyruvate-dependent sugar phosphotransferase system: purification and characterization of enzyme I. *J. Bacteriol.* **131**:988–996.

39. **Jinks, D. C., and L. L. Matz.** 1976. The reduced nicotinamide adenine dinucleotide "oxidase" of *Acholeplasma laidlawii* membranes. *Biochim. Biophys. Acta* **430**:71–82.

40. **Jinks, D. C., and L. L. Matz.** 1976. Purification of the reduced nicotinamide adenine dinucleotide dehydrogenase from membranes of *Acholeplasma laidlawii. Biochim. Biophys. Acta* **452**:30–41.

41. **Jinks, D. C., and R. N. McElhaney.** 1987. Method for exchange of the lipid environment of the membrane-bound (Na$^+$ + Mg^{2+})-ATPase of *Acholeplasma laidlawii* B. *Anal. Biochem.* **164**:331–335.

42. **Jinks, D. C., J. R. Silvius, and R. N. McElhaney.** 1978. Physiological role and membrane lipid modulation of the membrane-bound (Na$^+$ + Mg^{2+}) adenosine triphosphatase activity in *Acholeplasma laidlawii. J. Bacteriol.* **136**:1027–1036.

43. **Kapitanov, A. B., V. F. Ivonova, N. A. Belyaev, and M. Gunert.** 1982. Proteins of bacterial membranes. H$^+$-adenosine triphosphatase from *Acholeplasma laidlawii* cells. *Biokhimiya* **47**:575–581.

44. **Kapitanov, A. B., V. P. Noskova, and V. F. Ivanova.** 1980. Proteins of bacterial membranes. Purification of water-soluble ATPase from *Acholeplasma laidlawii. Biokhimiya* **45**:124–129.

45. **Konings, W. N., B. Poolman, and A. J. M. Driessen.** 1989. Bioenergetics and solute transport in *Lactococci. Crit. Rev. Microbiol.* **16**:419–476.

46. **Kundig, W., S. Ghosh, and S. Roseman.** 1964. Phosphate bound to histidine in a protein as an intermediate in a novel phosphotransferase system. *Proc. Natl. Acad. Sci. USA* **52**:1067–1074.

47. **Ladygina, V. G., V. L. Migoushina, T. P. Abaeva, A. P. Logatchev, and M. A. Tarshis.** 1977. Biochemical properties of mutants of *Acholeplasma laidlawii. Biokhimiya* **42**:151–158.

48. **Lala, A. K., T. M. Buttke, and K. Bloch.** 1979. On the role of the sterol hydroxyl group in membranes. *J. Biol. Chem.* **254**:10582–10585.

49. **Larraga, V., and S. Razin.** 1976. Reduced nicotinamide adenine dinucleotide oxidase activity in membranes and cytoplasm of *Acholeplasma laidlawii* and *Mycoplasma mycoides* subsp. *capri. J. Bacteriol.* **128**:827–833.

50. **Leblanc, G., and C. Le Grimellec.** 1979. Active K$^+$ transport in *Mycoplasma mycoides* var. *capri.* Net and unidirectional K$^+$ movements. *Biochim. Biophys. Acta* **554**:156–167.

51. **Leblanc, G., and C. Le Grimellec.** 1979. Active K$^+$ transport in *Mycoplasma mycoides* var. *capri.* Relationships between K$^+$ distribution, electrical potential and ATPase activity. *Biochim. Biophys. Acta* **554**:168–179.

52. **Le Grimellec, C., J. Cardinal, M.-C. Giocondi, and S. Carriere.** 1981. Control of membrane lipids in *Mycoplasma gallisepticum*: effect on lipid order. *J. Bacteriol.* **146**:155–162.

53. **Le Grimellec, C., and G. Leblanc.** 1978. Effect of membrane cholesterol on potassium transport in *Mycoplasma mycoides* var. *capri* (PG 3). *Biochim. Biophys. Acta* **514**:152–163.

54. **Le Grimellec, C., and G. Leblanc.** 1980. Temperature-dependent relationship between K$^+$ influx, Mg^{2+}-ATPase activity, transmembrane potential and membrane lipid composition in mycoplasma. *Biochim. Biophys. Acta* **599**:639–651.

55. **Lelong, I., B. Luu, M. Mersel, and S. Rottem.** 1988. Effect of 7β-hydroxycholesterol on growth and membrane composition of *Mycoplasma capricolum. FEBS Lett.* **232**:354–358.

56. **Lelong, I., M. H. Shirvan, and S. Rottem.** 1989. A cation/proton antiport activity in *Acholeplasma laidlawii. FEMS Microbiol. Lett.* **59**:71–76.

57. **Lewis, R. N. A. H., R. George, and R. N. McElhaney.** 1986. Structure-function investigations of the membrane $(Na^+ + Mg^{2+})$-ATPase from *Acholeplasma laidlawii* B; studies of reactive amino acid residues using group-specific reagents. *Arch. Biochem. Biophys.* **247**:201–210.

58. **Lewis, R. N. A. H., and R. N. McElhaney.** 1983. Purification and characterization of the membrane $(Na^+ + Mg^{2+})$-ATPase from *Acholeplasma laidlawii*. *Biochim. Biophys. Acta* **735**:113–122.

59. **Lieb, W. R., and W. D. Stein.** 1986. Simple diffusion across the membrane bilayer, p. 69–112. *In* W. D. Stein (ed.), *Transport and Diffusion across Cell Membranes.* Academic Press, Orlando Fla.

60. **Linker, C., and T. H. Wilson.** 1985. Cell volume regulation in *Mycoplasma gallisepticum*. *J. Bacteriol.* **163**:1243–1249.

61. **Linker, C., and T. H. Wilson.** 1985. Sodium and proton transport in *Mycoplasma gallisepticum*. *J. Bacteriol.* **163**:1250–1257.

62. **Linker, C., and T. H. Wilson.** 1985. Characterization and solubilization of the membrane-bound ATPase of *Mycoplasma gallisepticum*. *J. Bacteriol.* **163**:1258–1262.

63. **Macdonald, A. G., and A. R. Cossins.** 1983. Effects of pressure and pentanol on the phase transition in the membrane of *Acholeplasma laidlawii* B. *Biochim. Biophys. Acta* **730**:239–244.

64. **MacNaughton, W., and A. G. Macdonald.** 1982. Effects of pressure and pressure antagonists on the growth and membrane-bound ATPase of *Acholeplasma laidlawii* B. *Comp. Biochem. Physiol.* **72A**:405–414.

65. **Mahajan, S., R. N. A. H. Lewis, R. George, B. D. Sykes, and R. N. McElhaney.** 1988. Characterization of sodium transport in *Acholeplasma laidlawii* cells and in lipid vesicles containing purified *A. laidlawii* $(Na^+ + Mg^{2+})$-ATPase by using nuclear magnetic resonance spectroscopy and ^{22}Na tracer techniques. *J. Bacteriol.* **170**:5739–5746.

66. **Mahajan, S., R. N. A. H. Lewis, and R. N. McElhaney.** 1990. ATP-driven sodium transport in proteoliposomes reconstituted with the *Acholeplasma laidlawii* B $(Na^+ + Mg^{2+})$-ATPase. *Zentralbl. Bakteriol. Suppl.* **20**:670–673.

67. **McElhaney, R. N.** 1974. The effect of membrane lipid phase transitions on membrane structure and on the growth of *Acholeplasma laidlawii* B. *J. Supramol. Struct.* **2**:617–628.

68. **McElhaney, R. N.** 1974. The effect of alterations in the physical state of the membrane lipids on the ability of *Acholeplasma laidlawii* B to grow at various temperatures. *J. Mol. Biol.* **84**:145–157.

69. **McElhaney, R. N.** 1975. Membrane lipid, not polarized water, is responsible for the semipermeable properties of living cells. *Biophys. J.* **15**:777–784.

70. **McElhaney, R. N.** 1984. The relationship between membrane lipid fluidity and phase state and the ability of bacteria and mycoplasmas to grow and survive at various temperatures, p. 249–278. *In* M. Kates and L. Masen (ed.), *Biomembranes*, vol. 12. Academic Press, New York.

71. **McElhaney, R. N.** 1984. The structure and function of the *Acholeplasma laidlawii* plasma membrane. *Biochim. Biophys. Acta* **779**:1–42.

72. **McElhaney, R. N.** 1989. The influence of membrane lipid composition and physical properties on membrane structure and function in *Acholeplasma laidlawii*. *Crit. Rev. Microbiol.* **17**:1–32.

73. **McElhaney, R. N., J. de Gier, and L. L. M. van Deenen.** 1970. The effect of alterations in fatty acid composition and cholesterol content on the permeability of *Mycoplasma laidlawii* B cells and derived liposomes. *Biochim. Biophys. Acta* **219**:245–247.

74. **McElhaney, R. N., J. de Gier, and E. C. M. van der Neut-Kok.** 1973. The effect of alterations in fatty acid composition and cholesterol content on the nonelectrolyte permeability of *Acholeplasma laidlawii* B cells and derived liposomes. *Biochim. Biophys. Acta* **298**:500–512.

75. **McElhaney, R. N., and K. A. Souza.** 1976. The relationship between environmental temperature, cell growth, and the fluidity and physical state of the membrane lipids in *Bacillus stearothermophilus*. *Biochim. Biophys. Acta* **443**:348–359.

76. **Mugharbil, U., and V. P. Cirillo.** 1978. Mycoplasma phosphoenolpyruvate-dependent sugar phosphotransferase system: glucose-negative mutant and regulation of intracellular cyclic AMP. *J. Bacteriol.* **133**:203–209.

77. **Ne'eman, Z., I. Kahane, J. Kovartovsky, and S. Razin.** 1972. Characterization of the *Mycoplasma* membrane proteins. III. Gel filtration and immunological characterization of *Acholeplasma laidlawii* membrane proteins. *Biochim. Biophys. Acta* **266**:255–268.

78. **Ne'eman, Z., I. Kahane, and S. Razin.** 1971. Characterization of the *Mycoplasma* membrane proteins. II. Solubilization and enzyme activities of *Acholeplasma laidlawii* membrane proteins. *Biochim. Biophys. Acta* **249**:169–176.

79. **Ne'eman, Z., and S. Razin.** 1975. Characterization of the mycoplasma membrane proteins. V. Release and localization of membrane-bound enzymes in *Acholeplasma laidlawii*. *Biochim. Biophys. Acta* **375**:54–68.

80. **Panchenko, L. F., N. S. Fedotov, and M. A. Tarshis.** 1975. Transport properties of membrane vesicles from *Acholeplasma laidlawii*. II. Kinetic characteristics and specificity of glucose transport system. *Folia Microbiol.* (Prague) **20**:480–487.

81. **Panchenko, L. F., V. L. Migushina, N. S. Fedotov, and M. A. Tarshis.** 1973. Carbohydrate transport in *Mycoplasma laidlawii* cells. *Dokl. Akad. Nauk SSSR* **209**:213–216.

82. **Pecht, M., E. Giberman, A. Keysary, J. Yariv, and E. Katchalski.** 1972. Hydrolysis of alanine oligopeptides by an enzyme located in the membrane of *Mycoplasma laidlawii*. *Biochim. Biophys. Acta* **290**:267–273.

83. **Pollack, J. D.** 1975. Localization of reduced nicotinamide adenine dinucleotide oxidase activity in *Acholeplasma* and *Mycoplasma* species. *Int. J. Syst. Bacteriol.* **25**:108–113.

84. **Pollack, J. D., S. Razin, and R. C. Cleverdon.** 1965. Location of enzymes in *Mycoplasma*. *J. Bacteriol.* **90**:617–622.

85. **Postma, P. W., and J. W. Lengeler.** 1985. Phosphoenolpyruvate: carbohydrate phosphotransferase system of bacteria. *Microbiol. Rev.* **49**:232–269.

86. **Razin, S.** 1979. Membrane proteins, p. 289–322. *In* M. F. Barile and S. Razin (ed.), *The Mycoplasmas*, vol. 1. Academic Press, New York.

87. **Razin, S.** 1982. The mycoplasma membrane, p. 165–250. *In* B. K. Ghosh (ed.), *Organization of Prokaryotic Cell Membranes.* CRC Press, Boca Raton, Fla.

88. **Razin, S., L. Gottfried, and S. Rottem.** 1968. Amino acid transport in *Mycoplasma*. *J. Bacteriol.* **95**:1685–1691.

89. **Razin, S., A. Knyszynski, and Y. Lifshitz.** 1964. Nucleases of mycoplasma. *J. Gen. Microbiol.* **36**:323–332.

90. **Razin, S., and S. Rottem.** 1967. Role of carotenoids and cholesterol in the growth of *Mycoplasma laidlawii*. *J. Bacteriol.* **93**:1181–1182.

91. **Read, B. D., and R. N. McElhaney.** 1975. Glucose transport in *Acholeplasma laidlawii* B: dependence on the fluidity and physical state of the membrane lipids. *J. Bacteriol.* **123**:47–55.

92. **Reinards, R., J. Kubichki, and H.-D. Ohlenbusch.** 1981. Purification and characterization of NADH oxidase from membranes of *Acholeplasma laidlawii*, a copper-containing iron-sulfur flavoprotein. *Eur. J. Biochem.* **120**:329–337.

93. **Rigaud, J.-L., D. Lajeunesse, and C. Le Grimellec.** 1985. Surface potential changes on energization of myco-

plasma cell membranes. *Arch. Biochem. Biophys.* **242:**342–346.

94. **Rilfors, L. G., Wikander, and .Å Wieslander.** 1987. Lipid acyl chain-dependent effects of sterols in *Acholeplasma laidlawii* membranes. *J. Bacteriol.* **169:**830–838.

95. **Rodwell, A.** 1963. The steroid growth requirement of *Mycoplasma mycoides. J. Gen. Microbiol.* **32:**91–101.

96. **Rodwell, A. W., and J. E. Peterson.** 1971. The effect of straight-chain saturated, monoenoic and branched-chain fatty acids on growth and fatty acid composition of *Mycoplasma* strain Y. *J. Gen. Microbiol.* **68:**173–186.

97. **Romano, N., M. H. Shirvan, and S. Rottem.** 1986. Changes in membrane lipid composition of *Mycoplasma capricolum* affect the cell volume. *J. Bacteriol.* **167:**1089–1091.

98. **Romano, N., G. Tolone, and R. LaLicata.** 1982. Adenosine triphosphatase activity of *Ureaplasma urealyticum. Microbiologica* **5:**25–33.

99. **Romijn, J. C., L. M. G. van Golde, R. N. McElhaney, and L. L. M. van Deenen.** 1972. Some studies on the fatty acid composition of total lipids and phosphatidylglycerol from *Mycoplasma laidlawii* B and their relation to the permeability of intact cells of this organism. *Biochim. Biophys. Acta* **280:**22–32.

100. **Rottem, S.** 1979. Molecular organization of membrane lipids, p. 259–288. *In* M. F. Barile and S. Razin (ed.), *The Mycoplasmas*, vol. 1. Academic Press, New York.

101. **Rottem, S.** 1981. Cholesterol is required to prevent crystallization of *Mycoplasma arginini* phospholipids at physiological temperatures. *FEBS Lett.* **133:**161–164.

102. **Rottem, S., V. P. Cirillo, B. de Kruyff, M. Shinitzky, and S. Razin.** 1973. Cholesterol in mycoplasma membranes. Correlation of enzymic and transport activities with physical state of lipids in membranes of *Mycoplasma mycoides* var. *capri* adapted to grow with low cholesterol concentrations. *Biochim. Biophys. Acta* **323:**509–519.

103. **Rottem, S., and A. Greenberg.** 1975. Changes in composition, biosynthesis, and physical state of membrane lipids occurring upon aging of *Mycoplasma hominis* cultures. *J. Bacteriol.* **121:**631–639.

104. **Rottem, S., C. Linker, and T. H. Wilson.** 1981. Proton motive force across the membrane of *Mycoplasma gallisepticum* and its possible role in cell volume regulation. *J. Bacteriol.* **145:**1299–1304.

105. **Rottem, S., E. A. Pfendt, and L. Hayflick.** 1977. Sterol requirements of T-strain mycoplasmas. *J. Bacteriol.* **105:**323–330.

106. **Rottem, S., and S. Razin.** 1966. Adenosine triphosphatase activity of mycoplasma membranes. *J. Bacteriol.* **92:**714–722.

107. **Rottem, S., and S. Razin.** 1967. Uptake and utilization of acetate by mycoplasma. *J. Gen. Microbiol.* **48:**53–63.

108. **Rottem, S., and S. Razin.** 1969. Sugar transport in *Mycoplasma gallisepticum. J. Bacteriol.* **97:**787–792.

109. **Rottem, S., S. L. Trotter, and M. F. Barile.** 1977. Membrane-bound thioesterase activity in mycoplasmas. *J. Bacteriol.* **129:**707–713.

110. **Rottem, S., J. Yashouv, Z. Ne'eman, and S. Razin.** 1973. Composition, ultrastructure and biological properties of membranes from *Mycoplasma mycoides* var. *capri* cells adapted to grow with low cholesterol concentrations. *Biochim. Biophys. Acta* **323:**495–508.

111. **Saier, M. H.** 1977. Bacterial phosphoenolpyruvate: sugar phosphotransferase systems: structural, functional and evolutionary interrelationships. *Bacteriol. Rev.* **41:**856–871.

112. **Schiefer, H. G., and U. Schummer.** 1982. The electrochemical potential across mycoplasma membranes. *Rev. Infect. Dis.* **4:**S65–S70.

113. **Schiefer, H. G., U. Schummer, and U. Gerhardt.** 1979. Effect of cell-membrane active antimicrobial agents on membrane potential and viability of mycoplasma. *Curr. Microbiol.* **3:**85–88.

114. **Schneider, E., and K. Altendorf.** 1987. Bacterial adenosine 5'-triphosphate synthetase (F_1F_0): purification and reconstitution of F_0 complexes and the biochemical and functional characterization of their subunits. *Microbiol. Rev.* **51:**477–497.

115. **Schummer, U., and H. G. Schiefer.** 1980. A novel method for the determination of electrical potentials across cellular membranes. I. Theoretical considerations and mathematical approach. *Biochim. Biophys. Acta* **600:**993–997.

116. **Schummer, U., and H. G. Schiefer.** 1983. Electrophysiology of mycoplasma membranes. *Yale J. Biol. Med.* **56:**413–418.

117. **Schummer, U., and H. G. Schiefer.** 1986. Ion diffusion potentials across mycoplasma membranes determined by a novel method using a carbocyanine dye. *Arch. Biochem. Biophys.* **244:**553–562.

118. **Schummer, U., and H. G. Schiefer.** 1987. Transmembrane proton-motive potential of *Spiroplasma floricola. FEBS Lett.* **224:**79–82.

119. **Schummer, U., and H. G. Schiefer.** 1988. Membrane surface potential of *Spiroplasma floricola. FEBS Lett.* **236:**337–339.

120. **Schummer, U., H. G. Schiefer, and U. Gerhardt.** 1978. Mycoplasma membrane potential determined by a fluorescent probe. *Hoppe-Seyler's Z. Physiol. Chem.* **359:**1023–1025.

121. **Schummer, U., H. G. Schiefer, and U. Gerhardt.** 1979. Mycoplasma membrane potentials determined by potential-sensitive fluorescent dyes. *Curr. Microbiol.* **2:**191–194.

122. **Schummer, U., H.-G. Schiefer, and U. Gerhardt.** 1980. A novel method for the determination of electrical potentials across cellular membranes. II. Membrane potentials of acholeplasmas, mycoplasmas, streptococci and erythrocytes. *Biochim. Biophys. Acta* **600:**998–1106.

123. **Schummer, U., H. G. Schiefer, and U. Gerhardt.** 1981. The proton gradient across mycoplasma membranes. *Curr. Microbiol.* **5:**371–374.

124. **Shechter, E., L. Letellier, and T. Gulik-Krzywicki.** 1974. Relations between structure and function in cytoplasmic membrane vesicles isolated from an *Escherichia coli* fatty acid auxotroph. High-angle X-ray diffraction, freeze-etch microscopy and transport studies. *Eur. J. Biochem.* **49:**61–76.

125. **Shirvan, M. H., S. Schuldiner, and S. Rottem.** 1989. Role of Na$^+$ cycle in cell volume regulation of *Mycoplasma gallisepticum. J. Bacteriol.* **171:**4410–4416.

126. **Shirvan, M. H., S. Schuldiner, and S. Rottem.** 1989. Volume regulation in *Mycoplasma gallisepticum:* evidence that Na$^+$ is extruded via a primary Na$^+$ pump. *J. Bacteriol.* **171:**4417–4424.

127. **Silvius, J. R., D. C. Jinks, and R. N. McElhaney.** 1979. Effect of membrane lipid fluidity and phase state on the kinetic properties of the membrane-bound adenosine triphosphatase of *Acholeplasma laidlawii* B, p. 10–13. *In* D. Schlessinger (ed.), *Microbiology—1979.* American Society for Microbiology, Washington, D.C.

128. **Silvius, J. R., N. Mak, and R. N. McElhaney.** 1980. Why do prokaryotes regulate membrane lipid fluidity?, p. 213–221. *In* M. Kates and A. Kuksis (ed.), *Control of Membrane Fluidity.* Humana Press, Clifton, N.J.

129. **Silvius, J. R., N. Mak, and R. N. McElhaney.** 1980. Lipid and protein composition and thermotropic lipid phase behavior in fatty acid-homogeneous membranes of *Acholeplasma laidlawii* B. *Biochim. Biophys. Acta* **597:**199–215.

130. **Silvius, J. R., and R. N. McElhaney.** 1978. Lipid compositional manipulation in *Acholeplasma laidlawii* B. Effect of exogenous fatty acids on fatty acid composition

and cell growth when endogenous fatty acid production is inhibited. *Can. J. Biochem.* **56:**462–469.

131. **Silvius, J. R., and R. N. McElhaney.** 1980. Membrane lipid physical state and modulation of the (Na$^+$ + Mg^{2+})-ATPase activity in *Acholeplasma laidlawii* B. *Proc. Natl. Acad. Sci. USA* **77:**1255–1259.

132. **Silvius, J. R., B. D. Read, and R. N. McElhaney.** 1978. Membrane enzymes: artifacts in Arrhenius plots due to temperature dependence of substrate-binding affinity. *Science* **199:**902–904.

133. **Smith, P. F.** 1959. Cholesterol esterase activity of pleuropneumonia-like organisms. *J. Bacteriol.* **77:**682–689.

134. **Smith, P. F.** 1963. The carotenoid pigments of mycoplasma. *J. Gen. Microbiol.* **32:**307–319.

135. **Smith, P. F.** 1964. Relation of sterol structure to utilization in pleuropneumonia-like organisms. *J. Lipid Res.* **5:**121–125.

136. **Smith, P. F.** 1979. The composition of membrane lipids and lipopolysaccharides, p. 231–256. *In* M. F. Barile and S. Razin (ed.), *The Mycoplasmas*, vol. 1. Academic Press, New York.

137. **Smith, P. F., and C. U. Henrikson.** 1966. Growth inhibition of mycoplasmas by inhibitors of polyterpene biosynthesis and its reversal by cholesterol. *J. Bacteriol.* **91:**1854–1858.

138. **Steim, J. M., M. E. Tourtellotte, J. C. Reinert, R. N. McElhaney, and R. L. Rader.** 1969. Calorimetric evidence for the liquid-crystalline state of lipids in a biomembrane. *Proc. Natl. Acad. Sci. USA* **63:**104–109.

139. **Tarshis, M. A., A. G. Bekkouzjin, and V. G. Ladygina.** 1976. On the possible role of respiratory activity of *Acholeplasma laidlawii* cells in sugar transport. *Arch. Microbiol.* **109:**295–299.

140. **Tarshis, M. A., A. G. Bekkouzjin, and V. G. Ladygina, and L. F. Panchenko.** 1976. Properties of the 3-O-methyl-D-glucose transport system in *Acholeplasma laidlawii*. *J. Bacteriol.* **125:**1–7.

141. **Tarshis, M. A., N. S. Demikova, and V. L. Migoushina.**

142. **Tarshis, M. A., and A. B. Kapitanov.** 1978. Symport H$^+$/ carbohydrate transport into *Acholeplasma laidlawii* cells. *FEBS Lett.* **89:**73–77.

143. **Tarshis, M. A., V. L. Migoushina, and L. F. Panchenko.** 1973. On the phosphorylation of sugars in *Acholeplasma laidlawii*. *FEBS Lett.* **31:**111–113.

144. **Tarshis, M. A., V. L. Migoushina, L. F. Panchenko, N. S. Fedotov, and H. L. Bourd.** 1973. Studies of sugar transport in *Acholeplasma laidlawii*. *Eur. J. Biochem.* **40:**171–175.

145. **Tarshis, M. A., L. F. Panchenko, V. L. Migushina, and G. I. Bourd.** 1972. Active glucose transport in *Mycoplasma laidlawii*. *Biokhimiya* **37:**930–935.

146. **VanDemark, P. J., and P. Plackett.** 1972. Evidence for a phosphenolpyruvate-dependent sugar phosphotransferase in *Mycoplasma* strain Y. *J. Bacteriol.* **111:**454–458.

147. **van der Neut-Kok, E. C. M., J. De Gier, E. J. Middelbeek, and L. L. M. van Deenen.** 1974. Valinomycin-induced potassium and rubidium permeability of intact cells of *Acholeplasma laidlawii* B. *Biochim. Biophys. Acta* **332:**97–103.

148. **van Golde, L. M. G., R. N. McElhaney, and L. L. M. van Deenen.** 1971. A membrane-bound lysophospholipase from *Mycoplasma laidlawii* strain B. *Biochim. Biophys. Acta* **231:**245–249.

149. **van Zoelen, E. J. J., E. C. M. van der Neut-Kok, J. de Gier, and L. L. M. van Deenen.** 1975. Osmotic behavior of *Acholeplasma laidlawii* B cells with membrane lipids in liquid-crystalline and gel state. *Biochim. Biophys. Acta* **394:**463–469.

149a. **Wieslander, Å.** Personal communication.

150. **Wieslander, Å., and E. Selstam.** 1987. Acyl-chain-dependent incorporation of chlorophyll and cholesterol in membranes of *Acholeplasma laidlawii*. *Biochim. Biophys. Acta* **901:**250–254.

151. **Zilberstein, D., M. H. Shirvan, M. F. Barile, and S. Rottem.** 1986. The β-subunit of the F$_1$F$_0$-ATPase is conserved in mycoplasmas. *J. Biol. Chem.* **261:**7109–7111.

1978. Energetics of the active transport of carbohydrates into mycoplasma cells. *Biokhimiya* **43:**498–503.

16. Motility

HELGA KIRCHHOFF

INTRODUCTION

Motility is widely distributed among procaryotes. Three types of movement have been observed: motility by flagella, motility by axial filaments, and gliding motility (62, 101). The majority of motile procaryotes move by means of flagella. Bacteria with flagella occur in many groups of microorganisms, whereas motility by axial filaments is confined to spirochetes. Gliding motility is found in phototrophic cyanobacteria and related apochlorotic organisms, facultatively phototropic members of the family *Chloroflexaceae*, and myxobacteria (18, 84). Two types of motility have been described for mollicutes: gliding movement on solid surfaces covered with a film of fluid for several mycoplasma species (14, 55, 108), and a rotation about the helix axis and flexing of the cell body in fluid or semisolid medium for the helical spiroplasmas (8, 9).

Mollicutes are the smallest free-living procaryotes. Their genome is only about one-fifth to one-half the size of the *Escherichia coli* genome (82, 83), and it possesses very limited genetic information. There are many essential substances that mycoplasmas are unable to synthesize and must take from the host or the surrounding medium. Thus, it is remarkable that some mycoplasmas are motile, a property that requires a number of genes.

It has now been established that mycoplasmas have close evolutionary ties to the clostridia (120), many of which are also motile. Motility in clostridia is by means of flagella rather than by gliding or rotary and undulating motions, which indicates that the motility in mollicutes is a new development by these organisms. This is a notable achievement for organisms with such a small genome, highlighting the importance that this property must have for the organisms possessing it.

GLIDING MOTILITY

Gliding Mycoplasmas

The first description of gliding motility in mycoplasmas was given by Andrewes and Welch in 1946 (2) for a mycoplasma isolated from mice, later named *Mycoplasma pulmonis*. *M. pulmonis* is known to colonize the respiratory and genital tracts of mice and rats and to produce diseases in these locations. The observations of Andrewes and Welch (2) were confirmed in the 1960s by Nelson (76) and Nelson and Lyons (77). These authors found the movement to be surface dependent and restricted to freshly isolated mycoplasma strains.

Using cinematographic techniques for continuous observations of living mycoplasmas, Bredt (11–14), Bredt et al. (15, 16), and Erdmann (30a) detected gliding movement also for *M. pneumoniae*, the causative agent of human atypical pneumonia, and *M. gallisepticum*, which produces chronic respiratory diseases in poultry, and they presented a characterization of the

Helga Kirchhoff • Institut für Mikrobiologie und Tierseuchen, Tierärztliche Hochschule, D-3000 Hannover, Federal Republic of Germany.

gliding movement of *M. pneumoniae* (15, 16). Gliding movement has also been observed for *M. genitalium* (108) isolated from the human genital tract.

The most interesting organism among the gliding mycoplasmas is *M. mobile* 163K, isolated from the gills of a tench (55, 57), because its motility is much more efficient than that of the other gliding mycoplasmas. In addition, unlike the other gliding mycoplasmas, *M. mobile* glides best at room temperature (21°C), its optimal cultivation temperature, which greatly facilitates observations. Most of our knowledge about the gliding of mycoplasmas was obtained by observing this mycoplasma. Gliding motility has thus been observed in only 5 of the more than 100 mycoplasma and acholeplasma species described so far, i.e., *M. pulmonis*, *M. pneumoniae*, *M. genitalium*, *M. gallisepticum*, and *M. mobile*.

Morphological Characteristics of Gliding Mycoplasmas

Cell morphology

Gliding mycoplasmas differ from most nonmotile species by a special cell morphology exhibited by the majority of the organisms: a flask- or club-shaped cell form with a more or less defined terminal structure. In addition to cells with this typical form, filamentous and rounded cells are found in all gliding mycoplasma species, the number of such cells depending on the culture conditions and the age of the culture (92, 94).

The protruding terminal structure of *M. pulmonis*, which has been called a stalk (2, 77), is most often slightly thickened at the front end and can exceed the diameter of the cell considerably (17). Cells of *M. gallisepticum* have been described as pear shaped with a distinct hemispherical bleb structure on one end (66–68). The typical moving cell of *M. pneumoniae* appears elongated, consisting of a frontal projection (tip structure), a thicker body part, and a longer tail-like rear end (12, 14). Cells of *M. genitalium* are very similar to *M. pneumoniae* cells. They are more or less flask shaped, and their tip structure is often slightly broadened or truncated (115). The terminal structure of *M. mobile* has been called a headlike structure because of its similarity to a head clearly separated by a neck from the other part, the body of the cell. The length of the neck-like region differs among cells. The broadened headlike structure has the form of a rounded cone (55, 92, 94).

There are at least three other mycoplasma species with identical peculiarities: *M. alvi*, isolated from the intestinal and urogenital tracts of cows (42); *M. sualvi*, found in the intestinal and urogenital tracts of swine (43); and *M. pirum*, a tissue culture contaminant (29). These species also have a distinct terminal structure; gliding motility, however, has not been observed.

Ultrastructural peculiarities of gliding mycoplasmas

Electron microscopic studies have revealed that the motile mycoplasmas have two ultrastructural peculiarities which may play a role in motility: a surface layer, or nap, and a cytoskeleton.

A well-demarcated nap, in negatively stained preparations appearing as small peplomerlike particles or aggregations, has been observed on *M. pneumoniae*, *M. genitalium*, and *M. gallisepticum* cells. On *M. pneumoniae* and *M. genitalium* cells the nap is restricted to the terminal region (45, 115), which apparently is not the case with *M. gallisepticum* (66). A naplike outer layer, morphologically similar to the spikes of myxovirus, was observed on *M. pulmonis* cells (47). No surface nap has been defined on the cells of *M. mobile*, which has been investigated extensively (Fig. 1).

Cytoskeletal elements have been reported to be present in *M. pneumoniae*, *M. gallisepticum*, *M. genitalium*, and *M. mobile*. The terminal structures of *M. pneumoniae* (7, 12, 13, 40, 118, 125) and *M. genitalium* (115) contain an electron-dense, rodlike central core surrounded by adjacent electron-translucent material. The core of *M. pneumoniae* shows a distinct periodical striated structure suggesting the existence of substructures (7, 118, 125). In Triton X-100-treated *M. pneumoniae* cells, the core appeared to consist of parallel orientated microfilaments (38, 40). A bleblike structure was detected at the distal end. The proximal end was thickened to a basal node, where other fibers were inserted to form an irregular lattice in the cell body. The bleb of *M. gallisepticum* possesses a cytoskeleton consisting of two plates connected by filaments: a membrane-associated convex plate and an intracytoplasmic flat circular plate separating the bleb region from the so-called infrableb region (68, 72). In ultrathin sectioned cells of *M. mobile*, an electron-dense, membrane-associated inner layer in the area of the headlike structure and filamentous intracytoplasmic material could be demonstrated. In some sections, striated structures with regular periodicity were noticed (89a).

No ultrastructural details have been identified in electron micrographs of *M. pulmonis* cells (14). However, ultrastructural elements also have been observed in nonmotile mycoplasmas such as *M. alvi* (42) as well as in *M. mycoides* subsp. *mycoides*, *M. mycoides* subsp. *capri*, and *M. capri*, which have striated fibers called rho structures (86, 87). An extracellular, ruthenium red-staining surface layer, possibly involved in gliding motility, was demonstrated for *M. pneumoniae* (125), *M. gallisepticum* (107), and *M. mobile* (96).

Since actins or actinlike proteins mediate movement in all eucaryotes, from slime molds to the vertebrates (80), and in addition are highly conservative, it was reasonable to look for them in gliding mycoplasmas. The presence of an actinlike protein in *M. pneumoniae*, similar to rabbit muscle actin (α-actin) in molecular weight, solubility properties, and the ability to form filaments that could complex with heavy meromyosin, was described by Neimark (74, 75). Göbel et al. (40) also obtained evidence for an actinlike nature of the filaments observed by electron microscopy in *M. pneumoniae*, i.e., from their morphological and chemical properties, from their immunological reaction with antiactin antibodies, and from the binding of rhodamine-labeled phalloidin. The connection with myosin subfragments, however, could not be demonstrated. Rodwell et al. (88), on the other hand, could not find α-actin-like proteins in *M. pneumoniae* or several other mycoplasmas by high-resolution two-dimensional gel electrophoresis or by binding to DNase I, which is characteristic for eucaryotic actin. The con-

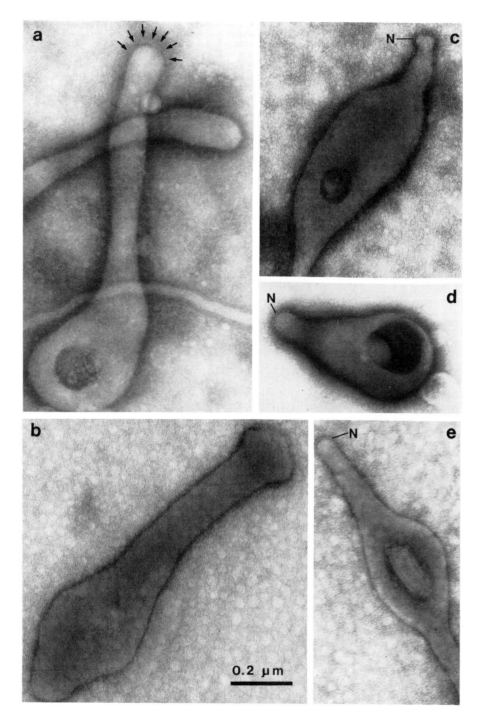

Figure 1. Electron micrographs of motile mycoplasmas, unfixed and negatively or positively stained with 2% ammonium molybdate. (a) *M. pulmonis* PG34. A protruding stalk which is slightly thickened at the front end can be seen; the surface layer is thin and amorphous. (b) *M. mobile* 163K. Note the well-demarcated, conspicuously broadened headlike structure with the form of a rounded cone; a surface layer is lacking. (c) *M. genitalium* G-37. The cell possesses a distinctly broadened and truncated tip, and the prominent terminal outer layer or nap (N) consists of small peplomerlike particles or aggregates. (d) *M. gallisepticum* PG31. Note the distinct bleb structure and the particulate surface nap (N), which apparently is not restricted to the terminal bleb. (e) *M. pneumoniae* FH. Note the distinguishing tapered terminus with its characteristic clearly demarcated particulate exterior nap (N) limited to the terminal tip region. (Courtesy of R. Rosengarten [58]; published with permission.)

troversy concerning the presence of actinlike substances in mycoplasmas is not yet resolved. Even Western immuno-blotting analysis by monoclonal antibodies directed against muscle protein, and investigations with genomic mycoplasma DNA fragments or mRNA by hybridization to an oligodeoxynucleotide probe complementary to the highly conserved phalloidin-binding site of filamentous eucaryotic actin, did not give unequivocal results (39). Thus, the question of whether actinlike proteins play a role in the gliding movement of mycoplasmas is still an open one.

Attachment

The precondition for gliding movement on surfaces is the ability to attach to surfaces. All gliding mycoplasmas are able to attach to glass and plastic material as well as to living cells such as erythrocytes, macrophages, epithelial cells, spermatozoa, and tissue culture cells (24, 33, 41, 49, 102, 109). Attachment, however, is not restricted to motile mycoplasmas, as it has been found in several nonmotile mycoplasmas (116).

Adherence occurs primarily by the terminal structure of the flask-shaped mycoplasmas. In *M. pneumoniae* and *M. genitalium*, the nap seems to play a special role in the attachment process. The nap of *M. pneumoniae* includes a trypsin-sensitive surface protein, designated P1 protein (59, 63), with a molecular mass of 169 kDa. The ability of *M. pneumoniae* to attach to erythrocytes and to glass is inhibited by a monoclonal antibody against the P1 protein (45, 60, 61, 63), providing evidence that the mechanism of attachment to erythrocytes and glass may operate at least in *M. pneumoniae* via identical or similar structures. The P1 protein is concentrated at the tip structure but is also present, although much less densely, on other parts of the membrane (4, 32). Besides the P1 protein, so-called accessory proteins have been found to be involved in the attachment process (6, 37, 50). Although P1 could not be demonstrated in *M. genitalium* and *M. gallisepticum* cells in previous investigations (5), in more recent studies (46) using a broad panel of monoclonal antibodies against the P1 protein, similarities between the P1 protein and a surface-exposed, 140-kDa protein located in the terminal structure of *M. genitalium* were observed. This protein, designated MgPa, is considered to be the counterpart of the P1 protein of *M. pneumoniae*. In the attachment of *M. mobile*, a protein (probably a glycoprotein) with a molecular mass of about 220 kDa seems to play the essential role. This protein was destroyed by concentrations of pronase and trypsin that did not affect the viability of the whole cell. The attachment protein of *M. mobile* seems to be different from the attachment proteins of *M. pneumoniae* and *M. gallisepticum*, since antisera against these two species did not inhibit the adherence of *M. mobile*, whereas a homologous antiserum did, and a monoclonal antibody against the adherence protein of *M. mobile* that prevented adherence of *M. mobile* to erythrocytes as well as to glass and plastic surfaces failed to suppress attachment of *M. pneumoniae* and *M. gallisepticum* to erythrocytes (32a). A detailed characterization of this protein remains to be performed. The attachment protein of *M. mobile* seems to occur on the whole cell surface, since *M. mobile* can attach with almost all parts of the cell (90, 103–105).

A highly variable surface antigen, called V-1 antigen, which showed an unusual multiple banding pattern after electrophoretic separation seems, because of its hydrophobic nature, to play an important role in the adherence of *M. pulmonis* (119).

Physiology of Gliding Motility

Characteristics of gliding motility of mycoplasmas

All of the gliding mycoplasmas are able to glide on glass or plastic material, but gliding occurs only on a solid-liquid interface, i.e., when the mycoplasma cells are in contact with a glass or plastic surface covered with broth medium. During gliding, organisms seem to adhere with all of the body surface that faces the glass or plastic surface. The cells become immotile when they lose surface contact. The only motion evident when cells were in suspension was Brownian movement. The cells do not glide at an air interface, or on bubbles of air, at the bottom of a hanging drop or on dry solid surfaces as observed with *M. mobile* (92). The gliding motility is temperature dependent, being optimal at the optimal cultivation temperatures of the gliding mycoplasmas.

Investigations by both dark-field and differential interference contrast microscopy revealed that *M. mobile* is able to glide on living cells also (34, 56, 95), as shown for bovine and ovine erythrocytes. Organisms coming into contact with erythrocytes enter the cell surface, cross the cells, or glide in irregular circles on the cell surface. Some mycoplasmas circle around the erythrocytes (Fig. 2). The other gliding mycoplasmas presumably are able to glide on cells also, since they can adhere to living cells. However, experimental proof will be difficult because of the much slower movement and the temperature requirements of these mycoplasmas, demanding time-lapse microcinematography and heated observation chambers.

In all gliding mycoplasmas described so far, the tip or headlike structures are always oriented in the direction of movement; the direction is never reversed. An occasional reversion of direction was observed only for filamentous forms of *M. pulmonis* (17, 77). Andrewes and Welch (2) noticed contractile waves along the stalk of moving *M. pulmonis* cells, and Bredt and Radestock (17) described the stalk of round cells and the body of elongated cells of *M. pulmonis* as highly flexible. No contractions or any other changes in cell shape have been described for moving cells of the other gliding mycoplasmas. Reversible changes of cell shape were observed, however, on dividing cells of *M. gallisepticum* (72) and *M. mobile* (94, 96). The ability to change cell shape has also been described for the nonmotile species *M. hominis*, *M. orale*, and *M. mycoides* (14).

The motility of *M. pneumoniae* and *M. mobile* seems to be a stable property. *M. pneumoniae* was cultivated for several hundred passages without impairment of movement (14). No significant changes in motility were observed during the first 150 passages of *M. mobile* on artificial medium. In further passages, the motility became gradually slower and was almost stopped by passage 240, obviously because of the development of a nonmotile mutant (unpublished observations). Electrophoretic analysis of the membranes

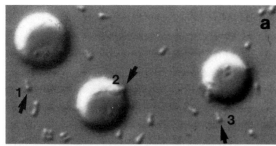

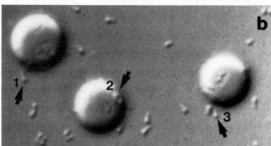

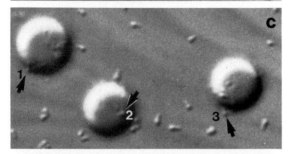

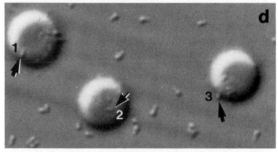

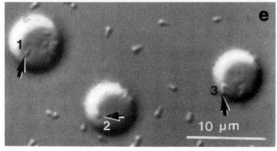

10 µm

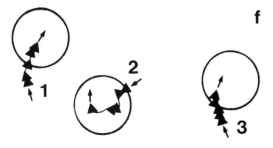

showed differences in the protein patterns between the low and high passages of *M. mobile*. The gliding capacity of *M. mobile* was not influenced by storage for several years at −20°C. In contrast, *M. pulmonis* is able to glide in low passages only (2, 17). Andrewes and Welch (2) were able to revive the loss of motility of *M. pulmonis* for some time by mouse passage, but after more subcultures, the loss of motility could not be prevented even by this method.

Velocity of gliding movement

The velocity achieved by the gliding mycoplasmas is quite variable (14, 55). The average and maximal speeds observed are presented in Table 1. Highest speeds (up to 7.7 µm/s) are reached by *M. mobile*, which is much more efficient than the other gliding mycoplasmas. The gliding velocity of *M. mobile* is 4 to 11 times faster than that of *M. pneumoniae* and *M. pulmonis*, up to 45 times faster than that of *M. genitalium*, and almost 100 times faster than that of *M. gallisepticum*. In addition, the gliding of *M. mobile* is not interrupted by resting periods, which is the case for all other gliding mycoplasmas. The percentage of the resting periods depends on the cultivation conditions (79, 81, 92). It is relatively small under optimal conditions and increases as living conditions become increasingly unfavorable. The most numerous and longest resting periods were observed for *M. gallisepticum*, the slowest of the gliding mycoplasmas detected so far. The gliding movement of *M. mobile* can be directly observed by microscopic examination of a simple native preparation at room temperature, using cell suspensions in common liquid culture medium, whereas demonstration of the movements of the other gliding mycoplasmas requires heated observation chambers and time-lapse microcinematography.

Movement patterns

The movement patterns of *M. pneumoniae*, *M. pulmonis*, and *M. mobile* seem to be similar, characterized by alternate linear and circular movements (14, 81, 92). The movement of *M. gallisepticum*, which is very slow (Table 1), is rather wriggling (14).

More detailed investigations with *M. pneumoniae* (81) and *M. mobile* (92) indicate that linear and circular movements occur under optimal conditions (suitable medium and temperature). These are characterized by permanent changes between straight motion and gliding in clockwise or counterclockwise curves, yielding irregular movement patterns. Under nonoptimal conditions (nonoptimal temperature, presence of antiserum), organisms tend to move in narrow circles without covering long distances or pass into trembling and tumbling movements characterized by frequent

Figure 2. (a to e) Photomicrographs of interference contrast microcinematographic frames showing three erythrocytes and gliding organisms of *M. mobile* 163K. The motility tracks of the three mycoplasma cells (1, 2, and 3) are followed from panel a to panel e. (f) Schematic presentation of the paths followed by the three cells. (Courtesy of R. Rosengarten [34]; published with permission.)

Table 1. Gliding velocities of mycoplasmas

Mycoplasma species	Avg speed (μm/s)	Maximum speed (μm/s)	Resting periods (%)[a]
M. pneumoniae	0.3–0.4	1.5–2.0	0–80
M. genitalium	0.1	ND[b]	ND
M. pulmonis	0.4–0.7	1	0–25
M. gallisepticum	0.03–0.05	0.15	40–80
M. mobile 163K	2.0–4.5	7.7	None

[a] Percentage of resting periods during time of observation.
[b] ND, not defined.

changes of direction as well as by short-term periods with reduced speed, resulting in zigzag movements. The zigzag movement is probably due to reduced surface adherence. It could be observed by light microscopy that the distal portion of *M. mobile* loses contact with the surface and oscillates free in the medium, so that the cells seem to glide only with their headlike structure, in contrast to the gliding with the whole body under normal and optimal conditions.

Cells of *M. mobile* glide individually as well as in multicellular configurations, either as pairs or small groups of three or more cells or as chainlike aggregations or microcolonies (56, 92, 95, 96). Such wandering groups arise by transient association of independently moving cells and rearrange constantly; existing groups enlarge, diminish, or break up, and new groups form. Electron microscopic investigations of adjacent cells of *M. mobile* showed that the surface layer of this organism may account for cell cohesiveness and the ability to form wandering groups (96). Multicellular wandering groups were observed mainly in dense cell populations with a high likelihood of cellular interactions. The contact between the gliding cells does not seem to be very close, for otherwise gliding pairs would not have produced double tracks on the photomicrographs during a long time exposure (Fig. 3). The cohesion force holding two cells together can be calculated to be approximately 3.0×10^{-8} μN, a value considerably less than the adhesion values calculated for the interaction of this organism with glass or erythrocytes (93). Organisms of pairs always dissociate first with their headlike structures, remaining in contact for a short time with their distal ends before moving away as individuals in different directions. Occasionally, elastic viscous connections between the separating cells could be observed, which became increasingly thinner and longer and finally disconnected, a

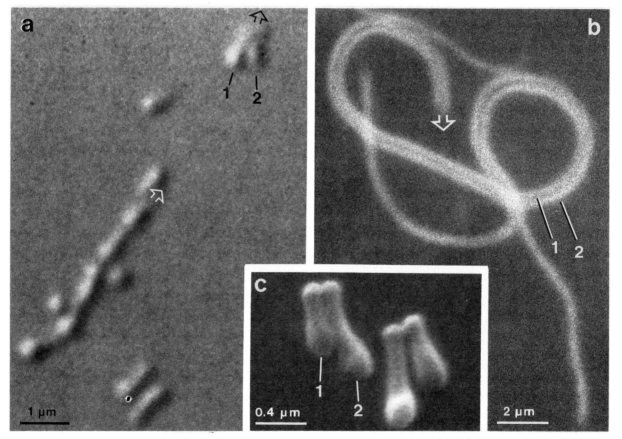

Figure 3. Group motility of *M. mobile*. Wandering groups representing chainlike aggregations (a) or groups of two cells aligned in parallel (indicated by 1 and 2 in panels b and c) are demonstrated by Nomarski interference contrast (a) and scanning electron (c) microscopy. Motility tracks of paired cells (1 and 2) obtained by prolonged-exposure dark-field photomicrography are shown in panel b. Arrows in panels a and b indicate the direction of cell-group movement. (Courtesy of R. Rosengarten.)

further indication for the presence of an extracellular slime layer (96). Movement in groups has not been observed for the other gliding mycoplasmas; they evidently glide as individual cells only.

Influence of environmental factors

The influence of environmental factors on gliding motility has been investigated primarily with *M. pneumoniae* (81) and *M. mobile* (79).

Nutrients. The composition of the culture medium does not seem to significantly affect gliding ability provided that it supports good growth and a sufficient rate of energy supply. A reduction of the serum content to 5% had only a slight effect on the gliding velocity of *M. pneumoniae* (81). Reduction of the yeast extract content to 5%, however, led to cessation of the gliding motility of *M. pneumoniae* after 1 h. Yeast extract obviously contains a substance necessary for constant movement. No effect on the gliding movement of *M. pneumoniae*, *M. gallisepticum*, and *M. mobile* was seen after the addition of 0.1% glucose (14, 81, 92).

Viscosity. With respect to the influence of the viscosity of the medium on gliding motility, there is a difference between *M. mobile* and the three other gliding mycoplasmas investigated. For *M. pneumoniae* (81), *M. gallisepticum* (30a), and *M. genitalium* (108), an increase of medium viscosity by addition of gelatin is the precondition for gliding movement, preventing detachment of the gliding cells from the glass or plastic surface. *M. pneumoniae* reached its highest velocity in medium containing 1 to 3% gelatin. Higher viscosities (for example, medium with 5% gelatin) reduced the speed and increased the percentage of resting periods (81). *M. mobile*, on the other hand, glides optimally in medium without gelatin. The addition of gelatin decreased the velocity of the movement. The difference in behavior of *M. mobile* and the other gliding mycoplasmas may be due to an adaptation to the different environmental conditions to which they are exposed. *M. pneumoniae*, *M. gallisepticum*, and *M. genitalium* colonize mucous membranes of the respiratory and genital tracts of warm-blooded animals, which represent a highly viscous environment, and *M. mobile* colonizes the gills of fish, an environment with much less viscosity.

Cultivation and observation time. A strong dependence of gliding motility on culture age could be shown for *M. mobile* (92), appearing as an increasing reduction of speed with increasing incubation time. The movements were fast and constant during the logarithmic growth phase and began to decrease at the beginning of the stationary phase, suggesting that the ability to move is correlated with the metabolic activity of the cells.

Other factors affecting the movement of *M. mobile* (92) were the observation time of the wet mount preparations and the density of the mycoplasmas in these preparations. The organisms became slower with increasing age of the preparations and with increasing density of the cell population resulting from multiplication. This process may be correlated with the deterioration of the living conditions for the mycoplasmas caused by the consumption of necessary nutrients, the accumulation of metabolic products, the inhibiting influence of the high-intensity light of the microscope lamp, and the evaporation of the suspending medium. Nevertheless, there was still a reduced movement even after an observation time of more than 8 h.

Temperature. A dependence on temperature was demonstrated for *M. pneumoniae* (81), which glides best at 37°C, and *M. mobile* (92), which shows optimal gliding capacity at room temperature. An influence of temperature on motility has been observed for *M. pulmonis*, which glides more slowly at 32°C but is able to move even at room temperature (14). Preliminary observations suggest a temperature dependence for the gliding movement of *M. gallisepticum* also (30a).

Gliding velocity is also influenced by the storage temperature, as shown for *M. mobile* (92). After storage at low temperatures (−20 and 4°C) and short (2-h) storage at 37°C, the cells were significantly slower and tended to move in narrow circles. After incubation for 1 h at room temperature, cells kept at low temperatures resumed motility at the normal level, whereas cells kept for 2 h at 37°C never resumed their initial speed. *M. mobile* dies after storage for 7 h at 37°C. Before death, however, cells pass through a period in which they multiply, as is visible from the growth curve (52). On the other hand, gliding movement is irreversibly reduced after incubation for 2 h at 37°C, i.e., within a period in which cells still multiply. This finding suggests that at least some of the components responsible for gliding movement are more sensitive to heat than is the whole cell.

Inhibitory substances. Several substances interacting with cell functions were investigated for their influence on gliding motility, using nontoxic concentrations of the various substances on *M. pneumoniae* (81) and *M. mobile* (79). For *M. pneumoniae*, gliding movements were characterized by evaluation of cinematographic pictures. Movements of *M. mobile* could be recorded photomicrographically by long exposures, resulting in so-called motility tracks, due to the much higher velocity of this species. It appeared in both investigations that the mycoplasmas not only became slower or nonmotile under the influence of the inhibitory substances but also changed their movement patterns by gliding in narrow circles.

The gliding motility of *M. pneumoniae* and *M. mobile* was significantly inhibited by mitomycin (2.5 and 0.4 μg/ml, respectively), acting on nucleic acid synthesis, and by p-chloromercuribenzoate (0.5 mM and 30 μg/ml, respectively) as well as iodoacetate (2.5 mM and 2 μg/ml, respectively), acting on energy metabolism, indicating that cell-derived energy and intact DNA or DNA synthesis is necessary for the gliding movement. Puromycin and chloramphenicol, antibiotics which inhibit protein synthesis, had no effect on the gliding motility of *M. pneumoniae* at a concentration of 10 μg/ml but inhibited significantly the motility of *M. mobile* at 100 and 125 μg/ml, concentrations that had no toxic effects on the viability of this organism. This finding suggests that the production of at least certain proteins is also required for movement. The concentrations used by Radestock and Bredt (81) may have been too low to cause an effect, or the effects caused may have been too small to be detected by cinematography. Either of these factors could also be the reason for the different results obtained with colchicine and cytochalasin B, agents shown to affect contractile elements

(36, 65). These agents did not inhibit the gliding motility of *M. pneumoniae* at a concentration of 10 or 50 μg/ml but significantly inhibited the gliding motion of *M. mobile* at a concentration of 6×10^3 or 2.5×10^2 μg/ml, although still not affecting the viability of *M. mobile*.

For *M. mobile*, agents acting on the cytoplasmic membrane were investigated for their motion-inhibiting effects. Gliding movement was affected by albumin (5×10^2 μg/ml), which inhibits adherence, possibly by attaching to hydrophobic membrane components (31); Ca^{2+} and Mg^{2+} ions, which in high (unphysiological) concentrations (10^5 μg/ml) also prevent adherence of the mycoplasmas; cholesterol (10^3 μg/ml) and procaine (1.25×10^3 μg/ml), which, like cholchicine, cause an increase in membrane fluidity, leading to changes in the arrangements of the membrane proteins or detachment of the membrane proteins from the cytoskeletal elements (79); EDTA (5.5×10^3 μg/ml), which chelates Ca^{2+} and Mg^{2+} ions from the membrane proteins (36, 100); 2-propanol (5×10^4 μg/ml), which denatures the proteins of the cytoplasmic membrane; KJ (5×10^3 μg/ml), which, as a so-called chaotropic substance, destroys cytoskeletal elements (79) and depolymerizes actinlike filaments as shown by Göbel et al. (40) for *M. pneumoniae*; and the surface-active compounds Triton X-100, Tego (ampholyte), and sodium dodecyl sulfate (SDS), which (i) increased the gliding velocity of *M. mobile* at lower concentrations and short incubation times, probably by virtue of the reduction of the surface tension, provoking a reduction of the frictional forces, and (ii) inhibited gliding movement at higher concentrations and longer incubation periods, leading to destruction of proteins of the cytoplasmic membrane, which must also be the proteins involved in gliding movement.

Antiserum. In the presence of homologous antibodies, gliding motility was significantly affected in *M. pneumoniae* (81) and *M. mobile* (92). The degree of inhibition depended on the antiserum concentration. As in the presence of other motility-inhibiting agents, *M. mobile* lost the ability to cover long distances and moved only in narrow circles. The transfer of antibody-treated *M. pneumoniae* cells to antibody-free medium restored motility to the normal level after about 2 h as a result of detachment of the antibodies. In investigations of *M. mobile* (unpublished observations) with use of monoclonal antibodies, motility and attachment to glass and plastic surfaces as well as to living cells were inhibited, suggesting that antibodies primarily prevent adherence.

Chemotaxis of Mycoplasmas

Chemotaxis, the movement of an organism toward or away from a chemical, has been observed in a variety of plants and animals and has also been shown for flagellated bacteria (1). Different opinions exist about the chemotactic behavior of gliding bacteria; this behavior has been described by some authors (35, 44, 71) but not by others (30).

Among the mollicutes, chemotaxis has been demonstrated for gliding mycoplasmas as well as for spiroplasmas. Early attempts to demonstrate chemotactic activities in gliding mycoplasmas failed because of the slow velocity of the movement of these mycoplasmas

and the lack of a suitable experimental system (81). The demonstration of chemotactic behavior was possible after the detection of *M. mobile* (55), which moves much faster than the other gliding mycoplasmas. Since the various experimental systems used to demonstrate chemotaxis in bacteria (1) were unsuitable for the investigation of mycoplasmas, new techniques had to be developed.

Chemotaxis of *M. mobile* could be demonstrated by two different approaches. The first investigation was based on the motility track technique of Vaituzis and Doetsch (117), which was modified by Daniels and Longland to demonstrate the chemotactic behavior of spiroplasmas (25). By this method, movements of the organisms are recorded photomicrographically by long exposures, resulting in motility tracks on the photographs. The procedure, however, had to be altered considerably to accommodate the special features of *M. mobile* (53). The tests were performed with special observation chambers, prepared by mounting coverslips (21 by 26 mm) on slides with paraffin at their longer edges. Concentration gradients were established by placing the substances to be tested along one of the two open sides of the chambers. Chemotaxis appeared as an alteration of the movement patterns of *M. mobile*. In the absence of chemoeffector substances, the cells appeared to move randomly in linear and circular courses, whereas in the presence of attractant gradients, the random-walk tracks were converted into almost straight lines, aligned parallel to the gradient (53, 56, 95) (Fig. 4). A definite positive chemotaxis to D-fructose, D-glucose, D-lactose, D-maltose, D-saccharose, L-arginine, and L-asparaginic acid, but not to D-arabinose, D-galactose, L-leucine, and L-tyrosine, was observed. Cells were also attracted by mucus from gills of a trout as well as by tracheal mucus of a piglet. The motility track technique was suitable to demonstrate positive chemotaxis but failed to show negative chemotaxis, i.e., movement away from a chemical. No straight alignment of the motility tracks could be observed in the opposite direction in the presence of substances without an attracting effect, and possible alterations in the courses of the motility tracks could not be quantified.

The second approach was performed with a Boyden chamber, originally developed for the demonstration of chemotaxis of polymorphonuclear leukocytes (10). The Boyden chamber used for the detection of chemotaxis of mycoplasmas consisted of a lower tank with 100-μl capacity and an upper tank with 250-μl capacity, separated by a filter membrane of 0.6-μm pore size (89). The mycoplasmas were applied to the lower tank, and the substances to be tested for their attractant properties were placed in the upper tank. Attracted organisms moved via the membrane into the upper tank, where they were counted by determination of CFU. The results obtained with this system varied considerably, and the method needs to be improved. There was, however, an unequivocal migration toward glucose and L-arginine, the two substances tested by this procedure. Chemotaxis could be shown not only for *M. mobile* but also for *M. pneumoniae* and *M. pulmonis*, which migrated toward the attractant into the upper tank also. However, the number of these organisms determined after 15 min was much lower than for *M.*

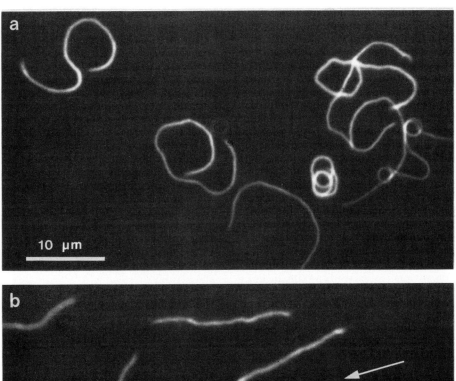

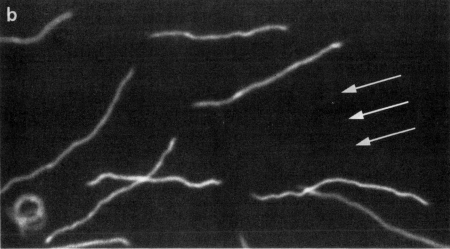

Figure 4. Positive prints of dark-field photomicrographs (10-s exposures) showing motility tracks of individual cells of *M. mobile* moving in random directions in nonflowing medium (a) and moving upstream in the presence of a current velocity gradient along streamlines (b). The flow direction is indicated by arrows. Similar pictures were obtained in investigations of chemotaxis: random walks in the absence of chemoeffector substances (as in panel a) and almost straight motility tracks in a concentration gradient of an attractant (as in panel b). (Courtesy of R. Rosengarten; published with permission of the Institut für den wissenschaftlichen Film, Göttingen, Germany.)

mobile, probably because of their much slower movement.

Rheotaxis of Mycoplasmas

Rheotaxis has been described for higher organisms such as fish (3) and higher organized cells such as spermatozoa (85). It was recently found (97) that *M. mobile*, the gliding mycoplasma isolated from the gills of a fish (55), possesses rheotactic properties also, being able to respond to mechanical stimuli of flow velocity gradients by moving preferentially upstream (56, 95). The rheotactic behavior could be demonstrated with special observation chambers similar to those used for the investigation of chemotaxis. A current velocity gradient across the chamber was induced by placing mi-

crodrops of medium along one open end of the chamber. The behavior of the mycoplasmas in the streaming medium was analyzed by taking interference contrast microcinematographic pictures. For velocity determinations, motility tracks on dark-field photomicrographs exposed for 10 to 40 s were evaluated.

It appeared that in nonflowing medium, the mycoplasma cells were unoriented, moving randomly in various directions. In flowing medium, 90 to 100% of the cells exhibited positive rheotaxis: they tended to move preferentially upstream, with a net migration toward the current (Fig. 4). The flow-induced orientation of the cells was strongly dependent on the local current velocity. A marked rheotactic reaction was observed for current velocities from 100 to 300 μm/s. In this case, the cells remained aligned toward the current for 10 to 23 s before they resumed their normal random movement. With decreasing current velocity values, the rheotactic behavior became less pronounced, and the number of cells that moved randomly tended to increase. At velocity values higher than 400 μm/s, the cells lost contact with the glass surface and rapidly drifted away with the current. The current velocity gradient along the direction of flow through the chamber decreased during the short duration of the experiments (30 to 60 s). Consequently, it is likely that the mycoplasma cells respond to temporal and spatial changes in current velocity rather than to absolute velocities. In 16 of the 33 experiments evaluated, the average gliding speed of the mycoplasmas exposed to a current increased significantly, from 1.79 to 2.29 μm/s ($P < 0.01$) (mean velocity values of 160 measurements). This enhancement of gliding speed in streaming medium suggests that the rheotactic response of *M. mobile* is a phenomenon not merely of orientation but also of increased activity. Indeed, taking into account the high frictional drag due to the opposing current, the energy expenditure of the cells must increase considerably to provide the observed gliding velocity.

M. mobile is the only procaryotic organism with rheotactic properties that has been described so far. It is remarkable that organisms as simple as mycoplasmas possess a physiological transduction system for processing mechanical information from the environment. *M. mobile* is a parasite in an aquatic environment, and its survival as a parasite depends on efficient dispersal mechanisms within and between its hosts. The ability to respond to the mechanical stimulus of a current velocity gradient may be an important factor in this respect and to a certain extent essential.

Energetic Aspects of Gliding Motility

Because of the relatively slow velocity reached by the gliding mycoplasmas *M. pneumoniae*, *M. pulmonis*, and *M. gallisepticum*, the question of whether gliding motility is an active or a passive process arose. To obtain an answer, Maniloff (64) assessed for a particle similar in shape and size to *M. pneumoniae* (i) the energy expenditure necessary for gliding movement for the observed mean velocity of *M. pneumoniae* and (ii) the two-dimensional root-mean-square velocity possible for the thermal energy available at 310 K (37°C). From the results obtained, Maniloff (64) suggested that thermal energy alone may be sufficient to drive the mycoplasma cell at the observed average velocity via a form of Brownian motion.

Maniloff developed his model for the average speed of *M. pneumoniae*. As shown in Table 2, the thermal energy available is in the same range as the calculated energy expenditure for the average speed of *M. pneumoniae*. The model is applicable for *M. gallisepticum* and *M. genitalium* also. It is, however, unsuitable to explain the gliding movement of *M. mobile* or *M. pulmonis* and the maximum velocity of *M. pneumoniae*. In addition, this model cannot answer the question of why only 5 of the more than 100 mycoplasma and acholeplasma species, all of about the same size, are able to glide. If the gliding motility of mycoplasmas is a biased Brownian motion, all mycoplasma species should have this property.

Table 2. Assessed rate of energy expenditure and thermal energy available per cell

Mycoplasma species	Energy expenditure (10^{-15} J/s) at:		Thermal energy (10^{-15} J/s)
	Avg velocity	Maximum velocity	
M. pneumoniae	3.34	109.16	4.28
M. genitalium	0.138		4.28
M. pulmonis	9.34	30.87	4.28
M. gallisepticum	0.024	0.336	4.28
M. mobile	46.05	293.49	4.07

Assessment of the energy expenditure and the velocity which can be expected due to Brownian movement (93) showed clearly that the movement of *M. pulmonis*, the maximum speed of *M. pneumoniae*, and especially the movement of *M. mobile* cannot be biased by Brownian motion (93). The energy required by *M. mobile* is about 11 times higher for the average speed and about 75 times higher for maximum speed than thermal energy can provide under the experimental conditions evaluated. Therefore, an active form of movement must be assumed. This assumption is valid also for the gliding movement of *M. pulmonis* and at least for the maximum velocity of *M. pneumoniae* (Table 2).

That at least *M. mobile* must depend on an active form of movement is evidenced also by its ability to transport sheep erythrocytes (90). This ability is impressive when one considers that the mass of an individual sheep erythrocyte is about 480 times as great as the mass of an individual *M. mobile* cell. Transport of the erythrocytes requires a considerable increase of energy input to the propulsive mechanism of *M. mobile*. The theoretically calculated propulsive energy is about 11 times as great as the energy expenditure calculated for an *M. mobile* cell gliding at the same velocity without an attached erythrocyte (90). This finding clearly shows the requirement for cell-derived energy. Finally, an active form of movement is also required for the chemotactic and rheotactic behavior observed in gliding mycoplasmas.

Mechanism of Gliding Motility

The mechanism of the gliding motility of mycoplasmas is still unknown. Investigations are very difficult because of the small size of the organisms, which are barely visible by light microscopy. Information was obtained predominantly from electron microscopic investigations, which cannot show vital functions, or from the reactions of the organisms to substances with known modes of action. The results of such investigations suggest that the gliding motility of mycoplasmas is an active, energy-consuming process, requiring an optimally operating cytoplasmic membrane and cytoskeletal elements.

An active form of movement, requiring a cellular energy source, can be assumed at least for the more rapidly gliding mycoplasmas *M. pneumoniae*, *M. pulmonis*, and particularly *M. mobile*. This ability was clearly indicated by calculation of the energy required for gliding (93) and could be demonstrated experimentally by inhibition of the gliding movement of *M. mobile* and *M. pneumoniae* (79, 81) by iodoacetate and *p*-chloromercuribenzoate, agents acting on energy metabolism, as well as by substances inhibiting the metabolic activity of the mycoplasma cells, i.e., agents acting on nucleic acid synthesis (mitomycin) or protein synthesis (puromycin and chloramphenicol). The strongest evidence for an active form of translocation comes from demonstrations of chemotaxis and rheotaxis, reactions which require cell-derived energy (18), and the ability of *M. mobile* to transport attached erythrocytes (90).

Cytoskeletal elements have been detected in ultrathin sections of the cells of *M. pneumoniae*, *M. gallisepticum*, *M. genitalium*, and *M. mobile*, but not *M. pulmonis*. The latter mycoplasma, however, exhibits contractile waves along the stalk during gliding (2), which is indirect proof for the existence of contractile elements. The temporary changes in cell shape observed during the division of *M. gallisepticum* (72) and *M. mobile* (96) also suggest the existence of contractile cytoskeletal elements. That cytoskeletal elements have also been found in nonmotile mycoplasmas (42, 86, 87) does not necessarily mean that these elements do not play a role in the movement of the gliding mycoplasmas. Contractile elements are required also for maintenance of the distinct but variable cell shape and the cell divisions in these wall-less procaryotes. Possibly, these structures are present only at different stages of phylogenetic development or are present in different quantities in motile and nonmotile mycoplasmas. Moreover, it cannot be completely excluded that the mycoplasmas exhibiting these structures are motile under certain conditions not yet defined.

Further evidence for the existence of cytoskeletal elements is provided by the inhibition of gliding movement by substances reacting with cytoskeletal elements or the cytoplasmic membrane, such as albumin, cytochalasin B, cholesterol, EDTA, 2-propanol, procaine, CaCl$_2$, MgCl$_2$, colchicin, KJ, and surface-active compounds (Triton X-100, Tego, and SDS) (79, 81). The inhibition of the movement by substances reacting with the cytoplasmic membrane suggests a close connection between the cytoplasmic membrane and the cytoskeleton. The effects of substances reacting with surface components of the cytoplasmic membrane and the action of specific antibodies on gliding motility cannot be fully substantiated. These agents also inhibit attachment. It is possible that the motility is inhibited by the prevention of attachment, which is a precondition for gliding movement.

The surface layer detected on the cells of *M. pneumoniae* (125), *M. gallisepticum* (107), and *M. mobile* (96) may play a role in adhesiveness and gliding motility. It is not unlikely that this polyanionic material has the same function as does the extracellular slime of the gliding bacteria: (i) mediating attachment of the cell to the substratum (69, 70) and (ii) allowing and facilitating the movement on that substratum (20) by reducing the friction between the contacted surfaces. These properties are characteristic of a temporary adhesive (48).

Not conclusively answered is the question of the presence of actinlike proteins in mycoplasmas. This question is of general interest with respect to the occurrence of actin in procaryotic cells. The more important question with respect to the motility of mycoplasmas is whether mycoplasmas possess a protein identical in function to actin. This protein could be quite different from actin in its biochemical and immunological properties. The available data indicate that mycoplasmas very likely possess such a protein.

Significance of Gliding Motility in Pathogenicity

Three of the five known gliding mycoplasmas are established pathogens, producing more or less severe diseases. These are *M. pneumoniae*, causing the so-called atypical human pneumonia that may be accompanied by several complications; *M. gallisepticum*, the agent of a respiratory disease in chickens and turkeys, occasionally combined with nervous system complications and arthritis; and *M. pulmonis*, primarily a murine respiratory pathogen but causing genital disease and arthritis also.

There are no definite data relating *M. genitalium* to infections of the human genitourinary tract from which it has been isolated. However, it seems likely that *M. genitalium* possesses pathogenic properties, because it produced an inflammatory cell response accompanied by an antibody response following vaginal inoculation in chimpanzees (110) and caused histopathological changes in the lungs of hamsters, including edema, congestion, and consolidation, after intratracheal inoculation (18a). In addition, *M. genitalium* is able to attach both to ciliary shafts and to the cell surface of the human fallopian tube epithelium, as shown by scanning electron microscopic examination (23).

Pathogenicity can be assumed also for *M. mobile* 163K, isolated from the gills of a tench (*Tinca tinca* L.) with red disease. *M. mobile* inhibited the ciliary activity in tracheal organ cultures and caused a complete exfoliation of the epithelial cells and a total destruction of the multi-layer epithelium in the tracheal organ cultures (103). It also caused heavy damage of the gill epithelium in gill organ cultures (104), as demonstrated by scanning and transmission electron microscopy. After intraperitoneal injection, *M. mobile* was able to colonize the gills, kidney, spleen, and air bladder of tenches (58) and carps (73a) and to produce pathological changes in the air bladder of carps, apparent as opaqueness, thickening, and adhesions with adjacent organs. Carps placed in culture supernatant of *M. mobile* showed symptoms of intoxication after 1 to 2 min, probably due to toxic metabolic products liberated by *M. mobile*.

The pathogenic properties of the motile mycoplasmas suggest that motility is a pathogenicity factor. Mycoplasmas generally are parasites of the epithelial cells of the respiratory and urogenital tract of humans and animals. There is no doubt that motile mycoplasmas can reach epithelial cells more easily than can nonmotile species, because they can better penetrate the mucous layer, probably by moving down the cilia, or the lamellae of the gills in the case of *M. mobile*. In doing so, their chemotactic capacities help them take the shortest way along the concentration gradient in the mucous layer generated by the steady secretion of substances from epithelial cells. The ability to glide on living cells (34) enables the mycoplasmas to invade intracellular spaces or membrane crypts of the epithelial cells, where they presumably find optimal living conditions and are protected from host defense reactions or drugs. Because of their ability to respond to chemical substances, gliding mycoplasmas probably can leave areas in which the environmental conditions have become unfavorable.

For *M. mobile* living in an aquatic environment as a parasite on the gills of fish, the ability to respond to the mechanical stimuli of flow velocity gradients by moving preferentially upstream may be an important factor or possibly even the precondition for survival, enabling the mycoplasma to overcome the increasing water flux in the gills.

Motility and especially motility in combination with chemotaxis and rheotaxis are advantageous for organisms in colonizing the host epithelia and therefore are true pathogenicity factors. However, there are many pathogenic mycoplasmas that are not dependent on the ability to move. Thus, motility is only one of the strategies developed by mycoplasmas to reach adequate living and growth conditions.

MOTILITY BY ROTATION AND UNDULATION

Motility of Spiroplasmas

Motility characterized by rotational and flexional movements is one of the distinctive properties of spiroplasmas. It was first described by Davis and Worley (28) for *Spiroplasma kunkelii*, the corn stunt organism, and by Cole et al. (22) for *S. citri*, the spiroplasma causing citrus stubborn disease. Further investigations showed that the other spiroplasmas are also motile. The motility of spiroplasmas can easily be observed in simple dark-field preparations by using $10\times$ lenses.

Davis and Worley (28) described the movements of *S. kunkelii* as rapid spinning about the long axis combined with flexional movements characterized by bending, flexing, and curling. Movements were observed in organisms floating free in the medium as well as in organisms attached with one end of the filament to the surface of a slide. Translational movement was not noticed. *S. citri* showed two types of movement, characterized by Cole et al. (22) as a rapid rotary or "screw" motion about the helix axis, which can be reversed and lead to minimal back-and-forth progress, and a slow undulation and bending of the filaments with slight rotation that does not causing translational movement.

Spiroplasmas are capable of translational movements when they are cultivated in semisolid medium (26, 28), such as medium with 0.5% carboxymethyl cellulose and 3% gelatin. Translational movements are characterized by rotations (mostly clockwise) and intermittent contractions, which can be initiated at any part of the helical cell. There is some evidence (25) that motion in a straight line is driven by rotation about the helix axis and that changes in direction are caused by flexing of the spiroplasma helix.

Translational movement could also be demonstrated by placing cells of *S. melliferum* BC-3 in the center of a agar plate, from which they migrated radially through the agar (0.6%, wt/vol), producing satellite colonies clearly visible after Dienes staining (26). Satellite colonies were formed also from *S. mirum* SMCA by cultivation in 1 to 2% agar medium (91). Organisms inoculated on the surface of the agar developed colonies in the depth of the agar and at the bottom of the petri dish, indicating their ability to migrate through the agar medium.

Movement of the spiroplasmas seems to be a very stable property. *S. mirum* was cultivated for more than 40 passages without a reduction in motility; in dark-field preparations, motility was very vigorous even after 8 h of observation (unpublished observations).

Morphological Characteristics of Spiroplasmas

Cell morphology

The most distinctive property of the spiroplasmas is their helical cell form. It is developed in situ, i.e., in the affected plants and animals, as well as in liquid cultures and colonies growing on solid medium (91). In addition to the helices, long nonhelical filaments, asteroid cells, and even coccoid cells can be observed. In vitro, the number of these cells increases with deterioration of the living conditions.

Spiroplasma helices show a clear morphological polarity characterized by a blunt and a tapered end. Investigations with insect cell cultures revealed that spiroplasmas are able to attach to cells and that the attachment site differs among the spiroplasma species. *S. citri* attaches by the blunt end, strain 277 attaches by either the blunt or the tapered end, and *S. apis* B31 attaches by the blunt end or any other point along the helix but never by the tapered end (8).

Ultrastructural features

Several investigations were performed to ascertain the structural basis for motility and helical morphology of spiroplasmas. An electron-dense layer (X layer) located on the cytoplasmic side of the cytoplasma membrane was noticed in ultra-thin sections of *S. citri* in one of the first investigations of spiroplasmas (22). Intracytoplasmic fibrillar ultrastructures could be detected when living cells were treated with detergents before embedment for ultra-thin sectioning (112, 121). Fibrils were found in the negatively stained, detergent-insoluble residues of the *Drosophila* spiroplasma (121), *S. citri* and *S. kunkelii* (124), *Spiroplasma* strain 277F (106), *S. melliferum* BC-3 (112), *S. floricola* 23-6 (27), and *S. floricola* OBMG (19). They were also detected in the nonhelical ASP strain of *S. citri*. Fibrils seem to be present in all spiroplasmas (113).

Individual fibrils are of various lengths, are 4 nm in diameter, and possess a striation repeat at 9 nm along their length that is dramatically displayed in the bundles (8, 112, 124). Polyacrylamide gel electrophoresis of density gradient-purified fibrils showed them to be composed of a 55-kDa protein (111). Antibodies against either native or SDS-denatured fibrillar protein obtained from *S. melliferum* BC-3 recognized a similar protein in Western blotting experiments of many but apparently not all of the spiroplasmas tested (112, 123).

The fibrils observed in the spiroplasmas are considered to play a role in maintaining the helical morphology and possibly in the motility of these organisms. This assumption was supported by the observation that the molecular weight of the fibril monomer is almost identical with the molecular weight of the tubulin subunit, which occurs in all eucaryotic cells forming the microtubuli via protofilaments, though there are differences in the physicochemical properties of these two proteins (8). At present, however, neither the structure nor the function of the spiroplasma fibrils is understood. Even the arrangement of the fibrils within the spiroplasma cell is not known with any certainty. Some evidence exists (19, 123, 124) that the fibrils are arranged in a single helical twisted band, apposed to the cytoplasmic face of the cytoplasmic membrane, continuously following the inner curves of the helical cell from one end to the other.

Spiroplasma proteins

Some special proteins that are considered to be involved in helicity and motility have been detected in spiroplasmas. The best known is spiralin, originally detected in *S. citri* as the most abundant protein of the cell membrane, representing more than 20% of the total membrane protein. It has a molecular weight of about 26,000 and is unusual in that it lacks methionine, histidine, and tryptophan (8). Proteins with compositions similar to that of to spiralin C189 were purified from other helical strains of *S. citri* (R8A2, Scaph, and SP-A), and spiralins with slightly different electrophoretic mobilities but similar immunological properties were found in all *S. citri* strains tested, including the nonhelical strain ASP1. Proteins identical to spiralin in solubility properties, electrophoretic mobility, and molecular weight and similar in amino acid composition were detected in *S. melliferum* BC-3 and B88. These proteins, however, had only a weak serological relationship with *S. citri* spiralin, and were therefore designated spiralinlike proteins (8).

Spiralin of *S. citri* and the spiralinlike proteins of the other spiroplasmas are amphiphilic integral membrane proteins, with a hydrophilic portion protruding on the membrane surface and a hydrophobic portion within the lipid bilayer. They are acylated with palmitate through ester bonds, which may support their insertion and anchoring in the lipid bilayer. Spiralin oligomers, probably mainly dimers, span the spiroplasma membrane (8).

One can assume that such dominant proteins as spiralin or the spiralinlike proteins play a role in the structure or function of the spiroplasma membrane and that they may be involved in maintaining the helical structure of the spiroplasmas. Interestingly, substantial amounts of a protein identical in molecular weight to the spiralinlike protein of *S. melliferum* BC-3 (26,000) are copurified with the fibrils of this spiroplasma strain (8). The true function of spiralin and the spiralinlike proteins, however, has not been ascertained so far.

Like the gliding mycoplasmas (74, 75), spiroplasmas were investigated for the presence of actin or actinlike proteins. The investigations performed so far provide more evidence for such proteins in spiroplasmas than in mycoplasmas. It could be shown that all strains of *S. citri* contain a protein similar to muscle actin in molecular weight (45,000), solubility at high but not low salt concentrations, and the ability to form a complex with myosin. This protein, however, did not bind DNase I, characteristic for eucaryotic actin, and its isoelectric point was slightly different from that of muscle actin (8).

Indications for the presence of actinlike proteins in spiroplasmas were also obtained by immunological investigations. Antiserum to SDS-denatured actin from invertebrate muscle reacted with proteins of *S. citri* (122), and a protein of *S. citri* with a molecular weight of 45,000 bound to rabbit immunoglobulin G directed against rabbit actin in immunoaffinity chromatography (73). In addition, a protein with a molecular weight of about 55,000 was detected in both the cytoplasmic and membrane fractions of *S. citri* to react by immunoblotting with antiactin antibodies (99). Hybridization of *S. citri* DNA cleaved with the restriction endonuclease *Hin*dIII with the entire yeast actin gene, however, yielded no unequivocal answer. Antibodies against the actinlike protein of *S. citri* R8A2 recognized proteins in all spiroplasmas investigated so far (8), indicating that all spiroplasmas may possess these proteins.

The data obtained show that spiroplasmas possess proteins that may be related to actin. However, it remains to be demonstrated that these proteins have the biological activities that have been characterized for the actin of eucaryotes.

Physiology of Spiroplasma Motility

Little is known about the physiology of spiroplasma motility. Like the gliding mycoplasmas, spiroplasmas show highest motility under optimal conditions. Changes of the pH values of the culture medium and alterations of the cultivation temperature to both higher and lower levels reduce motility, though the helical shape is retained (26).

Velocity

Spiroplasmas are capable of translational movements in viscous media only, and their velocity depends on the viscosity of the medium. Unlike flagellated bacteria (98) and gliding mycoplasmas (81, 92), which move more slowly in fluids with higher viscosities, spiroplasmas, like leptospiras (51), increase velocity with increasing viscosity of the medium, as shown for *S. melliferum* BC3 (26). Velocity was determined by two different methods: by timing organisms over a 10-μm path, using an eyepiece graticule and a stopwatch, and by measuring the motility tracks on films exposed for 10 s. Both methods revealed that *S. melliferum* BC-3 moves with a velocity of between 1 μm/s (in medium with about 0.1% methylcellulose) and 5 μm/s (in medium with 0.75% methylcellulose) (26).

Influence of inhibitory substances

Washed and suspended in phosphate-buffered sorbitol (a nonmetabolizable substrate), *S. melliferum* BC-3 cells were unable to move but in some cases resumed characteristic movement less than 30 s after addition of fructose (a fermentable substrate) (26). Motility also ceased after addition of inhibitors of glycolysis (sodium iodoacetate [10^{-4} M], sodium arsenate [10^{-4} M]) or membrane-bound ATPase (*N,N'*-dicyclohexylcarbodiimide [10^{-3} M]). This finding indicates that intact energy metabolism is necessary for motility. The helicity of the cells was not influenced in these investigations. By contrast, potassium cyanide (10^{-2} M), which inhibits respiration, and 2,4-dinitrophenol (10^{-3} M), an uncoupler of oxidative phosphorylation, had no discernible effects (26).

Chemotaxis of Spiroplasmas

Chemotaxis of spiroplasmas could be demonstrated by two different tests: determination of the number of organisms migrating into capillaries containing a range of concentrations of substances to be tested (26) and the motility track technique (25).

The capillary technique, commonly used to demonstrate chemotaxis in bacteria (1), allows the detection of both positive and negative chemotaxis. Positive chemotaxis appears as an increase and negative chemotaxis appears as a decrease in the number of organisms in the capillary compared with values for controls. Investigations were performed with *S. melliferum* (26), which was attracted by sugars (D-fructose, D-glucose, D-maltose, D-raffinose, and sucrose), several amino acids (L-alanine, L-aspartate, L-arginine, L-cysteine, L-glutamate, glycine, L-methionine, L-serine, and L-threonine), fetal calf serum, yeast extract, and PPLO broth. *S. melliferum* was repelled by hydrophobic amino acids (L-histidine, L-leucine, L-phenylalanine, L-proline, and L-valine), acidic metabolites (lactic acid), and heavy metals (CoCl$_2$). D-Xylose, L-lysine, L-asparagine, cyclic AMP, and sodium lactate (pH 7.0) neither attracted nor repelled spiroplasmas (26).

For the motility track technique, special observation chambers were constructed from slides and coverslips (25). Substances to be tested were dissolved in medium containing 1% agar and introduced into an open end of the chamber; the organisms, suspended in medium containing 0.13 or 0.25% methylcellulose, were placed at the other end. Like the attracted mycoplasmas, the attracted spiroplasmas produced essentially straight motility tracks, aligned perpendicular to the agar-liquid boundary in the observation chamber, as shown for L-methionine, L-serine, and PPLO broth, whereas in the absence of attractants, cells appeared to be moving randomly (25). Examination of individual spiroplasmas showed that in the absence of an attractant or repellent, the flexing frequency was constant at different points of the chamber, whereas in the presence of an attractant, the flexing frequency steadily decreased with increasing concentrations in the concentration gradient. From these observations, Daniels and Longland (25) suggested that straight motion is achieved by rotation about the helix axis and that changes of direction are caused by flexing of the spiroplasma helix.

Viscotaxis of Spiroplasmas

The ability of leptospiras to increase velocity with increasing viscosity was termed viscotaxis (78), i.e., migration in the direction of a viscosity gradient. Daniels and Longland (25) showed that the behavior of *S. melliferum* in viscous media is very similar to that of leptospiras; i.e., *S. melliferum* also possesses viscotactic capacities. This ability probably is of advantage for spiroplasmas in their natural habitats (i.e., the nectar of flowers, the phloem sieve tubes, and the tissues of arthropods), which are viscous, facilitating dispersal of the organisms in the host.

Mechanism of Spiroplasma Motility

Nothing is yet known about the mechanism of spiroplasma motility. As for mycoplasmas, however, there are some observations that allowing certain preliminary assumptions.

As a possible morphological basis for helicity and motility, the fibrils detected in several spiroplasmas are discussed. In extensive investigations using various chemical fixatives and freezing techniques for preserving ultrastructures, Charbonneau and Ghiorse (19) found that the fibrils in *S. floricola* OBMG are arranged as a band on the inner surface of the cytoplasmic membrane, and they proposed a model for its location. In this model, the helical fibril band is depicted as following the inner curves of the helical cell apposed to the cytoplasmic face of the membrane. Anchor points of the band were not indicated in the model because they could not be ascertained in the investigations. Indications for a ribbonlike arrangement of the fibrils were obtained also for *S. melliferum* BC-3 by Williamson et al. (123) and by Townsend and Plaskitt (114). Open is the question of whether the fibril band is contractile. If it is, it would be possible to explain the movements by contractions and extensions of this band as proposed for the axial filament of the spirochetes.

Nothing is known so far about the significance of the special proteins found in spiroplasmas (8). The question of whether spiralin or the spiralinlike proteins play any role in helicity or motility of the spiroplasmas is still unresolved. The same is true for the proteins exhibiting properties identical to those of actin. There is no doubt that spiroplasmas possess contractile structures, because their biological and physiological behavior requires such structures. There is, however, no indication as to the nature of these proteins. It is also evident that spiroplasmas, like gliding mycoplasmas, possess an active form of movement. This property appears clearly in their chemotactic and viscotactic behavior and in the inhibition of motility by agents acting on energy metabolism (26).

Significance of Motility in the Pathogenicity of Spiroplasmas

Spiroplasmas are parasites in plants, arthropods, and vertebrates, causing diseases in all of these hosts (9). In plants, spiroplasmas colonize predominantly the interior of phloem sieve tubes and the nectar of flowers. In arthropods, they are present in the salivary glands, the hemolymph, and several other tissues. From vertebrates, in which they occur only after experimental inoculation, spiroplasmas have been isolated from the blood, brain, eye, and several organs (9, 54).

Motility facilitates the dispersal of microorganisms generally and the spread of spiroplasmas in their hosts specifically. The restriction of translational movement to viscous media is probably an adaptation to the environments that spiroplasmas colonize, all of which are viscous. Dispersal in the host apparently is supported by the viscotactic and chemotactic behavior of the spiroplasmas. Viscotaxis may help them to move efficiently through natural-viscosity gradients in the host, for example, from external body cavities into body fluids and tissues, and the ability to respond to chemical gradients may be an important factor in the natural host cycle of the spiroplasmas, as pointed out by Daniels et al. (26). There are observations that in the concentration gradient of photosynthetic products existing in the phloem of plants between roots and shoots, spiroplasmas tend to migrate to the top of actively photosynthesizing plants and accumulate in the shoots, where they are ingested by feeding insects. The observed concentration of spiroplasmas in these tissues may favor acquisition by insects. Chemotaxis also could be responsible for the accumulation of spiroplasmas in the salivary glands of insects, whence they are discharged with saliva into plants.

As with mycoplasmas, motility is only one of the pathogenicity factors developed by spiroplasmas, since *S. citri* ASP1, which lacks helical morphology and motility, shows the same degree of pathogenicity as do the helical *S. citri* strains (113).

REFERENCES

1. Adler, J. 1975. Chemotaxis in bacteria. *Annu. Rev. Biochem.* **44:**341–356.
2. Andrewes, C. H., and F. V. Welch. 1946. A motile organism of the pleuropneumonia group. *J. Pathol. Bacteriol.* **58:**578–580.
3. Arnold, G. P. 1974. Rheotropism in fishes. *Biol. Rev. Camb. Philos. Soc.* **49:**515–576.
4. Baseman, J. B., R. M. Cole, D. C. Krause, and D. K. Leith. 1982. Molecular basis for cytadsorption of *Mycoplasma pneumoniae. J. Bacteriol.* **151:**1514–1522.
5. Baseman, J. B., D. L. Drouillard, D. K. Leith, and J. G. Tully. 1984. Absence of *Mycoplasma pneumoniae* cytadsorption protein P1 in *Mycoplasma genitalium* and *Mycoplasma gallisepticum. Infect. Immun.* **43:**1103–1105.
6. Baseman, J. B., J. Morrison-Plummer, D. Drouillard, B. Puleo-Scheppke, V. V. Tryon, and S. C. Holt. 1987. Identification of a 32-kilodalton protein of *Mycoplasma pneumoniae* associated with hemadsorption. *Isr. J. Med. Sci.* **23:**474–479.
7. Biberfeld, G., and P. Biberfeld. 1970. Ultrastructural features of *Mycoplasma pneumoniae. J. Bacteriol.* **102:**855–861.
8. Bové, J. M., P. Carle, M. Garnier, F. Laigret, J. Renaudin, and C. Saillard. 1989. Molecular and cellular biology of spiroplasmas. p. 243–364. *In* R. F. Whitcomb and J. G. Tully (ed.), *The Mycoplasmas*, vol. 5. *Spiroplasmas, Acholeplasmas, and Mycoplasmas of Plants and Arthropods.* Academic Press, New York.
9. Bové, J. M., and C. Saillard. 1979. Cell biology of spiro-

plasmas, p. 85–153. *In* M. F. Barile, S. Razin, J. G. Tully, and R. F. Whitcomb (ed.), *The Mycoplasmas*, vol 3. *Plant and Insect Mycoplasmas.* Academic Press, New York.
10. Boyden, S. 1962. The chemotactic effect of mixtures of antibody and antigen on polymorphonuclear leukocytes. *J. Exp. Med.* **115:**453–458.
11. Bredt, W. 1968. Motility and multiplication of Mycoplasma pneumoniae. A phase contrast study. *Pathol. Microbiol.* **32:**321–326.
12. Bredt, W. 1973. Motility of mycoplasmas. *Ann. N.Y. Acad. Sci.* **225:**246–259.
13. Bredt, W. 1974. Structure and motility. *Colloq. INSERM.* **33:**47–52.
14. Bredt, W. 1979. Motility, p. 141–145. *In* M. F. Barile, S. Razin, J. G. Tully, and R. F. Whitcomb (ed.), *The Mycoplasmas*, vol. 1. *Cell Biology.* Academic Press, New York.
15. Bredt, W., K. H. Höfling, and H. H. Heunert. 1970. *Mycoplasma pneumoniae* (Mycoplasmataceae): Bewegung, Vermehrung and Koloniebildung, Film E 1633. *In* G. Wolf (ed.), *Encyclopaedia Cinematographica.* Institut für den wissenschlaftlichen Film, Göttingen, Germany.
16. Bredt, W., K. H. Höfling, H. H. Heunert, and B. Milthaler. 1970. Messungen an beweglichen Zellen von *Mycoplasma pneumoniae. Z. Med. Mikrobiol. Immunol.* **156:**39–43.
17. Bredt, W., and U. Radestock. 1977. Gliding motility of *Mycoplasma pulmonis. J. Bacteriol.* **130:**937–938.
18. Burchard, R. P. 1981. Gliding motility of prokaryotes: ultrastructure, physiology, and genetics. *Annu. Rev. Microbiol.* **35:**497–529.
18a. Chandler, D. K. F., M. W. Grabowski, H. Yoshida, R. Harasawa, S. Razin, and M. F. Barile. 1990. Experimentally induced *Mycoplasma pneumoniae* and *Mycoplasma genitalium* pneumonias in hamsters. *IOM Lett.* **1:**156–157.
19. Charbonneau, D. L., and W. C. Ghiorse. 1984. Ultrastructure and location of cytoplasmic fibrils in *Spiroplasma floricola* OBMG. *Curr. Microbiol.* **10:**65–72.
20. Chosteron, J. W. F., R. G. E. Murray, and C. F. Robinow. 1961. Observation on the motility and structure of *Vitreoscilla. Can. J. Microbiol.* **7:**329–339.
21. Chu, H. P., and R. W. Horne. 1967. Electron microscopy of *Mycoplasma gallisepticum* and *Mycoplasma mycoides* using the negative staining technique and their comparison with myxovirus. *Ann. N.Y. Acad. Sci.* **143:**190–203.
22. Cole, R. M., J. G. Tully, T. J. Popkin, and J. M. Bové. 1973. Morphology, ultrastructure, and bacteriophage infection of the helical mycoplasma-like organism (*Spiroplasma citri* gen. nov. sp. nov.) cultured from "stubborn" disease of citrus. *J. Bacteriol.* **115:**367–386.
23. Collier, A. M., Y. L. Carson, P. C. Hu, S. S. Hu, C. H. Huang, and M. F. Barile. 1990. Attachment of *Mycoplasma genitalium* to the ciliated epithelium of human fallopian tubes. *Zentralbl. Bakteriol. Suppl.* **20:**730–732.
24. Collier, A. M., and W. A. Clyde, Jr. 1971. Relationships between *Mycoplasma pneumoniae* and human respiratory epithelium. *Infect. Immun.* **3:**694–701.
25. Daniels, M. J., and J. M. Longland. 1984. Chemotactic behaviour of spiroplasmas. *Curr. Microbiol.* **10:**191–194.
26. Daniels, M. J., J. M. Longland, and J. Gilbart. 1980. Aspects of motility and chemotaxis in spiroplasmas. *J. Gen. Microbiol.* **118:**429–436.
27. Davis, R. E., J.-M. Lee, and J. F. Worley. 1981. *Spiroplasma floricola*, a new species isolated from surfaces of flower of the tulip tree, *Liriodendron tulipifera* L. *Int. J. Syst. Bacteriol.* **31:**456–464.
28. Davis, R. E., and J. F. Worley. 1973. Spiroplasmas: motile, helical microorganism associated with corn stunt disease. *Phytopathology* **63:**403–408.
29. Del Giudice, R. A., J. G. Tully, D. L. Rose, and R. M. Cole. 1985. *Mycoplasma pirum* sp. nov., a terminal structured mollicute from cell cultures. *Int. J. Syst. Bacteriol.* **35:**285–291.

30. **Dworkin, M., and D. Eide.** 1983. *Myxococcus xanthus* does not respond chemotactically to moderate concentration gradients. *J. Bacteriol.* **154:**437–442.

30a.**Erdmann, T.** 1976. Untersuchungen zur Morphologie, Vermehrung und Beweglichkeit von *Mycoplasma gallisepticum.* M.D. thesis. Johannes Gutenberg Universität, Mainz, Germany.

31. **Feldner, J., and W. Bredt.** 1983. Differences in surface antigens within a given population of *Mycoplasma pneumoniae* or *Mycoplasma gallisepticum* as shown by monoclonal antibodies. *FEMS Microbiol. Lett.* **19:**17–22.

32. **Feldner, J., U. Göbel, and W. Bredt.** 1982. *Mycoplasma pneumoniae* adhesin localized to tip structure by monoclonal antibody. *Nature (London)* **298:**765–767.

32a.**Fischer, M.** 1988. Immunologische und biochemische Untersuchungen an der Membran von *Mycoplasma mobile* 163K. Ph.D. thesis. Universität Hannover, Hannover, Germany.

33. **Fischer, M., and H. Kirchhoff.** 1987. Interaction of *Mycoplasma mobile* 163K with erythrocytes. *Zentralbl. Bakteriol. Hyg. A* **266:**497–505.

34. **Fischer, M., H. Kirchhoff, R. Rosengarten, G. Kerlen, and K. H. Seack.** 1987. Gliding movement of *Mycoplasma* sp. nov. strain 163K on erythrocytes. *FEMS Microbiol. Lett.* **40:**321–324.

35. **Fluegel, W.** 1963. Fruiting chemotaxis in *Myxococcus fulvus* (Myxobacteria). *Proc. Minn. Acad. Sci.* **32:**120–123.

36. **Furcht, L. T., and R. E. Scott.** 1975. Effect of vinblastine sulfate, cholchicine and luminocolchicine on membrane organization of normal and transformed cells. *Cell Res.* **96:**271–282.

37. **Geary, S. J., M. G. Garbridge, and M. F. Gladd.** 1990. Utilization of a 100Kd human lung fibroblast receptor site to identify a 32 kDa *Mycoplasma pneumoniae* antigen involved on attachment. *Zentralbl. Bakteriol. Suppl.* **20:**697–700.

38. **Göbel, U.** 1983. Supramolecular structures in mycoplasmas. *Yale J. Biol. Med.* **56:**695–700.

39. **Göbel, U., M. M. Müller, and R. Maas.** 1990. Actin related DNA-sequences and proteins from motile mycoplasmas: a molecular puzzle. *Zentralbl. Bakteriol. Suppl.* **20:**335–344.

40. **Göbel, U., V. Speth, and W. Bredt.** 1981. Filamentous structures in adherent *Mycoplasma pneumoniae* cells treated with nonionic detergents. *J. Cell Biol.* **91:**537–543.

41. **Gorski, F., and W. Bredt.** 1977. Studies on the adherence mechanism of *Mycoplasma pneumoniae. FEMS Microbiol. Lett.* **1:**265–267.

42. **Gourlay, R. N., S. G. Wyld, and R. H. Leach.** 1977. *Mycoplasma alvi*, a new species from bovine intestinal and urogenital tracts of cows. *Int. J. Syst. Bacteriol.* **27:**86–96.

43. **Gourlay, R. N., S. G. Wyld, and R. H. Leach.** 1978. *Mycoplasma sualvi*, a new species from the intestinal and urogenital tracts of pigs. *Int. J. Syst. Bacteriol.* **28:**289–292.

44. **Ho, J., and H. D. McCurdy.** 1979. Demonstration of positive chemotaxis to cyclic GMP and 5′AMP in *Myxococcu xanthus* by means of a simple apparatus for generating practically stable concentration gradients. *Can. J. Microbiol.* **25:**1214–1218.

45. **Hu, P. C., R. M. Cole, Y. S. Huang, J. A. Graham, D. E. Gardner, A. M. Collier, and W. A. Clyde, Jr.** 1982. *Mycoplasma pneumoniae* infection: role of a surface protein in the attachment organelle. *Science* **216:**313–315.

46. **Hu, P. C., U. Schaper, A. M. Collier, W. A. Clyde, M. Horikawa, Y. S. Huang, and M. Barile.** 1987. A *Mycoplasma genitalium* protein resembling the *Mycoplasma pneumoniae* attachment protein. *Infect. Immun.* **55:**1126–1131.

47. **Hummeler, K., N. Tomassini, and L. Hayflick.** 1965. Ultrastructure of a mycoplasma (Negroni) isolated from human leukemia. *J. Bacteriol.* **90:**517–523.

48. **Humphrey, B. A., M. R. Dickson, and K. C. Marshall.** 1979. Physicochemical and in situ observations on the adhesion of gliding bacteria to surfaces. *Arch. Microbiol.* **120:**231–238.

49. **Jonas, T. C., S. Yeh, and J. G. Hirsch.** 1971. Studies on attachment and ingestion phases of phagocytosis of *Mycoplasma pulmonis* by mouse peritoneal macrophages. *Proc. Soc. Exp. Biol. Med.* **139:**464–470.

50. **Kahane, J., J. Granek, and A. Reich-Saada.** 1984. The adhesins of *Mycoplasma gallisepticum* and *Mycoplasma pneumoniae. Ann. Microbiol.* (Paris) **135A:**25–32.

51. **Kaiser, G. E., and R. N. Doetsch.** 1975. Enhanced translational motion of *Leptospira* in viscous environments. *Nature* (London) **255:**656–657.

52. **Kirchhoff, H., P. Beyene, M. Fischer, J. Flossdorf, J. Heitmann, B. Khattab, D. Lopatta, R. Rosengarten, G. Seidel, and C. Youseff.** 1987. *Mycoplasma mobile* sp. nov., a new species from fish. *Int. J. Syst. Bacteriol.* **37:**192–197.

53. **Kirchhoff, H., U. Boldt, R. Rosengarten, and A. Klein-Struckmeier.** 1987. Chemotactic response of a gliding mycoplasma. *Curr. Microbiol.* **15:**57–60.

54. **Kirchhoff, H., T. Kuwabara, and M. F. Barile.** 1981. Pathogenicity of *Spiroplasma* sp. strain SMCA in syrian hamster: clinical, microbiological and histological aspects. *Infect. Immun.* **31:**445–452.

55. **Kirchhoff, H., and R. Rosengarten.** 1984. Isolation of a motile mycoplasma from fish. *J. Gen. Microbiol.* **130:**2439–2445.

56. **Kirchhoff, A., and R. Rosengarten.** 1988. *Mycoplasma mobile*—morphology, multiplication and gliding motility. *Publ. Wiss. Film Sekt. Med. Sez. 7* **11/C1670:**1–13.

57. **Kirchhoff, H., R. Rosengarten, and C. Chercheletzi.** 1983. Isolation of mycoplasma from a tench (*Tinca tinca* L.). *Yale J. Biol. Med.* **56:**841–842.

58. **Kirchhoff, H., R. Rosengarten, W. Lotz, M. Fischer, and D. Lopatta.** 1984. Flask-shaped mycoplasmas: properties and pathogenicity for man and animals. *Isr. J. Med. Sci.* **20:**848–853.

59. **Krause, D. C., and J. B. Baseman.** 1982. *Mycoplasma pneumoniae* proteins that selectively bind to host cells. *Infect. Immun.* **37:**382–386.

60. **Krause, D. C., and J. B. Baseman.** 1983. Inhibition of *Mycoplasma pneumoniae* hemadsorption and adherence to respiratory epithelium by antibodies to membrane protein. *Infect. Immun.* **39:**1180–1186.

61. **Krause, D. C., D. K. Leith, R. M. Wilson, and J. B. Baseman.** 1982. Identification of *Mycoplasma pneumoniae* proteins associated with hemadsorption and virulence. *Infect. Immun.* **35:**809–817.

62. **Krieg, N. R., and J. G. Holt (ed.).** 1984. *Bergey's Manual of Systematic Bacteriology*, vol 1. Williams & Wilkins, Baltimore.

63. **Leith, D. K., and J. B. Baseman.** 1984. Purification of a *Mycoplasma pneumoniae* adhesin by monoclonal antibody affinity chromatography. *J. Bacteriol.* **157:**678–680.

64. **Maniloff, J.** 1979. Mycoplasma gliding may be a biased Brownian motion. *J. Theor. Biol.* **81:**617–620.

65. **Maniloff, J.** 1981. Cytoskeletal elements in mycoplasmas and other prokaryotes. *BioSystems* **14:**305–312.

66. **Maniloff, J., and H. Morowitz.** 1967. Ultrastructure and life cycle of *Mycoplasma gallisepticum* A5969. *Ann. N.Y. Acad. Sci.* **143:**59–65.

67. **Maniloff, J., and H. J. Morowitz.** 1972. Cell biology of the mycoplasmas. *Bacteriol. Rev.* **36:**263–290.

68. **Maniloff, J., H. J. Morowitz, and R. J. Barrnett.** 1965. Ultrastructure and ribosomes of *Mycoplasma gallisepticum. J. Bacteriol.* **90:**193–204.

69. **Marshall, K. C., and R. H. Cruickshank.** 1973. Cell surface hydrophobicity and the orientation of certain bacteria at interfaces. *Arch. Microbiol.* **91:**29–40.

70. **Marshall, K. C., R. Stout, and R. Mitchell.** 1971. Mecha-

nism of initial events in the sorption of marine bacteria to surfaces. *J. Gen. Microbiol.* **68:**337–348.

71. **McVittie, A., and S. A. Zahler.** 1962. Chemotaxis in *Myxococcus. Nature* (London) **194:**1299–1300.

72. **Morowitz, H. J., and J. Maniloff.** 1966. Analysis of the life cycle of *Mycoplasma gallisepticum. J. Bacteriol.* **91:**1638–1644.

73. **Mouches, C., A. Menara, B. Geny, D. Charlemagne, and J. M. Bové.** 1982. Synthesis of *Spiroplasma citri* protein specifically recognized by rabbit immunoglobulin to rabbit actin. *Rev. Infect. Dis.* **4**(Suppl):S277.

73a.**Naumann, W.** 1988. Pathogenicity of *M. mobile* 163K for carps. Thesis. Tierärztliche Hochschule, Hannover, Germany.

74. **Neimark, H.** 1983. Mycoplasma and bacterial proteins resembling contractile proteins: a review. *Yale J. Biol. Med.* **56:**419–423.

75. **Neimark, H. C.** 1977. Extraction of an actin-like protein from the prokaryote *Mycoplasma pneumoniae. Proc. Natl. Acad. Sci. USA* **74:**4041–4045.

76. **Nelson, J. B.** 1960. The behavior of murine PPLO in Hela cell cultures. *Ann. N.Y. Acad. Sci.* **79:**450–457.

77. **Nelson, J. B., and M. J. Lyons.** 1965. Phase-contrast and electron microscopy of murine strain of mycoplasma. *J. Bacteriol.* **90:**1750–1763.

78. **Petrino, M. G., and R. N. Doetsch.** 1978. "Viscotaxis", a new behavioural response of *Leptospira interrogans* (*biflexa*) strain B16. *J. Gen. Microbiol.* **109:**113–117.

79. **Piper, B., R. Rosengarten, and H. Kirchhoff.** 1987. The influence of various substances on the gliding motility of *Mycoplasma mobile* 163K. *J. Gen. Microbiol.* **133:**3193–3198.

80. **Pollard, T. D., and J. A. Cooper.** 1986. Actin and actin-binding proteins. A critical evaluation of mechanisms and functions. *Annu. Rev. Biochem.* **55:**987–1035.

81. **Radestock, U., and W. Bredt.** 1977. Motility of *Mycoplasma pneumoniae. J. Bacteriol.* **129:**1495–1501.

82. **Razin, S.** 1985. Molecular biology and genetics of mycoplasmas (*Mollicutes*). *Microbiol. Rev.* **49:**419–459.

83. **Razin, S., and E. A. Freundt.** 1984. The mycoplasmas, p. 740–798. *In* N. R. Krieg and J. G. Holt (ed.), *Bergey's Manual of Systematic Bacteriology*, vol. 1, Williams & Wilkins, Baltimore.

84. **Reichenbach, H.** 1981. Taxonomy of the gliding bacteria. *Annu. Rev. Microbiol.* **35:**339–364.

85. **Roberts, A. M.** 1970. Motion of spermatozoa in fluid streams. *Nature* (London) **228:**375–376.

86. **Rodwell, A. W., J. E. Peterson, and E. S. Rodwell.** 1973. Nature of striated structures in mycoplasma. *Ann. N.Y. Acad. Sci.* **225:**190–200.

87. **Rodwell, A. W., J. E. Peterson, and E. S. Rodwell.** 1974. Rho structures. *Colloq. INSERM.* **33:**43–46.

88. **Rodwell, A. W., E. S. Rodwell, and D. B. Archer.** 1979. Mycoplasmas lack a protein which closely resembles α-actin. *FEMS Microbiol. Lett.* **5:**235–238.

89. **Rosenbusch, J., M. Fischer, and H. Kirchhoff.** 1990. An experimental system for the detection of chemotaxis of mycoplasmas. *Zentralbl. Bakteriol. Suppl.* **20:**645–646.

89a.**Rosengarten, R.** 1985. Morphologische und feinstrukturelle sowie wachstums- und bewegungsphysiologische Untersuchungen an einer gleitenden Mycoplasemenart (*Mycoplasma* sp. nov. Stamm 163K). Ph.D. thesis. Universität Hannover, Germany.

90. **Rosengarten, R., M. Fischer, H. Kirchhoff, G. Kerlen, and K.-H. Seack.** 1988. Transport of erythrocytes by gliding cells of *Mycoplasma mobile* 163K. *Curr. Microbiol.* **16:**253–257.

91. **Rosengarten, R., and H. Kirchhoff.** 1983. Morphological studies on *Spiroplasma mirum* strain SMCA grown on modified Hayflick medium. *Yale J. Biol. Med.* **56:**901.

92. **Rosengarten, R., and H. Kirchhoff.** 1987. Gliding motility of *Mycoplasma* sp. nov. strain 163K. *J. Bacteriol.* **169:**1891–1898.

93. **Rosengarten, R., and H. Kirchhoff.** 1988. Energetic aspects of the gliding motility of mycoplasmas. *Curr. Microbiol.* **16:**247–252.

94. **Rosengarten, R., and H. Kirchhoff.** 1989. Growth morphology of *Mycoplasma mobile* 163K on solid surfaces: reproduction, aggregation and microcolony formation. *Curr. Microbiol.* **18:**15–22.

95. **Rosengarten, R., H. Kirchhoff, and Institut für den wissenschlaftlichen Film.** 1988. *Mycoplasma mobile*—morphology, multiplication and gliding motility, Film C1670. Institut für den wissenschlaftlichen Film, Göttingen, Germany.

96. **Rosengarten, R., H. Kirchhoff, G. Kerlen, and K. H. Seack.** 1988. The surface layer of *Mycoplasma mobile* 163K and its possible relevance to cell cohesion and group motility. *J. Gen. Microbiol.* **134:**275–281.

97. **Rosengarten, R., A. Klein-Struckmeier, and H. Kirchhoff.** 1988. Rheotactic behavior of a gliding mycoplasma. *J. Bacteriol.* **170:**989–990.

98. **Schneider, W. R., and R. N. Doetsch.** 1974. Effect of viscosity on bacterial motility. *J. Bacteriol.* **117:**696–701.

99. **Simoneau, P., and J. Labarère.** 1990. Immunochemical identification of an actin-like protein from *Spiroplasma citri. Zentralbl. Bakteriol. Suppl.* **20:**927–931.

100. **Singer, S. J., and G. L. Nicolson.** 1972. The fluid mosaic model of the structure of the cell membrane. *Science* **175:**720–731.

101. **Sneath, P. H. A., N. S. Mair, M. E. Sharpe, and J. G. Holt (ed.).** 1986. *Bergey's Manual of Systematic Bacteriology*, vol 2. Williams & Wilkins, Baltimore.

102. **Sobeslavsky, O., B. Prescott, and R. M. Chanock.** 1968. Adsorption of *Mycoplasma pneumoniae* to neuraminic acid receptors of various cells and possible role in virulence. *J. Bacteriol.* **96:**695–705.

103. **Stadtländer, C., and H. Kirchhoff.** 1988. The effects of *Mycoplasma mobile* 163K on the ciliary epithelium of tracheal organ cultures. *Zentralbl. Bakteriol. Hyg. A* **269:**355–365.

104. **Stadtländer, C., and H. Kirchhoff.** 1989. Gill organ culture of rainbow trout, *Salmo gairdneri* Richardson: an experimental model for the study of pathogenicity of *Mycoplasma mobile* 163K. *J. Fish Dis.* **12:**79–86.

105. **Stadtländer, C., and H. Kirchhoff.** 1990. Surface parasitism of the fish mycoplasma *Mycoplasma mobile* 163K on tracheal epithelial cells. *Vet. Microbiol.* **21:**339–343.

106. **Stalheim, O. H. V., A. E. Ritchie, and R. F. Whitcomb.** 1978. Cultivation, serology, ultrastructure, and virus-like particles of Spiroplasma 277F. *Curr. Microbiol.* **1:**365–370.

107. **Tajama, M., T. Yagihashi, and Y. Miki.** 1982. Capsular material of *Mycoplasma gallisepticum* and its possible relevance to the pathogenic process. *Infect. Immun.* **36:**803–833.

108. **Taylor-Robinson, D., and W. Bredt.** 1983. Motility of *Mycoplasma* strain G37. *Yale J. Biol. Med.* **56:**910.

109. **Taylor-Robinson, D., and R. J. Manchee.** 1967. Sperm-adsorption and spermagglutination by mycoplasmas. *Nature* (London) **215:**484–487.

110. **Taylor-Robinson, D., J. G. Tully, and M. F. Barile.** 1985. Urethral infection in male chimpanzees produced experimentally by *Mycoplasma genitalium. Br. J. Exp. Pathol.* **66:**95–101.

111. **Townsend, R., and D. B. Archer.** 1983. A fibril protein antigen specific to *Spiroplasma. J. Gen. Microbiol.* **129:**199–206.

112. **Townsend, R., D. B. Archer, and K. A. Plaskitt.** 1980. Purification and preliminary characterization of spiroplasma fibrils. *J. Bacteriol* **142:**694–700.

113. **Townsend, R., P. G. Markham, K. A. Plaskitt, and M. J. Daniels.** 1977. Isolation and characterization of a non-helical strain of *Spiroplasma citri. J. Gen. Microbiol.* **100:**15–21.

114. **Townsend, R., and K. A. Plaskitt.** 1985. Immunogold

localization of p55-fibril protein and p25-spiralin in spiroplasma cells. *J. Gen. Microbiol.* **131:**983–992.

115. **Tully, J. G., D. Taylor-Robinson, D. L. Rose, R. M. Cole, and J. M. Bové.** 1983. *Mycoplasma genitalium*, a new species from the human urogenital tract. *Int. J. Syst. Bacteriol.* **33:**387–396.

116. **Tully, J. G., and R. F. Whitcomb (ed.).** 1979. *The Mycoplasmas*, vol. 2. *Human and Animal Mycoplasmas.* Academic Press, New York.

117. **Vaituzis, Z., and R. N. Doetsch.** 1969. Motility tracks: technique for quantitative study of bacterial movement. *Appl. Microbiol.* **17:**584–588.

118. **Wall, F., R. M. Pfister, and N. L. Somersom.** 1983. Freeze-fracture confirmation of the presence of a core in the specialized tip structure of *Mycoplasma pneumoniae. J. Bacteriol.* **154:**924–929.

119. **Watson, H. L., D. K. Blalock, and G. H. Cassel.** 1990. Relationship of hydrophobicity of the V-1 antigen of *Mycoplasma pulmonis* to adherence. *Zentralbl. Bakteriol. Suppl.* **20:**650–654.

120. **Weisburg, W. G., J. G. Tully, D. L. Rose, J. P. Petzel, H. Oyaizu, D. Yang, L. Mandelco, J. Sechrist, T. G. Lawrence, J. van Etten, J. Maniloff, and C. R. Woese.** 1989. A phylogenetic analysis of the mycoplasmas: basis for their classification. *J. Bacteriol.* **171:**6455–6467.

121. **Williamson, D. L.** 1974. Unusual fibrils from the spirochete-like sex ratio organism. *J. Bacteriol.* **117:**904–906.

122. **Williamson, D. L., D. I. Blaustein, R. J. C. Levine, and M. J. Elfvin.** 1979. Anti-actin-peroxidase staining of the helical wall-free prokaryote *Spiroplasma citri. Curr. Microbiol.* **2:**143–145.

123. **Williamson, D. L., P. R. Brink, and G. W. Zieve.** 1984. Spiroplasma fibrils. *Isr. J. Med. Sci.* **20:**830–835.

124. **Williamson, D. L., and R. F. Whitcomb.** 1974. Helical, wall-free prokaryotes in *Drosophila*, leafhoppers, and plants. *Colloq. INSERM* **33:**283–290.

125. **Wilson, M., and A. M. Collier.** 1976. Ultrastructural study of *Mycoplasma pneumoniae* in organ culture. *J. Bacteriol.* **125:**332–339.

IV. MACROMOLECULE BIOSYNTHESIS AND GENETICS

17. DNA Replication and Repair

JACQUES LABARÈRE

INTRODUCTION

Although the enzymatic systems and mechanisms involved in DNA replication and repair are well known in bacteria such as *Escherichia coli*, this is not the case for the mollicutes. Despite abundant experimental data, much remains to be discovered before a comparative model of such systems may be established for the mollicutes.

Cellular division, DNA replication machinery, and repair systems appear to be less complex than in most other bacteria with larger genomes. This simplicity is correlated with phylogenetic data that strongly support the notion that the mollicutes arose by degenerative evolution from gram-positive eubacteria and involved severe reduction of the genetic information that was present in the bacterial ancestors. Mycoplasmas lack a cell wall, many metabolic pathways, and probably a great part of the molecular genetic machinery, especially in the DNA replication and repair systems.

By cloning and sequencing of the genes which code for the replication and repair enzymes or for their reg-

ulation, mutants that are defective for these functions will provide more information as to how these mechanisms work in the mollicutes and how they compare with the models from *E. coli*.

DNA REPLICATION

Cellular Division and Replication

In most species of mollicutes, cell division and DNA replication are not closely coordinated (96). Cytoplasmic division lags behind genome replication, resulting in the formation of multinucleate filamentous organisms which later transform into chains of cocci by first constricting around each of the chromosomes and disintegrating into single cocci (88).

For *Spiroplasma citri*, which grows in in vitro cultures from short elementary helices into longer parental helices that divide by constriction to again produce elementary helices (37), Garnier et al. determined the growth pattern of the membrane in order to study its

Jacques Labarère • Laboratoire de Génétique Moléculaire, Unviersité de Bordeaux II–INRA, Centre de Recherches Agronomiques de Bordeaux, BP 81, 33883 Villenave d'Ornon Cedex, France.

role in DNA replication (9, 37, 38). The elongation observed around the constriction zone may play a role in the segregation of DNA strands in the newly formed elementary helices (8, 38). In the tissues or cells of their hosts, the morphology of spiroplasmas is less simple; nonhelical forms were found (22, 58). Labeling of the nonhelical forms of *S. citri* with tritiated thymidine indicated that spiroplasmal DNA replication occurred within the insect cell; this is in contrast to the situation observed in vitro, where DNA replication occurred only in helical forms (9).

In *Mycoplasma gallisepticum*, cell division by binary fission is synchronous with DNA replication (84). Maniloff and Quinlan (65) showed that *M. gallisepticum* has specialized polar subcellular organelles consisting of a terminal bleb structure and an infrableb area connecting the bleb to the rest of the cell. Replication of these polar structures during the cell cycle leads to the cytologic appearance of a type of primitive mitotic cell division cycle (65). These authors then isolated a subcellular fraction (designated P2) which contains the DNA replication complex (66). Sonic treatment further fractionated the cell ghost and allowed partial purification, on sucrose density gradients, of a DNA replication complex attached to the cells' polar membrane-bleb-infrableb structures (66, 83, 84). The attachment of the DNA growing point to this area indicates that as for bacteria, membrane synthesis could act to segregate the DNA genome during division of the organism (66).

Replication Mechanism

In *Acholeplasma laidlawii* B, early work of Smith demonstrated that DNA replication is very similar to that observed in other bacteria (104). DNA replication of this species is semiconservative, proceeding unidirectionally from, at most, a few growing points. DNA which is replicated near the beginning of one generation is also preferentially replicated near the beginning of the following generation, supporting the notion of a sequential mode of replication. Results also suggest a less stable replication complex in *A. laidlawii* than in *E. coli* or *Bacillus subtilis*. It seems that the replication mechanism is less efficient in *A. laidlawii* than in other bacteria; nevertheless, results strongly suggest that *A. laidlawii* DNA is replicated throughout the generation time. Smith and Hanawalt also demonstrated the existence of a nonconservative DNA replication: about 1% of the *A. laidlawii* chromosome turns over per generation time (105).

Rodwell et al. (96) compared the labeling of lipids of *M. mycoides* in the part of the membrane to which DNA is attached with the labeling of lipids in the entire membrane. They found that there is no evidence for local lipid synthesis in this part of the membrane, but they considered their experiments inconclusive because of the high probability of lipid redistribution.

Using electron microscopy, Miyata and Fukumura (73) observed *M. capricolum* DNA-membrane complexes composed of cell ghosts or cell membrane fragments with short DNA fragments attached to them. The genomic DNA was found to be attached to the cell membrane at many sites which were distributed over the genome (60). It was hypothesized that only a few binding sites are involved in DNA replication, and the many other sites must therefore serve other functions, such as DNA segregation (60).

Wang et al. have localized the DNA replication origin region in the *M. capricolum* genome by using synchronous cultures of mutants and wild-type strains. DNA labeling experiments with a temperature-sensitive initiation-defective mutant suggested that the replication origin is located in a region composed of *Bam*HI fragments B8 and B9 and that the terminus is located in fragment B3 (112). They also showed that in wild-type cells, chloramphenicol inhibits the synthesis of a protein which is necessary for the initiation of DNA replication from the origin (112).

DNA Polymerases in Mollicutes

Although the DNA replication machinery is well known in *E. coli* and other procaryotes, the only well-characterized components of the DNA replication complex in mollicutes are the DNA polymerases. The number of DNA polymerases characterized varies with the family studied.

The early work of Mills et al. (69) demonstrated a single DNA polymerase in *M. orale* and *M. hyorhinis*; after partial purification, the molecular mass was 130 kDa and the enzyme had no exonuclease activity. The DNA polymerase of *M. orale* was fully purified and characterized by Boxer and Korn (12), who showed that this enzyme consists of a single protein of 116 kDa, possesses the catalytic properties exhibited by the eubacterial DNA polymerases, and is completely devoid of exo- and endo-DNase activities. The DNA polymerase of *M. orale* resembles *E. coli* polymerase I, but no $3' \rightarrow 5'$ exonuclease activity was demonstrated, so the nature of a proofreading function is unclear. By Coomassie blue staining, only a single protein band was observed for *M. orale* (molecular mass, 103 kDa) (12). The *M. mycoides* enzyme contained a major peptide with a molecular mass of 98 kDa and three smaller peptides (67). It seems well established that *Mycoplasma* species have only one DNA polymerase. The single enzyme described in *M. hyorhinis* and in *M. mycoides* is similar to the enzyme of *M. orale* (67, 69); however, the *M. mycoides* enzyme was strongly inhibited by N-ethylmaleimide (NEM), whereas the *M. orale* DNA polymerase was only weakly affected.

DNA polymerases of three species of mollicutes were isolated and characterized by Charron et al. (17, 18). They isolated first two (17) and then three (20) DNA polymerases in *S. citri* R8A2, in *S. melliferum* BC-3, and in *S. floricola* BNR1.

More complete investigation of the number and characteristics of these enzymes was undertaken by Maurel et al. (67); they confirmed the existence of a single DNA polymerase in *M. orale* and also demonstrated a single enzyme in *M. mycoides* and in *Ureaplasma urealyticum* (14, 67). In the genus *Acholeplasma*, three DNA polymerases were characterized (*Apol*1, *Apol*2, and *Apol*3); they were always detectable in *A. laidlawii* extracts but not always in extracts from *A. equifetale* and *A. oculi*, probably because of a too-weak specific activity. In *A. laidlawii*, a 142-kDa polypeptide was associated with *Apol*3 activity and 96-kDa polypeptide was associated with *Apol*2 activity (67).

Chromatographic, Catalytic, and Physical Properties of DNA Polymerases

Catalytic and physical properties of DNA polymerases have been studied by the Bébéar group (17, 18, 66a, 67), by Mills et al. (69), and by Boxer and Korn (12) and are summarized in Table 1.

DEAE-cellulose chromatography

The three DNA polymerases of *S. citri* (*Sc*A, *Sc*B, and *Sc*C) and of *S. floricola* (*Sf*A, *Sf*B, and *Sf*C) have different elution properties on DEAE-cellulose. *Sc*B and *Sf*A are not retained, and the others are retained with different affinities (20). *Apo*l1 of *A. laidlawii* is not retained on DEAE-cellulose, and in this way it resembles spiroplasma enzymes *Sc*B and *Sf*A. The *U. urealyticum* enzyme was retained on a DEAE-cellulose column, whereas the single enzymes of *M. orale* and *M. mycoides* were not (14, 67).

DNA-cellulose chromatography

The DNA polymerase from *U. urealyticum* is more strongly retained on a DNA-cellulose column than is that of *M. orale* or *M. hyorhinis* (67, 69). *Apo*l2 also has a very high affinity for DNA-cellulose (0.5 M KCl), which is probably the reason for the poor separation of this enzyme unless high-ionic-strength treatment is applied before extraction and cellular fractionation (67).

Sedimentation velocity

The sedimentation coefficient for the DNA polymerase from *M. mycoides* (98 kDa) is 4.7S, while that for the analogous enzyme from *M. orale* (103 kDa) is 5.2S (67). For the latter, the value estimated by Boxer and Korn is 5.6S (12), and its molecular mass is 116 kDa. In the DNA polymerase preparation from *M. orale*, silver nitrate staining shows several bands. Maurel et al. have shown that the DNA polymerase activity is related to the major band at 103 kDa (67). Only indirect evidence, such as the serological relationship with the major band from *M. orale* at 103 kDa, suggests that the DNA polymerase activity of *M. mycoides* is related to its major band at 98 kDa.

The sedimentation coefficient for the DNA polymerase from *U. urealyticum* is 5.9S, a value which suggests either a higher molecular weight than that of mycoplasma polymerases or an asymmetric protein conformation. Although we have no precise data on the molecular weight of this enzyme, the DNA polymerase activity appears to be linked to a 135-kDa polypeptide (67).

For *A. laidlawii*, the DNA polymerase sedimentation coefficients are 6S for *Apo*l1, 5S for *Apo*l2, and 6.4S for *Apo*l3, which correlates with their molecular masses of 100, 96, and 142 kDa, respectively.

There are not sufficient data to calculate the molecular masses of *S. citri* polymerases, but the molecular masses for mollicute DNA polymerases are generally close to those for DNA polymerase I from *E. coli* (109 kDa) or *B. subtilis* (115 kDa) and subunit A of DNA polymerase III from *E. coli* (132 kDa).

Sensitivity to NEM

*Sc*A, *Sf*A, and *Apo*l2 are not inhibited by NEM, a reagent that binds to SH groups of proteins. The DNA polymerases of *M. orale* and *Apo*l3 are slightly inhibited by NEM, whereas all other DNA polymerases are NEM sensitive (14, 17, 18, 67).

Effect of ethanol

*Apo*l1 and *Apo*l3 are highly stimulated by 10% ethanol, which may indicate their linkage to a hydrophobic part of the membrane. *Sc*A and *Sf*A are slightly stimulated by ethanol. DNA polymerases of *Mycoplasma* and *Ureaplasma* species are not sensitive or are weakly sensitive to ethanol (67), whereas the other DNA polymerases (*Sc*B, *Sc*C, *Sf*B, *Sf*C, and *Apo*l2) are inhibited by ethanol (17, 18, 67).

Effect of KCl

When the template in the DNA polymerase reaction mixture is poly(dA)-oligo(dT)$_{12}$, the *Sc*B and *Sc*C activities are inhibited by KCl. *Sc*B is more sensitive than *Sc*C, whereas the *Sc*A activity seems weakly stimulated at 25 mM KCl before being inhibited at higher concentrations (17, 18). On the other hand, with activated DNA or poly(dA-dT) as the template, a stimulatory effect is exerted on *Sc*A and *Sc*B at 80 to 100 mM KCl; with activated DNA, this stimulation could be increased by a factor of 3 (17).

Whatever the template in the reaction mixture, *Apo*l1 is always inhibited by KCl, while *Apo*l2 is stimulated at 50 mM with poly(dA)-oligo(dT)$_{12-18}$ and at 150 mM with activated DNA. *Apo*l3 is highly stimulated at moderate molarities of KCl before being inhibited as these molarities increase (67).

The *M. mycoides* enzyme is more sensitive to inhibition by KCl than are the *M. orale* and *U. urealyticum* polymerases. The *U. urealyticum* polymerase is stimulated at 100 mM KCl when the template is activated DNA (67).

Thermal sensitivity

In *S. citri*, *Sc*B is heat resistant, as is enzyme *Sf*A in *S. floricola* (18). In *A. laidlawii*, the heat-resistant enzyme is *Apo*l1. The DNA polymerases of *Mycoplasma* species seem to be heat resistant, whereas the DNA polymerase of *U. urealyticum* is slightly heat sensitive (67).

Exonuclease Activities Associated with DNA Polymerases

3'→5' exonuclease activities

Early studies on the DNA polymerases of *M. orale* and *M. hyorhinis* (11, 12, 70) did not show any exonuclease activity associated with their DNA polymerase activities. However, Maurel et al. (67) demonstrated 3'→5' exonuclease activity in DNA polymerase preparations from *M. mycoides* and *M. orale*. Among these activities is the capability of hydrolyzing double-stranded substrate in the presence of dTTP. A 3'→5'

Table 1. Properties of DNA polymerases in mollicutes

Property	S. citri			S. floricola			M. mycoides	M. orale	U. urealyticum	A. laidlawii		
	ScA	ScB	ScC	SfA	SfB	SfC				Apol1	Apol2	Apol3
Molecular mass (kDa)							98	103		100	96	142
Sedimentation velocity	6.3S	4.4S	4.5S				4.7S	5.2S	5.9S	6S	5S	6.4S
Thermal sensitivity (% of optimal) 46°C	62	100	22	100	35	52	95	100	70	100	33	18
49°C									70	50		
Affinity to DEAE-cellulose (M KCl for elution)	0.09	Not retained	0.30	Not retained	0.09	0.032	Not retained	Not retained	0.17	Not retained	0.15	0.28
Affinity to DNA-cellulose (M KCl for elution)	0.18	0.31	0.32	0.10	0.36	0.35	0.30	0.23	0.42	0.18	0.50	0.25
pH optimum range	8.1–8.2	8.1–8.3					7.5–8.5	7.5–8.5	7.0–7.5	8.1–8.7	7.7–8.5	8.1–8.5
Effect of KCl (% of optimal) 0 mM	95	100	100	100	100	100	100	95	100	100	84	49
25 mM	100	55	83	99	66	71	80	100	75	40	95	100
50 mM	65	25	65	89	51	54	35	78	48	10	100	81
100 mM	8	5	10	11	22	19	5	30	24	2	69	17
$MgCl$ (optimal concn [mM])	8	5	5	8	6	4	7.5–10	7.5–10	2.5–7.5	2.5–5	5–10	2.5
Inhibition by NEM	No	Yes	Yes	No	Yes	Yes	Yes	Weak	Yes	Yes	No	Weak
Effect of 10% ethanol (% of optimal)	115	30	60	115	49	78	100	95	90	240	85	600
Template primer [% relative to poly(dA)-oligo(dT)$_{12-18}$ taken as 100%] Activated DNA	90–130	16.5	11.5				65	81	32	175	28	270
Poly(dA-dT)	70–100	20–40	27	105	25	40	150	120	31	90	13	149
Poly(rA)-oligo(dT)[a]	1.5	1	1.3	1.2	2	1.3	2	1	8	1	11	1

[a] Poly(rA)-oligo(dT)$_{12-18}$ for Mycoplasma, Ureaplasma, and Acholeplasma species; poly(rA)-oligo(dT)$_{10}$ for Spiroplasma species.

exonuclease activity was also detected in the DNA polymerase preparation obtained from *U. urealyticum* as well as in the three DNA polymerases purified from *A. laidlawii* (67). However, Maurel et al. also showed that for *M. mycoides*, *M. orale*, and *A. laidlawii Apol*2, the $3'{\rightarrow}5'$ exonuclease and DNA polymerase activities were associated with two different polypeptides. This situation is comparable to that observed in the replicative enzyme of *E. coli*, DNA polymerase III holoenzyme, in which two subunits, the α subunit and the ϵ subunit, are responsible for DNA synthesis and for $3'{\rightarrow}5'$ exonuclease activities. However, whereas DNA polymerase and $3'{\rightarrow}5'$ exonuclease activities were separated in mycoplasma enzymes by nondenaturing polyacrylamide gel electrophoresis (PAGE), the subunits of the *E. coli* holoenzyme core comigrated when examined under the same conditions (67, 68, 82).

$5'{\rightarrow}3'$ exonuclease activities

In *M. mycoides*, Maurel et al. have found strong $5'{\rightarrow}3'$ exonuclease activity regardless of the template used (67). The nature of this activity has not yet been determined, but it seems to be related to a contaminant from the purification process rather than an activity of the DNA polymerase itself (67). No such activity has been observed in *M. orale* (12, 67).

The DNA polymerase from *U. urealyticum* appears to have some $5'{\rightarrow}3'$ exonuclease activity; however, it cannot yet be demonstrated reproducibly and does not seem to be closely associated with the activity of DNA polymerase (66a).

$5'{\rightarrow}3'$ exonuclease activity has been demonstrated for all three DNA polymerases for *A. laidlawii*; *Apol*1 prefers a single-stranded substrate, while *Apol*2 requires a double-stranded structure in order to hydrolyze its substrate (66a). In any case, there is no proof that the exonuclease activities found in mollicutes are intrinsic to their DNA polymerases rather than the products of contaminants.

Relationships between DNA Polymerases

S. melliferum BC-3 is serologically related to *S. citri*. Both spiroplasmas are members of serogroup I, *S. citri* representing subgroup I-1 and BC-3 representing subgroup I-2; *S. floricola* BNR1 is a member of serogroup III (48). Interestingly, each of the three DNA polymerases of *S. melliferum* seems to be similar to the respective enzyme of *S. citri* (8). However, the DNA polymerases of *S. floricola* show some differences from those of *S. citri*. The A enzyme isolated from *S. citri* or from *S. melliferum* was retained on DEAE-cellulose and required 0.09 M KCl for elution, whereas the enzyme from *S. floricola* was not retained. Furthermore, the heat-resistant enzyme is ScB in *S. citri*, whereas it is SfA in *S. floricola* (18).

The activity of the *M. orale* DNA polymerase was completely inhibited by homologous immune serum directed against this enzyme in amounts as small as 2 μg of protein (512-fold dilution), while undiluted preimmune serum had no effect. The *M. mycoides* DNA polymerase activity was not affected by anti-*M. orale* DNA polymerase immune serum (67). However, when the serological relationships are examined by immunoblotting, the immune serum directed against *M. orale* DNA polymerase detected not only the homologous enzyme but also the *M. mycoides* enzyme, thus demonstrating a serological relationship between the two polymerases (67).

In *Mycoplasma* and *Ureaplasma* species, DNA polymerases show a homogeneity of characteristics. The most important difference between *U. urealyticum* and *Mycoplasma* DNA polymerases was their chromatographic behavior on DEAE-cellulose columns: the *Ureaplasma* enzyme was retained, whereas the *Mycoplasma* enzyme was not. Moreover, an interesting property of *Ureaplasma* DNA polymerase was its optimal pH range (7.0 to 7.5), clearly lower than the optimal pH values for the other mycoplasma DNA polymerases studied (14).

None of the three DNA polymerases of *A. laidlawii* are affected by immune serum directed against the *M. orale* enzyme. Furthermore, immunoblotting did not detect any serological relationship between *A. laidlawii* and *M. orale* DNA polymerases (67). Antibodies against *Apol*1 and *Apol*2, produced in rabbits, inhibited the homologous DNA polymerase activity, but there was no heterologous cross-reaction. Similarly, there was no inhibition of *Spiroplasma* polymerase *Sc*B or of the single *M. orale* DNA polymerase by antibodies against *Apol*1 and *Apol*2 (67).

Comparison of mollicute DNA polymerases does not permit distinction between those from one genus and those from another. Thus, it is not possible to attribute precise roles in the cellular machinery to them, as has been done for *E. coli*. The *Sc*A enzyme resembles DNA polymerase I of *E. coli*, and *Sc*B is reminiscent of DNA polymerase III (inhibition by NEM and KCl, insensitivity to arabinosyl-CTP). In wild-type *E. coli*, the amount of polymerase I is far greater than that of polymerase III; with *S. citri*, there seem to be approximately the same amounts of *Sc*A and *Sc*B (17).

Nucleases

The existence of nucleases which hydrolyze DNA was first established by Razin et al. (91). Although not yet demonstrated, the endogenous nucleases of mollicutes may have functions in DNA repair and genetic recombination in addition to their role in restricting foreign DNA (see chapter 18).

Nucleases in acholeplasmas

All extracts of several acholeplasmas (*A. laidlawii* B and *A. equifetale*) and mycoplasmas (*M. arthritidis*, *M. pulmonis*, and *M. pneumoniae*) have DNase and endonuclease activities (81, 97). Using sucrose gradient centrifugation, Pollack and Hoffman found two to five peaks of endonuclease activity in *A. laidlawii* B (81). The variety of DNases in acholeplasmas has been verified by electrophoretic analysis of cell protein extracts from seven *Acholeplasma* species in agar gels containing DNA. Each species yielded a specific pattern of DNase-containing bands (97).

Maniloff and coworkers have reported that *A. laidlawii* K2 and JA1 are able to phenotypically modify and restrict mycoplasma viruses L2 (31, 63), L172 (32), and L51 (103). The *A. laidlawii* K2 cellular DNA and the L2 and L172 DNAs from virus grown on strain K2 contain both N^6-methyladenine (M^6Ade) and 5-methylcytosine (m^5Cyt), (32, 63), the latter in the nucleotide sequence GATC (32, 63). L51 DNA from virus grown on K2 also possesses GATm^{5}C (103). Sladek et al. have shown that *A. laidlawii* K2 restricts viral DNA containing the GATC sequence but does not restrict viral DNA containing the methylated sequence GATm^{5}C (103). They proposed that K2 possesses a restriction endonuclease that recognizes the GATC sequence and cleaves the DNA, but does not cleave it when the sequence contains m^{5}Cyt. Therefore, they hypothesized that K2 cells must also have a complementary methylating enzyme that methylates cytosine in the GATC sequence (103).

By contrast, *A. laidlawii* cellular DNA and L2 DNA from virus grown on JA1 contain no detectable methylated bases (32), but strain JA1 restricts viruses grown on strain K2 (31, 32, 63, 101, 103) and is able to restrict DNA containing m^{5}Cyt (103). Sladek and Maniloff demonstrated that JA1 possesses endonuclease activity (102). The partially purified enzyme cleaves not only DNA containing m^{5}Cyt but also DNA containing no methylated bases. One possible way to explain this unexpected result is that the JA1 endonuclease is a multisubunit enzyme containing one or more subunits which confer the specificity for DNA which contains methylcytosine, but this subunit(s) might become dissociated during purification (102).

Nucleases in spiroplasmas

The site-specific endonuclease *Sci*NI has been partially purified from *S. citri* by Stephens (108). This enzyme is an isoschizomer of *Hha*I, recognizes the sequence 5'GCGC-3', and cleaves between the first G and the adjacent C (whereas *Hha*I cleaves between the second G and the adjacent C). However, no correlation has been established between the *Sci*NI activity and restriction-modification systems, which strongly suggests the existence of other site-specific endonucleases in this organism.

Nucleases in mycoplasmas

Nuclease activity located in *M. pulmonis* membranes was first observed by Minion and Goguen (70). They proposed that this activity might be involved in the uptake of nucleic acid precursors from the environment and therefore might serve a vital function in the pathogenesis of this species. Linear DNA rather than supercoiled DNA was the preferred template for this nuclease, suggesting a strong exonuclease activity. The activity of the membrane nuclease was increased approximately 32-fold with the addition of 2.5 mM calcium and about 128-fold with the addition of 2.5 mM magnesium (71).

Minion and Tigges studied 11 strains of *M. pulmonis* and 14 species of mycoplasmas (71). All strains and species tested possessed nuclease activity but at various levels. The activity was low in *M. pulmonis* 5782 and UATB and in *A. laidlawii* PG8. The strongest activity was found in *M. pulmonis* PG34 and UABCT and in *M. bovis*, *M. bovoculi*, and *M. capricolum*. The sodium dodecyl sulfate-PAGE profiles of these species showed the presence of multiple nuclease bands with a diver-

sity of molecular weights in all mycoplasmal preparations (71).

TYPES OF DNA DAMAGE

Agents That Damage DNA

DNA damage in microorganisms is a complex, multistep process initiated by physicochemical attack on cells by radiation or chemicals to form various types of stable premutational lesions in DNA.

Nitrosoguanidine (*N*-methyl-*N*'-nitro-*N*-nitrosoguanidine), acriflavine, UV light, and gamma radiation have been used as mutagenic agents in mollicutes and to study DNA damage and repair.

DNA damage is easily estimated by survival curves obtained after action of the mutagenic agents. The most interesting findings are obtained with the survival curves after UV irradiation. These curves exhibit a shoulder followed by exponential inactivation or killing (1, 53, 54).

Nitrosoguanidine

Nitrosoguanidine is a highly mutagenic agent which often simultaneously induces mutations in several closely linked genes (41). As a consequence, clones selected for mutation in one gene have increased probabilities of carrying mutations in nearby genes. Nitrosoguanidine action also triggers repair activity (15). Repair plays an important role in survival after nitrosoguanidine treatment: error-prone repair is responsible for some of the mutations induced in stationary, starved cells (46). Nitrosoguanidine also induces an error-free repair mechanism, which in *E. coli* may involve DNA polymerase II and counteract both the lethal and mutagenic effects of the mutagenic agent (72). The advantage of nitrosoguanidine for sequential mutagenesis lies in the high mutation and survival rates obtained with well-synchronized cultures (16).

Nitrosoguanidine was used as a mutagenic agent in the search for hemadsorption-negative (HA$^-$) mutants of *M. pneumoniae* (35, 43), temperature-sensitive mutants of *M. pneumoniae* (107) and *M. gallisepticum* (55), and immunolysis-resistant mutants of *A. laidlawii* (21). The increases in the frequency of mutation obtained with nitrosoguanidine were of the same order of magnitude as those reported for other procaryotes (89).

Various experimental conditions were used for the mutation of mollicutes by nitrosoguanidine. Mugharbil and Cirillo incubated *M. capricolum* for 2 h in the presence of 100 µg of nitrosoguanidine per ml to obtain methylmannoside-resistant mutants (74). Liss incubated *A. laidlawii* for 30 min in the presence of 50 µg of nitrosoguanidine per ml to obtain conditional lethal mutants (56).

Acriflavine

Acriflavine hydrochloride was used by Chaudhuri et al. to study photodynamic inactivation and its repair in *Acholeplasma* and *Mycoplasma* species (19). For treatment, exponentially growing cells were harvested by centrifugation and resuspended to a final titer of 1

$\times$ 10^8 to 2 $\times$ 10^8 CFU/ml in buffer containing acriflavine at final concentrations of 0.5 to 10 µg/ml. Exposure to light resulted in photodynamic inactivation: loss in viability due to single-strand DNA breaks. *M. gallisepticum* is more sensitive than *A. laidlawii* to photodynamic inactivation (17).

Gamma radiation

Chelton et al. studied the sensitivity of *M. mycoides* subsp. *capri* to gamma radiation (20). The dose-response curve for the control cells is essentially linear over a dose range of 0 to 40 krad, with the cell viability decreasing by 20% for each 10 krad of irradiation. Incorporation of 5-bromouracil into DNA of this species is accompanied by an increase in the sensitivity of the organism to gamma radiation, as is generally the case with other organisms. When *M. mycoides* subsp. *capri* was grown in the presence of the analog 5-vinyluracil, it showed a threefold increase in sensitivity to gamma irradiation at 15 krad (20).

UV radiation

UV-induced pyrimidine dimers are a well-known class of lesions in procaryotic cells. Normally, a large fraction of these dimers, which are potentially lethal, are removed soon after irradiation by some mode of error-free repair. Premutational lesions, which escape error-free repair, may undergo a process of fixation or conversion to an informationally altered DNA base sequence through some mode of error-prone repair or recombination for which replication or protein synthesis may be required (33). UV-induced DNA damage also induces a variety of other processes, such as enhanced postreplication repair, inhibition of cell division, and prophage induction (59).

In *E. coli*, three operationally different regions of the UV radiation-induced mutation frequency response (MFR) curve have been identified. At the lowest fluences, the MFR curve is nonlinear and is probably proportional to the square of the fluence. This finding suggests a two-hit mechanism; one is a lesion blocking the synthesis of DNA and inducing SOS error-prone repair, and the other is assumed to be a premutational lesion. At intermediate fluences, the MFR curve is linear. This observation suggests that all cells in the population had received sufficient radiation for the full induction of error-prone repair, and thus premutational lesions produce mutations with one-hit kinetics. The third region shows an increased rate of mutagenesis, which suggests the induction of two lesions in proximity that result in additional mutations. This region was thought to reflect the increasing importance of two interacting lesions, such as overlapping daughter strand gaps (30, 100).

Mollicutes are more sensitive to UV irradiation than are other procaryotes (20, 36, 53, 54, 64). The A + T-rich genome of mollicutes could be expected to increase their sensitivity to UV irradiation because of the greater likelihood of thymidine dimerization (90). The mollicute most sensitive to UV irradiation seems to be *S. citri* (3, 54). It also appears to be more sensitive than other well-studied wild-type microorganisms: a surviving fraction of 0.1 is obtained in strain R8A2 with UV doses of 11, 8, and 6 J/m^2 for cells in the middle logarithmic, late logarithmic, and stationary phases of growth, respectively (54). Such a survival fraction is obtained with about 40 J/m^2 in *E. coli* (30), *M. gallisepticum* (39), and *A. laidlawii* (23, 39) or with 80 J/m^2 in *Saccharomyces cerevisiae* (44). In the same way, UV radiation has a high mutagenic effect on *S. citri* cells. For example, a UV fluence of 10 J/m^2 increased the spontaneous mutation frequency to xylitol resistance by a factor of 2,500. In *E. coli*, by comparison, 10 J/m^2 increases the frequency of spontaneous mutation from tryptophan auxotrophy to prototrophy only about 40-fold (30).

UV Sensitivity during Growth

A. laidlawii

Das et al. studied UV sensitivity of *A. laidlawii* B at various phases of the growth cycle (23). All survival curves have an initial shoulder and then are exponential. UV sensitivity increases with culture age and then decreases; maximum sensitivity was observed for cells collected at 14 to 22 h of growth, that is, from the middle to the late logarithmic phases of growth. This finding suggests that as in other microorganisms, the repair enzyme(s) concentration varies with growth in response to physiological changes in cellular metabolism (23, 29).

S. citri

In *S. citri*, survival curves of cells at different phases of growth have similar patterns (54). Labarère and Barroso (54) distinguished four parts for each curve: (i) an initial shoulder, (ii) an exponential decrease, (iii) a plateau, and (iv) a new exponential decrease. They can be grouped in two parts of classical appearance consisting of an initial shoulder followed by an exponential decrease (54). The same biphasic curves were also reported by Aoki et al. for human mycoplasmas (1), which suggests heterogeneity of the UV susceptibility in the cell population.

The second part of the survival curve in *S. citri* involves 10^{-3} to 10^{-4} of the cells that seem to be less sensitive to UV irradiation. The difference observed in UV sensitivity may be related to physiological rather than genetic differences (54).

For *S. citri*, only the slopes of the first linear part of the curves vary, indicating that the UV sensitivity of the organisms increases with culture age. The values of these slopes are 0.26 m^2/J for the middle logarithmic phase, 0.35 m^2/J for the late logarithmic phase, and 0.40 m^2/J for the stationary phase. Concomitantly, the mutagenic effect of UV irradiation clearly increases with the age of the organisms (54).

Methods for Mutagenesis

UV radiation

Cells used must be in the logarithmic phase of growth. Generally 20 ml of a culture (5 $\times$ 10^8 CFU/ml) is centrifuged, resuspended in 10 ml of UV buffer, and incubated for 20 min at room temperature. The UV buffer used by Labarère and Barroso is a phosphate buffer (pH 7.6) with 20 mM MgSO$_4$, 200 mM NaCl, 10^3 U of penicillin G per ml, and 50 Kunitz units of DNase I per ml (54). It is necessary to add DNase to all washed cell suspensions to eliminate the highly viscous cellular DNA released from broken cells (99). The cells are then centrifuged and incubated again under the same conditions.

Samples of 10 ml containing approximately 10^9 CFU/ml are irradiated in 50-mm uncovered petri dishes with constant magnetic stirring during UV exposure to allow effective irradiation of the organisms. The total UV fluence received by the cells (F) is calculated for each exposure time (T), using the formula $F = aT^2 + bx$ (a and b are parameters determined by lamp calibration), and UV radiation fluence rates are expressed in joules per square meter. Throughout all UV irradiation steps and mutant recovery, it is necessary to use yellow light to avoid photoreactivation (53, 54).

Nitrosoguanidine

Cells in the exponential growth phase were centrifuged, and the pellet was resuspended in liquid nutrient medium (10^9 CFU/ml) and incubated for 10 to 30 min, with nitrosoguanidine at the optimal growth temperature. Using 50 μg of nitrosoguanidine per ml and incubation at 37°C for 30 min, Liss obtained 50% cell death and optimal mutagenesis for *A. laidlawii* JA1 (56). Mugharbil and Cirillo used 100 μg of nitrosoguanidine per ml and incubated cells for 2 h at 37°C (74). Nitrosoguanidine has maximum stability in solution at about pH 5, but there is no evidence that this is the best pH for mutagenesis. Mutagenesis with nitrosoguanidine seems to be quantitatively related to the release of an unstable, mutagenic intermediate of nitrosoguanidine decomposition. Nitrosoguanidine is generally used at alkaline pH (26). After treatment, cells are harvested and washed three times in 5 volumes of liquid medium containing DNase. Abundant washing is important to completely eliminate the mutagenic agent and avoid accumulation of mutations in the organism.

Induced Mutants in Mollicutes

For selection of mutants, one problem related to mollicutes is that the complexity of the culture medium prevents isolation of auxotrophic or metabolic mutants. It is also difficult to select chromosomal antibiotic-resistant or amino acid analog-resistant mutants because of the frequency of extrachromosomal antibiotic resistant or amino acid analog-resistant mutants because of the frequency of extrachromosomal antibiotic resistance genes (47) and large amounts of competitive amino acids in the culture medium (10, 53).

Mutants in acholeplasmas

In *A. laidlawii*, after mutagenesis by nitrosoguanidine and plating on 2,3,5-triphenyltetrazolium bromide indicator agar containing glucose, Tarshis et al.

isolated a mutant strain defective in glucose transport (109).

Liss developed a technique for selecting conditional lethal mutants after mutagenesis by nitrosoguanidine (56). The method is based on growth of mycoplasmas on membrane filters and use of the replica plating technique. He obtained temperature-sensitive mutants of *A. laidlawii* that were able to grow at the permissive temperature of 30°C but not at the nonpermissive temperature of 38 and 22°C. The frequency of mutants was 10^{-4} for conditional lethal mutants at 38°C (compared with the spontaneous mutation frequency of 10^{-7}) and 10^{-6} for conditional lethal mutants at 22°C (compared with the spontaneous mutation frequency of 10^{-8}) (56).

Mutants in mycoplasmas

Avirulent HA$^-$ mutants were isolated from *M. pneumoniae* (35, 43). Changes in the mutants include loss of the specific external protein P1 and morphological changes at the tip terminus structure (5). The rate of spontaneous appearance of HA$^-$ mutants is so high (7 × 10^{-3}) that their definition as mutants has been questioned (51, 89). Feldner and Bredt reported that many of their nitrosoguanidine-induced HA$^-$ *M. pneumoniae* mutants reverted spontaneously to HA$^+$ during cloning, again casting doubts about their being true mutants (35). Temperature-sensitive mutants of *M. pneumoniae* were obtained by Steinberg et al. (107), and temperature-sensitive mutants of *M. gallisepticum* were obtained by Lam et al. (55). In *M. capricolum*, methylmannoside-resistant mutants were obtained after mutagenesis by nitrosoguanidine. These mutants grew on fructose but not on glucose and were defective in the phosphoenolpyruvate:sugar phosphotransferase system for glucose (74).

Mutants in spiroplasmas

UV irradiation was used by Labarère and Barroso to induce mutants in *S. citri* (53, 54). Toxic agent resistant (i.e., xylitol- and arsenic acid-resistant) mutants have been obtained. MFR curves for xylitol-resistant and arsenic acid-resistant mutants were linear for doses from 5 to 9 J/m^2, while nonlinear responses were observed outside these values. The nonlinear responses can reflect the existence of multihit processes in mutation fixation (53).

DNA REPAIR

Some Descriptive Terminology in the Field of DNA Repair

Repair of undamaged templates

DNA polymerases influence correct base pair formation during DNA synthesis prior to proofreading (60). Biochemical and genetic evidence supports the idea that the 3′→5′ exonuclease activities associated with *E. coli* polymerases play editing or proofreading roles to remove newly incorporated bases which pair improperly (34). When mismatched bases survive proofreading, they can still be removed via the methyl-instructed mismatch repair systems.

Repair of damaged templates

Injury to DNA is minimized by damage containment systems, and the measured spontaneous or induced mutation rates reflect the balance between damaging events and corrections or miscorrections. The efficiencies of such DNA repair systems are themselves subject to evolutionary pressures, and the rate of evolution of a species may be coupled to the efficiency and discrimination of its repair processes. Five types of systems can repair DNA damage.

Enzymatic photoreactivation. Enzymatic photoreactivation reverses the thymine dimerization of DNA. The process depends on a light-dependent DNA photolyase. This phenomenon should not be confused with a number of other light-dependent processes that do not involve enzymes and by which pyrimidine dimers can be monomerized (for example, direct photoreversal and sensitized photoreversal).

Excision-repair. Excision repair, a dark repair system, removes and replaces the damaged DNA sequences. In the incision step, the damaged sequence is recognized by an endonuclease that cleaves the DNA on the 5' side of the damage. In the excision step, a 5'→3' exonuclease removes a stretch of the damaged DNA. In the repair step, the resulting single-stranded region serves as a template for a DNA polymerase. Some forms of base damage can be excised by the action of DNA glycosylases which catalyze the hydrolysis of the N-glycosidic bonds linking bases to the deoxyribose-phosphate backbone. The apurinic-apyrimidinic endonucleases specifically recognize sites of base loss in DNA and incise DNA by catalyzing the hydrolysis of phosphodiester bonds at the sites of base loss. DNA ligase intervenes at the end of the repair. In *E. coli*, several enzymes involved in the excision repair are part of the SOS system and are constitutively present in the cell (52).

Retrieval system. In the retrieval system (also called postreplicative repair or recombinational repair), the daughter strand is generated by replication when the damage remains at the original site. This system overlaps with the activities involved in genetic recombination.

SOS response. In addition to the preceding repair systems, the cessation of DNA replication after damage induces an error-prone repair; this phenomenon is called the SOS response (57, 79, 111). The induction of the SOS response leads to an increased repair capacity of the cells. It should be noted that a number of genes involved in the SOS phenomenon are also involved in error-free repair systems such as excision repair and methyl-directed mismatch repair (52).

O^6-Methylguanine-DNA methyltransferase. O^6-Methylguanine-DNA methyltransferase has a highly efficient repair activity which removes small alkyl groups from the O-6 position of guanine and the O-6 position of thymine, restoring the bases to their original states (78).

DNA Repair in Acholeplasmas

Initial indications of the existence of both photoreactivation and dark repair mechanisms in *A. laid-lawii* were obtained by Folsome (36) and Smith and Hanawalt (105). These mechanisms were further studied by Das et al. (23). UV sensitivity and the degree of photoreversal vary with the growth phase and pass through a maximum at the middle to late logarithmic phase. The fact that cells between the middle and late logarithmic phases of growth are maximally photoreversible also points to the possibility of a greater amount or activity of photoreactivating enzymes. All survival curves have an initial shoulder and then are exponential. Das et al. (23) clearly established that dark repair exists in *A. laidlawii* B and that there is an overlap of photoreversal and liquid holding recovery, suggesting that both act on the same lesion. Cells also show a liquid holding recovery after irradiation. Effects of chloramphenicol and nalidixic acid on DNA repair were also studied. Chloramphenicol added either before or after UV irradiation reduces the liquid holding recovery by a factor of 10. Nalidixic acid (which blocks semiconservative DNA replication and repair synthesis in *E. coli*) has a similar effect if added before irradiation, but when added after irradiation, the reduction in recovery is much less. Hence, liquid holding recovery may involve a DNA repair enzyme(s).

Analysis of the DNA during recovery shows a gradual decrease in the molecular weight of single-stranded DNA during incubation after UV irradiation, indicating an increasing number of breaks, with 60% of the breaks induced by UV irradiation being repaired within 2 h (23). This finding implies an excision repair.

A. laidlawii JA1 and B have different UV irradiation parameters; the slope of the linear part of the survival curve was 77 m²/kJ for strain JA1 versus 200 m²/kJ for strain B, and the zero dose intercepts the linear part of the curve at about 3 for strain JA1 versus 8 to 10 for strain B (45). Measurement of dark repair in UV-irradiated JA1 cells showed that survival increased exponentially, and the maximum dark recovery was reached in about 45 min (39). *A. laidlawii* JA1 is similar in dark repair and photoreactivation kinetics to strain B (39). In *A. laidlawii* JA1, DNA synthesis was almost completely inhibited for about 1 h after irradiation, which is about the time required for maximum dark repair, and then resumed at the same rate as found for unirradiated control cells. Acriflavine and caffeine, agents known to inhibit excision repair by binding to DNA, abolished dark repair in UV-treated *A. laidlawii* cells (40).

Most *A. laidlawii* strains possess photoreactivation and excision repair mechanisms (23, 36, 105) and are also able to repair UV-irradiated mycoplasma viruses by host cell and UV reactivation (25). The former mode involves repair of viral DNA by the cells' excision repair system, and the latter suggests the presence of a UV-inducible repair system in these cells (25).

Nowak et al. (75) isolated a variant (REP⁻) of *A. laidlawii* JA1 that no longer allows growth of single-stranded DNA mycoplasma viruses but retains the ability to propagate double-stranded DNA mycoplasma viruses. This variant also exhibits an increased sensitivity to UV light (75). The phenotype of this variant is similar to that observed with *E. coli* rep-3 mutants (27).

DNA Repair in Mycoplasmas

Some mycoplasmas are deficient in DNA repair systems. No photoreactivation was detected in *M. buccale*, although this species possesses dark repair capabilities (1), but *M. gallisepticum* seems to lack both dark repair and photoreactivation (39). Thus, it is surprising that there are no data on higher mutation rates in *M. gallisepticum*. This species appears to be genotypically homogeneous, as judged by only slight variations among its strains in terms of DNA cleavage patterns (92) and antigenic structure or total cell protein composition (87, 95).

Ghosh et al. studied DNA synthesis after UV irradiation in *M. gallisepticum* (39). The survival curves of *M. gallisepticum* are almost exponential, and the final slope of the curve is 75 m²/kJ. The absence of a shoulder in the curve suggests that *M. gallisepticum* in not able to repair DNA damage (39). In UV-irradiated *M. gallisepticum* cells, DNA synthesis was reduced and there was no photoreactivation. The sedimentation rate of *M. gallisepticum* DNA did not change after irradiation or during holding. This observation, together with the decrease in DNA synthesis following irradiation, indicates that UV-induced pyrimidine dimers may not be excised in *M. gallisepticum* and may block further DNA synthesis (39). Using *Micrococcus luteus* UV-endonuclease, Ghosh et al. demonstrated that UV-irradiated *M. gallisepticum* DNA must contain pyrimidine dimers which the cell is unable to repair; therefore, the cell must lack a UV-endonuclease specific for pyrimidine dimers (39).

M. gallisepticum has been reported to lack both dark and light repair (39) and seems to be the only procaryote lacking excision repair and photoreactivation systems. Maniloff has hypothesized that the lack of a DNA repair mechanism(s) may lead to the accumulation of base changes more frequently in *M. gallisepticum* than in other procaryotes, consistent with the rapid evolution of the mollicutes (61). Experimental support for higher mutation rates in *M. gallisepticum* is not available, except for *M. gallisepticum* 16S rRNA (118, 119).

In *M. buccale*, only a dark repair system has been described (1). This repair is inhibited by acriflavine and caffeine, agents known to inhibit excision repair. Photoreactivation was not detected in this *Mycoplasma* species (1).

DNA Repair in Spiroplasmas

The UV sensitivity of *S. citri*, as for other mollicutes (42), may be due to the lack of some or all of the known DNA damage repair systems, or it may be that these systems are less efficient in *S. citri* than in wild-type *E. coli*. However, the highly mutagenic effect of UV irradiation makes it unlikely that *S. citri* lacks all of the DNA repair systems. In any case, *S. citri* appears to be too sensitive to UV radiation to possess both *rec*- and *uvr*-type repair systems.

In *S. citri*, the degree of liquid holding recovery obtained in the dark is low and the MFR is slightly increased by the recovery period. In contrast with the results obtained with *A. laidlawii*, this phenomenon takes place in *S. citri* with a noticeable delay of about

1 h (3), which suggests induction of an error-prone repair system of the SOS type under liquid holding conditions. Indeed, the mechanism that acts in liquid holding of *S. citri* cells cannot be related to the excision repair in other microorganisms, which is substantially error free (54).

Light exposure of the irradiated cells increases the survival fraction and decreases the mutation frequency. However, the maximum increase of the survival fraction (2.9-fold) and the maximum decrease of the mutant frequency (3.3-fold) were obtained when heavily irradiated (39 J/m²) cells were exposed to 3 h of light (3). It should be noted that the light exposure effect seems too low to be due to an effective enzymatic photoreactivation. Therefore, its effect on survival might be due to photoprotection and the antimutagenic effect of suppression of the SOS response.

In conclusion, the high lethal and mutation frequency responses of *S. citri* cells to UV radiation may be explained by (i) the absence of a cell wall, (ii) the absence or inefficiency of dark reactivation and of photoreactivation, and (iii) the induction of an error-prone system similar to the SOS system (54).

Photodynamic Inactivation and Its Repair

Photodynamic inactivation is the loss in viability observed when organic dye-treated cells are exposed to visible light and molecular oxygen. DNA lesions are known to occur during photodynamic inactivation (19). Chaudhuri et al. (19) showed that photodynamically induced damage in *A. laidlawii* can be repaired if the irradiated cells are incubated in the dark in buffer. Analysis of the DNA of these cells showed that photodynamic inactivation induces single-strand breaks which can be repaired during liquid holding (19). However, cells irradiated long enough to give extensive inactivation are unable to recover viability, and DNA analysis showed that in these cells, the DNA is progressively degraded during holding (19).

Repair of UV-Induced Damage in Mycoplasma Viruses

Repair of UV-induced DNA damage in viruses depends on two kinds of systems: host cell reactivation (HCR), which is primarily dependent on the host cell excision repair of UV-damaged viral DNA (13), and UV reactivation (UVR), which increases survival of UV-irradiated viruses when the virus is grown on a host that has been slightly irradiated before infection. In coliphages, it has been demonstrated that the UVR mechanism involves a UV-induced repair system that is distinct from the excision repair responsible for HCR or recombinational repair (6).

Repair by *A. laidlawii* cells of UV-induced damage in mycoplasma viruses has been investigated by Das et al. (24, 25). They demonstrated that *A. laidlawii* has both HCR and UVR mechanisms similar to those found in more complex cellular systems; the efficiency of these mechanisms is comparable to those for bacteriophages. HCR was observed for double-stranded but not for single-stranded DNA mycoplasma viruses, which is consistent with the excision repair involved in HCR (24, 25). UVR was observed with use of both single- and double-stranded DNA mycoplasma viruses, which may indicate that *A. laidlawii* possesses an inducible error-prone repair system (24, 25).

Postreplicative Repair

Postreplicative repair in *S. citri*

In *E. coli*, two independent pathways have been proposed for postreplicative repair, one dependent on the *recF* gene and the other dependent on the *recB*, *uvrD*, and *lexA* genes (7, 57). No postreplicative repair was directly demonstrated in spiroplasmas; however, the existence of spontaneous gene transfer, insensitive to DNase and needing a membrane fusion step, leading to stable recombinant strains strongly suggests the existence of recombinational enzymes and postreplicative repair (2, 4).

DNA methylation and postreplicative mismatch repair

In bacteria, methylation is involved in at least two phenomena: restriction-modification and postreplication mismatch repair. During semiconservative DNA replication, noncomplementary nucleotide residues can occasionally be incorporated into the newly synthesized daughter strand, and as a result, mismatched bases are incorporated into the daughter strand and must be corrected. Repair enzymes recognize and repair the growing daughter strand by its lack of methylation but will not repair the methylated parental strand.

Razin and Razin were the first to detect methylated bases in mycoplasmal DNA (85). They examined the DNAs of four *Mycoplasma* and one *Acholeplasma* species and demonstrated that the five species contained m^6Ade; in this respect, the mycoplasmal DNA resembles DNAs of other procaryotes. The extent of methylation of adenine residues ranged from 0.2% in *M. capricolum*, a value much lower than that found in other bacteria, to about 2% in *M. arginini* and *M. hyorhinis* (85). About 5.8% of the cytosine residues in *M. hyorhinis* DNA were also methylated (85). Strains may differ in methylation patterns, and these variations may depend on the growth of the organism (31, 89).

Nur et al. studied DNA methylation in spiroplasmas (76, 77) and detected m^5Cyt and/or m^6Ade in *S. citri*, *S. melliferum*, *S. floricola*, and *S. apis*. The extent of methylation was found to be influenced by the age of the culture (77); thus, m^6Cyt increases from 2.3% of total cytosine residues in the early logarithmic phase to 4.4% in the late logarithmic phase.

Methylase from *Spiroplasma* sp. strain MQ-1 differs from eucaryotic methylases by showing high activity on nonmethylated DNA duplexes, low activity on hemimethylated DNA duplexes, and no activity on single-stranded DNA, whereas eucaryotic enzymes prefer hemimethylated double- or single-stranded DNA as a substrate (86).

Nur et al. discovered that all CpG residues in *Spiroplasma* sp. strain MQ-1 DNA are methylated (77). They cloned and characterized the gene coding for the CpG DNA methylase (93). The structure of the *Spiroplasma* enzyme (M.*SssI*) is similar to that of other procaryotic cytosine DNA methylases. M.*SssI* methylates only CpG sequences, which are common to all mammalian DNA methylases (93). M.*SssI* is a de novo methylase and is equally active on unmethylated duplex DNA and hemimethylated duplex DNA, a typically procaryotic trait. M.*SssI* shows strong homology to all of the conserved regions of the procaryotic cytosine DNA methylases (93). The sequence specificity of M.*SssI* is identical to that of mammalian DNA methylases, but its substrate specificity is different from that of mammalian methylases. M.*SssI* shows only de novo activity, whereas the mammalian methylase is primarily a maintenance enzyme (94).

Sladek et al. have identified different restriction-modification systems in *A. laidlawii* K2 and JA1, and they reported, for the first time, a DNA restriction activity specific for a single base (102, 103). K2 cells protect their DNA by methylating cytosine to m^5Cyt in the sequence GATC; DNA is unprotected and restricted when the sequence GATC is unmethylated. JA1 cells have a new type of restriction-modification system; they restrict DNA containing m^5Cyt, and protection occurs when cytosine is not methylated (102, 103).

Uracil-DNA glycosylase

Uracil-DNA glycosylase is a DNA repair enzyme that specifically removes uracil residues from DNA. The uracil residues arise either by spontaneous deamination of dCMP residues or by misincorporation of deoxyuridine (dUTP) into the DNA by DNA polymerase. Organisms which are deficient in uracil-DNA glycosylase activity accumulate significant levels of uracil residues in their DNA and exhibit an elevated mutation frequency (50, 113).

Williams and Pollack reported that *M. gallisepticum* (31 mol% G+C), *M. capricolum* (25 mol% G+C), and *U. urealyticum* (26 mol% G+C) lack uracil-DNA glycosylase activity (115) and that all the members of the genera *Mycoplasma* and *Ureaplasma* lack dUTPase activity (114). They also showed that *M. lactucae* (30 mol% G+C) possesses uracil-DNA glycosylase activity. The enzyme has a pI of 6.4 and exists as a nonspherical monomeric protein with a molecular weight of 28,000 ± 1,200. The uracil-DNA glycosylase from *M. lactucae* was similar to uracil-DNA glycosylases from other procaryotic organisms with respect to pH optimum, substrate specificity, isoelectric point, insensitivity to inhibition by EDTA, shape, subunit composition and molecular weight, and stimulation by monovalent cations. Conversely, the uracil-DNA glycosylase from *M. lactucae* differed from other procaryotic uracil-DNA glycosylases in that it was more resistant to inhibition by the uracil-DNA glycosylase inhibitor PBS-2, by monovalent cations, and by the divalent cations Fe^{2+}, Zn^{2+}, and Co^{2+}. The K_m of the enzyme for uracil-containing DNA was 40 to 1,000 times greater than that reported for other uracil-DNA glycosylases from procaryotic organisms (116). Thus, the low G+C content of the DNA of some mollicutes may be related to a decreased ability to remove uracil residues from the DNA and would result in increased AT transition mutations and ultimately in a decrease in the G+C content of the DNA.

DNA REPLICATION AND REPAIR, AND PHYLOGENETIC RELATIONSHIPS

The limited data available thus far on mycoplasma DNA replication and repair suggest that these systems are simpler in mollicutes than in other bacteria.

The acholeplasmas, considered the first mollicutes to have arisen from eubacteria, have three DNA polymerases, as do the phylogenetically related eubacteria.

The three *Spiroplasma* species analyzed (*S. floricola*, *S. melliferum*, and *S. citri*) also have three DNA polymerases. In the mollicutes phylogenetic tree, spiroplasmas appear to have arisen from an early splitting of the *Acholeplasma* branch. In this respect, spiroplasmas also resemble their eubacterial ancestors.

In the mollicutes phylogenetic tree, mycoplasmas and ureaplasmas arise from the *Spiroplasma* branch by several independent genome reductions. The loss of two DNA polymerases from the *Spiroplasma* to the *Mycoplasma* and *Ureaplasma* species perhaps reflects the genome reductions from 1,500 to 1,700 kbp to 600 to 1,000 kbp associated with the origin of the *Mycoplasma* and *Ureaplasma* branches. The presence of a single DNA polymerase among the mycoplasmas and ureaplasmas causes constraints in their replication and repair. It would be helpful in understanding these processes if mutants could be isolated to confirm the existence of a single DNA polymerase activity or to demonstrate other activities.

The consequence of loss of exonuclease activity among the mycoplasmas could be the absence of excision repair and photoreactivation systems in *M. gallisepticum* and *S. citri*.

The G + C content of the DNA of mollicutes is among the lowest known. It has been proposed that the low G + C content of their DNA is due to an AT-biased mutation pressure, perhaps caused by variations in the amounts or activities of enzymes involved in DNA replication and repair (106, 115).

DNA repair in living organisms serves to reduce the level of spontaneous and induced mutations and provides a balance between change and maintenance of the genetic information of a species. The number of DNA lesions required for inactivation of a genome increases with increasing genome complexity (49, 110). This progressive radioresistance is believed to be due to increasing DNA repair capability (45). Since mollicutes are assumed to arise by degenerative evolution from gram-positive eubacteria (118, 119), it can be concluded that the process of inducible error-prone DNA repair has been maintained in these simplest of cells. This conclusion strengthens the idea of Devoret that among the induced functions, the inducible error-prone DNA repair system is probably the most important from the point of view of evolution (28). Moreover, it supports the assumption of rapid evolution in these microorganisms by the accumulation of base changes far more frequently than in other procaryotes (61, 62, 98, 118, 119). The high mutation rate would allow mollicutes to explore areas of evolutionary phase space requiring multiple compensating mutations (62, 118). Necessary and sufficient conditions for rapid evolution are an increased mutation rate and environmental stress (98).

REFERENCES

1. **Aoki, S., S. Ito, and T. Watanabe.** 1979. UV survival of human mycoplasmas: evidence of dark reactivation in *Mycoplasma buccale. Microbiol. Immunol.* **23**:147–158.
2. **Barroso, G., and J. Labarère.** 1988. Chromosomal gene transfer in *Spiroplasma citri. Science* **241**:959–961.
3. **Barroso, G., and J. Labarère.** 1990. DNA repair in UV-irradiated *Spiroplasma citri* cells, p. 885–887. *In* G. Stanek, G. H. Cassell, J. G. Tully, and R. F. Whitcomb (ed.), *Recent Advances in Mycoplasmology.* Gustav Fisher Verlag, New York.
4. **Barroso, G., J. C. Salvado, and J. Labarère.** 1990. Influence of genetic markers and of the fusing agent polyethylene glycol on chromosomal gene transfer in *Spiroplasma citri. Curr. Microbiol.* **20**:53–56.
5. **Baseman, J. B., R. M. Cole, D. C. Krause, and D. K. Leith.** 1982. Molecular basis for cytadsorption of *Mycoplasma pneumoniae. J. Bacteriol.* **151**:1514–1522.
6. **Blanco, M., and R. Devoret.** 1973. Repair mechanisms involved in prophage reactivation and UV-reactivation of UV-irradiated phage λ. *Mutat. Res.* **17**:293–305.
7. **Blanco, M., G. Herrera, P. Collado, J. E. Rebollo, and L. M. Botella.** 1982. Influence of Rec A protein on induced mutagenesis. *Biochimie* **64**:633–636.
8. **Bové, J. M.** 1984. Wall-less procaryotes of plants. *Annu. Rev. Phytopathol.* **22**:361–396.
9. **Bové, J. M., P. Carle, M. Garnier, F. Laigret, J. Renaudin, and C. Saillard.** 1989. Molecular and cellular biology of spiroplasmas, p. 243–364. *In* R. F. Whitcomb and J. G. Tully (ed.), *The Mycoplasmas*, vol. 5 Academic Press, New York.
10. **Bové, J. M., J. C. Vignault, M. Garnier, C. Saillard, O. Garcia-Jurado, C. Bové, and A. Nhami.** 1978. Mise en évidence de *Spiroplasma citri*, l'agent causal de la maladie du "Stubborn" des agrumes dans les pervenches (*Vinca rosea* L.) ornementales de la ville de Rabat, Maroc. *C.R. Acad. Sci.* **286**:57–60.
11. **Boxer, L. M.** 1981. Biochemical studies of DNA replication. I. A DNA polymerase from *Mycoplasma orale*. II. A DNA-dependent ATPase from KB cells. Dissertation. Université de Bordeaux II, Bordeaux, France.
12. **Boxer, L. M., and D. Korn.** 1979. Structural and enzymological characterization of the homogenous deoxyribonucleic acid polymerase from *Mycoplasma orale. Biochemistry* **18**:4742–4749.
13. **Boyle, J. M., and R. B. Setlow.** 1970. Correlation between host cell reactivation, ultraviolet reactivation and pyrimidine dimer excision in the DNA of bacteriophage λ. *J. Mol. Biol.* **51**:131–144.
14. **Buisson, C., A. Charron, D. Maurel, and C. Bébéar.** 1990. Purification and partial characterization of a single DNA polymerase from *Ureaplasma urealyticum*, p. 609–612. *In* G. Stanek, G. H. Cassell, J. G. Tully, and R. F. Whitcomb (ed.), *Recent Advances in Mycoplasmology.* Gustav Fisher Verlag, New York.
15. **Cerda-Olmedo, E., and P. C. Hanawalt.** 1967. Repair of DNA damaged by N-methyl-N'-nitro-N-nitrosoguanidine in *Escherichia coli. Mutat. Res.* **4**:369–371.
16. **Cerda-Olmedo, E., and R. Ruiz-Vazquez.** 1979. Nitrosoguanidine mutagenesis, p. 15–20. *In* O. K. Sebek, and A. I. Laskin (ed.), *Genetics of Industrial Microorganisms.* American Society for Microbiology, Washington, D.C.
17. **Charron, A., C. Bébéar, G. Brun, P. Yot, J. Latrille, and J. M. Bové.** 1979. Separation and partial characterization of two deoxyribonucleic acid polymerases from *Spiroplasma citri. J. Bacteriol.* **140**:763–768.
18. **Charron, A., M. Castroviejo, C. Bébéar, J. Latrille, and J. M. Bové.** 1982. A third DNA polymerase from *Spiroplasma citri* and two other spiroplasmas. *J. Bacteriol.* **149**:1138–1141.
19. **Chaudhuri, U., J. Das, and J. Maniloff.** 1978. Photody-

namic inactivation and its repair in mycoplasmas. *Biochim. Biophys. Acta* **544**:624–633.

20. **Chelton, E. T. J., A. S. Jones, and R. T. Walker.** 1979. The sensitivity of *Mycoplasma mycoides* var. *capri* cells to γ radiation after growth in a medium containing the thymine analogue 5-vinyluracil. *Biochem. J.* **181**:783–785.

21. **Dahl, J. S., C. E. Dahl, and R. P. Levine.** 1979. Role of lipid fatty acid composition and membrane fluidity in the resistance of *Acholeplasma laidlawii* to complement-mediated killing. *J. Immunol.* **123**:104–108.

22. **Daniels, M. J.** 1979. Mechanisms of spiroplasma pathogenicity, p. 209–227. *In* R. F. Whitcomb and J. G. Tully (ed.), *The Mycoplasmas*, vol. 3. Academic Press, New York.

23. **Das, J., J. Maniloff, and S. B. Bhattacharjee.** 1972. Dark and light repair in ultraviolet-irradiated *Acholeplasma laidlawii*. *Biochim. Biophys. Acta* **259**:189–197.

24. **Das, J., J. Maniloff, U. Chaudhuri, and A. Ghosh.** 1978. Repair of DNA in Mycoplasmas, p. 277–281. *In* P. C. Hanawalt, E. C. Freidberg, and C. F. Fox (ed.), *DNA Repair Mechanisms*. Academic Press, New York.

25. **Das, J., J. A. Novak, and J. Maniloff.** 1977. Host cell and ultraviolet reactivation of ultraviolet-irradiated mycoplasmaviruses. *J. Bacteriol.* **129**:1424–1427.

26. **Delic, V., D. A. Hopwood, and E. J. Friend.** 1970. Mutagenesis by N-methyl-N′-nitro-N-nitrosoguanidine (NTG) in *Streptomyces coelicolor*. *Mutat. Res.* **9**:167–182.

27. **Denhardt, D. T., M. Iwaya, and L. L. Larison.** 1972. The REP- mutation. II. Its effect on *Escherichia coli* and on the replication of bacteriophage ϕX174. *Virology* **49**:486–496.

28. **Devoret, R.** 1978. Inductible error-prone repair: one of the cellular responses to DNA damage. *Biochimie* **60**:1135–1140.

29. **Doskar, J., J. Chladkova, and V. Drasil.** 1977. Effects of UV radiation on *Acholeplasma laidlawii* S-2. *Folia Microbiol.* **22**:449–450.

30. **Doudney, C. O.** 1976. Complexity of the ultraviolet mutation frequency response curve in *Escherichia coli* B/r: SOS induction, one-lesion and two-lesion mutagenesis. *J. Bacteriol.* **128**:815–826.

31. **Dybvig, K., J. A. Nowak, T. L. Sladek, and J. Maniloff.** 1985. Identification of an enveloped phage, mycoplasma virus L172, that contains a 14-kilobase single-stranded DNA genome. *J. Virol.* **53**:384–390.

32. **Dybvig, K., D. Swinton, J. Maniloff, and S. Hattman.** 1982. Cytosine methylation of the sequence GATC in mycoplasma. *J. Bacteriol.* **151**:1420–1424.

33. **Eckardt, F., and R. H. Haynes.** 1977. Kinetics of mutation induction by ultraviolet light in excision-deficient yeast. *Genetics* **85**:225–247.

34. **Eisenstadt, E.** 1987. Analysis of mutagenesis, p. 1016–1033. *In* F. C. Neidhardt, J. L. Ingraham, K. B. Low, B. Magasanik, M. Schaechter, and H. E. Umbarger (ed.), *Escherichia coli and Salmonella typhimurium: Cellular and Molecular Biology*. American Society for Microbiology, Washington, D.C.

35. **Feldner, J., and W. Bredt.** 1983. Analysis of polypeptides of mutants of *Mycoplasma pneumoniae* that lack the ability to hemadsorb. *J. Gen. Microbiol.* **129**:841–848.

36. **Folsome, C. E.** 1968. Deoxyribonucleic binding and transformation in *Mycoplasma laidlawii*. *J. Gen. Microbiol.* **50**:43–53.

37. **Garnier, M., M. Clerc, and J. M. Bové.** 1981. Growth and division of spiroplasmas: morphology of *Spiroplasma citri* during growth in liquid medium. *J. Bacteriol.* **147**:642–652.

38. **Garnier, M., M. Clerc, and J. M. Bové.** 1984. Growth and division of *Spiroplasma citri*: elongation of elementary helices. *J. Bacteriol.* **147**:642–652.

39. **Ghosh, A., J. Das, and J. Maniloff.** 1977. Lack of repair of UV light damage in *Mycoplasma gallisepticum*. *J. Mol. Biol.* **116**:337–344.

40. **Ghosh, A., J. Das, and J. Maniloff.** 1978. Effect of acriflavine on ultraviolet inactivation of *Acholeplasma laidlawii*. *Biochim. Biophys. Acta* **543**:570–575.

41. **Guerola, N. J., J. L. Ingraham, and E. Cerda-Olmedo.** 1971. Induction of closely linked multiple mutations by nitrosoguanidine. *Nature* (London) **230**:122–125.

42. **Hanawalt, P. C.** 1972. Repair of genetic material in living cells. *Endeavour* **31**:83–87.

43. **Hansen, E. J., R. M. Wilson, W. A. Clyde, and J. B. Baseman.** 1981. Characterization of hemadsorption-negative mutants of *Mycoplasma pneumoniae*. *Infect. Immun.* **32**:127–136.

44. **Haynes, R. H., and B. A. Kunz.** 1981. DNA repair and mutagenesis in yeast, p. 371–414. *In* J. N. Strathern, E. W. Jones, and J. R. Broach (ed.), *The Molecular Biology of the Yeast Saccharomyces: Life Cycle and Inheritance*. Cold Spring Harbor Laboratory, Cold Spring Harbor, N.Y.

45. **Howard-Flanders, P.** 1968. DNA repair. *Annu. Rev. Biochem.* **37**:175–200.

46. **Ishii, Y., and S. Kondo.** 1975. Comparative analysis of deletion and base change mutabilities of *Escherichia coli* B strains differing in DNA repair capacity (wild type, *uvr* A, *pol* A, *rec* A) by various mutagens. *Mutat. Res.* **27**:27–44.

47. **John, G., P. M. Laufs, and H. Kolenda.** 1979. Molecular nature of two *Haemophilus influenzae* R factors containing resistances and the multiple integration of drug resistance transposons. *J. Bacteriol.* **138**:584–597.

48. **Junca, P., C. Saillard, J. Tully, O. Garcia-Jurado, J. R. Degorce-Dumas, C. Mouches, J. C. Vignault, R. Voegl, R. McCoy, R. Whitcomb, D. Williamson, J. Latrille, and J. M. Bové.** 1980. Caractérisation de spiroplasmes isolés d'insectes et de fleurs de France continentale, de Corse et du Maroc. Proposition pour une classification des spiroplasmes. *C.R. Acad. Sci. Ser. D* **290**:1209–1212.

49. **Kondo, S.** 1964. Variations in mutagenicity and radiation resistance with genome complexity and evolution. *Jpn. J. Genet.* **39**:179–198.

50. **Konrad, E. B., and L. R. Lehman.** 1975. Novel mutants of *Escherichia coli* that accumulate very small replicative intermediates. *Proc. Natl. Acad. Sci. USA* **71**:2150–2154.

51. **Krause, D. C., D. K. Leith, R. M. Wilson, and J. Baseman.** 1982. Identification of *Mycoplasma pneumoniae* proteins associated with hemadsorption and virulence. *Infect. Immunol.* **35**:809–817.

52. **Kushner, S. R.** 1987. DNA repair, p. 1044–1053. *In* F. C. Neidhardt, J. L. Ingraham, K. B. Low, B. Magasanik, M. Schaechter, and H. E. Umbarger (ed.) *Escherichia coli and Salmonella typhimurium: Cellular and Molecular Biology*. American Society for Microbiology, Washington, D.C.

53. **Labarère, J., and G. Barroso.** 1984. Ultraviolet irradiation mutagenesis and recombination in *Spiroplasma citri*. *Isr. J. Med. Sci.* **20**:826–829.

54. **Labarère, J., and G. Barroso.** 1988. Lethal and mutation frequency responses of *Spiroplasma citri* cells to UV irradiation. *Mutat. Res.* **210**:135–141.

55. **Lam, K. M., J. Rosen, and H. E. Alder.** 1984. Temperature-sensitive mutants of *Mycoplasma gallisepticum*. *J. Comp. Pathol.* **94**:1–8.

56. **Liss, A.** 1976. A novel method for isolation of conditional-lethal mutants of mycoplasma and mycoplasmaviruses. *Biochem. Biophys. Res. Commun.* **71**:235–240.

57. **Little, J. W., and D. W. Mount.** 1982. The SOS regulatory system of *Escherichia coli*. *Cell* **29**:11–22.

58. **Liu, H. Y., D. J. Gumpf, G. N. Oldfield, and E. C. Calavan.** 1983. The relationship of *Spiroplasma citri* and *Circulifer tenellus*. *Phytopathology* **73**:585–590.

59. **Livneh, Z.** 1983. Directed mutagenesis method for anal-

ysis of mutagen specificity: application to ultraviolet-induced mutagenesis. *Proc. Natl. Acad. Sci. USA* **80:**237–241.

60. **Loeb, L. A., and T. A. Kunkel.** 1982. Fidelity of DNA synthesis. *Annu. Rev. Biochem.* **51:**429–457.

61. **Maniloff, J.** 1978. Molecular biology of mycoplasma, p. 390–393. *In* D. Schlessinger (ed.), *Microbiology—1978.* American Society for Microbiology, Washington, D.C.

62. **Maniloff, J.** 1983. Evolution of wall-less prokaryotes. *Annu. Rev. Microbiol.* **37:**477–499.

63. **Maniloff, J., and J. Das.** 1975. Replication of Mycoplasmaviruses, p. 445–450. *In* M. Goulian, P. Hanawalt, and C. F. Fox (ed.), *DNA Synthesis and Its Regulation.* W. A. Benjamin, Reading, Mass.

64. **Maniloff, J., and H. J. Morowitz.** 1972. Cell biology of the mycoplasmas. *Bacteriol. Rev.* **36:**263–290.

65. **Maniloff, J., and D. C. Quinlan.** 1973. Biosynthesis and subcellular organization of nucleic acids in *Mycoplasma gallisepticum* strain A5969. *Ann. N.Y. Acad. Sci.* **225:**181–189.

66. **Maniloff, J., and D. C. Quinlan.** 1974. Partial purification of a membrane-associated deoxyribonucleic acid complex from *Mycoplasma gallisepticum. J. Bacteriol.* **120:**495–501.

66a.**Maurel, D.** Personal communication.

67. **Maurel, D., A. Charron, and C. Bébéar.** 1989. Mollicutes DNA polymerases: characterization of a single enzyme from *Mycoplasma mycoides* and *Ureaplasma urealyticum* and of three enzymes from *Acholeplasma laidlawii. Res. Microbiol.* **140:**191–205.

68. **McHenry, C. S., and W. Crow.** 1979. DNA polymerase III of *Escherichia coli*: purification and identification of subunits. *J. Biol. Chem.* **254:**1748–1753.

69. **Mills, L. B., E. J. Standbridge, W. D. Sedwick, and D. Korn.** 1977. Purification and partial characterization of the principal deoxyribonucleic acid polymerase from Mycoplasmatales. *J. Bacteriol.* **132:**641–649.

70. **Minion, F. C., and J. D. Goguen.** 1986. Identification and preliminary characterization of external membrane-bound nuclease activities in *Mycoplasma pulmonis. Infect. Immun.* **51:**352–354.

71. **Minion, F. C., and E. Tigges.** 1990. Nucleases of *Mycoplasma pulmonis* and other mycoplasmal species. *IOM Lett.* **1:**290–291.

72. **Miyaki, M. G., G. Sai, S. Katagiri, N. Akamatsu, and T. Ono.** 1977. Enhancement of DNA polymerase II activity in *E. coli* after treatment with N-methyl-N′-nitro-N-nitrosoguanidine. *Biochem. Biophys. Res. Commun.* **76:**136–141.

73. **Miyata, M., and T. Fukumura.** 1990. DNA-membrane association in *Mycoplasma capricolum. IOM Lett.* **1:**292–293.

74. **Mugharbil, U., and V. P. Cirillo.** 1978. Mycoplasma phosphoenolpyruvate-dependent sugar phosphotransferase system: glucose-negative mutant and regulation of intracellular cyclic AMP. *J. Bacteriol.* **133:**203–209.

75. **Nowak, J. A., J. Das, and J. Maniloff.** 1976. Characterization of an *Acholeplasma laidlawii* variant with a REP⁻ phenotype. *J. Bacteriol.* **127:**832–836.

76. **Nur, I., S. Razin, and S. Rottem.** 1985. Bilirubin incorporation into spiroplasma membranes and methylation of spiroplasma DNA. *Isr. J. Med. Sci.* **20:**1019–1021.

77. **Nur, I., M. Szyf, A. Razin, G. Glaser, S. Rottem, and S. Razin.** 1985. Eucaryotic and procaryotic traits of DNA methylation in spiroplasmas (mycoplasmas). *J. Bacteriol.* **164:**19–24.

78. **Olsson, M., and T. Lindahl.** 1980. Repair of alkylated DNA in *Escherichia coli*: methyl group transfer from O⁶- methylguanine to a protein cysteine residue. *J. Biol. Chem.* **255:**10569–10571.

79. **Ossanna, N., K. R. Peterson, and D. W. Mount.** 1986. Genetics of DNA repair in bacteria. *Trends Genet.* **2:**55–58.

80. **Poddar, S. K., S. P. Cadden, J. Das, and J. Maniloff.** 1985. Heterogenous progeny viruses are produced by a budding enveloped phage. *Intervirology* **23:**208–221.

81. **Pollack, J. D., and P. J. Hoffman.** 1982. Properties of nucleases of Mollicutes. *J. Bacteriol.* **152:**538–541.

82. **Pyle, L. E., and L. R. Finch.** 1988. Preparation and FIGE separation of infrequent restriction fragments from *Mycoplasma mycoides* DNA. *Nucleic Acids Res.* **16:**2263–2268.

83. **Quinlan, D. C., and J. Maniloff.** 1972. Membrane association of the deoxyribonucleic acid growing region in *Mycoplasma gallisepticum. J. Bacteriol.* **112:**1375–1381.

84. **Quinlan, D. C., and J. Maniloff.** 1973. Deoxyribonucleic acid synthesis in synchronously growing *Mycoplasma gallisepticum. J. Bacteriol.* **115:**117–120.

85. **Razin, A., and S. Razin.** 1980. Methylated bases in mycoplasmal DNA. *Nucleic Acids Res.* **8:**1383–1390.

86. **Razin, A., and M. Szyf.** 1984. DNA methylation patterns. *Biochim. Biophys. Acta* **782:**331–342.

87. **Razin, S.** 1968. Mycoplasma taxonomy studied by electrophoresis of cell proteins. *J. Bacteriol.* **96:**687–694.

88. **Razin, S.** 1978. The mycoplasmas. *Microbiol. Rev.* **42:**414–470.

89. **Razin, S.** 1985. Molecular biology and genetics of mycoplasmas (Mollicutes). *Microbiol. Rev.* **49:**419–455.

90. **Razin, S.** 1989. Molecular approach to mycoplasma phylogeny, p. 33–69. *In* R. F. Whitcomb and J. G. Tully (ed.), *The Mycoplasmas*, vol. 5. *Spiroplasmas, Acholeplasmas, and Mycoplasmas of Plants and Arthropods.* Academic Press, New York.

91. **Razin, S., A. Knyszynski, and Y. Lifshitz.** 1964. Nucleases of mycoplasma. *J. Gen. Microbiol.* **36:**323–331.

92. **Razin, S., J. G. Tully, D. L. Rose, and M. F. Barile.** 1983. DNA cleavage patterns as indicators of genetic heterogeneity among strains of *Acholeplasma and Mycoplasma* species. *J. Gen. Microbiol.* **129:**1935–1944.

93. **Renbaum, P., D. Abrahamove, A. Fainsod, G. G. Wilson, S. Rottem, and A. Razin.** 1990. Cloning, characterization, and expression in *Escherichia coli* of the gene coding for CpG DNA methylase from *Spiroplasma* sp. strain MQ1 (M.SssI). *Nucleic Acids Res.* **18:**1145–1152.

94. **Renbaum, P., S. Rottem, and A. Razin.** 1990. M.SssI, a CpG DNA methylase from Spiroplasma sp. strain MQ1. *IOM Lett.* **1:**87.

95. **Rhoades, K. R., M. Phillips, and H. W. Yoder, Jr.** 1974. Comparison of strains of *Mycoplasma gallisepticum* by polyacrylamide gel electrophoresis. *Avian Dis.* **18:**91–96.

96. **Rodwell, A. W., J. E. Peterson, and E. S. Rodwell.** 1972. Macromolecular synthesis and growth of mycoplasmas. *Excerpta Med.* **1972:**123–139.

97. **Roganti, F. S., and A. L. Rosenthal.** 1983. DNases of *Acholeplasma* spp. *J. Bacteriol.* **155:**802–805.

98. **Rogers, M. J., J. Simmons, R. T. Walker, W. G. Weisburg, C. R. Woese, R. S. Tanner, I. M. Robinson, D. A. Stahl, G. Olsen, R. H. Leach, and J. Maniloff.** 1985. Construction of the mycoplasma evolutionary tree from 5S rRNA sequence data. *Proc. Natl. Acad. Sci. USA* **82:**1160–1164.

99. **Rottem, S.** 1983. Harvest and washing of mycoplasmas, p. 221–223. *In* J. G. Tully and S. Razin (ed.), *Methods in Mycoplasmology*, vol. 1. Academic Press, New York.

100. **Sargentini, N. J., and K. C. Smith.** 1979. Multiple, independent components of ultraviolet radiation mutagenesis in *Escherichia coli* K-12 *uvrB5. J. Bacteriol.* **140:**436–444.

101. **Sladek, T. L., and J. Maniloff.** 1983. Polyethylene glycol-dependent transfection of *Acholeplasma laidlawii* with mycoplasma virus L2 DNA. *J. Bacteriol.* **155:**734–741.

102. **Sladek, T. L., and J. Maniloff.** 1987. Endonuclease from *Acholeplasma laidlawii* strain JA1 associated with *in*

vivo restriction of DNA containing 5-methylcytosine. *Isr. J. Med. Sci.* **23**:423–426.

103. **Sladek, T. L., J. A. Nowak, and J. Maniloff.** 1986. Mycoplasma restriction: identification of a new type of restriction specificity for DNA containing 5-methylcytosine. *J. Bacteriol.* **165**:219–225.

104. **Smith, D. W.** 1968. DNA replication in *Mycoplasma laidlawii* B. *Biochim. Biophys. Acta* **179**:408–421.

105. **Smith, D. W., and P. C. Hanawalt.** 1969. Repair replication of DNA in ultraviolet irradiated *Mycoplasma laidlawii* B. *J. Mol. Biol.* **46**:57–72.

106. **Stanbridge, E. J., and M. E. Reff.** 1979. The molecular biology of mycoplasmas, p. 157–185. *In* M. F. Barile and S. Razin (ed.), *The Mycoplasmas*, vol. 1. *Cell Biology*. Academic Press, New York.

107. **Steinberg, P., R. L. Horswood, and R. M. Chanock.** 1969. Temperature sensitive mutants of *Mycoplasma pneumoniae*. I. *In vitro* biologic properties. *J. Infect. Dis.* **120**:217–224.

108. **Stephens, M. A.** 1982. Partial purification and cleavage specificity of a site-specific endonuclease, *Sci*Ni, isolated from *Spiroplasma citri. J. Bacteriol.* **149**:508–514.

109. **Tarshis, M. A., V. G. Ladygina, and T. P. A. Abaeva.** 1976. *Acholeplasma laidlawii* mutant defective in glucose transport system. *FEBS Lett.* **71**:209–211.

110. **Terzi, M.** 1961. Comparative analysis of inactivation efficiency of radiation on different organisms. *Nature* (London) **191**:461–463.

111. **Walker, G. C.** 1985. Inducible DNA repair systems. *Annu. Rev. Biochem.* **54**:425–457.

112. **Wang, L., M. Miyata, and T. Fukumura.** 1990. Estimation of DNA replication origin region in *Mycoplasma capricolum* genome. *IOM Lett.* **1**:272–273.

113. **Warner, H. R., B. K. Duncan, C. Garrett, and J. Neuhard.** 1981. Synthesis and metabolism of uracil-containing deoxyribonucleic acid in *Escherichia coli. J. Bacteriol.* **145**:687–695.

114. **Williams, M. V., and J. D. Pollack.** 1984. Purification and characterization of a dUTPase from *Acholeplasma laidlawii* B-PG9. *J. Bacteriol.* **159**:278–282.

115. **Williams, M. V., and J. D. Pollack.** 1988. Uracil-DNA glycosylase activity. Relationship to proposed biased mutation pressure in the class *Mollicutes*, p. 440–444. *In* R. E. Moses and W. C. Summers (ed.), *DNA Replication and Mutagenesis*. American Society for Microbiology, Washington, D.C.

116. **Williams, M. V., and J. D. Pollack.** 1990. A mollicute (mycoplasma) DNA repair enzyme: purification and characterization of uracil-DNA glycosylase. *J. Bacteriol.* **172**:2979–2985.

117. **Woese, C. R.** 1987. Bacterial evolution. *Microbiol. Rev.* **51**:221–271.

118. **Woese, C. R., J. Maniloff, and L. B. Zablen.** 1980. Phylogenetic analysis of the mycoplasmas. *Proc. Natl. Acad. Sci. USA* **77**:494–498.

119. **Woese, C. R., E. Stackebrandt, and W. Ludwig.** 1985. What are mycoplasmas: the relationship of tempo and mode in bacterial evolution. *J. Mol. Evol.* **21**:305–316.

18. Mycoplasma DNA Restriction and Modification

JACK MANILOFF, KEVIN DYBVIG, and TODD L. SLADEK

INTRODUCTION

Restriction and Modification in Eubacteria

Restriction and modification was first described in 1953 for *Escherichia coli* on the basis of variation in coliphage plating efficiency as a function of the host cell strain used to grow the phage (3). About 10 years later, the molecular basis of restriction and modification was shown to involve specific DNA nucleases (restriction endonucleases) and methylases (modification methylases) which recognize the same DNA base sequences (reviewed in reference 1). At present, restriction-modification systems have been reported to exist in every major group of bacteria (27).

Bacteria with restriction and modification activity have a restriction endonuclease that cleaves DNA containing a specific base sequence. These bacteria also have a sequence-specific methylase that methylates specific adenine or cytosine residues in the restriction endonuclease recognition sequence, thereby blocking endonuclease binding and protecting cell DNA from cleavage by its own restriction endonuclease. In most cases, the methylated base is *N*-6-methyladenine (m⁶Ade) or 5-methylcytosine (m⁵Cyt), although in a few cases *N*-4-methylcytosine has been found (27).

The exceptions to this general mechanism are microorganisms in which the restriction endonuclease is specific for a sequence containing a methylated base and modification is the absence of these methylated sequences. This situation has been reported for (i) *Streptococcus pneumoniae*, in which the *Dpn*I restriction endonuclease recognition sequence is GmATC and DNA containing GmATC sites, but not GATC sites, is restricted (15, 16) (*Dpn*I isoschizomers have been reported in several other bacteria [27]); (ii) some *E. coli* strains, in which two restriction systems for m⁵Cyt-containing DNA have been reported, one for m⁵Cyt in the sequence RmC (R = A or G) and the other for m⁵Cyt in a sequence that has not been determined (24); and (iii) *Acholeplasma laidlawii* JA1, in which m⁵Cyt-containing DNA is restricted regardless of the m⁵Cyt-containing sequence (30; also reviewed below).

Restriction-Modification Systems

Three types of restriction-modification systems in eubacteria have been described (reviewed in reference 4).

Type II restriction-modification systems are biochemically the simplest and consist of two enzymes: a single polypeptide (generally present as a dimer) with endonucleolytic activity, and a monomeric modification methylase. The type II restriction endonuclease recognition site is usually a 4- to 6-bp palindromic sequence, and cleavage is either within this sequence or at a fixed distance no more than 12 bp from it. Over 1,350 type II restriction endonucleases, with representatives from every major eubacterial phylogenetic group, have been identified (27).

Jack Maniloff • Department of Microbiology and Immunology, University of Rochester, Medical Center Box 672, Rochester, New York 14642. **Kevin Dybvig** • Department of Comparative Medicine and Department of Microbiology, University of Alabama at Birmingham, Birmingham, Alabama 35294. **Todd L. Sladek** • Department of Genetics, School of Medicine, Case Western Reserve University, Cleveland, Ohio 44106.

Type III restriction-modification systems consist of bifunctional dimeric enzymes made up of different subunits. Endonucleolytic cleavage is ATP dependent, although ATP is not hydrolyzed during the cleavage reaction. The rate of cleavage is increased by S-adenosylmethionine (AdoMet), but in the presence of AdoMet, type III enzymes also function as modification methylases, with cleavage and methylation being competing reactions. The recognition sites are asymmetric 5- to 6-bp sequences, and cleavage is 25 to 30 bp from the recognition site. Only five type III enzymes have been described thus far: all from three species of bacteria, two from *E. coli* strains, two from *Haemophilus influenzae* strains, and one from a *Salmonella typhi* strain (27). These species are facultatively anaerobic gram-negative rod-shaped bacteria and are phylogenetically related as part of the γ-3 subgroup of the γ-purple branch of the bacterial phylogenetic tree (34). It is not known whether type III restriction-modification systems are limited to species on this single phylogenetic branch or whether there are type III enzymes in species on other branches. The problem has been the difficulty in detecting type III enzyme activity in crude cell lysates and the fact that there apparently has not yet been a systematic search of other bacterial genera for type III restriction-modification systems.

Type I restriction-modification systems consist of multimeric endonuclease and methylase enzymes. The restriction endonuclease contains three different subunits and requires both ATP (which is hydrolyzed during cleavage) and AdoMet. Type I enzyme recognition sites are in two parts, with a 3-bp upstream sequence separated from a 4- to 5-bp downstream sequence by a 6- to 8-bp spacer of nonspecific sequence. Cleavage is random and far (up to 7 kbp) from the recognition site. Type I methylases contain two of the three endonuclease subunits and require AdoMet. Thus far, only 13 type I restriction endonucleases have been identified, all from three closely related species of enteric bacteria: one from *Citrobacter freundii*, eight from *E. coli*, and four from *S. typhi*. These three species are phylogenetically related on a subline of the γ-3 subgroup of the γ-purple branch of the bacterial phylogenetic tree (34). As for type III restriction-modification systems, it is not known whether type I systems are limited to this single phylogenetic branch or whether there are type I enzymes in species on other bacterial phylogenetic branches.

Restriction and Modification in Mycoplasmas

As in the eubacteria, restriction and modification in mycoplasmas was first described as host-controlled variation in mycoplasma virus plating efficiencies (18). Subsequent studies (described below) have identified DNA restriction and methylation activities in *Acholeplasma*, *Spiroplasma*, *Mycoplasma*, and *Ureaplasma* species (Table 1). Those that have been characterized thus far have been type II restriction endonucleases. Hence, restriction and modification is widespread throughout the major phylogenetic branches of the eubacteria and mycoplasmas.

MYCOPLASMA RESTRICTION-MODIFICATION SYSTEMS

A. laidlawii K2

A. laidlawii K2 was found to restrict mycoplasma viruses containing unmethylated DNA, and DNAs from these cells and from mycoplasma viruses grown on these cells contain both m^{6}Ade and m^{5}Cyt (7). However, since both DNAs are resistant to *Sau*3AI (which cleaves at GATC and GmATC sites but not at GATmC sites) digestion and sensitive to *Mbo*I (which cleaves at GATC and GATmC sites but not at GmATC sites) digestion, all GATC sites in the DNAs of *A. laidlawii* K2 cells and viruses grown on strain K2 must be methylated to GATmC. Hence, it was proposed that *A. laidlawii* K2 restricts DNA containing GATC sequences with unmethylated cytosine residues and protects its DNA by methylating this site to GATmC (7). However, these studies could not rule out the possibility that the specificity of the *A. laidlawii* K2 restriction system was for DNA containing m^{6}Ade or m^{5}Cyt in some sequence other than GATC.

The specificity of the *A. laidlawii* K2 restriction system was determined by using *Acholeplasma* virus L51, which has a small single-stranded DNA genome containing a single GATC site (30). An L51 virus deletion mutant lacking the GATC site was constructed. By using viruses grown on host cells that do not methylate DNA, it was found that *A. laidlawii* K2 cells restrict wild-type L51 viruses (which contain a single GATC site) but do not restrict L51 deletion mutant viruses (which lack the GATC site). By using viruses grown on

Table 1. Mycoplasma restriction-modification DNA sequences

Mycoplasma	Restriction endonuclease	Restriction recognition sequence	Modified sequence	Reference
A. laidlawii K2	—[a]	GATC	GATmC	8
A. laidlawii JA1	—[a]	mC	C	30
S. citri ASP2	SciNI	G/CGC[b]	GmCGC[c]	31
M. fermentans	MfeI	C/AATTG[b]	—[d]	10
U. urealyticum 960	Uur960I	GC/NGC[d]	—[d]	6

[a] —, the restriction endonuclease for this restriction activity has not been isolated.
[b] The slash (/) marks the cleavage site.
[c] The conclusion that this is the modified sequence is discussed in the text.
[d] —, not determined.

K2 cells so that GATC sites were methylated to GATmC, it was found that strain K2 cells do not restrict either wild-type L51 viruses (which contain a single GATmC site) or L51 deletion mutant viruses.

Therefore, *A. laidlawii* K2 has a restriction system specific for DNA containing the sequence GATC, and host cell DNA is protected by methylation of cytosine in this sequence to m^5Cyt (30). Restriction systems specific for GATC are very common in eubacteria. Of the 86 isoschizomers that have been isolated, 50 are like *Mbo*I and cleave DNA at GATC sites but not at GmATC sites and 36 are like *Sau*3AI and cleave DNA at GATC sites but not at GATmC sites (references in reference 27). Hence, the *A. laidlawii* K2 restriction system specificity resembles that for restriction endonuclease *Sau*3AI.

Although the restriction activity of *A. laidlawii* K2 was originally identified on the basis of host-controlled restriction of *Acholeplasma* viruses (18), it was subsequently found that L3 virus, the *Acholeplasma* virus with the largest genome, is not restricted by strain K2 cells (30). Hence, L3 has evolved a mechanism to avoid the strain K2 restriction system. L3 virus contains linear double-stranded DNA of 39.4 kbp (13) and should contain about 150 GATC sites. However, L3 DNA has no cleavage sites for restriction endonuclease *Mbo*I (which cleaves at GATC and GATmC) or *Sau*3AI (which cleaves at GATC and GmATC) (30); hence, L3 virus DNA contains no GATC sites. Therefore, *Acholeplasma* virus L3 evolution has involved selective pressure for the loss of GATC sites, thereby allowing these viruses to escape host cell restriction. Similar selection against recognition sequences of host restriction systems has been found in a number of bacteriophages (14, 28).

A. laidlawii JA1

A. laidlawii JA1 cells restrict mycoplasma viruses grown on *A. laidlawii* strain K2 cells (18). However, the nature of the *A. laidlawii* JA1 restriction system presented a problem, because no methylated bases could be detected in DNAs from *A. laidlawii* JA1 cells or mycoplasma viruses grown on strain JA1 cells (7). The solution was suggested by the finding that whereas wild-type *Acholeplasma* virus L51 grown on strain K2 cells was restricted by strain JA1 cells, the L51 deletion mutant virus (lacking the single GATC site) grown on strain K2 cells was not restricted by strain JA1 cells. Since strain K2 cells have a modification methylase activity and methylate cytosine to m^5Cyt in the sequence GATC (30), the single GATC sequence in wild-type L51 virus grown on K2 cells is present as GATmC. This finding, together with the absence of methylated bases in strain JA1 cells, suggested that strain JA1 restricts DNA containing m^5Cyt and protects host cell DNA by the absence of m^5Cyt (30).

To investigate this possibility, unmethylated *Acholeplasma* virus L2 DNA (from virions grown on *A. laidlawii* JA1 cells) was methylated in vitro by specific DNA methylases and used in transfection experiments with *A. laidlawii* JA1 cells (30). L2 virus DNA that was unmethylated or contained m^6Ade was not restricted by strain JA1 cells. However, L2 virus DNA containing m^5Cyt in a variety of sequences was restricted by strain JA1 cells; these experiments investigated m^5Cyt in the dinucleotide sequences BmC (B = G or T or C) and mCB. Hence, *A. laidlawii* JA1 has a restriction system for m^5Cyt-containing DNA, independent of the sequence containing the m^5Cyt, and protects host cell DNA by the absence of methylated cytosine residues.

An endonuclease fraction has been identified in *A. laidlawii* JA1 extracts that is absent in a strain JA1 mutant (discussed below) lacking restriction activity (29). However, this endonuclease fraction cleaves both unmethylated and m^5Cyt-containing DNA, suggesting its restriction specificity has been lost during purification.

A. laidlawii JA1 Restriction and recA Mutants

A variant of *A. laidlawii* JA1, designated REP⁻, was isolated from a mottled plaque on a lawn on JA1 cells infected with a single-stranded DNA mycoplasma virus (20). Strain JA1 cells are hosts for a variety of double- and single-stranded DNA mycoplasma viruses, but REP⁻ cells can no longer propagate single-stranded DNA mycoplasma viruses, although they continue to be hosts for double-stranded DNA mycoplasma viruses (see chapter 3). REP⁻ cells have the same restriction-modification activity as do wild-type strain JA1 cells.

A. laidlawii 8195 was isolated as a spontaneous mutant of REP⁻ cells; strain 8195 cells retain the REP⁻ phenotype but have lost the strain JA1 restriction system (30). Since the JA1 restriction system is specific for m^5Cyt-containing DNA, the loss of the JA1 restriction system in strain 8195 was shown by the result that mycoplasma virus DNA containing m^5Cyt is restricted by strain JA1 cells but not by strain 8195 cells (30). Hence, strain 8195 cells should be useful hosts for mycoplasma gene transfer systems because there is no host cell restriction system to degrade incoming DNA.

Another surprising difference between strains JA1 and 8195 was found in recent studies in which the *recA* genes from both strains were cloned and sequenced (8). The sequences are identical except for a point mutation creating a stop codon in the coding region of the strain 8195 *recA* gene, which means that strain JA1 is probably *recA*⁺ and strain 8195 is probably *recA*. Strain 8195 is therefore an important host for cloning experiments because of its restriction-minus, RecA⁻ phenotype.

S. citri ASP2

A type II restriction endonuclease, *Sci*NI, has been purified from *Spiroplasma citri* ASP2 cells (31). *Sci*NI recognizes the sequence GCGC. Eleven isoschizomers have been identified in eubacteria; two have been shown (like *Sci*NI) to cleave after the first G (i.e., G/CGC), leaving a two-base 5′ overhang, and two cleave after the second G (i.e., GCG/C), leaving a two-base 3′ overhang (references in reference 27).

DNAs from *S. citri* ASP2 and *H. influenzae* (the source of the *Sci*NI isoschizomer restriction endonuclease *Hha*I) are not cleaved by *Sci*NI or *Hha*I (31), indicating that the same modification methylation protects cell DNA against *Sci*NI and *Hha*I. Since *Hha*I cleaves DNA containing GCGC but not GmCGC (references in reference 27), modification in *S. citri* ASP2 probably involves methylation of cytosine to m^{5}Cyt in the sequence GCGC to form GmCGC.

Although some *S. citri* strains have been found to restrict *Spiroplasma* viruses (31), it is not known whether *Sci*NI is responsible for these restriction activities.

M. fermentans

A type II restriction endonuclease, *Mfe*I, has been isolated from a *Mycoplasma fermentans* strain contaminating two T-cell lines (10). The *Mfe*I cleavage site is C/AATTG, leaving a four-base 5' overhang. No isoschizomer for this recognition sequence has been reported (27).

U. urealyticum 960

A type II restriction endonuclease, *Uur*960I, has been isolated from *Ureaplasma urealyticum* 960 (6). *Uur*960I cleaves the sequence GC/NGC. Four isoschizomers have been identified in eubacteria, all with the same cleavage site (references in reference 27). *U. urealyticum* 960 DNA has been found to be resistant to cleavage by restriction endonuclease *Uur*960I and one of the isoschizomers, *Fnu*4HI, suggesting that the same base modification is involved for protection from both *Uur*960I and *Fnu*4HI (6). However, the modification system for neither enzyme has been identified thus far.

Mycoplasma Methylases

Methylation in eubacteria

Many bacteria have sequence-specific methylases but lack restriction endonucleases with the same sequence specificity (4, 19). It has been suggested that some of these methylases may be remnants of restriction-modification systems that lost their restriction activity by mutation (4).

Methylation is not required for bacterial viability, since *E. coli* mutants with no detectable m^{6}Ade or m^{5}Cyt can be isolated (19). Similarly, the existence of an *A. laidlawii* strain with no detectable methylated bases (8) means methylated bases are not required for mycoplasma viability.

There have been a number of biological functions proposed for m^{5}Cyt and m^{6}Ade, in addition to protecting host cell DNA from its own restriction system (19): m^{5}Cyt residues are mutation hot spots, and m^{6}Ade appears to function in regulation of gene activity, DNA mismatch repair, and (at least in *E. coli*) initiation of DNA replication.

Methylation in mycoplasmas

With the exception of *A. laidlawii* JA1 (7), methylated bases have been detected in every mycoplasma examined: *A. laidlawii* K2 (7) and oral strain (25), *S. apis* (21), *S. citri* (21), *S. floricola* (21), *Spiroplasma* sp. strains MQ-1 and PPS1 (21), *M. arginini* (25), *M. capri-colum* (2, 25, 33), *M. hyopneumoniae* (5), *M. hyorhinis* (25), *M. mycoides* (2, 33), and *M. orale* (25). The methylated bases are m^{5}Cyt and m^{6}Ade, although only one of these methylated bases could be detected in some mycoplasmas and the extent of methylation is a function of culture age (21).

GATC is a common restriction-modification site in eubacteria (27) and must also be frequently restricted and/or modified in mycoplasmas, since this sequence has been found to be restricted in *A. laidlawii* K2 (30) and methylated in several mycoplasmas. *A. laidlawii* K2 methylates GATC to GATmC (30), and *M. hyopneumoniae* (5) and *M. mycoides* (2) methylate GATC to GmATC. The latter methylation is not universal for all strains of the *M. mycoides* cluster (2).

Further study of strains in the *M. mycoides* cluster has indicated that some of these strains contain a modification within the GGNCC sequences in their DNAs, because they are resistant to digestion by restriction endonucleases *Apa*I (recognition sequence GGGCCC) and *Sau*96I (recognition sequence GGNCC) (33). Confirmation that genomic DNAs of these strains contain *Apa*I digestion-resistant recognition sites has been obtained by demonstrating *Apa*I digestion of polymerase chain reaction amplification products of DNA from a tRNA gene cluster containing the GGGCCC sequence within a tRNA^{Ala} gene (34).

The only mycoplasma methylase to be purified and characterized thus far is *Spiroplasma* sp. strain MQ-1 cytosine methylase (26). This enzyme is a specific methylase for cytosine in the dinucleotide CG and has amino acid sequence homology to other cytosine methylases.

RESTRICTION-MODIFICATION SYSTEMS AND MYCOPLASMA EVOLUTION

Mycoplasmas have retained typical bacterial restriction-modification systems during their degenerate evolution from the gram-positive eubacteria (17, 32, 35). This appears somewhat surprising, since restriction-modification systems are not essential for eubacteria or mycoplasma cell survival (discussed above), and mycoplasma evolution involved significant reductions in genetic complexity (mycoplasma genomes are three- to sevenfold smaller than that of *E. coli* [see chapter 9]). Hence, there must have been selective pressure to keep restriction endonuclease and modification methylase genes during mycoplasma phylogeny.

Although restriction-modification systems may not be essential for bacterial survival, they may play an important role in bacterial evolution. Eubacterial restriction-modification systems are believed to have two functions: protection against bacteriophage infection (14) and promotion of mutation. Both restriction endonucleases and modification methylases may affect mutation frequency: restriction endonucleases by increasing recombination by cleaving foreign DNA and providing double-stranded DNA ends for recombination (23), and modification methylases by methylating cytosine residues to produce mutation hot spots (19). Hence, the selective pressure for retaining eubacterial restriction-modification systems may be a consequence of the increased evolutionary potential of cells with these systems.

Restriction-modification systems may play similar roles in mycoplasmas, perhaps explaining the rapid rate of mycoplasma evolution (17, 32, 35–37; also see chapter 33). In particular, the role of m⁵Cyt in creating mutation hot spots might be a major driving force in mycoplasma evolution. In most mycoplasma DNAs, m⁵Cyt is present at significantly higher molar ratios than is m⁶Ade (7, 21). Since mycoplasmas with low-G+C DNAs have higher G+C contents in coding regions than in noncoding regions (9, 11, 12, 22), m⁵Cyt residues (and hence mutation hot spots) may be concentrated in coding regions and, together with the relatively high mutation rate per base pair found in mycoplasmas (17, 35–37), increase the potential of specific mycoplasma DNA regions to explore a wide range of evolutionary possibilities.

The role of restriction-modification systems in promoting DNA base changes in eubacteria and mycoplasmas may be the selective pressure for retaining these systems during evolution of eubacteria and mycoplasmas. The effect may have been amplified in mycoplasmas because of the concentration of cytosine residues in mycoplasma coding regions and the high mycoplasma mutation rate, leading to an increase in mutation in these regions and consequent rapid evolution of the mycoplasmas.

Acknowledgments. We thank Lloyd Finch for his critical reading of and suggestions regarding the manuscript, and we thank Lloyd Finch and Jane Whitley for providing unpublished data.

REFERENCES

1. **Arber, W.** 1968. Host controlled restriction and modification of bacteriophage. *Symp. Soc. Gen. Microbiol.* **18:**296–314.
2. **Bergemann, A. D., J. C. Whitley, and L. R. Finch.** 1990. Taxonomic significance of differences in DNA methylation within the *Mycoplasma mycoides* cluster detected with restriction endonucleases *Mbo*I and *Dpn*I. *Lett. Appl. Microbiol.* **11:**48–51.
3. **Bertani, G., and J. J. Weigle.** 1953. Host controlled variation in bacterial viruses. *J. Bacteriol.* **65:**113–21.
4. **Bickle, T. A**. 1987. DNA restriction and modification systems, p. 692–696. *In* F. C. Neidhardt, J. L. Ingraham, K. B. Low, B. Magasanik, M. Schaechter, and H. E. Umbarger (ed.), *Escherichia coli and Salmonella typhimurium: Cellular and Molecular Biology.* American Society for Microbiology, Washington, D.C.
5. **Chan, H. W., and R. F. Ross.** 1984. Restriction endonuclease analyses of two porcine mycoplasma deoxyribonucleic acids: sequence-specific methylation in the *Mycoplasma hyopneumoniae* genome. *Int. J. Syst. Bacteriol.* **34:**16–20.
6. **Cocks, B. G., and L. R. Finch.** 1987. Characterization of a restriction endonuclease from *Ureaplasma urealyticum* 960 and differences in deoxyribonucleic acid modification of human ureaplasmas. *Int. J. Syst. Bacteriol.* **37:**451–453.
7. **Dybvig, K., D. Swinton, J. Maniloff, and S. Hattman.** 1982. Cytosine methylation of the sequence GATC in a mycoplasma. *J. Bacteriol.* **151:**1420–1424.
8. **Dybvig, K., and A. Woodward.** 1992. Cloning and DNA sequence of a mycoplasmal *recA* gene. *J. Bacteriol.* **174:**778–784.
9. **Frydenberg, J., and C. Christiansen.** 1985. The sequence of 16S rRNA from *Mycoplasma* strain PG50. *DNA* **4:**127–137.
10. **Halden, N. F., J. B. Wolf, and W. J. Leonard.** 1989. Identification of a novel site specific endonuclease produced by *Mycoplasma fermentans*: discovery while characterizing DNA binding proteins in T lymphocyte cell lines. *Nucleic Acids Res.* **17:**3491–3499.
11. **Inamine, J. M., T. P. Denny, S. Loechel, U. Schaper, C.-H. Huang, K. F. Bott, and P.-C. Hu.** 1988. Nucleotide sequence of the P1 attachment-protein gene of *Mycoplasma pneumoniae. Gene* **64:**217–229.
12. **Iwami, M., A. Muto, F. Yamao, and S. Osawa.** 1984. Nucleotide sequence of the *rrnB* 16S ribosomal RNA gene from *Mycoplasma capricolum. Mol. Gen. Genet.* **196:**317–322.
13. **Just, W., and G. Klotz.** 1990. Terminal redundancy and circular permutation of mycoplasma virus L3 DNA. *J. Gen. Virol.* **71:**2157–2162.
14. **Kruger, D. H., and T. A. Bickle.** 1983. Bacteriophage survival: multiple mechanisms for avoiding the deoxyribonucleic acid restriction systems of their hosts. *Microbiol. Rev.* **47:**345–360.
15. **Lacks, S., and B. Greenberg.** 1975. A deoxyribonuclease of *Diplococcus pneumoniae* specific for methylated DNA. *J. Biol. Chem.* **250:**4060–4066.
16. **Lacks, S., and B. Greenberg.** 1977. Complementary specificity of restriction endonucleases of *Diplococcus pneumoniae* with respect to DNA methylation. *J. Mol. Biol.* **114:**153–168.
17. **Maniloff, J**. 1983. Evolution of wall-less prokaryotes. *Annu. Rev. Microbiol.* **37:**477–499.
18. **Maniloff, J., and J. Das.** 1975. Replication of mycoplasmaviruses, p. 445–450. *In* M. Goulian, P. Hanawalt, and C. F. Fox (ed.), *DNA Synthesis and Its Regulation.* W. A. Benjamin, Reading, Mass.
19. **Marinus, M. G.** 1987. Methylation of DNA, p. 697–702. *In* F. C. Neidhardt, J. L. Ingraham, K. B. Low, B. Magasanik, M. Schaechter, and H. E. Umbarger (ed.), *Escherichia coli and Salmonella typhimurium: Cellular and Molecular Biology.* American Society for Microbiology, Washington, D.C.
20. **Nowak, J. A., J. Das, and J. Maniloff.** 1976. Characterization of an *Acholeplasma laidlawii* variant with a REP⁻ phenotype. *J. Bacteriol.* **127:**832–836.
21. **Nur, I., M. Szyf, A. Razin, G. Glaser, S. Rottem, and S. Razin.** 1985. Procaryotic and eucaryotic traits of DNA methylation in spiroplasmas (mycoplasmas). *J. Bacteriol.* **164:**19–24.
22. **Ohkubo, S., A. Muto, Y. Kawauchi, F. Yamao, and S. Osawa.** 1987. The ribosomal gene cluster of *Mycoplasma capricolum. Mol. Gen. Genet.* **210:**314–322.
23. **Price, C., and T. A. Bickle.** 1986. A possible role for DNA restriction in bacterial evolution. *Microbiol. Sci.* **3:**296–299.
24. **Raleigh, E. A., and G. Wilson.** 1986. *Escherichia coli* K-12 restricts DNA containing 5-methylcytosine. *Proc. Natl. Acad. Sci. USA* **83:**9070–9074.
25. **Razin, A., and S. Razin.** 1980. Methylated bases in mycoplasmal DNA. *Nucleic Acids Res.* **8:**1383–1390.
26. **Renbaum, P., D. Abrahamove, A. Fainsod, G. G. Wilson, S. Rottem, and A. Razin.** 1990. Cloning, characterization, and expression in *Escherichia coli* of the gene coding for the CpG DNA methylase from *Spiroplasma sp.* strain MQ1 (M Sss1). *Nucleic Acids Res.* **18:**1145–1152.
27. **Roberts, R. J.** 1990. Restriction enzymes and their isoschizomers. *Nucleic Acids Res.* **18**(Suppl.):2331–2365.
28. **Sharp, P. M.** 1986. Molecular evolution of bacteriophages: evidence of selection against the recognition sites of host restriction enzymes. *Mol. Biol. Evol.* **3:**75–83.
29. **Sladek, T. L., and J. Maniloff.** 1987. Endonuclease from *Acholeplasma laidlawii* strain JA1 associated with *in vivo*

restriction of DNA containing 5-methylcytosine. *Isr. J. Med. Sci.* **23:**423–426.

30. **Sladek, T. L., J. A. Nowak, and J. Maniloff**. 1986. Mycoplasma restriction: identification of a new type of restriction specificity for DNA containing 5-methylcytosine. *J. Bacteriol.* **165:**219–225.

31. **Stephens, M. A**. 1982. Partial purification and cleavage specificity of a site-specific endonuclease, *Sci*NI, isolated from *Spiroplasma citri. J. Bacteriol.* **149:**508–514.

32. **Weisburg, W. G., J. G. Tully, D. L. Rose, J. P. Petzel, H. Oyaizu, D. Yang, L. Mandelco, J. Sechrest, T. G. Lawrence, J. Van Etten, J. Maniloff, and C. R. Woese**. 1989. A phylogenetic analysis of the mycoplasmas: basis for their classification. *J. Bacteriol.* **171:**6455–6467.

33. **Whitley, J. C**. 1991. Genome organization in mycoplasmas. Ph.D. thesis. University of Melbourne, Parkville, Victoria, Australia.

34. **Whitley, J. C., S. Reid, and L. R. Finch**. Personal communication.

35. **Woese, C. R**. 1987. Bacterial evolution. *Microbiol. Rev.* **51:**221–271.

36. **Woese, C. R., J. Maniloff, and L. B. Zablen**. 1980. Phylogenetic analysis of the mycoplasmas. *Proc. Natl. Acad. Sci. USA* **77:**494–498.

37. **Woese, C. R., E. Stackebrandt, and W. Ludwig**. 1985. What are mycoplasmas: the relationship of tempo and mode in bacterial evolution. *J. Mol. Evol.* **21:**305–316.

19. Transcription and Translation

AKIRA MUTO, YOSHIKI ANDACHI, FUMIAKI YAMAO, REIJI TANAKA, and SYOZO OSAWA

INTRODUCTION

The mechanisms of bacterial transcription and translation have been extensively studied, mainly in *Escherichia coli*, whereas very little is known for mycoplasmas. Elucidation of the genetics of mycoplasmas, which is indispensable for understanding transcription and translation, has remained undeveloped until recently, mainly because of the difficulty of applying concepts of classical microbial genetics to these organisms. The recent development of recombinant DNA techniques has opened the way for analysis of mycoplasma genes. DNA sequences of various genes, including transcriptional and translational signals, have now become available, and knowledge of transcriptional and translational components (such as RNA polymerase, ribosomes, and tRNAs) has been accumulating.

This chapter describes the features of transcription and translation of mycoplasmas derived from these studies, focusing on *Mycoplasma capricolum*, the most extensively studied mycoplasma.

GENERAL FEATURES OF MYCOPLASMA GENES

Overall Composition of the Genome

The genome of mycoplasmas is distinguished by small size and the low G+C content (42, 54). Among members of the class *Mollicutes*, the sizes of *Acholeplasma*, *Spiroplasma*, and *Anaeroplasma* genomes are about 10^9 Da; those of *Mycoplasma* and *Ureaplasma* genomes are about 5×10^8 Da, the smallest of all known free-living organisms. The reported G+C contents of mycoplasma genomes range from 25 to 40%. Many mycoplasmas, including *M. capricolum*, have a G+C content as low as 25%, the lowest in eubacteria. Mycoplasmas are phylogenetically related to gram-positive bacteria such as *Bacillus* spp. and *Clostridium* spp. (22, 23, 57, 74, 75) and are regarded as degenerate forms of gram-positive bacteria. They seem to have evolved under two evolutionary constraints, to minimize genome size and G+C content (49).

The size of the genome reflects the number of genes encoded. A genome of 5×10^8 Da can code for about 650 proteins with an average molecular weight of 4×10^4, assuming that the genes are packed in the genome without spacers. However, the bacterial genome usually contains spacers, including various signals, that make up 20 to 30% of the total DNA. Therefore, the actual number of genes in *M. capricolum* may be estimated to be around 500. Two-dimensional polyacrylamide gel electrophoresis of the total proteins of *M. capricolum* shows about 350 protein spots, indicating that at least 350 genes for proteins are expressed in these cells (29). The average molecular weight of the *M. capricolum* proteins is about 4×10^4. Under the same conditions, the number of protein spots detected

Akira Muto, Yoshiki Andachi, and Syozo Osawa • Department of Biology, School of Science, Nagoya University, Furo-cho, Chikusa-ku, Nagoya 464-01, Japan.   **Fumiaki Yamao** • National Institute of Genetics, Mishima 411, Japan.   **Reiji Tanaka** • Aburahi Laboratories, Shionogi Ltd., Kouga, Shiga 520-34, Japan.

in *Escherichia coli* or *Bacillus subtilis* is more than 1,100. The number of expressed genes is a rough estimate of the number of proteins encoded.

All mycoplasma genomes so far analyzed have one or two sets of rRNA genes, with one gene each for 23S, 16S, and 5S rRNAs (1, 18). The *M. capricolum* genome contains 2 rRNA sets (60, 61), in contrast to 7 in *E. coli* (31, 34) and 10 in *B. subtilis* (35). *M. capricolum* has 30 genes encoding 29 tRNA species (3, 46), whereas *E. coli* carries 78 genes for 45 tRNA species (37) and *B. subtilis* contains at least 51 genes for 31 tRNA species (73). Thus, the number of mycoplasma rRNA and tRNA genes is also much lower than in other eubacteria. These data indicate that the *M. capricolum* genome contains about 400 genes, not far from the total number of the genes calculated from the genome size (about 500). This small number of genes is consistent with the view that mycoplasmas contain only a limited variety of genes, most of which must be indispensable for growth (43). The mycoplasma genome must have discarded many dispensable genes that were unnecessary for growth.

Gene Organization and Structure

The organizations and structures of many genes from various mycoplasma species have been analyzed by DNA cloning and sequencing methods. The two rRNA gene clusters, 30 tRNA genes, and a protein gene cluster including 20 ribosomal protein genes from *M. capricolum* have been cloned, and most parts of the genes, including flanking regions, have been sequenced (16, 27, 46, 51, 60). The organizations of these genes and gene clusters in the isolated clones are schematically shown in Fig. 1. The rRNA genes in the *rrnA* and *rrnB* clusters are in the order 5'-16S-23S-5S-3' (Fig. 1a), as in other eubacteria (27, 60). Each cluster is constructed as a transcription unit (operon). This organization of the rRNA operon seems to be conserved in most mycoplasma species (1, 18, 53) except *M. hyopneumoniae*, in which the 5S rRNA gene is separated from the 16S-23S rRNA operon in the genome (71). The tRNA genes, which often occur in the spacer region between 16S and 23S rRNA genes in other eubacteria, are absent in the mycoplasmas analyzed so far. Twenty-two of a total of thirty tRNA genes in *M. capricolum* are organized in five tRNA gene clusters consisting of nine, five, and four tRNA genes and two sets of two tRNA genes. Eight other tRNA genes are each present as a single operon (Fig. 1b). Clustering of tRNA genes is a common feature in many eubacteria, including several mycoplasma species (56, 58, 59, 64). The gene arrangement in most of the *M. capricolum* tRNA gene clusters reveals extensive similarity with that in *B. subtilis* (46). Figure 1c shows the organization of a large gene cluster that includes genes for 20 ribosomal proteins and 2 other proteins (51). The gene order in the cluster is essentially the same as that in the S10 and *spc* operons of *E. coli* (8). These facts indicate that the organizations and structures of genes indispensable for growth, such as those for rRNAs, tRNAs, and ribosomal proteins, have been highly conserved in mycoplasmas during evolution, despite a great reduction in the total number of genes.

The sequences of various parts of *M. capricolum* ge-

nome are also low in G + C, reflecting the low G + C content of genomic DNA. The spacer regions between the genes have the lowest G + C content (about 20%), and the protein genes have the second lowest (about 30%). The G + C contents of rRNA and tRNA genes are high (46 to 54%) compared with those of other regions of the genome, although they are lower than in the corresponding regions of other eubacteria (48). Thus, all regions of the *M. capricolum* genome contribute to the low G + C content of the genome.

The low G + C content of mycoplasma genomes may be largely brought about by AT-biased directional mutation pressure (AT pressure) that has been exerted on mycoplasma genomes (48, 67). During mycoplasma evolution, mutations predominantly replacing G·C pairs by A·T (or T·A) pairs must have occurred in the whole genome. Directional mutations must have occurred equally in all regions of the genome and then been subjected to selective constraints that usually operate to eliminate functionally deleterious changes (32). As a result, functionally less important regions of the genome evolve faster than more important ones, because many mutations in the former are nondeleterious, i.e., selectively neutral. Thus, AT pressure changes the G + C content of various regions of the genome in the same direction (A + T richness), but to different extents, depending on their functional importance. Since most parts of spacers are functionally the least important in the genome, mutations there are selectively neutral, and therefore the evolution rate from G·C to A·T pairs is higher than for other parts. The rRNA and tRNA genes are less variable because their transcripts are not translated, and most if not all rRNA and tRNA sequences are important for biological function. The protein genes are more variable than the stable RNA genes, because synonymous codon changes can occur without deleterious effect. The effect of AT pressure on the choice of synonymous codons is discussed below.

TRANSCRIPTION

RNA Polymerase

DNA-dependent RNA polymerase has been partially purified from several *Spiroplasma* species (15). The subunit composition of the enzyme from *Spiroplasma melliferum* analyzed by polyacrylamide gel electrophoresis reveals at least three major components of about 140, 130, and 38 kDa, which probably correspond to the *E. coli* RNA polymerase core enzyme subunits β (155 kDa), β' (145 kDa), and α (40 kDa), respectively. The partially purified *M. capricolum* enzyme fraction (77) also contains at least two large subunits of 130 to 140 kDa (unpublished data). Although no information is available for the σ subunit, the structure of mycoplasma RNA polymerase seems to resemble those of eubacteria such as *E. coli* and *B. subtilis*. In fact, several mycoplasma genes cloned in *E. coli* vector DNA are expressed in *E. coli* in in vivo as well as in vitro transcription systems (see below), suggesting that the enzymes of mycoplasmas and *E. coli* resemble each other both structurally and functionally.

The mycoplasmal RNA polymerase is apparently re-

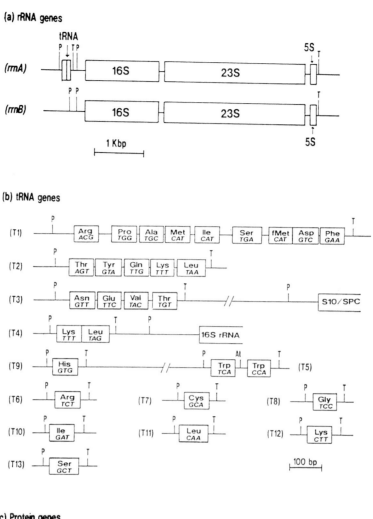

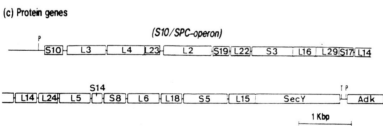

Figure 1. Organization of rRNA, tRNA, and protein genes of *M. capricolum*. (a) rRNA operons (60); (b) tRNA operons (46); (c) S10/*spc* operon (51). P, T, and At represent putative promoter, terminator, and attenuator sites, respectively.

sistant to rifampin, an antibiotic that blocks transcription initiation by binding to the β subunit of eubacterial RNA polymerase. Growth of various mycoplasma species is not inhibited by rifampin (4, 11, 12). Gadeau et al. (15) showed that partially purified RNA polymerases from *S. melliferm* and *S. apis* were at least 1,000 times less sensitive to rifampin in vitro than was *E. coli* RNA polymerase. The molecular basis of this insensitivity is unknown.

Promoter and Initiation

RNA polymerase recognizes a promoter sequence located upstream of a gene or operon and initiates tran-

scription. From compilations of DNA sequences of promoters from *E. coli*, the consensus promoter sequence, 5'-TTGACA-about 17 bp-TATAAT-5 to 9 bp-RNA start-3' has been deduced (20). The consensus TTGACA and TATAAT sequences are referred to as −35 and −10 sequences (or boxes), respectively.

The upstream regions of most cloned genes or operons from a variety of mycoplasma species contain promoterlike sequences resembling the *E. coli* −35 and −10 consensus sequences. In Fig. 2, the promoterlike sequences from all of the genes and operons of *M. capricolum* so far analyzed (Fig. 1) are aligned. The −10 sequences are well conserved in most cases, whereas the −35 regions are more variable. The space between the −10 and −35 boxes is 15 to 17 bp.

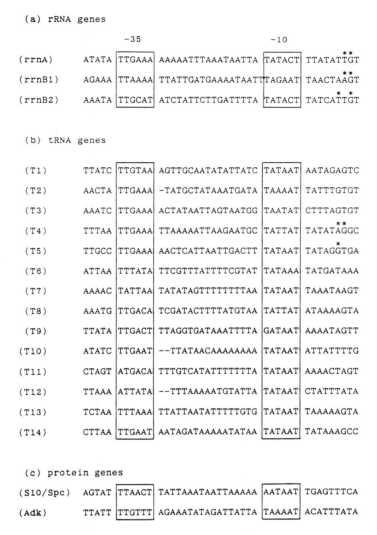

Figure 2. Promoters and transcription initiation sites. Putative −35 and −10 sequences are boxed. The initiation sites of RNA transcription are shown by asterisks (16, 70, 77).

The transcription initiation sites of the rRNA operons and some of the tRNA operons of *M. capricolum* have been analyzed by S1 mapping and/or primer extension methods, using in vitro-synthesized RNA or native mRNA fractions prepared from cell extracts (16, 53, 70, 77). The deduced initiation sites are indicated on the sequences in Fig. 2 (asterisks). All of the initiation sites are 6 to 8 bp downstream of the putative −10 boxes, as in the case of *E. coli*, suggesting that the *M. capricolum* RNA polymerase recognizes promoter sequences resembling those of *E. coli*. In fact, Gafny et al. (16) reported that the promoters of *M. capricolum rrnA* and a tRNA gene cluster were recognized by *E. coli* polymerase both in vivo and in vitro.

Termination and Attenuation

In *E. coli*, there appear to be two ways in which RNA polymerase can terminate transcription: (i) by passage across a special type of DNA sequence that specifies, in the RNA, a G + C-rich hairpin followed by a series of U residues (rho-independent-type termination) or (ii) by exposure of a paused transcription complex to the termination factor rho or other specific protein factors (rho-dependent-type termination) (76).

There are rho-independent terminator-like structures, consisting of a dyad-symmetrical sequence and a T cluster, downstream of all rRNA, tRNA, and ribosomal protein genes or gene clusters in *M. capricolum* (Fig. 3). However, the sequences forming the hairpin structures are A + T rich, in contrast to the G + C-rich sequences in *E. coli*. Analysis of in vitro transcription of the *M. capricolum* Trp tRNA gene cluster indicated that termination takes place at the T-stretch region soon after the dyad-symmetrical structure (77). Rho-independent terminator-like sequences have also been found in other mycoplasma genes (9, 13, 38, 56, 58, 59, 64), showing that this type of transcription termination is common in mycoplasmas, although it is not known whether rho-dependent-type termination is also used.

The genes for tRNA^Trp(UCA) and tRNA^Trp(CCA) in *M. capricolum* are arranged tandemly on the chromosome

(a) rRNA genes

(rrnA)   GCAAGCTGCCAGTT TATAAGAACCCTAGTGGTTCTTTTTTAATATATACTTGAATTA

(rrnB)   GCAAGCTGCCAGTT TATAAGAACCTTAGTGGTTCTTTTTTTTGTTTCTCTTTTTAAAA

(b) tRNA genes

(T1)   CCA CTTGAAATTAAAAAATCCAGTAGTCATAAGACTACTTTTTTTATTTTTATAACAT

(T2)   CCA TTTTGAAAATCAACATGCTATAAAAGGCATGTTTTTTTATTTTCTACTTTTTAAA

(T3)   CCA TTAGAAAATTCGAGCACTATAGTGCTCTTTATTTTTAAACAACCAA

(T4)   CCA ATTTTGAATTTAACCAGATTTTTCTGGTTTTTTATTTGAAATTTTAAAATGTTAT

(T5)   CCA AAGAAATAAAAAAAAACTGGAAATTCCAGTTTTTTTTATTCTTCTTCAATTGCAAC

(T6)   CCA TTTAGAATCATTAAAGAGCTAAGCTCTTTTTTTTTTTACGAAAAAA

(T7)   CCA TTTGAAAAATAAAAATAGTCGTTGACTATTTTTTTATTTTATTAAGTTATTAA

(T8)   CCA TTGAAAATAACAACAACACTTAGGTGTTGTTTTTTTATATTCAATCTTATA

(T9)   CCA TTTTGAAAACAACAAACAACACTTAGGTGTTGTTTTTTTATTTTTACTAATGAATG

(T10)   CCA TATGAATATTAATTTTGACACCAATTGGTGTCTTTTTTTTTTACTTTTTTTATATAA

(T11)   CCA ATTGATTATAAACTTGGAGAAATCCAAGTTTTTTATTTTTTTTATTCATTAGAATAA

(T12)   CCA TTTTTGATAACACAAAAAAAGACTTTTAAGTCTTTTTTTATTTTATACTTTAAAT

(T13)   CCA TTAGAAATTAAATAGACTACATAAGTAGTCTTTTTTTATTTTTAATTTTAATATA

(T5 att.) CCA TTTTGAAAGCAAATCACACTTTGTGTGATTTTTTTAT

(c) protein genes

(S10/spc) TCTCATATTTGA TAAAAAGCAATACGCCTTTTTTACTTTATTGTTATTTTATAT

Figure 3. Terminator and attenuator (att.). Dyad-symmetrical sequences are shown by arrows under the sequences (46, 51, 60).

as an operon (78) (Fig. 1). Promoter- and terminatorlike sequences are located upstream of the tRNA(UCA) gene and downstream of the tRNA(CCA) gene, respectively. In addition, there is a terminatorlike sequence, a dyad-symmetrical sequence followed by a stretch of T's in the 40-bp spacer between the two tRNA genes. In vitro transcription of the DNA fragment containing this operon with partially purified *M. capricolum* RNA polymerase produced two RNA transcripts of 240 and 120 bp. S1 mapping analysis showed that initiation of these two transcripts occurred at the same position, 10 bp upstream of the tRNA(CCA) gene (77). This finding indicates that the 240-bp transcript is a dimeric precursor molecule containing the two tRNA genes, while the 120-bp transcript is a precursor to tRNA(UCA). The amount of dimeric precursor is about one-fifth that of the monomeric precursor (77), which means that five times more tRNA(UCA) than tRNA(CCA) is produced. In fact, the intracellular level of tRNA(UCA) is 5 to 10 times as high as that of tRNA(CCA). The terminatorlike sequence between the two tRNA genes operates as an attenuator of transcription, and more than 80% of the transcripts that start from the initiation site are terminated by the structure.

Processing of RNA Gene Transcripts

There are complementary sequences at the 5' and 3' flanking regions of both the 16S and 23S rRNA genes

of *M. capricolum* (27, 70). Thus, within the putative primary transcript of the rRNA operon, two large stems may form by pairing of complementary sequences, with the 16S and 23S structural gene regions as loops (Fig. 4). Similar stem-loop structures have been found in the rRNA transcripts of *E. coli* (81) and *B. subtilis* (50, 66), and the stem regions have been suggested as possible substrates for a processing enzyme (RNase III) during rRNA maturation. Moreover, a 12-bp sequence is similar in the 16S and 23S stems (boxed in Fig. 4) and is also conserved in the rRNA operons of *Mycoplasma* sp. strain PG50 (53) and *M. hyopneumoniae* (69). One of the precursor rRNAs has been shown to start from a site in the repeated stem sequence in the 5' flanking region of the 16S rRNA gene of *rrnA* (indicated by an arrow in Fig. 4). Interestingly, a repeated stem structure with a very similar sequence is also present in *B. subtilis* (50, 66) and is where one of the processing sites is located. Thus, RNA processing signals as well as the processing enzyme(s) seem to be conserved between mycoplasmas and *B. subtilis*.

Regulation

Regulation of gene expression occurs mainly at the transcription initiation level. Most of the genes encoded in the mycoplasma genome seem to be essential for growth and thus are assumed to be expressed con-

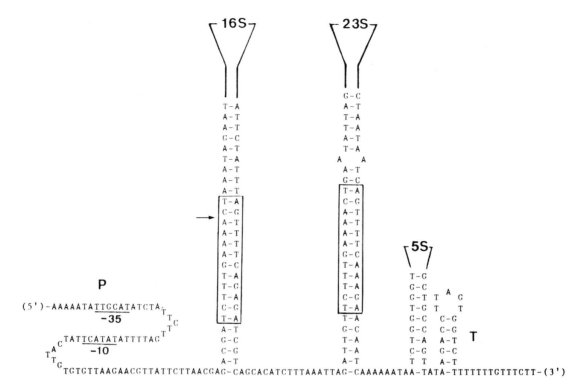

Figure 4. Possible secondary structure for the transcript of the *rrnB* gene cluster. The repeated stem structures are boxed. One of the processing sites is indicated by an arrow (16, 70). The promoterlike sequences (P; −35 and −10 boxes) and the terminatorlike sequence (T) are also shown.

stitutively. The refined switching mechanisms for transcriptional adaptation to environments, such as negative control by repressor molecules in *E. coli* and other eubacteria, may not be required in mycoplasmas. The major control in mycoplasmas might be quantitative regulation of the gene products rather than an on/off control switch for gene expression. In *E. coli*, intracellular amounts of many constitutively expressed gene products (such as rRNAs, tRNAs, ribosomal proteins, and RNA polymerase) are coordinately controlled depending on the growth rate of the cell (41). One of the major control elements for this regulation is believed to be guanosine tetraphosphate (ppGpp) or guanosine pentaphosphate (pppGpp), which operate as negative factors for transcription initiation (6, 41). In amino acid auxotrophic mutants of *E. coli*, synthesis of rRNA and tRNA is inhibited by deprivation of the required amino acid (stringent control), accompanied by simultaneous accumulation of ppGpp and pppGpp in the cell (6). Glaser et al. (17) reported that rRNA synthesis in *M. capricolum* was markedly inhibited by omission of an amino acid supplement from the partially defined medium and that ppGpp and pppGpp accumulated simultaneously. This result suggests that *M. capricolum* is also subject to negative stringent control homologous to that in *E. coli*. Since mycoplasmas, as parasites, may not usually face such a sudden change in environmental conditions, the physiological meaning of the observed phenomenon is unclear. It is possible, however, that the intracellular level of ppGpp or pppGpp plays some role in the coordinate regulation of constitutively ex-

pressed genes in mycoplasmas. In *E. coli*, a G + C-rich "discriminator" sequence between −7 and +1 from the transcription initiation site is reported to be required for repression of promoters by ppGpp (72). Neither rRNA nor tRNA genes of *M. capricolum* have G + C-rich sequences in their promoter regions (Fig. 2). The expression of *M. capricolum rrnA* is activated rather than repressed by high levels of ppGpp in *E. coli* (16), suggesting that the control mechanism involving ppGpp in *M. capricolum*, if any, may be different from that in *E. coli*.

The relative amounts of the 29 tRNA species in *M. capricolum* vary over 2 orders of magnitude (79). There is a positive correlation between the frequency of synonymous codons and the relative amount of corresponding isoacceptor tRNAs. Also, a strong correlation exists between the total amount of tRNA(s) for an amino acid and the amino acid composition of *M. capricolum* proteins; the higher the amino acid content in proteins, the higher the amount of tRNA(s) specifying the amino acid. The amount of tRNAs in the cell seems to be controlled so as to adapt to the amino acid usage in proteins, ensuring efficient growth of the cell. Since 28 of the 29 tRNA species of *M. capricolum* are each encoded by a single gene, the wide variety of the relative contents of tRNAs cannot be attributed to a dosage effect. The promoter efficiency of the genes might determine each tRNA level in the cell. However, the amounts of various tRNAs transcribed from the same operon are not equal in the cell; the order of the tRNA gene arrangement in the operon does not reflect the levels of the product tRNAs. These facts imply that intracellular tRNA levels are regulated not only by promoter efficiencies for different tRNA genes but also by other factors such as processing of tRNA precursors or degradation of the products (79).

TRANSLATION

Shine-Dalgarno Sequence

The 3'-terminal sequence of 16S rRNA of *M. capricolum* is 5'- −−−−−GAUCACCUCCUUU-3' (27), which is conserved among eubacteria. Base pairing between the 3' end of 16S rRNA and complementary sequences on mRNA upstream of the initiation codon (Shine-Dalgarno sequence) may be required for correct translation initiation on ribosomes (19, 62). Figure 5 lists the 5' termini and upstream sequences of all genes in the S10/*spc* operon of *M. capricolum*. Supporting this view, there is a three- to eight-base stretch of a probable ribosome binding sequence, complementary to the 3'-terminal sequence of 16S rRNA, upstream of the initiation codons. Probable Shine-Dalgarno sequences have also been found in the other mycoplasma species (9, 13, 38).

S10	AAATTAGTAAATTT<u>AGGAGG</u>TTAGT	ATG	GCAGAA
L3	TGATTATCAATT<u>AGGAGG</u>AAATAAA	ATG	AAAGGA
L4	AGTTCAAGCATAGTT<u>GAGGT</u>AAGAA	ATG	AAATTA
L23	TTGCAGTTG<u>AGGAGG</u>TATACGCATA	ATG	CATATC
L2	AGCGCATTAAATAG<u>AAAGGG</u>AAAAC	ATG	GCAATT
S19	ATAAG<u>AAAGGGAG</u>AATAGAAGATAAT	ATG	GCAAGA
L22	ATT<u>AGGTT</u>GGATAAGAACTTAAACA	ATG	GAAGCA
S3	AAAAATAAG<u>AAAGGA</u>TAGTTAGGAA	ATG	GGACAA
L16	CTAAT<u>AAAGGAGG</u>TAAAAGATAATT	ATG	TTACAA
L29	AATTTGTTAAAAG<u>AGGTG</u>AAAATTA	ATG	GCTAAA
L17	CTGATACT<u>AAAGGAG</u>AAACTAAATA	ATG	CAAAGA
L14	AACTTTATAAT<u>AGGAG</u>ATAAAAAAT	ATG	GATTCA
L24	GAAGTATTAT<u>AGGAGG</u>AACCAGATT	ATG	GGCAAA
L5	TAAATAAG<u>AAAGGA</u>AATAAATTAGT	ATG	AAATCA
S14	AAAATAGAAC<u>AAGGG</u>AGATATTATA	ATG	GCTAAA
S8	ATAGAAAGA<u>GAGA</u>AGATTCAAAAGT	ATG	ACAACA
L6	TTCATTTGATAAT<u>AGGAG</u>TTTAAAT	ATG	TCTCGT
L18	TACCAGAGCTT<u>AGGG</u>ATTACTAAGT	ATG	AAATTT
S5	GGT<u>AGAAGAG</u>ATTATGACTGAAGAA	ATG	AATGTA
L15	GAGTAGTAG<u>AAAGGAG</u>TCATAATTA	ATG	AAATTA
SecY	TGGGAGGAAAAGTA<u>GAGGTGA</u>TTTA	ATG	GTTATT
Adk	GTGCTATTAAA<u>AAAGGA</u>ATTTTATAT	ATG	AACATT

Figure 5. Translational signals. Probable ribosome binding (Shine-Dalgarno) sequences upstream of the protein genes in the S10/*spc* operon are underlined. The initiation codons of genes are boxed (51).

Codon Usage

The G+C content of the coding regions of protein genes in *M. capricolum* is 29%, much lower than that of the corresponding genes in *E. coli* (51%). All of the codons in the *M. capricolum* protein genes that have been sequenced are listed in Table 1 (3). The outstanding feature is the extremely high usage of the codons having A or U(T) at the codon third position (47, 51). More than 90% of codons end in A or U. As a result, codons ending in G or C are rarely used, except codon AUG for Met. Two codons, CUC and CGG, have not been found among the 6,413 codons examined. All initiation codons are AUG, and all stop codons are UAA and UAG (mostly UAA). This implies that *M. capricolum* preferentially uses A- or U-ending codons among synonymous codons, since most synonymous codons differ in the codon third position. The preferential use of A- and U-rich codons can also be seen at the first position among synonymous codons for Leu and Arg, which have six-codon degeneracy. Among six Leu codons, UUR (R = A or G) and CUN (N = U, C, A, or G), 82% of codons used in *M. capricolum* are UUR (mostly UUA). Similarly, AGR codons (mostly AGA) are much more frequently used (76%) than are CGN codons among synonymous Arg codons. The average G+C contents of the codon first and second positions in *M. capricolum* are 43 and 36%, respectively, significantly lower than those in *E. coli* (62 and 41%, respectively) (8). Thus, all codon positions in *M. capricolum* are biased to A and U richness compared with those in *E. coli* and many other bacteria (48).

Such a biased use of A- and U-rich codons may be largely brought about by AT pressure (discussed above). Directional mutations have occurred equally at all three codon positions. However, the silent codon positions, mainly the third and partly the first positions, evolve fastest, because many mutations at these positions are nondeleterious. Thus, the bias to A and U richness in *M. capricolum* is strongest in the third codon position and then in the first position (48). The second codon position is the most invariable, because mutations at this position always cause amino acid substitutions in proteins.

The outstanding feature in the codon usage of *M. capricolum* is that two codons deviate from the universal genetic code: codon UGA, from stop to Trp (78), and codon CCG, from Arg to unassigned (nonsense) (3). These changes are evidenced by the existence of a Trp tRNA having anticodon UCA, which pairs with codon UGA, and the absence of an Arg tRNA with anticodon CGG, respectively (see below). Codon UGA is used more frequently than UGG, and codon CGG has not been found (Table 1).

In several species in the genus *Mycoplasma* (*M. gallisepticum* [25, 26], *M. pneumoniae* [24, 25, 39], *M. genitalium* [25], *M. hyorhinis* [13], and *M. arginini* [38]) and in the genus *Spiroplasma* (*S. citri* [4, 9] and *Spiroplasma* sp. strain MQ-1 [55]), codon UGA is also used for Trp, suggesting that this change is common in all species in these two genera. On the other hand, *Acholeplasma laidlawii* does not use UGA as a Trp codon (68). It is not known whether species in the genera *Ureaplasma* and *Anaeroplasma* use UGA as a Trp codon. The change of codon CCG from Arg to nonsense has been reported only for *M. capricolum*.

Table 1. Codon usage in *M. capricolum*[a]

Amino acid (codon)	Position	Amino acid (codon)	Position	Amino acid (codon)	Position	Amino acid (codon)	Position
Phe (UUU)	269	Ser (UCU)	107	Tyr (UAU)	171	Cys (UGU)	41
Phe (UUC)	28	Ser (UCC)	1	Tyr (UAC)	24	Cys (UGC)	10
Leu (UUA)	433	Ser (UCA)	169	— (UAA)	—	Trp (UGA)	42
Leu (UUG)	22	Ser (UCG)	5	— (UAG)	—	Trp (UGG)	7
Leu (CUU)	36	Pro (CCU)	66	His (CAU)	72	Arg (CGU)	54
Leu (CUC)	0	Pro (CCC)	3	His (CAC)	22	Arg (CGC)	4
Leu (CUA)	62	Pro (CCA)	120	Gln (CAA)	256	Arg (CGA)	2
Leu (CUG)	1	Pro (CCG)	3	Gln (CAG)	10	Arg (CGG)	0
Ile (AUU)	480	Thr (ACU)	206	Asn (AAU)	440	Ser (AGU)	117
Ile (AUC)	56	Thr (ACC)	8	Asn (AAC)	78	Ser (AGC)	20
Ile (AUA)	111	Thr (ACA)	151	Lys (AAA)	730	Arg (AGA)	189
Met (AUG)	153	Thr (ACG)	1	Lys (AAG)	71	Arg (AGG)	3
Val (GUU)	284	Ala (GCU)	228	Asp (GAU)	294	Gly (GGU)	180
Val (GUC)	8	Ala (GCC)	3	Asp (GAC)	24	Gly (GGC)	5
Val (GUA)	157	Ala (GCA)	140	Glu (GAA)	373	Gly (GGA)	199
Val (GUG)	16	Ala (GCG)	4	Glu (GAG)	29	Gly (GGG)	16

[a] Data for 6,814 codons used in the genes in the *spc* operon (51) and other genes (3). —, not identified.

The G+C content of *M. pneumoniae* genomic DNA is about 40%, significantly higher than that of *M. capricolum* and most other mycoplasmas (25 to 35%). The average G+C content of an *M. pneumoniae* protein gene (the surface protein P1) is 53%, and that of the codon third position is 56% (24). Thus, codon usage is not significantly biased to A and U, in contrast to the case for *M. capricolum* and most other *Mycoplasma* species, although *M. pneumoniae* uses UGA as a Trp codon (24, 25, 39). Presumably, the AT pressure would have been weakened by increased GC pressure in the *M. pneumoniae* lineage during evolution. This would be a relatively recent event, because the G+C content observed for *M. pneumoniae* DNA is high among phylogenetically related mycoplasmas. The change of the UGA assignment from stop to Trp codon must have occurred before the separation of *M. pneumoniae* from other mycoplasmas, so that UGA has been retained as a Trp codon in this mycoplasma.

Ribosomes and Translation Factors

The mycoplasmas resemble typical eubacteria in having 70S ribosomes consisting of 50S and 30S subunits. The 50S subunit contains two rRNA species, 5S and 23S, and about 30 proteins, and the 30S subunit consists of 16S rRNA and about 20 proteins. The sequences of 5S and 16S rRNAs from various mycoplasma species have been determined and used to establish phylogenetic relationships of the mycoplasma species and eubacterial groups (14, 22, 23, 57, 74, 75) (see chapter 33). The length of 5S rRNA ranges from 104 bases in *U. urealyticum* to 113 bases in *Anaeroplasma* species (23, 57, 74), shorter than that of *B. subtilis* (116 bases) or *E. coli* (120 bases). The *M. capricolum* 5S rRNA is 107 bases and has 70 and 65% sequence identity to the *B. subtilis* and *E. coli* 5S rRNAs, respectively (23). The nucleotide sequence of 16S rRNA of the *M. capricolum rrnB* operon is 1,521 bases (27), showing 85 and 74% identity to that of *B. subtilis* (66) and *E. coli* (5), respectively. *M. capricolum* has about 30 ribosomal proteins in the 50S subunit and

about 20 in the 30S subunit (29). The molecular weights of these proteins range from 9,000 to 40,000, averaging about 15,000. Thus, the number and size of *M. capricolum* ribosomal proteins are not significantly different from those of eubacteria. The amino acid sequences of 20 ribosomal proteins of *M. capricolum* deduced from the DNA sequences of the genes (51) are similar to the corresponding *E. coli* sequences (8). The sequence homology varies from 61% (protein S19) to 37% (protein L4) (or from 78% [protein S19] to 52% [protein L24] when conservative amino acid substitutions are included), averaging 49% (63%). These data indicate that the structures of ribosomal components have been conserved between mycoplasmas and eubacteria.

tuf genes, encoding translation elongation factor Tu, from *M. gallisepticum* and *M. genitalium* show 71 and 69% amino acid sequence identity, respectively, to *E. coli tufB* (26, 40). The gene for elongation factor Ts was cloned from *S. citri*, revealing 46% amino acid sequence identity to *E. coli tsf* (9).

Two codon-specific protein factors participate in translation termination in *E. coli*. Release factor 1 (RF-1) recognizes stop codons UAA and UAG, and release factor 2 (RF-2) recognizes UGA and UAA (7). Since in many mycoplasma species, codon UGA is used for Trp and codons UAA and UAG are used for translation termination (stop), it remains to be determined whether RF-2 has been deleted, leaving RF-1 for UAA and UAG, or whether RF-2 has become specific to UAA.

tRNAs in *M. capricolum*

The sequences of all tRNA species and the genes for these tRNAs in *M. capricolum* are now available (2, 46, 78). Therefore, *M. capricolum* represents the first genetic system among all organisms and organelles for which complete sequences of all tRNAs have been determined at both the RNA and DNA levels. Figure 6 shows the sequences of these tRNAs, each of which can be arranged in a typical cloverleaf structure. Most of the consensus sequences for tRNAs are conserved in *M.*

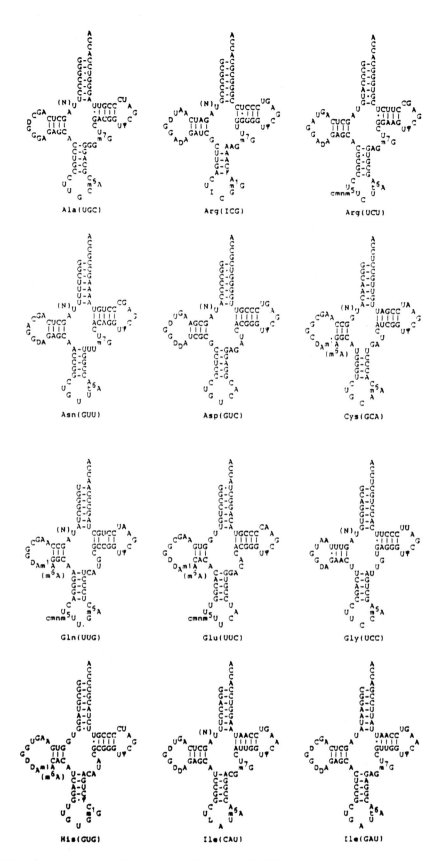

Figure 6. tRNAs of *M. capricolum*. Sequences of 29 species of tRNAs from *M. capricolum* shown in cloverleaf form, corrected from Fig. 2 in reference 3. Abbreviations for modified nucleosides: D, dihydrouridine; m⁶A, *N*⁶-methyladenosine; m⁷G, 7-methylguanosine; Ψ, pseudouridine; I, inosine; m¹G, 1-methylguanosine; cmnm⁵U, 5-carboxymethylaminomethyluridine; t⁶A, *N*-((9-β-D-ribofuranosylpurine-6-yl)carbamoyl)-threonine; m¹A, 1-methyladenosine; L, lysidine; Cm, 2′-*O*-methylcytidine; cmnm⁵Um, 5-carboxymethylaminomethyl-2′-*O*-methyluridine; N, uridine with unidentified modification. Residues in parentheses are the alternatives occurring at that position.

339

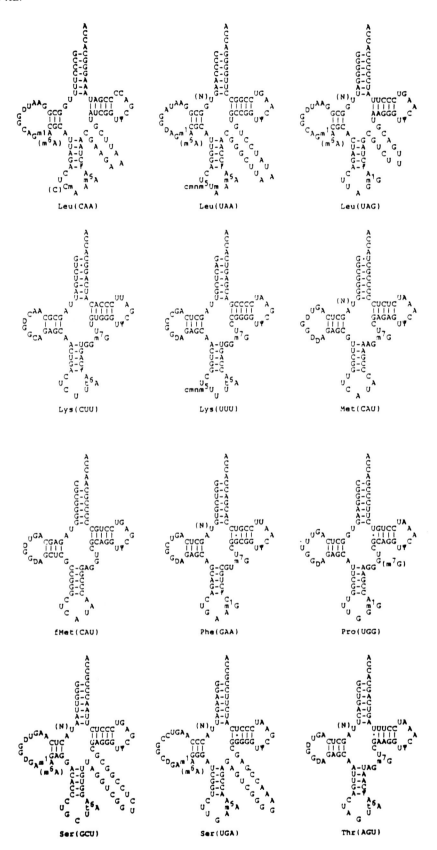

Figure 6. *Continued.*

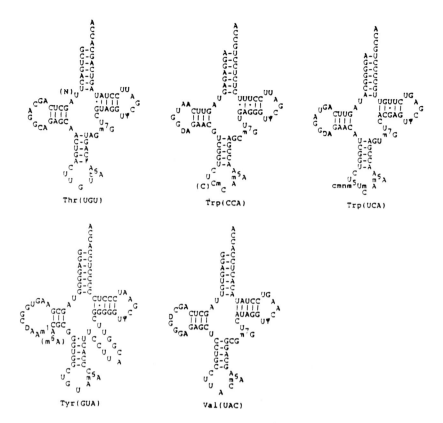

Figure 6. *Continued.*

capricolum tRNAs. A striking feature of *M. capricolum* tRNAs is that they contain fewer modified nucleosides than do eubacterial tRNAs. Five types of modification of the anticodon first nucleoside are found in *M. capricolum* (see next section and Table 2), while at least eight different modifications have been found in *E. coli* tRNAs (65). Unmodified nucleosides are used at the anticodon first position in 19 tRNA species. In *M. capricolum*, only 13 types of modified nucleosides are found in the total tRNAs, in contrast to 23 so far reported for *E. coli* (65). Thus, modified nucleosides are rare both in the anticodon first positions and elsewhere in the tRNAs. The 5'-terminal nucleoside of the TUC loop of all *M. capricolum* tRNAs is U unmodified, whereas the corresponding nucleoside of most tRNAs in eubacteria is ribothymidine (T) (65). Hence, the *M. capricolum* genome seems to have discarded the genes for many enzymes for tRNA nucleoside modifications as a result of pressures to minimize its genome size.

Anticodons and Codon Recognition Patterns

Anticodon composition and codon recognition patterns as deduced from the structures of *M. capricolum* tRNAs are different in many ways from those of eubacteria. There are two Met tRNAs, initiator and elongator, having the same anticodon, CAU; hence, the 29 *M. capricolum* tRNAs contain 28 different anticodons. This number is only a few more than the 24 in yeast mitochondria and much fewer than the number in *E. coli*, for which at least 45 tRNA species containing 39 anticodons have been deduced from tRNA gene sequences (37). These facts suggest that many tRNA

genes have been discarded in the evolution of mycoplasmas, allowing codons to be read by as small a number of anticodons as possible. Table 2 shows the deduced anticodon composition of *M. capricolum* in the codon table compared with those of *E. coli* and fungal mitochondria. There is a striking difference between *E. coli* and *M. capricolum* for the "family boxes," in which there are four codons for a single amino acid. In *E. coli*, four codons in family boxes are read by two anticodons, GNN and *UNN (*U represents a derivative of 5-hydroxyuridine or its equivalent), except for the Arg family box (see below). Anticodon GNN reads codons NNU and NNC, and anticodon *UNN reads codons NNU, NNA, and NNG by wobbling (80). Anticodon CNN is present in some boxes and reads only NNG codons. Strikingly, anticodons GNN and CNN do not exist in any of the eight family boxes in *M. capricolum*. Anticodon UNN, with U unmodified, is the sole anticodon for each of six family boxes in *M. capricolum*, excluding the Thr and Arg family boxes. Thus, the four synonymous codons in each of these six family boxes must be translated by a single anticodon, UNN, by four-way wobbling. UNN anticodons in family boxes also occur in *M. mycoides* (33, 59). This situation is analogous to that in most family boxes in various mitochondria (except plant mitochondria [Table 2] [21, 65]). In the Thr family box, in addition to anticodon UGU, there is a tRNA with anticodon AGU, with A unmodified, which, according to Crick's wobble rule, reads only codon ACU (10). An unmodified A residue at the anticodon first position occurs for yeast mitochondrial tRNA^Arg(ACG) (63) and *Aspergillus* mitochondrial tRNA^Gly(ACC) (36). *M. capricolum* tRNA^Thr(AGU) may be present to fulfill a heavy de-

Table 2. Anticodons in *M. capricolum*, *E. coli*, and fungal mitochondria[a]

Amino acid (codon)	M. c.	E. c.	Mit
Phe (UUU)	GAA	GAA	GAA
Phe (UUC)			
Leu (UUA)	UAA[c]	UAA[c]	UAA[f]
Leu (UUG)	CAA[h]	CAA	
Leu (CUU)[e]	UAG	GAG	UAG
Leu (CUC)[e]			
Leu (CUA)[e]		UAG[k]	
Leu (CUG)[e]		CAG	
Ile (AUU)	GAU	GAU	GAU
Ile (AUC)			
Ile (AUA)[e]	CAU[m]	CAU[m]	CAU[o]
Met (AUG)	CAU	CAU[q]	CAU
Val (GUU)	UAC	GAC	UAC
Val (GUC)			
Val (GUA)		UAC[d]	
Val (GUG)			

Amino acid (codon)	M. c.	E. c.	Mit
Ser (UCU)		GGA	
Ser (UCC)			
Ser (UCA)	UGA	UGA[d]	UGA
Ser (UCG)		CGA	
Pro (CCU)		GGG	
Pro (CCC)	UGG		UGG
Pro (CCA)		UGG[k]	
Pro (CCG)		CGG	
Thr (ACU)	AGU	GGU	
Thr (ACC)			
Thr (ACA)	UGU[k]	UGU	UGU
Thr (ACG)		CGU	
Ala (GCU)		GGC	
Ala (GCC)	UGC		UGC
Ala (GCA)			
Ala (GCG)		UGC[d]	

Amino acid (codon)	M. c.	E. c.	Mit
Tyr (UAU)	GUA	GUA[b]	GUA
Tyr (UAC)			
(UAA)			
(UAG)			
His (CAU)	GUG	GUG[b]	GUG
His (CAC)			
Gln (CAA)	UUG[f]	UUG[l]	UUG[k]
Gln (CAG)		CUG	
Asn (AAU)	GUU	GUU[b]	GUU
Asn (AAC)			
Lys (AAA)	UUU[f]	UUU[p]	UUU[f]
Lys (AAG)	CUU		CUU[r]
Asp (GAU)	GUC	GUC[b]	GUC
Asp (GAC)			
Glu (GAA)	UUC[f]	UUC[p]	UUC[k]
Glu (GAG)			

Amino acid (codon)	M. c.	E. c.	Mit
Cys (UGU)	GCA	GCA	GCA
Cys (UGC)			
Trp (UGA)[e]	UCA[c]	CCA	UCA[g]
Trp (UGG)	CCA[h]		
Arg (CGU)	ICG[i]	ICG[i]	U/ACG[j]
Arg (CGC)		CCG	
Arg (CGA)			
Ser (AGU)	GCU	GCU	GCU
Ser (AGC)			
Arg (AGA)	UCU[f]	UCU[n]	UCU[f]
Arg (AGG)		CCU	
Gly (GGU)		GCC	ACC[s]
Gly (GGC)	UCC	UCC[g]	UCC
Gly (GGA)		CCC	
Gly (GGG)			

[a] *M. capricolum* (M. c.) anticodons are from Andachi et al. (3). *E. coli* (E. c.) anticodons, including those from DNA sequences, are from Sprinzl et al. (65) and Komine et al. (37). Fungal mitochondrial (Mit) anticodons (*Saccharomyces cerevisiae*, *Neurospora crassa*, and *Aspergillus nidulans*), including those from DNA sequences, are from Sprinzl et al. (65).
[b] Modification of anticodon first nucleoside: queuosine.
[c] Modification of anticodon first nucleoside: cmnm5Um.
[d] Modification of anticodon first nucleoside: uridine-5-oxyacetic acid.
[e] CUN codons are for Thr and AUA is for Met in *S. cerevisiae* mitochondria. UGA codon is for stop in *E. coli*. CGG is probably an unassigned codon in *M. capricolum*.
[f] Modification of anticodon first nucleoside: cmnm5U.
[g] Modification of anticodon first nucleoside: unidentified.
[h] Modification of anticodon first nucleoside: partially 2'-O-methylcytidine.
[i] Modification of anticodon first nucleoside: inosine (I).
[j] ACG was reported only for *S. cerevisiae* mitochondria; UCG was reported for *A. nidulans* mitochondria.
[k] Probable modification of anticodon first nucleoside.
[l] Modification of anticodon first nucleoside: probably 2-thiouridine.
[m] Modification of anticodon first nucleoside: 4-amino-2-(N^6-lysino)-1-(β-D-ribofuranosyl)pyridinium (lysidine).
[n] Modification of anticodon first nucleoside: 5-methoxycarbonylmethyluridine.
[o] Two different genes for tRNAs with anticodon CAU were reported for *A. nidulans* mitochondria. Whether one of them has anticodon *CAU for codon AUA (Ile) is not known.
[p] Modification of anticodon first nucleoside: 5-methylaminomethyl-2-thiouridine.
[q] Modification of anticodon first nucleoside: N^4-acetylcytidine.
[r] Host nuclear origin.
[s] ACC (modification unknown) only for *A. nidulans* mitochondria.

mand for translation of codon ACU (2). In the Arg family box, three codons, CGU, CGC, and CGA, are read by anticodon ICG (I = inosine) by three-way wobbling, and codon CGG is read by anticodon CCG in *E. coli* and other eubacteria. Interestingly, only one tRNA, having anticodon ICG, has been found in the Arg family box in *M. capricolum*. In accordance with this finding, codon CGG has not been detected among the more than 6,800 codons in the *M. capricolum* genes that have been examined (Table 1), suggesting that CGG is an unassigned (nonsense) codon in *M. capricolum*. Perhaps strong AT pressure has converted all CGG codons to the synonymous codon CGU, CGA, or AGR by silent mutations. As a result, anticodon CCG may have become unnecessary and disappeared.

Two synonymous codons in all NNY-type (Y = U or C) two-codon sets (for Asn, Asp, Cys, His, Phe, Ser, and Tyr) in *M. capricolum* are translated by a single anticodon, GNN, with G unmodified. The G residue of these anticodons is sometimes modified to queuosine or 2′-O-methylguanosine in *E. coli* and other eubacteria (65). Two codons in NNR-type two-codon sets are translated by anticodon $^+$UNN ($^+$U represents a 5-methyl-2-thiouridine derivative [xm^{5}s^{2}U] or its equivalent), pairing mainly with NNA and weakly with NNG, in *E. coli*. The second anticodon CNN pairing only with NNG codons is present in some boxes. The U residue at the first anticodon position for NNR-type two-codon sets in *M. capricolum* is always modified; it is 5-carboxymethylaminomethyluridine (cmnm^{5}U) for Gln, Glu, Lys, and Arg, in contrast to xm^{5}s^{2}U (for Gln, Glu, and Lys) and 5-methoxycarbonylmethyluridine (for Gln, Glu, and Lys) and 5-methoxycarbonylmethyluridine (for Arg) in *E. coli*, and 5-carboxymethylaminomethyl-2′-O-methyluridine (cmnm^{5}Um) for Leu, as in the case of *E. coli* tRNA^{Leu}(UAA). Yeast mitochondria use cmnm^{5}U at the anticodon first position for at least three NNR-type two-codon sets (Table 2) (63).

In *M. capricolum*, tRNA^{Trp} has anticodon UCA, with the first anticodon nucleotide being modified to cmnm^{5}Um. The occurrence of tRNA^{Trp}(UCA), which reads UGA and UGG codons by wobbling, has been found only in mitochondria (21). In addition to these $^+$UNN anticodons, CNN anticodons are found in three NNR-type two-codon sets, Leu (CAA), Lys (CUU), and Trp (CCA). The anticodon first nucleosides of tRNA^{Leu} (CAA) and tRNA^{Trp}(CCA) are partially 2′-O methylated.

Both initiator and elongator tRNA^{Met} have an unmodified C residue at the anticodon first position, in contrast to *E. coli* elongator tRNA^{Met}, in which the first anticodon nucleoside C is N-4 acetylated. There are two tRNA^{Ile} species, tRNA^{Ile}(GAU) for codons AUU and AUC, and tRNA^{Ile}(*CAU) for codon AUA, where *C is 4-amino-2-(N^6-lysino)-1-(β-D-ribofuranosyl)pyrimidinium in *M. capricolum* (lysidine), as in *E. coli* (45).

In *M. capricolum*, of 61 amino acid codons, 57 are translated by a single anticodon. Only four codons, UUG (Leu), AAG (Lys), UGG (Trp), and ACU (Thr), may be read by two anticodons; nonobligate (redundant) anticodons for these codons are CAA (Leu), CUU (Lys), CCA (Trp), and AGU (Thr), respectively.

Anticodon composition and codon recognition patterns of *M. capricolum* resemble those of mitochondria rather than those of eubacteria (Table 2) as follows: (i) the use of UNN, with U unmodified, anticodons in

family boxes; (ii) the disappearance of nonobligate GNN and CNN anticodons; (iii) the presence of anticodon UCA that can read the universal stop codon UGA as a Trp codon; (iv) the use of cmnm^{5}U at the anticodon first position of tRNAs for NNR-type two-codon sets; and (v) the low content of modified nucleosides. There is a significant difference in that *M. capricolum* uses anticodon ICG for Arg codons CGU, CGC, and CGA as in the eubacteria, whereas these codons are usually read by a single anticodon UCG (sometimes ACG) in mitochondria. The mitochondrial genome is small, implying that like the mycoplasma genome, it has discarded many genes during evolution. The G+C content of mitochondrial DNA of simpler eucaryotes is very low, suggesting that strong AT pressure has been exerted at an early stage of mitochondrial evolution. Thus, the genomes of mitochondria and mycoplasmas seem to have developed under similar evolutionary constraints, gene economization and AT pressure, resulting in similarities in their tRNAs.

Evolution of the UGA Codon

All species belonging to the genera *Mycoplasma* and *Spiroplasma* so far analyzed use UGA as a Trp codon, whereas *A. laidlawii* does not (discussed above), suggesting that the code change, UGA from stop to Trp, occurred in the *Mycoplasma-Spiroplasma* lineage after separation of this phylogenetic branch from the *Acholeplasma* branch.

A. laidlawii contains a single Trp tRNA with anticodon CCA for the UGG codon, the gene for which is present as a single operon (Fig. 7a) (68). In *M. capricolum*, the genes of two Trp tRNAs are arranged tandemly in a single operon in the order tRNA^{Trp}(UCA)-tRNA^{Trp}(CCA), separated by a short (40-bp) spacer (Fig. 7b) (78). The tRNA^{Trp}(UCA) gene could have emerged by duplication of the tRNA^{Trp}(CCA) gene, since the two genes are closely related, both in their linkage on the chromosome and in their high sequence homology (78% identity).

Since tRNA^{Trp}(UCA) can translate both UGA and UGG codons by wobbling, tRNA^{Trp}(CCA) should no longer be needed in *M. capricolum*. tRNA^{Trp}(CCA) is found to be charged by Trp in cells much less than is tRNA^{Trp}(UCA), and the intracellular amount of tRNA^{Trp}(CCA) is 5 to 10 times lower than that of tRNA^{Trp}(UCA) (76) (see above). The tRNA^{Trp}(CCA) gene and its product in *M. capricolum* are apparently vestigial remnants. Inamine et al. (25) demonstrated that *M. pneumoniae* and *M. genitalium* contained a single Trp tRNA gene with anticodon UCA (Fig. 7c), showing that the tRNA^{Trp}(CCA) has disappeared in these species. Thus, the changes in the Trp tRNA genes in *A. laidlawii*, *M. capricolum*, and *M. genitalium* (Fig. 7) appear to represent evolutionary steps in the change of the anticodon from CCA to UCA. However, the appearance of UGA as a Trp codon simply by emergence of anticodon UCA is unlikely to have happened, because UGA must have been used as a stop codon in ancestral bacteria. It is likely that a series of changes led to the establishment of UGA as a regular Trp codon (28, 52). First, AT pressure would lead to the mutational conversion of the stop codon UGA to UAA. At this stage, the gene for RF-2, which recognizes UGA as stop

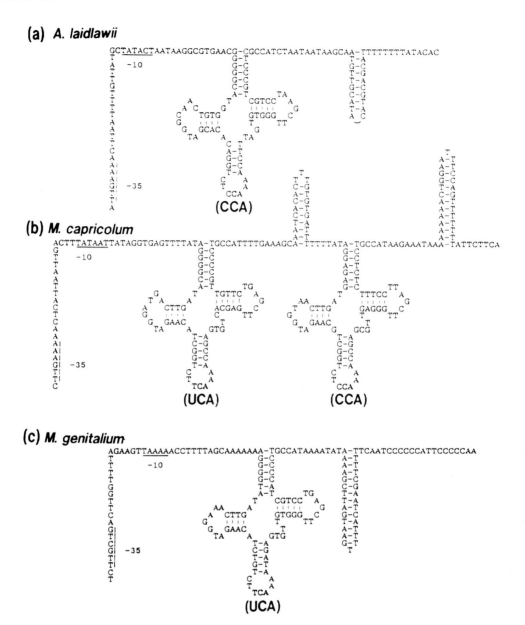

Figure 7. Evolution of Trp tRNA genes. Shown are the nucleotide sequences of Trp tRNA genes from *A. laidlawii* (68) (a), *M. capricolum* (78) (b), and *M. genitalium* (25) (c). Putative promoters (−35 and −10 boxes) and terminator or attenuator sequences (hairpin structures) are also shown.

codon, would have been deleted from the genome, so that UGA would have become unassigned (52a). Then, duplication of tRNA^{Trp}(CCA) must have occurred, followed by the mutational change of one of the duplicates to tRNA^{Trp}(UCA). The appearance of tRNA^{Trp}(UCA) enabled the UGG codon, under AT pressure, to mutate to UGA Trp codons. These evolutionary steps could have taken place by a series of silent (neutral) changes.

Translation In Vivo and In Vitro

Mycoplasma protein genes cloned into vector DNAs of *E. coli* can be expressed in *E. coli* cells. However, most genes are not fully expressed because UGA is a Trp codon in many mycoplasma species, whereas it is a stop codon in *E. coli*. Some ribosomal protein genes of *M. capricolum* (30) and the spiralin gene of *S. citri* (44) are fully expressed in *E. coli* because these proteins have no Trp residues. The DNA methylase gene of *Spiroplasma* sp. strain MQ-1 (M.*Sss*) is transcribed with its own promoter in *E. coli*, but translation of the entire message requires the use of an opal suppressor (55). So far, no vector DNA capable of expressing genes in mycoplasma cells is available.

Recent experiments by Oba et al. (49a) have shown that synthetic RNA-dependent peptide synthesis occurred in the S-30 fraction of *M. capricolum* as efficiently as in that of *E. coli*. Establishment of this in vitro translation system has opened the way to understanding the detailed mechanisms of mycoplasma translation.

REFERENCES

1. **Amikam, D., G. Glaser, and S. Razin.** 1984. Mycoplasmas (*Mollicutes*) have a low number of rRNA genes. *J. Bacteriol.* **158:**376–378.

2. **Andachi, Y., F. Yamao, M. Iwami, A. Muto, and S. Osawa.** 1987. Occurrence of unmodified adenine and uracil at the first position of anticodon in threonine tRNAs in *Mycoplasma capricolum. Proc. Natl. Acad. Sci. USA* **84:**7393–7402.

3. **Andachi, Y., F. Yamao, A. Muto, and S. Osawa.** 1989. Codon recognition patterns as deduced from sequences of the complete set of transfer RNA species in *Mycoplasma capricolum. J. Mol. Biol.* **209:**37–54.

4. **Bové, J. M., P. Carle, M. Garnier, F. Laigret, J. Renaudin, and C. Saillard.** 1989. Molecular and cellular biology of spiroplasmas, p. 243–364. *In* R. F. Whitcomb and J. G. Tully (ed.), *The Mycoplasmas*, vol. 5. Academic Press, Inc., New York.

5. **Brosius, J., M. L. Palmer, P. J. Kennedy, and H. F. Noller.** Complete nucleotide sequence of a 16S ribosomal RNA gene from *Escherichia coli. Proc. Natl. Acad. Sci. USA* **75:**4801–4805.

6. **Cashel, M., and K. E. Rudd.** 1987. The stringent response, p. 1410–1438. *In* F. C. Neidhardt, J. L. Ingraham, B. Magasanik, K. B. Low, M. Schaechter, and H. E. Umbarger (ed.), *Escherichia coli and Salmonella typhimurium: Cellular and Molecular Biology.* American Society for Microbiology, Washington, D.C.

7. **Caskey, C. T.** 1977. Peptide chain termination, p. 443–465. *In* H. Weissback and S. Pestka (ed.), *Molecular Mechanisms of Protein Biosynthesis.* Academic Press, Inc., New York.

8. **Cerretti, D. P., D. Dean, G. R. Davis, D. M. Bedwell, and M. Nomura.** 1983. The *spc* ribosomal protein operon of *Escherichia coli*: sequence and cotranscription of the ribosomal protein genes and a protein export gene. *Nucleic Acids Res.* **11:**2599–2616.

9. **Chevalier, C., C. Saillard, and J. M. Bové.** 1990. Organization and nucleotide sequences of the *Spiroplasma citri* genes for ribosomal protein S2, elongation factor Ts, spiralin, phosphofructokinase, pyruvate kinase, and an unidentified protein. *J. Bacteriol.* **172:**2693–2703.

10. **Crick, F. H. C.** 1966. Codon-anticodon pairing: the wobble hypothesis. *J. Mol. Biol.* **19:**548–555.

11. **Das, J., and J. Maniloff.** 1976. Replication of mycoplasma virus MVL51. V. Inhibition of viral synthesis by rifampin. *J. Virol.* **44:**877–881.

12. **Davis, J. W. and B. A. Hanna.** 1981. Antimicrobial susceptibility of *Ureaplasma urealyticum. J. Clin. Microbiol.* **13:**320–325.

13. **Dudler, R., C. Schmidhauser, R. W. Parish, E. H. Wettenhall, and T. Schmidt.** 1988. A mycoplasma high-affinity transport system and the *in vitro* invasiveness of mouse sarcoma cells. *EMBO J.* **7:**3963–3970.

14. **Frydenberg, J., and C. Christiansen.** 1985. The sequence of 16S rRNA from *Mycoplasma* strain PG50. *DNA* **4:**127–137.

15. **Gadeau, A.-P., C. Mouches, and J. M. Bové.** 1986. Probable insensitivity of mollicutes to rifampin and characterization of spiroplasmal DNA-dependent RNA polymerase. *J. Bacteriol.* **166:**824–828.

16. **Gafny, R., H. C. Hyman, S. Razin, and G. Glaser.** 1988. Promoters of Mycoplasma capricolum ribosomal RNA operons: identical activities but different regulation in homologous and heterologous cells. *Nucleic Acids Res.* **16:**61–76.

17. **Glaser, G., D. Amikam, and S. Razin.** 1981. Stable RNA synthesis and its control in *Mycoplasma capricolum. Nucleic Acids Res.* **9:**3641–3646.

18. **Göbel, U., G. H. Batler, and E. J. Stanbridge.** 1984. Comparative analysis of mycoplasma ribosomal RNA operons. *Isr. J. Med. Sci.* **20:**762–764.

19. **Gold, L., D. Pribnow, T. Schneider, S. Shinedling, B. S. Singer, and G. Stormo.** 1984. Translational initiation in prokaryotes. *Annu. Rev. Microbiol.* **35:**365–403.

20. **Hawley, D. K., and W. R. McClure.** 1983. Compilation and analysis of *Escherichia coli* promoter DNA sequences. *Nucleic Acids Res.* **11:**2237–2255.

21. **Heckman, J. E., J. Sarnoff, B. Alzner-DeWeerd, S. Yin, and U. L. RajBhandary.** 1990. Genetic code and codon reading patterns in *Neurospora crassa* mitochondria: novel features based on sequences of six mitochondrial tRNAs. *Proc. Natl. Acad. Sci. USA* **77:**3159–3163.

22. **Hori, H., and S. Osawa.** 1987. Origin and evolution of organisms as deduced from 5S ribosomal RNA sequences. *Mol. Biol. Evol.* **4:**445–472.

23. **Hori, H., M. Sawada, S. Osawa, K. Murao, and H. Ishikura.** 1981. The nucleotide sequence of 5S rRNA from *Mycoplasma capricolum. Nucleic Acids Res.* **9:**5407–5410.

24. **Inamine, J. M., T. P. Denny, S. Loechel, U. Schaper, C.-H. Huang, K. F. Bott, and P.-C. Hu.** 1988. Nucleotide sequence of the P1 attachment-protein gene of *Mycoplasma pneumoniae. Gene* **64:**217–229.

25. **Inamine, J. M., K.-C. Ho, S. Loechel, and P.-C. Hu.** 1990. Evidence that UGA is read as a tryptophan codon rather than as a stop codon by *Mycoplasma pneumoniae, Mycoplasma genitalium*, and *Mycoplasma gallisepticum. J. Bacteriol.* **172:**504–506.

26. **Inamine, J. M., S. Loechel, and P.-C. Hu.** 1989. Nucleotide sequence of the *tuf* gene from *Mycoplasma gallisepticum. Nucleic Acids Res.* **17:**10126.

27. **Iwami, M., A. Muto, F. Yamao, and S. Osawa.** 1984. Nucleotide sequence of *rrnB* 16S ribosomal RNA gene from *Mycoplasma capricolum. Mol. Gen. Genet.* **196:**317–322.

28. **Jukes, T. H.** 1985. A change in the genetic code in *Mycoplasma capricolum. J. Mol. Evol.* **22:**361–362.

29. **Kawauchi, Y., A. Muto, and S. Osawa.** 1982. The protein composition of *Mycoplasma capricolum. Mol. Gen. Genet.* **188:**7–11.

30. **Kawauchi, Y., A. Muto, F. Yamao, and S. Osawa.** 1984. Molecular cloning of ribosomal protein genes from *Mycoplasma capricolum. Mol. Gen. Genet.* **196:**521–525.

31. **Kenerly, M. E., E. A. Morgan, L. Post, and M. Nomura.** 1977. Characterization of hybrid plasmids carrying individual ribosomal ribonucleic acid transcription units of *Escherichia coli. J. Bacteriol.* **132:**931–949.

32. **Kimura, M.** 1983. *The Neutral Theory of Molecular Evolution.* Cambridge University Press, Cambridge.

33. **Kirpatrick, M. W., and R. T. Walker.** 1980. Nucleotide sequence of glycine tRNA from *Mycoplasma mycoides* sp. capri. *Nucleic Acids Res.* **8:**2783–2784.

34. **Kiss, A., B. Sain, and P. Venetialner.** 1977. The number of rRNA genes in *Escherichia coli. FEBS Lett.* **79:**77–79.

35. **Kobayashi, H., and S. Osawa.** 1982. The number of 5S rRNA genes in *Bacillus subtilis. FEBS Lett.* **141:**161–163.

36. **Kochel, H. G., C. M. Lazarus, N. Basak, and H. Kuntzel.** 1981. Mitochondrial tRNA gene clusters in *Aspergillus nidulans*: organization and nucleotide sequence. *Cell* **23:**625–633.

37. **Komine, Y., Y. Adachi, H. Inokuchi, and H. Ozeki.** 1990. Genomic organization and physical mapping of the transfer RNA genes in *Escherichia coli* K12. *J. Mol. Biol.* **212:**579–598.

38. **Kondo, K., H. Sone, H. Yoshida, T. Toida, K. Kanatani, Y.-M. Hong, N. Nishino, and J. Tanaka.** 1990. Cloning and sequence analysis of the arginine deaminase gene from *Mycoplasma arginini. Mol. Gen. Genet.* **221:**81–86.

39. **Loechel, S., J. M. Inamine, and P.-C. Hu.** 1989. Nucleo-

tide sequence of *deoC* gene of *Mycoplasma pneumoniae. Nucleic Acids Res.* **17**:801.

40. **Loechel, S., J. M. Inamine, and P.-C. Hu.** 1989. Nucleotide sequence of the *tuf* gene from *Mycoplasma genitalium. Nucleic Acids Res.* **17**:10127.

41. **Maaløe, O.** 1979. Regulation of the protein synthesizing machinery—ribosomes, tRNA, factors and so on, p. 487–542. *In* R. Goldberger (ed.), *Biological Regulation and Development*, vol. 1. *Gene Expression.* Plenum Publishing Corp., New York.

42. **Maniloff, J., and H. J. Morowitz.** 1972. Cell biology of mycoplasmas. *Bacteriol. Rev.* **36**:263–290.

43. **Morowitz, H. J.** 1967. Biological self-replicating system. *Prog. Theor. Biol.* **1**:35–58.

44. **Mouches, C., T. Candresse, C. Saillard, H. Wroblewski, and J. M. Bové.** 1985. Gene for spiralin, the major membrane protein of the helical Mollicute *Spiroplasma citri*: cloning and expression in *Escherichia coli. J. Bacteriol.* **164**:1094–1099.

45. **Muramatsu, T., S. Yokoyama, N. Horie, A. Matsuda, T. Ueda, Z. Yamaizumi, Y. Kuchino, S. Nishimura, and T. Miyazawa.** 1988. A novel lysine-substituted nucleoside in the first position of the anticodon of minor isoleucine tRNA from *Escherichia coli. J. Biol. Chem.* **263**:9261–9267.

46. **Muto, A., Y. Andachi, H. Yuzawa, F. Yamao, and S. Osawa.** 1990. The organization and evolution of transfer RNA genes of *Mycoplasma capricolum. Nucleic Acids Res.* **18**:5037–5043.

47. **Muto, A., Y. Kawauchi, F. Yamao, and S. Osawa.** 1984. Preferential use of A- and U-rich codons for *Mycoplasma capricolum* ribosomal proteins S8 and L6. *Nucleic Acids Res.* **12**:8209–8217.

48. **Muto, A., and S. Osawa.** 1987. The guanine and cytosine content of genomic DNA and bacterial evolution. *Proc. Natl. Acad. Sci. USA* **84**:166–169.

49. **Muto, A., F. Yamao, and S. Osawa.** 1987. The genome of *Mycoplasma capricolum. Prog. Nucleic Acid Res. Mol. Biol.* **34**:29–58.

49a. **Oba, T., Y Andachi, A. Muto, and S. Osawa.** 1991. CGG: an unassigned codon in *Mycoplasma capricolum. Proc. Natl. Acad. Sci. USA* **88**:921–925.

50. **Ogasawara, N., S. Moriya, and H. Yoshikawa.** 1983. Structure and organization of rRNA operons in the region of the replication origin of the *Bacillus subtilis* chromosome. *Nucleic Acids Res.* **11**:6301–6318.

51. **Ohkubo, S., A. Muto, Y. Kawauchi, F. Yamao, and S. Osawa.** 1987. The ribosomal protein gene cluster of *Mycoplasma capricolum. Mol. Gen. Genet.* **210**:314–322.

52. **Osawa, S., and T. H. Jukes.** 1989. Codon reassignment (codon capture) in evolution. *J. Mol. Evol.* **28**:271–278.

52a. **Osawa, S., A. Muto, T. H. Jukes, and T. Ohama.** 1990. Evolutionary changes in the genetic code. *Proc. R. Soc. London Ser. B* **241**:19–28.

53. **Rasmussen, O. F., J. Frydenberg, and C. Christiansen.** 1987. Analysis of the leader and spacer regions of the two rRNA operons of *Mycoplasma* PG50: two tRNA genes are located upstream of *rrnA. Mol. Gen. Genet.* **208**:23–29.

54. **Razin, S.** 1985. Moleclar biology and genetics of mycoplasmas (*Mollicutes*). *Microbiol. Rev.* **49**:419–455.

55. **Renbaum, P., D. Abrahamobe, A. Fainsod, G. G. Wilson, S. Rottem, and A. Razin.** 1990. Cloning, characterization, and expression in *Escherichia coli* of the gene coding for the CpG DNA methylase from *Spiroplasma* sp. strain MQ1 (M. Sss1). *Nucleic Acids Res.* **18**:1145–1152.

56. **Rogers, M., A. A. Steinmetz, and R. T. Walker.** 1985. The nucleotide sequence of a tRNA gene cluster from *Spiroplasma meliferum. Nucleic Acids Res.* **14**:3145.

57. **Rogers, M. J., J. Simmons, R. T. Walker, W. G. Weisburg, C. R. Woese, P. S. Tenner, I. M. Robinson, D. A. Stahl, G. Olsen, R. H. Leach, and J. Maniloff.** 1985. Construction

of the mycoplasma evolutionary tree from 5S rRNA sequence data. *Proc. Natl. Acad. Sci. USA* **82**:1160–1164.

58. **Samuelsson, T., P. Elias, F. Lustig, and Y. S. Guidy.** 1985. Cloning and nucleotide sequence analysis of transfer RNA genes from *Mycoplasma mycoides. Biochem. J.* **232**:223–228.

59. **Samuelsson, T., Y. S. Guidy, F. Lustig, T. Boren, and U. Lagerkvist.** 1987. Apparent lack of discrimination in the reading of certain codons in *Mycoplasma mycoides. Proc. Natl. Acad. Sci. USA* **88**:3166–3170.

60. **Sawada, M., A. Muto, F. Yamao, and S. Osawa.** 1984. Organization of ribosomal RNA genes in *Mycoplasma capricolum. Mol. Gen. Genet.* **196**:311–316.

61. **Sawada, M., S. Osawa, H. Kobayashi, H. Hori, and A. Muto.** 1982. The number of ribosomal RNA genes in *Mycoplasma capricolum. Mol. Gen. Genet.* **182**:502–502.

62. **Shine, J., and L. Dalgarno.** 1974. The 3′-terminal sequence of *Escherichia coli* 16S ribosomal RNA: complementarity to nonsense triplets and ribosome binding sites. *Proc. Natl. Acad. Sci. USA* **71**:1342–1346.

63. **Sibler, A.-P., G. Dirheimer, and R. P. Martin.** 1986. Codon reading patterns in *Saccharomyces cerevisiae* mitochondria based on sequences of mitochondrial tRNAs. *FEBS Lett.* **194**:131–138.

64. **Simoneau, P., R. Wenzel, R. Herrmann, and P.-C. Hu.** 1990. Nucleotide sequence of a tRNA cluster from *Mycoplasma pneumoniae. Nucleic Acids Res.* **18**:2814.

65. **Sprinzl, M., T. Hartmann, F. Meissner, J. Moll, and T. Vorderwulbecke.** 1987. Compilation of tRNA sequences and sequences of tRNA genes. *Nucleic Acids Res.* **15**:r53–r188.

66. **Stewart, G. C., and K. F. Bott.** 1983. DNA sequence of ribosomal RNA promoter for *B. subtilis* operon *rrnB. Nucleic Acids Res.* **11**:6289–6300.

67. **Sueoka, N.** 1962. On the genetic basis of variation and heterogeneity of DNA base composition. *Proc. Natl. Acad. Sci. USA* **48**:582–592.

68. **Tanaka, R., A. Muto, and S. Osawa.** 1989. Nucleotide sequence of tryptophan tRNA gene in *Acholeplasma laidlawii. Nucleic Acids Res.* **17**:5842.

69. **Taschke, C., and R. Herrmann.** 1985. Analysis of transcription and processing signals of the 16S–23S rRNA operon of *Mycoplasma hyopneumoniae. Mol. Gen. Genet.* **205**:434–441.

70. **Taschke, C., and R. Herrmann.** 1985. Analysis of transcription and processing signals in the 5′-regions of the two *Mycoplasma capricolum* rRNA operons. *Mol. Gen. Genet.* **212**:522–530.

71. **Taschke, C., M.-Q. Klinkert, J. Wolters, and R. Herrmann.** 1986. Organization of the ribosomal RNA genes in *Mycoplasma hyopneumoniae*: the 5S rRNA gene is separated from the 16S and 23S rRNA genes. *Mol. Gen. Genet.* **205**:428–433.

72. **Travers, A. A.** 1984. Conserved features of coordinately regulated *E. coli* promoters. *Nucleic Acids Res.* **12**:2605–2618.

73. **Vold, B. S.** 1985. Structure and organization of genes for transfer ribonucleic acid in *Bacillus subtilis. Microbiol. Rev.* **49**:71–80.

74. **Walker, R. T., E. T. J. Chelton, M. W. Kirpatrick, M. J. Roberts, and J. Simmons.** 1983. The nucleotide sequence of the 5S rRNA from *Spiroplasma species* BC3 and *Mycoplasma mycoides* subsp. *capri. Nucleic Acids Res.* **5**:57–70.

75. **Weisburg, W. G., J. G. Tully, D. L. Rose, J. P. Petzel, H. Oyaizu, D. Yang, L. Mandelco, J. Sechrest, T. G. Lawrence, J. Van Etten, J. Maniloff, and C. R. Woese.** 1989. A phylogenetic analysis of the mycoplasmas: basis for their classification. *J. Bacteriol.* **171**:6455–6467.

76. **Yager, T. D., and P. H. von Hippel.** 1987. Transcription elongation and termination in *Escherichia coli*, p. 1241–1275. *In* F. C. Neidhardt, J. L. Ingraham, B. Magasanik, K. B. Low, M. Schaechter, and H. E. Umbarger (ed.), *Escherichia coli and Salmonella typhimurium: Cellu-*

lar and Molecular Biology. American Society for Microbiology, Washington, D.C.

77. **Yamao, F., S. Iwagami, Y. Azumi, A. Muto, S. Osawa, N. Fujita, and A. Ishihama.** 1988. Evolutionary dynamics of tryptophan tRNAs in *Mycoplasma capricolum*. *Mol. Gen. Genet.* **212:**364–369.

78. **Yamao, F., A. Muto, Y. Kawauchi, M. Iwami, S. Iwagami, Y. Azumi, and S. Osawa.** 1985. UGA is read as tryptophan in *Mycoplasma capricolum*. *Proc. Natl. Acad. Sci. USA* **82:**2306–2309.

79. **Yamao, F., A. Muto, and S. Osawa.** 1989. The tRNA levels in bacterial cells as affected by amino acid usage in proteins. *Proc. Jpn. Acad. Ser. B* **65:**73–75.

80. **Yokoyama, S., T. Watababe, K. Murao, H. Ishikura, Z. Yamaizumi, S. Ninshimura, and T. Miyazawa.** 1985. Molecular mechanism of codon recognition by tRNA species with modified uridine in the first position of the anticodon. *Proc. Natl. Acad. Sci. USA* **82:**4905–4909.

81. **Young, R. A., and J. A. Steitz.** 1978. Complementary sequences 1700 nucleotides apart from a ribonuclease III cleavage site in *Escherichia coli* ribosomal precursor RNA. *Proc. Natl. Acad. Sci. USA* **75:**3593–3597.

20. Heat Shock Response

CHRISTOPHER C. DASCHER and JACK MANILOFF

INTRODUCTION

The potential to adapt to variations in environmental conditions is essential for the evolutionary survival of biological organisms. Failure to respond to changes in nutrients, toxins, radiation, temperature, and other growth conditions can compromise an organism's biological systems and reduce viability. Rapid temperature fluctuations are one of the most common types of environmental stress that organisms, especially free-living microorganisms, encounter. The cells' physiological systems must respond to the potential deleterious effects of a sudden increase in temperature (i.e., heat shock) to minimize damage caused by the heat shock and maintain normal cellular functions under the new environmental conditions.

The heat shock response has been demonstrated in every organism that has been studied and is characterized by the synthesis of a distinct set of proteins. These proteins constitute a defined regulon in *Escherichia coli*, the most extensively characterized heat shock system (reviewed in references 9 and 26). The *E. coli* heat shock regulon is controlled by a 32-kDa sigma factor that directs transcription of genes from specific heat shock promoter sequences (10, 11). Hence, heat shock (e.g., a temperature shift from 37 to 42°C) induces an immediate increase in the rate of synthesis of *E. coli* heat shock proteins. This is followed, in 10 to 20 min, by a decrease in the rate of heat shock protein synthesis to steady-state levels slightly higher than the initial pre-heat shock levels. Induction of the heat shock response has been correlated with a corresponding increase in thermal tolerance in *E. coli* (37). At present, 17 *E. coli* heat shock proteins with different degrees of inducibility following heat shock have been reported (reviewed in reference 26). Subsets of these proteins and some additional proteins can also be induced by other environmental stresses, such as organic solvents, nalidixic acid, viral infection, alkylating agents, and radiation (35). This phenomenon has led these proteins to be referred to as stress response proteins, reflecting their more generalized role in cellular function.

Mycoplasmas evolved from the eubacteria through a process of degenerate evolution (see chapter 33). The most striking change during mycoplasma phylogeny was the loss of a significant amount of genetic information. This reduction in genetic coding capacity resulted in the relatively small genome sizes of the mycoplasmas. Mycoplasma genome sizes range from about 600 to 1,700 kb (see chapter 9), with the smallest mycoplasma genomes approaching the theoretical genome size limit for a free-living organism (24).

In view of these observations, it has been of interest to learn whether mycoplasmas possess the apparently universal heat shock response or whether these organisms, during their phylogenetically selective loss of genetic information, were able to delete this function. Hence, Dascher and coworkers (7) carried out studies to measure mycoplasma thermal inactivation and to identify and characterize the heat shock response in mycoplasmas. In addition, preliminary data on mycoplasma heat shock proteins have been reported by Borchsenius et al. (3) and Sondergard-Anderson et al. (31). The data show that mycoplasmas have indeed conserved the heat shock response and that the mycoplasma heat shock response is very similar to that of other procaryotes, with some sequence conservation of specific heat shock proteins.

THERMAL INACTIVATION OF MYCOPLASMAS

The survival of *Acholeplasma laidlawii* and *Mycoplasma capricolum* cells at temperatures above their

Christopher C. Dascher and Jack Maniloff • Department of Microbiology and Immunology, University of Rochester, Medical Center Box 672, Rochester, New York 14642.

37°C optimal growth temperature has been studied (6, 7). For bacteria with first-order inactivation kinetics, thermal inactivation is quantitated in terms of two parameters, D and z (34). D is the time required, at a particular temperature, for a 10-fold reduction in survival fraction; z is the number of degrees required for a 10-fold change in D.

There is no measurable change in survival fraction of *A. laidlawii* JA1 when exponentially growing cultures at 32°C are shifted to 42°C (Fig. 1). However, when the shift-up is to 46, 47, or 48°C, there is thermal inactivation, with an initial shoulder followed by exponential inactivation (Fig. 1). This type of inactivation kinetics is characteristic of many bacteria, with a shoulder, presumably due to cell clumping, and subsequent first-order inactivation. The D and z parameters for *A. laidlawii* JA1 thermal inactivation have been calculated from the first-order inactivation curves (Table 1).

When exponentially growing cultures of *M. capricolum* California kid are shifted from 32°C to 42, 45, or 47°C, there is an initial increase in cell number, with the rate of increase being greater than the 140-min *M. capricolum* doubling time at 32°C (Fig. 2). At 42°C, the increase continues for at least 80 min, with an apparent first-order doubling time of 65 min. Larger rate increases are seen at 45 and 47°C, but these are followed by decreasing survival fraction values. The increase in CFU after shift-up to higher temperatures is probably due to disaggregation of the cell clumps characteristic of growing *M. capricolum* cultures. The low inactivation rates seen at later times at 45 and 47°C must, therefore, be the result of CFU increases due to clump disaggregation and CFU decreases due to thermal inactivation. The D and z parameters for *M. capricolum* California kid thermal inactivation have been calculated from the first-order inactivation curves (Table 1).

Although the moderate growth temperatures of mycoplasmas suggest that these organisms are mesophilic, their high D values (Table 1) resemble those of psychrophiles rather than mesophiles (34). This disparity may reflect differences between mycoplasmas

Table 1. Mycoplasma thermal inactivation parameters[a]

Mycoplasma	D (min)[b] at:				z (°C)[c]
	45°C	46°C	47°C	48°C	
A. laidlawii JA1		73.1	39.9	24.2	4.2
M. capricolum California kid	843.4		287.8		4.3

[a] Calculated from data in Fig. 1 and 2 (6).
[b] Time required for a 10-fold reduction in survival fraction (34).
[c] Number of degrees required for a 10-fold change in D (34).

and eubacteria in both morphology (e.g., the absence of cell walls in mycoplasmas) and biochemistry (e.g., the relative inefficiency of mycoplasma repair systems). The approximately 10-fold difference in *A. laidlawii* and *M. capricolum* D values may be due to the effects of medium composition on heat resistance (34) and the 2- to 3-fold-greater dimensions of *A. laidlawii* cells relative to *M. capricolum* cells, which give the former about a 10-fold-larger thermal inactivation target. In contrast to D values, which vary with experimental conditions, z values are fairly constant over a range of conditions (34). While the similarity of *A. laidlawii* and *M. capricolum* z values (Table 1) may be coincidental, they are close to the range of $z = 5$ to 20 found for most eubacteria (mesophiles, psychrophiles, and thermophiles) (34).

MYCOPLASMA HEAT SHOCK PROTEINS

Identification of Mycoplasma Heat Shock Proteins

The classic method for identifying heat shock proteins is to pulse-label nascent proteins in vivo in cells before and after a shift to a high temperature, followed by comparative analysis of these proteins by polyacrylamide gel electrophoresis (PAGE). This procedure has been used to identify heat shock-induced pro-

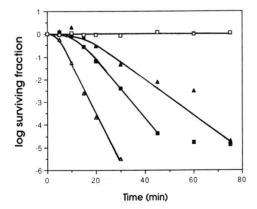

Figure 1. Thermal inactivation curves of *A. laidlawii* JA1 after shift-up of exponentially growing cultures from 32°C to various temperatures (6, 7). The logarithm of the surviving fraction of cells is plotted as a function of incubation time after shift-up to 42°C (□), 46°C (▲), 47°C (■), and 48°C (△).

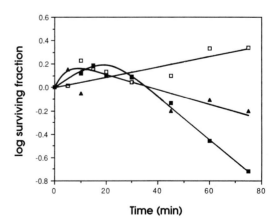

Figure 2. Thermal inactivation curves of *M. capricolum* California kid after shift-up of exponentially growing cultures from 32°C to various temperatures (6, 7). The logarithm of the surviving fraction of cells is plotted as a function of incubation time after shift-up to 42°C (□), 45°C (▲) and 47°C (■).

teins in *A. laidlawii* and *M. capricolum* (3, 7). In addition, Western immunoblotting was used to demonstrate an increased amount of a specific antigen in heat-shocked *M. pneumoniae* and *M. fermentans* (31).

A. laidlawii JA1 proteins show a typical heat shock response (Fig. 3). This *Acholeplasma* strain provides a good model for heat shock studies, because both total protein synthesis and total cell number do not change for at least 1 h following a temperature shift from 32 to 42°C (Fig. 1) (7). Following this temperature shift, at least 11 *A. laidlawii* JA1 heat shock proteins are synthesized, representing either synthesis of new proteins or increased synthesis of proteins already being synthesized at 32°C. Many protein bands visible in control cells (Fig. 3 lane a) show a marked decrease during heat shock (Fig. 3, lanes b to d). This observation is typical of heat shock in bacteria, since the heat shock response causes a redirection of the cells' transcription to genes with heat shock promoter sequences. However, the lack of mycoplasma genetic systems has prevented studies of whether mycoplasmas have a heat shock regulon with regulatory elements similar to those in *E. coli*.

Table 2 summarizes the mycoplasma heat shock proteins identified by Dascher et al. (7) by one-dimensional PAGE of pulse-labeled proteins from heat-shocked cells. This table compares proteins synthesized during heat shock for two *A. laidlawii* strains and *M. capricolum*. The heat shock proteins thus far identified in these mycoplasmas should be considered a minimum value of the potential number of mycoplasma heat shock proteins, since one-dimensional PAGE cannot resolve multiple proteins with similar molecular sizes.

Table 2. Mycoplasma heat shock proteins[a]

Protein (kDa)[b]	Mycoplasma			Identification[d]
	A. laidlawii JA1	*A. laidlawii* K2	*M. capricolum*[c]	
92	+	−	−	
87–90	+	−	+	
78	−	+	−	
75	+	−	+	
66–68	+	+	+	DnaK
56–57	+	+	−	GroEL(?)[e]
49–50	+	−	+	
39	+	−	−	
35–36	+	+	−	
29	+	+	−	
26–27	+	−	+	
20	+	−	−	

[a] Determined by PAGE analysis of pulse-labeled proteins in heat-shocked cells (7).
[b] Determinations have an experimental error of about ±3 kDa.
[c] *M. capricolum* cells also have a 105-kDa heat shock protein (7).
[d] The basis of identification is described in the text.
[e] There are no data on the presence or identity of GroEL in *M. capricolum*.

Optimal visualization of mycoplasma heat shock proteins varies according to the induction time and temperature used. Longer pulse times seem to be required to observe a heat shock response in mycoplasmas than in eubacteria, probably because of the relatively slow mycoplasma growth rates. This conclusion is illustrated by the 56-, 29-, and 27-kDa heat shock proteins in *A. laidlawii* JA1. These proteins are not apparent during the first 20 min of heat shock but are observed at later times as a result of their increased synthesis at 20 to 40 min after heat shock followed by a decrease in their synthesis to pre-heat shock levels at 40 to 60 min after heat shock (Fig. 1).

Borchsenius et al. (3) observed four major and several minor heat shock protein bands in an unidentified *A. laidlawii* strain. In their pulse-labeling experiments, heat shock was carried out for 90 min at 45°C. Under these conditions, the sizes of the major heat shock proteins observed were 78, 70, 62, and 17 kDa. These proteins probably correspond to a subset of the heat shock proteins observed in the two *Acholeplasma* strains examined by Dascher et al. (7) at 42°C. However, there is a significant decrease in *A. laidlawii* survival at 45°C (6). In view of the loss in *A. laidlawii* viability at 45°C, it is interesting that the four major heat shock proteins observed by Borchsenius et al. (3) are among the most prominent heat shock proteins observed at 42°C by Dascher et al. (7), i.e., the 75-, 66- to 68-, 56- to 57-, and 20-kDa proteins. The fact that these are the major heat shock proteins observed at 45°C may be indicative of their importance in maintaining cell viability under high thermal stress conditions.

Mycoplasma DnaK-Like Protein

One of the major heat shock proteins in procaryotes is a 69-kDa protein, which has been shown to be the *E. coli* DnaK protein (reviewed in references 9 and 26).

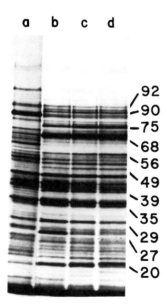

Figure 3. Autoradiogram of pulse-labeled proteins of *A. laidlawii* JA1 before and after heat shock, analyzed by sodium dodecyl sulfate-PAGE (6, 7). The labeling times and temperatures were as follows: lane a, 0 to 20 min at 32°C (control); lane b, 0 to 20 min at 42°C; lane c, 20 to 40 min at 42°C; and lane d, 40 to 60 min at 42°C. Each lane was loaded with total protein from 10^8 cells. The molecular masses (in kilodaltons) of the most prominent heat shock protein bands are marked.

The eucaryotic homolog, with significant sequence similarity to the DnaK protein, is the Hsp70 protein. In *E. coli*, the DnaK protein is synthesized constitutively as well as being a heat shock protein, is essential for phage lambda DNA replication (reviewed in reference 9), and may play a role in translocation of exported proteins (39). The DnaK protein also modulates and shuts down the *E. coli* heat shock response after initial activation of the regulon (33).

The mycoplasma 66- to 68-kDa heat shock protein cross-reacts with antibodies to the *E. coli* DnaK protein (7). In *A. laidlawii* and *M. capricolum*, this DnaK-like heat shock protein is also synthesized constitutively. The *A. laidlawii* 68-kDa and *E. coli* DnaK proteins are almost identical in size and degree of cross-reactivity to antibody to *E. coli* DnaK protein. However, the *M. capricolum* 66-kDa protein is slightly smaller in size and significantly less cross-reactive to antibody to the *E. coli* DnaK protein.

Studies with *M. hyopneumoniae*, the causative agent of mycoplasmal pneumonia in swine, suggest the mycoplasma DnaK-like protein may be an important antigenic determinant. It had been shown that prior infection of swine with *M. hyopneumoniae* confers resistance to reinfection, but vaccination with heat-inactivated *M. hyopneumoniae* does not protect from reinfection (16). Brooks and Faulds (4) found that convalescent (immune) swine produce antibody to an *M. hyopneumoniae* 74.5-kDa antigen, while swine injected with heat-inactivated *M. hyopneumoniae* lack antibody to this antigen. In addition, purified *M. hyopneumoniae* 74.5-kDa protein elicits a neutralizing antibody response, suggesting a possible role for it in protective immunity against *M. hyopneumoniae* infection. The gene coding for the 74.5-kDa protein has been cloned and sequenced, and it has been found to have 50% amino acid sequence similarity to the *E. coli* DnaK protein (4). Recent data indicate the 74.5-kDa protein is partially exposed on the cell surface (8). In *Chlamydia trachomatis*, a 70.6-kDa protein that has 71% amino acid sequence similarity to the *E. coli* DnaK protein also appears to be exposed at the cell surface (5). Hence, the DnaK-like protein may be a major antigenic determinant in mycoplasmas and other bacteria that lack a typical peptidoglycan-containing cell wall (such as *C. trachomatis*), in agreement with the suggestion that stress proteins may be important targets for the host immune response (38).

Mycoplasma GroEL-Like Protein

A common cross-reacting antigen (referred to as the bacterial common antigen) has been identified in over 60 different gram-positive and gram-negative eubacteria and archaebacteria; in all cases studied it was found to be a 58- to 65-kDa protein (references in reference 12). The gene for this protein has been cloned and sequenced from a wide range of procaryotic and eucaryotic species, and it was found to have a high degree of sequence similarity between species (25, 29). The common antigen was subsequently shown to be one of the stress response proteins: the GroEL protein in procaryotes and Hsp60 in eucaryotes (25, 29). In vivo and in vitro studies of the procaryotic and eucaryotic 58- to 60-kDa heat shock protein have led to its classification as a molecular chaperone, a family of proteins involved in protein folding, assembly, and transport across membranes (13).

Both the bacterial common antigen and the GroEL protein have been identified in mycoplasmas, but in separate studies. Sondergard-Anderson et al. (31) found that antibody to the common antigen of *Legionella micdadei* cross-reacts with a 62-kDa protein in *M. pneumoniae*, *M. fermentans*, and *M. genitalium*. Interestingly, both *M. pneumoniae* and *M. fermentans* required growth at 42°C for visualization of the common antigen, while *M. genitalium* common antigen could be observed when cells were grown at either 37 or 42°C. This difference may reflect a lower cross-reactivity of the *M. pneumoniae* and *M. fermentans* common antigen to the antiserum, as suggested by Western blots (e.g., Fig. 1 of reference 31), so that visualization of the common antigen in these species requires the increased abundance of heat shock proteins found at higher temperatures. Dascher et al. (7) showed that antibody to the *C. trachomatis* GroEL homolog, which cross-reacts with *E. coli* GroEL and the bacterial common antigen (1), cross-reacts with an *A. laidlawii* JA1 protein of about 60 kDa.

These data suggest that the 56- to 57-kDa heat shock protein identified in mycoplasma cells (7) is the mycoplasma GroEL-like protein, corresponding to the common antigen in mycoplasmas.

PHYSIOLOGICAL ASPECTS OF THE HEAT SHOCK RESPONSE IN MYCOPLASMAS

Heat Shock and Mycoplasma Virus Growth

Mycoplasma and *E. coli* heat shock systems differ in the effects of heat shock on phage yield. In *E. coli*, progeny coliphage production is increased when phages are grown at high temperatures on heat-shocked host cells (references in reference 36). However, no increase in progeny yield is observed when mycoplasma virus L2 (a temperate virus containing double-stranded DNA of 12 kb) is propagated at 42°C on heat-shocked *A. laidlawii* cells (7). This finding suggests *A. laidlawii* heat shock proteins are not limiting factors in L2 progeny virus yield.

Heat Shock and DNA Repair Systems

The relationship between mycoplasma DNA repair and heat shock systems has been investigated by studying host cell reactivation of UV-irradiated mycoplasma virus L2 (7). Increased reactivation was observed when UV-irradiated L2 virus was plated on UV-irradiated or heat-shocked *A. laidlawii* host cells. Hence, as in the bacteria, heat shock leads to both a heat shock response and SOS DNA repair in mycoplasmas.

DISCUSSION

Mycoplasmas have a heat shock response similar to that found in all living cells, both procaryote and eucaryote, studied thus far. The characteristic feature of these heat shock systems is an increased synthesis of a specific subset of proteins following a shift-up in temperature. The heat shock proteins carry out a variety of functions which must somehow protect the cells or repair damage caused by high temperatures. A critical aspect in defining the role of the heat shock system in mycoplasmas will be experiments to provide direct evidence that this system confers some degree of resistance to the deleterious effects of thermal stress. However, the heat shock response must be important in terms of natural selection, because mycoplasmas have retained heat shock systems during their degenerate evolution from the bacteria, even though doing so involved about a fivefold reduction in genetic complexity (see chapter 33).

Some heat shock proteins appear to be common to all species that have been investigated. Two such heat shock proteins are the 70-kDa DnaK-like protein (Hsp70 in eucaryotes) and the 60-kDa GroEL-like protein (Hsp60 in eucaryotes). Both of these proteins are present in the mycoplasma species studied thus far (4, 7, 31). Although no functional role can be assigned to these proteins in mycoplasmas, their functions in other systems suggest that they are essential for an optimal heat shock response. DnaK and GroEL are members of the chaperone class of proteins identified in procaryotes and eucaryotes (19, 28). Chaperone proteins are believed to be required for protein folding and assembly processes as well as for translocation of exported proteins. During heat shock, there may be an increased requirement for chaperone proteins to help cells cope with an increased burden of improperly folded proteins (17, 28).

The 60-kDa common antigen (i.e., the GroEL-like protein) appears to be an immunodominant antigen for a number of pathogenic bacterial species (12, 18, 20, 23). Studies with mycobacteria suggest that the common antigen may be a specific target for the γδ subset of T cells (14, 27). This result may have broad implications for host defense mechanisms: an antigenic target common among a number of bacteria might facilitate host immune surveillance, but it might also inadvertently trigger a host autoimmune response under certain conditions (18). Such an immune response may be an important determinant of mycoplasma pathogenicity and may explain reports of autoimmune reactions accompanying human *M. pneumoniae* infections (references in references 2 and 21).

In summary, the mycoplasma heat shock system has important implications for both mycoplasma biology and pathology. The general aspects of the mycoplasma heat shock response (described above) are similar to those of other bacterial heat shock systems, which means this system could not be deleted during the attrition in genetic complexity accompanying degenerate evolution of the mycoplasmas from the eubacteria. Future studies of the molecular biology of the mycoplasma heat shock system are needed to determine whether specific details of the eubacterial heat shock response were modified or simplified as a result of the limiting genome size constraint in the mycoplasmas.

The pathogenic role of microbial heat shock proteins may include protecting the pathogen during infection, serving as immunodominant pathogen antigens, and

inducing host autoimmune responses (reviewed in reference 15). There are indications of a relationship between heat shock proteins and pathogenicity in studies of invasive intracellular bacteria (references in reference 30). Mycoplasma-eucaryote interactions might be functionally equivalent to intracellular bacterium-eucaryote interactions because, although (with one important exception) mycoplasmas are not intracellular parasites, there is a close association between mycoplasma and host cell membranes (reviewed in reference 32), and the lack of a cell wall allows direct presentation of mycoplasma membrane-associated heat shock proteins for an immune response without the need for intracellular host cell processing. The single reported intracellular mycoplasma is the AIDS-associated mycoplasma, *M. fermentans* (*incognitus*) (22). These considerations and the known relationship between *M. pneumoniae* infection and autoantibodies (discussed above) indicate the need for specific investigations of the association between the mycoplasma heat shock response and mycoplasma pathogenicity.

Acknowledgments. We thank Sergei Borchsenius (Institute of Cytology, St. Petersburg, Russia) for sending us a preprint of his paper on mycoplasma heat shock and Daryl Faulds (Berlex Biosciences, South San Francisco, Calif.) for providing unpublished data on the *M. hyopneumoniae* DnaK-like protein.

REFERENCES

1. **Bavoil, P., R. S. Stephens, and S. Falkow**. 1990. A soluble 60 kiloDalton antigen of Chlamydia spp. is a homologue of *Escherichia coli* GroEL. *Mol. Microbiol.* **4**:461–469.
2. **Biberfeld, G**. 1985. Infection sequelae and autoimmune reactions in *Mycoplasma pneumoniae* infection, p. 293-311. *In* S. Razin and M. F. Barile (ed.), *The Mycoplasmas*, vol. 4. Academic Press, Inc., New York.
3. **Borchsenius, S. N., E. V. Budantseva, and M. S. Vonsky**. 1990. The heat-shock proteins of *Acholeplasma laidlawii*. *Zentralbl. Bakteriol. Suppl.* **20**:657–658.
4. **Brooks, E., and D. Faulds**. 1989. The *Mycoplasma hyopneumoniae* 74.5-kD antigen elicits neutralizing antibodies and shares sequence similarity with heat-shock proteins, p. 265–269. *In* R. A. Lerner, H. Ginsberg, R. M. Chanock, and F. Brown (ed.), *Vaccines 89: Modern Approaches to New Vaccines Including Prevention of AIDS*. Cold Spring Harbor Laboratory, Cold Spring Harbor, N.Y.
5. **Danilition, S. L., I. W. Maclean, R. Peling, S. Winston, and R. C. Brunham**. 1990. The 75-kilodalton protein of *Chlamydia trachomatis*: a member of the heat shock protein 70 family? *Infect. Immun.* **58**:189–196.
6. **Dascher, C. C., and J. Maniloff**. Unpublished data.
7. **Dascher, C. C., S. K. Poddar, and J. Maniloff**. 1990. Heat shock in mycoplsmas, genome-limited organisms. *J. Bacteriol.* **172**:1823–1827.
8. **Faulds, D. (Berlex Biosciences)**. 1991. Personal communication.
9. **Georgopoulos, C., D. Ang, A. Maddock, S. Raina, B. Lipinska, and M. Zylicz**. 1990. Heat shock response of *Escherichia coli*, p. 405–419. *In* K. Drlica and M. Riley (ed.), *The Bacterial Chromosome*. American Society for Microbiology, Washington, D.C.
10. **Gross, C. A., D. B. Strauss, J. W. Erickson, and T. Yura**. 1990. The function and regulation of heat shock proteins in *Escherichia coli*, p. 167–189. *In* R. I. Morimoto, A. Tissières, and C. Georgopoulos (ed.), *Stress Proteins in Biol-*

ogy and Medicine. Cold Spring Harbor Laboratory, Cold Spring Harbor, N.Y.

11. **Grossman, A. D., J. W. Erickson, and C. A. Gross.** 1984. The *htpR* gene product of *E. coli* is a sigma factor for heat-shock promoters. *Cell* **38**:383–390.

12. **Hansen, K., J. M. Bangsborg, H. Fjordvang, N. S. Pedersen, and P. Hindersson.** 1988. Immunochemical characterization of and isolation of the gene for a *Borrelia burgdorferi* immunodominant 60-kilodalton antigen common to a wide range of bacteria. *Infect. Immun.* **56**:2047–2053.

13. **Hemmingsen, S. M., C. Woolford, S. M. van der Vies, K. Tilly, D. T. Dennis, C. P. Georgopoulos, R. W. Hendrix, and J. Ellis.** 1988. Homologous plant and bacterial proteins chaperone oligomeric protein assembly. *Nature* (London) **333**:330–334.

14. **Janis, E. M., S. H. E. Kaufmann, R. H. Schwartz, and D. M. Pardoll.** 1989. Activation of γδ T cells in the primary immune response to *Mycobacteria tuberculosis*. *Science* **244**:713–716.

15. **Kaufmann, S. H. E.** 1990. Heat-shock proteins: a missing link in the host-parasite relationship? *Med. Microbiol. Immunol.* **179**:61–66.

16. **Kristensen, B., P. Paroz, J. Nicolet, M. Wanner, and A. L. de Weck.** 1981. Cell-mediated and humoral immune response in swine after vaccination and natural infection with *Mycoplasma hyopneumoniae*. *Am. J. Vet. Res.* **42**:784–788.

17. **Kusukawa, N., and T. Yura.** 1988. Heat shock protein GroE of *Escherichia coli*: key protective roles against thermal stress. *Genes Dev.* **2**:874–882.

18. **Lamb, J. R., V. Bal, J. B. Rothbarb, A. Mehlert, P. Mendez-Samperio, and D. B. Young.** 1989. The mycobacterial Groel stress protein: a common target of T-cell recognition in infection and autoimmunity. *J. Autoimmun.* **2**(Suppl.):93–100.

19. **LaRossa, R. A., T. K. VanDyk.** 1991. Physiological roles of the DnaK and GroE stress proteins: catalysts of protein folding or macromolecular sponges? *Mol. Microbiol.* **5**:529–534.

20. **Lehner, T., E. Lavery, R. Smith, R. van der Zee, Y. Mizushima, and T. Shinnick.** 1991. Association between the 65-kilodalton heat shock protein, *Streptococcus sanguis*, and the corresponding antibodies in Behçet's syndrome. *Infect. Immun.* **59**: 1434–1441.

21. **Lind, K., M. Hoeier-Madsen, and A. Wiik.** 1990. Mitotic spindle apparatus autoantibodies in *Mycoplasma pneumoniae* disease. *Zentralbl. Bakteriol. Suppl.* **20**:953–955.

22. **Lo, S.-C., M. S. Dawson, D. M. Wong, P. B. Newton, M. A. Sonoda, W. F. Engler, R. Y.-H. Wang, J. W.-K. Shih, H. J. Alter, and D. J. Wear.** 1989. Identification of *Mycoplasma incognitus* infection of patients with AIDS: an immunohistochemical, in situ hybridization and ultrastructural study. *Am. J. Trop. Med. Hyg.* **41**:601–616.

23. **Meeker, H. C., D. L. Williams, D. C. Anderson, T. P. Gillis, G. Schuller-Levis, and W. R. Levis.** 1989. Analysis of human antibody epitopes on the 65-kilodalton protein of *Mycobacteria leprae* by using synthetic peptides. *Infect. Immun.* **57**:3689–3694.

24. **Morowitz, H. J.** 1967. Biological self-replicating systems. *Prog. Theor. Biol.* **1**:35–38.

25. **Morrison, R. P., R. J. Belland, K. Lyng, and H. D. Caldwell.** 1989. Chlamydial disease pathogenesis: the 57-kD chlamydial hypersensitivity antigen is a stress response protein. *J. Exp. Med.* **170**:1271–1283.

26. **Neidhardt, F. C., and R. A. VanBogelen.** 1987. Heat shock response, p. 1334–1345. *In* F. C. Neidhardt, J. L. Ingraham, K. B. Low, B. Magasanik, M. Schaechter, and H. E. Umbarger (ed.), *Escherichia coli and Salmonella typhimurium: Cellular and Molecular Biology*, vol. 2. American Society for Microbiology, Washington, D.C.

27. **O'Brien, R. L., M. P. Happ, A. Dallas, E. Palmer, R. Kubo, and W. K. Born.** 1989. Stimulation of a major subset of lymphocytes expressing T cell receptor γδ by an antigen derived from Mycobacterium tuberculosis. *Cell* **57**:667–674.

28. **Pelham, H. R. B.** 1990. Functions of the hsp70 protein family: an overview, p. 287–299. *In* R. I. Morimoto, A. Tissières, and C. Georgopoulos (ed.), *Stress Proteins in Biology and Medicine*. Cold Spring Harbor Laboratory, Cold Spring Harbor, N.Y.

29. **Picketts, D. J., C. S. K. Mayanil, and R. S.R.S. Gupta.** 1989. Molecular cloning of a Chinese hamster mitochondrial protein related to the "chaperonin" family of bacterial and plant proteins. *J. Biol. Chem.* **264**:12001–12008.

30. **Sokolovic, Z., A. Fuchs, and W. Gobel.** 1990. Synthesis of species-specific stress proteins by virulent strains of *Listeria monocytogenes*. *Infect. Immun.* **58**:3582–3587.

31. **Sondergard-Anderson, J., J. S. Jensen, S. A. Uldum, and K. Lind.** 1990. Heat-shock protein in *Mycoplasma pneumoniae* shown by immunoblotting to be related to the bacterial common antigen. *J. Infect. Dis.* **161**:1039–1040.

32. **Stanbridge, E. J., and C.-J. Doersen.** 1978. Some effects that mycoplasmas have upon their infected host, p. 119–134. *In* G. J. McGarrity, D. G. Murphy, and W. W. Nichols (ed.), *Mycoplasma Infection of Cell Cultures*. Plenum Press, New York.

33. **Tilly, K., N. McKittrick, M. Zylicz, and C. Georgopoulos.** 1983. The *dnaK* protein modulates the heat-shock response of Escherichia coli. *Cell* **34**:641–646.

34. **Tomlins, R. I., and Z. J. Ordal.** 1976. Thermal injury and inactivation in vegetative bacteria, p. 153–190. *In* F. A. Skinner and W. B. Hugo (ed.), *Inhibition and Inactivation of Vegetative Microbes*. Academic Press, Inc., New York.

35. **Van Bogelen, R. A., P. M. Kelley, and F. C. Neidhardt.** 1987. Differential induction of heat shock, SOS, and oxidation stress regulons and accumulation of nucleotides in *Escherichia coli*. *J. Bacteriol.* **169**:26–32.

36. **Wiberg, J. S., M. F. Mowrey-McKee, and E. J. Stevens.** 1988. Induction of the heat shock regulon of *Escherichia coli* markedly increases production of bacterial viruses at high temperatures. *J. Virol.* **62**:234–245.

37. **Yamamori, T., and T. Yura.** 1982. Genetic control of heat-shock protein synthesis and its bearing on growth and thermal resistance in *Escherichia coli* K-12. *Proc. Natl. Acad. Sci. USA* **79**:860–864.

38. **Young, D., R. Lathigra, R. Hendrix, D. Sweeter, and R. A. Young.** 1988. Stress proteins are immune targets in leprosy and tuberculosis. *Proc. Natl. Acad. Sci. USA* **85**:4267–4270.

39. **Zimmerman, R., M. Sagstetter, M. J. Lewis, and H. Pelham.** 1988. Seventy-kilodalton heat shock proteins and an additional component from reticulocyte lysate stimulate import of M13 procoat protein into microsomes. *EMBO J.* **7**:2875–2880.

21. Gene Transfer

KEVIN DYBVIG

INTRODUCTION

The mycoplasmal genome is thought to be the smallest of any free-living cell. The minimal coding capacity of the genome provides a limited biosynthetic capability, necessitating the use of complex media to support growth. For most species, defined media have not been developed and auxotrophic mutants are unavailable. Genetic studies are further complicated by the fact that the genetic codes of most mycoplasmal species (*Acholeplasma laidlawii* [54] is the only known exception) are different from those of other bacteria (57). Despite these inherent difficulties, promising approaches for the development of mycoplasmal genetic systems have recently become available.

Primarily because of their close phylogenetic relationship and the lack of cell walls, there are important similarities between mycoplasmas and gram-positive bacterial protoplasts. In particular, artificial methods for genetic transformation of many mycoplasmas, using polyethylene glycol (PEG)-mediated procedures, have been described. Some transposons and plasmids of gram-positive bacterial origin function in mycoplasmas, and the few mycoplasmal plasmids that have been characterized to date probably replicate in a manner similar to that of many gram-positive bacterial plasmids. Some mycoplasmas have a gene transfer system that involves direct cell-to-cell contact, but it remains to be determined whether this phenomenon is similar to gram-positive bacterial conjugation.

TRANSFORMATION

Genetic transformation is often defined as nuclease-sensitive gene transfer, involving the uptake of naked DNA by the organism. It is a primary means for creating novel strains of bacteria by the introduction of new or mutated genes. Natural transformation occurs in some bacterial systems, but in many systems, transformation must be induced or promoted by various artificial treatments. Transformation of mycoplasmas has usually been promoted by artificial treatments involving either PEG or electroporation.

PEG-mediated transformation of gram-positive bacterial protoplasts was first described for streptomycetes (6). Transformation of streptomycetes is remarkably efficient; up to 80% of the CFU can be transformed by using saturating levels of DNA. The optimum concentration of PEG for transformation of streptomycetes is 20%. PEG can also promote fusion of *Streptomyces* protoplasts, but at higher PEG concentrations of about 50% (reviewed in reference 27). It is therefore thought that transformation and cell fusion of protoplasts are distinct processes.

The methodology for protoplast transformation of streptomycetes was first applied to *Bacillus subtilis* (10) and then to numerous other gram-positive bacterial systems. Sladek and Maniloff (51) first described PEG-mediated transformation of a mycoplasma (*A. laidlawii*) in transfection studies using DNA from mycoplasma virus L2. Subsequent studies established similar transformation protocols for *Spiroplasma* and *Mycoplasma* species. Unlike the efficient transformation described for streptomycetes and *B. subtilis*, PEG-mediated transformation of mycoplasmas is extremely inefficient. Most studies have used at least 5 μg of homogeneous DNA (viral or plasmid) per transformation, with reported frequencies generally ranging from 10^{-4} to 10^{-8} transformants per CFU.

Kevin Dybvig • Department of Comparative Medicine and Department of Microbiology, University of Alabama at Birmingham, Birmingham, Alabama 35294.

A. laidlawii

Transfection

Sladek and Maniloff (51) determined that transfection of A. laidlawii with L2 DNA was optimal at a PEG concentration of 36%. Using saturating concentrations of DNA (10 μg), the transfection frequency was 10^{-4}/CFU or 10^4/μg of DNA. PEG-mediated transfection of A. laidlawii by using DNA from mycoplasma viruses L1 (52) and L172 (21) has also been described, but attempts using DNA from mycoplasma virus L3 have been unsuccessful (30, 52). L1 DNA is a 4.5-kb single-stranded, circular molecule, L172 DNA is a 14-kb single-stranded, circular molecule, and L2 DNA is a 11.6-kb double-stranded, circular molecule (reviewed in reference 38). Transfection frequencies with L1, L172, and L2 DNAs are comparable, indicating that single-stranded and double-stranded DNAs are equally efficient at transformation. L3 DNA is a 39-kb double-stranded, linear molecule. Perhaps PEG-mediated transfection with L3 DNA was ineffective because of the large size of the molecule or because this DNA is linear (and more susceptible to exonucleases). As discussed below, transfection with L3 DNA has been achieved by another method, electroporation.

Transposon studies

Transformation of A. laidlawii has also been examined by using gram-positive transposon Tn916. Because of its very broad host range, Tn916 (11) has been useful for developing transformation methods for numerous microorganisms. Transformants are selected by using the transposon's tetracycline resistance determinant, tetM, as a marker. The tetM determinant usually results in a high level of tetracycline resistance, which allows for selection of transformants under conditions that have little if any background of spontaneous mutants. The Tn916-containing plasmid pAM120 (24) replicates in Escherichia coli but not in mycoplasmas, and transposition of Tn916 from the plasmid into the recipient chromosome is required for successful mycoplasma transformation. Dybvig and Cassell (19) described PEG-mediated transformation of A. laidlawii with pAM120 at a frequency of 10^{-6} transformants per CFU. The transposon was located at a diversity of sites within recipient chromosomes, suggesting that Tn916 will be useful as an insertional mutagen. One interpretation of studies with mycoplasma virus L3 DNA is that large DNAs are refractory to PEG-mediated transformation of mycoplasmas. However, pAM120 is also fairly large, about 26 kb (18), and the effect of DNA size on PEG-mediated transformation of mycoplasmas requires more study.

Transformation of A. laidlawii with pAM120 (19) occurred less efficiently than transfection with mycoplasma virus L2 DNA (51). One possible explanation for this difference is that transposition of Tn916 may not readily occur in every cell that is transformed. However, transformation with pAM120 was as efficient as transformation with tetM-containing plasmids that replicate in A. laidlawii (see studies below describing plasmid pKJ1), suggesting that transposition events do not limit transformation frequencies. Data from gram-positive bacterial systems indicate that transposition is induced when Tn916 is first introduced into a cell (11). This phenomenon, referred to as zygotic induction, probably occurs in mycoplasmas as well. Possibly other factors, such as expression of the tetM determinant or differences in medium preparation between laboratories, account for differences in transformation frequencies obtained with viral DNAs and tetM-containing plasmid DNAs.

Plasmid studies

Many plasmids isolated from gram-positive bacteria have extremely broad host ranges which include not only many genera of gram-positive bacteria but, in some cases, gram-negative bacteria as well. Because of the phylogenetic relationship between mycoplasmas and gram-positive bacteria, it is anticipated that some of these plasmids will be useful as mycoplasmal vectors. Initial examples of gram-positive bacterial plasmids that replicate in some mycoplasmas come from studies of streptococcal plasmids transformed into A. laidlawii.

Dybvig (15) has examined transformation of A. laidlawii with streptococcal plasmids pVA868 and pVA920. Plasmid pVA380-1 (33) is a 4.2-kb cryptic plasmid originally isolated from Streptococcus ferus, and several streptococcal cloning vehicles have been constructed by combining the origin of replication (ori) from this plasmid with various antibiotic resistance markers. Plasmids pVA868 and pVA920 contain the pVA380-1 ori combined with a tetracycline resistance determinant (tetM). Plasmid DNAs isolated from A. laidlawii that had been transformed with pVA868 or pVA920 were deletion derivatives of the parent plasmids. The deletion derivative of pVA868 (13.7 kb) was a 3.7-kb plasmid designated pKJ1 (15, 16). pKJ1 was stable in A. laidawii in the sense that additional deletions in the plasmid were not detected, and PEG-mediated transformation of A. laidlawii with pKJ1 occurred at a frequency of 10^{-6} transformants per CFU. The deletion derivative of pVA920 (12.2 kb) was a 10.3-kb plasmid designated pKJ3 (15, 16). In addition to the tetM determinant, pVA920 contains an erythromycin resistance determinant originally from streptococcal plasmid pAMβ1. The erythromycin resistance determinant was still present in pKJ3, and it rendered A. laidlawii cells resistant to this antibiotic. pKJ3 underwent additional deletions when transformed again into A. laidlawii. These deletions resulted in transformants that were resistant to tetracycline or erythromycin, depending on which antibiotic was used for selection, but not resistant to the other antibiotic. Plasmids pKJ1 and pKJ3 also exhibited a high degree of segregational instability when propagated in the absence of antibiotic selection.

Unlike pKJ3, pKJ1 is apparently stable in A. laidlawii (except for segregational instability), and it may be useful as a vector. pKJ1 has a unique HindIII site which should be available for cloning because it is located within sequences that are not involved with plasmid replication or antibiotic resistance. A plasmid consisting of pKJ1 combined with E. coli plasmid pUC18 at their respective HindIII sites has been constructed, but this chimeric molecule was unstable in both E. coli and A. laidlawii (17a). pKJ1 may nevertheless be useful as a Streptococcus-Acholeplasma shuttle vector; both pKJ1 and pKJ3 have retained the ability to replicate in streptococci (15). Unfortunately, pKJ1 may not be useful as a vector in *Mycoplasma* species, because attempts to transform *Mycoplasma pulmonis* (by using PEG-mediated methods described below) with plasmids containing the *ori* from pVA380-1 have thus far not been successful.

Recent studies by Sundstrom and Wieslander (53) have examined streptococcal plasmid pNZ18. Plasmid pNZ18, a 5.7-kb derivative of plasmid pNZ12, contains the *ori* from *Streptococcus lactis* plasmid pSH71, the kanamycin-neomycin resistance determinant from plasmid pUB110, and the chloramphenicol resistance determinant from plasmid pC194 (13). pNZ18 has an extremely broad host range; its *ori* functions in many gram-positive bacterial species as well as *E. coli*, and the finding that this plasmid replicates in *A. laidlawii* is not surprising. Transformation of *A. laidlawii* with pNZ18 occurred at a frequency of 10^{-7} transformants per CFU (53), and unlike pVA868 and pVA920, pNZ18 did not undergo deletions. The apparent stability of pNZ18 in *A. laidlawii* suggests that this plasmid will be an important vector in this system, and it likely will function in other mycoplasmas as well. For identification of *A. laidlawii* transformants containing pNZ18, selection with kanamycin or neomycin was effective. Some background of spontaneous mutants resistant to kanamycin were observed, but transformants containing pNZ18 were distinguishable from spontaneous mutants on the basis of colony morphology. *A. laidlawii* cells containing pNZ18 were not resistant to chloramphenicol, indicating that the plasmid's chloramphenicol acetyltransferase gene is not expressed in this system.

Mycoplasma Species

Transposon studies

Definitive evidence for transformation of *Mycoplasma* species came with the demonstration that transposon Tn*916* functions in these organisms (19). By using pAM120, PEG-mediated transformation has been established for several *Mycoplasma* species, including *M. pulmonis* (18, 19) *M. hyorhinis* (18), and *M. mycoides* subsp. *mycoides* (27a, 55, 56). Transformation of *M. pulmonis* and *M. hyorhinis* occurred at frequencies of 10^{-6} and 10^{-8} transformants per CFU, respectively. Whereas the optimal PEG concentration has not been determined for transformation of *M. hyorhinis*, transformation of *M. pulmonis* was optimal at 36% PEG at a frequency comparable to that for transformation of *A. laidlawii*. Transformation of *M. mycoides* subsp. *mycoides* also occurred at a frequency of 10^{-6}/CFU, but the optimal PEG concentration of 60 to 70% was surprisingly high (27a). With the *Mycoplasma* species studied to date, recipient chromosomes contain Tn*916* inserted at a diversity of sites, indicating that the transposon will be a useful mutagen. However, there is some evidence (18, 27a) that Tn*916* may sometimes transpose to secondary sites at high frequency, suggesting that some Tn*916*-generated mutants may be unstable.

PEG-mediated transformation of *M. pulmonis* has been examined by using another transposable element, staphylococcal transposon Tn*4001* (37). Tn*4001* (4.7 kb) is flanked by a 1.3-kb insertion element, IS*256*, and it encodes a bifunctional peptide specifying resistance to kanamycin and gentamicin (31, 32). Gentamicin resistance serves as the selectable marker in mycoplasmas. As with studies using Tn*916*, transformation with Tn*4001*-containing plasmids requires a transposition event. Transformation was successful with pISM1001, a 13.45-kb plasmid containing Tn*4001*, but not with pSK31, a 37.7-kb plasmid. As suggested from transfection studies with *A. laidlawii*, PEG-mediated transformation may be ineffective for large DNAs. Alternatively, pSK31 may be more susceptible to a host restriction-modification system than is pISM1001 or pAM120. Tn*4001*, like Tn*916*, may be a useful mutagen because it is inserted into the chromosome of transformed cells at a diversity of sites. Because IS*256* can apparently transpose independently of Tn*4001* in *M. pulmonis*, mutants may be generated by insertion of either of these transposable elements.

Integrative plasmids requiring homologous recombination

Impressive studies by Mahairas et al. have examined transformation of *M. pulmonis* in the absence of a transposable element or a plasmid capable of replication within the mycoplasma by relying on homologous recombination for incorporation of antibiotic resistance markers into recipient chromosomes (34, 36). Numerous plasmids that replicate in *E. coli* were constructed to contain either the gentamicin resistance determinant from Tn*4001* or the *tetM* gene from Tn*916*, combined with fragments of chromosomal DNA from *M. pulmonis*. Transformation of *M. pulmonis* resulted in insertion of the plasmid marker into the recipient chromosome at frequencies generally ranging from 10^{-4} to 10^{-6}/CFU. These results suggest the presence of high levels of homologous recombination, and they should provide a basis for introducing a variety of genes into *M. pulmonis* (34). Of particular importance is the capability of targeting specific genes to create mutations that can studied in vivo. Transformation frequencies were apparently affected by the specific chromosomal insert present on the plasmid, and transformation with plasmids containing large inserts (greater than 22 kb) was not successful. As with *A. laidlawii* studies, there is a suggestion that PEG-mediated transformation may be ineffective with large DNAs.

Plasmids that replicate in *Mycoplasma* species

The first cryptic *Mycoplasma* plasmid that was characterized is the 1.7-kb plasmid pADB201, isolated from *M. mycoides* subsp. *mycoides* (4, 5). Sequence data indicate homology between an open reading frame in pADB201 and the replication proteins of staphylococcal plasmid pE194 and streptococcal plasmid pLS1, indicating a commonality between these plasmids. Replication of pE194 and pLS1 is thought to involve intermediates containing single-stranded DNA (reviewed in reference 26), and pADB201 presumably has a similar mode of replication. In fact, by comparing the sequence of pADB201 with that of plasmids that replicate by a single-stranded mode, the putative *ori* for the plus strand of pADB201 has been identified (26). Because plasmids that replicate via single-stranded intermediates tend to undergo deletion events at high frequency (1, 22), it is likely that a vector developed from pADB201 would have some inherent problems with instability. Despite instability problems, many gram-positive bacterial plasmids that replicate via single-stranded intermediates have been successfully used as vectors; these include plasmids pUB110, pC194, pNZ12, pT181, pLS1, and pE194. Therefore, the potential of pADB201 as a vector warrants further examination.

Plasmid pKMK1 (1.85 kb) is a second cryptic plasmid isolated from *M. mycoides* subsp. *mycoides* (16, 20). The sequence of pKMK1 has recently been determined (27b). Sequence similarities between pKMK1 and other gram-positive bacterial plasmids, including pADB201, indicate that pKMK1 also replicates via single-stranded intermediates.

Spiroplasma Species

As with *Acholeplasma* species, transfection studies provided the basis for the first descriptions of PEG-mediated transformation of spiroplasmas. Transfection of *Spiroplasma melliferum* with single-stranded spiroplasma virus 4 DNA occurred at a frequency of 10^2 to 10^3 transfectants per µg of DNA (42, 43), and transfection of *S. citri* with single-stranded SVTS2 DNA occurred at a frequency of 10^5 transfectants per µg of DNA (40).

PEG-mediated transformation has also been examined by using plasmids (reviewed in reference 7) isolated from spiroplasmas. Spiroplasma plasmid pMH1 (7 kb) has been combined with a chloramphenicol acetyltransferase gene, from *E. coli* plasmid pBR328, under the control of a spiroplasma promoter (50). Transformation of this chimeric plasmid into *S. citri*, selecting for chloramphenicol resistance, resulted in transformants that contained plasmids related to pMH1. However, the plasmids isolated from the transformants had lost the ability to replicate in *E. coli*, and their mobility on agarose gels suggested that deletions had occurred. With passaging, these plasmids displayed segregational instability, and additional deletions were also observed. Similar plasmid instability was observed when *A. laidlawii* was transformed with streptococcal plasmids pVA868 and pVA920 (see above).

In another interesting transformation study, the involvement of a spiroplasma plasmid in acquisition of erythromycin resistance was examined (48). Plasmid pM42 (12.3 kb) is a cryptic plasmid related to pMH1 and is present as an extrachromosomal element in the erythromycin-sensitive *S. citri* strain M4$^+$. A spontaneous erythromycin-resistant mutant of strain M4$^+$ (designated strain M4 Er-1) was isolated, and pM42 DNA isolated from the mutant was transformed into the erythromycin-sensitive *S. citri* strain R8A2$^+$. Erythromycin-resistant transformants were obtained, but Southern blot analysis failed to detect extrachromosomal pM42 in the transformed cells. Instead, pM42 sequences were present at a specific site within the recipient chromosome. pM42 sequences were also present within the chromosome of strain M4 Er-1 but

not strain M4$^+$. These data suggest that the insertion of pM42 sequences into the *S. citri* chromosome can influence susceptibility of the cell to erythromycin.

Transformation of Mycoplasmas without PEG

Electroporation

Electroporation has been an effective method for transformation in many cell systems, both eucaryotic and procaryotic, that have been refractory to transformation by other methods. This method uses high-voltage electric field pulses to transiently increase membrane permeability, allowing uptake of DNA. With *E. coli*, electroporation has resulted in extremely high transformation frequencies ranging from 10^9 to 10^{10} transformants per µg of DNA (56). Unfortunately, electroporation of gram-positive bacterial protoplasts and mycoplasmas has resulted in transformation frequencies much lower than those reported for *E. coli*. However, because many parameters (e.g., the choice of buffer, voltage, pulse length, and cell concentration) affect transformation, electroporation of mycoplasmas may become more efficient as conditions are optimized.

Lorenz et al. (30) used electroporation to study transfection of *A. laidlawii*. Interestingly, trypsin treatment of the cells prior to electroporation increased the efficiency of transfection by about 10-fold. Trypsinization may have increased transformation efficiencies by inactivating nucleases, or it conceivably may have removed other cell surface proteins that interfere with DNA uptake. Electroporation of trypsin-treated *A. laidlawii* cells was about 10 times less efficient than traditional PEG methods for transfection with mycoplasma virus L1 DNA. However, electroporation was effective for transfection with mycoplasma virus L3 DNA, whereas PEG-mediated transfection with L3 DNA was not successful. Therefore, electroporation may be more effective than PEG for transformation using large DNA molecules, whereas PEG methods appear to be preferable for smaller DNAs. In another study, electroporation was successful for transfection of *S. citri* with SVTS2 DNA (39). In this case, electroporation was about as efficient as the PEG method for transformation. Electroporation has also been used, though at a frequency of only 10^{-10} transformants per CFU, for transformation of *M. mycoides* subsp. *mycoides* with pAM120 (56).

Other reports on transformation

Some reports have described transformation in the absence of PEG (or electroporation), but these results have been difficult to evaluate. Transformation of *M. hominis* cells made competent by treatment with divalent cations has been reported (9, 23), but this approach was not successful in another laboratory (46). Transfection of *A. laidlawii* with viral L1 DNA has been reported in the absence of PEG or other treatments involving divalent cations (28, 29), but subsequent transfection studies have required PEG (or electroporation) (30, 52). Transformation of *A. laidlawii* by using DNA from a neomycin-resistant strain of *A. laidlawii* in the absence of PEG or divalent ion treatment has also been reported (25). Similarly, some reports have described low-frequency transformation of spiroplasmas in the absence of PEG (12, 40, 48, 50). These studies suggest the possible existence of natural transformation systems in some mycoplasmas. However, even if natural transformation occurs, it would seem to be inefficient and difficult to reproduce.

MYCOPLASMAL MATING

It is advantageous for organisms to have some mechanism(s) for acquiring novel genes from the environment. Although there is little evidence of natural transformation systems in mycoplasmas, recent studies suggest that some mycoplasmas possess gene transfer systems that require cell-to-cell contact. The mechanism(s) of these gene transfer systems is unknown, and the lack of a cell wall may have allowed the evolution of systems that are unique to mycoplasmas. Gene transfer between mycoplasmas may be conjugationlike or involve other processes such as cell fusion. In addition to mating between mycoplasmas, these organisms can acquire DNA from walled bacteria via conjugative transposons.

Conjugal Transfer of Tn916 from Streptococcal Donors

Transfer of a conjugative DNA element, such as Tn916, is a likely mechanism for how some clinical isolates of M. hominis and Ureaplasma urealyticum initially acquired the tetM gene (44, 45, 47). As a laboratory method, conjugal transfer is usually more convenient than transformation for the introduction of Tn916 into bacteria because fewer manipulations are required and plasmid DNA does not need to be isolated. Tn916 has been transferred by conjugation from Enterococcus faecalis to numerous gram-positive bacteria. Tn916 is about 16.4 kb, and over half of its coding capacity is required for conjugal transfer (49). Transfer of Tn916 from E. faecalis into a mycoplasma was first examined by using M. hominis as the recipient (46). About 10^{-6} to 10^{-7} transconjugants per recipient CFU were obtained. It is now clear that conjugal transfer using E. faecalis as the donor will be an effective mechanism for introducing Tn916 into a variety of mycoplasmas. For example, conjugal transfer using M. pulmonis as the recipient occurred at a similar frequency of 10^{-6} to 10^{-7} transconjugants per recipient CFU (17). Tn916-mediated conjugation in bacilli can promote cotransfer of plasmids not harboring the transposon (41). Therefore, conjugative transposons may prove useful for transferring a variety of plasmids from gram-positive bacteria into mycoplasmas. To date, conjugal transfer of Tn916 by using a mycoplasma as donor has not been described.

Gene Transfer between Mycoplasmas

Spiroplasmas

Transfer of chromosomal DNA between S. citri cells has been examined by using resistance to arsenic acid,

vanadium oxide, and xylitol as markers (2, 3). DNase I-resistant gene transfer occurred in growth medium in the absence of PEG, and controls strongly argue that the mechanism was neither transformation nor transduction. The lack of a requirement for PEG indicates that gene transfer is distinct from the PEG-mediated cell fusion phenomenon described for gram-positive bacterial protoplasts. Gene transfer between spiroplasmas may involve either a different type of cell fusion not requiring PEG or a conjugationlike process. For observable mating to occur, cells resistant to one marker had to be incubated in nonselective medium with cells resistant to a second marker for more than 9 h prior to assays for resistance to both markers on selective medium. Colonies resistant to both markers were obtained at a frequency of 10^{-4} to 10^{-5}/CFU, and the phenotype of these colonies was stable for at least 20 generations of growth. Why mating required long incubation times in nonselective medium is unknown, but this amount of time may be required for the physical transfer of the marker, incorporation of the marker into the recipient chromosome by recombination, or expression of the resistant marker in the recombinant cell. Matings in which cells resistant to two markers were mixed with cells resistant to the third marker were unsuccessful. It is unclear why cells resistant to all three markers were unobtainable.

Mycoplasmas

Gene transfer between Mycoplasma cells has been studied in M. pulmonis by using the tetracycline resistance determinant from Tn916 and the gentamicin resistance determinant from Tn4001 as markers (35). Several strains with these antibiotic resistance markers located at a variety of chromosomal sites were constructed. These constructs were obtained by transforming cells with plasmids that inserted into the chromosome by homologous recombination, as described above. Genetic exchange in M. pulmonis occurred on agar surfaces at a frequency ranging from 3 $\times$ 10^{-4} to 6 $\times$ 10^{-8}/CFU, depending on the location and nature of the marker. DNA-DNA hybridization analysis showed that the resistance markers in the progeny strains were located in the same site as they were in the parent strains. Gene transfer apparently involved a trypsin-sensitive membrane protein, and transfer frequencies were usually reduced if one of the parent strains was preexposed to UV light at doses that decreased cell viability. However, strains containing Tn4001 were an exception. Lethal doses of UV irradiation of strains containing Tn4001 did not impair the ability of the cells to undergo gene transfer. The basis for why transfer involving nonviable cells occurred only when Tn4001 was present in the irradiated strain is unknown.

TRANSDUCTION

Although transduction has not been described for the mycoplasmas, the prevalence of viruses isolated from these organisms indicates that transduction is feasible and that it may occur in nature. Until recently, demonstration of transduction in the laboratory has been hampered by the lack of markers. The markers presently available (e.g., the *tetM* gene) should facilitate development of transducing systems.

CONCLUDING REMARKS

Despite the inherent difficulties in working with fastidious organisms with an unusual genetic code, significant progress is being made toward development of mycoplasmal gene transfer systems. The evolution of mycoplasmas indicates that gram-positive bacteria may be a valuable resource for development of mycoplasmal genetic tools. Initial successes along these lines have shown that some gram-positive bacterial transposons function in mycoplasmas. Many gram-positive bacterial plasmids may be capable of replication in mycoplasmas, and it should be possible to develop some of these plasmids into useful cloning vectors. In addition to the exciting approach of using gram-positive bacterial DNA elements as tools for studying mycoplasmas, DNA elements of mycoplasmal origin are becoming available. Numerous mycoplasma viruses have been isolated, and cryptic plasmids are now being identified as well. Exploitation of these genetic elements should rapidly advance our understanding of mycoplasmal molecular biology.

Acknowledgments. I acknowledge support from the National Institutes of Health (grant AI25640).

REFERENCES

1. **Ballester, S., P. Lopez, M. Espinosa, J. C. Alonso, and S. A. Lacks**. 1989. Plasmid structural instability associated with pC194 replication functions. *J. Bacteriol.* **171:**2271–2277.
2. **Barroso, G., and J. Labarère**. 1988. Chromosomal gene transfer in *Spiroplasma citri*. *Science* **241:**959–961.
3. **Barroso, G., J.-C. Salvado, and J. Labarère**. 1990. Influence of genetic markers and of the fusing agent polyethylene glycol on chromosomal gene transfer in *Spiroplasma citri*. *Curr. Microbiol.* **20:**53-56.
4. **Bergemann, A. D., and L. R. Finch**. 1988. Isolation and restriction endonuclease analysis of a mycoplasma plasmid. *Plasmid* **19:**68–70.
5. **Bergemann, A. D., J. C. Whitley, and L. R. Finch**. 1989. Homology of mycoplasma plasmid pADB201 and staphylococcal plasmid pE194. *J. Bacteriol.* **171:**593–595.
6. **Bibb, M. J., J. M. Ward, and D. A. Hopwood**. 1978. Transformation of plasmid DNA into *Streptomyces* at high frequency. *Nature* (London) **274:**398–400.
7. **Bové, J. M., P. Carle, M. Garnier, F. Laigret, J. Renaudin, and C. Saillard**. 1989. Molecular and cellular biology of spiroplasmas, p. 243–364. *In* R. F. Whitcomb and J. G. Tully (ed.), *The Mycoplasmas*, vol. 5. Academic Press, New York.
8. **Burdett, V., J. Inamine, and S. Rajagopalan**. 1982. Multiple tetracycline resistance determinants in *Streptococcus*, p. 155–158. *In* D. Schlessinger (ed.), *Microbiology—1982*. American Society for Microbiology, Washington, D.C.
9. **Cerone-McLernon, A. M., and G. Furness**. 1980. The preparation of transforming DNA from *Mycoplasma hominis* strain Sprott *tet*^r and quantitative studies of the factors affecting the genetic transformation of *Mycoplasma salivarium* strain S9*tet*^s to tetracycline resistance. *Can. J. Microbiol.* **26:**1147–1152.
10. **Chang, S., and S. N. Cohen**. 1979. High frequency transformation of *Bacillus subtilis* protoplasts by plasmid DNA. *Mol. Gen. Genet.* **168:**111–115.
11. **Clewell, D. B., and C. Gawron-Burke**. 1986. Conjugative transposons and the dissemination of antibiotic resistance in streptococci. *Annu. Rev. Microbiol.* **40:**635–659.
12. **Cole, R. M., W. O. Mitchell, and C. F. Garon**. 1977. *Spiroplasmavirus citri*. 3. Propagation, purification, proteins, and nucleic acid. *Science* **198:**1262–1263.
13. **de Vos, W. M.** 1987. Gene cloning and expression in lactic streptococci. *FEMS Microbiol. Rev.* **46:**281–295.
14. **Dower, W. J., J. F. Miller, and C. W. Ragsdale**. 1988. High frequency transformation of *E. coli* by high voltage electroporation. *Nucleic Acids Res.* **16:**6127–6145.
15. **Dybvig, K.** 1989. Transformation of *Acholeplasma laidlawii* with streptococcal plasmids pVA868 and pVA920. *Plasmid* **21:**155–160.
16. **Dybvig, K.** 1990. Mycoplasmal genetics. *Annu. Rev. Microbiol.* **44:**81–104.
17. **Dybvig, K.** 1990. Genetic manipulation of mycoplasmas, p. 43–46. *In* G. Stanek, G. H. Cassell, J. G. Tully, and R. F. Whitcomb (ed.), *Recent Advances in Mycoplasmology*. Gustav Fischer Verlag, Stuttgart.
17a. **Dybvig, K.** Unpublished data.
18. **Dybvig, K., and J. Alderete**. 1988. Transformation of *Mycoplasma pulmonis* and *Mycoplasma hyorhinis*: transposition of Tn*916* and formation of cointegrate structures. *Plasmid* **20:**33–41.
19. **Dybvig, K., and G. H. Cassell**. 1987. Transposition of gram-positive transposon Tn*916* in *Acholeplasma laidlawii* and *Mycoplasma pulmonis*. *Science* **235:**1392–1394.
20. **Dybvig, K., and M. Khaled**. 1990. Isolation of a second cryptic plasmid from *Mycoplasma mycoides* subsp. *mycoides*. *Plasmid* **24:**153–155.
21. **Dybvig, K., J. A. Nowak, T. L. Sladek, and J. Maniloff**. 1985. Identification of an enveloped phage, mycoplasma virus L172, that contains a 14-kilobase single-stranded DNA genome. *J. Virol.* **53:**384–390.
22. **Ehrlich, S. D., P. H. Noirot, M. A. Petit, L. Janniere, B. Michel, and H. te Riele**. 1986. Structural instability of *Bacillus subtilis* plasmids. p. 71–83. *In* J. K. Setlow and A. Hollaender (ed.), *Genetic Engineering*, vol. 8. Plenum Press, New York.
23. **Furness, G., and A. M. Cerone**. 1979. Preparation of competent single-cell suspensions of *Mycoplasma hominis tet*^s and *Mycoplasma salivarium tet*^s for genetic transformation to tetracycline resistance by DNA extracted from *Mycoplasma hominis tet*^r. *J. Infect. Dis.* **139:**441–451.
24. **Gawron-Burke, C., and D. B. Clewell**. 1984. Regeneration of insertionally inactivated streptococcal DNA fragments after excision of transposon Tn*916* in *Escherichia coli*. *J. Bacteriol* **159:**214–221.
25. **Goulay, J. L., J. C. Darbord, and A. Desvignes**. 1983. Étude comparative de la transformation et de la fusion induite par les polyéthyléneglycols chez *Acholeplasma laidlawii* B. *Can. J. Microbiol.* **30:**40–44.
26. **Gruss, A., and S. D. Ehrlich**. 1989. The family of highly interrelated single-stranded deoxyribonucleic acid plasmids. *Microbiol. Rev.* **53:**231–241.
27. **Hopwood, D. A.** 1981. Genetic studies with bacterial protoplasts. *Annu. Rev. Microbiol.* **35:**237–272.
27a. **King, K. W., and K. Dybvig**. 1991. Plasmid transformation of *Mycoplasma mycoides* subspecies *mycoides* is promoted by high concentrations of polyethylene glycol. *Plasmid* **26:**108–115.
27b. **King, K. W., and K. Dybvig**. Nucleotide sequence of *Mycoplasma mycoides* subspecies *mycoides* plasmid pKMK1. *Plasmid*, in press.
28. **Liss, A., and J. Maniloff**. 1972. Transfection mediated by *Mycoplasmatales* viral DNA. *Proc. Natl. Acad. Sci. USA* **69:**3423–3427.
29. **Liss, A., and J. Maniloff**. 1974. Effect of EDTA and competitive DNA on mycoplasmavirus transfection of *Acholeplasma laidlawii*. *Microbios* **11:**107–113.

30. **Lorenz, A., W. Just, M. da Silva Cardoso, and G. Klotz.** 1988. Electroporation-mediated transfection of *Acholeplasma laidlawii* with mycoplasma virus L1 and L3 DNA. *J. Virol.* **62:**3050–3052.

31. **Lyon, B. R., J. W. May, and R. A. Skurray.** 1984. Tn*4001*: a gentamicin and kanamycin resistance transposon in *Staphylococcus aureus. Mol. Gen. Genet.* **193:**554–556.

32. **Lyon, B. R., and R. A. Skurray.** 1987. Antimicrobial resistance of *Staphylococcus aureus*: genetic basis. *Microbiol. Rev.* **51:**88–134.

33. **Macrina, F. L., K. R. Jones, and P. H. Wood.** 1980. Chimeric streptococcal plasmids and their use as molecular cloning vehicles in *Streptococcus sanguis* (Challis). *J. Bacteriol.* **143:**1425–1435.

34. **Mahairas, G. G., C. Jian, and F. C. Minion.** 1990. Development of a cloning system in *Mycoplasma pulmonis. Gene* **93:**61–66.

35. **Mahairas, G. G., C. Jian, and F. C. Minion.** 1990. Genetic exchange of transposon and integrative plasmid markers in *Mycoplasma pulmonis. J. Bacteriol.* **172:**2267–2272.

36. **Mahairas, G. G., and F. C. Minion.** 1989. Transformation of *Mycoplasma pulmonis*: demonstration of homologous recombination, introduction of cloned genes, and preliminary description of an integrating shuttle system. *J. Bacteriol.* **171:**1775–1780.

37. **Mahairas, G. G., and F. C. Minion.** 1989. Random insertion of the gentamicin resistance transposon Tn*4001* in *Mycoplasma pulmonis. Plasmid* **21:**43–47.

38. **Maniloff, J.** 1988. Mycoplasma viruses. *Crit. Rev. Microbiol.* **15:**339–389.

39. **McCammon, S. L., E. L. Dally, and R. E. Davis.** 1990. Electroporation and DNA methylation effects on the transfection of *Spiroplasma*, p. 60–65. *In* G. Stanek, G. H. Cassell, J. G. Tully, and R. F. Whitcomb (ed.), *Recent Advances in Mycoplasmology*. Gustav Fischer Verlag, Stuttgart.

40. **McCammon, S. L., and R. E. Davis.** 1987. Transfection of *Spiroplasma citri* with DNA of a new rod-shaped spiroplasmavirus, p. 458–464. *In* E. L. Civerolo, A. Collmer, R. E. Davis, and A. G. Gillaspie (ed.), *Plant Pathogenic Bacteria*. Martinus Nijhoff Publishers, The Hague, The Netherlands.

41. **Naglich, J. G., and R. E. Andrews, Jr.** 1988. Tn*916*-dependent conjugal transfer of pC194 and pUB110 from *Bacillus subtilis* into *Bacillus thuringiensis* subsp. *israelensis. Plasmid* **20:**113–26.

42. **Pascarel-Devilder, M.-C., J. Renaudin, and J. M. Bové.** 1986. The spiroplasma virus 4 replicative form cloned in *Escherichia coli* transfects spiroplasmas. *Virology* **151:**390–93.

43. **Renaudin, J., M. C. Pascarel, M. Garnier, and J. M. Bové.** 1984. Characterization of spiroplasma virus group 4 (SV4). *Isr. J. Med. Sci.* **20:**797–799.

44. **Roberts, M. C.** 1990. Characterization of the Tet M determinants in urogenital and respiratory bacteria. *Antimicrob. Agents Chemother.* **34:**476–478.

45. **Roberts, M. C., and G. E. Kenny.** 1986. Dissemination of the *tetM* tetracycline resistance to *Ureaplasma urealyticum. Antimicrob. Agents Chemother.* **29:**350–352.

46. **Roberts, M. C., and G. E. Kenny.** 1987. Conjugal transfer of transposon Tn*916* from *Streptococcus faecalis* to *Mycoplasma hominis. J. Bacteriol.* **169:**3836–3839.

47. **Roberts, M. C., L. A. Koutsky, K. K. Holmes, D. J. LeBlanc, and G. E. Kenny.** 1985. Tetracycline-resistant *Mycoplasma hominis* strains contain streptococcal *tetM* sequences. *Antimicrob. Agents Chemother.* **28:**141–143.

48. **Salvado, J.-C., G. Barroso, and J. Labarère.** 1989. Involvement of a *Spiroplasma citri* plasmid in the erythromycin-resistance transfer. *Plasmid* **22:**151–159.

49. **Senghas, E., J. M. Jones, M. Yamamoto, C. Gawron-Burke, and D. B. Clewell.** 1988. Genetic organization of the bacterial conjugative transposon Tn*916. J. Bacteriol.* **170:**245–249.

50. **Simoneau, P., and J. Labarère.** 1990. Construction of chimeric antibiotic resistance determinants and their use in the development of cloning vectors for spiroplasmas, p. 66–74. *In* G. Stanek, G. H. Cassell, J. G. Tully, and R. F. Whitcomb (ed.), *Recent Advances in Mycoplasmology*. Gustav Fischer Verlag, Stuttgart.

51. **Sladek, T. L., and J. Maniloff.** 1983. Polyethylene glycol-dependent transformation of *Acholeplasma laidlawii* with mycoplasma virus L2 DNA. *J. Bacteriol.* **155:**734–741.

52. **Sladek, T. L., and J. Maniloff.** 1985. Transfection of REP⁻ mycoplasmas with viral single-stranded DNA. *J. Virol.* **53:**25–31.

53. **Sundstrom, T. K., and Å. Wieslander.** 1990. Plasmid transformation and replica filter plating of *Acholeplasma laidlawii. FEMS Microbiol. Lett.* **72:**147–152.

54. **Tanaka, R., A. Muto, and S. Osawa.** 1989. Nucleotide sequence of tryptophan tRNA gene in *Acholeplasma laidlawii. Nucleic Acids Res.* **17:**5842.

55. **Whitley, J. C., A. D. Bergemann, L. E. Pyle, B. G. Cocks, R. Youil, and L. R. Finch.** 1990. Genetic maps of mycoplasmas and Tn*916* insertion, p. 47–55. *In* G. Stanek, G. H. Cassell, J. G. Tully, and R. F. Whitcomb (ed.), *Recent Advances in Mycoplasmology*. Gustav Fischer Verlag, Stuttgart.

56. **Whitley, J. C., and L. R. Finch.** 1989. Location of sites of transposon Tn*916* insertion in the *Mycoplasma mycoides* genome. *J. Bacteriol.* **171:**6870–6872.

57. **Yamao, D., A. Muto, Y. Kawauchi, M. Iwami, S. Iwagami, Y. Azumi, and S. Osawa.** 1985. UGA is read as tryptophan in *Mycoplasma capricolum. Proc. Natl. Acad. Sci. USA* **82:**2306–2309.

22. Repetitive DNA Sequences

MARK A. McINTOSH, GANG DENG, JIANHONG ZHENG, and REBECCA V. FERRELL

INTRODUCTION

The concept of stability in the structure, organization, and expression of the bacterial chromosome has given way in recent years to the idea that many dynamic processes are at work to continually reorganize individual or global gene systems or to influence their expression in response to conditions encountered by the organism. This constant molecular reshuffling process ensures greater genomic flexibility to enable organisms to respond productively to unexpected fluctuations in environment or to adapt readily to the development of new growth opportunities or biological niches and, at the same time, offers some degree of protection against catastrophic changes that might be lethal if genomes were rigidly fixed in organization or expression.

The primary determinant underlying this reevaluation of chromosome structure and evolution was the discovery, in both procaryotes and eucaryotes, of repetitive DNA sequences that provided a wealth of DNA homologies, either scattered around the chromosome or capable of being mobilized between genomes, for the activity of specific recombination functions that drive genomic reordering (45). Principal among these sequences are elements designated insertion sequences (ISs) because of their propensity to create insertion mutations within the genome (17, 20, 25). ISs account for many other genetic alterations detected to date, including deletions, inversions, replicon fusions, and changes in gene expression. Recombination pathways similar to those utilized by ISs are also involved in plasmid and prophage integration events, most of which require duplicated sequences on both molecules to enhance their interactions. Additional recombination processes have led to gene duplications and amplifications, allowing the evolution of multigene families or repetitive partial coding sequences capable of combinatorial interactions among copies to elaborate considerable heterogeneity among the products (reviewed in references 11, 33, 37, and 62). Not all repetitive sequences appear to be involved in these diversity-generating devices. Small repetitive sequences of unknown origin seem to be scattered around the chromosome in many bacterial systems (24, 63) and have been suggested to influence such parameters as transcription, translation, mRNA stability, and organization of the bacterial nucleoid. It is reasonable to conclude, therefore, that enormous diversity at both the

Mark A. McIntosh, Gang Deng, Jianhong Zheng, and Rebecca V. Ferrell • Department of Molecular Microbiology and Immunology, School of Medicine, University of Missouri–Columbia, Columbia, Missouri 65212.

genome level and the gene activity level can be directly attributed to processes involving repetitive DNA.

The 70 to 80 species that make up the class *Mollicutes* have been categorized as an extremely diverse group of organisms (50) that have evolved at a rapid tempo (71, 72) from the low-G+C gram-positive branch that includes the genera *Clostridium*, *Lactobacillus*, *Bacillus*, and *Streptococcus* (51). This diversification is apparent in various morphological, biochemical, and serological characteristics of the organisms (16) and from comparisons of genetic conservation by hybridization experiments (61) or by direct sequence analysis of conserved genes, e.g., rRNA (51, 71, 72) and tRNA (74) genes. Moreover, individual strains within several mycoplasma species, including *Mycoplasma hyorhinis* (6, 18), display significant phenotypic and antigenic variability. Recently, the examination of intraspecies variabilities associated with isolated gene sequences from *M. hyorhinis* (14, 53, 67, 75) has elucidated important genomic structures that are expected to play a significant role in generating such diversity. These genetic structures are repetitive at the primary nucleotide sequence level and are analogous to documented eubacterial gene diversity-generating systems that apparently operate by directing recombination events that result in dramatic changes in gene structure, organization, and regulation. Examples of similar genetic and phenotypic variations in many other species are scattered throughout the mycoplasma literature; some currently being investigated at the molecular level implicate similar recombinational mechanisms between repetitive DNA sequences as the foundation underlying the observed genetic heterogeneity.

This chapter concentrates on distinctive examples from several mycoplasmas that provide a view (albeit probably limited at this particular time) of the spectrum of potential genomic alterations that may manifest themselves in observable and measurable phenotypic differences in this class of organisms. These examples focus on the involvement of repetitive DNA sequences in such phenomena as (i) genome interruptions by insertion and imprecise excision, (ii) gene duplication and diversification that might involve entire coding sequences or repetitive units within coding sequences, (iii) transposition of genetic sequences mediated by specific insertion sequences, and (iv) gene amplification phenomena.

SPIROPLASMA REPETITIVE SEQUENCES ASSOCIATED WITH EXTRACHROMOSOMAL DNA

Early evidence for the existence of repeated copies of specific DNA sequences within the limited genomes of various mycoplasma species was uncovered during the investigation of extrachromosomal DNA in several *Spiroplasma* species, especially *Spiroplasma citri* (39, 40, 43, 44, 48, 55). These studies strongly suggested that recombination events had occurred between these episomes and the *Spiroplasma* chromosome at a moderately high frequency and that these events resulted in the deposition of specific or random epigenetic sequences at one or more genomic locations. Mouches et al. (39) initially characterized two distinct plasmids of 8 kb (pM41) and 7 kb (pMH1) from individual *S. citri* strains and showed that whereas pMH1 was present only as extrachromosomal DNA in strain MH (39, 40), it could be found integrated at one or more sites within the chromosome of strain M4 and could be detected in limited copy numbers within the genomes of other *Spiroplasma* strains as well (40).

More recent studies (55) indicated that these integration events were specific and linked to phenotypic changes in these strains. *S. citri* M4$^+$ was shown to harbor two cryptic plasmids, pM41, identified previously, and a 12.3-kb plasmid designated pM42 and shown by hybridization analysis to be closely related to pMH1. M4 Er-1, a spontaneous erythromycin-resistant (Er^r) mutant of M4$^+$, also contained both plasmids, and following numerous subcultures, additional small (<4-kb) extrachromosomal molecules appeared. Hybridization analysis with pMH1 as a probe revealed that M4 Er-1, unlike its parent M4$^+$, contained several DNA fragments of 10 to 20 kb with homology to pMH1 and that the small episomes also strongly hybridized. These data suggested that the Er^r phenotype resulted from one or more recombination events that allowed pM42 to integrate into the *S. citri* M4$^+$ genome and that the appearance of these miniplasmids may have represented subsequent defective excision events, which produced a variety of deletion derivatives of pM42 that are likely self-replicating and left regions (perhaps specific) of pM42 in the chromosome as "scars" of the original integration event.

Accompanying experiments (55) provided evidence that it was the integration event itself that triggered the Er^r phenotype. The erythromycin-sensitive (Er^s) *S. citri* strain R8A2$^+$ was transformed to Er^r by using total DNA from M4 Er-1 or isolated pM42 plasmid DNA. Transformants did not contain extrachromosomal pM42-related sequences but rather resulted from its specific integration into one or two genomic locations. Moreover, all R8A2$^+$ cells, whether Er^s or Er^r, contained two fragments with some homology to pMH1, suggesting that through homologous recombination, these might represent the integration sites. The authors concluded that specific integration of a pM42 (or pMH1) sequence in both the M4$^+$ and R8A2$^+$ strains induced the Er^r phenotype, perhaps by providing an otherwise missing promoter sequence for a resident gene. Neither the plasmid nor chromosomal integration sites have been characterized as yet. However, there are many documented instances of portable homology regions, especially related to procaryotic insertion sequences, that serve as substrates for recombination mechanisms that produce chromosomal rearrangements, replicon fusions, and, perhaps particularly relevant in this case, modulation of adjacent gene expression by providing a mobile promoter (see reference 17 for a review). Whatever the mechanism, these observations clearly indicate that sequence-directed recombinational events between *S. citri* extrachromosomal DNA and its genome have resulted in (i) modulation of the phenotypic characteristics of the strains and (ii) the integration of plasmid-related sequences at one or more genomic sites within each organism.

A similar, but apparently unrelated, recombinational phenomenon was identified and characterized for *S. citri* R8A2 (Maroc) strains carrying a cryptic 8-

kb plasmid designated pRA1 (43, 44, 48). This plasmid has not been shown to bear any homology to those described above. Plasmid pRA1 was prevalent as extrachromosomal DNA in low-passage subclones, but persistent laboratory culturing resulted in increased chromosomal integration at multiple sites and correspondingly diminished epigenetic levels (43). Free and integrated sequences related to pRA1 were also detected in other *Spiroplasma* species, some genetically remote from *S. citri*. Data from hybridization analysis and from isolated subclones carrying chromosomal copies of the integrated pRA1-related sequences (43, 44) revealed that isolated regions of pRA1 had been integrated at multiple but specific sites in the *S. citri* chromosome. The authors suggested that these regions of homology may be as short as 50 bp in length and may be repeated 30 to 40 times per genome. It is not clear whether several regions of the pRA1 plasmid are capable of such recombinational interactions, since the initial report (43) documented hybridization to three separate regions of the plasmid, while the later study (44) suggested that the homology was limited to a single 3.7-kb *Eco*RI fragment. However, it was shown that two separate (but apparently adjacent) sequences from this specific region may be present in the *S. citri* genome at distinctly variable copy numbers (44). Subsequent evidence was presented that these same two sequences are also present in replicative form DNA from the *Spiroplasma* virus SV3 (48). This viral DNA has been shown to circularize and integrate in a site-specific manner into the host chromosome (10), suggesting the possibility that (i) pRA1 represents the replicative form of a virus related to SV3 (although perhaps defective in some *S. citri* strains) and/or (ii) the processes of integration (and perhaps excision) of pRA1 and SV3 occur by similar mechanisms and involve similar chromosomal and extrachromosomal DNA sequences. Since no data characterizing the inserted sequences themselves are available, it is not clear whether they represent mobile regions of homology like insertion sequences, some other type of repetitive DNA sequence analogous to repetitive extragenic palindromic sequences (63) or enterobacterial repetitive intergenic consensus sequences (24) found dispersed around the genomes in several procaryotic species, or simply a specific DNA sequence native to the pRA1 plasmid (or SV3 chromosome) that lies adjacent to its integration site and is therefore likely to be left behind in the genome as a result of a defective excision event upon induction of the prophage or integrated plasmid. Whatever the nature of these recombination events, their multiplicity had no obvious biological effects on the ability of these strains to grow in culture media; if anything, strains with greater levels of free pRA1 plasmid DNA grew more slowly and tended to lyse more frequently than did those containing significant numbers of inserted sequences.

REPETITION OF SPECIFIC PROTEIN-CODING SEQUENCES IN MYCOPLASMAS

The amplification and diversification of DNA sequences encoding proteins that have a significant role in the ability of a microorganism to adapt to its environment or interact productively with a host organism is a widespread phenomenon among pathogenic procaryotes, and examples are found in eucaryotic microorganisms as well. This repetition in coding sequence creates a repertoire of potential genetic variability that allows these organisms to rearrange their coding potential continually, creating the appearance of rapid phenotypic switches under favorable conditions or in response to host defense mechanisms or changing environmental stimuli. The genetic variety encumbered by these switch mechanisms is extensive and has been carefully reviewed in recent years (11, 37, 59). Most of these variable genetic systems are involved in the expression of microbial surface proteins expected to function directly in pathogen-host interactions. For example, outer membrane proteins of *Neisseria gonorrhoeae* responsible for pilus structure and phase variation (opacity protein) are involved in adhesion, colonization, and survival and are expressed from multiple gene families shown to undergo frequent gene conversion events (58, 62). In addition, the *Neisseria* H.8 lipoprotein antigen gene contains repetitive primary sequence structure that encodes multiple copies of a pentapeptide motif (73). Variant serotype antigens are produced in *Borrelia hermsii* (4) from a plasmid-encoded gene family that has been shown to undergo DNA rearrangements associated with differential gene expression; this phenomenon is analogous to variant surface glycoprotein rearrangements and expression characteristics in the trypanosomes (5). Also pertinent to this chapter on repetitive DNA structures is the class of surface proteins which use tandemly arrayed assortments of repetitive protein structure cassettes, including the streptococcal M proteins (15) and surface proteins of the rickettsias (2). The analysis of repetitive genetic structures producing variant mycoplasma surface proteins has only recently begun, but already two significant examples suggesting that similar recombinational mechanisms are functional in mycoplasma phenotypic and genetic variation have emerged.

The Adhesins of *M. pneumoniae* and *M. genitalium*

The P1 adhesin of *M. pneumoniae* has been implicated in the specific attachment of this organism to the human respiratory epithelium. Studies initially identifying P1-coding sequences by using oligonucleotide probes based upon primary amino acid sequence also revealed multiple chromosomal fragments bearing striking homology (26, 65). Independently, the search for repetitive DNA in *M. pneumoniae* chromosomal DNA libraries by cross-hybridization identified two sequences, RepMP1 and RepMP2, which were present in 8 to 10 copies per genome; RepMP2 was shown to represent a region of the P1 structural gene (70). These various investigations suggested that part or all of the P1 gene may be present in multiple copies, opening the prospect of gene rearrangements associated with its expression, as had been documented in other eubacteria. Hybridization experiments with probes from specific regions of the P1 structural gene revealed a mosaic of multicopy and unique domains interspersed along its coding length (64), presenting yet an additional opportunity for genetic rearrangements to dictate variant P1 surface proteins. However, no detectable variation of the P1 protein has been observed. The P1 gene probe was also used to identify and clone the corresponding adhesin protein gene from *M. genitalium* (27); genetic sequences encoding this MgPa protein also appear to occur in multiple copies, perhaps analogous to the situation with P1.

Other repetitive DNA sequences have also been identified in *M. pneumoniae* (7, 54, 70). RepMP1, a 300-bp sequence, was found frequently in association with RepMP2, the P1-associated repetitive sequence, except in the case of the authentic P1 structural gene, in which no associated copy of RepMP1 was found. In those associations, RepMP1 usually is separated from RepMP2 by an identical 400-bp sequence (70). No further definition of the nature of these repetitive sequences has been reported. Downstream of the P1 gene, but within the genetic operon encoding P1, is an open reading frame encoding a 130-kDa membrane protein that also contains a DNA sequence found repeated elsewhere in the genome; this sequence was designated SDC1 (7) and later RepMP5 (54). Ruland et al. (54) further characterized the *M. hyopneumoniae* P1-associated repetitive sequences and located their copies on a physical map of the genome. These data are described more fully in chapter 9.

The Variant Surface Lipoproteins of *M. hyorhinis*

Proteins displayed on the external membrane surface of *M. hyorhinis* have been extensively examined by immunochemical and biochemical methods (reviewed in chapter 28). These studies revealed a family of lipid-modified, surface-exposed polypeptides that were characterized by (i) size heterogeneity within a population of cells and (ii) antigenic diversity with respect to expression of variable epitopes. Superimposed upon the variation in protein structure and expression, colonies within the population were also observed to undergo a morphological phase variation not necessarily related to antigenic switching (52, 53). It was suggested that this phenotypic diversification could be attributed to alterations in the structure and expression of a set of related but variant lipoproteins (Vlps). Isolation and characterization of the Vlp structural genes (75) supported this hypothesis. A cluster of related but distinct *vlp* genes (*vlpA*, *vlpB*, and *vlpC*) encoded products that expressed conserved N-terminal domains for membrane translocation and lipid modification but variable C-terminal (externally exposed) domains capable of undergoing size variation by the amplification or deletion of repetitive intragenic coding sequences. These repetitive coding cassettes are represented by distinctive periodic amino acid sequences but retain structural properties and charge distribution. The overall organizational conservation among the genes of this cluster and significant regional sequence similarities strongly suggest that they arose as a result of uncharacterized gene duplication events and that their current association allows for the combinatorial expression, as well as phase and size variation, of the *M. hyorhinis* surface Vlps.

PROCARYOTIC ISs IN MYCOPLASMA SPECIES

Many examples of genomic variability or instability have been directly attributed to the class of repetitive DNA sequences known as ISs. These genetic entities have capacities for (i) promoting significant genome rearrangements, including deletions, inversions, and insertions, (ii) modifying gene expression, either up or down, as a result of their integration in or near structural genes, and (iii) sequestering and translocating genes as a result of recombinatorial interactions between duplicate copies flanking affected DNA sequences (reviewed extensively in references 17, 20, and 25). The variety of ISs is extensive, and the most thoroughly studied are found in bacteria, although they have been identified in the great majority of organisms examined. They have been characterized from both gram-negative (17) and gram-positive (41) eubacteria, and they have been grouped in classes based upon (i) nucleotide sequence homologies, (ii) conservation of structural and sequence features of their respective recombinases (the enzymes that mediate their mobility and many of the genetic alterations attributed to ISs), and (iii) the mechanisms that promote their duplication and transposition. Most ISs range in size from 800 to 2,500 bp and encode only the proteins necessary to catalyze these recombination events. In many instances, however, ISs are found flanking larger genetic sequences that encode factors detectable by their phenotypes (e.g., antibiotic resistance), creating compound transposable elements.

While there is at present no definitive evidence that the presence of ISs has a long-term evolutionary impact on the organization and expression of the bacterial genome, their propensity to produce many complex changes, physical rearrangements, and regulatory alterations cannot be expected to be entirely benign. These changes might be especially significant in the mycoplasmas for two reasons. First, their limited genomic capacities are hypothesized to have evolved by a degenerative process involving the selective elimination of genomic sequences that became superfluous as these organisms adapted to distinctive biological niches (50); such massive deletion events certainly could be mediated through recombination involving repetitive DNA. Second, many mycoplasma species have been characterized by significant phenotypic and genotypic heterogeneity that might be influenced by molecular interactions between individual copies of repetitive DNA sequences. Therefore, the identification and characterization of ISs resident in the limited mycoplasma genome may be one of perhaps several factors influencing the genomic diversification capability within these species.

Identification of Repetitive DNA in Swine Mycoplasmas

Interspecies Southern DNA hybridization was used to identify and isolate DNA sequences shared among mycoplasmas that are genetically distant but that inhabit a common animal host, namely, the swine mycoplasmas *M. hyorhinis* and *M. hyopneumoniae* (67). These shared sequences were also examined for distribution among a select group of mycoplasmas of widely disparate origins. DNA homologies detected by hybridization at moderate stringencies between chromosomal DNA of *M. hyorhinis* and *M. hyopneumoniae* were confined to rRNA genes and a specific set of sequences that have now been characterized in detail. These sequences were found at a restricted copy number in the *M. hyopneumoniae* genome but were present on numerous DNA fragments in all strains of *M. hyorhinis* tested. Copies of sequences from both species were isolated, and their homology was verified by limited nucleotide sequence analysis. DNA hybridization revealed that similar sequences were also present at a low copy number in the genome of *M. flocculare*, another species of swine origin, but were not detected in several other *Mycoplasma* species tested. These observations therefore defined a novel DNA sequence that is highly redundant in the genome of *M. hyorhinis* and was also found to be present in two other species that have the same animal host but are at best only distantly related among the mycoplasmas. One explanation is that the novel DNA sequence was distributed among these species by some uncharacterized interspecies genetic exchange process. It was also suggested (67) that the high copy number of this repetitive sequence (hereafter referred to as RS-1) in *M. hyorhinis* might play a role in promoting mutational processes (i.e., recombination, transposition, or other chromosomal rearrangements) that could contribute to the considerable intraspecies divergence characteristic of these organisms.

The RS-1 Nucleotide Sequence Reveals Structures Resembling Bacterial ISs

The nucleotide sequence of RS-1 was initially derived from the only two copies present in the *M. hyopneumoniae* genome, and it revealed structural features that allowed its categorization as a bacterial IS (14). These features included terminal repetitive structures, internal inverted repeat sequences that may affect the overall expression levels of RS-1, and a limited coding capacity, predicted from those particular sequences as two potential but independent open reading frames (ORFs). The DNA sequences from seven isolated copies from the *M. hyorhinis* chromosome have now been compiled (76), allowing a consensus primary sequence to be deduced; this sequence maintains these important structural features (summarized in Fig. 1),

albeit with some modification from those originally predicted on the basis of the previous data (14).

The RS-1 consensus nucleotide sequence is 1,513 bp long, although two variants, one each from the two mycoplasma species, contain identical 42-bp insertions in an interesting variable region of the predicted coding sequence (see below). There are other slight variations in these lengths that arise from small insertions and deletions in individual copies, and there are regions where significant numbers of base substitutions have accumulated, although overall the sequence is highly conserved. The termini of RS-1 are 28-bp inverted repetitive structures (designated LTR and RTR [left and right terminal repeats]; Fig. 1), with 23 of the residues conserved, and appear to be analogous to similar structures in many distinctive bacterial ISs (25), in which they are believed to function as components of the machinery required for IS mobilization.

In addition to the terminal repeat sequences, there are three internal inverted repeat sequences, which are distinct from one another. The 33-bp left internal inverted repeat (LIR) and the 40-bp right internal inverted repeat (RIR) are positioned near either end of RS-1 and would generate structures in an mRNA transcript that are analogous to *Escherichia coli* rho-independent transcription terminators (46), consisting of a G + C-rich stem-and-loop structure followed by a cluster of U residues. The position of the LIR in the coding strand is appropriate to prevent promiscuous transcription of coding sequences from outside the element, while the RIR in the noncoding strand would terminate transcription from adjacent genes in the opposite orientation, thus preventing the production of an antisense mRNA. These features have been suggested to play a significant role in maintaining the stability of ISs within bacterial genomes (66). The third internal inverted repeat (IIR) sequence contains 37 bp which could potentially form two different stable stem-loop structures; it is located within protein-coding sequences, but its potential function is unclear. All three of these sequences are highly conserved among all RS-1 copies and are predicted to form stable structures, with calculated free energies (69) of − 15 to − 20 kcal (1 cal = 4.184 J)/mol.

Translational Capability of RS-1

Bacterial ISs, because of their limited sizes, are restricted to encoding only those functions that mediate

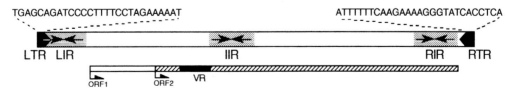

Figure 1. Structural organization of the mycoplasma RS-1 insertion sequence. The location, orientation, and nucleotide sequences of the terminal repetitive structures (LTR and RTR) are denoted. Approximate positions of the internal inverted repeat sequences (LIR, IIR, and RIR) are indicated. These structures are not represented to scale. A single long coding sequence is represented below the DNA structure. Two potential in-frame AUG start codons are indicated by the designations ORF1 and ORF2. The approximate position of a variable repetitive (VR) amino acid sequence displaying heptameric periodicity is noted within the protein sequence.

their mobility, thus enhancing their distribution and survival (17, 20, 25). The translational capability of the consensus RS-1 sequence was assessed, taking into account that many, if not all, mycoplasmas thus far examined utilize the opal codon (UGA) to incorporate tryptophan into the nascent polypeptide (see chapter 19). A single ORF spanning almost the entire length of RS-1 was deduced from the DNA sequence (76). This ORF could initiate translation from either of two AUG (Met) codons, both of which are preceded by appropriate ribosome binding sites (and are thus designated ORF1 and ORF2 for clarification in Fig. 1); it is not known whether one or both are utilized in these mycoplasmas. The ORF1 initiation codon is located just downstream of the LIR, providing an opportunity to regulate its expression as a consequence of the formation of this potential secondary structure. In addition, a promoter directing the transcription of ORF1 would have to be located just inside the left end of RS-1 to be effective. Such arrangements are found in other ISs (17, 20, 25); no evidence for control signals in RS-1 has been found. The longer ORF1 spans 1,422 bp and encodes a 474-residue polypeptide of approximately 56 kDa; the smaller ORF2 is 1,071 bp long and would produce a 357-amino-acid protein of 42.5 kDa. Both potential products are highly basically charged and have a potential for considerable α-helical structure.

It is interesting that of the nine RS-1 copies thus far analyzed, only one from *M. hyorhinis* has maintained all of the structural features of both the nucleotide and deduced amino acid sequences of the consensus element (76). This copy, designated G1135.2, may be significant in the original intraspecies and interspecies distribution of RS-1 because of its association with specific flanking sequences that may be extrachromosomal; these sequences are discussed more fully below. In all other copies thus far examined, insertions or deletions have created frameshift mutations, and some base substitutions have eliminated the potential AUG start codons or have created in-frame nonsense codons (e.g., Ferrell et al. [14] suggested two possible ORFs because of a nonsense codon in these copies that is not consensus). This observation suggests that in each case, the encoded protein product presumably required for RS-1 mobility has been inactivated. This situation is not atypical for organisms harboring multiple copies of a particular IS (25), since mobilization

could still be mediated in *trans* by functional copies of the coding sequence located elsewhere on the chromosome.

These sequence variations also provide "signatures" that allow the variants to be grouped according to the subsequent conservation of landmark substitutions. In particular, the two RS-1 copies from *M. hyopneumoniae* J share multiple signatures not found in any of the *M. hyorhinis* copies. This finding strongly suggests that one of these copies arose from the other by duplication and transposition, subsequent to the original introduction of RS-1 into this species, since even at the high mycoplasma mutation rate, the chance of identical substitutions occurring multiple times over this 1,500-bp length is vanishingly low. In addition, if the consensus RS-1 sequence reflects the original element, then both copies of RS-1 in *M. hyopneumoniae* J contain frameshift mutations that would prematurely truncate the presumed transposase protein (this led to the original prediction of two ORFs in RS-1 on the basis of these DNA sequences). If inactivation of RS-1 mobilization functions resulted from these mutations, the limited copy number of RS-1 in this species compared with *M. hyorhinis* (which may still maintain an original version) might be explained.

One very striking feature of the predicted product of the RS-1 coding sequence is a region just preceding the IIR sequence that is characterized by reasonably conserved DNA sequences specifying a seven-amino-acid periodicity within the polypeptide that suggests an amphipathic α-helical structure (14). This region is designated the variable repetitive region (Fig. 1) because in two copies of RS-1, one from either species, identical 42-bp insertions within this region produce a 14-residue expansion of the predicted peptide but maintain the periodicity of the structure (Fig. 2). This motif of repeated nonpolar residues at precisely spaced positions is characteristic of a coiled-coil protein configuration (35, 47), and the periodicity of leucine residues at seven-amino-acid intervals is reminiscent of leucine zipper dimerization domains found in several eucaryotic DNA-binding regulatory proteins (31). This region of heptameric periodicity also shows structural similarity to the α-helical domains of region A of the *Streptococcus pyogenes* M5 protein (34) and suggests that its genetic potential for expansion (or contraction) may result from similar recombination

```
Consensus

... leu ser val tyr GLU GLU LEU LYS LEU LEU ARG
                    GLU GLU ILE LYS LEU LEU LYS
                    LYS GLU ASN GLU VAL LEU LYS
                    LYS TRP LYS ALA LEU VAL GLU ile phe asp ser ...


J125-2

... ile ser val leu GLU LYS LEU LYS LEU LEU GLU
                    GLU LYS ASN ASN HIS PHE LYS
                    LYS ARG GLU LYS ASN LEU GLU
                    LYS GLU ILE LYS LEU LEU LYS
                    LYS GLU ILE GLU ALA LEU LYS
                    LYS TRP LYS ALA LEU VAL GLU ile phe asp ser ...
```

Figure 2. Comparison of heptameric repeat subunits from the RS-1 consensus polypeptide and the J125-2 insertion variant (from *M. hyopneumoniae*). The insertion of 14 residues into this region of the J125-2 variant (as a result of a 42-bp DNA insertion or duplication) conserves the periodicity of this predicted amphipathic α-helical domain. Periodic leucine residues are shown in bold.

pathways between repetitive sequences that generate size variation in these M-type proteins or in the variable repetitive sequence cassettes of the *M. hyorhinis* Vlp system (75).

RS-1 Belongs to the IS*3* Class of ISs

Data base searches have produced significant homologies (76) that allow RS-1 to be categorized in the group of ISs related to IS*3* (summarized in reference 17), isolated and characterized originally from *E. coli*. While considerable genetic drift has reduced the degree of similarity at the nucleotide level, by comparison of predicted coding sequences, RS-1 is very strongly related to IS*150* (57), an element discovered in *E. coli* K-12 as a frequent agent in insertional mutations (56). Significant protein homologies were also detected with ORFs from IS*3* (68), IS*3411* (28), IS*600* (36), isolated originally from *Shigella sonnei*, and IS*103* (21), considered to be a closely related variant of IS*150*. Table 1 summarizes the relevant structural characteristics of these IS3-related elements. The amino acid homologies between RS-1 and IS*150* are most striking if one considers ORF2 from RS-1 (Fig. 1) and ORFB from IS*150* (57); there are at best only limited regional homologies when the region separating ORF1 and ORF2 in RS-1 and the corresponding ORFA in IS*150* are compared, but these may also be significant, since the latter is encoded by a separate reading frame in IS*150* while the former represents a 117-residue in-frame extension of the N terminus of ORF2 in RS-1. Since the mechanism of IS3-mediated recombination as a function of its mobility, or the regulation of such, has not yet been elucidated, the functional importance of these homologous ORF regions is not presently understood.

It should be noted, however, that although there is considerable variation in the primary nucleotide sequences of these IS3-related elements, there is a striking similarity among all of them in the outermost sequences of their terminal repetitive structures (Table 2). Again, RS-1 bears the strongest resemblance to IS*150* at these sites. Since it has been established that recombinational mobility of ISs depends on the nature of these sequences, in conjunction with the corresponding recombinase function (17, 20, 25), these homologies further substantiate that RS-1 belongs to this group of mobile genetic elements and is closely related to the IS*150* subgroup.

While most of the procaryotic ISs related to IS*3* have been identified in association with gram-negative or-

ganisms, particularly the enteric species, a rather distant relative (i.e., bearing only very limited sequence homologies) has been isolated from *Lactobacillus casei* (60) and designated IS*L1*. Sequence comparisons reveal that RS-1 is clearly more closely related to its gram-negative counterparts than it is to IS*L1*, raising the question of where these particular isolates originated. However, other IS3-related sequences have recently been characterized from the AIDS-related mycoplasma, *M. fermentans* (*incognitus*) (23), and from *M. pulmonis* (4a). Sequence data from copies of these elements have revealed significant similarities with IS*3* (and RS-1) in coding regions. It is anticipated that as additional copies from these mycoplasma species are analyzed to provide a consensus sequence, very distinctive correlations will be apparent between them and other members of this IS class, including RS-1. It is clear from these investigations that ISs are likely to be found in many mycoplasma species, as they are in other eubacteria. However, it is too early to speculate on whether only limited groups of these sequences will be found or whether the same variety will be found in the gram-negative species.

Mycoplasma Genomic Sequences Flanking Individual RS-1 Copies

The majority of known ISs generate small, directly repeated duplications of the recipient DNA at the point of insertion (17), predictably as a consequence of a staggered cleavage of the target DNA by the IS recombinase enzyme. The extent of the duplication is a characteristic property of each IS and ranges from 2 to 13 bp; the IS*3* group generally duplicates 3 bp at its target site (Table 2). Figure 3 depicts the genomic sequences immediately flanking four copies of RS-1 from *M. hyorhinis*. Each is flanked by 3- to 7-bp directly repeated sequences, although in the copy designated G27, RS-1 appears to be integrated asymmetrically with respect to the apparent duplication (perhaps as a result of an uncharacterized defective recombination event). Another copy (not shown) appears to duplicate only one nucleotide (if any) at its target site. Generally speaking, the majority of RS-1 insertion events are similar to those of other IS3-like elements in that only 3 to 4 bp are duplicated.

The more striking observation relative to these genomic flanking sequences, however, is that each RS-1 element is centered between near-perfect palindromic sequences with 14- to 20-bp stem structures (Fig. 3). Moreover, there is a polarity to these palindromes relative to the coding strand of RS-1; the A-rich stem is always upstream, and the T-rich stem is downstream. The importance of these features to the mechanism of RS-1 insertion is not yet understood, but they appear to be consistent in all copies examined to date and thus may provide some sequence or structural recognition factor for the machinery that mediates RS-1 chromosomal integration.

The position and orientation of RS-1 relative to *M. hyorhinis* structural genes can also affect chromosomal organization and gene expression by rearranging genomic segments or modulating the expression of flanking genes. In particular, in two cases involving the position of RS-1, the P115 gene of clone G27 (42)

Table 1. IS3-related DNA sequences

Sequence name	Size (bp)	Target duplication (bp)	Inverted repeats (bp)	Source
RS-1	1,513	1–7	23/28	*M. hyorhinis, M. hyopneumoniae*
IS*3*	1,258	3	29/40	*E. coli*
IS*150*	1,443	3	22/31	*E. coli*
IS*3411*	1,309	3	23/25	Tn*3411, E. coli*
IS*600*	1,264	3	19/27	*Shigella sonnei*

Table 2. Terminal repetitive DNA sequences of the IS3 class

Sequence name	Inverted repeats
RS-1	L TGAgCAgATCCCCTTTTCcTagAAAAAT
	R TGAaCAtATCCCCTTTTCtTgaAAAAAT
IS3	L TGATCtTACCCAgc AATAgTGGACACgcGGC TAAGtGAG
	R TGATCcTACCCAcgtAATA TGGACACa GGCcTAAGcGAG
IS150	L TGTACTGcaCCCAttttGTTGGACGgaTcAAA
	R TGTACTGacCCCAaaaaGTTGGACagTtAAA
IS3411	L TGAACCGCCCCGGGaaTCCTGGAGA
	R TGAACCGCCCCGGGttTCCTGGAGA
IS600	L TGAGGTagcCTGagttTAaCGGACACT
	R TGAGGTgtaCTGgcaaTAgCGGACACT

and the uncharacterized P37 operon, presumed to encode substrate transport proteins (12), RS-1 copies are located immediately 3' to a protein-coding sequence and are positioned such that the RIR of RS-1 would predictably function as the transcription terminator for these genes. Furthermore, the palindrome in which RS-1 is inserted in the G27 genomic fragment (Fig. 3) may have been the original transcription terminator for the P115 gene (since it contains all of the requisite structural features), and the sequence flanking RS-1 near the P37 operon appears by preliminary analysis to be similar. Another RS-1 copy has been localized between the genes *vlpA* and *vlpB* (75), encoding two of the Vlps of *M. hyorhinis*. This copy is positioned such that its LIR may serve as the terminator for *vlpA* transcription and its RIR is oriented toward the *vlpB* promoter, but the overall features of the sequences flanking the insertion are similar to those described above (Fig. 3). No effect of this RS-1 on *vlp* gene expression has been observed, although it is intriguing that both IS3 and IS150 have been shown to activate adjacent gene expression through the activity of a promoter sequence positioned near the right end of the element and oriented outward (56, 57). These and other IS elements therefore represent mobile promoters capable of up-regulating flanking gene expression. Although there are sequences near the right end of RS-1 that very strongly resemble procaryotic promoters at both the consensus −10 region (TATAAT) and −35 region (TTGACA), with the appropriate spacing between these sequences (16 to 18 bp), no experiments delineating outward transcriptional activity have been reported.

While the current analysis of RS-1 positional effects

is limited in scope, it is interesting that no structural gene interruptions have been discovered. Assuming that most, if not all, mycoplasma structural genes are required for free-living or cell-associated growth (50) when dealing with such a limited genome size, then such integration events would have deleterious effects on survival of *M. hyorhinis* and would be selected against. Therefore, the cases examined to this point may represent only those events that are minimally disruptive. Only further analysis of the entire population of stable RS-1 insertions in the *M. hyorhinis* genome will address this question.

Distribution of RS-1 among the Swine Mycoplasmas

Hybridization studies (14, 67) indicated that RS-1 was present in multiple copies in all strains of *M. hyorhinis* examined, although hybridization pattern differences may define distinctive chromosomal locations in some individual instances (reflecting independent insertion events within specific populations) or may simply represent restriction enzyme cleavage polymorphisms. RS-1 gene probes also detected limited genomic copy numbers in all strains of *M. hyopneumoniae* tested except the ATCC type strain VPP11 (14), indicating that this strain did not harbor the IS element. Unexpectedly, however, when the probe was an 8-kb fragment from *M. hyopneumoniae* type strain J, which included two copies of RS-1 and approximately 5 kb of flanking DNA sequences, no homologous sequences were detected in VPP11 (14), suggesting that this entire RS-1 flanking region from strain J was nonessential. This observation was verified by

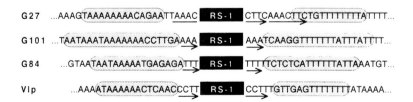

Figure 3. Comparison of genomic sequences flanking four individual copies of the RS-1 sequence. The designation of each isolate is given at the left. The RS-1 sequences are approximately 1,513 bp in length. Underlined sequences flanking RS-1 presumably represent nucleotide duplications that result from the RS-1 integration event. The shaded sequences are extensive palindromic sequences that are distinctive for each integration but show consistent characteristics from one example to another.

using a fragment of the original 8-kb probe but remote from either copy of RS-1. This probe still detected sequences in all other strains of *M. hyopneumoniae* and, furthermore, hybridized to a subset of the multiple RS-1 copies in *M. hyorhinis* strains (14). In addition, hybridization results with *M. flocculare* suggest that its restricted number of RS-1 sequences are associated with similar flanking sequences (77).

These data led to the suggestion (14) that some RS-1 copies are associated with a genetic sequence that is extrachromosomal in origin and that may represent all or part of an original integrated prophage or plasmid that was responsible for the dissemination of RS-1 among these mycoplasma species by a horizontal genetic transfer process. Subsequent genomic integration of this vector might perhaps have been analogous to those recombination events described earlier for the interactions between the *Spiroplasma* genome and its extrachromosomal DNA. Currently, no extrachromosomal plasmid molecules have been identified in either of these mycoplasma species. A lysogenic phage, Mhr1, was identified and preliminarily characterized (19), but it has not been able to be revived for analysis. Some strains of *M. hyorhinis* have been observed to exhibit a spontaneous plaquing phenotype, characteristic of induced prophages, when plated as confluent lawns on agar medium (51a). Assuming that this phenomenon can be stably reproduced, molecular probes specific for RS-1 and its flanking extrachromosomal sequences can be used to define possible interrelationships between them and the presumptive spontaneously induced viral particles.

Current efforts have determined that at least 4 kb of these specific RS-1 flanking sequences have been absolutely conserved between *M. hyorhinis* and *M. hyopneumoniae* (77), but there have also been considerable alterations (deletions and possible rearrangements or insertions) that would significantly affect the original organization and presumably the function of this surrounding region. It may be more than coincidental that the only consensus copy of RS-1 thus far identified (G1135.2) is one that is associated with this presumptive extrachromosomal DNA in *M. hyorhinis*. The presence of multiple RS-1 copies in this species, but restricted numbers in both other species, may also indicate that at least one of the RS-1 copies in *M. hyorhinis* is still capable of transposition, or was active for a longer time period after introduction, than were those copies introduced by whatever means into *M. hyopneumoniae* or *M. flocculare*. The multiple defects found in the coding sequences of both *M. hyopneumoniae* RS-1 copies support this position. These preliminary observations cannot presently be interpreted in terms of the potential origin of RS-1 elements in these three mycoplasma species or whether they gained entry into these organisms through a compatible genetic vector exchanged during periods of association within the common animal host.

A NOVEL REPETITIVE SEQUENCE (RS-2) FROM *M. HYORHINIS* ASSOCIATED WITH GENE AMPLIFICATION

Genomic Variation in a Mycoplasma Population as a Result of Gene Amplification

Evidence for a dramatic chromosomal alteration that resulted from a gene duplication event was uncovered during the examination of individual copies of the RS-1 insertion sequence from *M. hyorhinis* GDL-1 (this strain designation is defined in reference 6). One particular copy, first identified as G101 (14, 67), was isolated numerous times from a recombinant phage library, but the cloned genomic *Eco*RI fragments harboring this RS-1 varied considerably in size from approximately 13 kb to greater than 17 kb. Genetic mapping and hybridization experiments revealed that RS-1 was not responsible for this size heterogeneity, which was localized to a region some 2.5 kb upstream of RS-1 (9). This region (designated RS-2) was nearly 1.4 kb in size and was present in variable copy numbers, tandemly arranged within these cloned fragments. By using hybridization probes specific for RS-2, it was determined that all of the size-variant forms of this genomic fragment were present among the individual cells in the broth-cultured cell population that produced the chromosomal DNA used for library construction and Southern hybridization. Therefore, the arrangement of RS-2 as multiple copies of a 1.4-kb directly repeating unit suggests that these repeating units were generated via recombinational amplification and reduction events in the growing cell population, perhaps in response to some uncharacterized selective pressure, and that variation in the number of such repeating units likely results from interconversion of the signals that control these two reciprocal recombination processes.

Individual RS-2 genomic fragments containing variable repetitive units were sequenced to determine their molecular characteristics (9). Figure 4 summarizes structural features of three individual isolates containing two (G1020), three (G1042), or four (G1021) tandem copies of RS-2. This RS-2 sequence is 1,348 bp in length, and the multiple units are identical in sequence. Each unit is flanked by identical 20-bp cassette sequences, except that the leftmost cassette in each isolate is 6 bp longer than any subsequent cassettes (Fig. 5). This physical organization is analogous to similar configurations identified for recombinational gene amplification or reduction phenomena that result in modulation of gene dosage for metabolic purposes (i.e., in response to some selective pressure, stress, or stimulus) or that create multigene families (by duplication and divergence) in other organisms, both procaryotic and eucaryotic (8, 13, 33). It also suggests that the 20-bp cassettes represent the sites at which a specific duplication (recombination) event may occur. The cassette sequences (Fig. 5) are all characterized by two direct copies of a hexanucleotide sequence, TTCTTG, separated by three nucleotides except in the leftmost copy, where an additional six nucleotides, TTCTTC, are present. If these sequences represent the site of recombination in this amplication-reduction process controlling RS-2 copy number, these sequence features suggest that the hexanucleotide repeat may bind recombination factors or serve as the crossover point for such an event and that the variant cassette may reflect a previous slippage or mistake in such a mechanism. In most characterized gene amplification events, it is the initial tandem gene duplication that may occur by a specific process involving such small repetitive DNA sequences (8, 29, 33, 45), although no specific mechanism has been characterized. Subsequent duplications or deletions can occur

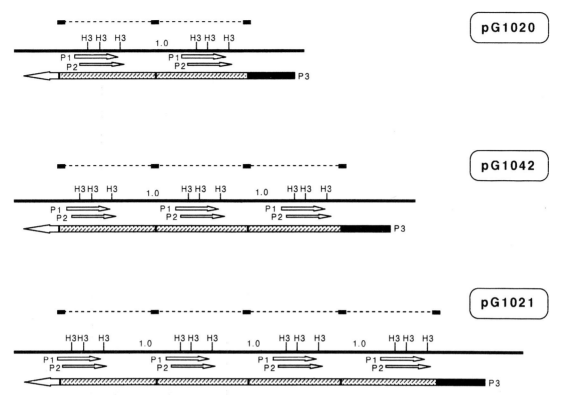

Figure 4. Organization and expression of three variant forms of RS-2 from individual populations of broth-grown *M. hyorhinis*. The genetic organization (including landmark *Hin*dIII restriction sites) is given for three variants: G1020, with two copies of RS-2; G1042, with three copies; and G1021, with four copies. The extent of the RS-2 sequence homology is given above the depicted DNA region as a dashed line. The black rectangles demarcating these sequences are repetitions of the 20-bp cassette sequence that may be involved in tandem duplication events. Potential protein-coding regions are noted below each structure. The P1 and P2 ORFs are overlapping and encoded by two separate reading frames of the upper strand; they are entirely contained within a single RS-2 unit so that amplification simply increases their gene dosage. The P3 ORF is encoded on the lower strand; it originates and terminates in unique sequences (dark and open bars) outside either end of RS-2. Duplication events maintain the reading frame, causing a repetition of an internal 456-residue cysteine-rich peptide domain (stippled bar).

by normal recombination pathways between homologous regions of the already duplicated genes.

Translational Capacity of RS-2

As depicted in Fig. 4, several ORFs can be deduced from the nucleotide sequence. On one strand, two possible overlapping ORFs encoding the proteins designated P1 and P2 are predicted, and both are completely contained within the 1,348-bp RS-2 sequence. The basically charged 20-kDa P1 protein is considerably hydrophobic and rich in histidine (11.8%) and cysteine (5.9%) residues. Data base homology searches revealed only limited similarities of unknown significance to a few nucleic acid-binding proteins, including RNA polymerase and reverse transcriptase. The P2 protein initiates downstream of P1 and from a distinct reading frame; this potential 23-kDa protein is also hydrophobic and contains numerous histidine and cysteine residues. Again, no extensive amino acid homologies were detected, although an interesting regional similarity was observed between P2 and the bacterial heavy-metal binding protein MerR (38). This region includes the strong positional conservation of a number of serine and aliphatic residues surrounding

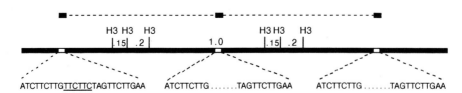

Figure 5. Nucleotide sequences of the 20-bp cassettes from the G1020 RS-2 gene region. The genetic organization is as depicted in Fig. 4. The open boxes represent the flanking cassettes, whose nucleotide sequences are given. A 6-bp insertion (underlined) is noted in the leftmost cassette.

a few cysteine residues in a region that has unknown significance to the functional activity of this group of proteins. While there is no obvious functional relevance to either of these potential ORFs at present, the predicted gene amplification results in the increase of gene dosage for P1 and P2 from two in G1020 to four in G1021. No clonal derivative of strain GDL-1 with only a single copy of RS-2 has been isolated.

Examination of the other strand revealed a very large ORF designated P3 that initiates in unique sequences flanking RS-2, extends entirely across it, and terminates in unique sequences on the opposite side of RS-2. Duplication of RS-2 maintains the reading frame and results in amplification of only the internal domains of the predicted product (Fig. 4). The P3 protein from G1020 would contain 1,187 residues, with a calculated mass of 135 kDa; the G1042 product would increase in length by 456 amino acids, bringing it to a size of 186.5 kDa; the G1021 P3 product predicted from these structures would be 238 kDa. The coding sequence within the RS-2 component of the P3 gene is extremely hydrophilic, acidic, and cysteine rich (each of the three potential P3 products contains 12% cysteine residues). It is these cysteine-rich domains that are highlighted in data base homology searches in that they exhibit highly significant similarities with domains in metal-binding proteins like the eucaryotic metallothioneins (1) and with metal-binding domains of complex eucaryotic proteins from the multigene family (3, 30, 32) that includes the fibronectin receptor, the β_2-laminins, and the β_1-integrins. These homologies are generally related to the distribution of cysteine residues to form a metal-binding cluster and therefore do not necessarily reflect functional similarities to any of these identified proteins other than the potential to bind metals. Therefore, the amplification of this particular P3 domain may be functionally significant to M. hyorhinis in increasing its biochemical potential to bind metal ions, either as a cofactor for its as yet uncharacterized biological function or as a detoxification mechanism to protect these organisms against the detrimental effects of heavy-metal buildup, as has been predicted for the small peptide metallothioneins (1). Although these sequence similarities do not elucidate the biological function that might be carried out by P3, antibodies to a recombinant form of this protein have been generated and have shown conclusively multiple proteins in M. hyorhinis bearing epitopes also expressed on the recombinant P3 peptide (9).

Clonal and Strain Variations in RS-2 Copy Number

The discrimination of multiple variants in RS-2 copy number within a broth-cultured population of M. hyorhinis GDL-1 suggested that the molecular process generating this variation was active within this population and that individual variants could be segregated. Therefore, broth-cultured cells were diluted and grown on agar plates to select individual colonies. Chromosomal DNAs from selected colonies were shown by DNA hybridization to contain predominantly one form of the RS-2 region, usually two or four copies of the 1.4-kb repetitive unit. Further limited clonal selection from any of these individual isolates

did not reveal any dramatic changes in copy number that might indicate either the frequency of these recombination events or the stimulus to initiate them.

No mycoplasmas examined other than M. hyorhinis hybridized with RS-2, but other broth-cultured strains of M. hyorhinis also contained RS-2-homologous sequences. The swine-derived strains SK76, PG29 and BTS-7 (6) showed only a single size variant within cultured populations; it is not clear whether this variant represents one or two copies of RS-2. However, a broth culture of strain GDL-2 (a continuously passaged tissue culture derivative [6]), like GDL-1, showed multiple hybridizing fragments, indicating variations in RS-2 copy number at least equivalent to that seen with GDL-1. These observations may prove fundamental to unraveling the process of RS-2 copy number variation and the signals to which it responds. For example, does continuous passage in broth culture trigger the amplification mechanism, or could tissue culture cell associations have some influence?

RS-2 therefore represents yet another dramatic example of continuous genomic variation within the species M. hyorhinis, which, along with documented changes in Vlp gene expression and antigenic variation and with potential genomic instability associated with multiple copies of RS-1, indicates that this species is in a constant state of genetic flux, allowing for rapid and continuous adaptation to potential changes in growth requirements or environmental conditions. RS-2 provides another significant opportunity in these unique organisms to investigate the potential for recombination mechanisms that drive their high rate of genomic diversity.

SUMMARY

This chapter has summarized observations from a variety of mycoplasmas that strongly implicate repetitive DNA sequences in the generation of genomic diversification in these organisms. It appears that despite their limited genomic capacities, mycoplasmas have incorporated into their genetic repertoire a variety of recombination systems that are based on interactions between repeated DNA units and perhaps specific recombinase enzymes so that they maintain a combinatorial flexibility that likely allows them to respond to fluctuating growth conditions. Examples of repetitive DNA structures found throughout the eubacteria, including ISs, repetitive peptide-encoding cassettes, and multigene families, are also found in mycoplasmas. There will likely be others recognized as well, as exemplified by the recent discovery by polymerase chain reaction methodology of a sequence from M. hyopneumoniae (22) that appears to be present in the genome in multiple copies but at a preliminary glance is not related to any of those already described. The identification and characterization of these repetitive DNA sequences will fuel many future efforts to understand genomic diversification in mycoplasmas catalyzed by specific recombination mechanisms mediating such processes as transposition and insertion, antigenic and phenotypic switching, and gene amplification.

It is now clearly apparent that the wide genetic heterogeneity that is prevalent not only among the multitude of mycoplasma species (61) but also among isolated strains within a given mycoplasma species (49) can be attributed to several genetic mechanisms, including a higher than normal mutation rate (72), and a variety of repetitive DNA structures that provide efficient substrates for recombination mechanisms, both general and site specific (45). These factors endow upon the mycoplasma genome a considerable degree of flexibility to produce random or directed DNA substitutions or rearrangements at a high frequency that, under the appropriate conditions of growth or host association, may offer a selective advantage to a subpopulation of cells, thereby allowing a rapid adaptive (or selective) response for these individuals. It is also assumed that under these circumstances, the great majority of genomic alterations attempted by the population as a whole will have no selective advantage or in fact will be detrimental to that particular cell's survival and will be diluted out of the population. In line with the hypothesis that mycoplasmas evolved by a degenerative process from a gram-positive predecessor, repetitive sequences placed strategically so as to flank clustered gene systems (transport operons, cell wall biosynthesis genes, etc.) could result in their extinction from the genome, a process that may have been favored during selective periods in their evolutionary development.

Acknowledgments. Our own work discussed in this chapter was supported in part by Public Health Service grant AR35587 from the National Institutes of Health. We thank our colleagues Kim S. Wise, Manijeh Heidari, Renate Rosengarten, and David Yogev for discussion and expertise relative to these studies.

REFERENCES

1. **Andersen, R. D., B. W. Birren, S. J. Taplitz, and H. R. Herschman.** 1986. Rat metallothionein-1 structural gene and three pseudogenes, one of which contains 5'-regulatory sequences. *Mol. Cell. Biol.* **6:**302–315.

2. **Anderson, B. E., G. A. McDonald, D. C. Jones, and R. L. Regnery.** 1990. A protective protein antigen of *Ricksettsia rickettsii* has tandemly repeated, near-identical sequences. *Infect. Immun.* **58:**2760–2769.

3. **Argraves, W. S., S. Suzuki, H. Arai, K. Thompson, M. D. Pierschbacher, and E. Ruoslahti.** 1987. Amino acid sequence of the human fibronectin receptor. *J. Cell Biol.* **105:**1183–1190.

4. **Barbour, A. G.** 1990. Antigenic variation of a relapsing fever *Borrelia* species. *Annu. Rev. Microbiol.* **44:**155–171.

4a. **Bhugra, B., and K. Dybvig.** 1992. Genomic rearrangments involving insertion elements present in *Mycoplasma pulmonis. Abstr. Gen. Meet. Am. Soc. Microbiol. 1992,* G14, p. 161.

5. **Borst, P., and G. A. M. Cross.** 1982. Molecular basis for trypanosome antigenic variation. *Cell* **29:**291–303.

6. **Boyer, M. J., and K. S. Wise.** 1989. Lipid-modified surface protein antigens expressing size variation within the species *Mycoplasma hyorhinis. Infect. Immun.* **57:**245–254.

7. **Colman, S. D., P. Hu, and K. F. Bott.** 1990. Prevalence of novel repeat sequences in and around the *P1* operon in the genome of *Mycoplasma pneumoniae. Gene* **87:**91–96.

8. **Cross, M., and R. Renkawitz.** 1990. Repetitive sequence involvement in the duplication and divergence of mouse lysozyme genes. *EMBO J.* **9:**1283–1288.

9. **Deng, G., and M. A. McIntosh.** Unpublished data.

10. **Dickinson, M. J., and R. Townsend.** 1985. Lysogenization of *Spiroplasma citri* by a type 3 spiroplasmavirus. *Virology* **146:**102–110.

11. **DiRita, V. J., and J. J. Mekalanos.** 1989. Genetic regulation of bacterial virulence. *Annu. Rev. Genet.* **23:**455–482.

12. **Dudler, R., C. Schmidhauser, R. W. Parish, R. E. H. Wettenhall, and T. Schmidt.** 1988. A mycoplasma high-affinity transport system and the *in vitro* invasiveness of mouse sarcoma cells. *EMBO J.* **7:**3963–3970.

13. **Edlund, T., and S. Normark.** 1981. Recombination between short DNA homologies causes tandem duplication. *Nature* (London) **292:**269–271.

14. **Ferrell, R. V., M. B. Heidari, K. S. Wise, and M. A. McIntosh.** 1989. A *Mycoplasma* genetic element resembling prokaryotic insertion sequences. *Mol. Microbiol.* **3:**957–967.

15. **Fischetti, V. A.** 1991. Streptococcal M protein. *Sci. Am.* **264:**32–39.

16. **Freundt, E. A., and D. G. Edward.** 1979. Classification and taxonomy, p. 1–42. *In* M. F. Barile and S. Razin (ed.), *The Mycoplasmas,* vol. 1. Academic Press, New York.

17. **Galas, D. J., and M. Chandler.** 1989. Bacterial insertion sequences, p. 109–162. *In* D. E. Berg and M. M. Howe (ed.), *Mobile DNA.* American Society for Microbiology, Washington, D.C.

18. **Gois, M., F. Kuksa, J. Franz, and D. Taylor-Robinson.** 1974. The antigenic differentiation of seven strains of *Mycoplasma hyorhinis* by growth-inhibition, metabolism-inhibition, latex-agglutination and polyacrylamide-gel-electrophoresis tests. *J. Med. Microbiol.* **7:**105–115.

19. **Gourlay, R. N., S. G. Wyld, and M. E. Poulton.** 1983. Some characteristics of Mycoplasma virus Hr1, isolated from and infecting *Mycoplasma hyorhinis. Arch. Virol.* **77:**81–85.

20. **Grindley, N. D. F., and R. R. Reed.** 1985. Transpositional recombination in prokaryotes. *Annu. Rev. Biochem.* **54:**863–896.

21. **Hall, B. G., L. L. Parker, P. W. Betts, R. F. DuBose, S. A. Sawyer, and D. L. Hartl.** 1989. IS*103,* a new insertion element in *Escherichia coli*: characterization and distribution in natural populations. *Genetics* **121:**423–431.

22. **Harasawa, R., K. Koshimizu, O. Takeda, T. Uemori, K. Asada, and I. Kato.** 1991. Detection of *Mycoplasma hyopneumoniae* DNA by the polymerase chain reaction. *Mol. Cell. Probes* **5:**103–109.

23. **Hu, W. S., R. Y.-H. Wang, R.-S. Liou, J. W.-K. Shih, and S.-C. Lo.** 1990. Identification of an insertion-sequence-like genetic element in the newly recognized human pathogen *Mycoplasma incognitus. Gene* **93:**67–72.

24. **Hulton, C. S. J., C. F. Higgins, and P. M. Sharp.** 1991. ERIC sequences: a novel family of repetitive elements in the genomes of *Escherichia coli, Salmonella typhimurium* and other enterobacteria. *Mol. Microbiol.* **5:**825–834.

25. **Iida, S., J. Meyer, and W. Arber.** 1983. Prokaryotic IS elements, p. 159–221. *In* J. A. Shapiro (ed.), *Mobile Genetic Elements.* Academic Press, New York.

26. **Inamine, J. M., T. P. Denny, S. Loechel, U. Schaper, C. Huang, K. F. Bott, and P. Hu.** 1988. Nucleotide sequence of the P1 attachment-protein gene of *Mycoplasma pneumoniae. Gene* **64:**217–229.

27. **Inamine, J. M., S. Loechel, A. M. Collier, M. F. Barile, and P. Hu.** 1989. Nucleotide sequence of the MgPa (*mgp*) operon of *Mycoplasma genitalium* and comparison to the P1 (*mpp*) operon of *Mycoplasma pneumoniae. Gene* **82:**259–267.

28. **Ishiguro, N., and G. Sato.** 1988. Nucleotide sequence of insertion sequence IS*3411,* which flanks the citrate utilization determinant of transposon Tn*3411. J. Bacteriol.* **170:**1902–1906.

29. **Karin, M., R. Najarian, A. Haslinger, P. Valenzuela, J. Welch, and S. Fogel.** 1984. Primary structure and transcription of an amplified genetic locus: the *CUP1* locus of yeast. *Proc. Natl. Acad. Sci. USA* **81:**337–341.

30. **Kishimoto, T. K., K. O'Connor, A. Lee, T. M. Roberts, and T. A. Springer.** 1987. Cloning of the β subunit of the leukocyte adhesion proteins: homology to an extracellular matrix receptor defines a novel supergene family. *Cell* **48:**681–690.

31. **Landschultz, W. H., P. F. Johnson, and S. L. McKnight.** 1988. The leucine zipper: a hypothetical structure common to a new class of DNA binding proteins. *Science* **240:**1759–1764.

32. **Larson, R. S., and T. A. Springer.** 1990. Structure and function of leukocyte integrins. *Immunol. Rev.* **114:**181–217.

33. **Maeda, N., and O. Smithies.** 1986. The evolution of multigene families: human haptoglobin genes. *Annu. Rev. Genet.* **20:**81–108.

34. **Manjula, B. N., S. D. Acharya, S. M. Mische, T. Fairwell, and V. A. Fischetti.** 1984. The complete amino acid sequence of a biologically active 197-residue fragment of M protein isolated from type 5 group A streptococci. *J. Biol. Chem.* **259:**3686–3693.

35. **Manjula, B. N., B. L. Trus, and V. A. Fischetti.** 1985. Presence of two distinct regions in the coiled-coil structure of the streptococcal Pep M5 protein: relationship to mammalian coiled-coil proteins and implications to its biological properties. *Proc. Natl. Acad. Sci. USA* **82:**1064–1068.

36. **Matsutani, S., H. Ohtsubo, Y. Maeda, and E. Ohtsubo.** 1987. Isolation and characterization of IS elements repeated in the bacterial chromosome. *J. Mol. Biol.* **196:**445–455.

37. **Meyer, T. F.** 1987. Molecular basis of surface antigen variation in *Neisseria. Trends Genet.* **3:**319–324.

38. **Misra, T. K., N. L. Brown, D. C. Fritzinger, R. D. Pridmore, W. M. Barnes, L. Haberstroh, and S. Silver.** 1984. Mercuric ion-resistance operons of plasmid R100 and transposon Tn*501*: the beginning of the operon including the regulatory region and the first two structural genes. *Proc. Natl. Acad. Sci. USA* **81:**5975–5979.

39. **Mouches, C., G. Barroso, and J. M. Bové.** 1983. Characterization and molecular cloning in *Escherichia coli* of a plasmid from the mollicute *Spiroplasma citri. J. Bacteriol.* **156:**952–955.

40. **Mouches, C., G. Barroso, A. Gadeau, and J. M. Bové.** 1984. Characterization of two cryptic plasmids from *Spiroplasma citri* and occurrence of their DNA sequences among various spiroplasmas. *Ann. Microbiol.* (Paris) **135A:**17–24.

41. **Murphy, E.** 1989. Transposable elements in gram-positive bacteria, p. 269–288. *In* D. E. Berg and M. M. Howe (ed.), *Mobile DNA.* American Society for Microbiology, Washington, D.C.

42. **Notarnicola, S. M., M. A. McIntosh, and K. S. Wise.** 1991. A *Mycoplasma hyorhinis* protein with sequence similarities to nucleotide-binding enzymes. *Gene* **97:**77–85.

43. **Nur, I., G. Glaser, and S. Razin.** 1986. Free and integrated plasmid DNA in spiroplasmas. *Curr. Microbiol.* **14:**169–176.

44. **Nur, I., D. J. LeBlanc, and J. G. Tully.** 1987. Short, interspersed, and repetitive DNA sequences in *Spiroplasma* species. *Plasmid* **17:**110–116.

45. **Petes, T. D., and C. W. Hill.** 1988. Recombination between repeated genes in microorganisms. *Annu. Rev. Genet.* **22:**147–168.

46. **Platt, T.** 1986. Transcription termination and the regulation of gene expression. *Annu. Rev. Biochem.* **55:**339–372.

47. **Presta, L. G., and G. D. Rose.** 1988. Helix signals in proteins. *Science* **240:**1632–1641.

48. **Ranhand, J. M., I. Nur, D. L. Rose, and J. G. Tully.** 1987. *Spiroplasma* species share common DNA sequences among their viruses, plasmids and genomes. *Ann. Inst. Pasteur/Microbiol.* **138:**509–522.

49. **Razin, S.** 1969. Structure and function in mycoplasma. *Annu. Rev. Microbiol* **23:**317–356.

50. **Razin, S.** 1985. Molecular biology and genetics of mycoplasmas (*Mollicutes*). *Microbiol. Rev.* **49:**419–455.

51. **Rogers, M. J., J. Simmons, R. T. Walker, W. G. Weisburg, C. R. Woese, R. S. Tanner, I. M. Robinson, D. A. Stahl, G. Olsen, R. H. Leach, and J. Maniloff.** 1985. Construction of the mycoplasma evolutionary tree from 5S rRNA sequence data. *Proc. Natl. Acad. Sci. USA* **82:**1160–1164.

51a.**Rosengarten, R.** Unpublished data.

52. **Rosengarten, R., and K. S. Wise.** 1990. Phenotypic switching in mycoplasmas: phase variation of diverse surface lipoproteins. *Science* **247:**315–318.

53. **Rosengarten, R., and K. S. Wise.** 1991. The Vlp system of *Mycoplasma hyorhinis*: combinatorial expression of distinct size variant lipoproteins generating high-frequency surface antigenic variation. *J. Bacteriol.* **173:**4782–4793.

54. **Ruland, K., R. Wenzel, and R. Herrmann.** 1990. Analysis of three different repeated DNA elements present in the P1 operon of *Mycoplasma pneumoniae*: size, number and distribution on the genome. *Nucleic Acids Res.* **18:**6311–6317.

55. **Salvado, J.-C., G. Barroso, and J. Labarère.** 1989. Involvement of a *Spiroplasma citri* plasmid in the erythromycin-resistance transfer. *Plasmid* **22:**151–159.

56. **Schwartz, E., C. Herberger, and B. Rak.** 1988. Second-element turn-on of gene expression in an IS*1* insertion mutant. *Mol. Gen. Genet.* **211:**282–289.

57. **Schwartz, E., M. Kröger, and B. Rak.** 1988. IS*150*: distribution, nucleotide sequence and phylogenetic relationships of a new *E. coli* insertion element. *Nucleic Acids Res.* **16:**6789–6802.

58. **Segal, E., P. Hagblom, S. H. Seifert, and M. So.** 1986. Antigenic variation in gonococcal pilus involves assembly of separated silent gene segments. *Proc. Natl. Acad. Sci. USA* **83:**2177–2188.

59. **Seifert, H. S., and M. So.** 1988. Genetic mechanisms of bacterial antigenic variation. *Microbiol. Rev.* **52:**327–336.

60. **Shimizu-Kadota, M., M. Kiwaki, H. Hirokawa, and N. Tsuchida.** 1985. ISL*1*: a new transposable element in *Lactobacillus casei. Mol. Gen. Genet.* **200:**193–198.

61. **Stanbridge, E. J., and M. E. Reff.** 1979. The molecular biology of mycoplasmas, p. 157–187. *In* M. F. Barile and S. Razin (ed.). *The Mycoplasmas*, vol. 1. Academic Press, New York.

62. **Stern, A., M. Brown, P. Nickel, and T. F. Meyer.** 1986. Opacity genes in *Neisseria gonorrheae*: control of phase and antigenic variation. *Cell* **47:**61–71.

63. **Stern, M. J., G. F.-L. Ames, N. H. Smith, E. C. Robinson, and C. F. Higgins.** 1984. Repetitive extragenic palindromic sequences: a major component of the bacterial genome. *Cell* **37:**1015–1026.

64. **Su, C.-J., A. Chavoya, and J. B. Baseman.** 1988. Regions of *Mycoplasma pneumoniae* cytadhesin P1 structural gene exist as multiple copies. *Infect. Immun.* **56:**3157–3161.

65. **Su, C.-J., V. V. Tryon, and J. B. Baseman.** 1987. Cloning and sequence analysis of cytadhesin P1 gene from *Mycoplasma pneumoniae. Infect. Immun.* **55:**3023–3029.

66. **Syvanen, M.** 1984. The evolutionary implications of mobile genetic elements. *Annu. Rev. Genet.* **18:**271–293.

67. **Taylor, M. A., R. V. Ferrell, K. S. Wise, and M. A. McIntosh.** 1988. Reiterated DNA sequences defining genomic diversity within the species *Mycoplasma hyorhinis. Mol. Microbiol.* **2:**665–672.

68. **Timmerman, K. P., and C.-P. D. Tu.** 1985. Complete sequence of IS*3. Nucleic Acids Res.* **13:**2127–2139.

69. **Tinoco, I., P. N. Borer, B. Dengler, M. D. Levine, O. C. Uhlenbeck, D. M. Crothers, and J. Gralla.** 1973. Improved estimation of secondary structure in ribonucleic acids. *Nature* (London) **246:**40–41.

70. **Wenzel, R., and R. Herrman.** 1988. Repetitive DNA sequences in *Mycoplasma pneumoniae. Nucleic Acids Res.* **16:**8337–8350.

71. **Woese, C. R.** 1987. Bacterial evolution. *Microbiol. Rev.* **51:**221–271.

72. **Woese, C. R., E. Stackebrandt, and W. Ludwig.** 1985. What are mycoplasmas: the relationship of tempo and mode in bacterial evolution. *J. Mol. Evol.* **21:**305–316.

73. **Woods, J. P., J. F. Dempsey, T. H. Kawula, D. S. Barritt, and J. G. Cannon.** 1989. Characterization of the neisserial lipid-modified azurin bearing the H.8 epitope. *Mol. Microbiol.* **3:**583–591.

74. **Yamao, F., A. Muto, Y. Kawauchi, M. Iwami, S. Iwagami, Y. Azumi, and S. Osaya.** 1985. UGA is read as tryptophan in *Mycoplasma capricolum. Proc. Natl. Acad. Sci. USA* **82:**2306–2309.

75. **Yogev, D., R. Rosengarten, R. Watson-McKown, and K. Wise.** 1991. Molecular basis of *Mycoplasma* surface antigenic variation: a novel set of divergent genes undergo spontaneous mutation of periodic coding regions and 5′ regulatory sequences. *EMBO J.* **10:**4069–4079.

76. **Zheng, J., R. V. Ferrell, M. B. Heidari, and M. A. McIntosh.** Unpublished data.

77. **Zheng, J., and M. A. McIntosh.** Unpublished data.

V. IDENTIFICATION AND TREATMENT OF PATHOGENIC MYCOPLASMAS

23. Mycoplasmas Which Infect Plants and Insects

ING-MING LEE and ROBERT E. DAVIS

INTRODUCTION

The term "mycoplasmas" is used as the trivial name for all members of the class *Mollicutes*. This class contains in vitro-cultivated cell wall-less procaryotes. Two types of cell wall-less organisms infect plants; one, termed spiroplasmas, is characteristically helical, and the other, termed mycoplasmalike organisms (MLOs), is nonhelical. Both infect insects, and evidence indicates that both belong to the class *Mollicutes* (reviewed in references 13, 72, 89 to 91, and 106).

The spiroplasmas were recognized as a new microbial entity in the early 1970s (27, 29, 30), when they were found to be associated with two plant diseases, corn stunt and citrus stubborn, and their insect vectors. The association of spiroplasmas with plants and their frequent occurrence in insects, including nonvector insects, are now well established (reviewed in references 5, 18a, 47, 127, and 128). The majority of spiroplasmas can be cultured in vitro without much difficulty (reviewed in references 13 and 47). Numerous spiroplasmas have been characterized and classified in the family *Spiroplasmaceae*, order *Mycoplasmatales*, class *Mollicutes* (reviewed in references 47, 127, and 128). To date, however, only three species, *Spiroplasma citri*, *S. kunkelii*, and *S. phoeniceum*, are known to be plant pathogenic (reviewed in reference 128). Biochemical methods in conjunction with serological assays have been generally used to identify and differentiate these three species of plant-pathogenic spiroplasmas (reviewed in references 13, 20, 22, 59, and 97). Spiroplasmas and their characteristics have been extensively reviewed elsewhere (5, 39, 127, 128).

Nonhelical MLOs are associated with plant diseases known as yellows diseases (reviewed in reference 99). Their presence in phloem of plants and in tissues of insect vectors has been demonstrated, most often by electron microscopy (16, 48, 54; reviewed in reference 99). MLOs are believed to cause more than 600 diseases in several hundred plant species (reviewed in reference 99). In contrast to plant-pathogenic spiroplasmas, thus far no MLO has been cultured in vitro (reviewed in references 7, 77, and 99). The term "MLO" refers to this type of organism's resemblance to animal mycoplasmas in morphology and ultrastructure. The phylogenetic relationship of MLOs with members of the *Mycoplasmatales* has been studied only recently, after recombinant DNA technology became available. On the basis of rRNA gene analysis, MLOs have been reported to be related to, but distinct from, animal mycoplasmas (62, 63, 71, 72, 89). MLOs may have a closer evolutionary link to *Acholeplasma* species (89–91).

Until recently, diagnosis of MLO-associated plant disease and classification of MLOs relied primarily on electron microscopy, or DNA staining of sieve cells of diseased plants, and on biological characteristics which included MLO-insect vector relationships, plant host range, and characteristic symptoms in MLO-infected host plants (reviewed in reference 99). The recent introduction of recombinant DNA and hybridoma technologies, however, has made it feasible to accurately identify and even classify MLOs. This chapter discusses primarily diagnostic detection and identification of MLOs and treatment of MLO-associated diseases, with emphasis on recent research.

IDENTIFICATION

Biological Properties

Morphology and ultrastructure

Prior to 1967, all yellows diseases of plants were presumed to be caused by viruses, although viruses could

Ing-Ming Lee and Robert E. Davis • Microbiology and Plant Pathology Laboratory, Agricultural Research Service, U.S. Department of Agriculture, Beltsville, Maryland 20705.

not be consistently visualized in diseased tissues or isolated from infected plants (20; reviewed in reference 99). Discovery that a nonviral type of agent was associated with yellows diseases resulted in a marked change in the classification of the pathogen sought as the probable causal agent. Morphology and ultrastructure are the properties of MLOs by which they were first recognized in the phloem of yellows-diseased plants (36). As seen in ultrathin sections, these organisms were surrounded only by a single "unit membrane" and lacked evidence of a rigid cell wall (reviewed in reference 5). In their minute size and generally rounded and pleomorphic shape, and in their internal ultrastructure consisting of granules the size of procaryotic ribosomes and strands presumed to be DNA, these phloem-dwelling organisms resembled the mycoplasmas already known to colonize humans and animals. Recognition of these morphological and ultrastructural properties as mycoplasmalike amounted, in effect, to a tentative classification of the MLOs along with mycoplasmas in the subsequently established class *Mollicutes*.

After the discovery of MLOs, many yellows diseases were examined for the presence of wall-less procaryotic organisms in infected plants and for the occurrence of such organisms in insect vectors capable of transmitting the causal pathogens. Ultrathin-section electron microscopy became a major avenue for assessing the probable cause of disease, linking the presence of MLOs in insects and in plant phloem with disease. Electron microscopy thus became an important means for detection of MLOs in infected hosts. This means of pathogen detection is still used today, usually in conjunction with other methods, both in determining the association of MLOs with diseases of unsolved etiology and in investigating new possible plant hosts of MLOs (16, 37, 48, 54).

In addition to electron microscopy, optical and fluorescence microscopic methods have been used to detect MLOs, particularly in plant tissues. The DAPI (4',6-diamidino-2-phenylindole·2HCl) (44, 114, 119) staining method has been widely applied. Similarly, the Dienes staining method has been used to detect MLOs in plants (31, 37). While these methods can provide evidence for the presence of an MLO in diseased plant tissues, they, like electron microscopy, do not indicate the identity of the detected MLO and therefore have been applied chiefly in studies of specific, known MLOs and in cases requiring general information about the association of MLOs with disease.

Examination by optical microscopy of sieve cells isolated from infected plants offers a unique method for observing MLOs (76) By this approach, the differing morphologies of MLOs, spiroplasmas, and a walled phloem-inhabiting procaryote have been compared (76). The method presents another means to determine the possible association of a procaryotic organism with disease and allows observations of the overall morphology of organisms in sieve cells. That the observed organisms are viable is indicated by successful in vitro culture of spiroplasmas from isolated sieve cells (78a). Detection of phloem-inhabiting pathogens is thus possible by examination of isolated sieve cells, and the method can distinguish, for example, between a nonhelical MLO and a helical spiroplasma, but it provides no information on the identity of the detected

organism beyond that indicated by its general morphology.

Symptoms

Collectively, plant diseases associated with the presence of MLOs in phloem typically exhibit an array of symptoms suggestive of profound disturbances in the normal balance of plant hormones. Because some of these symptoms are highly characteristic of MLO infection, their occurrence generally provides the first evidence indicating the possible presence of an MLO in diseased plants. Symptoms in plants include sterility of flowers, virescence (the development of green flowers and loss of normal flower color), phyllody (the development of floral parts into leafy structures), proliferation of auxiliary shoots resulting in a witches' broom appearance, generalized stunting, bunchy appearance of growth at the ends of stems, yellowing, necrosis in phloem, dieback of branches in woody plants, and generalized decline (reviewed in references 21 and 99). In some cases, certain disease symptoms seem to be mutually exclusive, and the diseases and their associated MLOs have been categorized, or classified, in whole or in part on the basis of symptoms (14, 37, 42, 98, 118; reviewed in references 61 and 99).

For example, Shiomi and Sugiura (118) have classified several yellows diseases of plants in Japan on the basis of transmission of the pathogen(s) by the leafhopper insect vector *Macrosteles orientalis* Virvaste, ability of the pathogen(s) to infect a common range of plant species, and the development of similar symptoms in infected plants. Kirkpatrick (61) has broadly classified several MLOs into two categories, virescence-inducing MLOs and decline-inducing MLOs, on the basis of symptoms exhibited in the plants with the respective diseases with which they are associated. Virescence diseases include aster yellows, beet leafhopper-transmitted virescence, stolbur, and clover proliferation, whereas decline diseases include western X-disease of stone fruits, apple proliferation, elm yellows, maize bushy stunt, and coconut lethal yellowing. As noted by Kirkpatrick (61), MLOs associated with decline diseases are associated not with virescence or phyllody but with the production of flowers reduced in size and normal or nearly normal in color, as observed either in the agronomic plant of interest or in the common experimental MLO host periwinkle (*Catharanthus roseus* (L.) G. Don). Since the virescent/phylloid flower symptom(s) and the symptom of reduced flower size but normal color appear to be mutually exclusive, these two categories may be important for understanding MLO-associated diseases.

Chiykowski and Sinha (14) similarly noted an apparent mutually exclusive occurrence of phyllody (and/or virescence) symptoms and symptoms of reduced flower size and color (without phyllody or virescence). They differentiated diseases with these two respective symptom syndromes into a category 1 (containing eastern aster yellows, western aster yellows, clover phyllody, and clover proliferation) and a category 2 (containing peach X-disease and clover yellow edge). As seen in Table 1, Chiykowski and Sinha's (14) classification of peach X-disease MLOs and clover yellow edge MLO into a single category (category 2) on the basis of disease symptoms is consistent with classifica-

Table 1. Classification of some MLOs in genomic strain clusters

MLO strain cluster designation	MLO strain	Associated disease	Geographic origin of MLO strain
Aster yellows			
Type I	BB	Tomato big bud	Arkansas
	CN1	Periwinkle little leaf 0–1	Connecticut
	CN13	Periwinkle little leaf 0–13	Connecticut
	OK1	Oklahoma aster yellows (western aster yellows)	Oklahoma
	NAY	Eastern aster yellows	Canada
	AY27	Alberta aster yellows (western aster yellows)	Canada
	NJAY	New Jersey aster yellows	New Jersey
Type II	AY1	Maryland aster yellows	Maryland
	OK3	Oklahoma aster yellows (western aster yellows)	Oklahoma
	NYAY	New York aster yellows	New York
	SAY2	Severe western aster yellows	California
	TLAY2	Tulelake western aster yellows	California
	DAY	Dwarf western aster yellows	California
	CY2	Chrysanthemum yellows	Italy
Type III	CPh	Clover phyllody	Canada
Elm yellows	EY1	Elm yellows	New York
	EY2	Elm yellows	New York
	ItaEY1	Elm yellows	Italy
Peach X-disease	WX	Peach X-disease	California
	CX	Peach X-disease	Ontario, Canada
	CYE	Clover yellow edge	Ontario, Canada
Paulownia witches' broom (tentative)	PaWB	Paulownia witches' broom	Taiwan
Beet leafhopper-transmitted virescence (tentative)	VR	Beet leafhopper-transmitted virescence	California
Clover proliferation (tentative)	CP	Clover proliferation	Alberta, Canada
	PWB	Potato witches' broom	Alberta, Canada
Ash yellows (tentative)	AshY	Ash yellows	New York

tion of these MLOs into a single genomic cluster on the basis of dot hybridizations with cloned DNA probes (87). That cluster is considered to be distinct from other clusters, including an aster yellows MLO genomic strain cluster (87). In addition, the placement by Chiykowski and Sinha (14) of eastern aster yellows MLO, western aster yellows MLO, and clover phyllody MLO into a single category (category 1) is consistent with our consideration of these three MLOs as members of the aster yellows MLO genomic strain cluster (79, 80). However, we have considered clover proliferation MLO to represent, along with potato witches' broom MLO, a genomic cluster probably distinct from the aster yellows MLO strain cluster, as judged from dot hybridization analyses of chromosomal DNA (79, 80, 85).

Distinctions among MLOs on the basis of flower symptoms probably reflect differences in MLO genetic determinants. We suggest, however, that such genetic determinants may be quite variable, even within closely related MLOs, and may not be indicative of distinctions at major taxonomic levels such as the MLO species level. The occurrence of both virescence-associated MLOs and reduced flower-associated MLOs as closely interrelated strains in the aster yellows strain cluster (79, 80) is consistent with the concept that induction of flower symptoms may be determined by relatively minor, highly variable genes in MLOs.

Classification of MLOs on the basis of symptoms characterizing plant infection by the MLOs could provide an important basis for fundamental investigations of MLOs. Such classification coupled with genetic studies conceivably could lead to identification of MLO genes determining symptom induction.

Host range

Both plants and insects serve as MLO hosts; MLOs are not known to exist in nature outside of living host tissues. MLOs multiply in and induce systemic infections in both plant and insect hosts. Symptoms of infection in insects have been studied in fewer cases than have symptoms in infected plants. Typically, insect infection results in reduced longevity and fecundity, but increased survival and reproduction on normally inhospitable host plants have been reported (95; reviewed in references 96 and 108). Ultrastructural aspects and cytopathology of MLO infections, and changes in feeding habits as a result of apparent MLO infection, have been described (95, 108; reviewed in references 96 and 108).

Development of a characteristic symptom syndrome in diseased plants, as noted above, and transmission of pathogens by phloem-feeding leafhoppers or psyllids have long been considered distinctive of the yellows diseases and their causal agents. When the causal pathogens were believed to be viruses, these biological properties collectively defined the plant yellows diseases and set the presumed causal viruses apart from other plant pathogens. These properties continue to be important in describing yellows diseases and attributes of the causal pathogens now that the pathogens are believed to be MLOs. In addition, the particular range of plant species susceptible to infection by a yellows disease pathogen and the identities of insect species capable of transmitting the pathogen from plant to plant are important properties by which the causal agents of yellows diseases have traditionally been identified and classified (41, 42, 51, 69, 70; reviewed in reference 107). These biological properties continue to distinguish yellows diseases in general from other types of diseases, they continue to be distinctive of the pathogens, now believed to be MLOs, and they have been used to identify and classify the presumptive MLO pathogens.

Experimentally determined plant host ranges and ranges of insect vector species are typically broader than those observed in nature (42, 69). Considerable overlap exists, particularly in experimentally determined plant host ranges. Chiykowski and Sinha (14) recently presented an interesting and informative discussion of these aspects of MLOs and MLO diseases, concluding that differentiation of MLOs on the basis of host range is of limited value. In work by these researchers, the transmission of western aster yellows MLO by the vector *Aphrodes bicinctus* depended on the identity of the plant species to which transmission was attempted. This insect acquired the MLO readily from aster and transmitted it efficiently to clover and chrysanthemum, but it did not readily transmit the MLO to aster. In transmission experiments involving clover phyllody MLO, aster was highly susceptible when inoculated by *Macrosteles fascifrons* but highly resistant when inoculated by *A. bicinctus*. Most plant species found susceptible to infection by peach X-disease MLO were also susceptible to infection by clover yellow edge MLO, but some differences in plant host ranges were observed. These differences possibly could be explained, as noted by Chiykowski and Sinha (14), by differences in vector feeding. The two MLOs could be distinguished from one another on the basis of vector specificity; for example, peach X-disease MLO but not clover yellow edge MLO was transmitted by *Scaphytopius acutus*. Peach X-disease MLOs were efficiently transmitted by *Paraphlepsius irroratus* whereas clover yellow edge MLO was inefficiently transmitted by this insect, and clover yellow edge MLO was efficiently transmitted by *Aphrodes bicinctus* but inconsistently transmitted by *P. irroratus*. Since similar symptoms were induced in infected plants and few biological properties distinguished the two MLOs, these authors placed peach X-disease MLO and clover yellow edge MLO into their category 2, principally on the basis of type of symptoms induced in infected plants. Consideration of these MLOs as belonging to one category is consistent with their placement by Lee et al. (87) into a single MLO strain cluster along with western X-disease MLO (see Table 1).

The range of plant species capable of serving as hosts for a given MLO and the range of insect species capable of transmitting the MLO are determined experimentally (14, 41, 69, 118). Under controlled conditions, healthy leafhoppers are permitted an acquisition access period on diseased plants during which the MLO is acquired by the feeding insect. This is followed by an incubation period during which the MLO multiplies in the insect prior to the insect's becoming inoculative, that is, capable of transmitting the MLO to a healthy plant. Although some nonvector insects may acquire an MLO by feeding (95, 96, 108), the identities of such species have not been utilized to aid in the identification or classification of MLOs. In practice, only a relatively small number of plant and insect species are tested as hosts and vectors of causal pathogens. This number is limited by, among other factors, difficulties in raising healthy leafhoppers of some species and by insect feeding preferences. Nevertheless, valuable information can be obtained from comparative studies of MLOs on the basis of their experimental transmission by a selected series of insect species to a specific range of plants. As in the case of symptom syndromes induced in infected plants, similarities and differences in species of insects transmitting MLOs and in species of plant hosts probably reflect genetic determinants in the MLOs as well as the genetics of plant and insect hosts.

It is interesting in this connection that the aster yellows MLO strain cluster (23, 78, 82) contains many MLOs that are transmitted by *Macrosteles* species and are capable of infecting the same general range of plant species (69). Admittedly, the feeding preference of a given insect species may be a major factor in determining ability of the insect to transmit an MLO to or from a given plant species. Thus, feeding preference could influence observed insect transmissibility and plant host range of an MLO, assuming that more suitable insect vectors are not used. However, since many MLO strains in the aster yellows MLO strain cluster appear to be similar in their insect transmission and plant host characteristics, it may be that the MLO genes influencing plant host range and transmissibility by insect species are less variable that those determining symptom induction, in view of the preceding discussion on symptoms.

Serological Assays

Plant-pathogenic spiroplasmas and many other spiroplasmas associated with insects (vectors or nonvectors), ticks, and flower surfaces have been cultured in vitro (reviewed in references 5, 7, 18a, and 128). Sensitive serological assays have been routinely used for identification and classification of these spiroplasmas (22, 59; reviewed in references 5, 13, 22, 59, and 97). The assays have been done with antisera or monoclonal antibodies (MAbs) prepared against cultivatable spiroplasmas. Such an approach has not been feasible for uncultured MLOs until recently, when partially purified MLOs have been used as immunogens (15, 58, 76, 92). Partial purification of MLOs from infected plants was first attempted by Sinha (reviewed in references 120 and 121) and later by others (15, 58, 76). Using partially purified MLO preparations (intact organisms or membrane fractions) as immunogens, antisera and MAbs have been raised against several MLOs, including aster yellows, clover phyllody, peach X-disease, primula yellows, western X-disease, grapevine flavescence doree, American tomato big bud, stolbur, maize bushy stunt, elm yellows, paulownia witches' broom, and ash yellows (4, 8, 11, 15, 38, 40, 45, 55, 57, 112; reviewed in reference 12).

Polyclonal antisera thus prepared often have relatively low specific titers and react with antigens from healthy plants or insect vectors, although antisera prepared from MLOs purified from insects may have less background reaction with healthy plant antigens (reviewed in references 12 and 61). For this reason, polyclonal antisera are not readily useful for differentiating MLOs. MAbs overcome problems encountered with polyclonal antisera. MAbs produced by hybridoma techniques are monospecific, each reacting with only one epitope of the selected antigen. Through appropriate screening procedures, antibodies that react with plant or insect contaminants in partially purified MLO preparations can be effectively eliminated. The high specificity and sensitivity of MAbs have greatly improved the reliability of immunoidentification techniques. MAbs are particularly useful to differentiate among closely related strains of MLOs. Since Lin and Chen (92) developed the first MAbs against New Jersey aster yellows MLO, several other MLO-specific MAbs have been produced (11, 15, 40, 45, 57, 123; reviewed in reference 12). Undoubtedly, use of MAbs will significantly facilitate identification and classification of uncultured MLOs. The following serological procedures are commonly applied for assaying MLOs.

ELISA

The enzyme-linked immunosorbent assay (ELISA) is highly sensitive and has been applied for identification and differentiation of plant-pathogenic spiroplasmas (13; reviewed in references 12 and 120). It has also been used to assay *S. citri* and *S. kunkelii* in leafhoppers and is sensitive enough to detect spiroplasmas in individual infected insects (13, 59; reviewed in reference 97). Recently, ELISA has been used to assay uncultured MLOs. The ELISA in conjunction with immunofluorescence microscopy using MAbs has become one of the most reliable means for diagnosis of MLO-induced diseases (13, 93; reviewed in reference 53).

Earlier attempts, using polyclonal antisera prepared from partially purified MLOs in ELISAs for identification of MLOs in infected plants, indicated that polyclonal antisera could not readily differentiate among some related MLO strains (reviewed in reference 120). With appropriate controls (for example, cross-absorbing antisera with healthy plant extracts prior to use in assays), these antisera clearly detected disease-specific antigens in infected plants and, in most cases, differentiated among distantly related MLOs (15, 38; reviewed in reference 120).

The use of MAbs has greatly improved both the specificity and sensitivity of the ELISA for MLOs. For example, Clark et al. (15) noted that the MAbs raised against primula yellows cross-reacted with a European strain of aster yellows but differentiated aster yellows from clover phyllody MLO. These latter two MLOs could not be differentiated with polyclonal antisera (reviewed in reference 120). As noted by Lin and Chen (92), MAbs raised against New Jersey aster yellows reacted only with this aster yellows strain. ELISA using MLO-specific MAbs has also been applied for

detection of MLOs in individual insect vectors (4; reviewed in reference 13).

Dot blot immunoassay

A dot blot immunoassay has been used for detection of spiroplasmas (reviewed in reference 13) and was recently used for diagnosis of MLO infection (4, 55). MLO antigens in crude extracts were first dot blotted on nitrocellulose membranes. The blots were reacted with mouse MAbs and detected with alkaline phosphatase-labeled goat anti-mouse immunoglobulin antibodies. Distinct purple precipitates on the blots indicated positive reactions. As noted by Hsu et al. (55), the sensitivity in these dot blot immunoassays was about 1.5 orders of magnitude greater than that of indirect ELISA, which usually exhibits higher background in negative controls. A simplified blotting procedure, tissue blotting, in which a freshly cut tissue surface is pressed directly on nitrocellulose membranes, was developed and applied for detection of plant virus and MLOs (94). In the tissue blotting technique, specific antigens on nitrocellulose membranes are immunologically visualized with enzyme-labeled antibodies. Examination of immunologically stained tissue blots of infected leaf tissue (cross sections) revealed that MLO antigens were restricted, in leaves, to phloem cells of midrib and secondary veins.

Dot blot immunoassays using tomato big bud MLO-specific MAbs were recently used to differentiate MLO strains in the aster yellows MLO strain cluster (Table 1) (86). These MAbs specifically reacted with tomato big bud MLO (designated a type I strain) and with all other type I strains in the aster yellows MLO strain cluster. No other MLOs reacted. The dot blot immunoassay can also be applied for detection of MLOs in insect vectors (40).

Immunofluorescence microscopy

Indirect immunofluorescence staining, usually in conjunction with the ELISA, has been widely applied for diagnosis of MLO infections (6, 57, 88, 121, 123, 125; reviewed in references 53 and 120). The immunofluorescence microscopy assay is very sensitive, specific, and simple to use to provide in situ detection of MLOs in sections of infected plant or insect tissues. Although polyclonal antisera can be used in this type of assay for detection of MLOs in infected tissues, for identification of an MLO of interest, or for differentiation among MLOs, use of MAbs is preferred. Immunofluorescence microscopy may be very useful for revealing the intracellular distribution of mycoplasmas at the light microscopy level (reviewed in reference 53).

ISEM

Immunosorbent electron microscopy (ISEM) has been used for detection of aster yellows MLO in preparations partially purified from infected tissues (reviewed in references 120 and 121). Grids coated with antiserum specifically trapped the aster yellows MLO in the preparations. ISEM has also been used to detect other MLOs (reviewed in reference 120). In addition, the ISEM technique appears to be promising for detection of MLOs in individual insect vectors (reviewed in references 120 and 121).

Nucleic Acid-Based Techniques

Recombinant DNA technology has made it possible to clone fragments of MLO chromosomal or extrachromosomal DNA (plasmids) from MLO-infected insects (18, 66) and plants (3, 9, 10, 19, 23–26, 34, 46, 49, 50, 67, 68, 71–74, 78, 81, 82, 84, 85, 87, 105, 113, 116, 124). The procedures used to enrich MLO titers in plant or insect extracts for production of MLO-specific MAbs have been adopted for preparation of MLO DNA-enriched extracts for molecular cloning. Kirkpatrick et al. (66) first successfully cloned DNA fragments from the insect vector *Colladonas montanus* (Van Duzee) infected with western X-disease MLO. Thus far, DNA fragments have been cloned from at least 20 MLO strains: Western X-disease (66, 87), Maryland aster yellows (78), maize bushy stunt (18), *Oenothera* virescence (113), apple proliferation (68), periwinkle little leaf 0-1 (23), elm yellows (81), tomato big bud (81, 82), clover proliferation (34, 84, 85), ash yellows (26), beet leafhopper-transmitted virescence (84, 116), Canada peach X-disease (87), walnut witches' broom (9, 10), paulownia witches' broom (125), pigeon pea witches' broom (50), lethal yellowing of palm (49), rice yellow dwarf (105), grapevine flavescence doree (19, 46), Italian periwinkle virescence (19), and blueberry stunt (124). Use of cloned MLO DNA fragments as molecular probes in DNA-DNA hybridization permits sensitive and specific detection of these MLOs in infected plant or insect tissues. Furthermore, cloned DNA probes of various MLOs can be used to evaluate the overall genetic interrelatedness among uncultured MLOs. This ability makes it possible, for the first time, to establish a genetically based MLO classification.

Dot hybridization assay

Cloned MLO DNAs or their complementary RNAs (83) used as probes (^{32}P labeled or labeled with nonradioactive biotin) have been applied widely in dot hybridization assays to detect and identify these pathogens in plant and insect hosts (1–3, 9, 10, 18, 23, 26, 32, 35, 52, 62, 66, 68, 78, 83, 85, 87, 105, 113, 115, 117). The sensitivity of MLO detection by dot hybridization assay seems to exceed that by the ELISA method, since the dot hybridization assay (using ^{32}P-labeled probes) readily detects MLOs in small groups and in individual leafhoppers (24, 66).

Cloned DNA probes have been used to evaluate the genetic relatedness of MLOs. For example, cloned DNA fragments (^{32}P labeled) of the western X-disease MLO showed relatively high homology with the DNA of MLOs associated with Eastern peach X-disease and peach yellows as well as pecan bunchy and walnut witches' broom disease. Little homology was found with DNA of any other MLOs tested (62). Plasmids (extrachromosomal DNA) of the western aster yellows MLO were found to have homology with plasmids from other plant-pathogenic MLOs (73, 74). By using a number of probes derived from various MLOs in dot hybridization assays, overall genetic interrelatedness among these MLOs can be investigated. With this ap-

proach, we have identified several strains of MLOs, including aster yellows MLO, which share extensive sequence homology with one another but have relatively little homology with other strains of MLO (23–25, 78, 81, 82). We proposed that those strains should be classified into a genomic group, termed the aster yellows genomic strain cluster (78). Subsequently, several distinct genomic strain clusters (Table 1), including the elm yellows MLO, peach X-disease MLO, and beet leafhopper-transmitted virescence MLO clusters, were identified on the basis of analyses by dot hybridizations (81, 84, 87). As more cloned MLO DNA probes from various sources become available for DNA hybridization assays, genetic characteristics, rather than insect transmission characteristics and phenotypic or pathological characteristics exhibited by infected hosts, will provide a more reliable basis for MLO classification. As noted by us (80) and others (75), the classification of MLOs on the basis of biological properties is not always consistent with their phylogenetic relationships.

RFLP

Restriction fragment length polymorphism (RFLP) analysis has been used for differentiation of closely related spiroplasmas (reviewed in reference 5). In conjunction with dot or Southern hybridization analysis, RFLP has recently been used for differentiation and classification of MLOs (19, 35, 75, 80, 84, 85, 87). Using cloned chromosomal DNA probes, derived from the severe strain of the western aster yellows MLO in Southern blot hybridization, and RFLP analysis, Kuske et al. (75) were able to differentiate among virescence-inducing MLOs from various sources. Three distinct groups were identified on the basis of RFLP patterns. Using dot hybridization and RFLP analyses, Lee et al. (85) and Deng and Hiruki (35) determined that the potato witches' broom MLO and the clover proliferation MLO are closely related strains of the same MLO. RFLP patterns of these latter two MLOs were almost identical, indicating very similar genomic organization. A comparative study of grapevine flavescence doree and southern European grapevine yellows by RFLP analysis revealed that these MLOs are related but distinct from each other (19). Recently, an extensive and systematic RFLP analysis was conducted to differentiate numerous strains in the aster yellows MLO strain cluster (80). Twenty-two probes derived from three MLO strains in this strain cluster were used in Southern hybridizations and RFLP analyses. Similarity coefficients derived from RFLP analyses indicated that strains in the aster yellows MLO strain cluster can be classified into three distinct genotypic groups: type I, type II, and type III (Table 1). Many strains, previously designated either eastern aster yellows or as western aster yellows MLO on the basis of biological properties, were reclassified. Some undesignated MLO strains and strains previously designated under other disease names (e.g., clover phyllody, chrythanthemum yellows, and tomato big bud) were reevaluated and designated members of the aster yellows MLO strain cluster. This classification is consistent with results from serological assays using MAbs (see above).

PCR

Relatively low titers and an uneven distribution of MLOs in plant hosts have been obstacles to accurate diagnosis of MLO-induced plant diseases. This problem is particularly important, for example, in screening for disease-free planting stocks. Highly sensitive means are required for routine detection and identification of MLOs in samples collected from symptomless or apparently healthy plants. Sensitive MLO detection is also important in identification of potential insect vector species. The polymerase chain reaction (PCR) assay, in which copies of target DNA fragments present in samples are extensively amplified, may provide the most sensitive means available for pathogen detection.

By using primer pairs designed on the basis of the sequence of an MLO DNA fragment, target DNA can be specifically amplified and detected by agarose or polyacrylamide gel electrophoresis and ethidium bromide staining. Preliminary results from our laboratory and others have shown the PCR assay to be valuable in MLO detection (33, 110, 111). PCR has been successfully applied for detection and identification of MLOs in crops (33, 111) and trees (e.g., elm and palm) in which MLO titers are relatively low and may not be readily detected by serological or DNA hybridization assays (48a, 78a). PCR has also been used to assay individual insect vectors and study MLO-vector interaction (126). By using multiple primer pairs constructed from several well-characterized key probes in PCR assays, various MLO strains, including closely related ones, can be readily differentiated (78a, 110, 111).

rRNA sequences

Studies by Lim and Sears (89), Kirkpatrick and Fraser (63), and Kuske and Kirkpatrick (72) on analysis of 16S rRNA sequences of *Oenothera* virescence, western X-disease, and western aster yellows MLOs, respectively, have indicated the phylogenetic status of the uncultured MLOs. The evidence that 16S rRNA genes from MLOs have greater sequence homology with the 16S rRNA genes of animal mycoplasmas than with those of any other procaryote has placed MLOs in the family *Mycoplasmatales*. Therefore, it appears that plant-inhabiting MLOs could be termed mycoplasmas, the trival name used for all members of the class *Mollicutes*. Additional studies by Lim et al. (90, 91) suggest that MLOs are distinct from animal *Mycoplasma* species and are more closely linked with the genus *Acholeplasma*, although the genome sizes of MLOs may be more similar to those of some *Mycoplasma* species (90, 106).

Comparative study of 16S rRNA genes from three strains of MLO has shown that two copies of 16S rRNA genes are present in the western aster yellows chromosome, whereas only one copy is present in western X-disease MLO, and that there is 89% sequence homology between these genes in western aster yellows and western X-disease MLO and 99.5% sequence homology between 16S rRNA genes of western aster yellows and *Oenothera* virescence MLOs (65).

Selected MLO-specific rRNA oligonucleotide sequences have been applied for detection and differentiation of MLOs in infected plant tissues (64). Recently, we have designed PCR primers on the basis of a 16S RNA gene sequence published by Lim and Sears (89) for the *Oenothera* virescence MLO. PCR utilizing these primers has identified and differentiated among MLOs. Two of the primer pairs specifically amplified a target DNA sequence of equal size in all MLO strains in the aster yellows MLO strain cluster, thus separating members of this cluster from all other MLOs examined and yielding cluster-specific reactions (78a).

This delineation of the aster yellows strain cluster MLOs from other MLOs by PCR coincides with our earlier delineation of this cluster by use of cloned random MLO DNA fragments as probes in hybridization assays.

TREATMENT

For control of mycoplasmas that infect plants and insect vectors, the primary concern is usually prevention rather than treatment. MLO-associated diseases are managed through planting clean (disease-free) stocks or disease-resistant varieties, through application of certain cultural practices (e.g., control of insect vectors), and through chemotherapy.

Clean Stock

Proper quarantine practice prevents importation of exotic mycoplasmas and potential insect vectors. Production of clean (or disease-free) stocks through shoot tip (51), callus (103), or meristem tissue culture (43, 51), sometimes in combination with either heat or antibiotic treatment (51), can eliminate MLOs from plants. Plant-pathogenic MLOs are generally heat labile (at 37°C) and are not present in plant meristems (6). A critical step is to ensure the absence of pathogens in treated material, traditionally by indexing through graft inoculation of sensitive indicator host plants.

Insect Vectors and Alternate Plant Hosts

Control of insect vectors can be important for effective regulation of MLO-induced diseases. No evidence indicates that MLOs are transmitted transovarially. Overwintering adult insect vectors often account for the initial disease incidence in early spring. Weed plant hosts of MLOs can act as sources of inoculum (14, 69; reviewed in reference 99) and are subjected to control in some cases. Culture practices such as manipulating planting dates (to escape infections by insect vectors) or applying insecticides (often systemic) to reduce insect populations can also be important factors for successful control of disease spread. To reemphasize, sensitive and reliable means for detection of MLOs are essential for identification of insect vectors or alternate plant hosts. For example, a highly useful application of the PCR technique in the future could be for indexing potential insect vectors for their MLO infection status and use of this information, along with data on insect migrations, to predict new disease outbreaks and MLO disease spread.

Resistance

Breeding of resistant varieties can provide an alternative approach to avoid devastating infectious MLOs. This potentially useful method of MLO disease control has been practiced in relatively few cases (60, 101, 102), such as to obtain eggplant resistant to little leaf disease (101), elm resistant to elm yellows (102), and coconut resistant to lethal yellowing (100). However, efficient breeding for disease resistance has long been hampered by lack of reliable and sensitive means to detect MLO infection.

Chemotherapy

In retrospect, it is interesting that as early as 1947, the antibiotic sensitivity of a yellows disease was reported, when viruses were believed to be the causal pathogens (122). The sensitivity of MLOs, and the diseases with which they are associated, to tetracycline antibiotics was well established in the pioneering work by Ishiie et al. (56) and in subsequent studies in the late 1960s and the 1970s (28; reviewed in reference 104). Treatment with tetracyclines for MLO disease control has been extended to a few crop plants, such as peach for control of X-disease, coconut for control of lethal yellowing, and sandal wood (*Santalum album*) for control of spike disease (reviewed in references 104 and 109).

Tetracycline antibiotics are usually applied to trees by using a pressure injection apparatus. In the case of peach, for example, treatment with as little as 0.5 to 1.0 g per tree once a year is effective and economical in control of X-disease (reviewed in reference 109).

CONCLUDING REMARKS

Traditionally, the association of an MLO with a plant disease has been inferred on the basis of disease symptoms, followed in some cases by treatment with tetracycline antibiotics and electron microscopy to determine the presence of MLOs in phloem tissues. These procedures, in effect, were used to identify, or classify, a pathogen as a probable MLO. Identification and differentiation of various MLOs associated with disease have long relied upon similarities and differences in MLO biological properties and characteristics of their associated diseases. The procedures to identify a presumed pathogen as an MLO, and reliance on biological properties to differentiate and identify an MLO, are time-consuming and not completely applicable to all MLOs. Biological properties of some MLOs are difficult to determine; for example, insect vectors of many MLOs are still unknown. The development of MLO-specific serological and DNA hybridization assays has provided rapid and reliable means for detection and identification of MLOs. These techniques have also made it feasible to investigate the genetic relatedness among various MLO strains, which has led to the establishment of a molecular genetic classification scheme.

MLOs are believed to cause diseases in several hundred plant species and are associated with numerous insects. These hosts undoubtedly harbor a broad array of MLOs. A classification scheme based on molecular genetics can permit a systematic process for identification of these pathogens. Investigation of genetic interrelationships among MLOs from various sources by using newly developed molecular assays has resulted in the recognition of several genomic strain clusters. Each cluster consists of MLO strains which share extensive nucleotide sequence homology with one another. Within a single cluster, the aster yellows MLO strain cluster, at least three genotypic groups, designated types I, II, and III, have been delineated.

Investigations of rRNA genes have indicated that MLOs are related to but distinct from animal mycoplasmas, possibly having a close evolutionary link with acholeplasmas. Known nucleotide sequences of highly conserved genes such as rRNA genes are useful for investigating evolutionary relationships. Conceivably, rRNA genes can provide a basis both for differentiating closely related strains and for developing molecular assays for universal detection of MLOs. Recently, we designed a pair of oligonucleotide primers, on the basis of an MLO 16S rRNA sequence, useful in PCR detection and identification of all members of the aster yellows MLO strain cluster. This delineation of an MLO genomic strain cluster by PCR coincides with our earlier delineation of the cluster by use of cloned random MLO DNA fragments as probes in hybridization assays and indicates a new approach for determining the cluster affinity of unknown MLOs.

Serological assays continue to play an important role in MLO identification. MAbs reveal sharing of single epitopes among related MLOs and thus appear to be highly useful for establishing identities between closely related MLOs. Polyclonal antisera can potentially reveal sharing of epitopes among a broader array of MLOs, although production of highly MLO-specific polyclonal antisera is still difficult. Although serological assays probably could be developed for MLO strain cluster definition, to date classification of MLOs into a system of strain clusters has been accomplished through DNA-based methods.

Future applications of DNA-based methods undoubtedly will include frequent use of PCR. We expect that PCR will enable very sensitive detection of MLOs and identification of cluster and subcluster (type) affiliations. Through the use of primer pairs derived from well-characterized cloned random fragment DNA probes or known gene nucleotide sequences, PCR should become an important tool for MLO identification and classification.

REFERENCES

1. **Bertaccini, A., R. E. Davis, and I.-M. Lee.** 1990. Distinctions among mycoplasmalike organisms (MLOs) in *Gladiolus, Ranunculus, Brassica,* and *Hydrangea* through detection with nonradioactive cloned DNA probes. *Phytopathol. Mediterr.* **29:**107–113.
2. **Bertaccini, A., R. E. Davis, I.-M. Lee, M. Conti, E. L. Dally, and S. M. Douglas.** 1990. Detection of chrysanthemum yellows mycoplasmalike organism by dot hybridization and Southern blot analysis. *Plant Dis.* **74:**40–43.
3. **Bonnet, F., C. Saillard, A. Kollar, E. Seemüller, F. Dosba, and J. M. Bové.** 1990. Molecular probes for the

apple proliferation MLO. *Zentralbl. Bakteriol. Suppl.* **20:**908–909.

4. **Boudon-Padieu, E., J. Larrue, and A. Caudwell.** 1989. ELISA and dot-blot detection of flavescence doree-MLO in individual leafhopper vectors during latency and inoculative state. *Curr. Microbiol.* **19:**357–364.

5. **Bové, J. M., P. Carle, M. Garnier, F. Laigret, J. Renaudin, and C. Saillard.** 1989. Molecular and cellular biology of spiroplasmas, p. 243–364. *In* R. F. Whitcomb and J. G. Tully (ed.), *The Mycoplasmas*, vol. 5. Academic Press, New York.

6. **Caudwell, A., E. Boudon-Padieu, J. Lherminier, Y. Schwartz, and P. Meignoz.** 1990. Current spread of the grapevine yellows and characterization methods for the MLO pathogen. *Zentralbl. Bakteriol. Suppl.* **20:**916–918.

7. **Chang, C. J.** 1989. Nutrition and cultivation of spiroplasmas, p. 201–241. *In* R. F. Whitcomb and J. G. Tully (ed.), *The Mycoplasmas*, vol. 5. Academic Press, New York.

8. **Chang, T. I., and T. A. Chen.** 1991. Utilization of monoclonal antibodies against elm yellows mycoplasmalike organisms in detection of elm yellows disease. *Phytopathology* **81:**121.

9. **Chen, J., and C. J. Chang.** 1991. Plasmid-like DNAs with a mycoplasma-like organism (MLO) and their seasonal occurrence. *Phytopathology* **81:**1169.

10. **Chen, J., C. J. Chang, R. Jarret, and N. Gawel.** 1992. Isolation and cloning of DNA fragments from mycoplasmalike organism associated with walnut witches'-broom disease. *Phytopathology* **82:**306–309.

11. **Chen, T. A., and X. F. Jiang.** 1988. Monoclonal antibodies against the maize bushy stunt agent. *Can. J. Mirobiol.* **34:**6–11.

12. **Chen, T. A., and Y. P. Jiang.** 1990. Progress in the detection of plant mycoplasmalike organisms by using monoclonal and polyclonal antibodies. *Zentralbl. Bakteriol. Suppl.* **20:**270–275.

13. **Chen, T. A., J. D. Lei, and C. P. Lin.** 1989. Detection and identification of plant and insect mollicutes, p. 393–424. *In* R. F. Whitcomb and J. G. Tully (ed.), *The Mycoplasmas*, vol. 5. Academic Press, New York.

14. **Chiykowski, L. N., and R. C. Sinha.** 1990. Differentiation of MLO diseases by means of symptomatology and vector transmission. *Zentralbl. Bakteriol. Suppl.* **20:**280–287.

15. **Clark, M. F., A. Morten, and S. L. Buss.** 1989. Preparation of mycoplasma immunogens from plants and a comparison of polyclonal and monoclonal antibodies made against primula yellows MLO-associated antigens. *Ann. Appl. Biol.* **114:**111–124.

16. **Cousin, M. T., A. K. Sharma, and S. Misra.** 1986. Correlation between light and electron microscopic observations and identification of mycoplasmalike organisms using consecutive 350 nm thick sections. *Phytopathol. Z.* **115:**368–374.

17. **Davis, M. J., M. Konai, and W.-C. Bak.** 1990. Electrophoretic separation of chromosomal DNA of mycoplasma-like organisms. *IOM Lett.* **1:**231–232.

18. **Davis, M. J., J. H. Tsai, R. L. Cox, L. L. McDaniel, and N. A. Harrison.** 1988. Cloning of chromosomal and extrachromosomal DNA of the mycoplasma-like organism that causes maize bushy stunt disease. *Mol. Plant-Microbe Interact.* **1:**295–302.

18a.**Davis, R. E.** 1981. The enigma of the flower spiroplasmas, p. 259–279. *In* K. Maramorosch and S. P. Raychaudhuri (ed.), *Mycoplasma Diseases of Trees and Shrubs.* Academic Press, Inc., New York.

19. **Davis, R. E., E. L. Dally, A. Bertaccini, R. Credi, R. Osler, V. Savino, E. Refatti, B. Di Terlizzi, M. Barba, and I.-M. Lee.** 1992. RFLP analyses and dot hybridization of chromosomal DNA distinguish two mycoplasmalike organisms (MLOs) associated with grapevine yellows disease. *Phytopathology* **82:**242.

20. **Davis, R. E., and I.-M. Lee.** 1982. Comparative properties of spiroplasmas and emerging taxonomic concepts—a proposal. *Rev. Infect. Dis.* **4**(Suppl.):122–128.

21. **Davis, R. E., and I.-M. Lee.** 1982. Pathogenicity of spiroplasmas, mycoplasmalike organisms, vascular-limited fastidious walled bacteria, p. 491–513. *In* M. S. Mount and G. H. Lacy (ed.), *Phytopathogenic Prokaryotes*, vol. 1. Academic Press, New York.

22. **Davis, R. E., I.-M. Lee, and L. K. Basciano.** 1979. Spiroplasmas: serological grouping of strains associated with plants and insects. *Can. J. Microbiol.* **25:**861–866.

23. **Davis, R. E., I.-M. Lee, S. M. Douglas, and E. L. Dally.** 1990. Molecular cloning and detection of chromosomal and extrachromosomal DNA of the mycoplasmalike organism (MLO) associated with little leaf disease in periwinkle (*Catharanthus roseus*). *Phytopathology* **80:**789–793.

24. **Davis, R. E., I.-M. Lee, S. M. Douglas, E. L. Dally, and N. D. DeWitt.** 1988. Cloned nucleic acid hybridization probes in detection and classification of mycoplasmalike organisms (MLOs). *Acta Hortic.* **234:**115–122.

25. **Davis, R. E., I.-M. Lee, S. M. Douglas, E. L. Dally, and N. DeWitt.** 1990. Development and use of cloned nucleic acid hybridization probes for disease diagnosis and detection of sequence homologies among uncultured mycoplasmalike organisms (MLOs). *Zentralbl. Bakteriol. Suppl.* **20:**303–307.

26. **Davis, R. E., I.-M. Lee, W. A. Sinclair, and E. L. Dally.** 1991. Cloned DNA probes specific for detection of a mycoplasmalike organism associated with ash yellows. *Mol. Plant-Microbe Interact.* **5:**163–169.

27. **Davis, R. E., and R. F. Whitcomb.** 1970. Evidence on possible mycoplasma etiology of aster yellows disease. I. Suppression of symptom development in plants by antibiotics. *Infect. Immun.* **2:**201–208.

28. **Davis, R. E., R. F. Whitcomb, and R. L. Steere.** 1968. Remission of aster yellows disease by antibiotics. *Science* **161:**793–795.

29. **Davis, R. E., and J. F. Worley.** 1973. Spiroplasma: motile, helical microorganism associated with corn stunt disease. *Phytopathology* **63:**403–408.

30. **Davis, R. E., J. F. Worley, R. F. Whitcomb, T. Ishijima, and R. L. Steere.** 1972. Helical filaments produced by a mycoplasma-like organism associated with corn stunt disease. *Science* **176:**521–523.

31. **Deeley, J., W. A. Stevens, and R. T. V. Fox.** 1979. Uses of Dienes' stain to detect plant diseases induced by mycoplasmalike organisms. *Phytopathology* **69:**1169–1171.

32. **Deng, S., and C. Hiruki.** 1990. The use of cloned DNA probes for diagnosis of noncultivable plant mollicutes. *Proc. Jpn. Acad.* **66:**58–61.

33. **Deng, S., and C. Hiruki.** 1990. Enhanced detection of a plant pathogenic mycoplasma-like organism by polymerase chain reaction. *Proc. Jpn. Acad.* **66:**140–144.

34. **Deng, S., and C. Hiruki.** 1990. Molecular cloning and detection of DNA of the mycoplasmalike organism associated with clover proliferation. *Can. J. Plant Pathol.* **12:**383–388.

35. **Deng, S., and C. Hiruki.** 1991. Genetic relatedness between two nonculturable mycoplasmalike organisms revealed by nucleic acid hybridization and polymerase chain reaction. *Phytopathology* **81:**1475–1479.

36. **Doi, Y. M., M. Teranaka, K. Yora, and H. Asuyama.** 1967. Mycoplasma or PLT-group-like microorganisms found in the phloem elements of plants infected with mulberry dwarf, potato witches' broom, aster yellows, or paulownia witches' broom. *Ann. Phytopathol. Soc. Jpn.* **33:**259–266.

37. **Errampalli, D., J. Fletcher, and P. L. Claypool.** 1991. Incidence of yellows in carrot and lettuce and characterization of mycoplasmalike organism isolates in Oklahoma. *Plant Dis.* **75:**579–584.

38. **Errampalli, D., J. Fletcher, and J. L. Sherwood.** 1989.

Production of monospecific polyclonal antibodies against the aster yellows mycoplasma-like organisms (AY MLO) of Oklahoma. *Phytopathology* **79**:1137.

39. **Freundt, E. A.** 1979. Isolation, characterization, and identification of spiroplasmas and MLOs, p. 1–34. *In* K. Maramorosch and S. P. Raychaudhuri (ed.), *Mycoplasma Diseases of Trees and Shrubs*. Academic Press, New York.

40. **Garnier, M., G. Martin-Gros, M. Iskra, L. Zreik, J. Gandar, A. Fos, and J. M. Bové.** 1990. Monclonal antibodies against the MLOs associated with tomato stolbur and clover phyllody. *Zentralbl. Bakteriol. Suppl.* **20**:263–269.

41. **Golino, D. A., G. N. Oldfield, and D. J. Gumpf.** 1987. Transmission characteristics of the beet leafhopper transmitted virescence agent. *Phytopathology* **77**:954–957.

42. **Granados, R. R., and R. K. Chapman.** 1968. Identification of some new aster yellows virus strains and their transmission by the aster leafhopper, *Macrosteles fascifrons. Phytopathology* **58**:1685–1692.

43. **Green, S. K., C. Y. Luo, and D. R. Lee.** 1989. Elimination of mycoplasma-like organisms from witches' broom infected sweet potato. *Phytopathol. Z.* **126**:204–212.

44. **Griffiths, H. M., W. A. Sinclair, I.-M. Lee, and R. E. Davis.** 1991. DAPI fluorescence versus DNA probes for detecting mycoplasmalike organisms in woody plants and insects. *Phytopathology* **81**:1210.

45. **Guo, J. R., T. A. Chen, and N. Loi.** 1991. Production of monoclonal antibodies against flavescence doree mycoplasma-like organism. *Phytopathology* **81**:1210.

46. **Guo, J. R., T. A. Chen, N. Loi, and R. C. Pearson.** 1992. Cloning of chromosomal DNA of the mycoplasmalike organism (ML) associated with grapevine flavescence doree. *Phytopathology* **82**:243.

47. **Hackett, K. J., and T. B. Clark.** 1989. Ecology of spiroplasmas, p. 113–200. *In* R. F. Whitcomb and J. G. Tully (ed.), *The Mycoplasmas*, vol. 5. Academic Press, New York.

48. **Haggis, G. H., and R. C. Sinha.** 1978. Scanning electron microscopy of mycoplasma-like organisms after freeze fracture of plant tissues affected with clover phyllody and aster yellows. *Phytopathology* **68**:677–680.

48a.**Hammond, R. W., R. E. Davis, and N. A. Harrison.** Unpublished data.

49. **Harrison, N. A., C. M. Bourne, R. L. Cox, J. H. Tsai, and P. A. Richardson.** 1992. DNA probes for detection of mycoplasmalike organisms associated with lethal yellowing disease of palms in Florida. *Phytopathology* **82**:216–224.

50. **Harrison, N. A., J. H. Tsai, C. M. Bourne, and P. A. Richardson.** 1991. Molecular cloning and detection of chromosomal and extrachromosomal DNA of mycoplasmalike organisms associated with witches'-broom disease of pigeon pea in Florida. *Mol. Plant-Microbe Interact.* **4**:300–307.

51. **Heintz, W.** 1989. Transmission of a new mycoplasma-like organism (MLO) from *Cuscuta odorata* (Ruiz. et Pav.) to herbaceous plants and attempts to its elimination in the vector. *Phytopathol. Z.* **125**:171–186.

52. **Hibben, C. R., W. A. Sinclair, R. E. Davis, and J. H. Alexander III.** 1991. Relatedness of mycoplasmalike organisms associated with ash yellows and lilac witches' broom. *Plant Dis.* **75**:1227–1230.

53. **Hiruki, C.** 1988. Immunofluorescence microscopy of yellows diseases associated with plant mycoplasmalike organisms, p. 193–203. *In* C. Hiruki (ed.), *Tree Mycoplasmas and Mycoplasma Diseases*. University of Alberta Press, Edmonton, Alberta, Canada.

54. **Hirumi, H., and K. Maramorosch.** 1973. Ultrastructure of the aster yellows agent. Mycoplasmalike bodies in sieve elements of *Nicotiana rustica. Ann. N.Y. Acad. Sci.* **225**:201–222.

55. **Hsu, H. T., I.-M. Lee, R. E. Davis, and Y. C. Wang.** 1990. Immunization for generation of hybridoma antibodies specifically reacting with plants infected with a mycoplasmalike organism (MLO) and their use in detection of MLO antigens. *Phytopathology* **80**:946–950.

56. **Ishiie, T., Y. Doi, K. Yora, and H. Asuyama.** 1967. Suppressive effects of antibiotics of tetracycline group on symptom development in mullberry dwarf disease. *Ann. Phytopathol. Soc. Jpn.* **33**:267–275.

57. **Jiang, Y. P., T. A. Chen, L. N. Chiykowski, and R. C. Sinha.** 1989. Production of monoclonal antibodies to peach eastern X-disease agent and their use in disease detection. *Can. J. Plant Pathol.* **11**:325–331.

58. **Jiang, Y. P., J. D. Lei, and T. A. Chen.** 1988. Purification of aster yellows agent from diseased lettuce using affinity chromatography. *Phytopathology* **78**:828–831.

59. **Jordan, R. L., M. Konai, I.-M. Lee, and R. E. Davis.** 1989. Species-specific and cross-reactive monoclonal antibodies to the plant-pathogenic spiroplasmas *Spiroplasma citri* and *S. kunkelii. Phytopathology* **79**:880–887.

60. **Keep, E.** 1989. Breeding red raspberry for resistance to diseases and pests. *Plant Breeding Rev.* **6**:245–321.

61. **Kirkpatrick, B. C.** 1989. Strategies for characterizing plant pathogenic mycoplasma-like organisms and their effects on plants, p. 241–293. *In* T. Kosuge and E. W. Nester (ed.), *Plant-Microbe Interactions, Molecular and Genetic Perspectives*, vol. 3. McGraw-Hill, New York.

62. **Kirkpatrick, B. C., G. A. Fisher, J. D. Fraser, and A. H. Purcell.** 1990. Epidemiological and phylogenetic studies on western X-disease mycoplasma-like organisms. *Zentralbl. Bakteriol. Suppl.* **20**:288–297.

63. **Kirkpatrick, B. C., and J. D. Fraser.** 1988. Cloning and partial sequence of the 16S ribosomal RNA gene from the western X-disease mycoplasma-like organism. *Phytopathology* **78**:1541.

64. **Kirkpatrick, B. C., and J. D. Fraser.** 1989. Detection and differentiation of mycoplasma-like organisms using MLO-specific ribosomal RNA oligonucleotide sequences. *Phytopathology* **79**:1206.

65. **Kirkpatrick, B. C., and C. R. Kuske.** 1990. Phylogeny of plant pathogenic mycoplasma-like organisms. *IOM Lett.* **1**:45–46.

66. **Kirkpatrick, B. C., D. C. Stenger, T. J. Morris, and A. H. Purcell.** 1987. Cloning and detection of DNA from a nonculturable plant pathogenic mycoplasma-like organism. *Science.* **238**:197–200.

67. **Kollar, A., and E. Seemüller.** 1989. Base composition of the DNA of mycoplasma-like organisms associated with various plant diseases. *Phytopathol. Z.* **127**:177–186.

68. **Kollar, A., E. Seemüller, F. Bonnet, C. Saillard, and J. M. Bové.** 1990. Isolation of the DNA of various plant pathogenic mycoplasma-like organisms from infected plants. *Phytopathology* **80**:233–237.

69. **Kunkel, L. O.** 1926. Studies on aster yellows. *Am. J. Bot.* **13**:646–705.

70. **Kunkel, L. O.** 1955. Cross protection between strains of yellows-type viruses. *Adv. Virus Res.* **3**:251–273.

71. **Kuske, C. R.** 1989. Molecular characterization of the western aster yellows mycoplasma-like organisms. Ph.D. thesis. University of California, Davis.

72. **Kuske, C. R., and B. C. Kirkpatrick.** 1989. Cloning and sequence analysis of the 16S ribosomal RNA gene of western aster yellows MLO (AY-MLO) *Phytopathology* **79**:1138.

73. **Kuske, C. R., and B. C. Kirkpatrick.** 1990. Isolation and characterization of plasmids from the western aster yellows mycoplasma-like organism. *J. Bacteriol.* **172**:1628–1633.

74. **Kuske, C. R., B. C. Kirkpatrick, J. M. Davis, and E. Seemüller.** 1991. DNA hybridization between western aster yellows mycoplasma-like organism plasmids and extrachromosomal DNA from other plant pathogenic

mycoplasma-like organisms. *Mol. Plant-Microbe Interact.* **4**:75–80.

75. **Kuske, C. R., B. C. Kirkpatrick, and E. Seemüller.** 1991. Differentiation of virescence MLOs using western aster yellows mycoplasma-like organism chromosomal DNA probes and restriction fragment length polymorphism analysis. *J. Gen. Microbiol.* **137**:153–159.

76. **Lee, I.-M., and R. E. Davis.** 1983. Phloem-limited prokaryotes in sieve elements isolated by enzyme treatment of disease plant tissues. *Phytopathology* **73**:1540–1363.

77. **Lee, I.-M., and R. E. Davis.** 1986. Prospects for *in vitro* culture of plant pathogenic mycoplasmalike organisms. *Annu. Rev. Phytopathol.* **24**:339–354.

78. **Lee, I.-M., and R. E. Davis.** 1988. Detection and investigation of genetic relatedness among aster yellows and other mycoplasma-like organisms by using cloned DNA and RNA probes. *Mol. Plant-Microbe Interact.* **1**:303–310.

78a. **Lee, I.-M., and R. E. Davis.** Unpublished data.

79. **Lee, I.-M., R. E. Davis, T. A. Chen, L. N. Chiykowski, J. Fletcher, and C. Hiruki.** 1989. Nucleic acid hybridization distinguishes MLO strain transmitted by *Macrosteles* spp., vectors of aster yellows agent. *Phytopathology* **79**:1137.

80. **Lee, I.-M., R. E. Davis, T.-A. Chen, L. N. Chiykowski, J. Fletcher, and C. Hiruki.** 1991. Classification of MLOs in the aster yellows MLO strain cluster on basis of RFLP analyses. *Phytopathology* **81**:1169.

81. **Lee, I.-M., R. E. Davis, and N. D. DeWitt.** 1988. Molecular cloning of and screening by a new method for DNA fragments from elm yellows (EY) and tomato big bud (BB) mycoplasmalike organisms (MLOs). *Phytopathology* **78**:1602.

82. **Lee, I.-M., R. E. Davis, and N. D. DeWitt.** 1990. Nonradioactive screening method for isolation of disease-specific probes to diagnose plant diseases caused by mycoplasma-like organisms. *Appl. Environ. Microbiol* **56**:1471–1475.

83. **Lee, I.-M., R. E. Davis, R. Hammond, and B. C. Kirkpatrick.** 1988. Cloned riboprobe for detection of a mycoplasmalike organism (MLO). *Biochem. Biophys. Res Commun.* **155**:443–448.

84. **Lee, I.-M., R. E. Davis, and C. Hiruki.** 1990. Beet leafhopper transmitted virescent and clover proliferation mycoplasmalike organisms (MLOs): two distinct strain types. *Phytopathology* **80**:958.

85. **Lee, I.-M., R. E. Davis, and C. Hiruki.** 1991. Genetic relatedness among clover proliferation mycoplasmalike organisms (MLOs) and other MLOs investigated by nucleic acid hybridization and restriction fragment length polymorphism analyses. *Appl. Environ. Microbiol.* **57**:3565–3569.

86. **Lee, I.-M., R. E. Davis, and H. T. Hsu.** 1990. Monoclonal antibodies against tomato big bud mycoplasmalike organism (MLO) distinguish a group of interrelated MLO strains within the "aster yellows" strain cluster. *Phytopathology* **80**:958.

87. **Lee, I.-M., D. E. Gundersen, R. E. Davis, and L. N. Chiykowski.** 1991. Peach X-disease mycoplasmalike organism (ML) genomic strain cluster. *Phytopathology* **81**:1169.

88. **Lherminier, J., T. Terwisscha Van Scheltinga, E. Boudon-Padieu, and A. Caudwell.** 1989. Rapid immunofluorescent detection of the grapevine flavescence doree mycoplasma-like organism in the salivary glands of the leafhopper *Euscelidius variegatus* KBM. *Phytopathol. Z.* **125**:353–360.

89. **Lim, P.-O., and B. B. Sears.** 1989. 16S rRNA sequence indicates that plant-pathogenic mycoplasmalike organisms are evolutionarily distinct from animal mycoplasmas. *J. Bacteriol.* **171**:5901–5906.

90. **Lim, P.-O., and B. B. Sears.** 1991. The genome size of a plant-pathogenic mycoplasmalike organism resembles those of animal mycoplasmas. *J. Bacteriol.* **173**:2128–2130.

91. **Lim, P.-O., B. B. Sears, and K. L. Klomparens.** 1992. Membrane properties of a plant-pathogenic mycoplasmalike organism. *J. Bacteriol.* **174**:682–686.

92. **Lin, C.-P., and T. A. Chen.** 1985. Monoclonal antibodies against the aster yellows agent. *Science* **227**:1233–1235.

93. **Lin, C.-P., and T. A. Chen.** 1986. Comparison of monoclonal antibodies and polyclonal antibodies in detection of the aster yellows mycoplasmalike organism. *Phytopathology* **76**:45–50.

94. **Lin, N. S., Y. H. Hsu, and H. T. Hsu.** 1990. Immunological detection of plant viruses and a mycoplasmalike organism by direct tissue blotting on nitrocellulose membranes. *Phytopathology* **80**:824–828.

95. **Maramorosch, K.** 1958. Beneficial effect of virus-diseased plants on non-vector insects. *Tijdschr. Pflantzieken* **64**:383–391.

96. **Maramorosch, K.** 1963. Arthropod transmission of plant viruses. *Annu. Rev. Entomol.* **8**:369–414.

97. **Markham, P. G.** 1988. Detection of mycoplasmas and spiroplasmas in insects, p. 157–177. *In* C. Hiruki (ed.), *Tree Mycoplasmas and Mycoplasma Diseases.* University of Alberta, Edmonton, Alberta, Canada.

98. **Marwitz, R.** 1990. Diversity of yellows disease agents in plant infections. *Zentralbl. Bakteriol. Suppl.* **20**:431–434.

99. **McCoy, R. E., A. Caudwell, C. J. Chang, T. A. Chen, L. N. Chiykowski, M. T. Cousin, G. T. N. Dale de Leeuw, D. A. Golino, K. J. Hackett, B. C. Kirkpatrick, R. Marwitz, H. Petzold, R. H. Sinha, M. Sugiura, R. F. Whitcomb, I. L. Yang, B. M. Zhu, and E. Seemüller.** 1989. Plant diseases associated with mycoplasma-like organisms, p. 545–560. *In* R. F. Whitcomb and J. G. Tully (ed.), *The Mycoplasmas*, vol. 5. Academic Press, New York.

100. **McCoy, R. E., F. W. Howard, J. H. Tsai, H. M. Donselman, D. L. Thomas, H. G. Basham, R. A. Atilano, F. M. Eskafi, L. Britt, and M. E. Collins.** 1983. Lethal yellowing of palms. *Univ. Fl. IFAS Agric. Exp. Stn. Tech. Bull.* **834**:1–100.

101. **Memane, S. A., and M. B. Joi.** 1987. Identification of sources of resistance to little leaf of bringjal. *J. Maharashtra Agric. Univ.* **12**:70–71.

102. **Mittempergher, L., A. Fagnani, F. Ferrini, and G. D'Agostino.** 1990. Elm yellows, a disease to be taken into consideration when breeding elm for disease resistance, p. 433–435. *In Proceedings of the 8th Congress of the Mediterranean Phytopathological Union.* Agadir, Morocco.

103. **Moellers, C., and S. Sarkar.** 1989. Regeneration of healthy plants from *Catharanthus roseus* infected with mycoplasma-like organisms through callus culture. *Plant Sci.* **60**:83–90.

104. **Nair, V. M. G.** 1988. Chemotherapeutic control of tree diseases, p. 217–237. *In* C. Hiruki (ed.), *Tree Mycoplasmas and Mycoplasma Diseases.* University of Alberta Press, Edmonton, Alberta, Canada.

105. **Nakashima, K., S. Kato, S. Iwanami, and N. Murata.** 1991. Cloning and detection of chromosomal and extrachromosomal DNA from mycoplasmalike organisms that cause yellow dwarf disease of rice. *Appl. Environ. Microbiol.* **57**:3570–3575.

106. **Neimark, H., and B. C. Kirkpatrick.** 1990. Isolation and size estimation of whole chromosomes from mycoplasma-like organisms. *Phytopathology* **80**:959.

107. **Ploaie, P. G.** 1981. Mycoplasmalike organisms and plant diseases in Europe, p. 61–104. *In* K. Maramorosch and K. F. Harris (ed.), *Plant Diseases and Vectors: Ecology and Epidemiology.* Academic Press, New York.

108. **Purcell, A. H.** 1988. Increased survival of *Dalbulus maidis*, a specialist on maize, on non-host plants in-

fected with molliculite plant pathogens. *Entomol. Exp. Appl.* **46**:187–196.

109. **Raju, B. C., and G. Nyland.** 1988. Chemotherapy of mycoplasma diseases of fruit trees, p. 207–216. *In* C. Hiruki (ed.), *Tree Mycoplasmas and Mycoplasma Diseases*. University of Alberta Press, Edmonton, Alberta, Canada.

110. **Schaff, D. A., I.-M. Lee, and R. E. Davis.** 1990. Sensitive detection of mycoplasma-like organisms (MLOs) by polymerase chain reactions (PCR). *Phytopathology* **80**:959.

111. **Schaff, D. A., I.-M. Lee, and R. E. Davis.** Unpublished data.

112. **Schwartz, Y., E. Boudon-Padieu, J. Grange, R. Meignoz, and A. Caudwell.** 1989. Monoclonal antibodies to the mycoplasma-like organism (MLO) responsible for grapevine flavescence doree. *Res. Microbiol.* **140**:311–324.

113. **Sears, B. B., P.-O. Lim, N. Holland, B. C. Kirkpatrick, and K. L. Klomparens.** 1989. Isolation and characterization of DNA from a mycoplasma-like organism. *Mol. Plant-Microbe Interact.* **2**:175–180.

114. **Seemüller, E.** 1976. Demonstration of mycoplasmalike organism in the phloem of trees with pear decline or proliferation symptoms by fluorescence microscopy. *Phytopathol. Z.* **85**:368–372.

115. **Shaw, M. E., and B. C. Kirkpatrick.** 1991. Identification and genetic variations among virescence-inducing MLOs in California. *Phytopathology* **81**:1168.

116. **Shaw, M. E., B. C. Kirkpatrick, and D. A. Golino.** 1990. Identification and characterization of plasmids present in the beet leafhopper transmitted virescence agent. *Phytopathology* **80**:985.

117. **Shaw, M. E., B. C. Kirkpatrick, and D. A. Golino.** 1991. Causal agent of tomato big bud disease in California is the beet leafhopper transmitted virescence agent. *Phytopathology* **81**:1210.

118. **Shiomi, T., and M. Sugiura.** 1984. Grouping of mycoplasma-like organisms transmitted by the leafhopper vector, *Macrosteles orientalis* Virvaste, based on host range. *Ann. Phytopathol. Soc. Jpn.* **50**:149–157.

119. **Sinclair, W. A., R. J. Iuli, A. T. Dyer, and A. O. Larsen.** 1989. Sampling and histological procedures for diagnosis of ash yellows. *Plant Dis.* **73**:432–435.

120. **Sinha, R. C.** 1988. Serological detection of mycoplasmalike organisms from plants affected with yellows diseases, p. 143–156. *In* C. Hiruki (ed.), *Tree Mycoplasmas and Mycoplasma Diseases*. University of Alberta Press, Edmonton, Alberta, Canada.

121. **Sinha, R. C., and L. N. Chiykowski.** 1990. Serological detection of MLOs in plants and vector leafhoppers using polyclonal antibodies. *Zentralbl. Bakteriol. Suppl.* **20**:276–279.

122. **Stoddard, E. M.** 1947. The X-disease of peach and its chemotherapy. *Conn. Agric. Exp. Stn. Bull.* **506**:1–19.

123. **Su, H. J.** Personal communication.

124. **Tang, W., and T. A. Chen.** 1992. Molecular cloning and detection of DNA for the mycoplasmalike organism associated with blueberry stunt disease. *Phytopathology* **82**:248.

125. **Tsai, M.-C., and H. J. Su.** Personal communication.

126. **Vega, F. E., R. E. Davis, P. Barbosa, E. Dally, A. Purcell, and I.-M. Lee.** Unpublished data.

127. **Whitcomb, R. F.** 1981. The biology of spiroplasmas. *Annu. Rev. Entomol.* **26**:397–425.

128. **Williamson, D. L., J. G. Tully, and R. F. Whitcomb.** 1989. The genus *Spiroplasma*, p. 71–111. *In* R. F. Whitcomb and J. G. Tully (ed.), *The Mycoplasmas*, vol. 5. Academic Press, New York.

24. Mycoplasma Diseases of Animals

JERRY W. SIMECKA, JERRY K. DAVIS, MAUREEN K. DAVIDSON, SUZANNE E. ROSS, CHRISTIAN T. K.-H. STÄDTLANDER, and GAIL H. CASSELL

INTRODUCTION

Animal mycoplasma and ureaplasma infections are of historic importance to mycoplasmology, in addition to causing significant health problems in commercial and experimental animals. In 1898, the very first mycoplasma described, *Mycoplasma mycoides* subsp. *mycoides*, was reported as the agent of contagious bovine pleuropneumonia (CBPP) in cattle (208) and was considered the type strain for mycoplasmas for many years (98). Subsequently, mycoplasmas and ureaplasmas have been isolated from almost every domestic and laboratory animal and are economically important in agriculture as well as in biomedical research. Infections are associated with diseases of the lung, genitourinary tract, joints, and other tissues and are useful as comparative models of similar diseases in humans. Thus, there has been, and continues to be, great emphasis in mycoplasmology on the pathogenesis, diagnosis, and treatment of mycoplasma diseases of animals.

This chapter briefly reviews the various mycoplasma diseases of animals. General features of the pathogenic mechanisms of mycoplasma diseases, including attachment, cell injury, and host responses to infection, are also presented. Finally, approaches to diagnosis of mycoplasma infections in animals are reviewed.

DESCRIPTION OF MYCOPLASMA DISEASES OF ANIMALS

Many different members of the genera *Acholeplasma*, *Mycoplasma*, and *Ureaplasma* have been isolated from animals, but the potential of many isolates to cause disease is unknown. We will concentrate our review of mycoplasma diseases on those described for mice and rats, ruminants (cattle, goats, and sheep), swine, and poultry (Table 1). Although many other animal species are affected by mycoplasma infections, many aspects of these diseases are similar to those discussed below.

Mice and Rats

Respiratory disease

Murine respiratory mycoplasmosis (MRM) is a disease of laboratory rats and mice caused by *M. pulmonis*; however, its expression is markedly influenced

Jerry W. Simecka, Suzanne E. Ross, Christian T. K.-H. Städtlander, and Gail H. Cassell • Department of Microbiology, University of Alabama at Birmingham, Birmingham, Alabama 35294. **Jerry K. Davis** • Departments of Comparative Medicine and Microbiology, University of Alabama at Birmingham, Birmingham, Alabama 35294. **Maureen K. Davidson** • Department of Comparative Medicine, University of Alabama at Birmingham, and Veterans Administration Medical Center, Birmingham, Alabama 35294.

Table 1. Mycoplasma diseases of animals

Host species	Mycoplasma species	Disease
Rats and mice	*Mycoplasma arthritidis*	Arthritis
	M. pulmonis	Murine respiratory mycoplasmosis, genital disease, and arthritis
Cattle	*M. alkalescens*	Arthritis
	M. bovigenitalium	Mastitis and genital disease
	M. bovirhinis	Mastitis
	M. bovis	Calf pneumonia, mastitis and arthritis
	M. bovoculi	Conjunctivitis
	M. californicum	Mastitis
	M. canadense	Mastitis
	M. dispar	Calf pneumonia and mastitis
	M. mycoides subsp. *mycoides*	Contagious bovine pleuropneumonia and arthritis
	Mycoplasma spp. group 7	Calf pneumonia and arthritis
	Ureaplasma spp.	Calf pneumonia, genital disease, and conjunctivitis
Goats	*M. putrefaciens*	Mastitis and arthritis
	Mycoplasma sp. strain GM790A	Mastitis
Sheep and goats	*M. capricolum*	Respiratory disease and arthritis
	M. agalactiae	Mastitis and arthritis
	M. mycoides subsp. *mycoides*	Pleuropneumonia and arthritis
	M. ovipneumoniae	Proliferative interstitial pneumonia (sheep); pneumonia (?) (goats)
	Mycoplasma sp. strain F38	Pleuropneumonia similar to classic caprine (contagious) pleuropneumonia
Sheep	*M. conjunctivae*	Conjunctivitis
Swine	*M. hyorhinis*	Pneumonia (?) and arthritis
	M. hyosynoviae	Arthritis
	M. hyopneumoniae	Enzootic pneumonia
Poultry	*A. axanthum*	Air sacculitis (geese)
	M. gallisepticum	Infectious air sacculitis (turkeys)
		Sinusitis (chickens)
		Arthritis
	M. iowae	Mild air sacculitis
	M. meleagridis	Air sacculitis
		Arthritis
	M. synoviae	Air sacculitis and arthritis (chickens, turkeys)

by a variety of environmental, host, and organismal factors. MRM, originally termed chronic murine respiratory disease, was recognized as one of the major diseases of laboratory rats and mice over 70 years ago, but more than 50 years were required before Koch's postulates were fulfilled for the etiology of MRM (194).

M. pulmonis has been isolated from other animals, but natural disease occurs only in rats and mice. Significant morbidity and mortality can occur, especially in animals used in long-term studies or in animals with subclinical infection exacerbated by various experimental procedures (44, 194). However, the most significant impact of *M. pulmonis* infection probably is through its interference with interpretation of research findings (44, 194). For example, infection with *M. pulmonis* can alter carcinogenesis, ciliary function, cell kinetics (44), neurogenic inflammation (200), natural killer (NK) cell activity (187, 188), and both local and systemic immune responses (44).

MRM provided a major impetus for the development of cesarean section and isolator maintenance technology for laboratory rodents; although these programs appear to have been successful in reducing the prevalence of *M. pulmonis* disease, they have failed to eliminate *M. pulmonis* infection (42, 84). Prevalence rates in the early to mid-1980s still ranged from 5 to 20% in barrier-maintained colonies. Although there have not been any reports from large-scale screening programs of rodent colonies in more recent years, infection with *M. pulmonis* still occurs in well-managed, barrier-maintained colonies (70). Preferred sites are the respiratory tract, nasopharynx, and middle ear (82). Transmission is thought to be by aerosol or intra-uterine infection between cagemates, including from dam to offspring, and between adjacent cages in holding rooms or isolators (62).

M. pulmonis respiratory disease usually is clinically silent in both rats and mice (194) except in the terminal stages of the disease. Characteristic microscopic lesions occur throughout the respiratory tract and include neutrophils in the airways, hyperplasia of mucosal epithelium, and a lymphoid response in the submucosa. Rhinitis, otitis media, laryngitis, tracheitis, bronchitis, bronchiectasis, and alveolitis are common and can be either acute or chronic. Pulmonary abscesses sometimes occur, and rarely pleuritis and emphysema are found. The most characteristic features are lymphoid hyperplasia and chronic inflammation (39). While *M. pulmonis* alone can reproduce all of the lesions of MRM, these mycoplasmas often are found in association with other pathogens, which may result in increased lesion severity as seen with Sendai or sialodacryoadenitis virus (249–251).

Both the organism and host factors influence the severity and susceptibility to disease. Not all strains of *M. pulmonis* produce severe respiratory disease in mice and rats (83). Furthermore, different strains of rats and mice are not equally susceptible to virulent organisms (85, 88, 90, 248). Differences among strains of animals appear to be related to differences in host responses after infection, which will be discussed in later sections.

Genital disease

Mycoplasma genital disease is better understood in mice and rats than in other animals because of the widespread use of rats and mice in biomedical research. The demand for axenic, gnotobiotic, and pathogen-free animals for research has provided many opportunities for study of murine mycoplasmosis both in naturally occurring infections and in experimental infections in the natural hosts.

M. pulmonis and *M. arthritidis* have been isolated from the genital tracts of both rats and mice (11, 29, 38, 70, 81), whereas *M. muris* (201) has been isolated only from mice. The incidence of genital infections with these organisms is unknown because commercial breeders cull any animals that are not breeding, usually without determining the cause of the low birth rate. Although there have been few studies involving natural infections, *M. pulmonis* is known to cause naturally occurring genital disease in both rats and mice (11, 70). *M. pulmonis* was isolated in pure cultures from genital tract lesions in a conventional colony of LEW rats that had undergone a reduction in breeding efficiency. Genital tract disease essentially identical to the natural disease was produced by intravenous inoculation of *M. pulmonis* into pathogen-free F344 rats, thus fulfilling Koch's postulates. A 50% reduction in breeding efficiency was also seen (38). Genital infections and vertical transmission in utero have been implicated in *M. pulmonis* isolations from cesarian section-derived rats (70).

Gross lesions in the rat and mouse genital tracts are more common in females; distention of the ovarian bursae with clear straw-colored fluid is the most common lesion. Secondary oophoritis is present in most mice that have purulent salpingitis. Many animals show evidence of a low-grade metritis, while endometritis is found in a small number of animals. Underdeveloped and partially resorbed fetuses sometimes occur. Gross genital tract lesions are rare in males and are limited to atrophied testes and enlarged ductus deferens.

M. pulmonis genital lesions are found both in conjunction with and independently of respiratory lesions. Both natural and experimental infections result in what appears to be a slowly progressing, chronic disease. As is often seen in MRM, there is little correlation between clinical signs and pathological alterations. One of the most noteworthy features of the genital disease is the lack of uniformity of lesions observed in animals of the same age from the same colony. Many naturally infected animals are colonized in the lower genital tract, but only a few are colonized in the upper genital tract. This finding suggests that complex host-parasite interactions may allow a commensal mycoplasma from the lower genital tract to invade the upper tract only under certain circumstances.

The significance of isolations of *M. arthritidis* and *M. muris* from the genital tracts of laboratory rodents is not clear. No naturally occurring diseases have been reported, so one must assume that genital disease due to these species alone is not a significant problem, at least in laboratory animals. However, given the known effects of mycoplasmas on many host systems, the potential importance of infection with any mycoplasma species in laboratory mice and rats cannot be ignored. These genital tract isolations certainly illustrate the fact that one cannot rely on cesarian section derivation to eliminate mycoplasmas from a rodent breeding colony.

Arthritis

Spontaneous polyarthritis in rats can result from infection with *M. arthritidis* (61), although known natural cases are rare (44). The organism is often found in rat colonies, but animals rarely show signs of arthritic disease. Experimental infection of rats with large intravenous doses of *M. arthritidis* results in an acute polyarthritis which usually subsides in about 50 days (61). The disease can affect all four extremities and result in hind limb paralysis due to involvement of the vertebral articulations. The arthritic joints are characterized by swelling, redness, and tenderness. There is a large influx of neutrophils into the synovial membranes and adjacent tissues. Although the disease is usually transient, genetic differences in rat strains can affect the susceptibility to chronic arthritis (19).

Experimental intravenous infection of mice with *M. arthritidis* results in the development of a chronic arthritis which resembles rheumatoid arthritis in humans (61). Early after infection, the disease is characterized by edema, an influx of neutrophils into the periarticular region, and a mild increase in the numbers of synoviocytes. The disease progresses from an intense infiltration of the synovial membrane and adjacent tissues to a massive proliferation of the synovial membrane, with a pronounced villus hypertrophy and mononuclear cell and neutrophil infiltration. In the later stages, collagen deposition and destruction of cartilage become apparent. The disease often subsides 3 to 6 months after infection but can recur.

M. pulmonis, although more commonly associated with respiratory and genital disease of rats and mice as described earlier, can also induce arthritis. In mice, arthritis due to *M. pulmonis* is less suppurative but resembles the chronic stages of disease due to *M. arthritidis* (52, 130). As with *M. arthritidis* disease, the severity of *M. pulmonis* arthritis can vary over time. Intravenous injection of organisms into F344 rats produces a mild tenosynovitis (43), although severity may vary among strains of rats.

Injection of either *M. arthritidis* or *M. pulmonis* into the knee joints of rabbits can produce arthritis which progresses similarly to that seen in the mouse, from acute to chronic inflammation (297). The disease can last for months, but organisms can be recovered only up to 4 weeks after infection. By immunofluorescent staining, immune complexes are found within the joint tissue (297, 298).

Ruminants

Respiratory disease

Cattle. There is convincing evidence that various mycoplasma species are involved in at least some cases of calf pneumonia. Mycoplasmas also have been implicated in pneumonia of feeder cattle, but the evidence is less convincing and remains primarily epizoological (197, 237).

(i) CBPP. *M. mycoides* subsp. *mycoides* is the etiologic agent of CBPP, which affects both cattle and water buffalo. This disease has been eradicated from North America, Europe, and Australia but is still common in some underdeveloped nations (121, 217, 291). CBPP probably is the most economically important mycoplasma disease in the world.

CBPP is difficult to produce experimentally, indicating that unknown factors in addition to *M. mycoides* are likely to be involved in expression of disease (121). Susceptible cattle become infected by inhaling aerosol droplets, after which there is an incubation period of about 3 to 8 weeks. Morbidity can be as high as 100% in susceptible herds, with up to 50% mortality. After recovery, animals are likely to be carriers of the organism and have chronic lung lesions sometimes not detectable either clinically or by serology.

There is a septicemic phase of CBPP, with lesions induced in the kidneys and placenta. Respiratory lesions of CBPP are unlike those of most mycoplasma respiratory diseases (149), with neutrophilic exudation in the airways, necrosis, and edema in regional lymph nodes, edema of the interlobular septa, and serous exudation into the pleural cavity. These changes intensify and develop into copious serofibrinous pleuritis, consolidation of the lungs, and necrosis of the regional lymph nodes. Alveoli are filled with large amounts of fluid, often containing fibrin. If the animal survives, a pattern similar to that for other chronic respiratory mycoplasmoses is superimposed, and various degrees of peribronchial, perivascular, and interseptal lymphoid infiltration occur.

(ii) Endemic calf pneumonia. Endemic calf pneumonia is a high-mortality pneumonia that primarily affects housed dairy calves (31). Viruses, especially bovine respiratory syncytial virus and parainfluenza type 3 virus, can initiate the disease and by themselves may result in extensive, and sometimes fatal, lung damage. Respiratory viral infections are followed by secondary mycoplasmal and bacterial invasion of the lower respiratory tract, which increases the extent and severity of lung damage. Poor-quality housing, most importantly bad ventilation, will increase the severity of pneumonia outbreaks and may be more important than viral infections in exacerbating endemic calf pneumonia.

Three of the many mycoplasma species isolated from calves (121, 269), *M. bovis*, *M. dispar*, and *Ureaplasma dispar*, can be pathogenic in the absence of viruses or other agents, as shown in experimental infections of gnotobiotic calves (105, 119, 125, 135, 137, 287). *M. bovis* causes the most severe lesions and highest mortality, but disease outbreaks with this organism are sporadic (32, 105, 119, 125, 135, 137). Both *M. bovis* and *U. dispar* produce a "cuffing" pneumonia, the most common form, characterized by mononuclear cell infiltration in both peribronchiolar and alveolar regions. *M. dispar* produces interstitial pneumonia with mononuclear infiltrates of the alveolar wall but no prominent peribronchiolar cuffing. This organism also frequently causes mild superficial and asymptomatic infections of the respiratory mucosa (307). The pathological picture is usually complicated by superimposed infection with other bacteria. For example, mixed infections of *M. bovis* and *Pasteurella multocida* are frequently exudative, and mixed infections of *M. bovis* and *Haemophilus somnus* are often necrotic (32).

Sheep and goats. (i) CCPP. Contagious caprine pleuropneumonia (CCPP) is one of the most economically important diseases in goats and is widely distributed (15, 69, 214, 215, 221). The causative agents are members of the *M. mycoides* subsp. *mycoides* group and include *M. mycoides* subsp. *capri*, *M. mycoides* subsp. *mycoides* large-colony type, and F38-like strains. All have been isolated from natural outbreaks, and all are capable of producing disease experimentally, although strain F38 may be the most virulent (20, 67, 74, 206, 235, 292). With strain F38, morbidity can be up to 100%, and mortality ranges from 60 to 100%. In general, lesions and signs of CCPP resemble those of CBPP except that polyarthritis is more common and necrotic sequestra are less common.

(ii) Nonprogressive interstitial pneumonia in sheep. In the early 1970s, *M. ovipneumoniae* was shown to be involved in naturally occurring pneumonia of lambs (4, 36). The disease is worldwide in occurrence. *M. ovipneumoniae* has been isolated from healthy sheep (28, 150), and asymptomatic ewes are apparently the main source of infection for lambs. Upper respiratory tract colonization can occur as early as 1 to 2 days after birth. The pneumonia, apparently related to the decline of colostral antibody, develops between 5 and 10 weeks of age. Other factors such as stocking density and management practices influence the incidence and severity within a flock. In housed flocks, 40% or more of the lambs may be affected; outbreaks may also occur in older lambs that are stressed. Clinically, the pneumonia is characterized by moist cough, sneezing, copious clear mucoid discharge from the nose, intolerance to exercise, and poor weight gain. Clinical signs decrease by 12 weeks of age, but even at 16 weeks there are pneumonic lesions characterized by proliferation of alveolar cells, nodular lymphoid hyperplasia, and peribronchial and perivascular lymphoid cell cuffing (103). Such lesions are inconsistent, which may be due to the existence of different strains of *M. ovipneumoniae* (157) or to the presence of other bacteria (most often *Pasturella haemolytica* biotype A) which can exacerbate the disease (156).

Mastitis

Mastitis due to mycoplasmas has been reported in virtually all mammals but is of greatest economic importance in cows, goats, and sheep (33). Numerous mycoplasma species have been isolated from both healthy and affected animals under a wide variety of conditions, but Koch's postulates have been fulfilled for relatively few mycoplasma species in their natural hosts.

Bovine mastitis has been shown to be caused by *M. bovigenitalium*, *M. bovirhinis*, *M. bovis*, *M. californicum*, *M. canadense*, and *M. dispar* (114, 118, 123, 151–153). *M. bovis* is considered to be the most important of all the mycoplasmal mastitis-producing organisms (118). Ureaplasmas have also been shown to cause experimental mastitis in cows, but natural disease has not been reported.

Mycoplasmal mastitis in sheep and goats is usually a manifestation of contagious agalactia, caused by *M. agalactiae*, but may also be caused by *M. capricolum* and *M. mycoides* subsp. *mycoides* (large colony) (66, 69, 76, 118). Mastitis in goats has also been attributed to *M. putrefaciens* and to a new mycoplasma strain, GM790A (77).

In general, mastitis transmission is horizontal. Infection occurs via the teat and may be directly related to trauma, poor husbandry, or milking technique. Apparently, organisms can be isolated for long periods of time from asymptomatic animals, only to have active disease appear at a later date. Infection can vary from subclinical to extreme involvement of the entire udder, with subsequent rapid spread throughout a herd. In some cases, mycoplasmas can be passed to nursing infants via colostrum or milk, resulting in serious infections in the offspring (118). Definitive diagnosis is based on culture and identification of the organism(s) from a sample of milk collected aseptically. Newer serological and molecular diagnostic techniques have been developed, but none have been adequately field tested to assess their clinical usefulness, especially in areas where infection with one or more pathogenic mycoplasmas is prevalent.

Genital disease

The role of *Mycoplasma* and *Ureaplasma* species in diseases of the genital tract of cattle is not clear, as other potential pathogens are often coisolated from animals with disease (281). Mycoplasmas have been isolated from the genital tracts of cattle, sheep, and goats (66, 120), and experimental inoculation of some of these organisms results in disease, but few natural cases have been reported. *M. bovigenitalium* infections in cattle may be the exception (120). Experimentally, *M. bovigenitalium* causes granular vulvovaginitis in females (10, 93, 120, 246) and can infect bulls (218, 220). *U. diversum* also is capable of causing disease in cows (94), and both organisms can decrease fertility under experimental conditions (178, 246). The significance of these agents in naturally occurring disease is unknown, however.

Arthritis

In cattle, there is no doubt that *M. bovis* is the cause of mastitis and pneumonia, but it should also be considered an arthritogenic agent in cows and calves. Arthritis develops most often in conjunction with mastitis or pneumonia (120). There are reports of joint infections, which seem to be the sole disease manifestation (133), but subclinical infections of other sites may have gone unrecognized (117).

Disease first appears as lameness and painful swollen joints (61, 245). The disease is characterized by tendovaginitis, peritendonitis, and synovitis with multiple joints affected. The synovial fluid of arthritic animals is highly fibrinous and coagulates after removal. Experimental infections with *M. bovis* can result in destruction of cartilage and development of fibrotic lesions within the joint. As with other mycoplasma-induced arthritides, there is variability in the severity and outcome of arthritis due to *M. bovis*. Some animals develop only mild disease and recover, but others develop chronic arthritis with a tendency to relapse.

Although *M. bovis* is the most recognized arthritogenic agent in cattle, other mycoplasmas have been isolated from arthritic cattle. *Mycoplasma* species group 7 has been isolated from joint fluids of cases of bovine arthritis (3, 256). The ability to experimentally produce arthritis was demonstrated first by injection of this agent into a joint of a calf and later by intravenous inoculation of this organism (120). *M. alkalescens* has also been suggested to be a rare cause of arthritis in calves (17, 301). Bennett and Jasper (17) demonstrated that inoculation of *M. alkalescens* into the joints of calves can induce arthritis, but intravenous injection of the organism does not result in the development of disease. Thus, the organism is probably not highly pathogenic but may be an opportunistic agent subject to host and environmental factors.

M. mycoides subsp. *mycoides* has been implicated in arthritis in cattle and goats (15, 72, 97, 236). In cattle, administration of live *M. mycoides* subsp. *mycoides* by intubation resulted in lameness and swollen joints (129). Some resolution of swelling at the joints was noticed by 70 days after infection. Although this finding suggests that ingestion of *M. mycoides* subsp. *mycoides* may result in arthritis, it is unclear whether this is truly a significant problem in cattle. However, in goats, arthritis is consistently a predominant finding in infection with *M. mycoides* subsp. *mycoides*. Fatal polyarthritis and septicemia of kids and arthritis associated with pneumonia and/or mastitis in adult goats and kids occur in natural infections (15, 72, 97). Experimental infection of goats produces polyarthritis (14, 234). The arthritis is characterized as fibrinopurulent with severe destruction of cartilage and tenosynovitis, sometimes so severe and painful that the animals will lean or lie down (72, 97).

M. capricolum can cause severe arthritis as a predominant lesion in goats and sheep. *M. capricolum* was probably the causal agent of a severe arthritis without lung disease in an outbreak in goats described by Cordy et al. (65, 68). The disease became so severe that many of the animals preferred to stand for long periods or, if they lay down, were unable to rise. The disease was characterized as a fibrinopurulent arthritis which was more severe in younger kids. Since this outbreak of *M. capricolum* arthritis disease, other cases of similar disease have been reported in goats (21) and sheep (274, 277). Histologically, serofibrinous synovitis, bursitis, and tendovaginitis are features of the disease. Experimental infection with *M. capricolum* confirmed the role of this agent in arthritic disease. Experimentally, the disease can be transmitted through contact or ingestion of the organisms (73, 75,

277). In general, *M. capricolum* and *M. mycoides* subsp. *mycoides* cause nearly identical diseases in goats, with septicemia leading to pyrexia, high morbidity and mortality, pneumonia, mastitis, and arthritis.

M. putrefaciens has been isolated from goats with arthritis and can have a devastating effect on goat herds. In one report, there was an outbreak of mastitis and arthritis in a herd of goats from which pure cultures of *M. putrefaciens* were recovered from joints and other tissues (75). As a result, almost all of the 700 goats had to be destroyed. *M. putrefaciens* can produce a polyarthritis after experimental inoculation (76); however, some strains may not be very arthritogenic (73).

M. agalactiae can also cause arthritis, but usually as a secondary infection (66). Contagious agalactia is characterized by keratoconjunctivitis, mastitis, and pneumonia. Organisms may be recovered from the blood for a short time during which they can localize to joints, resulting in the development of a painful arthritis.

Conjunctivitis

Infectious keratoconjunctivitis occurs in cattle, sheep, and goats. The disease is characterized by blepharospasm, conjunctivitis, lacrimation, and various degrees of corneal opacity and ulceration. Although *Moraxella bovis* is the most common cause of these problems in cattle, both *Ureaplasma* species and *M. bovoculi* (138, 232, 233) can produce conjunctivitis and transient corneal opacity by themselves and increase the severity of conjunctivitis due to *Moraxella bovis*. In sheep, *M. conjunctivae* is the most common cause and will produce disease experimentally (100, 155, 191, 283). In goats, conjunctivitis is usually due to *M. agalactiae*, but *M. conjunctivae* can cause similar lesions.

Swine

Respiratory disease

Enzootic pneumonia of swine is a chronic, clinically mild respiratory disease characterized by a dry, persistent cough, retarded growth rate, poor weight gain, and a high incidence of lesions in slaughter pigs (154, 211, 222, 302). Enzootic pneumonia occurs worldwide, and morbidity is high (30 to 80% of all pigs), but mortality is essentially zero. *M. hyopneumoniae*, the causative agent, was not isolated until 1965 (115, 196), probably because it is one of the most difficult mycoplasmas to grow on artificial media. *M. hyorhinis* is commonly found in the respiratory tract of healthy pigs and, at least experimentally, can produce lung lesions almost identical to those induced by *M. hyopneumoniae* (9, 112). In addition, enzootic pneumonia is frequently complicated by other bacteria and viruses, both of which can exacerbate the severity of the disease (49, 308). Common predisposing factors for disease flare-ups are changes in weather and transient viral infections (154, 211, 222, 303).

Although pigs of all ages are susceptible, pigs within a herd usually become infected within the first few weeks of life. The incidence of lung lesions is highest in 2- to 4-month-old pigs. Coughing is the most common clinical sign and is most obvious when the pigs are active. Histologically, lesions of the alveoli are characterized first by neutrophils; later, lymphocytes and macrophages predominate (16, 113). Constant features are hyperplasia of bronchiolar epithelium, perivascular and peribronchiolar lymphoid cuffing, and progressive and persistent lymphoid hypertrophy.

Arthritis

M. hyosynoviae, a recognized cause of arthritis in growing pigs, is frequently reported in the United States but less often in other parts of the world (61, 106, 242, 304). The disease likely has a high morbidity but low mortality. *M. hyosynoviae* commonly colonizes nasal passages and pharynges of adult pigs; these pigs act as reservoirs of infection, which results in the recurrence of disease in successive crops of pigs (238, 240). Generally, pharyngeal infection is first detected in pigs at 6 to 8 weeks of age. However, joint disease develops mostly in 3- to 6-month-old pigs and is characterized by a sudden onset of acute lameness persisting for 3 to 10 days. There is usually gradual improvement, but some animals become progressively more lame and may be unable to rise. *M. hyosynoviae* arthritis is nonsuppurative without polyserositis. Sometimes fibrin flakes are present in joint fluid. The disease can lead to the destruction of periarticular cartilage, but the articular surfaces often remain normal.

M. hyosynoviae arthritis has been reproduced by experimental infection of pigs (239, 241). However, two other studies did not reproduce the disease. Intranasal inoculation of gnotobiotic pigs with a pig-adapted clone of *M. hyosynoviae* led to infection in various organs but not joints (112). Furlong and Turner (106) gave 10-week-old pigs 2×10^{10} organisms from a cloned culture. The animals did not develop arthritis, although the organisms were recovered from various sites, including joints. The negative results from the last two studies are likely due to the use of cloned organisms which have lost virulence. Also, some strains of *M. hyosynoviae* are more invasive than others and may be more likely to produce arthritis (304).

The most common agent of polyserositis in pigs is *M. hyorhinis*; these animals usually also develop an arthritis due to this agent. It is a more serious problem in the United States (2 to 5% of the pigs) than in other parts of the world (304). Following intraperitoneal inoculation of *M. hyorhinis*, piglets developed polyserositis and arthritis. As the polyserositis progresses, pleural, pericardial, and peritoneal adhesions develop; the piglets recover but are commonly retarded in development. *M. hyorhinis* also causes a proliferative arthritis which is characterized by mononuclear cell infiltration and pannus production, with bone and cartilage destruction. The arthritis process can continue for many months, but eventually an inactive fibrotic lesion develops.

There is a genetic component to the *M. hyorhinis* arthritis, since Piney Woods strain miniature swine develop a less severe disease than do Yorkshire pigs when similarly infected (12). All animals from both breeds develop similar disease within the first month. The miniature pigs gradually recover after several months, while the Yorkshire pigs progress to a chronic arthritis. The reason for the differences between these two breeds is unclear, but it may be linked to their immunological responses to the organism.

Poultry

Respiratory disease

Respiratory disease in domestic poultry has a complex etiology in which various species of mycoplasmas are only a single, albeit crucial, factor. There is a marked interaction between mycoplasma, respiratory viruses, and bacteria, especially *Escherichia coli* (127, 160, 175, 228, 247, 265, 270). Environmental factors, especially dust and ammonia, also are important in lesion incidence and severity (160, 162, 265). One of three mycoplasma species, *M. gallisepticum*, *M. meleagridis*, and *M. synoviae*, is usually involved in the initiation of the disease complex, often in conjunction with a respiratory virus. While each of these organisms has distinctive epidemiological features and tends to produce a different spectrum of lesions, mixed infections occur (227). In addition, there is considerable variation in virulence among strains of each organism (223, 230). All three organisms can be transmitted through the egg, as well as horizontally, within an infected flock, and *M. meleagridis* can also be transmitted sexually.

When only mycoplasmas are involved, infection is often subclinical or mild (170). Clinical disease with mycoplasmas alone occurs most often when young birds become infected with more virulent strains (160). All three species of mycoplasmas often affect organs other than the respiratory tract (see below); only with *M. gallisepticum* do respiratory lesions predominate.

M. gallisepticum infection is commonly designated chronic respiratory disease in chickens and infectious sinusitis in turkeys. Similar conditions are seen in pheasants, chukar partridges, coturnix quail, and peacocks (95, 160). The disease is found worldwide and is most severe in large commercial operations. In the United States, most breeder flocks are free of *M. gallisepticum*, and outbreaks are due to lateral transmission from infected chickens. In other parts of the world, egg transmission is a major route of infection. The infection may be dormant in an infected chick until it is stressed, then aerosol transmission occurs, and the infection spreads throughout the flock. Crowding, cold weather, live virus vaccination, or natural virus infection may initiate active disease. The epithelium of the air passages is most susceptible to infection. Affected birds may show various degrees of respiratory distress, including rales, coryza, sneezing, and nasal discharge. In turkeys, swelling of the paranasal sinuses is common. Feed efficiency and weight gain are reduced, and in laying flocks, birds fail to reach peak egg production.

Typically, in uncomplicated cases, morbidity is high and mortality is low. There is hypertrophy and hyperplasia of respiratory epithelium, including cells of the mucous glands (210, 290). An infiltration of lymphoid cells leading to follicle formation in the lamina propria and heterophilic exudation in the airways are common. Lymphoid follicles also appear in the walls of the air sacs. If complicated by *E. coli*, extensive pneumonia and air sacculitis are common, along with fibrino-purulent pericarditis and perihepatitis (127). In turkeys, the upper respiratory tract lesions predominate, with less tendency to develop the complicated lower tract syndrome.

M. meleagridis rarely causes respiratory disease in adult turkeys, but air sacculitis in embryos, poults, and young turkeys up to 10 weeks of age is common (270). *M. meleagridis* infection is a true venereal disease, and the organism is found worldwide. While turkeys are the most common host, the organism can also occur in Japanese quail and peacocks. There is a marked difference in the pathogenicity of various strains of *M. meleagridis*, but characteristically, there is thoracic air sacculitis with thickening, turbidity, and caseous exudate in 1-day-old poults. This condition extends to the abdominal air sacs in 1 to 3 weeks and then recedes with age. While tracheitis may occur and lesions may spread to the lungs, sinusitis does not occur. Air sac lesions consist of epithelial hyperplasia and hypertrophy, along with edema and lymphoid infiltration leading to lymphofollicular foci.

Respiratory lesions in *M. synoviae* infections usually occur in younger birds and are often the result of combined mycoplasmal and viral infection, typically Newcastle disease, or infectious bronchitis (134, 265). With the exception of sinusitis, respiratory lesions are especially rare in turkeys (270).

Genital disease

Many mycoplasmas have been isolated from the genital tracts of many different avian species (164), but the significance is known for only a few species. *M. gallisepticum* and *M. synoviae*, in both chickens and turkeys, and *M. meleagridis* in turkeys are the most frequently isolated. Transmission of these three mycoplasmas is horizontal via aerosols and vertically through the egg, and the organism has been isolated from the oviduct of females and the semen of males. *M. meleagridis* is unusual in that it can be spread venereally, with both males and females harboring the organism in the cloaca. Subclinical infections can occur, with only a drop in egg production, hatchability, or viability of newly hatched chicks. Salpingitis can be experimentally induced with *M. gallisepticum* and is sometimes seen in broiler females at meat inspection, but it may not be due solely to *M. gallisepticum* infection. In general, while vertical transmission of avian-pathogenic mycoplasmas via eggs is not uncommon and can have serious effects on the offspring, genital tract disease due to these organisms is rare.

Arthritis

The development of mycoplasmal arthritis in poultry is most commonly associated with infection by *M. synoviae* (161, 163). Disease occurs in both chickens and turkeys and may be acute or chronic. Clinically, lameness and swelling of the joints are obvious, especially in chickens. Regression can occur following acute disease, but it may also evolve into a chronic and progressive condition.

Under natural conditions, disease can appear around 1 week after infection of chicks in ova, but disease has been reported within 2 to 3 days after footpad or intravenous injection (163). The disease is characterized by tendovaginitis, synovitis, and osteoarthritis. There is edema and a marked infiltration of mononuclear cells and plasma cells in the tendon sheaths, periarticular tissue, and synovial membranes along with hyperplasia of the synovial cells. Synovial membranes may show villus formation, and destruction of the articular cartilage can eventually occur.

M. gallisepticum and *M. meleagridis* have also been implicated as arthritogenic agents in poultry. *M. gallisepticum* infection can occasionally produce a mild arthritis, but it usually is a result of septicemia following respiratory infection (190). Histologically, the disease is similar to that described for *M. synoviae*. Destruction of cartilage is rarely seen with *M. gallisepticum* arthritis, and a limited number of joints are affected, whereas arthritis due to *M. synoviae* often affects multiple sites. In turkeys, a mild synovitis and arthritis may result from intravenous inoculation of *M. meleagridis* (163). However, clinical joint disease does not always follow infection with *M. meleagridis*, and the organism is usually associated with respiratory disease and/or stunting of growth.

Others

While the host species discussed above are victims of the most economically important diseases caused by mycoplasmas, they probably do not represent the full spectrum. Mycoplasmas have also been isolated from other animal species with disease, including horses, dogs, cats, and wild animals in association with lung, genital, joint, and eye diseases (141). The significance of many of these isolations is uncertain, with many likely to represent only commensal or opportunistic infections. On the other hand, many mycoplasmas causing mild or transient disease in a variety of hosts may be underdiagnosed.

General Features and Summary

From the foregoing discussion, it can be seen that several factors are remarkably constant among animal mycoplasmas. As has been emphasized, most mycoplasmas isolated from animals are not known to cause disease, and those that cause disease do so inconsistently. Most mycoplasma diseases are influenced by a variety of host and environmental factors. This pattern is especially prominent in MRM in laboratory rats and mice, epizootic pneumonia and polyserositis of swine, and the entire complex of genital and respiratory diseases caused by mycoplasmas in poultry. Second, there is a remarkable degree of variability in pathogenicity among mycoplasma strains of the same species. In most animal mycoplasma diseases, avirulent strains occur naturally, and at least some animals can carry the organisms with no signs of disease until they are stressed. In fact, with the exception of CBPP and CCPP, mycoplasma disease is rarely fatal. Conversely,

the host seldom is capable of quickly eliminating the organism. Furthermore, in almost all mycoplasma diseases, the host response, usually lymphocyte infiltration, is an integral part of lesion production. Almost invariably, the host and the mycoplasma reach a state of balance which can persist for long periods of time in the absence of outside interference. How this balance is reached, how it is maintained on a cellular and molecular level, and the long-term consequences are questions which have yet to be completely answered. However, it seems certain that there has been a long evolutionary association between mycoplasmas and their hosts and that these organisms are well adapted to their ecological niche. Thus, aspects of pathogenicity should preferentially be studied in the natural host. In addition, findings from in vitro studies must be confirmed in vivo before full credence can be given.

PATHOGENIC MECHANISMS

The pathogenesis of mycoplasma disease is a complex process influenced by the genetic background of both the host and the organism, environmental factors, and the presence of other infectious agents. Although many virulence factors have been suggested for various mycoplasmas, there is no clear case of cause and effect between these factors and pathogenicity. This lack of knowledge can be partly attributed to our inability to specifically alter or transfer genetic material to manipulate proposed virulence traits. However, there are a number of attributes of mycoplasmas that are likely to affect disease pathogenicity, including the ability to attach, to cause cell injury, to vary phenotype at a high frequency, and to modulate and resist the host immune response.

The Organism

Attachment

Most mycoplasmas are extracellular parasites whose pathogenic potential supposedly stems from membrane-membrane interactions with host cells, especially epithelial cells of the respiratory and urogenital tracts. Thus, there has been an intense interest in examining mechanisms of attachment of mycoplasmas to host cells in order to understand the initial steps of disease pathogenesis and perhaps to devise treatments based on inhibition of adherence. Also, mycoplasmas are metabolically deficient, so the close interaction probably contributes to survival by allowing the mycoplasmas to acquire needed nutrients directly from host cells. As there is an excellent review of mycoplasma adherence by Razin (224), we will briefly summarize what is known about attachment of the animal mycoplasmas.

The mechanisms of adherence of *M. gallisepticum* to host cells are the best understood among all of the animal mycoplasmas, with many similarities to the human pathogen *M. pneumoniae*. By electron microscopy, an apparent attachment organelle or tip structure has been identified (173, 192, 226, 275, 294), and both species bind to sialoglycoproteins (23, 111, 166). There is some serological cross-reaction and homology between adhesins of *M. pneumoniae* and *M. gallisepticum*, as demonstrated by using antisera (50, 71) and cytoadhesin genes as probes (71). In addition, a 100-kDa glycoprotein from human lung fibroblasts was identified as a receptor for *M. gallisepticum*, *M. pneumoniae*, and *M. genitalium* but not for *M. pulmonis* (107). This receptor binds to a 139-kDa protein of *M. gallisepticum*, a 32-kDa protein of *M. pneumoniae*, and a 190-kDa protein of *M. genitalium*. Thus, there is likely heterogeneity in the structural elements of the adhesins in this group of mycoplasmas even though there is functional homology.

There may be other animal mycoplasmas which share the functional properties of adherence with *M. gallisepticum*. *M. synoviae* has also been reported to have morphological and physiological features like those of *M. gallisepticum*, including neuraminidase-sensitive receptors on host cells (293). *M. dispar* has also been reported to have neuraminidase-sensitive receptors on sheep erythrocytes (23), but no tip structure or bleb has been described for this mycoplasma. *M. alvi* seems to possess a tip when attached to the mucosal surface of the intestine (173). Additional work is needed to strengthen the similarities in adherence mechanisms among these mycoplasmas and identify other mycoplasmas which fall into this group.

It is clear that other animal mycoplasmas do not have the same characteristic attachment mechanisms. *M. pulmonis*, for example, can attach to a wide variety of eucaryotic cells (47, 167, 177, 204), but no consistent evidence for a specialized attachment structure has been found in examinations of infected tracheal and genital epithelium (47, 267). Thus, attachment by *M. pulmonis* appears to be a more generalized interaction between the surfaces of the organism and host cells, but it is possible that attachment of *M. pulmonis* to other cell types is mediated by a specialized structure (6). Also in contrast to *M. gallisepticum*, sialic acid is not involved in adsorption of *M. pulmonis* (7, 167), and the receptor isolated from fibroblasts which binds *M. gallisepticum* does not interact with *M. pulmonis* (107). However, one study suggested that heterogeneity may exist between receptors on host cells for *M. pulmonis* (7). Attachment of *M. pulmonis* to rat synovial cells was reduced by treatment of those cells with formaldehyde or glutaraldehyde, but attachment to mouse synovial cells was unchanged after similar treatment. Thus, the mechanisms of attachment, or at least the characteristics of the components of this process, may vary between species of animals or between tissues.

Motility of mycoplasmas may contribute to the adherence process in vivo. Freshly isolated strains of *M. pulmonis* demonstrate motility (25), and it has been suggested that the mycoplasmas with attachment structures, *M. gallisepticum* and *M. pneumoniae*, are also motile (224). The perceived role of motility of mycoplasmas in attachment is twofold: (i) to aid the mycoplasma in penetrating the mucus layer of the respiratory and urogenital tracts to facilitate attachment to the underlying epithelial cells, and (ii) to orient mycoplasmas with attachment structures to encourage the interaction of the tip or bleb with the epithelial cell surface.

Cell injury and cytopathic effects

Although adherence is important in infection, it is unlikely that infection alone can produce the wide va-riety of effects seen in mycoplasma disease. Damage to host tissues, due directly or indirectly to mycoplasma infections, is probably the initiator of the disease process. The mechanisms involved in the production of cell injury are not well understood in most cases, but it is clear that several mycoplasmas have the capability to directly cause cell injury. Another possibility is that immune or inflammatory responses to mycoplasma infection can contribute to cell injury through "innocent bystander" damage.

Mycoplasma-induced cell injury is not a uniform process. In in vitro cultures of tracheal rings from chicks, hamsters, mice, or rats, the first cytopathic effect after mycoplasmal infection is an inhibition of ciliary activity (ciliostasis). There is correlation between ciliostasis and tissue injury seen after infection with *M. gallisepticum*, *M. mycoides* subsp. *capri*, *M. mycoides* subsp. *mycoides*, *M. dispar*, *M. hyorhinis*, *M. mobile*, *M. meleagridis*, *M. pulmonis*, and *M. fermentans* (192, 266). However, mycoplasmas can differ in the degree of ciliostasis induced, severity of tissue injury, and type of tissue injury (5). For example, *M. pulmonis* infection of tracheal rings in vitro results in an extensive and sequential destruction of each of the cell layers of the epithelium similar to that found in vivo after experimental infection of mice (267). In contrast, *M. fermentans*-induced ciliostasis results only in loss of cilia, without exfoliation of respiratory cells (268). In addition, some mycoplasmas show the potential to invade deeper areas of the tracheal tissue, i.e., the lamina propria (e.g., *M. fermentans* strains [268] and *M. bovis* [148]). Thus, mycoplasmas are heterogeneous in the types of cell injury seen in disease. Even when the individual steps in disease pathogenesis are similar between mycoplasma infections, the result of the total package of virulence factors may result in distinctive progression of cell injury and disease.

Mycoplasmal parasitism of host cells may contribute to cell injury through deprivation of nutrients, alteration of host cell components and metabolites, and the production of toxic substances. Lack of certain de novo synthetic pathways means that mycoplasmas must acquire host components for survival. Mycoplasmas produce a number of enzymes, such as phospholipases, proteases, and nucleases, that probably play a major role in this process (18). However, phospholipases and proteases could also contribute to damage of cell membranes. Nucleases have been suggested to increase the chances of genetic alteration of host cells leading to autoimmune response (296), but the viability of this hypothesis is questionable. One possible mechanism of injury that has not been clearly addressed is the disruption of normal cellular function through direct membrane interaction by possible activation of host cell second-messenger systems. Further studies are needed to demonstrate a clearer role for each of these activities in virulence.

Mycoplasmal production of hydrogen peroxide has also been suggested to play a role in cell injury and disease. Many mycoplasmas, including *M. mycoides* subsp. *capri*, *M. pulmonis*, *M. arthritidis*, *M. neurolyticum*, *M. gallinarum*, *M. gallisepticum*, *M. bovigenitalium*, and *M. felis*, are able to secrete hydrogen peroxide (60). hydrogen peroxide released in direct proximity to the host cell membrane may lead to oxidative stress (i.e., oxidation of membrane lipids and glutathione).

In support of this view, hydrogen peroxide can cause hemolysis (60). Also, the damage to tracheal tissue in culture by *M. mycoides* subsp. *capri* is inhibited by the addition of catalase (48). Catalase-deficient mice are more sensitive to *M. pulmonis* infection, suggesting that peroxide production in vivo contributes to the virulence of *M. pulmonis* (27). (Interestingly, peroxide is also toxic to *M. pulmonis*, and the presence of host catalase may promote growth and survival of *M. pulmonis* after infection [27].) The role of peroxide secretion by mycoplasmas in catalase-normal animals is unknown, but given the intimate association between mycoplasmas and host cells, even minute quantities of peroxide might be injurious. Thus, the potential pathogenic effect of in vivo peroxide production by mycoplasmas remains an area of interest.

Toxins produced by some mycoplasmas may also play an important role in disease pathogenesis. In an effort to demonstrate toxin production, Lloyd (195) placed diffusion chambers containing *M. mycoides* into the peritoneal cavities of rabbits. These chambers became encapsulated in tissue, with necrosis evident adjacent to the filter membranes. No tissue necrosis and substantially less encapsulation occurred after implantation of chambers filled with media alone. Subsequently, diffusion chambers containing *M. mycoides* were implanted intramuscularly into cattle (34). Tissue necrosis was evident in these studies; however, in contrast to the rabbit, there was also a large connective tissue response. These results suggest that *M. mycoides* produces a diffusible toxin. Although the toxin's role in disease has not been proven, these results are consistent with the connective tissue capsule seen around necrotic tissue in natural cases of CBPP. The nature of the toxin has not been fully characterized; however, a pyrogenic response in rabbits has been described for a galactan extracted from *M. mycoides* (295). It is possible that this galactan is a component of the diffusible toxin of *M. mycoides*.

Other mycoplasmas have been shown to produce toxins. A neurotoxin has been described for a variant of *M. gallisepticum* which can cause encephalitis in turkeys (181). Intravenous injection of viable *M. gallisepticum* results in damage to arteries of the brains of turkeys (285). The neurotoxic effect requires viable organisms and is not an exotoxin. Also, an inflammatory toxin has been extracted from *M. bovis* (109). The holotoxin in the cell membrane is a glycoprotein; however, the polysaccharide portion is toxic. This toxin increases vascular permeability and activates complement. The toxin, when infused into the bovine udder, produced an eosinophilic mastitis characteristic of *M. bovis* infection. Thus far, the role of this toxin has not been examined in respiratory disease due to *M. bovis*, but it seems likely that the toxin does contribute to the pathogenesis of this disease. Toxic components have been described for other mycoplasmas such as *M. arthritidis* (172, 180), *M. hyopneumoniae* (110) and *M. neurolyticum* (286). In addition, endotoxinlike lipopolysaccharides have been found for a number of avirulent organisms (253), and similar components may also be present in pathogenic organisms.

Variability in mycoplasma phenotype

In general, mycoplasma strains appear to be highly variable in their phenotypes, and many strains within the same species differ in the ability to cause disease after experimental infection. In addition, mycoplasmas can rapidly lose their virulence through passage in artificial media. High-frequency variation in colony morphology and surface antigens has been demonstrated in *M. pulmonis*, *M. hyorhinis*, and ureaplasmas (96) (a more detailed description of variation in antigens of mycoplasmas is presented in chapter 28). For *M. pulmonis*, the variation in a major surface antigen, V-1, has been characterized by Watson et al. (299). This antigen varies structurally in molecular weight and charge as seen by two-dimensional electrophoresis. Differences can be seen between subclones from the same strain and among subclones derived from a primary subclone. The structural variation in the antigen not only occurs in vitro but has also been demonstrated in vivo after experimental infection (276). Ongoing work by Watson et al. (300) has demonstrated that variation in V-1 can affect the type and severity of lung disease in mice after experimental infection. Thus, it is likely that similar variable antigens from other pathogenic mycoplasmas also influence virulence and account for differences seen between strains of organisms or after passage in culture.

The mechanisms by which high-frequency variation of this group of antigens can affect virulence are unknown. As these are surface antigens, they are likely to influence mycoplasma-host cell interactions, especially as the surface charge of the organism can be altered. Because of this, the organisms may be able to adapt to different conditions present during disease pathogenesis and alter their ability to attach to host cell types. However, there is no clear evidence that the structural variation of antigens on mycoplasmas results in the loss of immunological recognition, similar to that described for parasites.

Host Responses

Nonspecific defense mechanisms

Virulence of mycoplasmas appears to be related to the ability of the organisms to evade nonspecific defense mechanisms (79, 144). Nonspecific defense mechanisms are not as well understood as adaptive immunity; still, innate bactericidal activity is a primary defense against bacterial invasion. In the lungs, for example, mucociliary clearance and intrapulmonary killing are the major processes responsible for nonspecific resistance (126). Alveolar macrophages are generally thought to be the principal mediators of intrapulmonary killing of bacteria. Alveolar lining material (165, 185), neutrophils (216, 289), nonspecific opsonins such as fibronectin, serum components, and complement (131, 213), and unidentified fluid factors (64, 209) also are involved in intrapulmonary killing.

Noncellular factors. While a number of noncellular mycoplasmacidal factors have been reported, few of them have been specifically identified. Dialyzable mycoplasmacidal factors occur in the respiratory tract and in milk whey, but their significance has been questioned since mycoplasma resistance to these factors does not appear to be related to strain virulence or species specificity (140, 142). The only nonspecific factor that has a confirmed role is complement. While complement is also involved in antibody- and macrophage-mediated killing of mycoplasmas (22, 102, 280, 282), several species of mycoplasmas, including *M. pneumoniae*, *M. mycoides*, *M. meleagridis*, *M. canis*, and *M. gallisepticum*, directly activate complement through either the classical or alternative pathway and are susceptible to lysis by activated complement (24, 26, 30, 136, 198, 235, 254, 263). Furthermore, there are host differences in the mycoplasmacidal effect of complement, and genetically deficient mice lacking the fifth component of complement develop more severe mycoplasma-induced arthritis than do normal mice (171).

Phagocytes. Most pathogenic mycoplasmas are exposed to both neutrophils and macrophages during the course of infection. As might be expected, the interactions between mycoplasmas and phagocytes have been studied by numerous investigators.

(i) Neutrophils. Studies of interactions between mycoplasmas and neutrophils are somewhat contradictory. There is no evidence for phagocytosis by neutrophils in the absence of antibody (121, 147, 257, 284). In fact, mycoplasmas adhering to the surface of neutrophils may inhibit cellular function, including phagocytosis of other bacteria (284, 288). While mycoplasmas appear to be killed in vitro by neutrophils following opsonization by specific antibody (139, 279), neutrophil-rich exudates are incapable of clearing *M. pulmonis* from the peritoneal cavity of mice whereas macrophage exudates can do so (145).

(ii) Macrophages. The interactions of mycoplasmas with macrophages have been studied extensively, and the overall impression from in vitro experiments is that macrophages are incapable of ingesting mycoplasmas in the absence of specific antibody. This has been shown for *M. pulmonis* (87, 158, 280), *M. bovis* (139, 145), *M. dispar*, *M. agalactiae* (147), *M. ovipneumoniae* (2), and *M. arthritidis* (58) in several different in vitro culture systems. In the absence of opsonins, electron microscopic studies have shown that *M. pulmonis* (159) and *M. ovipneumoniae* (2) attach to the surface of macrophages but are not ingested. At least for *M. pulmonis*, resistance to ingestion is trypsin sensitive, suggesting the presence of an antiphagocytic surface protein (159). Once mycoplasmas are ingested, killing is rapid (102); there also is some evidence that macrophages may be able to kill surface-associated mycoplasmas through release of hydrolytic enzymes and activated complement components (282). Only the interaction of rat alveolar macrophages and *M. pulmonis* differs from this general scenario. In vitro, rat alveolar macrophages are capable of exerting a mycoplasmastatic effect, but this effect cannot be further enhanced by addition of immune serum (87). This in vitro capability of rat alveolar macrophages agrees with in vivo studies that demonstrate a more efficient removal of *M. pulmonis* from the alveoli of rat lungs than from those of mouse lungs (46).

Recent in vivo studies suggest that specific antibody is not necessary for killing of mycoplasmas in the lung. Efficient intrapulmonary killing of *M. pulmonis* occurs in the lungs of naive C57BL/6N mice in the absence of specific antibody (219). Although we have not yet been able to demonstrate in vitro killing of *M. pulmonis* in the absence of antibody, we have found that the cellular fraction of bronchoalveolar lavages can kill the organism in vitro if allowed to associate with the mycoplasmas in the lungs (80, 86). More than 95% of the cells recovered by bronchoalveolar lavage from *M. pulmonis*-infected animals are macrophages by morphological and immunological criteria, and the majority of cell-associated mycoplasmas in lavages were on or within alveolar macrophages. Furthermore, in vivo exposure to NO_2 damages the macrophage population, and recovery of in vivo intrapulmonary killing mechanisms parallels recovery from macrophage damage.

From the studies discussed above, it is evident that there are factors present or cellular interactions that occur in vivo and have yet to be identified which are critical for intrapulmonary killing of mycoplasmas by macrophages. It is not known what factors are present during in vivo association of macrophages to mycoplasmas that are not present in in vitro macrophage cultures, but the required factors are present in the naive lung and are not derived from serum transudates. Macrophage activation through direct and indirect interactions with mycoplasmas may also be critical (92, 174, 255, 271–273), but it is unclear why in vitro studies do not mimic the type of activation of macrophages that possibly occurs in vivo. However, killing by macrophages with specific immune serum suggests that killing requires opsonization; thus, it is likely that the lungs contain a nonspecific opsonin(s). Complement is one possible opsonin (24); other nonspecific opsonins have been identified for other bacteria and may also be involved in killing of mycoplasmas.

The interaction of mycoplasmas and macrophages may also increase susceptibility to other bacteria. For example, alveolar macrophages from pigs inoculated with *M. hyopneumoniae* have higher phagocytic capability than do those from control pigs (37). However, phagocytosis was depressed for *Actinobacillosis pleuropneumoniae* when macrophages were infected with *M. hyopneumoniae* and challenge exposed with *A. pleuropneumoniae* 2 and 4 weeks later. Thus, *M. hyopneumoniae* infection may suppress phagocytic responses to a secondary pathogen. If similar phenomena occur in other mycoplasma infections, this may partially explain why mycoplasma-infected animals are predisposed to secondary bacterial infections.

NK cells. Respiratory infection with *M. pulmonis* activates NK cell activity in both the spleen and lung between 3 and 7 days postinfection (168, 187, 188). Furthermore, NK cells inhibit growth of mycoplasmas in vitro (188), and treatment of mice with anti-NK cell antibody decreases clearance of *M. pulmonis* from the circulation (188). Activation of NK cells is apparently due to mycoplasma-induced release of gamma interferon, as treatment of mice with anti-gamma interferon reduces clearance. Also, we have shown that mycoplasmas can enhance NK cell activity (99); however, the significance of NK cell enhancement in disease is uncertain. The maximum NK cell activity in vivo is seen at 3 days postinfection with *M. pulmonis* (187, 188), but the maximum intrapulmonary killing of *M. pulmonis* occurs within the first 24 h following aerosol exposure to the organism (219). In fact, organism numbers in the lungs are increasing by day 3 postinfection. This finding suggests that NK cells may be more important in limiting the spread of certain mycoplasma infections than in clearance of the organism from the site of infection.

Adaptive immunity

The development of immunity to mycoplasmas can protect animals, as demonstrated by the ability to vaccinate for many mycoplasma diseases in animals (reviewed in reference 13). Both antibody and cellular immune responses have been described, but immune responses are not always efficient in either protection or recovery from infection. For example, immunization with *M. pulmonis* and *M. hyopneumoniae* confers only partial protection from disease in rats and pigs respectively, with organisms readily isolated from the tissues of challenged animals. Also, infected animals can become asymptomatic carriers of pathogenic mycoplasmas, allowing the maintenance of infection. Many aspects of immunity and mycoplasma infections have been reviewed by Howard and Taylor (146). In this section, we will highlight some of the major concepts in the immunology of mycoplasma diseases as well as present some new information.

Antibody responses are thought to be critical in protection or recovery from some mycoplasma diseases. Resistance can be conferred by passive transfer of antibody prior to infection. This is true for *M. pulmonis* infections of mice, *M. arthritidis* infections in rats and mice, and *M. hyorhinis* and *M. hyopneumoniae* infections in pigs (146). Although *M. mycoides* subsp. *mycoides* infections in cattle may also be protected by passive transfer of convalescent serum, it is unclear whether antibody is the major factor responsible, as nonimmune serum can confer partial protection (120). Some mycoplasma diseases, including those caused by *M. pulmonis* in rats, *M. gallisepticum* in chickens, and *M. meleagridis* in turkeys, are not affected by passively given antibody (146). In addition, local antibody production may be more reflective of disease resistance. For example, immunity to *M. bovis* correlates better with the presence of antibody in lung washings than with the presence of antibody in serum. Another function of antibody production in disease pathogenesis may be to limit the dissemination of infection to other tissues (260).

Systemic antibody responses to mycoplasmas have been studied extensively. Serum immunoglobulin M (IgM) responses are usually detected first after infection of rats or mice with *M. pulmonis* (45, 260) or of cattle with *M. bovis* (143). Serum IgG responses are usually detected next, but this may vary with the mycoplasma, the host, and the route of infection. For example, IgA responses in serum are detected prior to IgG responses in rats intranasally infected with *M. pulmonis* (260), while IgG is detected much earlier in *M. pulmonis* infection of mice (45) and *M. bovis* infection of cattle (143). There may also be some preference for the production of particular immunoglobulin subclasses. We have shown that the specific serum IgG response in F344 rats after immunization with *M. pulmonis* antigen is predominantly IgG2b (258). However, LEW rats do not show a similar preference for production of IgG2b antibody. These results are consistent with what we have described after infection of LEW and F344 rats with *M. pulmonis* (260). Preference for a particular IgG subclass has also been described

for *M. bovis* in cattle, in which IgG1 subclass antibody predominates after infection (140). This antibody subclass also mediates killing of *M. bovis* by macrophages but not neutrophils, while IgG2 is effective for both (139). Thus, the regulation and development of IgG subclass responses are probably important in defense mechanisms against many mycoplasma diseases.

Regional immunity is an important component of immune responses during disease pathogenesis. Immunity to *M. bovis* and *M. dispar* mastitis in cattle is stronger and persists longer in previously infected mammary glands than in the other glands in the same cow (120, 124). Also, many of the mycoplasma diseases are characterized by large infiltrations of mononuclear cells, including T and B lymphocytes, which may be involved in localized immune responses to mycoplasmas and may influence the progression of disease. The presence of antibody specific for mycoplasmas has been detected in lung, genitourinary tract secretions, and milk from animals infected with mycoplasmas (45, 140, 142, 169, 203). Antibody in colostrum may protect piglets from *M. hyopneumoniae* disease (176). In lungs of animals infected with *M. pulmonis*, *M. bovis*, and *M. hyopneumoniae*, antibody-producing (plasma) cells are present (45, 142, 203), but these studies did not examine the specificity of antibody produced. In rats experimentally infected with *M. pulmonis*, lymph nodes of the upper respiratory tract are the initial and major sites of antibody production throughout the course of disease (261, 262). Subsequently, anti-*M. pulmonis* antibody-forming cells appear in nasal passages, lungs, lung-associated lymph nodes, and spleens. Thus, antibody responses specific for mycoplasma do develop in the region of disease and may in some cases have a greater effect on disease pathogenesis.

Although vaccination demonstrates that acquired immunity to mycoplasmas can prevent disease, immune responses can in some cases also contribute to pathogenesis. Cattle given *M. bovoculi* antigen parenterally prior to infection developed more severe conjunctivitis than did naive animals (232), suggesting that immunity can have a detrimental effect. In addition, T cells contribute to the severity of arthritis due to *M. synoviae* infection in chickens, while B cells are involved in resistance (182). Rats and mice that are deficient in T cells also develop less severe respiratory disease than do immunocompetent animals after infection with *M. pulmonis* (91, 309). Also, differences in the proportion of T-helper cells in rats strains appear to be related to the severity of *M. pulmonis* lung disease (89); a larger proportion of T-helper cells is found in lymphoid tissues from the most susceptible rats. Still, passive transfer of immune splenic lymphocytes is protective in rats infected with *M. pulmonis*, and T cells may be protective in these studies (38, 186). T cells may therefore have conflicting roles in some mycoplasma diseases. Different T-cell subsets may also have different effects on the pathogenesis of mycoplasma diseases, as has been described for leishmaniasis and T-helper subsets in mice (252). Antibody responses may also contribute to disease through the formation of immune complexes, as has been demonstrated for mycoplasma-induced arthritis (297, 298).

Several questions about adaptive immunity and mycoplasma diseases remain. The development and regulation of cellular responses, especially local or regional immune responses, need to be further examined. In addition, the role of T-cell subsets in disease pathogenesis needs to be explored, particularly in relationship to pathogenesis and resistance to mycoplasma disease. Finally, it is unclear how mycoplasma infections can persist despite the presence of intense immune and inflammatory responses. This information will be useful both in understanding the pathogenesis of mycoplasma diseases and in developing treatments and vaccines.

Nonspecific interactions with host defenses

Many pathogenic and nonpathogenic mycoplasmas (*Acholeplasma laidlawii*, *M. arginini*, *M. arthritidis*, *M. canis*, *M. felis*, *M. fermentans*, *M. gallisepticum*, *M. hominis*, *M. hyorhinis*, *M. neurolyticum*, *M. pneumoniae*, *M. pulmonis*, *M. synoviae*, and *Spiroplasma citri*, for example) have mitogenic properties and can activate lymphocytes nonspecifically (55). Different species may polyclonally activate B cells, T cells, or both. This property has been demonstrated both in vitro and in vivo (55), and antibody responses to nonrelated antigens can be demonstrated (262, 305). Furthermore, the control mechanisms for lymphocyte activation of *M. arthritidis* mitogen are well described (51, 53, 54, 56), and those for *M. pulmonis* mitogen are beginning to be understood. Most of what is known has been learned in vitro; these studies have been reviewed previously (39, 55) and so will not be discussed in detail here. New developments include the recognition that *M. arthritidis* mitogen is similar to so-called superantigens (54) and that mycoplasmas, especially *M. pulmonis*, can induce increased expression of Ia antigen on B lymphocytes and macrophages and can produce chemotactic substances for host cells (243, 244, 271).

A crucial question is whether or not nonspecific, polyclonal lymphocyte activation plays any role in mycoplasma disease. Even for *M. pulmonis* and *M. arthritidis*, the two organisms best studied in regard to nonspecific lymphocyte activation, the answer is uncertain. For *M. pulmonis*, rat strains which give the strongest mitogenic response to the organism develop the most severe respiratory lesions (89, 259). Furthermore, administration of mitogenic *M. pulmonis* induces pulmonary lesions characterized by lymphoid infiltration, prominently in the alveolar region rather than in the bronchial region, as occurs with natural disease (207). Interpretation of these experiments is complicated by the fact that mitogenic preparations are also antigenic, but it has been shown in other systems that exposure of the respiratory tract to both mitogens and antigens results in more severe lesions than does exposure to either alone (306). LEW rats develop greater in vitro lymphocyte responses to *M. pulmonis* mitogen than do F344 rats (89), which correlates with the increased susceptibility to *M. pulmonis* respiratory disease (89, 259). This finding suggests that *M. pulmonis* mitogen may contribute to disease pathogenesis, especially as the lesions are characterized by an dramatic increase in mononuclear cells along the respiratory tract. However, LEW rats also develop more severe respiratory disease than do F344 rats after infection with viruses (Sendai and sialodacryoadenitis viruses) and intratracheal inoculation of bleomycin

(202). Thus, it is unlikely that all of these phenomena are directly related to nonspecific lymphocyte activation, which indicates that responses to *M. pulmonis* mitogen are not responsible for the observed differences in disease severity between LEW and F344 rats.

The role of nonspecific activation by *M. arthritidis* in disease pathogenesis also remains unclear. Early studies indicated that mouse strains whose lymphocytes were nonresponsive to the mitogen (C57BL/6 [*H-2^b*]) were less susceptible to the arthritogenic and toxic effects of viable *M. arthritis* than were mouse strains whose lymphocytes were responsive (59). In later studies, it was shown that the correlation was good for toxicity and lymphocyte responsiveness to *M. arthritidis* mitogen, but no association was found between arthritis and lymphocyte responses (57). Thus, responses to *M. arthritidis* mitogen are not critical to development of arthritis, but it is still possible that they contribute to the pathology of the lesions.

One suggested consequence of polyclonal activation may be the development of autoimmune responses. These responses have been demonstrated in humans infected with *M. pneumoniae* but thus far have not been documented for any mycoplasma infection in animals. However, little experimental effort has been expended to address this question in animal systems. Another potential consequence of polyclonal activation is altered immune responses to non-cross-reacting antigens. Both enhancement and suppression have been documented following infection with *M. pulmonis* and *M. arthritidis* (1, 189, 278). Suppression of responses to unrelated antigens may be related to disruption of immunoregulation (39), but this has not been demonstrated in vivo.

Induction of increased major histocompatibility complex expression, especially class II (Ia), on macrophages has been demonstrated for a number of mycoplasmas, including the murine species *M. pulmonis* and *M. arthritidis* (271). Both murine myelomonocytic cell lines and primary bone marrow-derived macrophages increased class II gene expression and surface expression of the gene product in response to a stable membrane component of the organism. *M. pulmonis* can also up-regulate class II expression on resting murine B lymphocytes, by an as yet undetermined mechanism (243). Hyperexpression of Ia on macrophages and B cells may prepare them for interaction with T-helper cells (179). Ia induction by mycoplasmas is polyclonal and non-antigen specific and thus may lead to an increased potential for response to self antigens and autoimmunity. Alternatively, increased class II expression due to mycoplasmas might promote a more efficient immune response to the organism by increasing macrophage and B-cell cooperation with T-helper lymphocytes. Interestingly, *M. pulmonis* mitogen-stimulated rat B lymphocytes entered cell cycle only after increasing expression of Ia, suggesting that Ia hyperexpression may be a necessary event for B-cell proliferation (243).

A consistent finding described here and elsewhere in a variety of mycoplasma infections, especially of the lungs and joints of many host species, is the accumulation of large numbers of mononuclear cells, especially in chronic stages of disease. Little is known about the recruitment of lymphocytes and macrophages to such sites of chronic inflammation, but a number of factors are likely to be involved. These include direct chemotactic activity of the organism for inflammatory cells; the production of active intermediates from host components such as complement; and the release of chemotactic factors from host cells, either as a result of mycoplasma- or inflammation-mediated tissue damage or through production by mycoplasma-activated host cells.

We have examined the role of *M. pulmonis* in in vitro inflammatory cell recruitment and demonstrated a novel chemoattractant activity for naive rat B lymphocytes and macrophages mediated by surface membrane proteins of *M. pulmonis* (244). Furthermore, the major variable surface antigen of *M. pulmonis*, V-1 (299), possesses this in vitro B-lymphocyte recruitment activity to a marked degree. This may have in vivo significance in the early and unusually persistent peribronchiolar and perivascular infiltrates of mononuclear cells seen in rats with chronic MRM. Furthermore, *M. pulmonis* mitogen-activated rat serum, likely containing chemotactic complement subcomponents, was chemotactic for rat macrophages and neutrophils, suggesting that at least one indirect mechanism of recruitment may be mediated by mycoplasma proteins (244). Type strains of two other pathogenic murine species, *M. arthritidis* and *M. neurolyticum*, did not appear to possess similar in vitro chemotactic activity for rat B and T lymphocytes or macrophages (244).

In summary, mycoplasmas are able to modulate immune responses without regard to antigen specificity. Nonspecific lymphocyte activation may be involved in disease pathogenesis through release of lymphokines such as interferon, changes in cell surface markers, and autoimmune responses, but clear evidence that these in vitro phenomena occur in disease in response to mycoplasmal mitogen is lacking. In addition, mitogenic components of mycoplasmas may function through stimulation of host cells, not necessarily lymphocytes, to increase production of needed nutrients and thereby contribute to the in vivo survival of the organisms (259). Evidence of genetic linkage between virulence and mitogenicity also would provide strong support. Finally, the availability of gene probes and in situ hybridization techniques offers the possibility of direct demonstration that nonspecifically stimulated lymphocytes produce inflammatory mediators in the diseased tissue. Until such evidence is available, it should be remembered that hyperresponsiveness to nonspecific stimuli may be a marker of a more general defect in host responses and not be directly related to disease production per se. Also, mycoplasma production of chemotactic factors may also have an effect in vivo. Thus, nonspecific interactions of mycoplasmas with the host defense system can potentially have important contributions to disease pathogenesis, especially as many mycoplasma infections are chronic and the cumulative effect may be substantial. However, additional work in this area is needed to demonstrate the significance of these phenomena in vivo.

DIAGNOSIS OF MYCOPLASMA INFECTIONS

Diagnosis of mycoplasma infections generally falls into two categories: isolation and identification of mycoplasmas from diseased tissues, and serological tests. However, isolation of a mycoplasma, even a pathogenic one, from a diseased tissue does not necessarily imply a causal relationship, and positive serological tests in areas that have endemic pathogenic mycoplasmas may not be useful because animals may have been exposed to the organism and developed an immune response to it without disease. We will focus on general principles for diagnosing mycoplasma infections rather than on specifics for each disease or species because the latter have been reviewed in depth elsewhere (41, 68, 78, 104, 116, 122, 132, 164, 212, 242).

Diagnosis of mycoplasma infections in clinically ill animals is not difficult, and any of the procedures discussed below will suffice. However, clinically ill animals may be rare with good management and husbandry practices, making diagnostic challenges of (i) the detection of subclinical infections, which often have very small numbers of organisms present, and (ii) differentiation between pathogenic mycoplasma species and those that are considered commensals.

Health surveillance programs should be designed with at least a 95% chance of detecting at least one infected animal at a given prevalence of infection. The sample size (number of animals) to be tested is of critical importance and can be determined mathematically, assuming that a truly random sample can be obtained, that the prevalence of the infection is known or can be estimated, and that the detection method approximates 100% accuracy (41, 63). As shown in Table 2, if one assumes that 40% of the animals in a population are infected with an agent, there is a 99% probability that 1 infected animal will be detected in a random sample of 10 animals. However, detection of 1 infected animal in a population with a 1% prevalence rate would require testing a random sample of over 200 animals (63). Since diagnosis of infection is much more difficult in such a population than in heavily infected populations, we will focus on these more difficult populations, since techniques that can detect infection in asymptomatic animals will surely work for animals with lesions.

Table 2. Minimal number of samples needed to detect infections

Incidence of infection (%)	Sample size necessary for confidence limit of[a]:	
	95%	99%
5	60	90
10	29	44
15	19	24
20	14	21
25	11	16
30	9	13
40	6	9
50	5	7

[a] Minimum number of animals that must be sampled to detect infectious agents at the indicated prevalence rates within the population. Samples must be taken with complete randomization from a population of 100 or more animals. The disease must show no age or sex predilection.

Culture

Culture remains the primary diagnostic aid for animal mycoplasma diseases. Mycoplasmas are fastidious organisms with many ecological niches in vivo. The general principle in culturing mycoplasmas is to mimic the ecological niche of the organism as closely as possible. Therefore, there are many different mycoplasma media, each designed to optimize growth of one or a few species. In general, each contains a nutrient-rich base and serum, plus antimicrobial agents to inhibit the growth of other bacteria. Although the general formulas are similar for all mycoplasmas, the details vary greatly and can heavily influence one's success in isolating specific organisms. It is a fairly common experience that isolation of fastidious mycoplasmas directly from animals can be much more difficult than growing laboratory-adapted stock cultures. Some mycoplasma strains prefer broth; others of the same species may prefer agar. Some strains require repeated blind subculturing to additional mycoplasma media before they will grow in vitro. Some investigators have reported strains that are so tissue adapted that they will grow only in cell culture systems. Since mycoplasmas have a propensity to colonize mucosal surfaces, samples are usually obtained from respiratory and urogenital tracts, joints, eyes, and mammary glands. For best results, multiple sites within the host should be sampled. One should pick the sites of predilection within the host, if known, plus as many other sites as possible.

Theoretically, one organism will grow and give a positive culture. However, in our hands, about 400 CFU/ml of sample is the limit of detection under most circumstances. Fewer organisms can be isolated, if extreme care is taken, but the cost of such measures is prohibitive (as much as $1,000 per rat or mouse). Even then, culture is relatively insensitive; up to 30% of pathogen-free rats experimentally infected with doses of 10^6 CFU of *M. pulmonis* were negative by culture at 28 days postinfection (82). As a comparison, some of the studies using genetic probes report sensitivity in the range of 10^3 to 10^5 CFU (108, 183, 193, 199, 225, 229), and with the polymerase chain reaction, detection may be sensitive to about 10 CFU (128,184).

Isolation, cultivation, and positive identification of mycoplasmas are difficult and may take 4 weeks or more. The media are expensive, and for animals with subclinical infections, multisite samples are required. Since we do not know the preferred natural sites for many of the animal mycoplasmas, it is impossible to know whether or not one has sampled a site that is likely to harbor organisms. In summary, culture is mandatory for verification of other methods but is a poor screening technique because false-negative results are common.

Histopathology

Gross lesions are inconsistent in many mycoplasma diseases. Examination of tissues, especially lungs, nasal passages, joints, and mammary glands, for microscopic lesions is much more useful. However, even microscopic lesions are rare or minimal in animals infected with low numbers of organisms. Thus, histopathology is insensitive and requires special training to interpret the results. Mild infections are easily overlooked unless one studies multiple tissues and is very familiar with minor changes in host tissues. In addition, lesions are usually suggestive rather than diagnostic.

Detection of Mycoplasma Antigen in Tissues

Immunofluorescence and immunoperoxidase methods for detection of mycoplasma antigen in tissues have been described (41, 68, 78, 104, 116, 122, 132, 164, 212, 242), and both methods work well in animals that are heavily infected. However, these methods usually require special processing of the tissues and experienced personnel to interpret the results. As we have demonstrated with experimentally infected rats, the ability to detect *M. pulmonis* in tissues is directly related to the number of organisms present (82). In animals infected with 10^3 CFU or less, immunofluorescence detected less than 50% of infected animals, and even this degree of success required examination of the trachea, larynx, and lungs. Examination of a single site gave a much lower success rate. In addition, following low-dose experimental inoculation, the majority of *M. pulmonis* organisms localized in the nasal passages (82), a site notoriously difficult to examine by immunofluorescence. Decalcification is required before sectioning of the nasal passages, and *M. pulmonis* antigen often is not detectable following this procedure. In addition, the organism usually can be cultivated readily from animals that are positive by immunofluorescence.

ELISA

Traditional methods of serological diagnosis of mycoplasma infections, such as complement fixation, hemagglutination, hemagglutination inhibition, and metabolic inhibition, have been widely used to diagnose and confirm clinical cases of mycoplasma disease. However, these tests are relatively insensitive and depend on antibody function. In well-managed herds or flocks, both the prevalence of infected animals and the numbers of organisms per animal are usually low. This situation makes detection by serological methods very difficult. We have used the enzyme-linked immunosorbent assay (ELISA) for *M. pulmonis* for many years and will use examples from our experience with that test to illustrate important principles and limitations of ELISAs (40, 78).

The ELISA for mycoplasma infections in rodents has proven to be the best serological test for screening large numbers of rodents. The test is relatively inexpensive to run, sensitive, rapid, and mycoplasma genus specific. In addition, animals do not have to be killed to obtain enough blood for the test. However, the assay currently available cannot distinguish among mycoplasma species, and quality control of the assay, as with all serological assays, is critical for reliable results.

In its simplest form, the ELISA is performed by allowing mycoplasma antigen to absorb nonspecifically to a solid phase (usually a 96-well microtiter plate) and then adding sequentially the serum sample, the secondary conjugated antibody, and the enzyme substrate, with adequate washing between steps (101). The assay is completed by developing the colored product of the enzyme reaction, and reactions are read either on a spectrophotometer or by visual inspection. Although the kit form of the mycoplasma ELISA is usually interpreted subjectively, the semiquantitative data obtained by determining the intensity of the color change spectrophotometrically provide better discrimination of positive and negative results, which is especially important in monitoring barrier-maintained colonies. A semiquantitative assay is relatively inexpensive and can easily be established in any laboratory with a 96-well plate spectrophotometer. Detection of early infection and infection due to small numbers of organisms can be improved with the use of specific anti-*M. pulmonis* IgM. Following experimental inoculation of specific-pathogen-free rats with 10 CFU of *M. pulmonis*, the IgM ELISA detects 17% of exposed animals, compared with 7% for the IgG assay, and the comparable figures for inoculation with 10^3 CFU are 24 versus 13% (82).

The ELISA has many advantages, but it depends on the ability of the animal to produce specific antibody. In very young or very old animals, and in T- and B-cell-deficient rodents, antibody production may be minimal or completely lacking. Also, there may be a delay in antibody production to subclinical infections, resulting in a 1- to 3-month lag time during which infected animals cannot be detected by serological methods.

Unfortunately, other major problems remain with the use of the ELISA as a diagnostic method for mycoplasmas. First, the quality control procedures necessary to ensure reliable results are rigorous. Different laboratories using this assay use different antigen preparations, different solid-phase supports, different reagents, and variations in incubation times. All of these factors affect the test and have led to a lack of agreement in test results between laboratories. The most crucial problem, however, is cross-reactions among the mycoplasmas (8, 35, 40, 78, 205, 264). For example, all of the murine mycoplasmas share some common antigens; these appear to be particularly troublesome in trying to discriminate *M. pulmonis* infection from *M. arthritidis* or *M. muris* infection. Several methods have been attempted to improve the species specificity of the murine mycoplasma ELISA. These include the development of an *M. arthritidis* ELISA, use of immunoblots to verify ELISA results, blocking of cross-reactive antibodies with rabbit antisera, precipitation of cross-reactive antibodies with heterologous organisms, and removal of cross-reactive antigens by affinity chromatography. All of the methods to improve species specificity have proven difficult to standardize, and with the exception of immunoblots, these stop-gap measures are not helpful in the diagnosis of mixed infections.

Immunoblots

Immunoblots (Western blots) have been widely used as specific tests to identify a large number of infec-

tions, including AIDS. For immunoblots, the proteins of an organism are separated by one-dimensional electrophoresis and transferred to nitrocellulose. Sera with antibody react with these separated antigens, which are revealed by using enzyme-linked secondary antibodies and the appropriate substrate. While immunoblots are relatively expensive, time-consuming, technically complicated, and impractical for screening large numbers of samples, this is the preferred method for achieving a specific diagnosis in a barrier maintained colony in which there are a few ELISA-positive animals. We use immunoblots only to achieve a specific diagnosis when ELISA results indicate that a given colony is infected with one of the murine mycoplasmas. This approach is based on the assumption that sera from infected animals should recognize more protein antigens from the infecting organism than from any of the other murine mycoplasmas. If the pattern of bands is sufficiently complex, i.e., 10 or more bands are present, it is relatively easy to make a specific diagnosis. Furthermore, dual infections can be recognized by the presence of a complex banding pattern to more than one organism. However, in about 50% of cases, fewer than four bands are seen with any antigen, or only the bands known to be cross-reacting proteins are present. From results of long-term monitoring of a barrier-maintained colony, the pattern seen with any single animal's serum often begins as one to four bands, and complete patterns develop only after the animal has been infected for several months (70).

Recommendations

At the present time, there is no fully satisfactory diagnostic test for mycoplasma infection in animals that is applicable to all situations. The combination of diagnostic tests chosen must be adapted to the desired goal, and the results must be interpreted with caution. The easiest situation in which to make a diagnosis is a conventional herd, flock, or colony. For example, virtually all conventional rodent colonies are infected with *M. pulmonis*, and these infections are easily detected by several methods. Agreement between cultural and ELISA results in these rodent colonies is approximately 98%. Screening of a well-run, virtually disease-free herd or flock or a barrier-maintained rat or mouse colony is much more difficult. These animals are housed in a well-managed facility containing no agents known to exacerbate mycoplasma infections and in which most of the animals are sold or used at weaning. If a mycoplasma is present, only a small number of the animals may be actually infected, and those that are infected will have few organisms. The ELISA should be the test of choice for initial screening of these populations for mycoplasma infection. Breeding populations should be monitored monthly by including as many animals of all subpopulations as possible. Breeding animals, preferably retired breeders, should be tested by both the IgG and IgM ELISA for mycoplasmas of interest.

If positive animals are found, one must decide whether to eliminate all mycoplasma-infected animals or just specific ones. If one decides to exclude only specific mycoplasmal species, then some species-discriminatory test is necessary. Multiple-site sampling for culture of the most commonly isolated species and immunoblots of the serum against all of the appropriate mycoplasma species are possible verification methods. Neither of these methods works in all instances, but use of the ELISA backed up by culture and immunoblots gives about an 80% chance of identifying *M. pulmonis* if it is present. If no pathogenic mycoplasma is identified in the population, one should continue to retest animals monthly until definite identification of the mycoplasmal species involved is obtained. If one decides that no mycoplasmas are desired in the colony, genital tract infection introduces an additional problem. Even cesarian section derivation to eliminate the organisms may be difficult or impossible. Finding mycoplasma-free foster mothers for the animals may also be difficult.

Obviously, an assay sensitive enough to detect low-level mycoplasma infections needs to be developed. Two possibilities that seem feasible with current technology are specific mycoplasma antigen detection assays or polymerase chain reaction using specific primers. Unfortunately, it will probably require at least 2 to 5 years for such assays to be developed and adequately field tested. Until that time, a combination of the techniques described for detection is recommended.

SUMMARY

An understanding of the pathogenic processes associated with mycoplasma infections in animals may lead to new approaches to the treatment and control of mycoplasma diseases, not only in animals but also in humans. Mycoplasma disease can vary from subtle, low-level disease that affects only breeding to overt severe disease that results in pain and, in some cases, death of the host. It is clear that host and environmental factors influence the development of disease. Mycoplasmas establish intimate contact with host cells, which may lead to cell injury through production of toxic substances or deprivation of nutrients. The variability of mycoplasma phenotypes, including surface antigens, may account for changes in virulence which can result in different patterns of disease with the same species of organisms. The mechanisms by which mycoplasmas survive despite the presence of intense inflammatory and immune responses are unclear. The host responses to mycoplasma infection can be protective; however, many times they either are ineffective or actually contribute to the disease process. Diagnosis of mycoplasma infections in animals can be difficult, as low-level infections can be present in well-maintained animals without clinical signs. These diseases can be treated with antibiotics, but vaccines which prevent disease or, ideally, infection are needed. By taking into account the concepts outlined in this review, we should be able to develop vaccines to a particular mycoplasma which specifically induce effective host responses that inhibit early steps in disease pathogenesis. These concepts include the limitations of current diagnostic techniques and interactions with environmental factors and other infectious agents, which will affect interpretation of studies on the efficacy of any vaccine for an animal mycoplasma.

REFERENCES

1. **Aguila, H. N., W. C. Lai, Y. S. Lu, and S. P. Pakes.** 1988 Experimental *Mycoplasma pulmonis* infection of rats suppresses humoral but not cellular immune response. *Lab. Anim. Sci* **38**:138–142.

2. **Al, K. A., and M. R. Alley.** 1983. Electron microscopic studies of the interaction between ovine alveolar macrophages and *Mycoplasma ovipneumoniae in vitro. Vet. Microbiol.* **8**:571–584.

3. **Alexander, P. G., K. J. Slee, S. McOrist, L. Ireland, and P. J. Coloe.** 1985. Mastitis in cows and polyarthritis and pneumonia in calves caused by Mycoplasma species bovine group 7. *Aust. Vet. J.* **62**:135–136.

4. **Alley, M. R., and J. K. Clarke.** 1979. The experimental transmission of ovine chronic non-progressive pneumonia. *N.Z. Vet. J.* **27**:217–220.

5. **Araake, M.** 1982. Comparison of ciliostasis by mycoplasmas in mouse and chicken tracheal organ cultures. *Microbiol. Immunol.* **26**:1–14.

6. **Araake, M., M. Yayoshi, and M. Yoshioka.** 1984. Electron microscopic studies on the attachment of *Mycoplasma pulmonis* to mouse synovial cells cultured in vitro. *Microbiol. Immunol.* **28**:379–384.

7. **Araake, M., M. Yayoshi, and M. Yoshioka.** 1985. Attachment of *Mycoplasma pulmonis* to rat and mouse synovial cells cultured *in vitro. Microbiol. Immunol.* **29**:601–607.

8. **Armstrong, C. H., M. J. Freeman, and F. L. Sands.** 1987. Cross-reactions between *Mycoplasma hyopneumoniae* and *Mycoplasma flocculare*—practical implications for the serodiagnosis of mycoplasmal pneumonia of swine. *Isr. J. Med. Sci.* **23**:654–656.

9. **Armstrong, C. H., A. B. Scheidt, H. L. Thacker, L. J. Runnels, and M. J. Freeman.** 1984. Evaluation of criteria for the postmortem diagnosis of mycoplasmal pneumonia of swine. *Can. J. Comp. Med.* **48**:278–281.

10. **Ball, H. J., D. Armstrong, S. Kennedy, and W. J. McCaughey.** 1990. Experimental intrauterine inoculation of cows at oestrus with *Mycoplasma bovigenitalium. Vet. Rec.* **126**:486.

11. **Banerjee, A. K., A. F. Angulo, V. A. A. Polak, and A. M. Kershof.** 1985. Naturally occurring genital mycoplasmosis in mice. *Lab. Anim.* **19**:275–276.

12. **Barden, J. A., J. L. Decker, D. W. Dalgard, and R. G. Aptekar.** 1973. *Mycoplasma hyorhinis* swine arthritis. III. Modified disease in Piney Woods swine. *Infect. Immun.* **8**:887–890.

13. **Barile, M. F.** 1985. Immunization against mycoplasma infections, p. 451–492. *In* S. Razin and M. F. Barile (ed.), *The Mycoplasmas*, vol. 4. Academic Press, New York.

14. **Bar-Moshe, B., E. Rapapport, and J. Brenner.** 1984. Vaccination trials against *Mycoplasma mycoides* subsp. *mycoides* (large-colony-type) infection in goats. *Isr. J. Med. Sci.* **20**:972–974.

15. **Bar-Moshe, B., and E. Rapapport.** 1981. Observations on *Mycoplasma mycoides* subsp. *mycoides* infection in Saanen goats. *Isr. J. Med. Sci.* **17**:537–539.

16. **Baskerville, A.** 1972. Development of the early lesions in experimental enzootic pneumonia of pigs: an ultrastructural and histological study. *Res. Vet. Sci.* **13**:570–578.

17. **Bennett, R. H., and D. E. Jasper.** 1978. *Mycoplasma alkalescens*-induced arthritis in dairy calves. *J. Am. Vet. Med. Assoc.* **172**:484–488.

18. **Bhandari, S., and P. J. Asnani.** 1989. Characterization of phospholipase A_2 of mycoplasma species. *Folia Microbiol.* **34**:294–301.

19. **Binder, A., K. Gartner, H. J. Hedrich, W. Hermanns, H. Kirchhoff, and K. Wonigeit.** 1990. Strain differences in sensitivity of rats to *Mycoplasma arthritidis* ISR 1 infection are under multiple gene control. *Infect. Immun.* **58**:1584–1590.

20. **Bolske, G., A. Engvall, L. H. Renstrom, and M. Wierup.**

1989. Experimental infections of goats with *Mycoplasma mycoides* subspecies *mycoides*, LC type. *Res. Vet. Sci.* **46**:247–252.

21. **Bolske, G., H. Msami, N. E. Humlesjo, H. Ern, and L. Jonsson.** 1988. *Mycoplasma capricolum* in an outbreak of polyarthritis and pneumonia in goats. *Acta Vet. Scand.* **29**:331–338.

22. **Bredt, W.** 1975. Phagocytosis by macrophages of *Mycoplasma pneumoniae* after opsonization by complement. *Infect. Immun.* **12**:695–696.

23. **Bredt, W., J. Feldner, and I. Kahane.** 1981. Adherence of mycoplasmas to cells and inert surfaces: phenomena, experimental models and possible mechanisms. *Isr. J. Med. Sci.* **17**:586–588.

24. **Bredt, W., M. Kist, and E. Jacobs.** 1981. Phagocytosis and complement actions. *Isr. J. Med. Sci.* **17**:637–640.

25. **Bredt, W., and U. Radestock.** 1977. Gliding motility of *Mycoplasma pulmonis*. *J. Bacteriol.* **130**:937–938.

26. **Bredt, W., B. Wellek, H. Brunner, and M. Loos.** 1977. Interactions between *Mycoplasma pneumoniae* and the first components of complement. *Infect. Immun.* **15**:7–12.

27. **Brennan, P. C., and R. N. Feinstein.** 1969. Relationship of hydrogen peroxide production by *Mycoplasma pulmonis* to virulence for catalase-deficient mice. *J. Bacteriol.* **98**:1036–1040.

28. **Brogden, K. A., D. Rose, R. C. Cutlip, H. D. Lehmkuhl, and J. G. Tully.** 1988. Isolation and identification of mycoplasmas from the nasal cavity of sheep. *Am. J. Vet. Res.* **49**:1669–1672.

29. **Brown, M. B., and L. Reyes.** 1991. Immunoglobulin class- and subclass-specific responses to *Mycoplasma pulmonis* in sera and secretions of naturally infected Sprague-Dawley female rats. *Infect. Immun.* **59**:2181–2185.

30. **Brunner, H., S. Razin, A. R. Kalica, and R. M. Chanock.** 1971. Lysis and death of *Mycoplasma pneumoniae* by antibody and complement. *J. Immunol.* **106**:907–916.

31. **Bryson, D. G.** 1985. Calf pneumonia. *Vet. Clin. North Am. Food Anim. Pract.* **1**:237–257.

32. **Buchvarova, Y., and A. Vesselinova.** 1989. On the aetiopathogenesis of mycoplasma pneumonia in calf. *Arch. Exp. Veterinaermed.* **43**:685–689.

33. **Bushnell, R. B.** 1984. Mycoplasma mastitis. *Vet. Clin. North Am. Large Anim. Pract.* **6**:301–312.

34. **Buttery, S. H., G. S. Cottew, and L. C. Lloyd.** 1980. Effect of soluble factors from *Mycoplasma mycoides* subsp. *mycoides* on the collagen content of bovine connective tissue. *J. Comp. Pathol.* **90**:303–314.

35. **Buttery, S. H., and J. R. Etheridge.** 1971. Observations on the cross reaction between *Mycoplasma pneumoniae* antigen and bovine antisera to *Mycoplasma mycoides* var. *mycoides*. *Aust. J. Exp. Biol. Med. Sci.* **49**:233–236.

36. **Carmichael, L. E., T. D. St. George, N. D. Sullivan, and N. Horsfall.** 1972. Isolation, propagation, and characterization studies of an ovine Mycoplasma responsible for proliferative interstitial pneumonia. *Cornell Vet.* **62**:654–679.

37. **Caruso, J. P., and R. F. Ross.** 1990. Effects of *Mycoplasma hyopneumoniae* and *Actinobacillus (Haemophilus) pleuropneumoniae* infections on alveolar macrophage functions in swine. *Am. J. Vet. Res.* **51**:227–231.

38. **Cassell, G. H.** 1982. Derrick Edward Award lecture. The pathogenic potential of mycoplasmas: *Mycoplasma pulmonis* as a model. *Rev. Infect. Dis.* **4**(Suppl.):S18–S34.

39. **Cassell, G. H., W. A. Clyde, Jr., and J. K. Davis.** 1985. Mycoplasmal respiratory infections, p. 65–106. *In* S. Razin and M. F. Barile (ed.), *The Mycoplasmas*, vol. 4. *Mycoplasma Pathogenicity*. Academic Press, New York.

40. **Cassell, G. H., N. R. Cox, J. K. Davis, M. B. Brown, F. C. Minion, and J. R. Lindsey.** 1986. State of the art detection methods for rodent mycoplasmas, p. 143–160. *In* T. E. Hamm, Jr. (ed.), *Complications of Viral and Mycoplasmal Infections in Rodents to Toxicology Research and Testing*. Hemisphere Press, Washington, D.C.

41. **Cassell, G. H., M. K. Davidson, J. K. Davis, and J. R. Lindsey.** 1983. Recovery and identification of murine mycoplasmas, p. 129–142. *In* J. G. Tully and S. Razin (ed.), *Methods in Mycoplasmology*, vol. 2. *Diagnostic Mycoplasmology*. Academic Press, New York.

42. **Cassell, G. H., J. K. Davis, N. R. Cox, M. K. Davidson, and J. R. Lindsey.** 1984. *Mycoplasma pulmonis* detection in rodents: lessons for diagnosis in other species. *Isr. J. Med. Sci.* **20**:859–865.

43. **Cassell, G. H., J. K. Davis, J. R. Lindsey, B. C. Cole, and M. W. Hartley.** 1981. Arthritis of rats and mice: implications for man. *Isr. J. Med. Sci.* **17**:608–615.

44. **Cassell, G. H., J. K. Davis, J. W. Simecka, J. R. Lindsey, N. R. Cox, S. E. Ross, and M. Fallon.** 1986. Mycoplasma infections: disease pathogenesis, implications for biomedical research and control, p. 87–130. *In* P. N. Bhatt, R. O. Jacoby, H. C. Morse III, and A. E. New (ed.), *Viral and Mycoplasma Infections of Laboratory Rodents: Effects on Biomedical Research*. Academic Press, Orlando, Fla.

45. **Cassell, G. H., J. R. Lindsey, and H. J. Baker.** 1974. Immune responses of pathogen-free mice inoculated intranasally with *Mycoplasma pulmonis*. *J. Immunol.* **112**:124–136.

46. **Cassell, G. H., J. R. Lindsey, R. G. Overcash, and H. J. Baker.** 1973. Murine mycoplasma respiratory disease. *Ann. N.Y. Acad. Sci.* **225**:395–412.

47. **Cassell, G. H., W. H. Wilborn, S. H. Silvers, and F. C. Minion.** 1981. Adherence and colonization of *Mycoplasma pulmonis* to genital epithelium and spermatozoa in rats. *Isr. J. Med. Sci.* **17**:593–598.

48. **Cherry, J. D., and D. Taylor-Robinson.** 1970. Growth and pathogenesis of *Mycoplasma mycoides* var. *capri* in chicken embryo tracheal organ cultures. *Infect. Immun.* **2**:431–438.

49. **Ciprian, A., C. Pijoan, T. Cruz, J. Camacho, J. Tortora, G. Colmenares, R. R. Lopez, and M. de la Garcia.** 1988. *Mycoplasma hyopneumoniae* increases the susceptibility of pigs to experimental *Pasteurella multocida* pneumonia. *Can. J. Vet. Res.* **52**:434–438.

50. **Clyde, W. A., Jr., and P. C. Hu.** 1986. Antigenic determinants of the attachment protein of *Mycoplasma pneumoniae* shared by other pathogenic mycoplasma species. *Infect. Immun.* **51**:690–692.

51. **Cole, B. C., R. A. Daynes, and J. R. Ward.** 1982. Stimulation of mouse lymphocytes by a mitogen derived from *Mycoplasma arthritidis*. III. Ir gene control of lymphocyte transformation correlates with binding of the mitogen to specific Ia-bearing cells. *J. Immunol.* **129**:1352–1359.

52. **Cole, B. C., L. Golightly Rowland, and J. R. Ward.** 1975. Arthritis of mice induced by *Mycoplasma pulmonis*: humoral antibody and lymphocyte responses of CBA mice. *Infect. Immun.* **12**:1083–1092.

53. **Cole, B. C., D. R. Kartchner, and D. J. Wells.** 1989. Stimulation of mouse lymphocytes by a mitogen derived from *Mycoplasma arthritidis*. VII. Responsiveness is associated with expression of a product(s) of the V beta 8 gene family present on the T cell receptor alpha/beta for antigen. *J. Immunol.* **142**:4131–4137.

54. **Cole, B. C., D. R. Kartchner, and D. J. Wells.** 1990. Stimulation of mouse lymphocytes by a mitogen derived from *Mycoplasma arthritidis* (MAM). VIII. Selective activation of T cells expressing distinct V beta T cell receptors from various strains of mice by the "superantigen" MAM. *J. Immunol.* **144**:425–431.

55. **Cole, B. C., Y. Naot, E. J. Stanbridge, and K. S. Wise.** 1985. Interactions of mycoplasmas and their products with lymphoid cells *in vitro*, p. 204–258. *In* S. Razin and M. F. Barile (ed.), *The Mycoplasmas*, vol. 4. Academic Press, New York.

56. **Cole, B. C., and R. N. Thorpe.** 1984. I-E/I-C region-associated induction of murine gamma interferon by a haplotype-restricted polyclonal T-cell mitogen derived from *Mycoplasma arthritidis*. *Infect. Immun.* **43**:302–307.

57. **Cole, B. C., R. N. Thorpe, L. A. Hassell, L. R. Washburn, and J. R. Ward.** 1983. Toxicity but not arthritogenicity of *Mycoplasma arthritidis* for mice associates with the haplotype expressed at the major histocompatibility complex. *Infect. Immun.* **41**:1010–1015.

58. **Cole, B. C., and J. R. Ward.** 1973. Interaction of *Mycoplasma arthritidis* and other mycoplasmas with murine peritoneal macrophages. *Infect. Immun.* **7**:691–699.

59. **Cole, B. C., J. R. Ward, and L. Golightly-Rowland.** 1973. Factors influencing the susceptibility of mice to *Mycoplasma arthritidis*. *Infect. Immun.* **7**:218–225.

60. **Cole, B. C., J. R. Ward, and C. H. Martin.** 1968. Hemolysin and peroxide activity of mycoplasma species. *J. Bacteriol.* **95**:2022–2033.

61. **Cole, B. C., L. R. Washburn, and D. Taylor-Robinson.** 1985. Mycoplasma-induced arthritis. p. 108–150. *In* S. Razin and M. F. Barile (ed.), *The Mycoplasmas*, vol. 4. *Mycoplasma Pathogenicity*. Academic Press, New York.

62. **Committee on Infectious Diseases of Mice and Rats. Institute of Laboratory Animal Resources. Commission on Life Sciences. National Research Council.** 1991. *Infectious Diseases of Mice and Rats*. National Academy Press, Washington, D.C.

63. **Committee on Long Term Holding of Laboratory Rodents.** 1976. Long term holding of laboratory rodents. *ILAR News* **19**:L1–L25.

64. **Coonrod, J. D., R. L. Lester, and L. C. Hsu.** 1984. Characterization of the extracellular bactericidal factors of rat alveolar lining material. *J. Clin. Invest.* **74**:1269–1279.

65. **Cordy, D. R., H. E. Adler, and R. Yamamoto.** 1955. A pathogenic pleuropneumonia-like organism from goats. *Cornell Vet.* **45**:50–68.

66. **Cottew, G. S.** 1979. Caprine-ovine mycoplasmas, p. 103–133. *In* J. G. Tully and R. F. Whitcomb (ed.), *The Mycoplasmas*, vol. 2. *Human and Animal Mycoplasmas*. Academic Press, New York.

67. **Cottew, G. S.** 1979. Pathogenicity of the subspecies mycoides of *Mycoplasma mycoides* for cattle, sheep and goats. *Zentralbl. Bakteriol. Orig Reihe A* **245**:164–170.

68. **Cottew, G. S.** 1983. Recovery and identification of caprine and ovine mycoplasmas, p. 91–104. *In* J. G. Tully, and S. Razin (ed.), *Methods in Mycoplasmology*, vol. 2. *Diagnostic Mycoplasmology*. Academic Press, New York.

69. **Cottew, G. S.** 1984. Overview of mycoplasmoses in sheep and goats. *Isr. J. Med. Sci.* **20**:962–964.

70. **Cox, N. R., M. K. Davidson, J. K. Davis, J. R. Lindsey, and G. H. Cassell.** 1988. Natural mycoplasmal infections in isolator-maintained LEW/Tru rats. *Lab. Anim. Sci.* **38**:381–388.

71. **Dallo, S. F., and J. B. Baseman.** 1990. Cross-hybridization between the cytoadhesin genes of *Mycoplasma pneumoniae* and *Mycoplasma genitalium* and genomic DNA of *Mycoplasma gallisepticum*. *Microb. Pathog.* **8**:371–375.

72. **DaMassa, A. J., D. L. Brooks, and H. E. Adler.** 1983. Caprine mycoplasmosis: widespread infection in goats with *Mycoplasma mycoides* subsp *mycoides* (large-colony type). *Am. J. Vet. Res.* **44**:322–325.

73. **DaMassa, A. J., D. L. Brooks, and C. A. Holmberg.** 1984. Pathogenicity of *Mycoplasma capricolum* and *Mycoplasma putrefaciens*. *Isr. J. Med. Sci.* **20**:975–978.

74. **DaMassa, A. J., D. L. Brooks, and C. A. Holmberg.** 1986. Induction of mycoplasmosis in goat kids by oral inoculation with *Mycoplasma mycoides* subspecies *mycoides*. *Am. J. Vet. Res.* **47**:2084–2089.

75. **DaMassa, A. J., D. L. Brooks, C. A. Holmberg, and A. I. Moe.** 1987. Caprine mycoplasmosis: an outbreak of mastitis and arthritis requiring the destruction of 700 goats. *Vet. Rec.* **120**:409–413.

76. **DaMassa, A. J., C. A. Holmberg, and D. L. Brooks.** 1987. Comparison of caprine mycoplasmosis caused by *Mycoplasma capricolum*, *Mycoplasma mycoides* subsp. *mycoides*, and *Mycoplasma putrefaciens*. *Isr. J. Med. Sci.* **23**:636–640.

77. **DaMassa, A. J., E. R. Nascimento, M. I. Khan, R. Yamamoto, and D. L. Brooks.** 1991. Characteristics of an unusual mycoplasma isolated from a case of caprine mastitis and arthritis with possible systemic manifestations. *J. Vet. Diagn. Invest.* **3**:55–59.

78. **Davidson, M. K., J. K. Davis, G. P. Gambill, G. H. Cassell, and J. R. Lindsey.** Mycoplasmas of laboratory rodents. *In* H. W. Whitford (ed.), *Laboratory Diagnosis of Mycoplasmosis in Animals*. Iowa State University Press, Ames, in press.

79. **Davidson, M. K., J. K. Davis, J. R. Linsey, and G. H. Cassell.** 1988. Clearance of different strains of *Mycoplasma pulmonis* from the respiratory tract of C3H/HeN mice. *Infect. Immun.* **56**:2163–2168.

80. **Davidson, M. K., J. K. Davis, T. R. Schoeb, J. W. Simecka, and J. R. Lindsey.** Unpublished data.

81. **Davidson, M. K., J. R. Lindsey, M. B. Brown, G. H. Cassell, and G. A. Boorman.** 1983. Natural *Mycoplasma arthritidis* infection in mice. *Curr. Microbiol.* **8**:205–208.

82. **Davidson, M. K., J. R. Lindsey, M. B. Brown, T. R. Schoeb, and G. H. Cassell.** 1981. Comparison of methods for detection of *Mycoplasma pulmonis* in experimentally and naturally infected rats. *J. Clin. Microbiol.* **14**:646–655.

83. **Davidson, M. K., J. R. Lindsey, R. F. Parker, J. G. Tully, and G. H. Cassell.** 1988. Differences in virulence for mice among strains of *Mycoplasma pulmonis*. *Infect. Immun.* **56**:2156–2162.

84. **Davis, J., G. H. Cassell, G. Gambill, N. Cox, H. Watson, and M. Davidson.** 1987. Diagnosis of murine mycoplasmal infections by enzyme-linked immunosorbent assay (ELISA). *Isr. J. Med. Sci.* **23**:717–722.

85. **Davis, J. K., and G. H. Cassell.** 1982. Murine respiratory mycoplasmosis in LEW and F344 rats. Strain differences in lesion severity. *Vet. Pathol.* **19**:280–293.

86. **Davis, J. K., M. K. Davidson, T. R. Schoeb, and J. R. Lindsey.** 1992. Decreased intrapulmonary killing of *Mycoplasma pulmonis* after short term exposure to NO$_2$ is associated with damaged alveolar macrophages. *Am. Rev. Respir. Dis.* **145**:406–411.

87. **Davis, J. K., K. M. Delozier, D. K. Asa, F. C. Minion, and G. H. Cassell.** 1980. Interactions between murine alveolar macrophages and *Mycoplasma pulmonis* in vitro. *Infect. Immun.* **29**:590–599.

88. **Davis, J. K., R. F. Parker, H. White, D. Dziedzic, G. Taylor, M. K. Davidson, N. R. Cox, and G. H. Cassell.** 1985. Strain differences in susceptibility to murine respiratory mycoplasmosis in C57BL/6 and C3H/HeN mice. *Infect. Immun.* **50**:647–654.

89. **Davis, J. K., J. W. Simecka, J. S. Williamson, S. E. Ross, M. M. Juliana, R. B. Thorp, and G. H. Cassell.** 1985. Nonspecific lymphocyte responses in F344 and LEW rats: susceptibility to murine respiratory mycoplasmosis and examination of cellular basis for strain differences. *Infect. Immun.* **49**:152–158.

90. **Davis, J. K., R. B. Thorp, P. A. Maddox, M. B. Brown, and G. H. Cassell.** 1982. Murine respiratory mycoplasmosis in F344 and LEW rats: evolution of lesions and lung lymphoid cell populations. *Infect. Immun.* **36**:720–729.

91. **Denny, F. W., D. Taylor-Robinson, and A. C. Allison.** 1972. The role of thymus-dependent immunity in *Mycoplasma pulmonis* infections in mice. *J. Med. Microbiol.* **5**:327–336.

92. **Dietz, J. N., and B. C. Cole.** 1982. Direct activation of

the J774.1 murine macrophage cell line by *Mycoplasma arthritidis*. *Infect. Immun.* **37**:811–819.

93. **Doig, P. A.** 1981. Bovine genital mycoplasmosis. *Can. Vet. J.* **22**:339–343.

94. **Doig, P. A., H. L. Ruhnke, and N. C. Palmer.** 1980. Experimental bovine genital ureaplasmosis. II. Granular vulvitis, endometritis and salpingitis following uterine inoculation. *Can. J. Comp. Med.* **44**:259–266.

95. **do Nascimento, M. da G., and E. R. do Nascimento.** 1986. Infectious sinusitis in coturnix quails in Brazil. *Avian Dis.* **30**:228–230.

96. **Dybvig, K., J. W. Simecka, H. L. Watson, and G. H. Cassell.** 1989. High-frequency variation in *Mycoplasma pulmonis* colony size. *J. Bacteriol.* **171**:5165–5168.

97. **East, N. E., A. J. DaMassa, L. L. Logan, D. L. Brooks, and B. McGowan.** 1983. Milkborne outbreak of *Mycoplasma mycoides* subspecies *mycoides* infection in a commercial goat dairy. *J. Am. Vet. Med. Assoc.* **182**:1338–1341.

98. **Edward, D. G. ff., and E. A. Freundt.** 1956. The classification and nomenclature of organisms of the pleuropneumoniae group. *J. Gen. Microbiol.* **14**:197–207.

99. **Egan, M., S. E. Ross, G. H. Cassell, and J. W. Simecka.** 1991. Unpublished data.

100. **Egwu, G. O., W. B. Faull, J. M. Bradbury, and M. J. Clarkson.** 1989. Ovine infectious keratoconjunctivitis: a microbiological study of clinically unaffected and affected sheep's eyes with special reference to *Mycoplasma conjunctivae*. *Vet. Rec.* **125**:253–256.

101. **Engvall, E., and P. Permann.** 1972. Enzyme-linked immunosorbent assay ELISA. III. Quantitation of specific antibodies by enzyme labeled anti-immunoglobulin in antigen coated tubes. *J. Immunol.* **109**:129–135.

102. **Erb, P., and W. Bredt.** 1979. Interaction of *Mycoplasma pneumoniae* with alveolar macrophages: viability of adherent and ingested mycoplasmas. *Infect. Immun.* **25**:11–15.

103. **Foggie, A., G. E. Jones, and D. Buxton.** 1976. The experimental infection of specific pathogen free lambs with *Mycoplasma ovipneumoniae*. *Res. Vet. Sci.* **21**:28–35.

104. **Freundt, E. A.** 1981. General principles of laboratory diagnosis of mycoplasma infections. *Isr. J. Med. Sci.* **17**:641–643.

105. **Friis, N. F.** 1980. *Mycoplasma dispar* as a causative agent in pneumonia of calves. *Acta Vet. Scand.* **21**:34–42.

106. **Furlong, S. L., and A. J. Turner.** 1975. The isolation of *Mycoplasma hyosynoviae* and exposure of pigs to experimental infection. *Aust. Vet. J.* **51**:291–293.

107. **Geary, S. J., M. G. Gabridge, R. Intres, D. L. Draper, and M. F. Gladd.** 1989. Identification of mycoplasma binding proteins utilizing a 100 kilodalton lung fibroblast receptor. *J. Recept. Res.* **9**:465–478.

108. **Geary, S. J., M. F. Gladd, and M. G. Gabridge.** 1990. Species-specific biotinylated DNA probe for *M. gallisepticum*, p. 864–866. *In* G. Stanek, G. H. Cassell, J. G. Tully, and R. F. Whitcomb (ed.), *Recent Advances in Mycoplasmology*. Gustav Fischer Verlag, New York.

109. **Geary, S. J., M. E. Tourtellotte, and J. A. Cameron.** 1981. Inflammatory toxin from *Mycoplasma bovis*: isolation and characterization. *Science* **212**:1032–1033.

110. **Geary, S. J., and E. M. Walczak.** 1983. Cytopathic effect of whole cells and purified membranes of *Mycoplasma hyopneumoniae*. *Infect. Immun.* **41**:132–136.

111. **Glasgow, L. R., and R. L. Hill.** 1980. Interaction of *Mycoplasma gallisepticum* with sialyl glycoproteins. *Infect. Immun.* **30**:353–361.

112. **Gois, M., and F. Kuksa.** 1974. Intranasal infection of gnotobiotic piglets with *Mycoplasma hyorhinis*: differences in virulence of the strains and influence of age on the development of infection. *Zentralbl. Veterinaermed. Reike B* **21**:352–361.

113. **Gois, M., F. Kuksa, and F. Sisak.** 1977. Experimental infection of gnotobiotic piglets with *Mycoplasma hyo-*

114. **Gonzalez, R. N., D. E. Jasper, T. B. Farver, R. B. Bushnell, and C. E. Franti.** 1988. Prevalence of udder infections and mastitis in 50 California dairy herds. *J. Am. Vet. Med. Assoc.* **193**:323–328.

115. **Goodwin, R. F., A. P. Pomeroy, and P. Whittlestone.** 1967. Characterization of *Mycoplasma suipneumonia*: a mycoplasma causing enzootic pneumonia of pigs. *J. Hyg.* (London) **65**:85–96.

116. **Gourlay, R. N.** 1981. Laboratory diagnosis of animal mycoplasma infections. *Isr. J. Med. Sci.* **17**:645–655.

117. **Gourlay, R. N.** 1981. Mycoplasma-induced arthritis in farm animals. *Isr. J. Med. Sci.* **17**:626–627.

118. **Gourlay, R. N.** 1981. Mycoplasmosis in cattle, sheep and goats. *Isr. J. Med. Sci.* **17**:531–536.

119. **Gourlay, R. N., and S. B. Houghton.** 1985. Experimental pneumonia in conventionally reared and gnotobiotic calves by dual infection with *Mycoplasma bovis* and *Pasteurella haemolytica*. *Res. Vet. Sci.* **38**:377–382.

120. **Gourlay, R. N., and C. J. Howard.** 1979. Bovine mycoplasmas, p. 50–102. *In* J. G. Tully and R. F. Whitcomb (ed.), *The Mycoplasmas*, vol. 2. *Human and Animal Mycoplasmas*. Academic Press, New York.

121. **Gourlay, R. N., and C. J. Howard.** 1982. Respiratory mycoplasmosis. *Adv. Vet. Sci. Comp. Med.* **26**:289–332.

122. **Gourlay, R. N., and C. J. Howard.** 1983. Recovery and identification of bovine mycoplasmas, p. 81–90. *In* J. G. Tully and S. Razin (ed.), *Methods of Mycoplasmology*, vol. 2. *Diagnostic Mycoplasmology*. Academic Press, New York.

123. **Gourlay, R. N., C. J. Howard, and J. Brownlie.** 1972. The production of mastitis in cows by the intramammary inoculation of T-mycoplasmas. *J. Hyg.* (London) **70**:511–521.

124. **Gourlay, R. N., C. J. Howard, and J. Brownlie.** 1975. Localized immunity in experimental bovine mastitis caused by *Mycoplasma dispar*. *Infect. Immun.* **12**:947–950.

125. **Gourlay, R. N., L. H. Thomas, and S. G. Wyld.** 1989. Increased severity of calf pneumonia associated with the appearance of *Mycoplasma bovis* in a rearing herd. *Vet. Rec.* **124**:420–422.

126. **Green, G. M., and E. Goldstein.** 1966. A method for quantitating intrapulmonary bacterial inactivation by individual animals. *J. Lab. Clin. Med.* **68**:669–677.

127. **Gross, W. B.** 1990. Factors affecting the development of respiratory disease complex in chickens. *Avian Dis.* **34**:607–610.

128. **Harasawa, R., K. Koshimizu, T. Uemori, O. Takeda, K. Asada, and I. Kato.** 1990. The polymerase chain reaction for *Mycoplasma pulmonis*. *Microbiol. Immunol.* **34**:393–395.

129. **Harbi, M. S., and M. M. Salih.** 1979. Artificial reproduction of arthritis in calves by intubation of a virulent strain of *Mycoplasma mycoides* subsp. *mycoides*. *Vet. Rec.* **104**:194.

130. **Harwick, H. J., A. D. Mahoney, G. M. Kalmanson, and L. B. Guze.** 1976. Arthritis in mice due to infection with *Mycoplasma pulmonis*. II. Serological and histological features. *J. Infect. Dis.* **133**:103–112.

131. **Heidbrink, P. J., G. B. Toews, G. N. Gross, and A. K. Pierce.** 1982. Mechanisms of complement-mediated clearance of bacteria from the lung. *Am. Rev. Respir. Dis.* **125**:517–520.

132. **Hill, A. C.** 1983. Recovery and identification of mycoplasmas from other laboratory animals (including primates), p. 143–148. *In* J. G. Tully and S. Razin (ed.), *Methods in Mycoplasmology*, vol. 2. *Diagnostic Mycoplasmology*. Academic Press, New York.

133. **Hjerpe, C. A., and H. D. Knight.** 1972. Polyarthritis and synovitis associated with *Mycoplasma bovimastitidis* in feedlot cattle. *J. Am. Vet. Med. Assoc.* **160**:1414–1418.

134. **Hopkins, S. R., and Yoder, H. W., Jr.** 1984. Increased incidence of airsacculitis in broilers infected with *Mycoplasma synoviae* and chicken-passaged infectious bronchitis vaccine virus. *Avian Dis.* **28**:386–396.

135. **Houghton, S. B., and R. N. Gourlay.** 1983. Synergism between *Mycoplasma bovis* and *Pasteurella haemolytica* in calf pneumonia. *Vet. Rec.* **113**:41–42.

136. **Howard, C. J.** 1980. Variation in the susceptibility of bovine mycoplasmas to killing by the alternative complement pathway in bovine serum. *Immunology* **41**:561–568.

137. **Howard, C. J.** 1983. Mycoplasmas and bovine respiratory disease: studies related to pathogenicity and the immune response—a selective review. *Yale J. Biol. Med.* **56**:789–797.

138. **Howard, C. J.** 1984. Animal ureaplasmas: their ecological niche and role in disease. *Isr. J. Med. Sci.* **20**:954–957.

139. **Howard, C. J.** 1984. Comparison of bovine IgG1, IgG2 and IgM for ability to promote killing of *Mycoplasma bovis* by bovine alveolar macrophages and neutrophils. *Vet. Immunol. Immunopathol.* **6**:321–326.

140. **Howard, C. J., J. Brownlie, R. N. Gourlay, and J. Collins.** 1975. Presence of a dialysable fraction in normal bovine whey capable of killing several species of bovine mycoplasmas. *J. Hyg.* (London) **74**:261–270.

141. **Howard, C. J., and R. N. Gourlay.** 1978. Mycoplasmas of animals. *Sci. Prog.* **65**:313–329.

142. **Howard, C. J., R. N. Gourlay, and G. Taylor.** 1978. Defence mechanisms in calves against respiratory infections with mycoplasmas, p. 317–325. *In* W. B. Martin (ed.), *Respiratory Defenses in Cattle.* Martinus Nijhoff, The Hague, The Netherlands.

143. **Howard, C. J., K. R. Parsons, and L. H. Thomas.** 1986. Systemic and local immune responses of gnotobiotic calves to respiratory infection with *Mycoplasma bovis.* *Vet. Immunol. Immunopathol.* **11**:291–300.

144. **Howard, C. J., and G. Taylor.** 1979. Variation in the virulence of strains of *Mycoplasma pulmonis* related to susceptibility to killing by macrophages *in vitro. J. Gen. Microbiol.* **114**:289–294.

145. **Howard, C. J., and G. Taylor.** 1983. Interaction of mycoplasmas and phagocytes. *Yale J. Biol. Med.* **56**:643–648.

146. **Howard, C. J., and G. Taylor.** 1985. Humoral and cell-mediated immunity, p. 259–292. *In* S. Razin and M. F. Barile (ed.), *The Mycoplasmas,* vol. 4. Academic Press, New York.

147. **Howard, C. J., G. Taylor, J. Collins, and R. N. Gourlay.** 1976. Interaction of *Mycoplasma dispar* and *Mycoplasma agalactiae* subsp. *bovis* with bovine alveolar macrophages and bovine lacteal polymorphonuclear leukocytes. *Infect. Immun.* **14**:11–17.

148. **Howard, C. J., L. H. Thomas, and K. R. Parsons.** 1987. Comparative pathogenicity of *Mycoplasma bovis* and *Mycoplasma dispar* for the respiratory tract of calves. *Isr. J. Med. Sci.* **23**:621–624.

149. **Hudson, J. R.** 1971. Contagious bovine pleuropneumonia. FAO Agricultural Studies no. 86. Food and Agricultural Organization, Rome.

150. **Ionas, G., A. J. Mew, M. R. Alley, J. K. Clarke, A. J. Robinson, and R. B. Marshall.** 1985. Colonisation of the respiratory tract of lambs by strains of *Mycoplasma ovipneumoniae. Vet. Microbiol.* **10**:533–539.

151. **Jasper, D. E.** 1981. Bovine mycoplasmal mastitis. *Adv. Vet. Sci. Comp. Med.* **25**:121–257.

152. **Jasper, D. E., J. T. Boothby, and C. B. Thomas.** 1987. Pathogenesis of bovine mycoplasma mastitis. *Isr. J. Med. Sci.* **23**:625–627.

153. **Jasper, D. E., J. D. Dellinger, M. H. Rollins, and H. D. Hakanson.** 1979. Prevalence of mycoplasmal bovine mastitis in California. *Am. J. Vet. Res.* **40**:1043–1047.

154. **Jericho, K. W.** 1986. Pathogenesis of mycoplasma pneumonia of swine. *Can. J. Vet. Res.* **50**:136–137.

155. **Jones, G. E., A. Foggie, A. Sutherland, and D. B. Harker.** 1976. Mycoplasmas and ovine keratoconjunctivitis. *Vet. Rec.* **99**:137–141.

156. **Jones, G. E., J. S. Gilmour, and A. G. Rae.** 1982. The effect of *Mycoplasma ovipneumoniae* and *Pasteurella haemolytica* on specific pathogen-free lambs. *J. Comp. Pathol.* **92**:261–266.

157. **Jones, G. E., J. S. Gilmour, and A. G. Rae.** 1982. The effects of different strains of *Mycoplasma ovipneumoniae* on specific pathogen-free and conventionally-reared lambs. *J. Comp. Pathol.* **92**:267–272.

158. **Jones, T. C., and J. G. Hirsch.** 1971. The interaction in vitro of *Mycoplasma pulmonis* with mouse peritoneal macrophages and L-cells. *J. Exp. Med.* **133**:231–259.

159. **Jones, T. C., R. Minick, and L. Yang.** 1977. Attachment and ingestion of mycoplasmas by mouse macrophages. II. Scanning electron microscopic observations. *Am. J. Pathol.* **87**:347–358.

160. **Jordan, F. T.** 1972. The epidemiology of disease of multiple aetiology: the avian respiratory disease complex. *Vet. Rec.* **90**:556–562.

161. **Jordan, F. T.** 1981. Mycoplasma-induced arthritis in poultry. *Isr. J. Med. Sci.* **17**:622–625.

162. **Jordan, F. T.** 1985. Gordon memorial lecture: people, poultry and pathogenic mycoplasmas. *Br. Poult. Sci.* **26**:1–15.

163. **Jordan, F. T. W.** 1979. Avian mycoplasmas, p. 1–49. *In* J. G. Tully and R. F. Whitcomb (ed.), *The Mycoplasmas,* vol. 2. *Human and Animal Mycoplasmas.* Academic Press, New York.

164. **Jordan, F. T. W.** 1983. Recovery and identification of avian mycoplasmas, p. 69–80. *In* J. G. Tully and S. Razin (ed.), *Methods in Mycoplasmology,* vol. 2. *Diagnostic Mycoplasmology.* Academic Press, New York.

165. **Juers, J. A., R. M. Rogers, J. B. McCurdy, and W. W. Cook.** 1976. Enhancement of bactericidal capacity of alveolar macrophages by human alveolar lining material. *J. Clin. Invest.* **58**:271–275.

166. **Kahane, I., J. Granek, and A. Reisch Saada.** 1984. The adhesins of *Mycoplasma gallisepticum* and *M. pneumoniae. Ann. Microbiol.* **135A**:25–32.

167. **Kahane, I., S. Pnini, M. Banai, J. B. Baseman, G. H. Cassell, and W. Bredt.** 1981. Attachment of mycoplasmas to erythrocytes: a model to study mycoplasma attachment to the epithelium of the host respiratory tract. *Isr. J. Med. Sci.* **17**:589–592.

168. **Kamiyama, T., M. Saito, and M. Nakagawa.** 1991. Effects of *Mycoplasma pulmonis* infection and exposure to nitrogen dioxide on activities of natural killer cells and macrophages of the mouse. *Jikken Dobutsu* **40**:255–257.

169. **Katsura, T., M. Kanamori, O. Kitamoto, and S. Ogata.** 1985. Protective effect of colostrum in *Mycoplasma pneumoniae* infection induced in infant mice. *Microbiol. Immunol.* **29**:883–894.

170. **Kerr, K. M., and N. O. Olson.** 1967. Pathology in chickens experimentally inoculated or contact-infected with *Mycoplasma gallisepticum. Avian Dis.* **11**:559–578.

171. **Keystone, E., R. D. Taylor, C. Pope, G. Taylor, and P. Furr.** 1978. Effect of inherited deficiency of the fifth component of complement on arthritis induced in mice by *Mycoplasma pulmonis. Arthritis Rheum.* **21**:792–797.

172. **Kirchhoff, H., A. Binder, M. Runge, B. Meier, R. Jacobs, and K. Busche.** 1989. Pathogenetic mechanisms in the *Mycoplasma arthritidis* polyarthritis of rats. *Rheumatol. Int.* **9**:193–196.

173. **Kirchhoff, H., R. Rosengarten, W. Lotz, M. Fischer, and D. Lopatta.** 1984. Flask-shaped mycoplasmas: properties and pathogenicity for man and animals. *Isr. J. Med. Sci.* **20**:848–853.

174. **Kirchner, H., W. Nicklas, D. Giebler, K. Keyssner, R. Berger, and E. Storch.** 1984. Induction of interferon gamma in mouse spleen cells by culture supernatants of *Mycoplasma arthritidis. J. Interferon Res.* **4**:389–397.

175. **Kleven, S. H., C. S. Eidson, and O. J. Fletcher.** 1978. Airsacculitis induced in broilers with a combination of *Mycoplasma gallinarum* and respiratory viruses. *Avian Dis.* **22**:707–716.

176. **Kobisch, M., L. Quillien, J. P. Tillon, and H. Wroblewski.** 1987. The *Mycoplasma hyopneumoniae* plasma membrane as a vaccine against porcine enzootic pneumonia. *Ann. Inst. Pasteur Immunol.* **138**:693–705.

177. **Kohn, D. F., and N. Chinookoswong.** 1981. Cytadsorption of *Mycoplasma pulmonis* to rat ependyma. *Infect. Immun.* **34**:292–295.

178. **Kreplin, C. M., H. L. Ruhnke, R. B. Miller, and P. A. Doig.** 1987. The effect of intrauterine inoculation with *Ureaplasma diversum* on bovine fertility. *Can. J. Vet. Res.* **51**:440–443.

179. **Kriger, J.** 1988. Studies on the capacity of intact cells and purified Ia from different B cell sources to function in antigen presentation to T cells. *J. Immunol.* **140**:338–394.

180. **Kruger, M., B. Patel, and H. Kirchhoff.** 1984. Toxic properties of the *Mycoplasma arthritidis* ISR-1 membrane. *Ann. Microbiol.* **135A**:103–109.

181. **Kumars, M., R. E. Dierks, J. A. Newman, C. J. Pfow, and B. S. Pomeroy.** 1963. Airsacculitis in turkeys. I. A study of airsacculitis in day-old poults. *Avian Dis.* **7**:376–385.

182. **Kume, K., Y. Kawakubo, C. Morita, E. Hayatsu, and M. Yoshioka.** 1977. Experimentally induced synovitis of chickens with *Mycoplasma synoviae*: effects of bursectomy and thymectomy on course of the infection for the first four weeks. *Am J. Vet. Res.* **38**:1595–1600.

183. **Kunita, S., E. Terada, A. Ghoda, Y. Sakurai, H. Suzuki, T. Takakura, and N. Kagiyama.** 1989. A DNA probe for specific detection of *Mycoplasma pulmonis*. *Jikken Dobutsu* **38**:215–219.

184. **Kunita, S., E. Terada, K. Goto, and N. Kagiyama.** 1990. Sensitive detection of *Mycoplasma pulmonis* by using the polymerase chain reaction. *Jikken Dobutsu* **39**:103–107.

185. **LaForce, P. M., W. J. Kelly, and G. L. Huber.** 1978. Inactivation of staphylococci by alveolar macrophages with preliminary observations on the importance of alveolar lining material. *Rev. Respir. Dis.* **108**:784–790.

186. **Lai, W. C., M. Bennett, Y. S. Lu, and S. P. Pakes.** 1991. Vaccination of Lewis rats with temperature-sensitive mutants of *Mycoplasma pulmonis*: adoptive transfer of immunity by spleen cells but not by sera. *Infect. Immun.* **59**:346–350.

187. **Lai, W. C., M. Bennett, S. P. Pakes, V. Kumar, D. Steutermann, I. Owusu, and A. Mikhael.** 1990. Resistance to *Mycoplasma pulmonis* mediated by activated natural killer cells. *J. Infect. Dis.* **161**:1269–1275.

188. **Lai, W. C., S. P. Pakes, Y. S. Lu, and C. F. Brayton.** 1987. *Mycoplasma pulmonis* infection augments natural killer cell activity in mice. *Lab. Anim. Sci.* **37**:299–303.

189. **Lai, W. C., S. P. Pakes, I. Owusu, and S. Wang.** 1989. *Mycoplasma pulmonis* depresses humoral and cell-mediated responses in mice. *Lab. Anim. Sci.* **39**:11–15.

190. **Lamas da Silva, J. M., and H. E. Adler.** 1969. Pathogenesis of arthritis induced in chickens by *Mycoplasma gallisepticum*. *Pathol. Vet.* **6**:385–395.

191. **Langford, E. V.** 1971. Mycoplasma and associated bacteria isolated from ovine pink-eye. *Can. J. Comp. Med.* **35**:18–21.

192. **Levisohn, S.** 1984. Early stages in the interaction between *Mycoplasma gallisepticum* and the chick trachea, as related to pathogenicity and immunogenicity. *Isr. J. Med. Sci.* **20**:982–984.

193. **Levisohn, S., H. Hyman, D. Yogev, and S. Razin.** 1990. The use of a specific DNA probe for detection of *Mycoplasma gallisepticum* in infected poultry, p. 489–493. *In* G. Stanek, G. H. Cassell, J. G. Tully, and R. F. Whitcomb (ed.), *Recent Advances in Mycoplasmology*. Gustav Fischer Verlag, New York.

194. **Lindsey, J. R., H. J. Baker, R. G. Overcash, G. H. Cassell, and C. E. Hunt.** 1971. Murine chronic respiratory disease. Significance as a research complication and experimental production with *Mycoplasma pulmonis*. *Am. J. Pathol.* **64**:675–708.

195. **Lloyd, L. C.** 1966. Tissue necrosis produced by *Mycoplasma mycoides* in intraperitoneal diffusion chambers. *J. Pathol. Bacteriol.* **92**:225–229.

196. **Mare, C. J., and W. P. Switzer.** 1966. Virus pneumonia of pigs: propagation and characterization of a causative agent. *Am. J. Vet. Res.* **27**:1687–1693.

197. **Martin, S. W., K. G. Bateman, P. E. Shewen, S. Rosendal, J. G. Bohac, and M. Thorburn.** 1990. A group level analysis of the associations between antibodies to seven putative pathogens and respiratory disease and weight gain in Ontario feedlot calves. *Can. J. Vet. Res.* **54**:337–342.

198. **Matsumoto, M., and R. Yamamoto.** 1973. Demonstration of complement-dependent and independent systems in immune inactivation of *Mycoplasma meleagridis*. *J. Infect. Dis.* **127**(Suppl.):S43–S51.

199. **Matsuzaki, M., R. Harasawa, F. Kimizuka, and K. Koshimizu.** 1989. A non-radioactive DNA probe for the detection of *Mycoplasma pulmonis* in murine mycoplasmosis. *Microbiol. Immunol.* **33**:129–132.

200. **McDonald, D. M., T. R. Schoeb, and J. R. Lindsey.** 1991. *Mycoplasma pulmonis* infections cause long-lasting potentiation of neurogenic inflammation in the respiratory tract of the rat. *J. Clin. Invest.* **87**:787–799.

201. **McGarrity, G. H., D. L. Rose, V. Kwiatkowski, A. S. Dion, D. M. Phillips, and J. G. Tully.** 1983. *Mycoplasma muris*, a new species from laboratory mice. *Int. J. Syst. Bacteriol.* **33**:350–355.

202. **McIntosh, J. C., J. W. Simecka, S. E. Ross, J. K. Davis, T. Schoeb, and G. H. Cassell.** Rodent strains with a difference in susceptibility to bleomycin-induced interstitial fibrosis apparently related to regulation of the inflammatory response. Submitted for publication.

203. **Messier, S., R. F. Ross, and P. S. Paul.** 1990. Humoral and cellular immune responses of pigs inoculated with *Mycoplasma hyopneumoniae*. *Am. J. Vet. Res.* **51**:52–58.

204. **Minion, F. C., G. H. Cassell, S. Pnini, and I. Kahane.** 1984. Multiphasic interactions of *Mycoplasma pulmonis* with erythrocytes defined by adherence and hemagglutination. *Infect. Immun.* **44**:394–400.

205. **Morrison-Plummer, J., S. F. Dallo, A. Lazzell, J. R. Horton, V. Tryon, and J. B. Baseman.** 1990. Characterization of an antigenic determinant shared by *Mycoplasma pneumoniae*, *Mycoplasma genitalium*, *Mycoplasma gallisepticum*, and *Acholeplasma laidlawii*, p. 210–220. *In* G. Stanek, G. H. Cassell, J. G. Tully, and R. F. Whitcomb (ed.), *Recent Advances in Mycoplasmology*. Gustav Fischer Verlag, New York.

206. **Nakagawa, M., W. D. Taylor, and R. J. Yedloutschnig.** 1976. Pathology of goats and sheep experimentally infected with *Mycoplasma mycoides* var. *capri*. *Natl. Inst. Anim. Health Q.* (Tokyo) **16**:65–77.

207. **Naot, Y., S. Davidson, and E. S. Lindenbaum.** 1981. Mitogenicity and pathogenicity of *Mycoplasma pulmonis* in rats. I. Atypical interstitial pneumonia induced by mitogenic mycoplasmal membranes. *J. Infect. Dis.* **143**:55–62.

208. **Nocard, E., and E. R. Roux.** 1898. Le microbe de la peripneumonie. *Ann. Inst. Pasteur* (Paris) **12**:240–262.

209. **Nugent, K. M., and R. L. Fick.** 1987. Candidacidal factors in murine bronchoalveolar lavage fluid. *Infect. Immun.* **55**:541–546.

210. **Nunoya, T., M. Tajima, T. Yagihashi, and S. Sannai.** 1987. Evaluation of respiratory lesions in chickens induced by *Mycoplasma gallisepticum*. *Nippon Juigaku Zasshi* **49**:621–629.

211. **Oboegbulem, S. I.** 1981. Enzootic pneumonia of pigs: a review. *Bull. Anim. Health Prod. Afr.* **29**:269–274.

212. **Ogata, M.** 1983. Recovery and identification of canine and feline mycoplasmas, p. 105–110. *In* J. G. Tully and S. Razin (ed.), *Methods in Mycoplasmology*, vol. 2. *Diagnostic Mycoplasmology*. Academic Press, New York.

213. **Oishi, K., M. Yamamoto, T. Yoshida, M. Ide, and K. Matsumoto.** 1986. Opsonic activity of plasma fibronectin for *Staphyloccocus aureus* by human alveolar macrophages: inefficacy of trypsin-sensitive staphyloccocal fibronectin receptor. *Tohoki J. Exp. Med.* **149**:95–102.

214. **Okoh, A. E., and M. Y. Kaldas.** 1980. Contagious caprine pleuropneumonia in goats in Gumel Nigeria. *Bull. Anim. Health Prod. Afr.* **28**:97–102.

215. **Okoh, A. E., and R. A. Ocholi.** 1986. Disease associated with *Mycoplasma mycoides* subspecies *mycoides* in sheep in Nigeria. *Vet. Rec.* **118**:212.

216. **Onofrio, J. M., G. B. Toews, M. F. Lipscomb, and A. K. Pierce.** 1983. Granulocyte-alveolar macrophage interaction in the pulmonary clearance of *Staphylococcus aureus*. *Am. Rev. Respir. Dis.* **127**:335–341.

217. **Osiyemi, T. I.** 1981. The eradication of contagious bovine pleuropneumonia in Nigeria: prospects and problems. *Bull. Anim. Health Prod. Afr.* **29**:95–97.

218. **Panagala, V. S., C. E. Hall, N. T. Caveney, D. H. Lein, and A. J. Winter.** 1982. *Mycoplasma bovigenitalium* in the upper genital tract of bulls: spontaneous and induced infections. *Cornell Vet.* **72**:292–303.

219. **Parker, R. F., J. K. Davis, D. K. Blalock, R. B. Thorp, J. W. Simecka, and G. H. Cassell.** 1987. Pulmonary clearance of *Mycoplasma pulmonis* in C57BL/6N and C3H/HeN mice. *Infect. Immun.* **55**:2631–2635.

220. **Parsonson, I. M., A. J. M. Al, and K. McEntee.** 1974. *Mycoplasma bovigenitalium*: experimental induction of genital disease in bulls. *Cornell Vet.* **64**:240–264.

221. **Pearson, J. E., N. W. Rokey, R. Harrington, S. J. Proctor, and D. R. Cassidy.** 1972. Contagious caprine pleuropneumonia in Arizona. *J. Am. Vet. Med. Assoc.* **161**:1536–1538.

222. **Pointon, A. M., D. Byrt, and P. Heap.** 1985. Effect of enzootic pneumonia of pigs on growth performance. *Aust. Vet. J.* **62**:13–18.

223. **Power, J., and F. T. Jordan.** 1976. A comparison of the virulence of three strains of *Mycoplasma gallisepticum* and one strain of *Mycoplasma gallinarum* in chicks, turkey poults, tracheal organ cultures and embryonated fowl eggs. *Res. Vet. Sci.* **21**:41–46.

224. **Razin, S.** 1985. Mycoplasma adherence, p. 161–203. *In* S. Razin an M. F. Barile (ed.), *The Mycoplasmas*, vol. 4. *Mycoplasma Pathogenicity*. Academic Press, New York.

225. **Razin, S., D. Amikam, and G. Glaser.** 1984. Mycoplasmal ribosomal RNA genes and their use as probes for detection and identification of Mollicutes. *Isr. J. Med. Sci.* **20**:758–761.

226. **Razin, S., M. Banai, H. Gamliel, A. Pollack, W. Bredt, and I. Kahane.** 1980. Scanning electron microscopy of mycoplasmas adhering to erythrocytes. *Infect. Immun.* **30**:538–546.

227. **Rhoades, K. R.** 1977. Turkey sinusitis: synergism between *Mycoplasma synoviae* and *Mycoplasma meleagridis*. *Avian Dis.* **21**:670–674.

228. **Rhoades, K. R.** 1981. Turkey airsacculitis: effect of mixed mycoplasmal infections. *Avian Dis.* **25**:131–135.

229. **Roberts, M. C., M. Hooton, W. Stamm, K. K. Holmes, and G. E. Kenny.** 1987. DNA probes for the detection of mycoplasmas in genital specimens. *Isr. J. Med. Sci.* **23**:618–620.

230. **Rodriguez, R., and S. H. Kleven.** 1980. Pathogenicity of two strains of *Mycoplasma gallisepticum* in broilers. *Avian Dis.* **24**:800–807.

231. **Romvary, J., J. Rozsa, L. Stipkovits, and J. Meszaros.** 1977. Incidence of diseases due to *Mycoplasma bovis* in a cattle herd. II. Experimental therapy of the pneumoarthritis syndrome of calves. *Acta Vet. Acad. Sci. Hung.* **27**:39–45.

232. **Rosenbusch, R. F.** 1987. Immune responses to *Mycoplasma bovoculi* conjunctivitis. *Isr. J. Med. Sci.* **23**:628–631.

233. **Rosenbusch, R. F., and W. U. Knudtson.** 1980. Bovine mycoplasmal conjunctivitis: experimental reproduction and characterization of the disease. *Cornell Vet.* **70**:307–320.

234. **Rosendal, S.** 1981. Experimental infection of goats, sheep and calves with the large colony type of *Mycoplasma mycoides* subsp. *mycoides*. *Vet. Pathol.* **18**:71–81.

235. **Rosendal, S.** 1984. Pathogenetic mechanisms of *Mycoplasma mycoides* subsp. *mycoides* septicemia in goats. *Isr. J. Med. Sci.* **20**:970–971.

236. **Rosendal, S., H. Ern, and D. S. Wyand.** 1979. *Mycoplasma mycoides* subspecies *mycoides* as a cause of polyarthritis in goats. *J. Am. Vet. Med. Assoc.* **175**:378–380.

237. **Rosendal, S., and S. W. Martin.** 1986. The association between serological evidence of mycoplasma infection and respiratory disease in feedlot calves. *Can. J. Vet. Res.* **50**:179–183.

238. **Ross, R. F.** 1973. Predisposing factors in *Mycoplasma hyosynoviae* arthritis in swine. *J. Infect. Dis.* **127**(Suppl.):S84–S86.

239. **Ross, R. F., S. E. Dale, and J. R. Duncan.** 1973. Experimentally induced *Mycoplasma hyorhinis* arthritis of swine: immune response to 26th postinoculation week. *Am. J. Vet. Res.* **34**:367–372.

240. **Ross, R. F., and M. L. Spear.** 1973. Role of the sow as a reservoir of infection for *Mycoplasma hyosynoviae*. *Am. J. Vet. Res.* **34**:373–378.

241. **Ross, R. F., W. P. Switzer, and J. R. Duncan.** 1971. Experimental production of *Mycoplasma hyosynoviae* arthritis in swine. *Am. J. Vet. Res.* **32**:1743–1749.

242. **Ross, R. F., and P. Whittlestone.** 1983. Recovery and identification of porcine mycoplasmas, p. 115–128. *In* J. G. Tully and S. Razin (ed.), *Methods in Mycoplasmology*, vol. 2. *Diagnostic Mycoplasmology*. Academic Press, New York.

243. **Ross, S. E., J. K. Davis, and G. H. Cassell.** 1990. Induction of hyper Ia antigen expression on F344 rat B lymphocytes by *Mycoplasma pulmonis* mitogen, p. 584–592. *In* G. Stanek, G. H. Cassell, J. G. Tully, and R. F. Whitcomb (ed.), *Recent Advances in Mycoplasmology*. Gustav Fischer Verlag, New York.

244. **Ross, S. E., J. W. Simecka, G. P. Gambrill, J. K. Davis, and G. H. Cassell.** 1992. *Mycoplasma pulmonis* possesses a novel chemoattractant for B lymphocytes. *Infect. Immun.* **60**:669–674.

245. **Ryan, M. J., D. S. Wyand, D. L. Hill, M. E. Tourtellotte, and T. J. Yang.** 1983. Morphologic changes following intraarticular inoculation of *Mycoplasma bovis* in calves. *Vet. Pathol.* **20**:472–487.

246. **Saed, O. M., and A. J. M. Al.** 1983. Infertility in heifers caused by pathogenic strain of *Mycoplasma bovigenitalium*. *Cornell Vet.* **73**:125–130.

247. **Saif, Y. M., P. D. Moorhead, and E. H. Bohl.** 1970. *Mycoplasma meleagridis* and *Escherichia coli* infections in germfree and specific-pathogen-free turkey poults: production of complicated airsacculitis. *Am. J. Vet. Res.* **31**:1637–1643.

248. **Saito, M., M. Nakagawa, T. Muto, and K. Imaizumi.** 1978. Strain difference of mouse in susceptibility to *Mycoplasma pulmonis* infection. *Nippon Juigaku Zasshi* **40**:697–705.

249. **Saito, M., M. Nakagawa, E. Suzuki, K. Kinoshita, and K. Imaizumi.** 1981. Synergistic effect of Sendai virus on *Mycoplasma pulmonis* infection in mice. *Nippon Juigaku Zasshi* **43**:43–50.

250. **Schoeb, T. R., K. C. Kevin, and J. R. Lindsey.** 1985. Exacerbation of murine respiratory mycoplasmosis in

gnotobiotic F344/N rats by Sendai virus infection. *Vet. Pathol.* **22**:272–282.

251. **Schoeb, T. R., and J. R. Lindsey.** 1987. Exacerbation of murine respiratory mycoplasmosis by sialodacryoadenitis virus infection in gnotobiotic F344 rats. *Vet. Pathol.* **24**:392–399.

252. **Scott, P., E. Pearce, A. W. Cheever, R. L. Coffman, and A. Sher.** 1989. Role of cytokines and CD4+ T-cell subsets in the regulation of parasite immunity and disease. *Immunol. Rev.* **112**:161–182.

253. **Seid, R. C., Jr., P. F. Smith, G. Guevarra, H. D. Hochstein, and M. F. Barile.** 1980. Endotoxin-like activities of mycoplasmal lipopolysaccharides. *Infect. Immun.* **29**:990–994.

254. **Sethi, K. K., and M. Teschner.** 1969. A study on the role of complement in the immune inhibition of mycoplasmal growth. *Z. Immunitaetsforsch.* **138**:458–474.

255. **Sher, T., S. Rottem, and R. Gallily.** 1990. *Mycoplasma capricolum* membranes induce tumor necrosis factor alpha by a mechanism different from that of lipopolysaccharide. *Cancer Immunol. Immunother.* **31**:86–92.

256. **Shiel, M. J., P. J. Coloe, B. Worotniuk, and G. W. Burgess.** 1982. Polyarthritis in a calf associated with a group 7 Mycoplasma infection. *Aust. Vet. J.* **59**:192–193.

257. **Simberkoff, M. S., and P. Elsbach.** 1971. The interaction *in vitro* between polymorphonuclear leukocytes and mycoplasma. *J. Exp. Med.* **134**:1417–1430.

258. **Simecka, J. W., and G. H. Cassell.** 1987. Serum antibody and cellular responses in LEW and F344 rats following immunization with *Mycoplasma pulmonis* antigen. *Infect. Immun.* **55**:731–735.

259. **Simecka, J. W., J. K. Davis, and G. H. Cassell.** 1987. Specific vs. nonspecific immune responses in murine respiratory mycoplasmosis. *Isr. J. Med. Sci.* **23**:485–489.

260. **Simecka, J. W., J. K. Davis, and G. H. Cassell.** 1989. Serum antibody does not account for differences in the severity of chronic respiratory disease caused by *Mycoplasma pulmonis* in LEW and F344 rats. *Infect. Immun.* **57**:3570–3575.

261. **Simecka, J. W., P. Patel, J. K. Davis, and G. H. Cassell.** 1989. Upper respiratory tract is the major site of antibody production in mycoplasmal induced disease. *Reg. Immunol.* **2**:385–389.

262. **Simecka, J. W., P. Patel, J. K. Davis, S. E. Ross, P. Otwell, and G. H. Cassell.** 1991. Specific and nonspecific antibody responses in different segments of the respiratory tract in rats infected with *Mycoplasma pulmonis*. *Infect. Immun.* **59**:3715–3721.

263. **Slavik, M. F., S. D. Maruca, and J. K. Skeeles.** 1982. Detection of inhibitors in chicken tracheal washings against *Mycoplasma gallisepticum*. *Avian Dis.* **26**:118–126.

264. **Spooner, R. K., D. Thirkell, and G. E. Jones.** 1990. Strain specific and cross reactive determinants of *Mycoplasma ovipneumoniae*, p. 647–650. *In* G. Stanek, G. H. Cassell, J. G. Tully, and R. F. Whitcomb (ed.), *Recent Advances in Mycoplasmology.* Gustav Fischer Verlag, New York.

265. **Springer, W. T., C. Luskus, and S. S. Pourciau.** 1974. Infectious bronchitis and mixed infections of *Mycoplasma synoviae* and *Escherichia coli* in gnotobiotic chickens. I. Synergistic role in the airsacculitis syndrome. *Infect. Immun.* **10**:578–589.

266. **Städtlander, C., and H. Kirchhoff.** 1988. The effects of *Mycoplasma mobile* 163 K on the ciliary epithelium of tracheal organ cultures. *Zentralbl. Bakteriol. Mikrobiol. Hyg. Reihe A.* **269**:355–365.

267. **Städtlander, C. T. K.-H., H. L. Watson, J. W. Simecka, and G. H. Cassell.** 1991. Cytopathic effects of *Mycoplasma pulmonis* in vivo and in vitro. *Infect. Immun.* **59**:4201–4211.

268. **Städtlander, C. T. K.-H., H. L. Watson, J. W. Simecka, and G. H. Cassell.** *In vivo* and *in vitro* cytopathogenicity

of *Mycoplasma fermentans* (including strain incognitus). *Clin. Infect, Dis.*, in press.

269. **Stalheim, O. H.** 1983. Mycoplasmal respiratory diseases of ruminants: a review and update. *J. Am. Vet. Med. Assoc.* **182**:403–406.

270. **Stipkovits, L.** 1979. The pathogenicity of avian mycoplasmas. *Zentralbl. Bakterol. Reihe Orig. A* **245**:171–183.

271. **Stuart, P. M., G. H. Cassell, and J. G. Woodward.** 1989. Induction of class II MHC antigen expression in macrophages by Mycoplasma species. *J. Immunol.* **142**:3392–3399.

272. **Stuart, P. M., G. H. Cassell, and J. G. Woodward.** 1990. Differential induction of bone marrow macrophage proliferation by mycoplasmas involves granulocyte-macrophage colony-stimulating factor. *Infect. Immun.* **58**:3558–3563.

273. **Sugama, K., K. Kuwano, M. Furukawa, Y. Himeno, T. Satoh, and S. Arai.** 1990. Mycoplasmas induce transcription and production of tumor necrosis factor in a monocytic cell line, THP-1, by a protein kinase C-independent pathway. *Infect. Immun.* **58**:3564–3567.

274. **Swanepoel, R., S. Efstratiou, and N. K. Blackburn.** 1977. *Mycoplasma capricolum* associated with arthritis in sheep. *Vet. Rec.* **101**:446–447.

275. **Tajima, M., T. Nunoya, and T. Yagihashi.** 1979. An ultrastructural study on the interaction of *Mycoplasma gallisepticum* with the chicken tracheal epithelium. *Am. J. Vet. Res.* **40**:1009–1014.

276. **Talkington, D. F., M. T. Fallon, H. L. Watson, R. K. Thorp, and G. H. Cassell.** 1989. *Mycoplasma pulmonis* V-1 surface protein variation: occurrence in vivo and association with lung lesions. *Microb. Pathog.* **7**:429–436.

277. **Taoudi, A., D. W. Johnson, D. Kheyyali, and H. Kirchhoff.** 1987. Pathogenicity of *Mycoplasma capricolum* in sheep after experimental infection. *Vet. Microbiol.* **14**:137–144.

278. **Taurog, J. D., S. L. Leary, M. A. Cremer, M. L. Mahowald, and G. P. Sandberg.** 1984. Infection with *Mycoplasma pulmonis* modulates adjuvant- and collagen-induced arthritis in Lewis rats. *Arthritis Rheum.* **27**:943–946.

279. **Taylor, G., and C. J. Howard.** 1980. Interaction of *Mycoplasma pulmonis* with mouse peritoneal macrophages and polymorphonuclear leucocytes. *J. Med. Microbiol.* **13**:19–30.

280. **Taylor, G., and C. J. Howard.** 1981. Protection of mice against *Mycoplasma pulmonis* infection using purified mouse immunoglobulins: comparison between protective effect and biological properties of immunoglobulin classes. *Immunology* **43**:519–525.

281. **Taylor, R. D.** 1984. Ureaplasmas as a cause of disease in man and animals: fact or fancy? *Isr. J. Med. Sci.* **20**:843–837.

282. **Taylor, R. D., H. U. Schorlemmer, P. M. Furr, and A. C. Allison.** 1978. Macrophage secretion and the complement cleavage product C3a in the pathogenesis of infections by mycoplasmas and L-forms of bacteria and in immunity to these organisms. *Clin. Exp. Immunol.* **33**:486–494.

283. **ter-Laak, E. A., B. E. Schreuder, T. G. Kimman, and D. J. Houwers.** 1988. Ovine keratoconjunctivitis experimentally induced by instillation of *Mycoplasma conjunctivae*. *Vet. Q.* **10**:217–224.

284. **Thomas, C. B., E. P. Van, L. J. Wolfgram, J. Riebe, P. Sharp, and R. D. Schultz.** 1991. Adherence to bovine neutrophils and suppression of neutrophil chemiluminescence by *Mycoplasma bovis*. *Vet. Immunol. Immunopathol.* **27**:365–381.

285. **Thomas, L.** 1967. The neurotoxins of *M. neurolyticum* and *M. gallisepticum*. *Ann. N.Y. Acad. Sci.* **143**:218–224.

286. **Thomas, L., F. Aleu, M. W. Bitensky, M. Davidson, and B. Gesner.** 1966. Studies of PPLO infection. II. The neu-

rotoxin of *Mycoplasma neurolyticum. J. Exp. Med.* **124:**1067–1082.

287. **Thomas, L. H., C. J. Howard, E. J. Stott, and K. R. Parsons.** 1986. *Mycoplasma bovis* infection in gnotobiotic calves and combined infection with respiratory syncytial virus. *Vet. Pathol.* **23:**571–578.

288. **Thomsen, A. C., and I. Heron.** 1979. Effect of mycoplasmas on phagocytosis and immunocompetence in rats. *Acta Pathol. Microbiol. Scand. Sect. C* **87:**67–71.

289. **Toews, G. B., W. C. Vial, and E. J. Hansen.** 1985. Role of C5 and recruited neutrophils in early clearance of nontypable *Haemophilus influenzae* from murine lungs. *Infect. Immun.* **50:**207–212.

290. **Trampel, D. W., and O. J. Fletcher.** 1981. Light microscopic, scanning electron microscopic, and histomorphometric evaluation of *Mycoplasma gallisepticum*-induced airsacculitis in chickens. *Am. J. Vet. Res.* **42:**1281–1289.

291. **Trichard, C. J., P. A. Basson, J. J. Van der Lugt, and E. P. Jacobsz.** 1989. An outbreak of contagious bovine pleuropneumonia in the Owambo Mangetti area of South West Africa/Namibia: microbiological, immunofluorescent, pathological and serological findings. *Onderstepoort J. Vet. Res.* **56:**277–284.

292. **Truscott, R. B., and G. G. Finley.** 1985. Studies on *Mycoplasma mycoides* subsp. *mycoides* (LC) in lambs and calves. *Can. J. Comp. Med.* **49:**233–234.

293. **Tully, J. G., D. Taylor-Robinson, D. L. Rose, R. M. Cole, and J. M. Bové.** 1983. *Mycoplasma genitalium*, a new species from the human urogenital tract. *Int. J. Syst. Bacteriol.* **33:**387–396.

294. **Uppal, P. K., and H. P. Chu.** 1977. Attachment of *Mycoplasma gallisepticum* to the tracheal epithelium of fowls. *Res. Vet. Sci.* **22:**259–260.

295. **Villemot, J. M., A. Provot, and R. Quelval.** 1962. Endotoxin from *Mycoplasma mycoides. Nature* (London) **193:**906–907.

296. **Vincze, S., G. Klein, and H. Altmann.** 1975. Deoxyribonuclease activity in the serum and spleen of rats with mycoplasma induced arthritis. *Z. Rheumatol.* **34:**49–54.

297. **Washburn, L. R., B. C. Cole, M. I. Gelman, and J. R. Ward.** 1980. Chronic arthritis of rabbits induced by my-

coplasmas. I. Clinical microbiologic, and histologic features. *Arthritis Rheum.* **23:**825–836.

298. **Washburn, L. R., B. C. Cole, and J. R. Ward.** 1980. Chronic arthritis of rabbits induced by mycoplasmas. II. Antibody response and the deposition of immune complexes. *Arthritis Rheum.* **23:**837–845.

299. **Watson, H. L., L. S. McDaniel, D. K. Blalock, M. T. Fallon, and G. H. Cassell.** 1988. Heterogeneity among strains and a high rate of variation within strains of a major surface antigen of *Mycoplasma pulmonis. Infect. Immun.* **56:**1358–1363.

300. **Watson, H. L., J. W. Simecka, A. L. Yancey, and G. H. Cassell.** Unpublished data.

301. **Whithear, K. G.** 1983. Isolation of *Mycoplasma alkalescens* from cases of polyarthritis in embryo-transplant calves. *Aust. Vet. J.* **60:**191–192.

302. **Whittlestone, P.** 1973. Enzootic pneumonia of pigs (EPP). *Adv. Vet. Sci. Comp. Med.* **17:**1–55.

303. **Whittlestone, P.** 1976. Effect of climatic conditions on enzootic pneumonia of pigs. *Int. J. Biometeorol.* **20:**42–48.

304. **Whittlestone, P.** 1979. Porcine mycoplasmas, p. 133–176. *In* J. G. Tully and R. F. Whitcomb (ed.), *The Mycoplasmas,* vol. 2. *Human and Animal Mycoplasmas.* Academic Press, New York.

305. **Williamson, J. S., J. K. Davis, and G. H. Cassell.** 1986. Polyclonal activation of rat splenic lymphocytes after in vivo administratino of *Mycoplasma pulmonis* and its relation to in vitro response. *Infect. Immun.* **52:**594–599.

306. **Willoughby, W. F., J. B. Willoughby, and G. F. Gerberick.** 1985. Polyclonal activators in pulmonary immune disease. *Clin. Rev. Allergy* **3:**197–216.

307. **Woldehiwet, Z., B. Mamache, and T. G. Rowan.** 1990. Effects of age, environmental temperature and relative humidity on the colonization of the nose and trachea of calves by Mycoplasma spp. *Br. Vet. J.* **146:**419–424.

308. **Yagihashi, T., T. Nunoya, T. Mitui, and M. Tajima.** 1984. Effect of *Mycoplasma hyopneumoniae* infection on the development of *Haemophilus pleuropneumoniae* pneumonia in pigs. *Nippon Juigaku Zasshi* **46:**705–713.

309. **Yancey, A., J. W. Simecka, P. Patel, G. H. Cassell, and J. K. Davis.** Unpublished data.

25. Mycoplasmas Which Infect Humans

DUNCAN C. KRAUSE and DAVID TAYLOR-ROBINSON

OVERVIEW

Over 30 years have passed since it was first suggested that a mycoplasma was the causative agent of diseases in humans (169). During this time, Koch's postulates have been fulfilled for two species, *Mycoplasma pneumoniae* and *Ureaplasma urealyticum*, which cause primary atypical pneumonia and nongonococcal urethritis (NGU), respectively. Furthermore, significant progress has been made in elucidating the basic biology of these microbes, as well as the molecular and cellular nature of their interactions with humans. At the same time, other mycoplasma species have been identified as part of the normal human flora, where their presence seems inconsequential or beneficial rather than detrimental. Between these two extremes is a nebulous area where the rela-tionship between mollicutes and humans remains poorly defined. This area includes, for example, associations between *M. hominis* and *M. genitalium* and urogenital disease, a possible role for *U. urealyticum* in spontaneous abortions and low-birth-weight deliveries, and the identification of potentially new mycoplasmas as possible cofactors in the pathology of AIDS. We provide here an overview of the relationships between humans and mycoplasmas, focusing on the species involved and the nature of the interactions. More detailed accounts of specific features of these interactions are provided in other chapters of this volume.

MYCOPLASMAS AS RESIDENT FLORA

Mycoplasma species which have been isolated from humans to date are listed in Table 1; most of the spe-

Duncan C. Krause • Department of Microbiology, University of Georgia, Athens, Georgia 30602. **David Taylor-Robinson** • Division of Sexually Transmitted Diseases, Clinical Research Centre, Watford Road, Harrow, Middlesex HA1 3UJ, United Kingdom.

Table 1. Mycoplasmas isolated from humans[a]

Species	Anatomical location	Occurrence
Acholeplasma laidlawii	Oropharynx	Rare
Mycoplasma arthritidis	Urogenital	Questionable
M. buccale	Oropharynx	Uncommon
M. faucium	Oropharynx	Uncommon
M. fermentans	Urogenital	Uncommon
	Systemic	Uncommon (?)
M. genitalium	Urogenital	Uncommon (?)
	Respiratory tract	Uncommon (?)
M. hominis	Urogenital	Common
	Respiratory tract	Uncommon (?)
M. lipophilum	Oropharynx	Rare
M. orale	Oropharynx	Widespread
M. pneumoniae	Oropharynx, lower respiratory tract	Uncommon
	Urogenital	Very rare
M. primatum	Oropharynx	Rare
	Urogenital	Rare
M. salivarium	Oropharynx	Widespread
	Urogenital	Rare
Ureaplasma urealyticum	Urogenital	Common
	Respiratory tract	Uncommon

[a] Adapted from reference 245.

cies indicated constitute part of the normal flora. Mycoplasmas commonly found as resident flora of the human oropharynx are thought to reside primarily in the gingival crevices (138). The two most common species are *M. salivarium* and *M. orale*; one or both have been isolated from as many as 84% of a study group (140), and both can probably be found in all humans. Less frequent isolates likewise considered resident flora include *M. buccale*, *M. faucium*, *M. primatum*, *M. lipophilum*, *M. fermentans*, *M. hominis*, *Acholeplasma laidlawii*, and *U. urealyticum*. However, considering the fastidious nature of mycoplasmas, the low frequency of isolation must be interpreted carefully. Failure to meet the nutritional needs of the mycoplasmas could limit successful culture.

Mycoplasmas are also common inhabitants of the human urogenital tract. *M. hominis*, *M. fermentans*, and *U. urealyticum* have all been isolated from the urogenital tract of healthy individuals and therefore might be considered resident flora. However, as detailed below, some of the species indicated are found both in healthy individuals and in association with disease. This complicates enormously attempts to clarify the etiological role of these mycoplasmas in disease. Factors to be considered in assessing their pathogenic potential include site(s) of colonization in the urogenital tract, numbers present, and perhaps strain differences.

M. PNEUMONIAE

History

M. pneumoniae, which causes tracheobronchitis and primary atypical pneumonia, was the first myco-plasma for which an etiological role in disease in humans was demonstrated. The first descriptions of primary atypical pneumonia as a clinical syndrome appeared in the late 1930s, with the recognition that some cases of pneumonia failed to respond to therapy with sulfonamides or penicillin (93, 215). The infectious nature of primary atypical pneumonia was demonstrated by Eaton and colleagues (72), who described the transmission of the disease to cotton rats and hamsters. Eaton's agent, as it came to be called, proved to be filterable, suggesting initially that it was a virus. From their observation of tiny coccobacilli in chicken bronchial tissue infected with sputum from patients with primary atypical pneumonia, Marmion and Goodburn suggested that Eaton's agent was similar to the agent of bovine pleuropneumonia, i.e., a mycoplasma (169).

Koch's postulates were fulfilled for Eaton's agent in 1961 with the transmission of the disease to human volunteers via laboratory-isolated organisms (46). Shortly thereafter, the first growth of Eaton's agent on artificial medium was reported (45), and subsequently this agent was named (44).

Cell Biology

Growth and morphology

M. pneumoniae grows over a temperature range of 30 to 39°C, with an optimum of approximately 36 to 38°C (86). Laboratory culture requires a complex medium generally containing a fresh yeast dialysate and horse serum. When grown on inert surfaces such as plastic tissue culture flasks or glass prescription bottles, wild-type mycoplasmas tend to grow attached to the surface (246, 274). *M. pneumoniae* strains incapable of hemadsorption or attachment to mammalian cells in tissue or organ culture (77, 101, 134, 153) adhere very poorly to inert surfaces. Growth on solid medium generally requires 7 to 10 days of culture. Colony morphology varies according to the extent of adaptation to artificial medium, with fresh isolates often appearing dome shaped, lacking the peripheral halo that gives medium-adapted colonies their characteristic fried-egg appearance (86).

M. pneumoniae is typically pleomorphic, but morphology appears to be growth phase dependent. Studies by dark-field light microscopy and transmission and scanning electron microscopy reveal that the organisms assume a spherical form in young cultures, become branched and filamentous with time, and then revert to asymmetrical rounded forms in declining cultures (18, 126). Small bodies approximately 1 μm in diameter have been described in cultures of *M. pneumoniae* as well as those of other mycoplasmas, but their origin is not clear. Bredt has suggested that these forms may be the result of cell degeneration during culture (27). Alternatively, they may represent growth medium components (25).

Ultrastructure

One terminus of filamentous *M. pneumoniae* cells possesses a distinctly tapered appearance, as seen by scanning electron microscopy in Fig. 1A. By transmis-

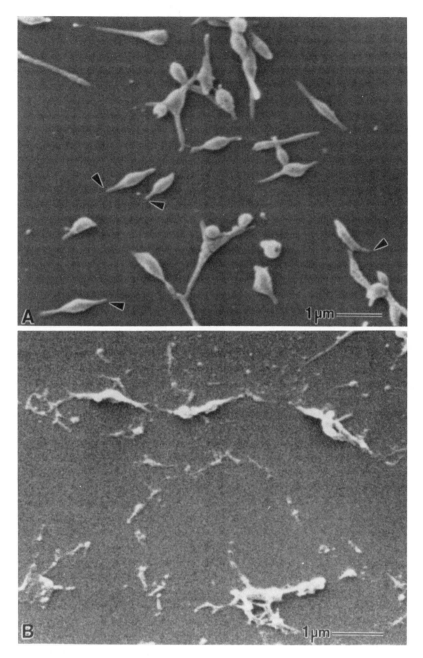

Figure 1. Scanning electron micrographs of *M. pneumoniae* cells and triton shells. (A) Whole mycoplasmas, with terminal structures indicated with arrows; (B) triton shells remaining following removal of the cell membrane with Triton X-100. (Courtesy of M. Stevens.)

sion electron microscopy, the terminal structure is seen as an extension of the cell and bound by the cell membrane. The interior of the terminus consists of a longitudinally oriented, electron-dense core which is separated from the cell membrane on either side by a clear zone (18). A fibrillar meshwork radiates in a less organized manner from the base of the central core into the rest of the cell (296). Cytochemical analysis suggests that the core structure contains basic protein but no nucleic acid and is organized with a degree of periodicity (303).

The terminal structure appears to function in sev-

eral capacities in *M. pneumoniae*. The description of cells branching at one end to yield two parallel terminal structures suggests a role in replication (18). Mycoplasma replication appears to proceed by binary fission, with the tip structure duplicated early in the cycle and subsequently functioning to draw the progeny apart during cell division (18). Second, *M. pneumoniae* exhibits gliding motility, with the differentiated terminus the leading end, followed by the thicker cell body, and with an elongated tail extending behind the body (26, 28, 213). Third, when examined in infected respiratory epithelial tissue, filamentous

M. pneumoniae cells appear oriented parallel to the ciliary shafts and anchored to the host cell surface by the terminal structure (55, 57, 58). Further evidence that the terminal structure serves as an attachment organelle comes from the observation that two putative adhesin proteins appear to be preferentially clustered in the mycoplasma membrane around the terminal structure (see below). The terminal structure would therefore appear to be a multifunctional organelle. This conclusion is consistent with the observation that a mycoplasma strain attenuated by broth passage and unable to adhere to erythrocytes or tracheal epithelium is also nonmotile (30).

Mycoplasma motility, directed changes in cell morphology, the ability to selectively cluster a membrane protein at a defined site on the cell surface, and ultrastructural observations all suggest cytoskeletal structure and function in *M. pneumoniae*. Removal of the mycoplasma membrane with the nonionic detergent Triton X-100 (Fig. 1B) reveals a lattice of filamentous material assuming the same general shape of the cell. This matrix is analogous to cytoskeletal structures observed in mammalian cells processed in the same manner (95, 174). What appears to be the core of the tip structure is visible, with a length of up to 300 nm and a width of 40 nm. A meshwork of 5-nm-wide filaments radiates through the remainder of the cell. Analysis by sodium dodecyl sulfate-polyacrylamide gel electrophoresis (SDS-PAGE) reveals a complex protein composition to the Triton X-100-insoluble material (triton shell), with over 20 different protein bands detected (125, 253, 254).

Attempts to define contractile material further have yielded inconclusive results. Using butanol, Neimark extracted from *M. pneumoniae* a protein that resembles eucaryotic actin in its molecular weight, solubility characteristics, ability to form 5- to 6-nm-diameter filaments in the presence of ATP and Mg^{2+}, and ability to bind vertebrate heavy meromyosin (191). However, no mycoplasma proteins coelectrophorese with α-actin on O'Farrell two-dimensional polyacrylamide gels, and no mycoplasma proteins of approximately 42,000 Da have a high affinity for DNase I, as does actin (225). The cytadhesin P1 and cytadherence accessory proteins HMW1 through HMW5 partition in the Triton X-100-insoluble fraction (125, 253, 254) (see below). Otherwise, the molecular components of the mycoplasma cytoskeleton remain poorly defined, and their organization is essentially unexplored.

Physiology

Mycoplasma physiology is discussed in detail elsewhere in this volume, and only the differential characteristics of the species (86) will be considered here. *M. pneumoniae* is capable of catabolizing glucose or mannose but will not hydrolyze arginine as a carbon and energy source. Tetrazolium reduction occurs anaerobically or aerobically, and hydrogen peroxide (248) and the superoxide anion (160) are by-products of glucose catabolism, resulting in complete hydrolysis of erythrocytes when overlaid in agarose on mycoplasma colonies.

M. pneumoniae lacks many common enzyme systems having iron as a cofactor, such as tricarboxylic acid cycle components or a complete electron transport chain containing cytochromes (202, 204). Iron has been detected in the mycoplasma membrane (14), however, and mycoplasmas are thought to employ a truncated electron transport system to generate energy. While an absolute requirement for iron has yet to be demonstrated, recent studies reveal that a mechanism exists for iron acquisition by *M. pneumoniae* through lactoferrin (285). This glycoprotein functions in the sequestration and transport of iron in mucosal secretions. *M. pneumoniae* binds lactoferrin in a manner dependent upon time, temperature, and concentration. While the contribution of lactoferrin binding to virulence has yet to be established, the utilization of lactoferrin or transferrin as a source for iron is a feature shared by several other pathogens that colonize mucosal surfaces (176, 199, 201).

Molecular biology

M. pneumoniae possesses a single circular chromosome of double-stranded DNA that has a G + C content of 39 to 41 mol% and is apparently typically procaryotic in every respect except perhaps size and codon usage. DNA renaturation studies indicate a genome size of only 720 kb (3). More recent analyses utilizing pulsed-field gel electrophoretic separation of large DNA fragments generated by infrequently cutting restriction endonucleases place the genome size at 774 to 849 kb (135, 299, 300), or approximately one-sixth the size of the *Escherichia coli* chromosome (130, 243). Analysis of *M. pneumoniae* protein profiles by two-dimensional polyacrylamide gel electrophoresis reveal a total of 161 polypeptides, as identified by staining with Coomassie brilliant blue (102). This number can be extended to 225 by employing the more sensitive approach of fluorography after intrinsic labeling of proteins with [^{35}S]methionine (Fig. 2). While this number begins to approach the total predicted by

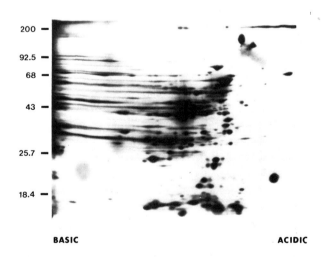

Figure 2. Profile of *M. pneumoniae* proteins following two-dimensional polyacrylamide gel electrophoresis. Mycoplasma proteins were labeled intrinsically with [^{35}S]methionine, separated in the first dimension by isoelectric focusing and in the second dimension by SDS-PAGE, and visualized by fluorography. Protein size standards in kilodaltons are indicated, as are the acidic and basic ends of the gel.

Morowitz as a minimum requirement for life as a free-living entity (183a), it reflects only approximately one-third the coding capacity of the genome, raising questions about the potential induction of additional mycoplasma proteins under the seemingly more demanding conditions of infection, as opposed to life in a nutrient-rich culture medium.

Comparison of cleavage patterns following treatment of *M. pneumoniae* DNA with restriction endonucleases that cleave the DNA frequently indicates considerable strain homogeneity (43) relative to that observed with a number of other mycoplasmas, such as the avian pathogen *M. gallisepticum* (129). More recent findings, however, suggest that *M. pneumoniae* strains may fall into two groups, based on their restriction sites around the gene for the cytadhesin protein P1 (65). The extent of the mycoplasma genome involved in these differences remains to be determined, however.

As a field, the molecular biology of *M. pneumoniae* remains in its infancy. The complex nutritional requirements of this organism have precluded the isolation of auxotrophic mutants. The only mutants available to date are a temperature-sensitive growth mutant (252) and nitrosoguanidine-derived mutants defective in cytadherence (77, 101, 103). To date, there have been no reports of the successful transformation of *M. pneumoniae*, though other mycoplasmas have been transformed (see chapter 21), and no plasmids or phages have been reported for *M. pneumoniae*.

Physical maps of the *M. pneumoniae* chromosome have been generated for *Xho*I, *Apa*I, *Not*I, and *Sfi*I sites, and several functional loci have been established (135, 299, 300). However, no classic genetic maps exist, except to the extent that mycoplasma genes have been localized on physical maps, by using as probes either the cloned genes themselves or cloned and defined genes from other bacteria. Our knowledge of *M. pneumoniae* genetics stems almost exclusively from the study of cloned genes, including the gene for the cytadhesin P1 (114, 117, 256), the cytadherence accessory proteins HMW3 (193) and HMW1 (131a), several tRNAs (240), and *deoC* (158). Nucleotide sequence analysis of cloned *M. pneumoniae* genes indicates that both UGG and UGA are utilized as codons for tryptophan. Unlike *M. capricolum*, however, *M. pneumoniae* does not seem to possess tRNAs for each, suggesting that the tRNA for UGA recognizes the UGG codon by wobble (115). Mycoplasma transcriptional and translational signals are discussed in detail in chapter 19.

Clinical Aspects of Infection

Most bacterial pneumonias (i.e., typical pneumonias) have an abrupt, often rigorous onset, involving a productive cough which generates a purulent sputum that is often "rusty" with pneumococcal pneumonia, together with high fever, chest consolidation and rales, pleuritic chest pain, and stiffness in the neck (105). Mycoplasma (atypical) pneumonia is characterized by flulike symptoms, including generalized aches and discomfort, headache, chills, and a dry cough. However, symptoms are typically chronic in both onset and recovery (as opposed to the acute onset of influenza). Often chest X rays are more impressive than expected,

revealing an interstitial pattern mostly affecting the lower lobes (52, 53). The nondescript and somewhat chronic nature of the disease prompted the nickname "walking pneumonia," reflecting the contrast with the more typical, life-threatening bacterial pneumonias. While *M. pneumoniae* is the leading cause of pneumonia in the age group that includes older children and young adults (68, 84), it is important to note that there are other causes of atypical pneumonia. Infections by influenza viruses A and B, respiratory syncytial virus, adenovirus, parainfluenza virus, cytomegalovirus, *Chlamydia pneumoniae*, *Chlamydia psittaci*, *Coxiella burnetii*, *Legionella* spp., *Histoplasma capsulatum*, *Coccidioides immitis*, and *Pneumocystis carinii* can present as atypical pneumonia (105).

Mycoplasma infections usually involve the nasopharynx, throat, trachea, bronchus, and bronchioles, while the alveoli generally are spared (52). Additional symptoms can include a low-grade fever, malaise, rhinorrhea, otitis media, pharyngitis, and bronchitis, but usually no chest pain (164). The most common manifestation of infection is not pneumonia but rather a tracheobronchitis (53). Symptoms commonly vary from one patient to the next. Antibiotic therapy often hastens abatement of symptoms, but surprisingly, organisms remain present for an extended time (52, 242). Antibiotic therapy is discussed in greater detail in chapter 31. Asymptomatic and repeated silent infections have been documented, most frequently in adults, suggesting that some degree of immunity may contribute to the failure of clinical symptoms to appear (83a). Limited epidemiological surveys suggest that approximately 20% of all *M. pneumoniae* infections may be asymptomatic (53).

Extrapulmonary manifestations have been reported but are rare. These include the induction of autoantibodies and cold hemagglutinins, neurological complications, cardiolipin and cardiac complications, gastrointestinal symptoms, and dermatological sequelae (17, 188). The diverse nature of these symptoms suggests an immunopathological etiology. While *M. pneumoniae* is generally not regarded as invasive, it has been isolated from extrapulmonary sites such as joints (123, 272), skin lesions (159), and pericardial fluid and blood (190).

Diagnosis of *M. pneumoniae* infections is generally a matter of ruling out alternatives, taking into account the patient's age and background and the physical examination, including X rays (53). Culture is difficult because of the organism's complex nutritional requirements and slow rate of growth and the potential for overgrowth by other microbes in the specimens. As a result, very few laboratories attempt to culture *M. pneumoniae*, and with an incubation period of 7 to 10 days, direct culture is generally useful only for retrospective purposes. Because of the rather nondescript, flulike nature of symptoms, patients often do not seek medical attention immediately. This delays the collection of a serum sample to the point that a true acute-phase–convalescent-phase serum pair is not available for assessment of a rise in antibody titers. Serodiagnosis is discussed in greater detail in chapter 30.

The difficulty in making a rapid and accurate diagnosis of *M. pneumoniae* infections has likewise precluded a broad assessment of incidence in the general population. Current understanding of the incidence and epidemiology of *M. pneumoniae* infections has been extrapolated from studies of limited sample size (68, 84, 149, 164, 192). Several conclusions can be drawn from these longitudinal surveys. (i) *M. pneumoniae* infections appear to be endemic, with cases arising year round and the only seasonal fluctuation seen as perhaps a slight increase in the late summer and early fall. The average annual rate for mycoplasma pneumonia in all age groups was 0.5 to 5.0/1,000 population per year, representing up to 30% of all pneumonias in the general population. The highest attack rate is seen in the 5- to 9-year age group. The rate declines until approximately age 25 and then rises again slightly in the 30- to 40-year age group and may reflect exposure through family contact with infected children. Mycoplasma pneumonia is rare in infants and in adults over 50 years.

(ii) Close contact appears to be necessary for *M. pneumoniae* infections to spread. While the efficiency of transmission among close contacts is very high, spread does not occur rapidly, often requiring several weeks for passage among family members. The organisms remain in the respiratory tract for prolonged periods, even after symptoms subside, and this feature may contribute to the endemic nature of the disease.

(iii) In addition to smouldering endemic *M. pneumoniae* infections, there are cyclic epidemics. These outbreaks occur in 4- to 7-year cycles and have been described in the United States, Japan, the United Kingdom, and Denmark. Since 1972, however, the cyclic trend in Denmark has changed, with a significant decrease until 1986, when a major epidemic occurred. This change in pattern may reflect sociologic changes, as the number of children in day care has increased. It will be interesting to observe whether this trend proves to be more widespread.

Pathogenesis

The pathogenesis of *M. pneumoniae* infections is perhaps the most thoroughly characterized of the host-parasite interactions involving mycoplasmas. Despite significant advances in this area over the last two decades, there remain rather large voids in our understanding of mycoplasma virulence factors. An overview of the pathogenesis of *M. pneumoniae* infections in humans follows. For a more detailed description, the reader is referred to chapter 27.

It is important that the model system to be used for the assessment of virulence factors be clearly defined. Several experimental systems have been described for the examination of *M. pneumoniae* virulence in vivo, including but not limited to hamsters, cotton rats, guinea pigs, and chimpanzees. The hamster model has generally been the most popular, for experimental infections in hamsters appear to mimic natural infections in humans in many ways, and because no mycoplasmas have been described as part of the normal flora of the hamster respiratory tract (63). The mycoplasmas colonize the respiratory epithelium, especially via their differentiated terminal structure (58). Histopathological features in humans and hamsters are similar, involving a perivascular and peribronchial infiltration of mononuclear leukocytes, with occasional intraluminal exudate primarily of neutro-phils (63). Furthermore, even after resolution of pneumonia in both humans and hamsters, the mycoplasmas remain in the respiratory tract for extended periods (63). There are at least three noteworthy differences in the hamster model, however: the absence of a nonproductive cough or other overt symptoms, the lack of lateral spread of the disease, and the less chronic nature of the pneumonia compared with that in untreated human disease (34).

The chimpanzee would appear to provide a more accurate model for *M. pneumoniae* infections, for the chimpanzee displays many of the symptoms seen in humans and can transmit the disease horizontally (5). However, cost and availability tend to limit the use of nonhuman primate models.

At least three factors seem to contribute to the pathogenesis in *M. pneumoniae* infections: (i) adherence of invading mycoplasmas to the respiratory epithelium, (ii) localized host cell injury, and (iii) what might be viewed as an overaggressive or inappropriate immune response, resulting in immunopathology.

M. pneumoniae cytadherence

Mucociliary action provides a very effective first line of defense against infection of the respiratory mucosa. *M. pneumoniae* adherence to host cells (cytadherence) allows the mycoplasma to resist removal from the respiratory tract and hence effectively colonize the respiratory epithelium. Cytadherence may also be important from a nutritional perspective. Considering the limited biosynthetic capabilities of *M. pneumoniae*, positioning of the mycoplasma cells in close proximity to the host cell surface may facilitate nutrient acquisition from that microenvironment (47).

The cytadherence phenotype of *M. pneumoniae* is easily monitored on the basis of the ability of mycoplasma colonies to adsorb erythrocytes (hemadsorption). Hemadsorption probably has no bearing on natural infections because *M. pneumoniae* is usually noninvasive. However, this trait generally correlates with the capacity to adhere to respiratory epithelium, thereby making colony screening a convenient indicator (Fig. 3).

The critical role of cytadherence in virulence is reflected by the inability of noncytadhering strains resulting from broth passage of a clinical isolate (153), chemical mutagenesis (103), or spontaneous phase variation (133, 134) to infect and cause disease in experimentally infected hamsters. Examination of desquamated epithelial cells in sputum samples from patients with confirmed *M. pneumoniae* infections reveals that the mycoplasmas are commonly oriented perpendicular to the host cell surface and anchored to it by the tapered tip structure (58). The same is true of experimentally infected trachea and lung tissue from hamsters (58). It is not entirely clear to what extent this orientation reflects the distribution of the adhesin, as opposed to morphologic constraints placed on the mycoplasmas by the ciliary shafts. When incubated with nonciliated regions of tracheal explant cultures or with erythrocytes, conditions in which *M. pneumoniae* need not contend with penetration between cilia to reach the cell surface, mycoplasma adherence is not limited to the terminal organelle (36, 91). Furthermore, immunoelectron microscopy using polyclonal antibodies to the adhesin P1 demonstrates that this

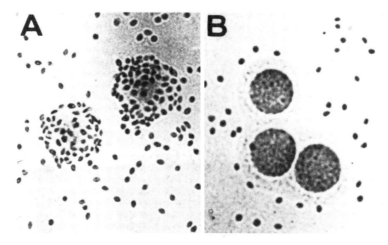

Figure 3. Hemadsorption by wild-type and cytadherence-negative phase variants of *M. pneumoniae*. Mycoplasmas were cultured for 7 days on PPLO agar plates, incubated with a suspension of chicken erythrocytes in saline, washed gently, and examined microscopically. (A) Wild-type *M. pneumoniae*; (B) phase variant.

protein is likewise not limited exclusively to the tip region but scattered elsewhere on the mycoplasma surface, though less densely than at the tip (8).

Two putative adhesins have been identified for *M. pneumoniae*: protein P1 (8, 78, 109, 110, 132) and a 32-kDa protein (11, 12). Furthermore, recent studies suggest that there are two different types of receptor populations on host cells: sialoglycoproteins and sulfated glycolipids (137, 216). The molecular properties of *M. pneumoniae* adhesins and receptors are considered in much greater detail in chapter 27.

While mycoplasmas are generally considered simple microorganisms, the process of *M. pneumoniae* adherence to host cells has proven to be anything but simple. The presence of at least two different adhesin populations on *M. pneumoniae* only begins to reflect the multifactorial nature of the cytadherence process. A broth passage-attenuated *M. pneumoniae* strain, unable to cytadhere, possesses the adhesin P1 but lacks three other proteins present in the wild-type parent and designated A, B, and C (72, 85, and 37 kDa, respectively) (102). Characterization of cytadherence-negative mutants derived by nitrosoguanidine treatment (77, 101) has expanded further the list of proteins putatively associated with cytadherence.

M. pneumoniae also exhibits in vitro a spontaneous, high-frequency loss and reacquisition of the ability to cytadhere (133, 134). The spontaneously arising noncytadhering strains were originally described as mutants. However, they arise at a high frequency which is more reminiscent of phase variation than mutation. Cytadherence phase variation is not unique to *M. pneumoniae* and has been described for a variety of bacterial pathogens of mucosal surfaces, including *E. coli*, *Neisseria gonorrhoeae*, and *Bordetella pertussis* (1, 187, 298).

The spontaneous loss of cytadherence by *M. pneumoniae* is accompanied by one of at least four changes in protein expression; the proteins involved are summarized in Table 2. In more than half of the 22 phase variants characterized, loss of cytadherence was accompanied by the loss of five high-molecular-weight proteins, designated HMW1 through HMW5 (134,

253). Proteins A, B, and C (described above) were absent in four variants, while four other variants lacked the 30-kDa protein adhesin (11, 12, 63a). A single variant lacked A, B, C, and P1. In each case, reversion to a cytadherence-positive phenotype was accompanied by the reacquisition of a normal complement of proteins (133).

It is tempting to speculate that all of the proteins listed in Table 2 function in cytadherence, in view of their coordinate loss or reacquisition in conjunction with phenotypic switching. However, as multiple virulence factors can be globally regulated (reviewed in reference 81), one must be cautious in assuming a cause-and-effect relationship. Nevertheless, progress has been made in ascertaining how some of these proteins may contribute to the adherence process. For example, protein P1 is widely scattered on the mycoplasma surface but also densely clustered about the terminal structure on wild-type *M. pneumoniae* cells. However, the loss of A, B, and C or HMW1 through HMW5 (and simultaneous loss of cytadherence and virulence) is accompanied by the inability to cluster P1 at the terminus. This finding suggests that one or more protein in each group may be necessary to maintain the proper distribution or disposition, or both, of P1 in the mycoplasma membrane. Furthermore, HMW1 through HMW5 partition in the cytoskeletonlike triton-insoluble fraction of *M. pneumoniae* (253, 254). The cosedimentation of these proteins with the other components in the triton shell by sucrose density gradient centrifugation (254) suggests that they are components of a complex, high-molecular-weight scaffolding structure.

Recent studies have demonstrated that HMW3 localizes exclusively to the attachment organelle (254a), where it might interact directly with P1, P30, or both. Analysis of the deduced amino acid sequences of P1 and P30 reveals homologous proline-rich domains at the carboxy terminus having a high content of basic amino acids (63a, 114, 256). Conversely, HMW3 possesses an internal proline-rich domain having a high content of acidic residues (194a). Thus, complementary charge interactions could promote a direct associ-

Table 2. Proteins associated with *M. pneumoniae* cytadherence

Protein	Size(s) (kDa)	Function or features	Reference(s)
P1	169	Adhesin; concentrated at tip; phase variable rarely; component of triton shell, though not exclusively	8, 78, 109, 110, 125, 132
P30	30	Adhesin; concentrated at tip; phase variable	11, 12, 63a
A	72	Phase variable	102, 103, 133, 134
B	85	Phase variable; accessible to peroxidase-mediated radioiodination	102, 103, 133, 134
C	37	Phase variable	102, 103, 133, 134
HMW1, HMW4	210, 215	Almost identical antigenically; phase variable; components of triton shell; membrane protein localizing in filamentous extensions	133, 134, 254
HMW2	190	Phase variable; component of triton shell; may be component of HMW5	133, 134, 253, 254
HMW3	140	Phase variable; component of triton shell and localized exclusively to attachment organelle; may migrate anomalously by SDS-PAGE	133, 134, 194, 194a, 254, 254a
HMW5	>340	Phase variable; disulfide-linked dimer of two 190-kDa subunits, one or both of which may be HMW2	253

ation between HMW3 and P1 and/or P30 in the attachment organelle (194a).

The molecular basis for phenotypic switching is only now being addressed, and studies in progress may ultimately clarify both the "how" and the "why." Nucleotide sequence analysis of the variant lacking A, B, C, and P1 has revealed a single base change in the P1 structural gene resulting in a nonsense mutation (255). It is not clear whether this is the only change in this variant and, if it is, how such a change would result in the simultaneous loss of A, B, and C. The coordinate loss and reacquisition of A, B, C, and P1 with phenotypic switching would suggest that a single molecular event is involved. However, no progress has been made in the cloning and analysis of the genes for A, B, and C. The genes for HMW1 and HMW3 have been cloned (131a, 193), and they map to adjacent regions of the *M. pneumoniae* chromosome. The level at which their expression is regulated has not yet been defined.

It is not known whether phenotypic switching of *M. pneumoniae* cytadherence is an in vitro curiosity or occurs during natural infections. Two explanations come to mind to account for how the mycoplasmas might benefit from the reversible loss of the capacity to cytadhere. (i) The temporary loss of cytadherence may facilitate exit from the host as a first step in initiating a new infection. (ii) Alternatively, cytadherence phase variation may contribute to the development of a carrier state in some individuals, for example, by disguising certain antigens such as the immunodominant protein P1.

Toxicity for respiratory epithelium

Microscopic examination of sputum samples reveals mycoplasmas attached to degenerating epithelial cells (58), prompting speculation that the infection leads to host cell dysfunction and death. Likewise, hamster and fetal human tracheal rings infected in vitro exhibit ciliary dysfunction and desquamation (55, 57, 59). At the ultrastructural level, freeze fracture/electron microscopy reveals that ciliary dysfunction is accompanied by alterations in the distribution of host cell membrane particles (39), including a necklace struc-

ture encircling the cilia at the base of the shaft, that is thought to be important in the regulation of ciliary motion (94). These observations correlate well with clinical findings, as ciliary clearance in the respiratory tract can remain depressed for extended periods following *M. pneumoniae* infections (38). These cytopathological changes are accompanied at the biochemical level by changes in host cell metabolism and macromolecular synthesis, as detailed in chapter 27.

Hydrogen peroxide and superoxide are the normal by-products of *M. pneumoniae* metabolism (160, 247, 248), resulting from the incomplete reduction of oxygen by a truncated electron transport system. It has been suggested that the accumulation of these oxygen metabolites in the extracellular milieu could overwhelm normal host cell mechanisms for defense against peroxidative injury (54). On the other hand, considering the biosynthetic limitations of the mycoplasma and the need to acquire specific nutrients from the microenvironment of the respiratory mucosa, parasitism could contribute to host cell dysfunction. Finally, there is evidence suggesting that mycoplasma membranes can physically perturb the host cell membrane (92), and this could likewise contribute to host cell injury. *M. pneumoniae* cytotoxicity is discussed in more detail in chapter 27.

Immune Response

Nonspecific factors

Much of the success of *M. pneumoniae* as a pathogen can be attributed in part to its resistance to several nonspecific defense mechanisms. Mucociliary clearance is an important first line of defense against infection in the respiratory tract. However, motility and the capacity to cytadhere allow *M. pneumoniae* to resist this defense mechanism. Furthermore, professional phagocytes are ineffective in removing the mycoplasmas in the absence of opsonins. Internalization and destruction are achieved following opsonization by antibodies (29, 205) or complement (29). Finally, *M. pneumoniae* is susceptible to complement-mediated cytolysis, but only upon activation by the classical pathway (36).

Specific immunity

Infections lead to the production of both circulating and secretory antibodies specific for mycoplasma antigens. In adults, the usual course of serum antibody appearance is immunoglobulin M (IgM), IgG, and IgA (16, 80). IgA is the predominant antibody class in respiratory secretions, though IgG and IgM have also been detected (20, 111). It is not clear whether the latter two classes reflect seepage accompanying inflammation or actual secretion. Immunity to *M. pneumoniae* infection correlates better with the presence of IgA antibodies in respiratory secretions than with serum antibody levels (35, 80). Nevertheless, immunity can be successfully transferred via serum in hamsters (104). Presumably, protective antibodies serve to enhance removal of the mycoplasmas by phagocytes, block adhesin-receptor interactions in cytadherence, or both. *M. pneumoniae* antigens appear to have mitogenic properties (19), and these may contribute to the histopathology and extrapulmonary complications.

The contribution of cellular mechanisms to immunity remains unclear. T-cell-depleted hamsters were impaired in their ability to clear mycoplasmas following experimental infection (258). However, these animals also exhibited significantly less lung histopathology, suggesting that the cellular immune response may also be detrimental. This conclusion is supported by two observations: (i) the development of delayed-type hypersensitivity in humans to *M. pneumoniae* correlates with disease severity (178), and (ii) mycoplasma-specific hilar lymphocytes apparently migrate to the bronchial airways in guinea pigs after infection with *M. pneumoniae* (119).

The identities of mycoplasma target antigens for humoral and cellular immune responses to infection are becoming clearer. Complement-fixing antibodies recognize glycolipid antigens on the mycoplasma surface (214). Radioimmunoprecipitation and Western immunoblot methodologies have identified several prominent protein immunogens, including the major adhesin P1 (111, 144). Approaches for the identification of antigens that initiate a cell-mediated response have lagged behind those for humoral responses. However, Jacobs et al. have recently established a T-cell epitope on the adhesin protein P1 (119).

Immunomodulation by components of *M. pneumoniae* and immunopathological sequelae associated with infection are discussed in detail in chapter 27. Vaccine development is addressed in chapter 29.

M. HOMINIS

History

Discovery

The first report (70) of the isolation of a mycoplasma from a human subject was in 1937. The organisms were recovered, apparently in pure culture, from an abscess of Bartholin's duct. Of course, there was no identification of *Mycoplasma* species at that time, but the organisms were probably *M. hominis* because this is the large-colony-forming species most frequently recovered from the genital tract.

Problems over nomenclature

In 1955, there were formal proposals (74, 85) to establish three species of mycoplasmas associated with humans: *M. hominis*, *M. fermentans*, and *M. salivarium*. The name *M. hominis* was proposed for genital strains that grew throughout a semisolid medium, usually produced a markedly granular growth, showed a weak and variable reduction of methylene blue, and did not produce acid from glucose. Morphologically, the strains were seen as very short and sparsely branched filaments. *M. hominis* was subdivided (74) into serologically distinct types 1 and 2. These types were also antigenically unrelated to *M. fermentans* and *M. salivarium*, but none of these mycoplasmas had been compared serologically with any of the animal species of *Mycoplasma* known at that time. However, in 1964 it was pointed out (146) that strain Campo, the representative strain of *M. hominis* type 2, was indistinguishable by the complement fixation test from five strains of *M. arthritidis* isolated from rats. The identity of strain Campo, and of two other strains tentatively classified as *M. hominis* type 2, with *M. arthritidis* was soon confirmed by agglutination and growth inhibition tests (75). In consequence, the classification of strain Campo and similar presumptive human genital strains as *M. hominis* type 2 was withdrawn (75). The true source of rat mycoplasmas in cultures derived from the human genital tract remains obscure, but the most likely explanation is that they were laboratory contaminants.

Cell Biology

Morphology and structure

Studies (220) of the morphology of *M. hominis* have shown that the cells resemble those of small coccoid or ovoid bacteria; the microstructure of the organism is compatible with reproduction by fission. Although dividing forms with equal-size lobes are common, filamentous cells, which are usually short but occasionally attain a length of up to 30 μm, and replicating buds sometimes occur, perhaps in response to suboptimal growth conditions. Data based on morphometric analysis have shown that cells of *M. hominis* ATCC 14027 have average dimensions of 0.27 by 0.74 μm and a mean diameter of 0.42 μm. The volume of an *M. hominis* cell has been calculated to be only about 60% of that of *U. urealyticum* T-960, a species that has a mean cell diameter of 0.5 μm. By transmission electron microscopy, the membrane of *M. hominis* is characteristically triple layered, as described in detail in chapters 6 through 8. The cytoplasm is filled with ribosomes and nuclear material, the ribosomes having a maximal size of about 17.5 nm (221) and being typical of 70S bacterial ribosomes (122).

Physiology

M. hominis metabolizes arginine (292). A possible mechanism is the three-step arginine dihydrolase pathway involving arginine deaminase and ornithine carbamoyltransferase. However, the former is only induced (79), and its late emergence may indicate that the pathway is not used until some other energy-yielding metabolite has been exhausted. A second pathway for the production of energy has been proposed (124) and involves the generation of ATP from ADP through two enzymes found in *M. hominis* (292), phosphate acetyltransferase and acetate kinase. Other enzymes described in *M. hominis* include NADH oxidase, thymidine kinase, ATPase, adenosine phosphorylase, RNase, DNase, phospholipase A, and aminopeptidase, the latter four being membrane bound (292).

M. hominis does not hydrolyze urea, ferment glucose or other carbohydrates, produce phosphatase or "film and spots" on agar, reduce tetrazolium salts, or digest gelatin or casein (86). Peroxide production by *M. hominis* is poor, yielding only partial lysis (alpha hemolysis or "greening") of guinea pig erythrocytes suspended over mycoplasma colonies (247). In addition, colonies of *M. hominis* do not hemadsorb (86).

Molecular biology

The G + C content of *M. hominis* DNA is 27.3 to 33.7 mol% (20). The mass of the *M. hominis* genome is 4.5 × 10^8 Da, or 680 (range, 630 to 750) kb; thus, the genome sizes of different strains may vary by about 100 kb (7). Christiansen et al. (49) analyzed the DNA of five *Mycoplasma* species, including *M. hominis*, and found that there was very low level homology (<0.5%). However, a 2.6% homology between *M. hominis* and *M. salivarium* was indicative of a quite separate identity but, nevertheless, a distant relationship. In addition, Christiansen et al. analyzed DNA from various strains of *M. hominis* for restriction fragment length polymorphism, using as a probe part of the *atp* operon of *Mycoplasma* strain PG50 (48). The *M. hominis* strains exhibited considerable polymorphism; although some groupings were observed, they were not conserved, thus further demonstrating the heterogeneity of *M. hominis* (50). A genetic map of *M. hominis* was constructed recently by hybridization with gene-specific probes (141); the genome contains two rRNA loci separated by more than 95 kb.

Molecular approaches to the detection of *M. hominis* have not been much exploited. In one study (217), a whole chromosomal DNA probe had poor sensitivity, detecting only 9 (56%) of 16 culture-positive specimens. It did, however, have much greater specificity, with only 2 of 128 culture-negative specimens being probe positive. A commercial DNA probe directed against mycoplasmal rRNA (Mycoplasma T.C.; Gen-Probe), used particularly for detecting mycoplasmas contaminating cell cultures, is capable of detecting *M. hominis* but is not specific for it. So far, the polymerase chain reaction (PCR) has not been used.

Clinical Aspects of Infection

The fact that *M. hominis*, like *U. urealyticum* (discussed below), is found as part of the normal flora of the human urogenital tract has complicated significantly clarification of the role of these species in disease. Nevertheless, indirect evidence reflects pathogenic potential for these species, as manifested in a variety of ways.

Urogenital tract disease and associated disorders

Although *M. hominis* occurs frequently in the lower genitourinary tract, it has been isolated from the upper urinary tract only in patients with symptoms of acute infection (283), and often with the development of a significant antibody response (284). Overall, *M. hominis* is thought to be involved in about 5% of cases of acute pyelonephritis in humans, and obstruction or instrumentation of the urinary tract may be a predisposing factor.

When it became clear that *Gardnerella vaginalis* was probably not the sole agent involved in the etiology of bacterial vaginosis (BV), a number of workers investigated the possible role of *M. hominis*. Pheifer et al. (200) isolated *M. hominis* from 63% of a group of symptomatic women with an abnormal vaginal discharge (compatible with a diagnosis of BV), compared with 10% of a similar group of women without abnormal findings. Similar observations have been made by other workers (196, 275), with qualitative and quantitative increases in *M. hominis* and higher levels of serum IgG antibody against *M. hominis* among women with BV (196). While there seems no doubt that *M. hominis* is associated with BV (166), whether it makes a real contribution to the pathological process is still unclear.

Pelvic inflammatory disease (PID) is a disease of multifactorial etiology, occurring iatrogenically or naturally from infection with various bacteria, principally *Chlamydia trachomatis* and, to a lesser extent, *N. gonorrhoeae*. *M. hominis* has been isolated from the endometrium and from the fallopian tubes of about 10% of women with salpingitis diagnosed by laproscopy (167), and its role is supported by specific antibody responses (168, 177). However, some (151) have found antibody responses to the mycoplasma only in patients who had evidence of chlamydial or gonococcal salpingitis and, on this basis, did not regard it as a primary pathogen. Overall, despite some doubts, *M. hominis* seems a likely cause of PID, although the exact proportion of cases attributable to it is unknown. As there are several indications that *M. hominis* has a primary pathogenic role in some cases of acute PID, it would be reasonable to believe that this mycoplasma has the potential for causing infertility as a consequence of tubal disease. Indeed, antibody to *M. hominis* has been found three times more often in infertile women following PID than in a control group of women (183). Nevertheless, the extent to which infertility may be attributed to *M. hominis* after *M. hominis*-associated PID is unknown, as is the role of this mycoplasma in unexplained infertility.

M. hominis has been isolated from amniotic fluids of women with severe chorioamnionitis who subsequently experienced preterm labor (40). Furthermore, the organisms, together with the bacteria found in BV, have been isolated significantly more often from the lower genital tract of women experiencing preterm delivery than they have from women who delivered normally (142), raising the possibility that the mycoplasmas together with the other microflora contribute to the prematurity. *M. hominis* likewise has been isolated from the blood of about 10% of women with postabortion fever and with postpartum fever, but not from afebrile women who have abortions or from normal pregnant women. In addition, antibody responses have been detected in about half of the women who become febrile but in few of those who remain afebrile. Thus, the evidence (275) indicates that *M. hominis* causes some cases of postabortion and postpartum fever.

Diseases of the newborn

M. hominis has been suggested as a possible cause of the respiratory distress syndrome, and in one case, infection of amniotic fluid by this mycoplasma after rupture of the membranes appeared to be responsible (275). In another case, this mycoplasma seemed to be the cause of respiratory distress, fever, and pneumonia occurring within a few hours of birth. Isolation from blood was accompanied by an antibody response, and the infant responded slowly to tetracycline (291). The few reported cases of meningitis in which *M. hominis* has been isolated from cerebrospinal fluid or brain have resulted presumably from infection in utero or from colonization at birth with subsequent infection (293). Invasion is liable to occur in premature infants, particularly if they have respiratory disease. In addition, infection seems to be more likely if there is an anatomical abnormality, such as spina bifida, and the possibility should be considered in cases of neonatal central nervous system disease in which the results of routine bacteriological staining and culture techniques are negative.

Extragenital infections

Extragenital infections by *M. hominis* have often been discovered fortuitously by growth on blood agar and in routine blood cultures. A review (161) of 36 cases of extragenital infections involving *M. hominis* revealed that they fall into five categories: septicemia, joint infection, central nervous system infection, respiratory infection, and wound infection, particularly after surgery. For example, sternal wound infections in heart or lung transplant patients appear particularly common (251), and infection of replaced heart valves has been recorded (139, 212). Few patients were found to be healthy prior to infection; most were debilitated, had major disruptions of anatomical barriers, or were immunocompromised. The latter patients were particularly at risk. Thus, *M. hominis*-induced suppurative arthritis has been seen in individuals with hypogammaglobulinemia (277) and polyarthritis, with recovery of both *M. hominis* and *U. urealyticum* in a kidney allograft patient on an immunosuppressive regimen (270).

Experimental Infections in Animals

Experimental studies lend some support to the observations made for humans. *M. hominis* inoculated into the urethra or vagina of male or female grivet monkeys, respectively, produced no clinical or serological signs of inflammation (181). On the other hand, inoculation of *M. hominis* into the upper genital tract (180) produced parametritis and salpingitis, with a serological response in which antibodies persisted for 60 days or longer (181). In addition, an acute septic arthritis was induced experimentally in a chimpanzee inoculated intra-articularly with a strain of *M. hominis* isolated from a patient with septic arthritis (6). The arthritis lasted for 5 weeks, after which the animal was resistant to rechallenge. A laboratory reference

strain did not cause disease in another chimpanzee. Studies in mice are discussed below.

Pathogenesis

Adherence

Adherence of erythrocytes to colonies of *M. hominis* (hemadsorption) does not occur (86), although attachment of the organisms to erythrocytes in suspension has been reported (118). However, numerous observations of adherence of *M. hominis* organisms to eucaryotic cells, including human WiDr cells (intestinal carcinoma), MRC-5 cells (human embryonic lung fibroblasts), and HeLa cells (cervical carcinoma) (118), have been made. Trypsin and pronase treatment of *M. hominis* markedly reduced attachment, suggesting that surface proteins of *M. hominis* play a role in its attachment to mammalian cells. Further evaluation (170) has revealed that monoclonal antibodies against surface-localized 108- and 31-kDa antigens inhibit adherence to HeLa cells, completely and partially, respectively. There is evidence that the organisms bind to sulfagalactolipid receptors on the cells, with no binding occurring upon removal of the sulfate group (152). Different attachment activities of *M. hominis* strains isolated from different infected sites of patients with a variety of diseases have been described (118) and may be relevant to the virulence of the strains.

Toxicity

Inoculation of *M. hominis* into tracheal and fallopian tube organ cultures reveals no clear cytopathic effects by conventional light microscopy (257). However, alterations in cellular morphology (detected by scanning electron microscopy) and ciliary wave pattern have been detected after infection by some strains of *M. hominis* (4, 257). It has been speculated (4, 257) that ciliary swelling and clubbing in fallopian tube organ cultures might be due to the production of ammonia by the organisms. There is, however, no direct support for this notion or for believing that ammonia production by *M. hominis* might contribute to the changes seen in BV. On the other hand, the depletion of arginine by arginine-metabolizing mycoplasmas growing in eucaryotic cell cultures has been shown to affect cell metabolism by inhibiting cytopathic changes caused by viruses that are arginine dependent (241). Furthermore, the membrane-bound enzymes of *M. hominis*, phospholipase and aminopeptidase, may have potential host cell-destroying properties (292).

Hormones

Colonization of the genital tract of mice by *M. hominis* is dependent on hormone treatment. *M. hominis* organisms were recovered persistently from the vagina of almost 90% of estradiol-treated mice (90), the reproductive cycle being arrested in the estrous phase; in contrast, the organisms were isolated transiently from only 10.5% of mice not treated with estradiol. Treatment with progesterone, which induced the diestrous phase of the cycle, did not render any of the mice susceptible to vaginal colonization. Vaginal colonization persisted for more than 200 days in some mice, and there was evidence of spread to the uterine horns and ovaries. Infection was not associated with a polymorphonuclear leukocyte response, but an antibody response to *M. hominis* was detected in almost half of the mice. Although there was proliferation also of the endogenous vaginal bacteria, this was not necessary for colonization of the vagina by *M. hominis* because germ-free, estradiol-treated mice also became colonized vaginally, with multiplication and spread of the organisms to the upper genital tract (88). The importance of estradiol was shown further by giving infected mice progesterone, which changed the reproductive cycle to the diestrous phase and rapidly eradicated the organisms (265).

Immune cell activation

It seems likely that the direct effect of *M. hominis* on cells is insufficient to account for the pathological changes that are associated with infection by this mycoplasma. Mycoplasma-mediated lymphocytotoxicity reactions against allogeneic and syngeneic fibroblast target cells have been shown to be dependent on the presence of viable *M. hominis* organisms (2). However, the significance of mitogenicity in the pathogenic process remains to be determined.

Immune Response

Antigenic relationships

In early studies (106), two membrane antigens were identified as proteins on the basis of their lability and susceptibility to proteolytic enzymes; a third antigen, stable to 100°C and relatively stable to both pronase and trypsin, was also found to exist. Since then, the proteinaceous nature of the predominant membrane antigens has been confirmed (147), and more than 80 proteins have been detected (51), some of which are probably lipoproteins. Numerous investigators have demonstrated extensive antigenic heterogeneity (33, 51). In addition, among strains isolated from the synovial exudates of a septic arthritis patient over a 6-year period, there was some evidence of antigenic variation (227). Strain differences are attributable to surface antigens and similarities to cytoplasmic soluble antigens. Lin (147) was able to detect 7 to 14 different strain-specific antigens, but no common surface antigens, in each of seven *M. hominis* strains that were suggested as being of different serovars. Although this suggestion has not been taken further, the need to use more than one strain in serodiagnostic studies, because of heterogeneity, has to be recognized. *M. hominis* is, of course, serologically distinct from other *Mycoplasma* species, although some antigens are shared with other arginine-utilizing species, including *M. arthritidis*, *M. buccale*, *M. faucium*, *M. fermentans*, *M. orale*, *M. primatum*, and *M. salivarium*.

Specific immunity

In addition to antibody responses to *M. hominis* in experimentally inoculated animals, responses have been recorded in the human clinical situation. For ex-

ample, a fourfold or greater rise in the titer of serum indirect hemagglutinating antibody to *M. hominis* was noted from 9 to between 34 and 47 days after laparoscopy of patients with acute salpingitis (168). The induction of class-specific antibodies to *M. hominis* can only be inferred; an increase in serum IgM was noted in one-third of patients with acute salpingitis, concentrations of IgG and IgA being normal or only slightly raised. Indirect hemagglutinating antibody to *M. hominis* was found in nearly all of the patients who had an increased serum IgM concentration but in few of those with a normal IgM concentration, although IgM specifically directed against *M. hominis* was not sought (165).

Subjects with pyelonephritis were found to have developed indirect hemagglutinating antibody to *M. hominis* in urine (284), as measured by an immunofluorescence test; IgA antibody appeared shortly before IgG, while IgM was usually absent. This observation apart, however, information on local secretory antibody responses to *M. hominis* is lacking.

Cell-mediated immune responses detectable by lymphocyte transformation were reported in female grivet monkeys that had developed salpingitis following inoculation of *M. hominis* directly into the oviducts (180) as well as in a group of women with PID attributed to *M. hominis* (232).

U. UREALYTICUM

History

Discovery in men with nongonococcal urethritis

Organisms which produced very small colonies (7 to 15 μm in diameter), referred to as tiny-form PPLO colonies, were first isolated from men with primary and recurrent NGU by Shepard (234). He also described and illustrated the structure of these colonies (234) and later provided a detailed account (237) of the discovery of the organisms, which were ascribed subsequently to a new genus and species, *Ureaplasma urealyticum* (238).

Metabolism of urea

The fact that *U. urealyticum* is unique among the mycoplasmas of human origin in metabolizing urea was discovered independently by Purcell et al. (207) and by Shepard (235) and reported in 1966. This finding was the key to being able more easily to detect and isolate ureaplasmas, as *U. urealyticum* organisms became known trivially, and it formed the basis of a test that was developed to detect antibodies against them (207). In addition, it was instrumental in the discovery of ureaplasmas in other animal species (261, 271, 273).

Nomenclature

Organisms that produced the tiny-form colonies were referred to originally as T strains (T = tiny) and later as T-strain mycoplasmas or T-mycoplasmas. The observations mentioned above, particularly that of urea metabolism, stimulated other workers to examine the organisms, and within the next decade, much new information on their basic biology and serology accrued. Gradually, a consensus developed that these organisms warranted a distinct taxonomic position within the order *Mycoplasmatales*. In 1974, an international cooperative effort among those working with the organisms resulted in a proposal (238), subsequently ratified, that there should be a new genus and species designation, *Ureaplasma urealyticum*, within the then current classification scheme. Since then, four other species, *U. diversum*, *U. gallorale*, *U. felinum*, and *U. cati*, have been designated for ureaplasmas isolated from bovine, avian, and feline species.

Cell Biology

Structure and chemical composition

Cells of *U. urealyticum* and those of ureaplasmas of other animal species after culture for 18 to 24 h are morphologically similar to cells of other mycoplasmas. By most staining methods, they appear as dense, round to ovoid elements about 330 nm in diameter, with a range of 100 to 850 nm (271); morphometric analysis indicates a mean diameter of about 500 nm (220). The cells are seen singly and in various combinations; by phase-contrast microscopy, they have been seen to occur singly or in pairs. Pleomorphic forms, such as branching filaments, occur in older cultures, but less frequently than in cultures of other members of the family *Mycoplasmataceae*. In electron micrographs of ultrathin sections and of negatively stained preparations, the cells are usually round, with a diameter ranging from 120 to 1,000 nm; filamentous forms up to 2,000 nm in length and 50 to 300 nm wide have been seen by some workers (22). Organelles usually associated with motility have not been detected by electron microscopy, in keeping with the lack of observable motility. *U. urealyticum*, like other mycoplasmas, is bounded by a single membrane, 7.5 to 10 nm thick, with no distinguishable cell wall. However, an extramembranous layer, 20 to 30 nm thick, has been observed (224) by ruthenium red staining, and structures morphologically similar to short pili have been seen radiating from the membrane surface (22). The extramembranous layer was found to contain glucosyl-like residues, and purified membranes from several strains of *U. urealyticum* were reported to contain between 1 and 7% carbohydrate, the sugars being mannose, galactose, and glucose (301). These membrane-associated hexoses are in the form of lipoglycans (244). The fatty acid composition of the ureaplasma membrane varies from that of other species in that larger proportions of free fatty acids and phosphatidic acid are present in ureaplasmas, and phosphatidylethanolamine and diaminohydroxy polar lipid have also been identified (239, 244). *U. urealyticum* membranes also contain cholesterol, and as would be expected, the cells are susceptible to lysis by digitonin (239).

Antigenic relationships

The existence of at least eight distinct serovars among strains of ureaplasmas of human origin (21)

posed a problem at the time the genus *Ureaplasma* was described (238), but the temptation to give each serovar a separate species designation was resisted. This decision seemed amply justified, since other serovars were subsequently defined; a total of 14 have now been described (271). However, further study of the serovars indicated that they could be allocated to two separate groups or clusters (A and B) on the basis of protein profiles by one- and two-dimensional polyacrylamide gel electrophoresis (271, 286). Additional support for the two distinct seroclusters was obtained by genetic techniques, utilizing DNA homology and restriction endonuclease patterns (271, 286). Group A contains serovars 2, 4, 5, 7, 8, 9, 10, 11, 12, and 13, and group B contains serovars 1, 3, 6, and 14. Serovars of *U. urealyticum* are antigenically distinct from all other known mycoplasmas and from ureaplasmas isolated from other animal species (271, 282), those from chimpanzees being closest antigenically (282).

Physiology

U. urealyticum and indeed other members of the genus *Ureaplasma* are unique in their ability to metabolize urea through the enzyme urease (207, 235, 239, 261, 271). In addition, the possession of at least 24 other enzymes has been reported (69, 203, 239, 271). However, ureaplasmas do not metabolize arginine and apparently are nonfermentative (203), and they are also metabolically unusual in that, unlike all other mycoplasmas, they do not have any detectable oxygen-dependent NADH oxidase activity (203). Since *U. urealyticum* seems to lack the conventional mechanisms for ATP generation (energy synthesis), it has been proposed (226) that ATP may be generated as a result of urea hydrolysis producing an electrical potential through NH_4^+ diffusion across the ureaplasma membrane. Others, however, have suggested a possible way in which ATP could be generated through pyruvate metabolism (67).

Ureaplasmas of human and animal origin lyse erythrocytes from several animal species (238, 239, 261, 271). The hemolysin is soluble and is probably peroxide, although it has not always been possible to inhibit hemolysis with catalase (239). The possibility that strains of *U. urealyticum* produce a toxin was suggested by Furness (87), who proposed that the accumulation of a catalase-resistant, thermostable, and dialyzable factor was responsible for the abrupt cessation of growth in liquid medium. However, the identity of this toxic factor is unknown.

Molecular biology

The G+C content of the DNA of *U. urealyticum* ranges from 26.9 to 28.0 mol% (271). Although this narrow range suggests genetic homogeneity among the various strains and serovars, the genome size varies quite widely and corresponds to the two serovar clusters. Thus, the genome size of the four serovars in one cluster (group B) is about 760 kb, while the size in the other cluster (group A) ranges from 880 to 1,140 kb (222). The urease and both serotype 8- and serocluster-specific antigens of *U. urealyticum* have been described, and monoclonal antibodies against these proteins have been developed (280, 281). There has not been uniform agreement about the nature of the urease; some believe it to be a dimer comprising subunits of 75 kDa each (228), while others (280) have strong evidence that it is a hexamer consisting of three subunits, one of 72 kDa containing nickel, one of 14 kDa, and one of 11 kDa. A fragment of chromosomal DNA from *U. urealyticum*, shown to be homologous with urease genes from other procaryotes, was cloned in *E. coli* and sequenced (23). Analysis of the sequence revealed three consecutive open reading frames; the deduced polypeptides had molecular masses of 11.2, 13.6, and 66.6 kDa, values reasonably consistent with the size of the three subunits of purified native urease. The three polypeptides were closely homologous with the subunits of some other bacterial ureases and with the single polypeptide of the urease of the jack bean.

Clinical Aspects of Infection

Detection

The most sensitive method of isolating *U. urealyticum* and other ureaplasmas consists of inoculation of a specimen into liquid medium and subsequent subculture to liquid and agar media (218, 236, 260, 271, 273). Colonies sometimes fail to develop or are not seen when a specimen is plated directly on agar medium, whereas the organisms are detected in liquid medium, taking advantage of their urease activity. Small colonies are due to lack of surface peripheral growth which results in the absence of a classical fried-egg appearance and renders them difficult to recognize. However, improved buffered medium has resulted in colonies of diameter 60 μm or even greater, and manganous sulfate or calcium chloride, both sensitive indicators of ammonia, may be added to the agar medium to aid in detection (239, 260, 271). On such medium, ureaplasmas form dark brown colonies.

A solid-phase enzyme immunoassay based on a monoclonal antibody to the urease enzyme of *U. urealyticum* has enabled the 14 serotypes to be detected (260), but so far, the sensitivity of the procedure has been insufficient to detect ureaplasmas in clinical specimens reliably.

A whole-chromosome DNA probe prepared from serovar 8 of *U. urealyticum* hybridized with all of the serovars tested (serovars 1 to 9) but not with several other mycoplasmas or bacteria sometimes found in the genitourinary tract (217). However, in tests on urethral specimens from men, the probe showed a lack of sensitivity, particularly with culture-positive specimens containing <10^3 CFU/ml. The probe was also positive for a significant number of the culture-negative specimens, suggesting either nonspecificity or defective culturing. The PCR that has been developed for *U. urealyticum* (24, 302) may provide the ultimate in sensitivity but awaits clinical evaluation.

NGU in men and women

The results of human (263) and animal inoculation studies and observations on immunocompromised patients (270) provide strong evidence that *U. urealyticum* is a cause of nonchlamydial NGU in men, and carefully controlled antibiotic (61) and serological (32) studies lend support to this contention. However, the proportion of ureaplasma-induced cases is unknown, and the occurrence of urethral ureaplasmas in healthy men suggests that only certain serovars are pathogenic or that predisposing factors, such as a lack of mucosal immunity, exist in those who develop disease. It is plausible that *U. urealyticum* could be responsible for some cases of the acute urethral syndrome in women, but the evidence obtained so far is weak (231, 250).

Prostatitis and epididymitis

It is likely that ureaplasmas can gain access to the prostate during an acute ureaplasmal infection of the urethra (263), but whether their isolation more frequently and in greater numbers from patients with acute urethroprostatitis than from controls (37) indicates that they cause acute inflammation of the prostate is debatable, even though patients with >10^3 organisms in expressed prostatic fluid have been reported to respond to tetracycline therapy (37). *U. urealyticum* has not been isolated from prostatic biopsy specimens taken from patients with chronic abacterial prostatitis (71). In contrast, ureaplasmas were recovered directly from the epididymis of a patient suffering from nonchlamydial, nongonococcal acute epididymo-orchitis who developed specific antibody and responded to tetracycline therapy (120). It seems that the organisms may be an infrequent cause of this disease.

Urinary tract involvement

Infection stones are induced by the urease of certain bacteria, mostly *Proteus* species, that degrade urea. In addition, ureaplasmas by virtue of their urease, induce crystallization of struvite and calcium phosphates in urine in vitro (98) and produce calculi in animal models (see below). Ureaplasmas have also been found more frequently in the urine and in the stones of patients with infection stones than in patients with metabolic stones (98). Although this finding suggests that ureaplasmas may have a causal role, they are likely to be implicated far less often than other urease-positive bacteria (100). There is no evidence suggesting that *U. urealyticum* is involved in causing pyelonephritis.

Reproductive tract disease and associated disorders

U. urealyticum has been isolated directly from the affected fallopian tubes in PID but usually together with other known pathogens (275). In addition, the rather negative results of serological tests, and studies of the inoculation of subhuman primates and fallopian tube organ cultures, do not support a causal role (275). The possibility that *U. urealyticum* might play an important part in involuntary infertility in humans was first raised more than 20 years ago, but the association remains speculative. Although ureaplasmas are associated with altered sperm motility, a finding reaffirmed recently (175), specimens from fertile and infertile subjects contain ureaplasmas with similar frequencies, and the results of comparative treatment trials do not imply that these organisms are important (259, 275).

U. urealyticum and *M. hominis* have been isolated

from amniotic fluids of women with severe chorioamnionitis who subsequently experienced preterm labor (40, 83). Ureaplasmas have also been isolated more frequently from spontaneously aborted fetuses and from stillborn and premature infants than from induced abortions or normal full-term infants (275). The recovery of organisms from aborted fetuses is not due entirely to superficial contamination, since the organisms have been isolated from internal organs. However, despite persuasive individual case reports of infection causing chorioamnionitis and abortion, the problem of whether abortion occurs because ureaplasmas invade the fetus and cause its death, or whether death for some other reason is followed by invasion, remains a mystery. It is true that the results of some serological and therapeutic studies tend to support a role for ureaplasmas (209, 275), but antibody responses may be seen also during a normal pregnancy, and the number of patients treated has been small.

There is an association between genital mycoplasmas, particularly *U. urealyticum*, and low birth weight in some but not all populations (127, 260, 275). The association is supported by serological data (127, 275) and by a double-blind placebo-controlled trial of erythromycin in which women given the drug in the third trimester delivered larger babies than did those given a placebo (127, 172, 275). It is feasible that the organisms cause chorioamnionitis in the later stages of pregnancy and that this results in impaired fetal nutrition, early labor, or both. However, it cannot be concluded that genital mycoplasmas are directly responsible for low birth weight because it is possible that there is selective colonization of women who are predisposed to smaller babies.

Ureaplasmas have been isolated from the blood of a small proportion of women with postpartum fever (76), and it seems that these organisms, like *M. hominis*, might induce fever by causing endometritis.

Disease of the newborn

U. urealyticum occasionally causes respiratory disease in the newborn (40, 210), the infections often being acquired in utero. Ureaplasmas, in particular, appear to be involved in respiratory disease of very low birth weight infants. Thus, infants of <1,000 g, from whom ureaplasmas were isolated from tracheal aspirates within the first 24 h after birth, were found to be twice as likely to die or to develop chronic lung disease as uninfected infants of similar birth weight or those of >1,000 g (41).

U. urealyticum, in addition to *M. hominis*, is able to invade the cerebrospinal fluid and seems particularly liable to do so in the first few days of life in premature infants with respiratory disease or hydrocephalus (293, 294). Meningitis may occur and run a mild subclinical course, or there may be more severe neurological damage. Although some investigators (293) consider *M. hominis* and ureaplasmas to be common causes of central nervous system infection in neonates, others (99, 233) have found them to be quite rare.

Extragenital infections

A few individuals with hypogammaglobulinemia develop suppurative arthritis, and it seems that *U. ure-*

alyticum, in particular, is responsible (270, 277). The organisms may be isolated from the joints, and the arthritis may persist for many months, despite antibiotic and anti-inflammatory treatment and administration of specific antiserum. The arthritis in hypogammaglobulinemia is not to be confused with that occurring after a genital infection in immunocompetent patients. This condition is probably reactive (Reiter's disease), and evidence for the involvement of ureaplasmas is immunological. The arthritis in hypogammaglobulinemic patients has been associated sometimes with subcutaneous abscesses, persistent urethritis, and chronic urethrocystitis/cystitis, ureaplasmas having been isolated from all of the inflammatory sites involved (270). In contrast, *U. urealyticum* does not seem to be responsible as often as *M. hominis* for causing disease in patients on immunosuppressive therapy. However, polyarthritis with recovery of both *M. hominis* and *U. urealyticum* was seen in a kidney allograft patient on an immunosuppressive regimen (270). Evidence that *U. urealyticum* is involved in AIDS is lacking.

Experimental Infections in Animals

Some of the results of inoculating animals experimentally are in keeping with clinical observations. *U. urealyticum* after multiple passage in vitro failed to stimulate a urethral cellular response in male chimpanzees (276) or in male grivet monkeys (181). On the other hand, intraurethral inoculation of unpassaged ureaplasmas produced a polymorphonuclear leukocyte response in male chimpanzees which was only a little less intense than the response to chlamydiae (261a).

Inoculation of the bladder of rats with *U. urealyticum* results in the production of struvite calculi (279). In addition, *U. urealyticum* multiplied and survived for at least 3 weeks after inoculation into the experimentally obstructed upper urinary tract of dogs and caused severe chronic interstitial nephritis accompanied by an antibody response (136).

Disease was not produced in the reproductive tract of female grivet monkeys after inoculation with *U. urealyticum* (179, 181). However, it has been possible to colonize the vagina and upper genital tract of mice, but only after first treating them with estradiol (89, 264). This model may be useful in looking at possible differences in the pathogenicity of ureaplasma strains, the role of the immune system in preventing colonization, and the effect of antibiotics.

Pneumonia occurs in newborn mice following intranasal inoculation with *U. urealyticum* (295). The disease resolves spontaneously, but exposure to 80% oxygen increases the inflammatory response, and then death often occurs (62). The relevance to human infant pneumonia and the respiratory distress syndrome is obvious.

Intra-articular inoculation of a chimpanzee with a strain of *U. urealyticum* isolated originally from a patient with agammaglobulinemia produced severe arthritis lasting for 1 month; reinoculation after resolution produced less severe disease (6). In contrast, a well-passaged laboratory reference strain caused minimal disease in another chimpanzee. These observations may imply that ureaplasmas will produce arthritis in the immunocompetent human counterpart if they gain access to the joint, the arthritis seen in hypogammaglobulinemic patients simply being a result of easier transport to the joint.

Pathogenesis

Adherence

As the first step in pathogenesis, it is relevant that *U. urealyticum* attaches to erythrocytes and to other eucaryotic cells. Hemadsorption has been demonstrated, at first only with guinea pig erythrocytes and only by colonies of serovar 3 of *U. urealyticum* (238, 239, 271). Subsequently, however, it was shown that colonies of other serovars hemadsorb (223) and that the organisms attach to erythrocytes in suspension (229). In addition, colonies of six different strains of ureaplasmas of human origin adsorbed HeLa cells from suspension, colonies of some ureaplasma strains more vigorously than others (163), and the organisms have also been observed to adsorb to HeLa and other cell monolayers (173). There is evidence (152) that the receptor on these cells is a sulfogalactolipid and that removal of the sulfate group leads to loss of binding. The lipoglycan on the ureaplasmal membrane may be important in the process.

Metabolites

It is not clear which, if any, of the various enzyme activities (203, 239, 271) of *U. urealyticum* might be important. Local changes in pH and the production of NH_4^+ due to the metabolism of urea cannot be discounted, nor can the toxinlike product (87), mentioned previously, which may have been responsible, at least partially, for the loss of ciliary activity brought about by ureaplasmas in bovine oviduct organ cultures (249). These factors could also account for the cytopathic changes seen in ureaplasma-infected cell cultures (171) and for chromosomal aberrations in infected human lymphocyte cultures (189). Peroxide also should not be forgotten, since it is probably responsible for the lysis of erythrocytes caused by ureaplasmas (238, 239, 261, 271).

IgA protease activity is postulated as an important virulence factor of some mucosal pathogens and has been demonstrated for *U. urealyticum*, with specificity for IgA1 (219). The significance depends on the unknown protective capacity of this immunoglobulin at the mucosal surface.

Hormones

As for *M. hominis*, one can render female mice susceptible to *U. urealyticum* colonization of the vagina and upper genital tract by first treating the mice with estradiol (89, 264); the mechanism is not understood, but the phenomenon could be relevant to the altered recovery of ureaplasmas from the genital tract of women (275) as a result of contraception, menstruation, and pregnancy.

Immune cellular aspects and HLA types

The ability of *U. urealyticum* to stimulate and recruit lymphocytes in the inflammatory process is largely unknown, although their suggested role in the etiology of reactive arthritis has been proposed (82). The ability of neutrophils to phagocytose *U. urealyticum* has been shown by chemiluminescence and by electron microscopy (297). The organisms were not killed even in the presence of complement, and in the absence of antibody, which is likely in hypogammaglobulinemia, the neutrophils would seem to have little defensive role and may even aid dissemination.

There are no data on the possible role of tissue antigens (HLA types) in the pathogenic process apart from those of a recent study (66); a monoclonal antibody to an HLA-B27 synthetic polypeptide reacted strongly with a cytoplasmic peptide (70 to 72 kDa) of the 14 serovars of *U. urealyticum*. The possible significance of this finding in patients with sexually acquired reactive arthritis, in whom this HLA type occurs often, is evident, since cross-reactivity between ureaplasmal antibody and the antigen could occur.

Immune Response

Humoral

The results of immunoblotting with human sera and rabbit antisera have suggested the possibility of nonprotein antigens of *U. urealyticum* also being involved in the immune response (108). In men with acute NGU, a fourfold or greater rise or fall in the titer of antibody to ureaplasmas, detected by an enzyme immunoassay or by metabolism inhibition, was seen in sera collected 10 to 35 days after the first samples (32); 10 of 12 patients had a change in the titer of IgM, suggesting an active infection. These findings are supported by some of those from volunteer and animal experimentation. Thus, a serum antibody response to *U. urealyticum*, measured by metabolism inhibition, was seen to develop in two subjects in the month after they had been inoculated intraurethrally with ureaplasmas (263), a similar observation being made in studies of male chimpanzees inoculated intraurethrally (261a). In addition, a fourfold ureaplasmal antibody response was seen in a patient with acute epididymitis and was a complementary diagnostic feature (120).

Antibody responses measured by an immunoassay were observed in dogs in which interstitial nephritis had been induced by experimental inoculation of *U. urealyticum* (136). Ureaplasmal antibody titers, measured by metabolism inhibition, fourfold greater in the fetus than in the mother, were found three times more often in aborted fetuses than in healthy ones (211, 275), a finding taken to mean that a sizeable proportion of fetuses were infected sufficiently to have produced antibody; whether the organisms caused the fetal death is open to question. In addition, antibody to some ureaplasmas has been detected at birth in higher titers in the sera of neonates with respiratory distress than in the sera of normal infants, and some have a higher titer than does the maternal antibody, suggesting infection in utero (208, 275). Serological results have also been used to support the role of *U. urealyticum* in low birth weight; women who developed a fourfold or greater antibody titer rise had a low-birth-weight rate of 30%, whereas women who did not have such a rise had a low-birth-weight rate of 7.3% (127, 275).

Cell mediated

Information relating to *U. urealyticum* infections is sparse. Blast transformation of lymphocytes from two male volunteers infected intraurethrally with ureaplasmas was not detected (263). Since lymphocyte transformation responses indicate previous in vivo exposure and sensitization to an antigen, the test has been used in attempts to implicate organisms in the etiology of disease. In this regard, mononuclear synovial cells from some patients with sexually acquired reactive arthritis (Reiter's disease) had a greater response to *U. urealyticum* in a lymphocyte transformation assay than did cells from patients with enteric Reiter's disease or those from patients with rheumatoid arthritis (82), suggesting a role for ureaplasmas in the sexually acquired form of the arthritis.

M. GENITALIUM

History

Dark-field microscopy of fresh urethral smears from patients with NGU, some of whom are infected by chlamydiae, ureaplasmas, *M. hominis*, and other microorganisms, sometimes reveals motile spiral forms. These are not *Treponema pallidum* but resemble spiroplasmas in appearance. In view of this finding, urethral swabs from 13 men with NGU attending the sexually transmitted disease clinic at St. Mary's Hospital, Paddington, London, in 1980 were expressed in sucrose-phosphate transport medium containing 10% heat-inactivated fetal calf serum. These specimens were transported in liquid nitrogen by one of us (D. Taylor-Robinson) to J. G. Tully's laboratory at the National Institutes of Health, Bethesda, Md., where they were inoculated into SP-4 medium (260). Spiroplasmas were not isolated, but specimens from two of the men yielded two strains, G-37 and M-30, of a glucose-fermenting mycoplasma (278, 287). These strains and a third were recovered in Taylor-Robinson's laboratory from the same specimens after they had been refrozen and transported back. Strains G-37 and M-30 were found to be closely related but different serologically from all other known mycoplasmas, and this finding resulted in the proposal that they should be regarded as belonging to a new species, *M. genitalium* (288).

Subsequent to the recovery of *M. genitalium* from the male urethra, there was an interval of several years, during which time some of its features and disease-producing capacity in animals were defined, before it was detected in specimens from the respiratory tract (9). Specimens taken from the respiratory tract of marine recruits in the United States in 1968 were found to contain *M. pneumoniae* and were stored at −70°C. Eighteen years later, 4 of 16 specimens were found also to contain *M. genitalium*. However, the frequency of occurrence of *M. genitalium* in the respiratory tract and, indeed, in the urogenital tract has yet to be established.

Cell Biology

Morphology and specialized structure

Dark-field microscopy of *M. genitalium* cultures shows small coccoid bodies, but details cannot be resolved. However, by electron microscopy, several mycoplasmas, of which *M. genitalium* is one, are seen to have specialized structures at one or both ends (128). Thus, *M. genitalium* is predominantly flask shaped (287, 288), the terminal portion being involved in attachment to cell surfaces. The dimensions have been calculated (288) to be as follows: length, 0.6 to 0.7 μm; and width, 0.3 to 0.4 μm at the broadest part and 0.06 to 0.08 μm at the tip. In addition, small projections (78 nm), similar to but somewhat coarser than those on myxoviruses, may be seen extending distally from the tip of *M. genitalium* (287, 288) for about 40 to 60% of its length and may facilitate attachment. Transmission electron microscopy of sections of the organisms shows the characteristic triple-layered membrane, 7.5 to 10 nm wide, the middle layer of which is less electron dense than the other two. In addition, the terminal structure exhibits an internal feature (288) similar to that seen in *M. pneumoniae*.

Motility

The specialized terminal structure of *M. genitalium* may be involved in motion, since the organisms exhibit gliding motility in which they move tip first (262). Many of them move in circles, often but not exclusively in a clockwise direction. The speed averages about 0.1 μm/s, which is slower than that recorded for *M. pneumoniae* but faster than that of *M. gallisepticum*.

Physiology

M. genitalium metabolizes glucose but not arginine or urea (278, 287, 288). It therefore acidifies medium in which it is growing, causing a reduction in pH which may be used for its detection (260). Growth is optimal at 37°C, and colonies develop best in an atmosphere of nitrogen–5% CO_2. Growth is inhibited by 0.05% thallium acetate (278, 288), whereas that of *M. pneumoniae* is not. *M. genitalium* does not produce phosphatase or film and spots on agar, but it does reduce tetrazolium anaerobically (weakly aerobically) and exhibits colony hemadsorption (288).

Molecular biology

The G + C content of the DNA of *M. genitalium* is 32.4 ± 1.0 mol%. Recently, a physical and partial genetic map of the *M. genitalium* genome was constructed, revealing it to be approximately 600 kb, or among the smallest genomes reported for a self-replicating procaryote (60). The adhesin gene of *M. genitalium* has been cloned and sequenced (64). The complete gene was found to contain 4,335 nucleotides coding for a protein of 159,668 Da, and considerable homology was found with the sequence of the P1 adhesin gene of *M.*

pneumoniae. For example, about 48% of the coding sequence of the adhesin gene of *M. genitalium* is 60 to 70% homologous with the sequence of the P1 gene. Confirmation of the *M. genitalium* adhesin gene sequence and its extensive homology with that of *M. pneumoniae* came from an independent study (116) in which a 10.4-kb region of the attachment gene of *M. genitalium* was cloned through the use of P1-derived DNA probes and subsequently sequenced.

The need for a rapid and sensitive means of detecting *M. genitalium* has stimulated attempts to develop a DNA probe. The fact that the DNA sequence of *M. genitalium* is 8% homologous with that of *M. pneumoniae* (305) may cause difficulty in obtaining a specific probe. However, a ^{32}P-labeled 20-kbp insert of cloned *M. genitalium* DNA yielded no or very weak hybridization signals in dot blots with nonhomologous DNAs, at concentrations 1,000-fold greater than the minimal concentration of homologous DNA giving a hybridization signal (113). This probe, therefore, seems to be specific for *M. genitalium*, detecting 100 pg of its DNA, but its potential needs to be tested on clinical samples. On the other hand, a nick-translated whole-genome DNA probe for *M. genitalium*, detecting as little as 50 to 100 pg of DNA per dot blot, has been used clinically (107). The stringency of hybridization was such that there was no cross-hybridization with *M. pneumoniae* DNA, and the probe gave positive results with 30% of urethral samples from homosexual men with NGU. Subsequently, the PCR has been developed by at least three groups of workers, each group amplifying different fragments of the attachment protein (MgPa) of *M. genitalium* (15, 121, 198). In each case, the *M. genitalium* DNA gave a characteristic PCR product which was not seen with DNA from any other source. As little as 10^{-15} g of *M. genitalium* DNA could be detected by one group (198), and it was found in the vagina of progesterone-treated mice inoculated with *M. genitalium* organisms at a time when they could not be cultured from this site but was not found in mice that were not colonized. In addition, the method has been used clinically. Thus, in Denmark (121), genital specimens from 3 of 26 men and 5 of 74 women that had been submitted for culture of *C. trachomatis* were PCR positive, as were about 20% of specimens taken from the lower genital tract of women attending a clinic for sexually transmitted diseases in England (197).

Clinical Aspects of Infection

As mentioned previously, *M. genitalium* was isolated originally from the urethra of 3 of 13 men with NGU (278, 287). Subsequently, attempts were made to isolate *M. genitalium* from the urethra and anal canal of other men with NGU (266). Urethral specimens from 5 of 18 heterosexual men produced acidity of SP-4 liquid medium after prolonged incubation at 37°C. These color changes were subcultured either once or twice but were not proven unequivocally to be due to *M. genitalium* and therefore can be regarded only as presumptive evidence for the presence of this mycoplasma. Nevertheless, the possibility exists that *M. genitalium* is present in the urethra of at least one-quarter of men with NGU. There is also similar presumptive evidence for the presence of *M. genitalium* in some swab specimens taken from the anal canal of men with NGU (266). This could happen merely as a result of contamination from the urogenital tract. On the other hand, the possibility exists that *M. genitalium* could reside primarily in the alimentary tract and secondarily in the urogenital tract. This view gains strength from the knowledge that *M. genitalium* has morphological features in common with those of *M. alvi* and *M. sualvi*, mycoplasmas which have been isolated from both the alimentary and genital tracts of cattle and pigs, respectively (96, 97).

The detection of *M. genitalium* in the lower genital tract of women has been mentioned above.

There have been no attempts to detect or isolate *M. genitalium* from the upper genital tract of women with salpingitis, but there are serological data (150, 182), some of which are compatible with *M. genitalium* causing the disease in a small proportion of patients. Thus, 31 women with acute PID, in whom serum antibodies to *C. trachomatis* and *M. hominis* could not be detected, were examined for antibodies to *M. genitalium* by a microimmunofluorescence technique; 40% of them had a fourfold or greater change in the titer of antibody during the 1 month after the onset of disease (182).

The association of *M. genitalium* with AIDS is covered in chapter 32.

Experimental Infections in Animals

Male and female animals have been inoculated urogenitally with *M. genitalium* (269). Mice and hamsters were susceptible only if treated with progesterone. Male rhesus monkeys (*Macaca mulatta*) were resistant, and male cynomolgus monkeys (*Macaca fascicularis*) were not as sensitive as male chimpanzees (*Pan troglodytes*); in one experiment, 9 of 11 of these animals developed an obvious genital tract infection, some shedding organisms for more than 18 weeks (289). *M. genitalium* was recovered from the blood of two of the monkeys when large numbers of organisms were in the urethra. Most of the chimpanzees colonized with the organisms had increased numbers of polymorphonuclear leukocytes in the genital tract and developed a fourfold or greater antibody response. Female squirrel monkeys (*Saimiri sciureus*) and female tamarins (*Saguinus mystax*) exhibited low-level genital tract infections following intravaginal inoculation, whereas marmosets (*Callithrix jacchus*) (267) and chimpanzees developed prolonged infections; thus, female chimpanzees shed organisms for 12 to 15 weeks (289). Marmosets and grivet monkeys (*Cercopithecus aethiops*) developed salpingitis with antibody responses after intraoviduct inoculation, and baboons (*Papio anubis*) developed parametritis after intracervical inoculation (269). The results provide unequivocal evidence that *M. genitalium* is pathogenic in the urogenital tract of subhuman primates and indicate that the microorganism could have a role in human genital tract disease.

The introduction of *M. genitalium* into the Syrian hamster lung by the intratracheal route has resulted in colonization and pneumonia (42). This is of interest in view of the recovery of *M. genitalium* from the human respiratory tract (9).

Pathogenesis

Adherence

The ability of *M. pneumoniae* to bind to erythrocytes is well known, and the same is true of *M. genitalium*, the adhesin (MgPa) appearing to be the counterpart of the P1 adhesin protein of *M. pneumoniae* (112, 185). Erythrocytes from chickens, guinea pigs, humans, rabbits, and sheep have been compared in order to monitor the extent of *M. genitalium* adherence, with guinea pig and sheep erythrocytes providing the most consistent results (10). Pretreatment of erythrocytes with neuraminidase reduced binding of *M. genitalium* by about 60%, whereas binding of *M. pneumoniae* was decreased by more than 80%. One group of investigators found that adsorption of erythrocytes (human type O) to *M. genitalium* colonies was abolished if the erythrocytes were treated with neuraminidase, and another group (10) found that the pattern of adsorption was influenced by the conditions under which the colonies developed. Binding of guinea pig erythrocytes to *M. pneumoniae* colonies occurred over the entire surface irrespective of whether the colonies developed aerobically or anaerobically. Binding to *M. genitalium* colonies grown anaerobically was greater than binding to those grown aerobically and most extensive if the colonies formed anaerobically in the presence of pyruvate, mannitol, and hemin.

M. genitalium has also been shown to adhere to Vero monkey kidney cells in vitro (288) and to the cilia, as well as the surface, of human fallopian tube epithelial cells (56), attachment being mediated via the terminal tip structure. Attachment to fallopian tube cells could be inhibited either by treating the organisms with trypsin, which removes the MgPa protein, or by preincubating them with a monoclonal antibody raised against the MgPa protein. Such observations indicate the important role of the MgPa protein in attachment of *M. genitalium* to human tissues and confirm that this protein is the counterpart of the P1 protein of *M. pneumoniae*. Whether *M. genitalium* uses long-chain sialo-oligosaccharides on host cells as receptors, as does *M. pneumoniae*, remains to be determined.

Hormones

The response of small laboratory animals to genital tract challenge with *M. genitalium* is different from that of the subhuman primates. Thus, treatment of female mice and hamsters with progesterone is a prerequisite for the successful establishment of genital tract colonization with *M. genitalium* (264), which can then be maintained for several weeks. Treatment with estradiol is ineffective. Whether the hormone stimulates receptors to which the organisms become attached as a means of facilitating colonization has yet to be determined.

Immune Response

Antigenic relationships

Although the results of serological tests, principally disk growth inhibition, showed that *M. genitalium* was distinct from all other known mycoplasmas (288), some antigenic cross-reactivity with *M. pneumoniae* soon became apparent. This was seen first in the complement fixation test (148) and later, to a lesser extent, in the metabolism inhibition test (268). Subsequently, an antigenic relationship with *M. pirum* was demonstrated (143), indicating that a serological technique which discriminates completely between infection by the flask-shaped mycoplasmas may be difficult to develop. Reasons for the cross-reactions have been sought by Western blot analysis of monoclonal antibodies generated against the mycoplasmas. Proteins of *M. genitalium* cross-reactive with *M. pneumoniae* have been identified (184). These include cytoplasmic antigens and a 140-kDa species-specific attachment protein (termed MgPa by one group [112]) which, while appearing to be immunodominant, functions similarly to the P1 protein (170 kDa) of *M. pneumoniae* (112) and shares cross-reactive epitopes with it (185).

Humoral

An antibody response has been detected in most of the animals inoculated with *M. genitalium* (269, 289), features being the rather late response of both males and females and the microimmunofluorescence test sometimes proving more sensitive than the metabolism inhibition test for detecting a response. Antibody in convalescent-phase sera from infected chimpanzees reacted strongly with the 140-kDa protein (184).

Antibody responses to *M. genitalium* were seen in 3 of 10 heterosexual men with NGU from whom a second serum sample was obtained 14 days after the first (266); in one other patient, a response was noted 9 months after the NGU and therefore was perhaps unrelated to the disease.

Previous mention has been made of the antibody response to *M. genitalium* in women with PID (182), with many of the responses occurring 1 month after hospital admission. Clearly, conventional collection of a convalescent-phase serum 2 weeks after the first may be too early to detect an antibody response, and thought should be given to obtaining widely spaced sera. This notion is reinforced by the finding (269, 289), mentioned above, of late antibody responses in some monkeys developing genital tract infections after inoculation with *M. genitalium*.

M. FERMENTANS

M. fermentans, first isolated from the urogenital tract (227a), has been regarded, as indicated before, as occurring infrequently at this site (245, 260). It is a known contaminant of cell cultures and in the 1970s was suggested, but never proven, to be a cause of rheumatoid arthritis (245). However, the tenuous association of *M. fermentans* with human disease needs to be reconsidered in the light of recent events.

Using immunohistochemical, DNA hybridization, and electron microscopic techniques, Lo and coworkers found a mycoplasma in AIDS patients as well as in non-AIDS patients dying of an acute disease (154–157). This agent was originally thought to be viral in nature (156), as judged by its initial detection following the supposed transfection of NIH 3T3 cells with Kaposi's sarcoma DNA taken from an individual with AIDS. However, subsequent hybridization analysis using probes specific for *E. coli* rRNA revealed the procaryotic nature of the agent. Its identity as a mycoplasma was implicated from hybridization studies using as probes DNA from representative mycoplasma species, and the agent was subsequently grown on a medium developed for the culture of fastidious mycoplasmas (290).

This mycoplasma was tentatively designated *M. incognitus* originally (155), but DNA hybridization revealed >90% relatedness to *M. fermentans*, and comparisons of restriction endonuclease digestion patterns of mycoplasma DNA, protein profiles by one-dimensional polyacrylamide gel electrophoresis, and susceptibilities to specific antisera, as measured by metabolism inhibition, suggest that *M. incognitus* is a strain of *M. fermentans* (230).

At the current time, there are more questions than answers regarding the *"incognitus"* strain of *M. fermentans* (13). From a biologic perspective, perhaps its most striking as well as controversial feature relates to its original isolation as a result of what was reported as transfection. The molecular events that would be necessary for the production and assembly of a mycoplasma, or any procaryote, following transfection of extracted DNA into eucaryotic cells are unprecedented. Furthermore, the possibility of an undetected contaminating mycoplasma in the NIH 3T3 cells remains difficult to dismiss. Nevertheless, the actual origin of the cultured mycoplasma agent does not seem to minimize the significance of observations regarding its association with human disease. What remains unclear, however, is whether this association is merely coincidental or reflects a primary or secondary role in pathogenesis. The latter conclusion of some primary or secondary role seems to be supported (i) by the observation by Lemaître et al. of antibiotic inhibition of cytopathology of human immunodeficiency virus-infected CEM cells (145), (ii) by the further detection of *M. fermentans* in the blood of human immunodeficiency virus-positive patients by use of the polymerase chain reaction (103a), and (iii) by a striking association of *M. fermentans* with AIDS-associated nephropathy (13a).

Clearly, these observations on *M. fermentans* and its association with AIDS have provided an exciting new twist to the realm of mycoplasmas, their molecular biology, and their interactions with humans. These experimental findings have opened the door to several intriguing new avenues of research. The subject of mycoplasmas and AIDS is considered in greater detail in chapter 32.

REFERENCES

1. **Abraham, J. M., C. S. Freitag, J. R. Clements, and B. I. Eisenstein.** 1985. An invertible element of DNA controls phase variation of type 1 fimbriae of *Escherichia coli*. *Proc. Natl. Acad. Sci. USA* **82:**5724–5727.
2. **Aldridge, K. E., B. C. Cole, and J. R. Ward.** 1977. *Mycoplasma*-dependent activation of normal lymphocytes: induction of a lymphocyte-mediated cytotoxicity for allogeneic and syngeneic mouse target cells. *Infect. Immun.* **18:**377–385.
3. **Bak, A. L., F. T. Black, C. Christiansen, and E. A. Freundt.** 1969. Genome size of mycoplasmal DNA. *Nature* (London) **224:**1209–1210.
4. **Baldetorp, B., P.-A. Mårdh, and L. Weström.** 1983. Studies on ciliated epithelia of the human genital tract. *Sex. Transm. Dis.* **10**(Suppl.)**:**363–365.
5. **Barile, M. F., M. W. Grabowski, P. J. Snoy, and D. K. F. Chandler.** 1987. Superiority of the chimpanzee animal model to study pathogenicity of known *Mycoplasma pneumoniae* and reputed mycoplasma pathogens. *Isr. J. Med. Sci.* **23:**556–560.
6. **Barile, M. F., P. J. Snoy, L. M. Miller, M. W. Grabowski, D. K. F. Chandler, A. Blanchard, T. M. Cunningham, L. D. Olson, and A. P. Guruswamy.** 1990. Mycoplasma-induced septic arthritis in chimpanzees, p. 389–393. *In* G. Stanek, G. H. Cassell, J. G. Tully, and R. F. Whitcomb (ed.), *Recent Advances in Mycoplasmology.* Gustav Fischer Verlag, Stuttgart.
7. **Barlev, N. A., and S. N. Borchsenius.** 1990. Gradual distribution of mycoplasma genome sizes. *IOM Lett.* **1:**238–239.
8. **Baseman, J. B., R. M. Cole, D. C. Krause, and D. K. Leith.** 1982. Molecular basis for cytadsorption of *Mycoplasma pneumoniae*. *J. Bacteriol.* **151:**1514–1522.
9. **Baseman, J. B., S. F. Dallo, J. G. Tully, and D. L. Rose.** 1988. Isolation and characterization of *Mycoplasma genitalium* strains from the human respiratory tract. *J. Clin. Microbiol.* **26:**2266–2269.
10. **Baseman, J. B., K. L. Daly, L. B. Trevino, and D. L. Drouillard.** 1984. Distinctions among pathogenic human mycoplasmas. *Isr. J. Med. Sci.* **20:**866–869.
11. **Baseman, J. B., D. L. Drouillard, D. K. Leith, and J. Morrison-Plummer.** 1985. Role of *Mycoplasma pneumoniae* adhesin P1 and accessory proteins in cytadsorption, p. 18–23. *In* S. E. Mergenhagen and B. Rosan (ed.), *Molecular Basis of Oral Microbial Adhesion.* American Society for Microbiology, Washington, D.C.
12. **Baseman, J. B., J. Morrison-Plummer, D. Drouillard, B. Puleo-Scheppke, V. V. Tryon, and S. C. Holt.** 1987. Identification of a 32-kilodalton protein of *Mycoplasma pneumoniae* associated with hemadsorption. *Isr. J. Med. Sci.* **23:**474–479.
13. **Baseman, J. B., and R. L. Quackenbush.** 1990. Preliminary assessment of AIDS-associated mycoplasma. *ASM News* **56:**319–323.
13a.**Bauer, F. A., D. J. Wear, P. Angritt, and S.-C. Lo.** 1991. *Mycoplasma fermentans* (incognitus strain) infection in the kidneys of patients with acquired immunodeficiency syndrome and associated nephropathy. *Hum. Pathol.* **22:**63–69.
14. **Bauminger, E. R., S. G. Cohen, F. Labenski DeKanter, A. Levy, S. Ofer, M. Kessel, and S. Rottem.** 1980. Iron storage in *Mycoplasma capricolum*. *J. Bacteriol.* **141:**378–381.
15. **Bernet, C., B. de Barbeyrac, A. Vekris, F. Bauduer, M. Garret, J. Bonnet, and C. Bébéar.** 1990. Detection of *M. pneumoniae* and *M. genitalium* by PCR. *IOM Lett.* **1:**153–154.
16. **Biberfeld, G.** 1968. Distribution of antibodies within 19S and 7S immunoglobulins following infection with *Mycoplasma pneumoniae*. *J. Immunol.* **100:**338–347.
17. **Biberfeld, G.** 1985. Infection sequelae and autoimmune reactions in *Mycoplasma pneumoniae* infection, p. 293–311. *In* S. Razin and M. F. Barile (ed.), *The Mycoplasmas*, vol. 1. Academic Press, Orlando, Fla.
18. **Biberfeld, G., and P. Biberfeld.** 1970. Ultrastructural features of *Mycoplasma pneumoniae*. *J. Bacteriol.* **102:**855–861.
19. **Biberfeld, G., and E. Gronowicz.** 1976. *Mycoplasma pneumoniae* is a polyclonal B-cell activator. *Nature* (London) **261:**238–239.
20. **Biberfeld, G., and G. Sterner.** 1971. Antibodies in bronchial secretions following natural infection with *Myco-*

plasma pneumoniae. Acta Pathol. Microbiol. Scand. **79:** 599–605.

21. **Black, F. T.** 1973. Modifications of the growth inhibition test and its application to human T-mycoplasmas. *Appl. Microbiol.* **25:**528–533.

22. **Black, F. T., A. Birch-Andersen, and E. A. Freundt.** 1972. Morphology and ultrastructure of human T mycoplasmas. *J. Bacteriol.* **111:**254–259.

23. **Blanchard, A.** 1990. Urease genes in *Ureaplasma urealyticum. IOM Lett.* **1:**82.

24. **Blanchard, A., and M. Gautier.** 1990. Detection of *Ureaplasma urealyticum* by using the polymerase chain reaction. *IOM Lett.* **1:**149.

25. **Boatman, E. S.** 1979. Morphology and ultrastructure of the Mycoplasmatales, p. 63–102. *In* M. F. Barile and S. Razin (ed.), *The Mycoplasmas,* vol. 1. Academic Press, New York.

26. **Bredt, W.** 1968. Growth morphology of *Mycoplasma pneumoniae* strain FH on glass surface. *Proc. Soc. Exp. Biol. Med.* **128:**338–340.

27. **Bredt, W.** 1970. Experimentelle Untersuchen über Morphologie und Vermehrung der beim menschen vorkommenden Mycoplasma unter besonderer Berücksichtigung von *Mycoplasma hominis. Z. Med. Mikrobiol. Immunol.* **155:**248–274.

28. **Bredt, W.** 1973. Motility of mycoplasma. *Ann. N.Y. Acad. Sci.* **225:**246–250.

29. **Bredt, W.** 1975. Phagocytosis by macrophages of *Mycoplasma pneumoniae* after opsonization by complement. *Infect. Immun.* **12:**694–695.

30. **Bredt, W.** 1979. Motility, p. 141–155. *In* M. F. Barile and S. Razin (ed.), *The Mycoplasmas,* vol 1. Academic Press, New York.

31. **Bredt, W., and D. Bitter-Suermann.** 1975. Interactions between *Mycoplasma pneumoniae* and guinea pig complement. *Infect. Immun.* **11:**497–504.

32. **Brown, M. B., G. H. Cassell, D. Taylor-Robinson, and M. C. Shepard.** 1983. Measurement of antibody to *Ureaplasma urealyticum* by an enzyme-linked assay and detection of antibody responses in patients with nongonococcal urethritis. *J. Clin. Microbiol.* **17:**288–295.

33. **Brown, M. B., F. C. Minion, J. K. Davis, D. G. Pritchard, and G. H. Cassell.** 1983. Antigens of *Mycoplasma hominis. Sex. Transm. Dis.* **10**(Suppl.):247–255.

34. **Brunner, H.** 1981. *Mycoplasma pneumoniae* infections. *Isr. J. Med. Sci.* **17:**516–523.

35. **Brunner, H., H. B. Greenberg, W. D. James, R. L. Horswood, R. B. Couch, and R. M. Chanock.** 1973. Antibody to *Mycoplasma pneumoniae* in nasal secretions and sputa of experimentally infected human volunteers. *Infect. Immun.* **8:**612–620.

36. **Brunner, H., H. Krauss, H. Schaar, and H.-G. Schiefer.** 1979. Electron microscopic studies on the attachment of *Mycoplasma pneumoniae* to guinea pig erythrocytes. *Infect. Immun.* **24:**906–911.

37. **Brunner, H., W. Weidner, and H.-G. Schiefer.** 1983. Quantitative studies on the role of *Ureaplasma urealyticum* in non-gonococcal urethritis and chronic prostatitis. *Yale J. Biol. Med.* **56:**545–550.

38. **Camner, P. C., C. Jarstrand, and K. Philipson.** 1978. Tracheobronchial clearance 5–15 months after infection with *Mycoplasma pneumoniae. Scand. J. Infect. Dis.* **10:** 33–35.

39. **Carson, J. L., A. M. Collier, and S.-C. S. Hu.** 1980. Ultrastructural observations on cellular and subcellular aspects of experimental *Mycoplasma pneumoniae* disease. *Infect. Immun.* **29:**1117–1124.

40. **Cassell, G. H., R. O. Davis, K. B. Waites, M. B. Brown, P. A. Marriott, S. Stagno, and J. K. Davis.** 1983. Isolation of *Mycoplasma hominis* and *Ureaplasma urealyticum* from amniotic fluid at 16–20 weeks of gestation: potential effect on outcome of pregnancy. *Sex. Transm. Dis.* **10**(Suppl.):294–302.

41. **Cassell, G. H., K. B. Waites, D. T. Crouse, P. T. Rudd, K. C. Canupp, S. Stagno, and G. R. Cutter.** 1988. Association of *Ureaplasma urealyticum* infection of the lower respiratory tract with chronic lung disease and death in very-low-birth-weight infants. *Lancet* **ii:**240–245.

42. **Chandler, D. K. F., M. W. Grabowski, H. Yoshida, R. Harasawa, S. Razin, and M. F. Barile.** 1990. Experimentally-induced *Mycoplasma pneumoniae* and *Mycoplasma genitalium* pneumonias in hamsters. *IOM Lett.* **1:** 156–157.

43. **Chandler, D. K. F., S. Razin, E. B. Stephens, R. Harasawa, and M. F. Barile.** 1982. Genomic and phenotypic analyses of *Mycoplasma pneumoniae* strains. *Infect. Immun.* **38:**604–609.

44. **Chanock, R. M., L. Dienes, M. D. Eaton, D. G. Edward, E. A. Freundt, L. Hayflick, J. F. P. Hers, K. E. Jensen, C. Liu, B. P. Marmion, H. E. Morton, M. A. Mufson, P. F. Smith, N. L. Somerson, and D. Taylor-Robinson.** 1963. *Mycoplasma pneumoniae:* proposed nomenclature for atypical pneumonia organism (Eaton agent). *Science* **140:**662.

45. **Chanock, R. M., L. Hayflick, and M. F. Barile.** 1962. Growth on artificial medium of an agent associated with atypical pneumonia and its identification as a PPLO. *Proc. Natl. Acad. Sci. USA* **48:**41–49.

46. **Chanock, R. M., D. Rifkind, H. M. Kravetz, V. Knight, and K. M. Johnson.** 1961. Respiratory disease in volunteers infected with Eaton agent; a preliminary report. *Proc. Natl. Acad. Sci. USA* **47:**887–890.

47. **Chen, Y.-Y., and D. C. Krause.** 1988. Parasitism of hamster trachea epithelial cells by *Mycoplasma pneumoniae. Infect. Immun.* **56:**570–576.

48. **Christiansen, C., G. Christiansen, and O. F. Rasmussen.** 1987. Heterogeneity of *Mycoplasma hominis* as detected by a probe for *atp* genes. *Isr. J. Med. Sci.* **23:**591–594.

49. **Christiansen, C., E. Hansen, and G. Christiansen.** 1983. The genetic relation between *Mycoplasma hominis* and other mycoplasma species. *Sex. Transm. Dis.* **10:** 230–231.

50. **Christiansen, G., S. Ladefoged, S. Hauge, S. Birkelund, and H. Andersen.** 1990. Use of monoclonal antibodies for detection of gene and antigen variation in *Mycoplasma hominis,* p. 535–545. *In* G. Stanek, G. H. Cassell, J. G. Tully, and R. F. Whitcomb (ed.), *Recent Advances in Mycoplasmology.* Gustav Fischer Verlag, Stuttgart.

51. **Christiansson, A., and P.-A. Mårdh.** 1983. Chemical composition and ultrastructure of *Mycoplasma hominis. Sex. Transm. Dis.* **10**(Suppl.):240–243.

52. **Clyde, W. A., Jr.** 1979. *Mycoplasma pneumoniae* infections of man, p. 275–306. *In* J. G. Tully and R. F. Whitcomb (ed.), *The Mycoplasmas,* vol. 2. Academic Press, New York.

53. **Clyde, W. A., Jr.** 1983. *Mycoplasma pneumoniae* respiratory disease symposium: summation and significance. *Yale J. Biol. Med.* **56:**523–521.

54. **Cohen, G., and N. L. Somerson.** 1967. *Mycoplasma pneumoniae:* hydrogen peroxide secretion and its possible role in virulence. *Ann. N.Y. Acad. Sci.* **143:**85–87.

55. **Collier, A. M., and J. B. Baseman.** 1973. Organ culture techniques with mycoplasmas. *Ann. N.Y. Acad. Sci.* **225:** 277–289.

56. **Collier, A. M., J. L. Carson, P. C. Hu, S. S. Hu, C. H. Huang, and M. F. Barile.** 1990. Attachment of *Mycoplasma genitalium* to the ciliated epithelium of human fallopian tubes, p. 730–732. *In* G. Stanek, G. H. Cassell, J. G. Tully, and R. F. Whitcomb (ed.), *Recent Advances in Mycoplasmology.* Gustav Fischer Verlag, Stuttgart.

57. **Collier, A. M., and W. A. Clyde, Jr.** 1971. Relationships between *Mycoplasma pneumoniae* and human respiratory epithelium. *Infect. Immun.* **3:**694–701.

58. **Collier, A. M., and W. A. Clyde, Jr.** 1974. Appearance of *Mycoplasma pneumoniae* in lungs of experimentally

infected hamsters and sputum from patients with natural disease. *Am. Rev. Respir. Dis.* **110:**765–773.

59. **Collier, A. M., W. A. Clyde, Jr., and F. W. Denny.** 1969. Biologic effects of *Mycoplasma pneumoniae* and other mycoplasmas from man on hamster tracheal organ culture. *Proc. Soc. Exp. Biol. Med.* **132:**1153–1158.

60. **Colman, S. D., P.-C. Hu, W. Litaker, and K. F. Bott.** 1990. A physical map of the *Mycoplasma genitalium* genome. *Mol. Microbiol.* **4:**683–687.

61. **Coufalik, E. D., D. Taylor-Robinson, and G. W. Csonka.** 1979. Treatment of non-gonococcal urethritis with rifampicin as a means of defining the role of *Ureaplasma urealyticum. Br. J. Vener. Dis.* **55:**36–43.

62. **Crouse, D. T., G. H. Cassell, and K. Waites.** 1990. Role of hyperoxia in ureaplasmal-induced respiratory disease in premature infants. *IOM Lett.* **1:**61–62.

63. **Dajani, A. S., W. A. Clyde, Jr., and F. W. Denny.** 1965. Experimental infection with *Mycoplasma pneumoniae* (Eaton's agent). *J. Exp. Med.* **121:**1071–1084.

63a.**Dallo, S. F., A. Charoya, and J. B. Baseman.** 1990. Characterization of the gene for a 30-kilodalton adhesin-related protein of *Mycoplasma pneumoniae. Infect. Immun.* **58:**4163–4165.

64. **Dallo, S. F., A. Chavoya, C-J. Su, and J. B. Baseman.** 1989. DNA and protein sequence homologies between the adhesins of *Mycoplasma genitalium* and *Mycoplasma pneumoniae. Infect. Immun.* **57:**1059–1065.

65. **Dallo, S. F., J. R. Horton, C. J. Su, and J. B. Baseman.** 1990. Restriction fragment length polymorphism in the cytadhesin P1 gene of human clinical isolates of *Mycoplasma pneumoniae. Infect. Immun.* **58:**2017–2020.

66. **Davis, J. W., D. Espinosa, K. Williams, V. Kissel, and F. C. Cabello.** 1990. *Ureaplasma* proteins react with a monoclonal antibody produced against an HLA-B27 antigen. *IOM Lett.* **1:**283.

67. **Davis, J. W., J. T. Manolukas, B. E. Capo, and J. D. Pollack.** 1990. Pyruvate metabolism and the absence of a tricarboxylic acid cycle in *Ureaplasma urealyticum*, p. 666–669. *In* G. Stanek, G. H. Cassell, J. G. Tully, and R. F. Whitcomb (ed.), *Recent Advances in Mycoplasmology.* Gustav Fischer Verlag, Stuttgart.

68. **Denny, F. W., W. A. Clyde, Jr., and W. P. Glezen.** 1971. *Mycoplasma pneumoniae* disease: clinical spectrum, pathophysiology, epidemiology, and control. *J. Infect. Dis.* **123:**74–94.

69. **de Silva, N. S., and P. A. Quinn.** 1986. Phospholipase A and C activity in *Ureaplasma urealyticum. Pediatr. Infect. Dis.* **5:**350.

70. **Dienes, L., and G. Edsall.** 1937. Observations on the L-organism of Klieneberger. *Proc. Soc. Exp. Biol. Med.* **36:**740–744.

71. **Doble, A., B. J. Thomas, P. M. Furr, M. M. Walker, J. R. W. Harris, R. O. Witherow, and D. Taylor-Robinson.** 1989. A search for infectious agents in chronic abacterial prostatitis using ultrasound guided biopsy. *Br. J. Urol.* **64:**297–301.

72. **Eaton, M. D., G. Meiklejohn, and W. van Herick.** 1944. Studies on the etiology of primary atypical pneumonia. A filterable agent transmissible to cotton rats, hamsters, and chicken embryos. *J. Exp. Med.* **79:**649–668.

73. **Edward, D. G.** 1947. A selective medium for pleuropneumonia-like organisms. *J. Gen. Microbiol.* **1:**238–243.

74. **Edward, D. G.** 1955. A suggested classification and nomenclature for organisms of the pleuropneumonia group. *Int. Bull. Bacteriol. Nomencl. Taxon.* **5:**85–93.

75. **Edward, D. G., and E. A. Freundt.** 1965. A note on the taxonomic status of strains like 'Campo', hitherto classified as *Mycoplasma hominis*, type 2. *J. Gen. Microbiol.* **41:**263–265.

76. **Eschenbach, D. A.** 1986. *Ureaplasma urealyticum* as a cause of postpartum fever. *Pediatr. Infect. Dis.* **5**(Suppl.):258–261.

77. **Feldner, J., and W. Bredt.** 1983. Analysis of polypeptides of mutants of *Mycoplasma pneumoniae* that lack the ability to hemadsorb. *J. Gen. Microbiol.* **129:**841–848.

78. **Feldner, J., U. Göbel, and W. Bredt.** 1982. *Mycoplasma pneumoniae* adhesin localized to tip structure by monoclonal antibody. *Nature* (London) **298:**765–767.

79. **Fenske, J. D., and G. E. Kenny.** 1976. Role of arginine deiminase in growth of *Mycoplasma hominis. J. Bacteriol.* **126:**501–510.

80. **Fernald, G. W.** 1979. Humoral and cellular immune responses to mycoplasmas, p. 399–423. *In* J. G. Tully and R. F. Whitcomb (ed.), *The Mycoplasmas*, vol. 2. Academic Press, Orlando, Fla.

81. **Finlay, B. B., and S. Falkow.** 1989. Common themes in microbial pathogenicity. *Microbiol. Rev.* **53:**210–230.

82. **Ford, D. K.** 1986. Synovial lymphocyte responses show that ureaplasmas cause sexually transmitted reactive arthritis. *Pediatr. Infect. Dis.* **5**(Suppl.):353.

83. **Foulon, W., L. De Catte, M. De Waele and A. Naessens.** 1990. Early placental abruption associated with *Ureaplasma urealyticum* infections, p. 734–735. *In* G. Stanek, G. H. Cassell, J. G. Tully, and R. F. Whitcomb (ed.), *Recent Advances in Mycoplasmology.* Gustav Fischer Verlag, Stuttgart.

83a.**Foy, H. M., J. T. Grayston, G. E. Kenny, E. R. Alexander, and R. McMahan.** 1966. Epidemiology of *Mycoplasma pneumoniae* infection in families. *J. Am. Med. Assoc.* **197:**859–866.

84. **Foy, H. M., G. E. Kenny, M. K. Cooney, and I. D. Allan.** 1979. Long-term epidemiology of infections with *Mycoplasma pneumoniae. J. Infect. Dis.* **139:**681–687.

85. **Freundt, E. A.** 1955. The classification of the pleuropneumonia group of organisms (Borrelomycetales). *Int. Bull. Bacteriol. Nomencl. Taxon.* **5:**67–78.

86. **Freundt, E. A., and S. Razin.** 1984. Mycoplasma, p. 742–770. *In* N. R. Krieg and J. G. Holt (ed.), *Bergey's Manual of Systematic Bacteriology*, vol. 1. Williams & Wilkins, Baltimore.

87. **Furness, G.** 1973. T-mycoplasmas. Factors affecting their growth, colonial morphology, and assay on agar. *J. Infect. Dis.* **128:**703–709.

88. **Furr, P. M., C. M. Hetherington, and D. Taylor-Robinson.** 1989. The susceptibility of germ-free, oestradiol-treated, mice to *Mycoplasma hominis. J. Med. Microbiol.* **30:**233–236.

89. **Furr, P. M., and D. Taylor-Robinson.** 1989. The establishment and persistence of *Ureaplasma urealyticum* in oestradiol-treated female mice. *J. Med. Microbiol.* **29:**111–114.

90. **Furr, P. M., and D. Taylor-Robinson.** 1989. Oestradiol-induced infection of the genital tract of female mice by *Mycoplasma hominis. J. Gen. Microbiol.* **135:**2743–2749.

91. **Gabridge, M. G., M. J. Bright, and H. R. Richards.** 1982. Scanning electron microscopy of *Mycoplasma pneumoniae* on the membrane of individual ciliated tracheal cells. *In Vitro* **18:**55–62.

92. **Gabridge, M. G., C. K. Johnson, and A. M. Cameron.** 1974. Cytotoxicity of *Mycoplasma pneumoniae* membranes. *Infect. Immun.* **10:**1127–1134.

93. **Gallagher, J. R.** 1941. Acute pneumonitis: a report of 87 cases among adolescents. *Yale J. Biol. Med.* **13:**663–678.

94. **Gilula, N. B., and P. Satir.** 1972. The ciliary necklace: a ciliary membrane specialization. *J. Cell Biol.* **53:**494–509.

95. **Göbel, U., V. Speth, and W. Bredt.** 1981. Filamentous structures in adherent *Mycoplasma pneumoniae* cells treated with nonionic detergents. *J. Cell Biol.* **91:**537–543.

96. **Gourlay, R. N., S. G. Wyld, and R. H. Leach.** 1977. *Mycoplasma alvi*, a new species from bovine intestinal and urogenital tracts. *Int. J. Syst. Bacteriol.* **27:**86–96.

97. **Gourlay, R. N., S. G. Wyld, and R. H. Leach.** 1978. *Mycoplasma sualvi*, a new species from the intestinal and urogenital tracts of pigs. *Int. J. Syst. Bacteriol.* **28:**289–292.

98. **Grenabo, L., H. Hedelin, and S. Pettersson.** 1988. Urinary infection stones caused by *Ureaplasma urealyticum*: a review. *Scand. J. Infect. Dis.* **53**(Suppl.):46–49.

99. **Guruswamy, A. P., D. F. Welch, K. E. Corff, and L. Guruswamy.** 1990. Genital mycoplasmas in the cerebrospinal fluid of infants with suspected sepsis—a survey. *IOM Lett.* **1**:414–415.

100. **Guruswamy, A., D. F. Welch, and V. Spaan.** 1990. Bacteriuria in patients with urinary tract stones: role of ureaplasma, p. 739–741. *In* G. Stanek, G. H. Cassell, J. G. Tully, and R. F. Whitcomb (ed.), *Recent Advances in Mycoplasmology.* Gustav Fischer Verlag, Stuttgart.

101. **Hansen, E. J., R. M. Wilson, and J. B. Baseman.** 1979. Isolation of mutants of *Mycoplasma pneumoniae* defective in hemadsorption. *Infect. Immun.* **23**:903–906.

102. **Hansen, E. J., R. M. Wilson, and J. B. Baseman.** 1979. Two-dimensional gel electrophoretic comparison of proteins from virulent and avirulent strains of *Mycoplasma pneumoniae. Infect. Immun.* **24**:468–475.

103. **Hansen, E. J., R. M. Wilson, W. A. Clyde, Jr., and J. B. Baseman.** 1981. Characterization of hemadsorption-negative mutants of *Mycoplasma pneumoniae. Infect. Immun.* **32**:127–136.

103a. **Hawkins, R. E., L. S. Rickman, S. H. Vermund, and M. Carl.** 1992. Association of mycoplasma and human immunodeficiency virus infection: detection of amplified *Mycoplasma fermentans* DNA in blood. *J. Infect. Dis.* **165**:581–585.

104. **Hayatsu, E.** 1978. Acquired immunity to *Mycoplasma pneumoniae* in hamsters. *Microbiol. Immunol.* **22**:181–195.

105. **Helms, C. M.** 1985. Differential diagnosis, p. 85–92. *In Mycoplasmas as Agents of Human Disease.* Windermere Communications, Inc., Waukegan, Ill.

106. **Hollingdale, M. R., and R. M. Lemcke.** 1972. Membrane antigens of *Mycoplasma hominis. J. Hyg.* **70**:85–98.

107. **Hooton, T. M., M. C. Roberts, P. L. Roberts, K. K. Holmes, W. E. Stamm, and G. E. Kenny.** 1988. Prevalence of *Mycoplasma genitalium* determined by DNA probe in men with urethritis. *Lancet* **i**:266–268.

108. **Horowitz, S. A., L. Duffy, B. Garrett, J. Stephens, J. K. Davis, and G. H. Cassell.** 1986. Can group- and serovar-specific proteins be detected in *Ureaplasma urealyticum? Pediatr. Infect. Dis.* **5**:325–331.

109. **Hu, P.-C., R. M. Cole, Y. S. Huang, J. A. Graham, D. E. Gardner, A. M. Collier, and W. A. Clyde, Jr.** 1982. *Mycoplasma pneumoniae* infection: role of a surface protein in the attachment organelle. *Science* **216**:313–315.

110. **Hu, P.-C., A. M. Collier, and J. B. Baseman.** 1977. Surface parasitism by *Mycoplasma pneumoniae* of respiratory epithelium. *J. Exp. Med.* **145**:1328–1343.

111. **Hu, P.-C., C. H. Huang, A. M. Collier, and W. A. Clyde, Jr.** 1983. Demonstration of antibodies to *Mycoplasma pneumoniae* attachment protein in human sera and respiratory secretions. *Infect. Immun.* **41**:437–439.

112. **Hu, P.-C., U. Schaper, A. M. Collier, W. A. Clyde, Jr., M. Horikawa, Y.-S. Huang, and M. F. Barile.** 1987. A *Mycoplasma genitalium* protein resembling the *Mycoplasma pneumoniae* attachment protein. *Infect. Immun.* **55**:1126–1131.

113. **Hyman, H. C., D. Yogev, and S. Razin.** 1987. DNA probes for detection and identification of *Mycoplasma pneumoniae* and *Mycoplasma genitalium. J. Clin. Microbiol.* **25**:726–728.

114. **Inamine, J. M., T. P. Denny, S. Loechel, U. Schaper, C.-H. Huang, K. F. Bott, and P.-C. Hu.** 1988. Nucleotide sequence of the P1 attachment-protein gene of *Mycoplasma pneumoniae. Gene* **64**:217–229.

115. **Inamine, J. M., K.-C. Ho, S. Loechel, and P.-C. Hu.** 1990. Evidence that UGA is read as a tryptophan codon rather than as a stop codon by *Mycoplasma pneumoniae, Mycoplasma genitalium,* and *Mycoplasma gallisepticum. J. Bacteriol.* **172**:504–506.

116. **Inamine, J. M., S. Loechel, A. M. Collier, M. F. Barile, and P.-C. Hu.** 1989. Nucleotide sequence of the *MgPa* (*mgp*) operon of *Mycoplasma genitalium* and comparison to the *P1* (*mpp*) operon of *Mycoplasma pneumoniae. Gene* **82**:259–267.

117. **Inamine, J. M., S. Loechel, and P.-C. Hu.** 1988. Analysis of the nucleotide sequence of the *P1* operon of *Mycoplasma pneumoniae. Gene* **73**:175–183.

118. **Izumikawa, K., D. K. F. Chandler, M. W. Grabowski, and M. F. Barile.** 1987. Attachment of *Mycoplasma hominis* to human cell cultures. *Isr. J. Med. Sci.* **23**:603–607.

119. **Jacobs, E., R. Röck, and L. Dalehite.** 1990. A B cell-, T cell-linked epitope located on the adhesin of *Mycoplasma pneumoniae. Infect. Immun.* **58**:2464–2469.

120. **Jalil, N., A. Doble, C. Gilchrist, and D. Taylor-Robinson.** 1988. Infection of the epididymis by *Ureaplasma urealyticum. Genitourin. Med.* **64**:367–368.

121. **Jensen, J. S., J. S. Andersen, S. A. Uldum, and K. Lind.** 1990. Polymerase chain reaction for the detection of *Mycoplasma pneumoniae* and *Mycoplasma genitalium. IOM Lett.* **1**:386–387.

122. **Johnson, J. D., and J. Horowitz.** 1971. Characterization of ribosomes and RNAs from *Mycoplasma hominis. Biochim. Biophys. Acta* **247**:262–279.

123. **Johnston, C. L. W., A. D. B. Webster, D. Taylor-Robinson, G. Rapaport, and G. R. V. Hughes.** 1983. Primary late-onset hypogammaglobulinemia associated with inflammatory polyarthritis and septic arthritis due to *Mycoplasma pneumoniae. Ann. Rheum. Dis.* **42**:108–110.

124. **Kahane, I., S. Razin, and A. Muhlrad.** 1978. Possible role of acetate kinase in ATP generation in *Mycoplasma hominis* and *Acholeplasma laidlawii. FEMS Microbiol. Lett.* **3**:143–145.

125. **Kahane, I., S. Tucker, D. K. Leith, J. Morrison-Plummer, and J. B. Baseman.** 1985. Detection of the major adhesin P1 in triton shells of virulent *Mycoplasma pneumoniae. Infect. Immun.* **50**:944–946.

126. **Kammer, G. M., J. D. Pollack, and A. S. Klainer.** 1970. Scanning-beam electron microscopy of *Mycoplasma pneumoniae. J. Bacteriol.* **104**:499–502.

127. **Kass, E. H., J.-S. Lin, and W. M. McCormack.** 1986. Low birth weight and maternal colonization with genital mycoplasmas. *Pediatr. Infect. Dis.* **5**(Suppl.):279–281.

128. **Kirchhoff, H., R. Rosengarten, W. Lotz, M. Fischer, and D. Lopatta.** 1984. Flask-shaped mycoplasmas: properties and pathogenicity for man and animals. *Isr. J. Med. Sci.* **20**:848–853.

129. **Kleven, S. H., G. F. Browning, D. M. Bulach, E. Ghiocas, C. J. Morrow, and K. G. Whithear.** 1988. Examination of *Mycoplasma gallisepticum* strains using restriction endonuclease DNA analysis and DNA-hybridization. *Avian Pathol.* **17**:559–570.

130. **Kohara, Y., K. Akiyama, and K. Isono.** 1987. The physical map of the whole *E. coli* chromosome: application of a new strategy for rapid analysis and sorting of a large genomic library. *Cell* **50**:495–508.

131. **Kok, T.-W., G. Varkanis, B. P. Marmion, J. Martin, and A. Esterman.** 1988. Laboratory diagnosis of *Mycoplasma pneumoniae* infection. 1. Direct detection of antigen in respiratory exudates by enzyme immunoassay. *Epidemiol. Infect.* **101**:669–684.

131a. **Krause, D. C., and K. K. Lee.** 1991. Juxtaposition of the genes encoding *Mycoplasma pneumoniae* cytadherence accessory proteins HMW1 and HMW3. *Gene* **107**:83–89.

132. **Krause, D. C., and J. B. Baseman.** 1983. Inhibition of *Mycoplasma pneumoniae* hemadsorption and adherence to respiratory epithelium by antibodies to a membrane protein. *Infect. Immun.* **39**:1180–1186.

133. **Krause, D. C., D. K. Leith, and J. B. Baseman.** 1983. Reacquisition of specific proteins confers virulence in *Mycoplasma pneumoniae. Infect. Immun.* **39**:830–836.

134. **Krause, D. C., D. K. Leith, D. K. Wilson, and J. B. Baseman.** 1982. Identification of *Mycoplasma pneumoniae*

proteins associated with hemadsorption and virulence. *Infect. Immun.* **35**:809–817.

135. **Krause, D. C., and C. B. Mawn.** 1990. Physical analysis and mapping of the *Mycoplasma pneumoniae* chromosome. *J. Bacteriol.* **172**:4790–4797.

136. **Krieger, J. N., and G. E. Kenny.** 1986. Evidence for pathogenicity of *Ureaplasma urealyticum* for the upper urinary tract derived from animal models. *Pediatr. Infect. Dis.* **5**(Suppl.):319–321.

137. **Krivan, H. C., L. D. Olson, M. F. Barile, V. Ginsburg, and D. D. Roberts.** 1989. Adhesion of *Mycoplasma pneumoniae* to sulfated glycolipids and inhibition by dextran sulfate. *J. Biol. Chem.* **264**:9283–9288.

138. **Kumagai, K., T. Iwabuchi, Y. Hinuma, K. Yuri, and N. Ishida.** 1971. Incidence, species, and significance of *Mycoplasma* species in the mouth. *J. Infect. Dis.* **123**:16–21.

139. **Kundsin, R. B., and L. Cohn.** 1990. *Mycoplasma hominis*: isolation from a heart valve, p. 743–744. *In* G. Stanek, G. H. Cassell, J. G. Tully, and R. F. Whitcomb (ed.), *Recent Advances in Mycoplasmology.* Gustav Fischer Verlag, Stuttgart.

140. **Kundsin, R. B., and J. Praznik.** 1967. Pharyngeal carriage of mycoplasma species in healthy young adults. *J. Epidemiol.* **86**:579–583.

141. **Ladefoged, S., B. Brock, and G. Christiansen.** 1990. Physical and genetic maps of the genome of five strains of *Mycoplasma hominis. IOM Lett.* **1**:253–254.

142. **Lamont, R. F., D. Taylor-Robinson, J. S. Wigglesworth, P. M. Furr, R. T. Evans, and M. G. Elder.** 1987. The role of mycoplasmas, ureaplasmas and chlamydiae in the genital tract of women presenting in spontaneous early preterm labour. *J. Med. Microbiol.* **24**:253–257.

143. **Leach, R. H., A. Hales, P. M. Furr, D. L. Mitchelmore, and D. Taylor-Robinson.** 1987. Problems in the identification of *Mycoplasma pirum* isolated from human lymphoblastoid cell cultures. *FEMS Microbiol. Lett.* **44**:293–297.

144. **Leith, D. K., L. B. Trevino, J. G. Tully, and J. B. Baseman.** 1983. Host discrimination of *Mycoplasma pneumoniae* proteinaceous immunogens. *J. Exp. Med.* **157**:502–514.

145. **Lemaître, M., D. Guétard, Y. Hénin, L. Montagnier, and A. Zerial.** 1990. Protective activity of tetracycline analogs against the cytopathic effect of human immunodeficiency virus in CEM cells. *Res. Virol.* **141**:5–16.

146. **Lemcke, R. M.** 1964. The serological differentiation of *Mycoplasma* strains (pleuropneumonia-like organisms) from various sources. *J. Hyg.* **62**:199–219.

147. **Lin, J.-S.** 1980. An antigenic analysis for membranes of *Mycoplasma hominis* by cross-absorption. *J. Gen. Microbiol.* **116**:187–193.

148. **Lind, K.** 1982. Serological cross-reactions between "*Mycoplasma genitalium*" and *M. pneumoniae. Lancet* **ii**:1158–1159.

149. **Lind, K., and M. W. Bentzon.** 1988. Changes in the epidemiological pattern of *Mycoplasma pneumoniae* infections in Denmark. *Epidemiol. Infect.* **101**:377–386.

150. **Lind, K., and G. B. Kristensen.** 1987. Significance of antibodies to *Mycoplasma genitalium* in salpingitis. *Eur. J. Clin. Microbiol.* **6**:205–207.

151. **Lind, K., G. B. Kristensen, A. C. Bollerup, P. Ladehoff, S. Larsen, A. Marushak, P. Rasmussen, J. Rolschau, I. Skoven, T. Sørensen, and I. Lind.** 1985. Importance of *Mycoplasma hominis* in acute salpingitis assessed by culture and serological tests. *Genitourin. Med.* **61**:185–189.

152. **Lingwood, C. A., and P. A. Quinn.** 1990. Common sulfogalactolipid receptor for mycoplasmas associated with infertility. *IOM Lett.* **1**:108–109.

153. **Lipman, R. P., and W. A. Clyde, Jr.** 1969. The interrelationship of virulence, cytadsorption, and peroxide formation in *Mycoplasma pneumoniae. Proc. Soc. Exp. Biol. Med.* **131**:1163–1167.

154. **Lo, S.-C., M. S. Dawson, P. B. Newton III, M. A. Sonoda, J. W.-K. Shih, W. F. Engler, R. Y.-H. Wang, and D. J. Wear.** 1989. Association of the virus-like infectious agent originally reported in patients with AIDS with acute fatal disease in previously healthy non-AIDS patients. *Am. J. Trop. Med. Hyg.* **41**:364–376.

155. **Lo, S.-C., J. W.-K. Shih, P. B. Newton III, D. M. Wong, M. M. Hayes, J. R. Benish, D. J. Wear, and R. Y.-H. Wang.** 1989. Virus-like infectious agent (VLIA) is a novel pathogenic mycoplasma: *Mycoplasma incognitus. Am. J. Trop. Med. Hyg.* **41**:586–600.

156. **Lo, S.-C., J. W.-K. Shih, N.-Y. Yang, C.-Y. Ou, and R. Y.-H. Wang.** 1989. A novel virus-like infectious agent in patients with AIDS. *Am. J. Trop. Med. Hyg.* **40**:213–226.

157. **Lo, S.-C., R. Y.-H. Wang, P. B. Newton III, N.-Y. Yang, M. A. Sonoda, and J. W.-K. Shih.** 1989. Fatal infection of silver leaf monkeys with a virus-like infectious agent (VLIA) derived from a patient with AIDS. *Am. J. Trop. Med. Hyg.* **40**:399–409.

158. **Loechel, S., J. M. Inamine, and P.-C. Hu.** 1989. Nucleotide sequence of the *deo*C gene of *Mycoplasma pneumoniae. Nucleic Acids Res.* **17**:581.

159. **Lyell, A., A. M. Gordon, H. M. Dick, and R. G. Sommerville.** 1967. Mycoplasmas and erythema multiforme. *Lancet* **i**:1116–1118.

160. **Lynch, R. E., and B. C. Cole.** 1980. *Mycoplasma pneumoniae*: a pathogen which manufactures superoxide but lacks superoxide dismutase. *Proc. Fed. Eur. Biochem. Soc. Symp.* **62**:49–56.

161. **Madoff, S., and D. C. Hooper.** 1990. Nongenitourinary tract infections in adults caused by *Mycoplasma hominis*: a review, p. 373–378. *In* G. Stanek, G. H. Cassell, J. G. Tully, and R. F. Whitcomb (ed.), *Recent Advances in Mycoplasmology.* Gustav Fischer Verlag, Stuttgart.

162. **Manchee, R. J., and D. Taylor-Robinson.** 1969. Studies on the nature of receptors involved in attachment of tissue culture cells to mycoplasmas. *Br. J. Exp. Pathol.* **50**:66–75.

163. **Manchee, R. J., and D. Taylor-Robinson.** 1969. Enhanced growth of T-strain mycoplasmas with *N*-2-hydroxyethylpiperazine-*N'*-2-ethanesulfonic acid buffer. *J. Bacteriol.* **100**:78–85.

164. **Mansel, J. K., E. C. Rosenow III, T. F. Smith, and J. W. Martin, Jr.** 1989. *Mycoplasma pneumoniae* pneumonia. *Chest* **95**:639–646.

165. **Mårdh, P.-A.** 1970. Increased serum levels of IgM in acute salpingitis related to the occurrence of *Mycoplasma hominis. Acta Pathol. Microbiol. Scand. Sect. B* **78**:726–732.

166. **Mårdh, P.-A., and E. Holst.** 1990. Should *Mycoplasma hominis* be regarded as a STD agent or a bacterial vaginosis-associated organism?—elaboration of an hypothesis and presentation of study data, p. 234–238. *In* G. Stanek, G. H. Cassell, J. G. Tully, and R. F. Whitcomb (ed.), *Recent Advances in Mycoplasmology.* Gustav Fischer Verlag, Stuttgart.

167. **Mårdh, P.-A., and L. Weström.** 1970. Tubal and cervical cultures in acute salpingitis with special reference to *Mycoplasma hominis* and T-strain mycoplasmas. *Br. J. Vener. Dis.* **46**:179–186.

168. **Mårdh, P.-A., and L. Weström.** 1970. Antibodies to *Mycoplasma hominis* in patients with genital infections and in healthy controls. *Br. J. Vener. Dis.* **46**:390–397.

169. **Marmion, B. P., and G. M. Goodburn.** 1961. Effect of an inorganic gold salt on Eaton's primary atypical pneumonia agent and other observations. *Nature* (London) **189**:247–248.

170. **Mathiesen, S. L., S. Birkelund, and G. Christiansen.** 1990. Analysis of membrane proteins in *Mycoplasma hominis. IOM Lett.* **1**:288–289.

171. **Mazzali, R., and D. Taylor-Robinson.** 1971. The behav-

iour of T-mycoplasmas in tissue culture. *J. Med. Microbiol.* **4:**125–138.

172. **McCormack, W. M., B. Rosner, Y.-H. Lee, A. Munoz, D. Charles, and E. H. Kass.** 1987. Effect on birth weight of erythromycin treatment of pregnant women. *Obstet. Gynecol.* **69:**202–207.

173. **McGarrity, G. J., and H. Kotani.** 1986. *Ureaplasma*-eukaryotic cell interactions *in vitro. Pediatr. Infect. Dis.* **5:** 316–318.

174. **Meng, K. E., and R. M. Pfister.** 1980. Intracellular structures of *Mycoplasma pneumoniae* revealed after membrane removal. *J. Bacteriol.* **144:**390–399.

175. **Meseguer, M., M. M. Ferrer, P. Caballero, R. Núñez, C. Redondo, V. M. Arrieta, and L. Rafael.** 1990. Changes in semen parameters by incubation with *Ureaplasma urealyticum* strains, p. 745–749. *In* G. Stanek, G. H. Cassell, J. G. Tully, and R. F. Whitcomb (ed.), *Recent Advances in Mycoplasmology.* Gustav Fischer Verlag, Stuttgart.

176. **Mickelsen, P. A., E. Blackman, and P. F. Sparling.** 1982. Ability of *Neisseria gonorrhoeae, Neisseria meningitidis,* and commensal *Neisseria* species to obtain iron from lactoferrin. *Infect. Immun.* **35:**915–920.

177. **Miettinen, A., J. Paavonen, E. Jansson, and P. Leinikki.** 1983. Enzyme immunoassay for serum antibody to *Mycoplasma hominis* in women with acute pelvic inflammatory disease. *Sex. Transm. Dis.* **10**(Suppl.):289–293.

178. **Mizutani, H., H. Mizutani, T. Kitayama, A. Hayakawa, E. Nagayama, J. Kato, K. Nakamura, E. Tamura, and T. Izuchi.** 1971. Delayed hypersensitivity in *Mycoplasma pneumoniae* infections. *Lancet* **i:**186–187.

179. **Møller, B. R., F. T. Black, and E. A. Freundt.** 1981. Attempts to produce gynaecological disease in grivet monkeys with *Ureaplasma urealyticum. J. Med. Microbiol.* **14:** 475–478.

180. **Møller, B. R., and E. A. Freundt.** 1978. Experimental infection of the genital tract of female grivet monkeys by *Mycoplasma hominis. Zentralbl. Bakteriol. Parasitenkd. Infektionskr. Hyg. Abt. 1 Orig. Reihe A* **241:**218.

181. **Møller, B. R., and E. A. Freundt.** 1983. Monkey animal model for study of mycoplasmal infections of the urogenital tract. *Sex. Transm. Dis.* **10**(Suppl.):359–362.

182. **Møller, B. R., D. Taylor-Robinson, and P. M. Furr.** 1984. Serological evidence implicating *Mycoplasma genitalium* in pelvic inflammatory disease. *Lancet* **i:** 1102–1103.

183. **Møller, B. R., D. Taylor-Robinson, P. M. Furr, B. Toft, and J. Allen.** 1985. Serological evidence that chlamydiae and mycoplasmas are involved in infertility of women. *J. Reprod. Fertil.* **73:**237–240.

183a.**Morowitz, H. J.** 1984. The completeness of molecular biology. *Isr. J. Med. Sci.* **20:**750–753.

184. **Morrison-Plummer, J., D. H. Jones, K. Daly, J. G. Tully, D. Taylor-Robinson, and J. B. Baseman.** 1987. Molecular characterization of *Mycoplasma genitalium* species-specific and cross-reactive determinants: identification of an immunodominant protein of *M. genitalium. Isr. J. Med. Sci.* **23:**453–457.

185. **Morrison-Plummer, J., A. Lazzell, and J. B. Baseman.** 1987. Shared epitopes between *Mycoplasma pneumoniae* major adhesin protein P1 and a 140-kilodalton protein of *Mycoplasma genitalium. Infect. Immun.* **55:** 49–56.

186. **Mufson, M. A., W. M. Ludwig, R. H. Purcell, T. R. Cate, D. Taylor-Robinson, and R. M. Chanock.** 1965. Exudative pharyngitis following experimental *Mycoplasma hominis* type 1 infection. *JAMA* **192:**1146–1152.

187. **Murphy, G. L., and J. G. Cannon.** 1988. Genetics of surface protein variation in *Neisseria gonorrhoeae. BioEssays* **9:**7–11.

188. **Murray, H. W., H. Masur, L. B. Senterfit, and R. B. Roberts.** 1975. The protean manifestations of *Myco-*

plasma pneumoniae infections in adults. *Am. J. Med.* **58:** 229–242.

189. **Naessens, A., L. Hens, G. Dierickx, S. Lauwers, and I. Liebaers.** 1990. Influence of infection with *Ureaplasma urealyticum* on the chromosomal aberration rate of human lymphocytes. *IOM Lett.* **1:**334–335.

190. **Naftalin, J. M., G. Wellish, Z. Kanana, and D. Diengott.** 1974. *Mycoplasma pneumoniae* septicemia. *JAMA* **228:** 565.

191. **Neimark, H. C.** 1977. Extraction of an actin-like protein from the prokaryote *Mycoplasma pneumoniae. Proc. Natl. Acad. Sci. USA* **74:**4041–4045.

192. **Niitu, Y.** 1983. *M. pneumoniae* respiratory diseases: clinical features—children. *Yale J. Biol. Med.* **56:** 493–503.

193. **Oatman, E. S.** 1979. Morphology and ultrastructure of the Mycoplasmatales, p. 63–102. *In* M. F. Barile and S. Razin (ed.), *The Mycoplasmas,* vol. 1. Academic Press, New York.

194. **Ogle, K. F., K. K. Lee, and D. C. Krause.** 1991. Cloning and analysis of the gene encoding the cytadherence phase-variable protein HMW3 from *Mycoplasma pneumoniae. Gene* **97:**69–75.

194a.**Ogle, K. F., K. K. Lee, and D. C. Krause.** 1992. Nucleotide sequence analysis reveals novel features of the phase-variable cytadherence accessory protein HMW3 of *Mycoplasma pneumoniae. Infect. Immun.* **60:** 1633–1641.

195. **Olson, L., S. Shane, C. Renshaw, and M. Barile.** 1990. Antigenic variability of surface proteins of *M. hominis. IOM Lett.* **1:**106–107.

196. **Paavonen, J., A. Miettinen, C. E. Stevens, K. C. S. Chen, and K. K. Holmes.** 1983. *Mycoplasma hominis* in nonspecific vaginitis. *Sex. Transm. Dis.* **10**(Suppl.):271–275.

197. **Palmer, H. M., C. B. Gilroy, E. J. Claydon, and D. Taylor-Robinson.** 1991. Detection of *Mycoplasma genitalium* in the genitourinary tract of women by the polymerase chain reaction. *Int. J. STD AIDS* **2:**261–263.

198. **Palmer, H. M., C. B. Gilroy, P. M. Furr, and D. Taylor-Robinson.** 1991. Development and evaluation of the polymerase chain reaction to detect *Mycoplasma genitalium. FEMS Microbiol. Lett.* **77:**199–204.

199. **Peterson, K. M., and J. F. Alderete.** 1984. Iron uptake and increased intracellular enzyme activity follow host lactoferrin binding by *Trichomonas vaginalis* receptors. *J. Exp. Med.* **160:**398–410.

200. **Pheifer, T. A., P. S. Forsyth, M. A. Durfee, H. M. Pollock, and K. K. Holmes.** 1978. Non-specific vaginitis: role of *Haemophilus vaginalis* and treatment with metronidazole. *N. Engl. J. Med.* **298:**1429–1434.

201. **Pidcock, K. A., J. A. Wooten, B. A. Daley, and T. L. Stull.** 1988. Iron acquisition by *Haemophilus influenzae. Infect. Immun.* **56:**721–725.

202. **Pollack, J. D.** 1979. Respiratory pathways and energy-yielding mechanisms, p. 187–211. *In* M. F. Barile and S. Razin (ed.), *The Mycoplasmas,* vol. 1. Academic Press, Orlando, Fla.

203. **Pollack, J. D.** 1986. Metabolic distinctiveness of ureaplasmas. *Pediatr. Infect. Dis.* **5**(Suppl):305–307.

204. **Pollack, J. D., A. J. Merola, M. Platz, and R. L. Booth.** 1981. Respiration associated components of *Mollicutes. J. Bacteriol.* **146:**907–913.

205. **Powell, D. A., and W. A. Clyde, Jr.** 1975. Opsonin-reversible resistance of *Mycoplasma pneumoniae* to in vito phagocytosis by alveolar macrophages. *Infect. Immun.* **11:**540–550.

206. **Pratt, B.** 1990. Automated blood culture systems: detection of *Mycoplasma hominis* in SPS-containing media, p. 778–781. *In* G. Stanek, G. H. Cassell, J. G. Tully, and R. F. Whitcomb (ed.), *Recent Advances in Mycoplasmology.* Gustav Fischer Verlag, Stuttgart.

207. **Purcell, R. H., D. Taylor-Robinson, D. Wong, and R. M.**

Chanock. 1966. Color test for the measurement of antibody to T-strain mycoplasmas. *J. Bacteriol.* **92:**6–12.

208. **Quinn, P. A.** 1986. Evidence of an immune response to *Ureaplasma urealyticum* in perinatal morbidity and mortality. *Pediatr. Infect. Dis.* **5**(Suppl.):282–287.

209. **Quinn, P. A.** 1990. Clinical trial of erythromycin in ureaplasma positive women for the prevention of spontaneous abortion and stillbirth. *IOM Lett.* **1:**444–445.

210. **Quinn, P. A., J. E. Gillan, T. Markestad, M. A. St. John, A. Daneman, K. I. Lie, H. C. Li, E. Czegledy-Nagy, and A. Klein.** 1985. Intrauterine infection with *Ureaplasma urealyticum* as a cause of fatal neonatal pneumonia. *Pediatr. Infect. Dis.* **4:**538–543.

211. **Quinn, P. A., A. B. Shewchuk, J. Shuber, K. I. Lie, E. Ryan, M. Sheu, and M. L. Chipman.** 1983. Serologic evidence of *Ureaplasma urealyticum* infection in women with spontaneous pregnancy loss. *Am. J. Obstet. Gynecol.* **145:**245–250.

212. **Quinn, P. A., I. Stewart, S. J. Landis, and J. Butany.** 1990. Aortic ring abscess associated with *Mycoplasma hominis* following prosthetic valve insertion, p. 712–714. *In* G. Stanek, G. H. Cassell, J. G. Tully, and R. F. Whitcomb (ed.), *Recent Advances in Mycoplasmology.* Gustav Fischer Verlag, Stuttgart.

213. **Radestock, U., and W. Bredt.** 1977. Motility of *Mycoplasma pneumoniae. J. Bacteriol.* **129:**1495–1501.

214. **Razin, S., B. Prescott, G. Caldes, W. D. James, and R. M. Chanock.** 1970. Role of glycolipids and phosphatidylglycerol in the serological activity of *Mycoplasma pneumoniae. Infect. Immun.* **1:**408–416.

215. **Reimann, H. A.** 1938. An acute infection of the respiratory tract with atypical pneumonia. *JAMA* **111:**2377–2384.

216. **Roberts, D. D., L. D. Olson, M. F. Barile, V. Ginsburg, and H. C. Krivans.** 1989. Sialic acid-dependent adhesion of *Mycoplasma pneumoniae* to purified glycoproteins. *J. Biol. Chem.* **264:**9289–9293.

217. **Roberts, M. C., M. Hooton, W. Stamm, K. K. Holmes, and G. E. Kenny.** 1987. DNA probes for the detection of mycoplasmas in genital specimens. *Isr. J. Med. Sci.* **23:**618–620.

218. **Robertson, J. A.** 1978. Bromothymol blue broth: improved medium for detection of *Ureaplasma urealyticum* (T-strain *Mycoplasma*). *J. Clin. Microbiol.* **7:**127–132.

219. **Robertson, J. A.** 1986. Potential virulence factors of *Ureaplasma urealyticum. Pediatr. Infect. Dis.* **5**(Suppl.):322–324.

220. **Robertson, J. A., M. Alfa, and E. S. Boatman.** 1983. Morphology of the cells and colonies of *Mycoplasma hominis. Sex. Transm. Dis.* **10:**232–239.

221. **Robertson, J., M. Gomersall, and P. Gill.** 1975. *Mycoplasma hominis*: growth, reproduction, and isolation of small viable cells. *J. Bacteriol.* **124:**1007–1018.

222. **Robertson, J. A., L. Pyle, J. Kakulphimp, G. W. Stemke, and L. R. Finch.** 1990. The genomes of the genus *Ureaplasma. IOM Lett.* **1:**72–73.

223. **Robertson, J. A., and R. Sherburne.** 1990. The phenomenon of haemadsorption by colonies of *Ureaplasma urealyticum. IOM Lett.* **1:**336.

224. **Robertson, J., and E. Smook.** 1976. Cytochemical evidence of extramembranous carbohydrates on *Ureaplasma urealyticum* (T-strain mycoplasma). *J. Bacteriol.* **128:**658–660.

225. **Rodwell, A. W., E. S. Rodwell, and D. B. Archer.** 1979. Mycoplasmas lack a protein which closely resembles α-actin. *FEMS Microbiol. Lett.* **5:**235–238.

226. **Romano, N., R. La Licata, and D. R. Alesi.** 1986. Energy production in *Ureaplasma urealyticum. Pediatr. Infect. Dis.* **5**(Suppl.):308–312.

227. **Rottem, S., and S. Razin.** 1973. Membrane lipids of *Mycoplasma hominis. J. Bacteriol.* **113:**565–571.

227a.**Ruiter, M., and H. M. M. Wentholt.** 1952. The occurrence of a pleuropneumonia-like organism in fuso-spirillary infections of the human genital mucosa. *J. Invest. Dermatol.* **18:**313–325.

228. **Saada, A.-B., V. Deutsch, and I. Kahane.** 1990. The urease of *Ureaplasma urealyticum.* Purification and study with a monoclonal antibody, p. 678–680. *In* G. Stanek, G. H. Cassell, J. G. Tully, and R. F. Whitcomb (ed.), *Recent Advances in Mycoplasmology.* Gustav Fischer Verlag, Stuttgart.

229. **Saada, A., Y. Terespolsky, Y. Beyth, and I. Kahane.** 1990. Adherence of *Ureaplasma urealyticum* (U.u.) to human erythrocytes (RBC) and bovine fallopian tube mucosa cell culture (FTMCC). *IOM Lett.* **1:**339–340.

230. **Saillard, C., P. Carle, J. M. Bové, C. Bébéar. S.-C. Lo, J. W.-K. Shih, R. Y.-H. Wang, D. L. Rose, and J. G. Tully.** 1990. Genetic and serologic relatedness between *Mycoplasma fermentans* strains and a mycoplasma recently identified in tissues of AIDS and non-AIDS patients. *Res. Virol.* **141:**385–396.

231. **Schiefer, H. G., and W. Weidner.** 1990. Urethral syndrome in women: aetiologic and cytologic studies, p. 756–757. *In* G. Stanek, G. H. Cassell, J. G. Tully, and R. F. Whitcomb (ed.), *Recent Advances in Mycoplasmology.* Gustav Fischer Verlag, Stuttgart.

232. **Sethi, K. K.** 1985. *Mycoplasma hominis* und entzündliche Erkrankungen des Beckens. In-vitro-Stimulation der Leukozyten bei Exposition gegen *M. hominis. Muench. Med. Wochenschr.* **117:**1045–1046.

233. **Shaw, N. J., B. C. Pratt, and A. M. Weindling.** 1989. Ureaplasma and mycoplasma infections of the central nervous system in preterm infants. *Lancet* **ii:**1530–1531.

234. **Shepard, M. C.** 1954. The recovery of pleuropneumonia-like organisms from negro men with and without nongonococcal urethritis. *Am. J. Syph. Gonorrhea Vener. Dis.* **38:**113–124.

235. **Shepard, M. C.** 1966. Human mycoplasma infections. *Health Lab. Sci.* **3:**163–169.

236. **Shepard, M. C.** 1983. Culture media for ureaplasmas, p. 137–146. *In* S. Razin and J. G. Tully (ed.), *Methods in Mycoplasmology,* vol. 1. Academic Press, New York.

237. **Shepard, M. C.** 1986. *Ureaplasma urealyticum:* history and progress. *Pediatr. Infect. Dis.* **5**(Suppl.):223–231.

238. **Shepard, M. C., C. D. Lunceford, D. K. Ford, R. H. Purcell, D. Taylor-Robinson, S. Razin, and F. T. Black.** 1974. *Ureaplasma urealyticum* gen. nov., sp. nov: proposed nomenclature for the human T (T-strain) mycoplasma. *Int. J. Syst. Bacteriol.* **24:**160–171.

239. **Shepard, M. C., and G. K. Masover.** 1979. Special features of ureaplasmas, p. 451–494. *In* M. F. Barile and S. Razin (ed.), *The Mycoplasmas,* vol. 1. Academic Press, New York.

240. **Simoneau, P., R. Wenzel, R. Herrmann, and P.-C. Hu.** 1990. Nucleotide sequence of a tRNA cluster from *Mycoplasma pneumoniae. Nucleic Acids Res.* **18:**2814.

241. **Slack, P. M., and D. Taylor-Robinson.** 1973. The influence of mycoplasmas on the cytopathic effect of varicella virus. *Arch. Virusforsch.* **42:**88–95.

242. **Smith, C. B., W. T. Friedewald, and R. M. Chanock.** 1967. Shedding of *Mycoplasma pneumoniae* after tetracycline and erythromycin therapy. *N. Engl. J. Med.* **276:**1172–1175.

243. **Smith, C. L., J. G. Econome, A. Schutt, S. Klco, and C. R. Cantor.** 1987. A physical map of the *Escherichia coli* K12 genome. *Science* **236:**1448–1453.

244. **Smith, P. F.** 1986. Mass cultivation of ureaplasmas and some applications. *Pediatr. Infect. Dis.* **5**(Suppl.):313–315.

245. **Somerson, N. L., and B. C. Cole.** 1979. The mycoplasma flora of human and nonhuman primates, p. 191–216. *In* J. G. Tully and R. F. Whitcomb (ed.), *The Mycoplasmas,* vol. 2. Academic Press, New York.

246. **Somerson, N. L., W. D. James, B. E. Walls, and R. M. Chanock.** 1967. Growth of *Mycoplasma pneumoniae* on a glass surface. *Ann. N.Y. Acad. Sci.* **143:**384–389.

247. **Somerson, N. L., D. Taylor-Robinson, and R. M. Chanock.** 1963. Hemolysin production as an aid in the identification and quantification of Eaton agent (*Mycoplasma pneumoniae*). *Am. J. Hyg.* **77:**122–128.

248. **Somerson, N. L., B. E. Walls, and R. M. Chanock.** 1965. Hemolysin of *Mycoplasma pneumoniae*: tentative identification as a peroxide. *Science* **150:**226–228.

249. **Stalheim, O. H. V., S. J. Proctor, and J. E. Gallagher.** 1976. Growth and effects of ureaplasmas (T mycoplasmas) in bovine oviductal organ cultures. *Infect. Immun.* **13:**915–925.

250. **Stamm, W. E., K. Running, J. Hale, and K. K. Holmes.** 1983. Etiologic role of *Mycoplasma hominis* and *Ureaplasma urealyticum* in women with the acute urethral syndrome. *Sex. Transm. Dis.* **10**(Suppl.):318–322.

251. **Steffensen, D. O., J. S. Dummar, M. S. Granick, A. W. Pasculle, B. P. Griffith, and G. H. Cassell.** 1987. Sternotomy infections with *Mycoplasma hominis*. *Ann. Intern. Med.* **106:**204–208.

252. **Steinberg, P., R. L. Horswood, and R. M. Chanock.** 1969. Temperature sensitive mutants of *Mycoplasma pneumoniae*. I. In vitro biologic properties. *J. Infect. Dis.* **120:**217–224.

253. **Stevens, M. K., and D. C. Krause.** 1990. Disulfide-linked protein associated with *Mycoplasma pneumoniae* cytadherence phase variation. *Infect. Immun.* **58:**3430–3433.

254. **Stevens, M. K., and D. C. Krause.** 1991. Localization of the *Mycoplasma pneumoniae* cytadherence-accessory proteins HMW1/4 in the cytoskeleton-like triton shell. *J. Bacteriol.* **173:**1041–1050.

254a.**Stevens, M. K., and D. C. Krause.** 1992. Cytadherence-accessory protein HMW3 of *Mycoplasma pneumoniae* is a component of the attachment organelle. *J. Bacteriol.* **174:**4265–4274.

255. **Su, C. J., A. Chavoya, and J. B. Baseman.** 1989. Spontaneous mutation results in loss of the cytadhesin (P1) of *Mycoplasma pneumoniae*. *Infect. Immun.* **57:**3237–3239.

256. **Su, C. J., V. V. Tryon, and J. B. Baseman.** 1987. Cloning and sequencing analysis of cytadhesin P1 gene from *Mycoplasma pneumoniae*. *Infect. Immun.* **55:**3023–3029.

257. **Swenson, C. E., J. P. Banks, and J. Schachter.** 1983. Organ culture studies with *Mycoplasma hominis*. *Sex. Transm. Dis.* **10**(Suppl.):355–358.

258. **Taylor, G., D. Taylor-Robinson, and G. W. Fernald.** 1974. Reduction in the severity of *Mycoplasma pneumoniae*-induced pneumonia in hamsters by immunosuppressive treatment with anti-thymocyte sera. *J. Med. Microbiol.* **7:**343–348.

259. **Taylor-Robinson, D.** 1986. Evaluation of the role of *Ureaplasma urealyticum* in infertility. *Pediatr. Infect. Dis.* **5**(Suppl.):262–265.

260. **Taylor-Robinson, D.** 1989. Genital mycoplasma infections, p. 501–523. *In* F. N. Judson (ed.), *Clinics in Laboratory Medicine*, vol. 9. *Sexually Transmitted Diseases.* The W. B. Saunders Co., Philadelphia.

261. **Taylor-Robinson, D.** 1990. The Mycoplasmatales: *Mycoplasma, Ureaplasma, Acholeplasma, Spiroplasma* and *Anaeroplasma*, p. 664–681. *In* M. T. Parker and B. I. Duerden (ed.), *Topley and Wilson's Principles of Bacteriology, Virology and Immunity. Systematic Bacteriology*, 8th ed., vol. 2. Edward Arnold, London.

261a.**Taylor-Robinson, D.** Unpublished data.

262. **Taylor-Robinson, D., and W. Bredt.** 1983. Motility of mycoplasma strain G37. *Yale J. Biol. Med.* **56:**910.

263. **Taylor-Robinson, D., G. W. Csonka, and M. J. Prentice.** 1977. Human intra-urethral inoculation of ureaplasmas. *Q. J. Med.* **46:**309–326.

264. **Taylor-Robinson, D., and P. M. Furr.** 1990. Hormones influence genital mycoplasma infections. *IOM Lett.* **1:**63.

265. **Taylor-Robinson, D., and P. M. Furr.** 1990. Elimination of mycoplasmas from the murine genital tract by hormone treatment. *Epidemiol. Infect.* **105:**163–168.

266. **Taylor-Robinson, D., P. M. Furr, and N. F. Hanna.** 1985. Microbiological and serological study of non-gonococcal urethritis with special reference to *Mycoplasma genitalium*. *Genitourin. Med.* **61:**319–324.

267. **Taylor-Robinson, D., P. M. Furr, and C. M. Hetherington.** 1982. The pathogenicity of a newly discovered human mycoplasma (strain G37) for the genital tract of marmosets. *J. Hyg.* **89:**449–455.

268. **Taylor-Robinson, D., P. M. Furr, and J. G. Tully.** 1983. Serological cross reactions between *Mycoplasma genitalium* and *M. pneumoniae*. *Lancet* **i:**527.

269. **Taylor-Robinson, D., P. M. Furr, J. G. Tully, M. F. Barile, and B. R. Møller.** 1987. Animal models of *Mycoplasma genitalium* urogenital infection. *Isr. J. Med. Sci.* **23:**561–564.

270. **Taylor-Robinson, D., P. M. Furr, and A. D. B. Webster.** 1986. *Ureaplasma urealyticum* in the immunocompromised host. *Pediatr. Infect. Dis.* **5**(Suppl.):236–238.

271. **Taylor-Robinson, D., and R. N. Gourlay.** 1984. The Mycoplasmas. Genus II. Ureaplasma, p. 770–775. *In* N. R. Krieg and J. G. Holt (ed.), *Bergey's Manual of Systematic Bacteriology*, vol. 1. Williams & Wilkins, Baltimore.

272. **Taylor-Robinson, D., J. M. Gumpel, A. Hill, and A. J. Swannell.** 1978. Isolation of *Mycoplasma pneumoniae* from synovial fluid of a hypogammaglobulinemic patient in a survey of patients with inflammatory polyarthritis. *Ann. Rheum. Dis.* **37:**180–182.

273. **Taylor-Robinson, D., D. A. Haig, and M. H. Williams.** 1967. Bovine T-strain mycoplasma. *Ann. N.Y. Acad. Sci.* **143:**517–518.

274. **Taylor-Robinson, D., and R. J. Manchee.** 1967. Adherence of mycoplasma to glass and plastic. *J. Bacteriol.* **94:**1781–1782.

275. **Taylor-Robinson, D., and P. E. Munday.** 1988. Mycoplasmal infection of the female genital tract and its complications, p. 228–247. *In* M. J. Hare (ed.), *Genital Tract Infection in Women.* Churchill Livingstone, Edinburgh.

276. **Taylor-Robinson, D., R. H. Purcell, W. T. London, and D. L. Sly.** 1978. Urethral infection of chimpanzees by *Ureaplasma urealyticum*. *J. Med. Microbiol.* **11:**197–202.

277. **Taylor-Robinson, D., B. J. Thomas, P. M. Furr, and A. C. Keat.** 1983. The association of *Mycoplasma hominis* with arthritis. *Sex. Transm. Dis.* **10:**191–198.

278. **Taylor-Robinson, D., J. G. Tully, P. M. Furr, R. M. Cole, D. L. Rose, and N. F. Hanna.** 1981. Urogenital mycoplasma infections of man: a review with observations on a recently discovered mycoplasma. *Isr. J. Med. Sci.* **17:**524–530.

279. **Texier-Maugein, J., M. Clerc, A. Vekris, and C. Bébéar.** 1987. *Ureaplasma urealyticum*-induced bladder stones in rats and their prevention by flurofamide and doxycycline. *Isr. J. Med. Sci.* **23:**565–567.

280. **Thirkell, D., A. D. Myles, B. L. Precious, J. S. Frost, J. C. Woodall, M. G. Burdon, and W. C. Russell.** 1989. The urease of *Ureaplasma urealyticum*. *J. Gen. Microbiol.* **135:**315–323.

281. **Thirkell, D., A. D. Myles, and W. C. Russell.** 1989. Serotype 8- and serocluster-specific surface-expressed antigens of *Ureaplasma urealyticum*. *Infect. Immun.* **57:**1697–1701.

282. **Thirkell, D., A. D. Myles, and D. Taylor-Robinson.** 1990. A comparison of four major antigens in five human and several animal strains of ureaplasmas. *J. Med. Microbiol.* **32:**163–168.

283. **Thomsen, A. C.** 1978. Occurrence of mycoplasmas in urinary tracts of patients with acute pyelonephritis. *J. Clin. Microbiol.* **8:**84–88.

284. **Thomsen, A. C.** 1978. Mycoplasmas in human pyelonephritis: demonstration of antibodies in serum and urine. *J. Clin. Microbiol.* **8:**197–202.

285. **Tryon, V., and J. B. Baseman.** 1987. The acquisition of human lactoferrin by *Mycoplasma pneumoniae*. *Microb. Pathog.* **3**:1–7.

286. **Tully, J. G., and D. Taylor-Robinson.** 1986. Taxonomy and host distribution of the ureaplasmas. *Pediatr. Infect. Dis.* **5**(Suppl.):292–295.

287. **Tully, J. G., D. Taylor-Robinson, R. M. Cole, and D. L. Rose.** 1981. A newly discovered mycoplasma in the human urogenital tract. *Lancet* **i**:1288–1291.

288. **Tully, J. G., D. Taylor-Robinson, D. L. Rose, R. M. Cole, and J. M. Bové.** 1983. *Mycoplasma genitalium*, a new species from the human urogenital tract. *Int. J. Syst. Bacteriol.* **33**:387–396.

289. **Tully, J. G., D. Taylor-Robinson, D. L. Rose, P. M. Furr, C. E. Graham, and M. F. Barile.** 1986. Urogenital challenge of primate species with *Mycoplasma genitalium* and characteristics of infection induced in chimpanzees. *J. Infect. Dis.* **153**:1046–1054.

290. **Tully, J. G., D. Taylor-Robinson, D. L. Rose, P. M. Furr, and D. A. Hawkins.** 1983. Evaluation of culture media for the recovery of *Mycoplasma hominis* from the human urogenital tract. *Sex. Transm. Dis.* **10**:256–260.

291. **Unsworth, P. F., D. Taylor-Robinson, E. E. Shoo, and P. M. Furr.** 1985. Neonatal mycoplasmaemia: *Mycoplasma hominis* as a significant cause of disease? *J. Infect.* **10**:163–168.

292. **Vinther, O.** 1983. Biochemistry of *Mycoplasma hominis*. *Sex. Transm. Dis.* **10**(Suppl.):244–246.

293. **Waites, K. B., N. R. Cox, D. T. Crouse, J. C. McIntosh, and G. H. Cassell.** 1990. Mycoplasma infections of the central nervous system in humans and animals, p. 379–386. *In* G. Stanek, G. H. Cassell, J. G. Tully, and R. F. Whitcomb (ed.), *Recent Advances in Mycoplasmology.* Gustav Fischer Verlag, Stuttgart.

294. **Waites, K. B., P. T. Rudd, D. T. Crouse, K. C. Canupp, K. G. Nelson, C. Ramsey, and G. H. Cassell.** 1988. Chronic *Ureaplasma urealyticum* and *Mycoplasma hominis* infections of central nervous system in preterm infants. *Lancet* **ii**:17–21.

295. **Waites, K. B., P. T. Rudd, C. T. Smedberg, L. B. Duffy, and G. H. Cassell.** 1986. A model of *Ureaplasma urealyticum* pneumonia in the newborn mouse. *Pediatr. Infect. Dis.* **5**(Suppl.):351–352.

296. **Wall, F., R. M. Pfister, and N. L. Somerson.** 1983. Freeze-fracture confirmation of the presence of a core in the specialized tip structure of *Mycoplasma pneumoniae.* *J. Bacteriol.* **154**:924–929.

297. **Webster, A. D. B., P. M. Furr, N. C. Hughes-Jones, B. D. Gorick, and D. Taylor-Robinson.** 1988. Critical dependence on antibody for defense against mycoplasmas. *Clin. Exp. Immunol.* **71**:383–387.

298. **Weiss, A. A., and S. Falkow.** 1984. Genetic analysis of phase change in *Bordetella pertussis. Infect. Immun.* **43**:263–269.

299. **Wenzel, R., and R. Herrmann.** 1988. Physical mapping of the *Mycoplasma pneumoniae* genome. *Nucleic Acids Res.* **16**:8323–8336.

300. **Wenzel, R., and R. Herrmann.** 1989. Cloning of the complete *Mycoplasma pneumoniae* genome. *Nucleic Acids Res.* **17**:7029–7043.

301. **Whitescarver, J., F. Castillo, and G. Furness.** 1975. The preparation of membranes of some human T-mycoplasmas and the analysis of their carbohydrate content. *Proc. Soc. Exp. Biol. Med.* **150**:20–22.

302. **Willoughby, J. J., M. G. Burdon, D. Thirkell, D. Taylor-Robinson, and W. C. Russell.** 1990. Use of a pair of PCR primers to detect *Ureaplasma* species in diagnostic situations. *IOM Lett.* **1**:467.

303. **Wilson, M. H., and A. M. Collier.** 1976. Ultrastructural study of *Mycoplasma pneumoniae* in organ culture. *J. Bacteriol.* **125**:332–339.

304. **Yogev, D., S. Levisohn, S. H. Kleven, D. Halachmi, and S. Razin.** 1988. Ribosomal RNA gene probes to detect intraspecies heterogeneity in *Mycoplasma gallisepticum* and *Mycoplasma synoviae. Avian Dis.* **32**:220–231.

305. **Yogev, D., and S. Razin.** 1986. Common deoxyribonucleic acid sequences in *Mycoplasma genitalium* and *Mycoplasma pneumoniae* genomes. *Int. J. Syst. Bacteriol.* **36**:426–430.

26. Mycoplasmas and Tissue Culture Cells

GERARD J. McGARRITY, HITOSHI KOTANI, and GARY H. BUTLER

INTRODUCTION

In any review of mycoplasmal pathogenesis, it is appropriate to cover the natural habitat of the organisms under consideration. The question of "natural habitat" poses a dilemma in any discussion of cell culture mycoplasmas, for mycoplasmas are not supposed to reside in cell cultures, and investigators who utilize cell cultures wish they never did. However, the paper by Robinson and colleagues in 1956 on the first reported incidence of unintentional mycoplasmal infection (MI) of cell cultures changed that (53). Since then, literally hundreds of papers have documented cell culture infection by various mycoplasmal species as well as mycoplasmal effects on virtually every cell culture parameter. Along with perplexing cell and molecular biologists, biochemists, and others who work with cell culture systems, these publications have yielded interesting and often valuable information on mycoplasmal physiology and pathogenesis as well as interactions with their cell culture hosts.

In vivo, mycoplasmas have an affinity for plasma cell membranes, and this preference is often observed in vitro (Fig. 1). According to Phillips, there is a space of approximately 40 Å between the procaryotic mycoplasma plasma membrane and the membrane of its eucaryotic host (48). It should not be surprising that in those species that exhibit strong cytoadsorption, e.g., *Mycoplasma hyorhinis*, significant cytopathology, including membrane damage, can occur. This close association between parasite and host plasma membranes is unusual; it is not seen in bacterial (except for L-form bacterial), viral, or rickettsial infections.

Mycoplasmas have low genomic molecular weights, which places obvious restrictions on the number of gene products elaborated. Mycoplasmas in cell cultures utilize medium components or cell culture products for their own metabolism, particularly nucleic acid and cholesterol metabolism. In mycoplasma-infected cell cultures, significant alterations in host nucleic acid metabolism and chromosomal aberrations are often observed.

General Considerations

Most of the early reports on MI of cell cultures described effects on fibroblast cells. While these reports were of interest in the description of cell culture artifacts, their value in understanding mycoplasmal pathogenesis was limited. Typically, mycoplasmas were associated with nonfibroblast cells in vivo, lymphocytes, and especially epithelial cells. With the development of additional differentiated cell culture systems, more reports appeared on the interactions of mycoplasmas and various types of lymphoblastoid cells. Other mycoplasma-infected cell culture models have also been used. In recent years, many reports have been published on effects of MI of cell cultures. Effects on many parameters, ranging from mycoplasmal enzymes (9) to effects of MI on reverse transcriptase (RT) (65) and to reduced immunoreactivity of varicella-zoster viral proteins by *M. hyorhinis* but not *M. orale*, have been published (17). The most significant work has been on the effects of MI on lymphoblastoid cells, mycoplasmal transformation of mammalian cells, and the emergence of *M. fermentans* as a major isolate from cell cultures as well as a possible cofactor in the pathogenesis of AIDS. These areas will receive major treatment in this review.

Characteristics of mycoplasma-infected cells

There are more mycoplasmas than cultured cells in an infected culture (39)! Typically, 10^7 to 10^8 myco-

Gerard J. McGarrity and Hitoshi Kotani • Genetic Therapy, Inc., 19 Firstfield Road, Gaithersburg, Maryland 20878.
Gary H. Butler • Coriell Institute for Medical Research, Camden, New Jersey 08103.

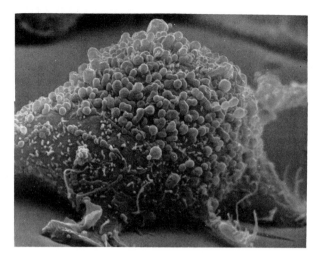

Figure 1. Scanning electron micrograph of mouse RAG cells infected with *M. hyorhinis* (magnification, ×2,000). (Courtesy of D. M. Phillips, Population Council, New York, N.Y.)

plasma CFU per ml of supernatant of medium is observed in an infected culture. In a confluent monolayer culture in a 25-cm^2 flask, the total yield of cultured cells is on the order of 1×10^6 to 5×10^6. With a minimum of 5.0 ml of medium, at least 5×10^7 mycoplasmas are present in the supernatant medium. Additional organisms are adsorbed onto the cultured cells.

Table 1 lists some characteristics of mycoplasma-infected cells. The presence of such large numbers of organisms and the significant alterations that they produce in the culture medium and, most significantly, in the host cells render infected cells wholly unacceptable in any research or diagnostic procedure.

EFFECTS OF MYCOPLASMAS ON CULTURED CELLS

How do mycoplasmas exert their effects on cell cultures? At least two mechanisms are possible. First, mycoplasmas can produce metabolic products that directly interact with their cell culture hosts. Second, they can deplete the cell culture medium of an essential component. The lack of this component can be detrimental to the host. The available data clearly suggest that the second possibility is by far the more likely.

Table 1. Characteristics of mycoplasma-infected cell cultures

Characteristic	Value
Mycoplasma cells/ml of supernatant medium	10^7–10^8
Approx. no. of mycoplasma gene products	550[a]–1,100[b]
Mycoplasma DNA/host cell DNA	About 25%
Mycoplasma protein/host cell protein	About 25%
Effects on cell culture	Unpredictable

[a] For *Mycoplasma* species.
[b] For *Acholeplasma* species.

In 1978, Barile et al. reported that 17 different mycoplasma species had been isolated from cell cultures (1). That list did not include *M. pirum*, first isolated from cell cultures by Del Giudice et al. (10). However, assay of more than 35,000 cell cultures in our laboratory indicates that five species, *M. hyorhinis*, *M. orale*, *M. arginini*, *M. fermentans*, and *Acholeplasma laidlawii*, account for more than 95% of the isolates (unpublished data).

Reviews on the effects that mycoplasmas exert on their cell culture hosts have been published elsewhere (7, 39, 40). This chapter presents an update of more recently published data, especially on differentiated cell cultures, with emphasis on lymphoblastoid cells and their modulation via various cytokines.

Interaction with Lymphoblastoid Cells in Culture

A broad variety of mycoplasmas have been shown to be mitogenic for mammalian lymphocytes. Cole et al. have reviewed the mycoplasma species and host lymphocytes (7). Mycoplasmas that have been shown to be mitogenic include *M. pneumoniae*, *M. fermentans*, *M. hominis*, *A. laidlawii*, *M. pulmonis*, *M. arthritidis*, *M. neurolyticum*, *M. hyorhinis*, *M. synoviae*, *M. felis*, *M. gallisepticum*, *M. canis*, *M. hyosynoviae*, *M. arginini*, *M. orale*, and *Spiroplasma citri*. Host species have included human, mouse, rat, and guinea pig. At least some studies have demonstrated that the mitogenesis did not reflect an anamnestic response, since lymphocytes from axenic animals, in studies using *M. pulmonis* and *M. arthritidis*, also responded, as did individuals with no demonstrable humoral antibody (reviewed in reference 7).

Typically, mycoplasmal mitogens have not been well characterized. The presence of lipopolysaccharides (LPSs) and lipoglycans cannot be excluded from many mycoplasmal preparations. Yiu and Yamazaki showed that ordinary lipids present in lipoproteins in eucaryotic cell membranes can induce cell growth in macrophages (69). In our laboratory, Butler et al. showed that proteinase K-treated *M. hyorhinis* extracts, delipidated by methanol-chloroform, had greater specific mitogenic activity than did delipidated extracts not treated with protease (Fig. 2) (5). The biphasic nature of the extract curve suggested that at least two mitogens were present. The protein-free methanol-chloroform lipid fraction recovered from these extracts also showed significant mitogenic activity (data not shown). Extracts were negative for endotoxin by the *Limulus* amoebocyte lysate test. The proteinase K-treated extracts contained a 40-kDa protease-resistant protein that was not digested by up to 100 µg of proteinase K per ml for 24 h (Fig. 3). The protein/lipid ratios in extracts and whole organisms increased with age, and this increase correlated with the appearance of the 40-kDa resistant protein. However, a causal relationship between lipid content and proteinase K resistance remains to be directly demonstrated. Tests in our laboratory showed that the 40-kDa *M. hyorhinis* proteinase K-resistant protein was not immunologically related to the mouse or hamster prions. This finding and differences in molecular mass differentiated the *M. hyorhinis* proteinase K-resistant protein from the spiroplasmal proteinase K-resistant

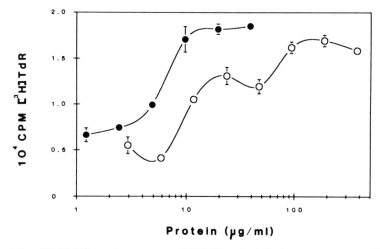

Figure 2. [^{3}H]thymidine ([^{3}H]TdR) uptake response of BALB/c splenic leukocytes mitogenically stimulated with partially delipidated *M. hyorhinis* extract (○) or partially delipidated proteinase K-treated extracts containing the 40-kDa proteinase K-resistant protein (●).

proteins, reported by Bastian et al. to be immunologically related to prions and similar in size (2).

Different mycoplasma species can either inhibit or stimulate lymphocyte mitogenesis (7, 44, 64). It is likely that some species may exhibit both inhibitory and mitogenic effects for lymphocytes. Effects on T and B lymphocytes have been extensively reported. Such effects have been seen with whole mycoplasma organisms, culture supernatants, mycoplasmal extracts, and purified mitogens. In most cases, however, precise mechanisms have not been defined. A problem in many publications is that the infecting organism was not identified.

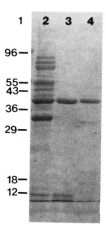

Figure 3. Sodium dodecyl sulfate-polyacrylamide gel electrophoresis of *M. hyorhinis* BTS-7 extracts. Samples were reduced with 2-mercaptoethanol, boiled, and analyzed on sodium dodecyl sulfate–12.5% polyacrylamide gels. Lanes: 1, M_r markers (indicated in thousands); 2, *M. hyorhinis* 3-[(3-cholamidopropyl)-dimethyl-ammonio]-1-propanesulfonate (CHAPS) extract; 3, *M. hyorhinis* CHAPS extract treated with 5 μg of proteinase K per ml for 24 h; 4, *M. hyorhinis* CHAPS extract treated with 100 μg of proteinase K per ml for 24 h.

B Lymphocytes

Hendershot and Levitt (18) showed that MI significantly altered the synthesis and the expression of specific immunoglobulins in the B-lymphocyte cell lines Daudi, LBN-2, and F4. *M. hominis* altered specific immunoglobulin gene expression in these cells (18). MI significantly reduced the ratio of membrane to secretory μ heavy chain in all three cell lines. Immunoglobulin M (IgM) synthesis increased 50 to 100% after *M. hominis* infection. Another significant finding was that MI altered the association of light chains with heavy chains. Reexpression of μ chains on the surface of B-lymphoblastoid cells was delayed in mycoplasma-infected cultures. The authors cautioned that inconsistent reports on immunoglobulin synthesis and alteration of B-cell line phenotypes in the literature might be explained by undetected MI.

In related studies, Sitia et al. showed that *M. fermentans* induced the murine B-lymphoma line I.29 to differentiate into plasma cells (58). In these studies, differentiating cells lost membrane-bound immunoglobulins and the level of cytoplasmic immunoglobulin increased. Levels of IgA secretion also increased significantly. The putative mitogen from *M. fermentans* in this culture acted similarly to LPS but was distinct. LPSs have not been reported in *M. fermentans*.

M. arginini could stimulate growth of B, but not T, lymphocytes that were pretreated with LPS (55). The organism was as effective as LPS in promotion of immunoglobulin secretion.

Williamson et al. showed that the in vivo response of rat strains LEW and F344 mimicked the in vitro response to *M. pulmonis* (67). LEW rat lymphocytes were more responsive than F344 lymphocytes in terms of plaque-forming cells.

Working with Fc receptor-bearing hybridomas, Lemke et al. showed that *M. arginini* infection led to apparent Fc receptor activity (28). Although this induction occurred with *M. arginini*, *M. orale* failed to induce the Fc receptor. This specificity was apparently due to a lectin present in *M. arginini* that bound antibody. *M. orale* lacked the lectin. The authors suggested that binding of antibodies to certain mycoplasma species may influence pathogenesis by masking the mycoplasma cells with the host's own immunoglobulins. This phenomenon, coupled with the observation that mycoplasmas can polyclonally activate B cells, could be a potentially important consideration for diseases such as rheumatoid arthritis.

Several groups have shown that certain mycoplasmas contain IgA proteases. Robertson et al. (52) and Killian et al. (20) independently showed that *Ureaplasma urealyticum* contained IgA protease activity. These proteases may be virulence factors for pathogenic bacteria, especially those that are found on epithelial surfaces, similar to findings for mycoplasmas. Kapatais-Zoumbos et al. demonstrated protease A activity in 28 strains of *U. urealyticum* but failed to demonstrate activity in *M. pneumoniae*, *M. genitalium*, and *M. hominis* (19). While protease activity has been clearly demonstrated, it is not clear whether the enzymes are immunoglobulin specific or whether they can also cleave other proteins.

Different mycoplasma species can have different qualitative effects on the same parameter. Oredipe et al. reported reduced antibody affinity and decreased number of antigenic receptor sites in one mycoplasma-infected human colorectal carcinoma cell culture, but they found a four- to fivefold increase in number of receptors and decreased antibody affinity in another infected culture (45). Unfortunately, the mycoplasmas were not identified, which renders precise interpretation difficult.

T Lymphocytes

Mycoplasmas have also been shown to be mitogenic for T lymphocytes. The archetype of mycoplasma-T lymphocyte interaction has been the *M. arthritidis* mitogen (MAM) exquisitely developed by Cole and colleagues. They have characterized the MAM in a series of papers, some of which were reviewed in 1985 (7,39); more recent studies are described in chapter 28.

Table 2 summarizes mycoplasma induction of various cytokines. Of particular interest are the papers by Beck et al. (3) and Birke et al. (4). Beck and colleagues demonstrated in a murine model that all lymphoma cells that induced acid-labile interferon (gamma interferon [IFN-γ]) in a mixed lymphocyte tumor cell assay were infected with mycoplasmas (3). Interferon was also induced by cell-free supernatants of mycoplasma-infected tumor cell cultures. Unfortunately, the mycoplasma was not identified. However, in the same study, these workers showed that *A. laidlawii* and *M. pneumoniae* induced IFN in a murine spleen cell culture.

Birke et al. performed similar studies in human tumor cells (4). Four melanoma cell lines and one ovarian carcinoma line infected with *M. orale* induced heat- and acid-stable leukocyte IFN (IFN-α). *M. orale*-infected lines were more susceptible to natural killer (NK) cell-mediated lysis than were mycoplasma-free cultures. However, these results did not unequivocally show that NK cell lysis was entirely due to MI of target cells, since some lysis occurred in the absence of myco-

Table 2. Mycoplasmal induction of cytokines

Mycoplasma species	Cytokine or activity	Reference
Many	Interferon	7 (review)
A. laidlawii, *M. pneumoniae*	NK cell targets	3
M. orale	NK cell targets	4
M. fermentans	IL-6	51
M. orale	TNF	14
M. gallisepticum	TNF	14
M. capricolum	TNF	14
S. floricola	TNF	14
S. melliferum	TNF	14
M. orale	IL-1, IL-6, TNF	21
M. arginini	IL-1, IL-6, TNF	21
M. hyorhinis	IL-1, IL-6, TNF	21
M. salivarium	IL-1, IL-6, TNF	21
M. gallisepticum	IL-1, IL-6, TNF	21
A. laidlawii	IL-1, IL-6, TNF	21
M. pneumoniae	IL-2	21
M. fermentans	PMNG[a] stimulation	25
M. orale	PMNG stimulation	25
M. buccale	PMNG stimulation	25

[a] PMNG, polymorphonuclear granulocytes.

plasmas. In the *M. orale*-human tumor cell system, cell-free supernatants did not induce IFN in human leukocytes.

Birke et al. also hypothesized that mycoplasmas may render cells susceptible to NK cell killing targets in vivo (4). An unidentified mycoplasma was shown to trigger the release of soluble cytotoxic factors from human peripheral blood lymphocytes. Release of these soluble cytotoxic factors occurred only with concanavalin A and mycoplasmas. These authors also concluded that mycoplasmas can play a crucial role in induction of human soluble cytotoxic factors and, like Beck et al. (3), noted that the premise that these factors are the lytic mediators in NK cell mediated cytotoxicity needs to be reevaluated.

In a subsequent study, Wayner and Brooks showed that MI of tumor cells also induced NK cell activity (66). The organism involved in some cases was identified as *M. orale*. Mycoplasmas from other cell lines used in this study were not identified. These workers showed that YAC-1α cells stimulated a splenic cytotoxic factor in mouse splenic cells. Cell-free supernatants of mycoplasma-infected cell cultures were mitogenic for CBA cells and induced the cytotoxic factor directly. Induction could be obtained both from the mycoplasma cells and from the supernatant medium. Perhaps some of these findings could be attributable to arginine depletion, since excess arginine abrogated up to 20% of the cytotoxic activity determined at 18 h.

The specific mediator was not identified. However, IFN produced by activated lymphocytes is one possibility. Peter et al. (46, 47) described a lymphotoxinlike mediator obtained from cell supernatants that augmented NK cell activity against cultured human melanoma targets. The mediator was eventually identified as IFN and was produced as a direct result of *M. orale* infection.

Demczuk et al. (11) studied the effect of an unidentified mycoplasma on transcription of interleukin-1α (IL-1α) and IL-1β. MI reduced steady-state levels of IL-

1α and IL-1β mRNAs in the A431 human squamous carcinoma line but had no effect on expression in U937 cells.

Sinaglia et al. showed that MI inhibited growth of an IL-2-dependent murine cytotoxic T-cell line, as measured by uptake of tritiated thymidine (57). The authors speculated that inhibition was due to mycoplasmal cleavage of thymidine via pyrimidine nucleoside phosphorylases.

Teh et al. showed similar effects in a murine IL-2-dependent T-cell line following infection with *M. hyorhinis* (62). This infection suppressed induction of cytotoxic responses to alloantigens. In a follow-up study, these workers characterized the suppressive factor as a 200-kDa protein that was found in mycoplasma-infected cell culture supernatants and was not present in uninfected controls (63). This factor did not inhibit the proliferation of human tumor cell lines, and its actions were not reversed by addition of excess IL-2. Cytotoxicity was apparent as early as 2 h after addition to the culture. The factor was resistant to heating at 60°C for 1 h and incubation at pH 2 or 12 for 4 h. It was sensitive to protease. Interestingly, Lau et al. reported a factor, termed suppressor-activating factor, produced by a human T-cell line (26). Its activity was similar to that reported by Teh et al. (63). However, the factor of Lau et al. appeared later in infection than did the one described by Teh et al. In the study by Lau et al., mycoplasmal assays apparently were not performed.

Stuart et al. described how *M. arginini* infection induced Ia antigen on a murine myelomonocytic cell line, WEHI-3 (61). Viable and nonviable *M. arginini* induced class II major histocompatibility complex (MHC) antigen to levels approaching those induced by IFN. Nonviable *M. arginini* likewise produced levels of class II mRNA equivalent to or exceeding those produced by IFN-α. Class I H2, K, and D surface antigens were unaffected by MI. The specific mycoplasma mediator of this induction was not identified. These results are of interest since several mycoplasma species, but not *M. arginini*, have been associated with autoimmune diseases. Activation by macrophages, reported to occur by *M. orale* (36), is one possibility. In a follow-up paper, Stuart et al. showed that *M. arthritidis*, *M. pulmonis*, *M. hominis*, and *M. pneumoniae* also induced class II MHC antigen (60). Tumang et al. demonstrated that MAM, like other microbial toxins, could act as a superantigen (64). This group of antigens, which bind to class II MHC molecules and activate selected T cells by virtue of T-cell receptor variable gene usage, may induce a similar form of T-helper cell–B-cell interaction. MAM bound to the surface of resting B cells was an effective means of activating superantigen-reactive T-helper cells that triggered polyclonal immunoglobulin production by the superantigen-bearing B-cell population.

In related studies, Carrington and Ward reported the conversion from a class II-positive to a class II-negative phenotype following eradication of *M. hyorhinis* (6). However, these authors concluded that use of the antibiotic BM cycline was responsible for this conversion. However, in light of the data presented by Stuart et al. (60), these conclusions should be reevaluated. It is at least as likely that the *M. hyorhinis* originally rendered the cells class II positive and that fol-lowing mycoplasmal eradication, this effect was reversed by the disappearance of mycoplasmas.

Cytokine Induction

Many of the effects on cell induction reported above are likely mediated by cytokines. There are numerous reports on direct activation of cytokines by mycoplasmas. It has long been recognized that many mycoplasmas induce IFN. Cole et al. (7) have summarized how mycoplasmas, and even mycoplasma viruses, can induce IFN-α or IFN-γ. To date, only *M. arthritidis* has been shown to induce both IFN species. In addition to having antiviral effects, IFN plays important functions in regulation of key host cell responses. It is possible, and even likely, that much of the mycoplasmal induction of cytokines is mediated by IFN. Tumor necrosis factor (TNF) induction is another possibility.

Quentmeier et al. showed that *M. fermentans* induced IL-6 in murine macrophages and human monocytes (51). The effect of this action was to cause differentiation of cytolytic T cells. A high-molecular-weight material with an apparent molecular mass of 1.5×10^6 Da was responsible. This material was not mitogenic for murine splenic cells, but it stimulated the release of IL-6 from murine macrophages. These authors stated that TNF and arachidonic acid were also induced. Their data show, however, that IL-6 was the key cytokine: formation of cytotoxic T lymphocytes was inhibited by anti-IL-6 antibody. This may be a possible mechanism in rheumatoid arthritis, often linked to at least a partial etiology by mycoplasmas. On the other hand, Gallily et al. implicated TNF as the mediator in macrophage-mediated lysis of tumor cells by lysates of *M. orale* (14). Lysis was inhibited by anti-TNF antibody. Other mycoplasmas that induced TNF were *M. gallisepticum*, *M. capricolum*, and, to a lesser extent, *S. floricola* and *S. melliferum*. It was significant that not all cell killing was mediated by soluble TNF in this study. These authors suggested the use of *M. orale* or its responsible macrophage-activated component as a possible therapeutic agent for human cancer. *M. arthritidis* also induced macrophage activation, but the mechanism was not reported (12).

In a related study, Krause et al. showed that *M. fermentans*, *M. orale*, and *M. buccale* achieved comparable levels of human polymorphonuclear granulocyte stimulation (25). Six strains of *M. hominis* were slightly less efficient, and *M. pneumoniae* produced approximately one-third the level of *M. fermentans*. In fact, the authors speculated that the reduced stimulation of polymorphonuclear granulocytes by *M. pneumoniae* and *U. urealyticum* might be related to the pathogenicity of these organisms.

Kita has presented preliminary results demonstrating that *M. pneumoniae*, *M. orale*, *M. arginini*, *M. hyorhinis*, *M. salivarium*, *M. gallisepticum*, and *A. laidlawii* induce a variety of cytokines (21). All of these species induced IL-1β, IL-6, and TNF-α in human lymphocyte cultures. IL-2 was induced only by *M. pneumoniae*. IFN was induced by five of the seven species tested. In subsequent collaboration with our laboratory, Kita showed that proteinase K digests of *M. salivarium*, *M. arginini*, *M. orale*, and *M. hyorhinis* induced IL-1β, IL-6, and TNF-α. *M. salivarium* and *M. orale* induced IFN.

Mycoplasma Transformation of Cell Cultures

Among the myriad reported effects of cell culture mycoplasmas, one of the more intriguing is that of cell transformation. In 1966, MacPherson and Russell reported that mycoplasmas mediated transformation of low-passage BHK cells (BHK-21, clone 13) (37). The transformation consisted of loss of growth control and altered morphology which consisted of "multinucleated giant cells, epitheloid cells, round cells and long spindle-shaped cells growing in disarray like polyoma transformed cells." *M. hominis* was isolated from all these cultures. However, the etiologic role of *M. hominis* in this transformation was not established in this publication. Significantly, the authors also reported corynebacteria in these cultures concomitantly with mycoplasmas. It was unclear in this publication whether the diagnosis of corynebacteria was based on microscopic observation or isolation on media. The authors did report that corynebacteria were not detected in mycoplasma broth or on mycoplasma agar. Antibiotic treatment eliminated *M. hominis*, but the transformed phenotype persisted. It was not clear whether the corynebacteria persisted after antibiotic treatment.

In separate experiments reported in the same publication (37), *M. fermentans* PG18, *M. hominis* PG21 and PG27, *M. orale* I and II, and *M. pneumoniae* Eaton FH all produced transformation in BHK-21 cells, as demonstrated by growth in soft agar. *M. salivarium* failed to transform. However, in all cases except *M. fermentans*, the cells returned to their original morphology (in contrast to the studies discussed above with another wild-type strain of *M. hominis*). The authors noted that ". . . some of our BHK21 cultures, apparently transformed by mycoplasmas no longer release mycoplasmas in detectable numbers." They concluded that ". . . perhaps mycoplasmas, like Rous sarcoma virus can exist in defective forms as an obligate cell parasite" (37). In 1965, Somerson and Cook observed that *M. orale* suppressed growth of Rous sarcoma virus in cell cultures (59).

In a subsequent paper, Russell et al. showed that *M. fermentans*-transformed cells had increased tumorigenicity for random-bred Syrian hamsters (54). *M. fermentans* could not be isolated from these cultures, and the control, untreated BHK-21 cells also produced tumors, albeit at a lower frequency. In two experiments, *M. fermentans*-infected BHK-21 cells produced tumors in 11 of 11 treated Syrian hamsters. Mycoplasma-free, control BHK-21 cells produced tumors in 4 of 11 Syrian hamsters. Unfortunately, mycoplasma broth was not included as a control. It was shown that tumor induction in Syrian hamsters was dose dependent: the number of cells required to produce tumors in 50% of the animals was between 10^2 and 10^3 for *M. fermentans*-infected BHK-21 cells and between 10^5 and 10^6 for control cells.

The same level of tumorigenicity of *M. fermentans*-infected BHK-21 cells was achieved when heat-killed organisms (56°C for 1 h) were used. *M. orale* type II also increased tumorigenicity (9 of 11 animals). On the basis of these considerations, it is difficult to interpret the results. It is unclear whether selection of a subpopulation of BHK-21 cells could have occurred as a result of mycoplasma infection or whether there was an effect due to mycoplasma medium.

The failure of Russell et al. to isolate mycoplasmas from these cultures is puzzling (54). It could be due to a different stage of parasitism of the mycoplasmas, as the authors suggested, or to a failure of the mycoplasma medium. Ponten and MacPherson (50) reported the failure to recover three different mycoplasma species from chicken embryo fibroblasts inoculated with mycoplasmas, including *A. laidlawii*.

Furness and Whitescarver described unsuccessful attempts to isolate *M. hominis* from BSC-1, a monkey kidney cell line (13). After treatment of *M. hominis*-infected BSC-1 cells with antibiotics, mycoplasmas could not be recovered on agar medium. However, the authors reported that mycoplasmas could be observed by electron microscopy. Structures resembling mycoplasmas were seen in close proximity to viable cells and only rarely were associated with vacuolated and necrotic cells. The authors also noted that mycoplasmas and viable BSC-1 cells were often seen touching each other.

We reported similar failures to recover ureaplasmas from infected cell cultures (23). Inoculation of *U. urealyticum* T-960 and the simian T-167-2 strain of ureaplasma into HeLa, murine 3T6, and monkey CV-1 cells resulted in infection, as evidenced by immunoperoxidase staining for ureaplasmas, fluorescent DNA staining using Hoechst 33258, and growth on T agar. Significantly, both strains in all three cell lines failed to grow in Edward-Hayflick medium. These ureaplasmas did not grow on mycoplasma agar with aerobic or anaerobic incubation. Ureaplasma strains T-960 and T-167-2 grew on Edward-Hayflick medium before inoculation into cell cultures.

We have reported that *S. mirum* SMCA transforms mouse NIH 3T3 cells (22, 24). Transformation was documented by loss of contact inhibition, growth in soft agar, and tumor production in athymic mice. Extensive studies have shown that these effects are not due to artifacts of the experimental system such as viral contamination of the fetal bovine serum, mislabeling of cell cultures, or spontaneous transformation. *S. mirum* was present in the cytoplasm of all transformed cells examined. These organisms were not in membrane-bound vacuoles, suggesting that organisms entered the cell by diacytosis. Typically, mycoplasmas are not intracellular. Elimination of spiroplasmas from spiroplasma-transformed 3T3 (ST-3T3) cells by antibiotics did not affect the transformed phenotype. DNA from ST-3T3 cells transformed CV-1 monkey kidney cells. DNA from these cells transformed other CV-1 cells and produced tumors in athymic mice. SMCA DNA did not transform CV-1 cells.

ST-3T3 cells contained a major excretory protein at a level similar to that in virally transformed cells. Levels of this protein (measured in cpm) were 3,753 for ST-3T3 cells, 3,348 for Kirsten virus-transformed 3T3 cells, and 283 for normal 3T3 cells. Spiroplasma proteins were not detected in spiroplasma-cured ST-3T3 cells by immunofluorescence or by Western immunoblotting. Dot and Southern blots were performed on 10 to 40 µg of DNA from spiroplasma-free ST-3T3 cells, using SMCA chromosomal DNA as the probe. No hybridization was observed, suggesting that SMCA DNA did not integrate into the chromosomal DNA of ST-

3T3 cells. We have shown that all three strains of *S. mirum* produce statistically significant syncytium formation in a variety of cell cultures, including human retina, rat eye lens, and rabbit eye lens cell cultures (22). This effect has been also found in respiratory epithelial cells of rats in *M. pulmonis* infection, both in lungs and in nasal passages (reviewed in reference 7).

Spiroplasma transformation differs from transformation by oncogenic viruses. The failure to detect spiroplasmal DNA in ST-3T3 cells may reflect (i) absence of the DNA, (ii) insufficient assay sensitivity, (iii) the fact that transformation is actually a contamination by either spontaneously or virally transformed 3T3 cells, or (iv) other mechanisms. However, we have been able to molecularly distinguish ST-3T3 cells from normal 3T3 cells as well as from virally and spontaneously transformed 3T3 cells.

M. fermentans Infection of Cell Cultures

Currently, *M. fermentans* is one of the most common isolates from cell cultures in our laboratory. The organism has generated considerable interest because of published reports of interactions with various lymphoblastoid cells and because of its putative association with AIDS.

This laboratory currently assays more than 6,000 cell cultures each year for mycoplasmas. Most of these cultures originate from several cell repositories that the Coriell Institute maintains for the National Institute of General Medical Sciences, the National Institute of Aging, the National Institute of Mental Health, and several private organizations. The overall incidence of MI is low, 5% or less. This relatively low incidence reflects the type of cell cultures being assayed, which are primary cultures or lines that are in early passage. Five mycoplasma species (*M. hyorhinis*, *M. orale*, *M. arginini*, *M. fermentans*, and *A. laidlawii*) account for more than 98% of our isolates. For the period from 1972 to 1983, we detected *M. fermentans* only six times in more than 10,000 cell cultures. For the period 1984 to 1990, *M. fermentans* was detected in 63 cell cultures. It now is responsible for 18 to 22% of our isolates. Over the past 7 years, 31 laboratories have contributed cell cultures infected with *M. fermentans*. It is not always possible to identify the type of cell culture being assayed. However, it appears that human lymphoblastoid cells, including T-cell lymphomas, predominate. Whether the significant increase in *M. fermentans* isolations since 1984 reflects a common source of infection (i.e., one laboratory supplying many others with infected materials) is unknown, but is unlikely, given the diversity of sources and investigational areas represented in our assays.

Can *M. fermentans* be a contaminant in primary peripheral blood specimens? Data from reports of Murphy et al. suggest that this is the case (42, 43). In their summary paper (42), they showed that 5 of 180 normal children (2.8%) had mycoplasmas (primarily *M. fermentans*) in the blood or bone marrow. Mycoplasmas were isolated from children with cancer at an incidence of 4.1% (48 of 1,174) (calculated from Table 6 of reference 42). Mycoplasmas were not isolated from 17 normal adults. The incidence from adults with cancer was 2.2%. The finding by these authors that cell cul-

tures were fourfold more effective for the isolation of mycoplasmas than were artificial media demonstrates that these strains are more fastidious than other *M. fermentans* isolates or that artificial media have significant inhibitors. On several occasions, three or four blind passages were necessary in cell cultures to allow primary isolation. It is noteworthy that the microbiological medium used in those studies was not significantly different from the medium now in use, with the exception of SP-4.

Where do these *M. fermentans* strains come from? Can they be contaminants from peripheral blood specimens used to establish T- and B-cell lines? According to the data of Murphy et al. (42, 43), this is a possibility. However, these isolations were from normal or leukemic children or from leukemic adults. Over the past 17 years, investigators have sent the Coriell Institute more than 5,000 primary B-lymphocyte cell lines for assay. These specimens came to the repositories as blood specimens and were then established as cell cultures. Blood samples were separated on Ficoll-Hypaque columns, centrifuged, and washed prior to Epstein-Barr virus transformation, at which time they were assayed for mycoplasmas. Of these more than 5,000 specimens, only one was positive for a mycoplasma, identified as *M. fermentans*. The assays did not sample T cells, since the cells would not have proliferated under these conditions. However, these tests indicate that *M. fermentans* is not a common isolate from peripheral blood.

Lo and colleagues published a series of papers on the detection of an agent from various tissues derived from AIDS patients (29–35). In the first of these papers, Lo and Liotta reported that NIH 3T3 cells transfected with Kaposi's sarcoma DNA derived from an AIDS patient produced malignant transformation and tumor production in athymic mice (32). An agent was visualized in these cultures and subsequently identified as a mycoplasma (33). Lo initially referred to this agent as *M. incognitus*, believing that it was a previously unrecognized species (31). It has now been shown that this agent is *M. fermentans* (56).

The major conclusions of the papers of Lo et al. were as follows. (i) A cell-free preparation of mycoplasmal DNA transfected NIH 3T3 cells. These cells, in turn, produced tumors in athymic mice. (ii) This mycoplasmal DNA preparation apparently gave rise to the mycoplasmal organism, *M. fermentans*. (iii) This strain (and perhaps other strains) of *M. fermentans* grow intracellularly in various cells in vivo. (iv) The strains of *M. fermentans* derived from AIDS patients, except strain sb_{51}, resist cultivation in cell-free media. (v) *M. fermentans* has been detected by immunological or genetic probes in AIDS patients. (vi) *M. fermentans*, when inoculated into silver leaf monkeys, produced no symptoms for 6 months, at which time weight loss and wasting occurred, resulting in death in 7 to 9 months. (vii) *M. fermentans* was detected in all of six non-AIDS patients who died with acute flulike illnesses. These patients came from different geographic areas.

These reports were originally received with some skepticism (68), especially with respect to the original isolation of the mycoplasma from Kaposi's sarcoma. The results postulated that the cell-free phenol extract from the Kaposi's tissue contained, intact, the genetic information necessary to generate the whole mycoplasma organism which, in turn, transformed 3T3 cells. Under this scenario, it is not clear whether the DNA or the intact organism transformed the 3T3 cells. Lo originally referred to this agent as a viruslike infectious agent (VLIA) (30). An 8.6-kb cloned probe and a 2.2-kb cloned probe detected specific VLIA sequences in DNA isolated from 7 of 10 AIDS patients. VLIA infection was detected in many tissues, including spleen, liver, brain, lymph node, and blood mononuclear cells, but was not detected in non-AIDS patients.

In a subsequent paper, VLIA was also detected in six patients from different geographic areas who had acute flulike illnesses. All were negative for *M. pneumoniae*, and all died in 1 to 7 weeks (30). Histopathological lesions of extensive necrosis in tissues from these patients were positive for VLIA by immunohistochemistry. Tissues were also positive by in situ hybridization for VLIA. Of interest was the fact that these patients did not belong to any of the known groups at high risk for contracting AIDS. The authors stated that VLIA may cause an extensive infection in apparently healthy subjects without eliciting the usual inflammatory response.

VLIA was eventually identified as a mycoplasma. Lo et al. originally referred to the agent as *M. incognitus* and showed it to be both an arginine utilizer and glucose fermenter, similar to *M. fermentans* (33). The organism generally failed to grow in conventional mycoplasmal media. An exception was the sb$_{51}$ strain, which grew poorly in modified SP-4 medium.

Saillard et al. identified the *M. incognitus* isolate as *M. fermentans* (56) by genomic, protein, and serologic analyses. *M. incognitus* isolate was compared with two strains of *M. fermentans*; genomic relatedness was greater than 90%, indicating that the isolate is a strain of *M. fermentans*. Polyacrylamide gel electrophoresis and restriction fragment length polymorphism profiles of the isolate reinforced its designation as *M. fermentans*.

Lemaître et al. showed that with tetracycline and chlortetracycline treatment of human immunodeficiency virus (HIV)-infected CEM cells, cytopathogenicity disappeared, suggesting the presence of a tetracycline-sensitive agent (27). Mycoplasmas were eventually detected in these cultures (68).

More recently, Lo et al. reported that *M. fermentans* significantly inhibited RT activity in HIV-1-infected A.301 T lymphocytes (35). RT inhibition occurred immediately after inoculation of supernatants containing *M. fermentans*, suggesting that mycoplasmal products could be responsible for the inhibition. Vasudevachari et al. reported that *M. hyorhinis* also inhibited RT activity in a system of HIV-1 and peripheral blood mononuclear cells (65). In this study, cultures that were RT negative but positive for syncytium formation were positive for p24 enzyme-linked immunosorbent assay activity. Lo et al. speculated that mycoplasma nucleases could be responsible for the inhibition of RT. Marcus and Yoshida characterized a double-stranded RNase (dsRNase) from a strain of *M. hyorhinis* isolated from cell cultures (38). These authors surveyed 12 different mycoplasma species for dsRNase. *A. laidlawii* yielded the most activity, 1,420 U/ml. *M. arginini, M. hyorhinis, M. gallisepticum, S. citri, M. neurolyticum, M. melaleuca, M. pneumoniae, M. capricolum*, Mycoplasma sp. strain PPAV, *S. apis*,

and *M. bovis* all had activity. Organisms propagated in Friis medium had significantly lower amounts of dsRNase than did the same number of organisms grown in SP-4 medium. These authors speculated that the dsRNase reported earlier in avian cells may have been mycoplasmal in origin. Mycoplasmal dsRNase may also have been responsible for reduced IFN induction by poly(rI)·poly(rC) and perhaps even by viruses (reviewed in reference 7).

Halden et al. described a specific restriction endonuclease produced by *M. fermentans* MT-2/NJW (15). The restriction enzyme (*Mfe*I) cuts at the recognition sequence C/AATG and was isolated initially from human T-lymphocyte Jurkat cells. It was eventually identified in broth-propagated *M. fermentans*. This is the first enzyme with this recognition sequence.

One characteristic common to the *M. fermentans* transformation reported by Lo et al. (31) and the *S. mirum* transformation described by Kotani et al. (22) was intracellular localization of mycoplasmas. Intracellular localization of mycoplasmas together with the absolute requirement of these organisms for nucleic acid precursors could result in altered nucleic acid and related metabolism in the cytoplasm of the host cell. According to a review by Meuth, such alterations have led to mutations in other systems (41). In a cell already primed toward transformation, such as 3T3, transformation is not an unlikely event.

In an interesting paper, Plagemann and Woffendin reported that MI produced an increased salvage of deoxyadenosine, which was more than 10-fold that of mycoplasma-free controls (49). Mycoplasmal phosphorylases convert deoxyadenosine to adenine and ultimately into ribonucleotides and RNA. The organism was identified as *M. orale*. In this case, it was assumed that deoxyadenosine transport into mycoplasmas was also sensitive to dipyridamole, similar to results for mammalian cells. Cells reported to be affected were P388 and L1210 cells. However, other mammalian cell lines expressing this pathway in vitro would likely also be affected.

CONCLUSION

While the traditional view of cell culture mycoplasmas has focused on these organisms as the ideal cell culture nuisance, data yielding an interesting glimpse of these wall-less procaryotes are now accumulating. The diverse interchanges that these organisms exhibit with lymphocytes and the cytokines that they trigger, the finding that mycoplasmas can reside intracellularly, and the tantalizing possibility that they may have some association with AIDS open up truly expanded horizons with which to study mycoplasma-eucaryotic cell relationships. In a bizarre sense, the method of study to define this will be—cell cultures.

REFERENCES

1. **Barile, M. F., H. E. Hopps, and M. Grabowski.** 1978. Incidence and sources of mycoplasma contamination: a brief review, p. 35–46. *In* G. J. McGarrity, D. G. Murphy, and W. W. Nichols (ed.), *Mycoplasma Infection of Cell Culture.* Plenum Press, New York.

2. **Bastian, F., R. Jennings, and W. Gardner.** 1987. Antiserum to scrapie-associated fibril protein cross reacts with *Spiroplasma mirum* fibril protein. *J. Clin. Microbiol.* **25:**2430–2431.

3. **Beck, J., H. Engler, H. Brunner, and H. Kirchner.** 1980. Interferon production in cocultures between mouse spleen cells and tumor cells. Possible role of mycoplasmas in interferon induction. *J. Immunol. Methods* **38:**63–73.

4. **Birke, C., H. H. Peter, U. Langenberg, J. P. Werner, J. Muller-Hermes, H. Peters, J. Heitmann, W. Leibold, H. Dallugge, E. Krapf, and H. Kirchner.** 1981. Mycoplasma contamination in human tumor cell lines: effect on interferon induction and susceptibility to natural killing. *J. Immunol.* **127:**94–98.

5. **Butler, G. H., H. Kotani, L. Kong, M. Frick, S. Evancho, E. J. Stanbridge, and G. J. McGarrity.** 1991. Identification and characterization of proteinase K-resistant proteins in mollicutes. *Infect. Immun.* **59:**1037–1042.

6. **Carrington, M. N., and F. E. Ward.** 1988. Conversion of a melanoma cell line from an HLA class II positive to negative phenotype after treatment with anti mycoplasma drugs. *Hum. Immunol.* **22:**275–282.

7. **Cole, B. C., Y. Naot, E. J. Stanbridge, and K. S. Wise.** 1985. Interactions of mycoplasmas and their products with lymphoid cells *in vitro*, p. 204–258. *In* S. Razin and M. F. Barile (ed.), *The Mycoplasmas*, vol. 4. Academic Press, New York.

8. **Cole, B. C., G. J. Sullivan, R. A. Daynes, I. A. Sayed, and J. R. Ward.** 1982. Stimulation of mouse lymphocytes by a mitogen derived from *Mycoplasma arthritidis*. II. Cellular requirements for T cell transformation mediated by a soluble mycoplasma mitogen. *J. Immunol.* **128:**2013–2018.

9. **Constantopoulos, G., and G. J. McGarrity.** 1989. Activities of aspartate and alanine transferase in the Mollicutes *A. laidlawii* MG, *M. pneumoniae* FH, and *M. salivarium* VV. *Curr. Microbiol.* **19:**213–216.

10. **Del Giudice, R. A., J. G. Tully, D. L. Rose, and R. M. Cole.** 1985. *Mycoplasma pirum* sp. nov., a terminal structured mollicute from cell cultures. *Int. J. Syst. Bacteriol.* **35:**285–291.

11. **Demczuk, S., C. Baumbergeer, B. Mach, and J. M. Dayer.** 1988. Differentiated effects of *in vitro* mycoplasma infection on interleukin-1α and β mRNA expression in U939 and A431 cells. *J. Biol. Chem.* **263:**13039–13045.

12. **Dietz, J. M., and B. C. Cole.** 1982. Direct activation of the J774.1 murine macrophage cell line by *Mycoplasma arthritidis*. *Infect. Immun.* **37:**811–819.

13. **Furness, G., and J. Whitescarver.** 1975. Adaptation of *Mycoplasma hominis* to an obligate parasitic existence in monkey kidney cell culture. *Proc. Soc. Exp. Biol. Med.* **149:**427–432.

14. **Gallily, R., T. Sher, P. Ben-av, and J. Loewenstein.** 1989. Tumor necrosis factor a mediator of *Mycoplasma orale*-induced tumor cell lysis by macrophages. *Cell. Immunol.* **121:**146–153.

15. **Halden, N. F., J. B. Wolf, and W. J. Leonard.** 1989. Identification of a novel site specific endonuclease produced by *Mycoplasma fermentans*: discovery while characterizing DNA binding protein in T lymphocyte cell lines. *Nucleic Acids Res.* **17:**3491–3499.

16. **Hammel-Berrey, G. A., and Z. Brahmu.** 1987. Relevance of soluble cytotoxic factors generated by mycoplasma contaminated targets to natural killer cell mediated killing. *Hum. Immunol.* **20:**33–46.

17. **Harper, D. R., H. O. Kangro, S. Argent, and R. B. Heath.** 1988. Reduction in immunoreactivity of varicella-zoster virus proteins induced by mycoplasma contamination. *J. Virol. Methods* **20:**65–72.

18. **Hendershot, L., and D. Levitt.** 1985. Effects of mycoplasma contamination on immunoglobulin biosynthesis by human B lymphoblastoid cell lines. *Infect. Immun.* **49:**36–39.

19. **Kapatais-Zoumbos, K., D. K. F. Chandler, and M. F. Barile.** 1985. Survey of immunoglobulin A protease activity among selected species of *Ureaplasma* and *Mycoplasma*: specificity for host immunoglobulin A. *Infect. Immun.* **47:**704–709.

20. **Killian, M., M. B. Brown, T. A. Brown, E. A. Freundt, and G. H. Cassell.** 1984. Immunoglobulin A1 protease activity in strains of *Ureaplasma urealyticum*. *Acta Pathol. Microbiol. Immunol. Scand. Sect. B* **1:**61.

21. **Kita, M.** 1990. Induction of cytokines by mycoplasmas in human lymphocyte culture. *Tissue Culture Res. Commun.* **9:**64.

22. **Kotani, H., G. H. Butler, and G. J. McGarrity.** 1990. Malignant transformation by *Spiroplasma mirum*, p. 14–152. *In* G. Stanek (ed.), *Recent Advances in Mycoplasmology*. Gustav Fisher Verlag, New York.

23. **Kotani, H., and G. J. McGarrity.** 1986. Ureaplasma infection of cell cultures. *Infect. Immun.* **52:**437–444.

24. **Kotani, H., D. M. Phillips, and G. J. McGarrity.** 1986. Malignant transformation of NIH-3T3 and CV-1 cells by a helical mycoplasma, *Spiroplasma mirum* SMCA. *In Vitro* **22:**756–762.

25. **Krause, R., U. Ullmann, and C. Wagener.** 1988. *In vitro* influence of mycoplasma species on the stimulation of human polymorphonuclear granulocytes. *Zentralbl. Bakteriol. Hyg. Reihe A* **270:**228–236.

26. **Lau, C. Y., E. Y. Wang, D. Li, S. Budy-Tymkewycz, V. Visconti, and A. Ashague.** 1985. Mechanism of action of a suppressor-activating factor (SAF) produced by a human T-cell line. *J. Immunol.* **134:**3155–3162.

27. **Lemaître, M., D. Guétard, Y. Hénin, L. Montagnier, and A. Zerial.** 1990. Protective activity of tetracycline analogs against the cytopathic effect of the human immunodeficiency virus in CEM cells. *Res. Virol.* **141:**5–16.

28. **Lemke, R., R. Krause, J. Lorenzen, and B. Havesteen.** 1985. Mycoplasma infection of cell lines can stimulate the expression of Fc receptors by binding of the carbohydrate moiety of antibodies. *Eur. J. Immunol.* **15:**442–447.

29. **Lo, S.-C.** 1986. Isolation and identification of a novel virus from patients with AIDS. *Am. J. Trop. Med. Hyg.* **35:**675–676.

30. **Lo, S.-C., M. S. Dawson, P. B. Newton III, M. A. Sonoda, J. W.-K. Shih, W. F. Engler, R. Y.-H. Wang, and D. J. Wear.** 1989. Association of the virus-like infectious agent originally reported in patients with AIDS with acute fatal disease in previously healthy non-AIDS patients. *Am. J. Trop. Med. Hyg.* **41:**364–376.

31. **Lo, S.-C., M. S. Dawson, D. M. Wong, P. B. Newton III, M. A. Sonoda, W. F. Engler, R. Y.-H. Wang, J. W.-K. Shih, H. J. Alter, and D. J. Wear.** 1989. Identification of *Mycoplasma incognitus* infection in patients with AIDS: an immunohistochemical, in situ hybridization and ultrastructural study. *Am. J. Trop. Med. Hyg.* **41:**601–616.

32. **Lo, S.-C., and L. A. Liotta.** 1985. Vascular tumors produced by NIH/3T3 cells transfected with human AIDS Kaposi's sarcoma DNA. *Am. J. Pathol.* **118:**7–13.

33. **Lo, S.-C., J. W.-K. Shih, P. B. Newton III, D. M. Wong, M. M. Hayes, J. R. Benish, D. J. Wear, and R. Y.-H. Wang.** 1989. The virus-like infectious agent (VLIA) is a novel pathogenic mycoplasma: *Mycoplasma incognitus*. *Am. J. Trop. Med. Hyg.* **41:**586–600.

34. **Lo, S.-C., J. W.-K. Shih, N.-Y. Wang, C.-Y. Ou, and R. Y.-H. Wang.** 1984. A novel virus-like infectious agents in patients with AIDS. *Am. J. Trop. Med. Hyg.* **40:**213–226.

35. **Lo, S.-C., S. Tsai, J. R. Benish, J. W.-K. Shih, D. J. Wear, and D. M. Wong.** 1990. Enhancement of the HIV-1 cytocidal effects in CD4+ lymphocyte by the AIDS-associated mycoplasma. *Science* **251:**1074–1076.

36. **Lowenstein, J., and R. Gallily.** 1984. Studies on the mechanism of macrophage-mediated tumor cell lysis induced by *Mycoplasma orale*. *Isr. J. Med. Sci.* **20:**895–897.

454   McGARRITY ET AL.

37. **MacPherson, I., and W. Russell.** 1966. Transformation in hamster cells mediated by mycoplasmas. *Nature* (London) **210:**1343–1345.

38. **Marcus, P. I., and I. Yoshida.** 1990. Mycoplasmas produce double-stranded ribonuclease. *J. Cell. Physiol.* **143:**416–419.

39. **McGarrity, G. J., and H. Kotani.** 1985. Cell culture mycoplasmas, p. 353–390. *In* S. Razin and M. Barile (ed.), *The Mycoplasmas*, vol. 4. Academic Press, New York.

40. **McGarrity, G. J., V. Vanaman, and J. Sarama.** 1984. Cytogenetic effects of mycoplasmal infection of cell cultures: a review. *In Vitro* **20:**1–18.

41. **Meuth, M.** 1989. The molecular basis of mutation induced by deoxyribonucleoside triphosphate pool imbalances in mammalian cells. *Exp. Cell Res.* **181:**305–316.

42. **Murphy, W. H., C. Bullis, L. Da-Bick, R. Heyn, and C. J. D. Zarafonetis.** 1970. Isolation of mycoplasma from leukemic and nonleukemic patients. *J. Natl. Cancer Inst.* **45:**243–251.

43. **Murphy, W. H., C. Bullis, I. J. Ertel, and C. J. D. Zarafonetis.** 1967. Mycoplasma studies of human leukemia. *Ann. N.Y. Acad. Sci.* **143:**544–556.

44. **Naot, Y., and H. Ginsburg.** 1978. Activation of B lymphocytes by mycoplasma mitogen(s). *Immunology* **34:**715–720.

45. **Oredipe, O. A., R. F. Barth, J. H. Rotaru, G. H. Hinkle, and Z. Steplenski.** 1990. Alteration in monoclonal antibody affinity and antigenic receptor site expression on mycoplasma-infected human colorectal cancer cells. *Proc. Soc. Exp. Biol. Med* **194:**301–307.

46. **Peter, H. H., H. Dalleuge, R. Zawatsky, S. Euler, W. Leibold, and H. Kirchner.** 1980. Human peripheral null lymphocyte. II. Production of type-1 interferon upon stimulation with tumor cells, herpes simplex virus and *Corynebacterium parvum. Eur. J. Immunol.* **10:**547–555.

47. **Peter, H. H., R. F. Eife, and J. R. Kalden.** 1976. Spontaneous cytotoxicity of SCMC of normal human lymphocytes against a human melanoma cell line: a phenomenon due to a lymphotoxin-like mediator. *J. Immunol.* **116:**342–348.

48. **Phillips, D. M.** 1978. Detection of mycoplasma contamination of cell cultures by electron microscopy, p. 105–118. *In* G. J. McGarrity, D. G. Murphy, and W. W. Nichols (ed.), *Mycoplasma Infection of Cell Cultures.* Plenum Press, New York.

49. **Plagemann, P. G. W., and C. Woffendin.** 1990. Mycoplasma contamination alters 2'-deoxyadenosine metabolism in deoxycoformycin treated mouse leukemia cells. *J. Cell Biochem.* **43:**161–172.

50. **Ponten, J., and I. MacPherson.** 1966. Interference with Rous sarcoma virus focus formation by a mycoplasma like factor prsent in human cell cultures. *Ann. Med. Exp. Fenn.* **44:**260–264.

51. **Quentmeier, H. E., Schmitt, H. Kirchhoff, W. Giate, and P. F. Muhbradt.** 1990. *Mycoplasma fermentans* derived high molecular weight material induces interleukin-6 release in cultures of murine macrophages and human monocyes. *Infect. Immun.* **58:**1273–1280.

52. **Robertson, J. A., M. E. Stemler, and G. W. Stemke.** 1984. Immunoglobulin A protease activity of *Ureaplasma urealyticum. J. Clin. Microbiol.* **19:**255–258.

53. **Robinson, L. B., R. H. Wichelhausen, and B. Roizman.** 1956. Contamination of human cell cultures by pleuropneumonia-like organism. *Science* **128:**1147–1148.

54. **Russell, W. C., J. S. F. Niven, and L. D. Berman.** 1968. Studies on the biology of the mycoplasma-induced "stimulation" of BHK21-C13 cells. *Int. J. Cancer* **3:**191–202.

55. **Ruuth, E., and E. Lundgren.** 1986. Enhancement of immunoglobulin secretion by the lymphokine-like activity of a *Mycoplasma arginini* strain. *Scand. J. Immunol.* **23:**575–580.

56. **Saillard, C., P. Carle, J. M. Bové, C. Bébéar, S.-C. Lo, J. W.-K. Shih, R. Y.-H. Wang, D. L. Rose, and J. G. Tully.** 1990. Genetic and serologic relatedness between *Mycoplasma fermentans* strains and a mycoplasma recently identified in tissues of AIDS and non-AIDS patients. *Res. Virol.* **141:**385–395.

57. **Sinaglia, F., and K. W. Talmadge.** 1985. Inhibition of [^{3}H]thymidine incorporation by *Mycoplasma arginini*-infected cells due to enzymatic cleavage of the nucleoside. *Eur. J. Immunol.* **15:**692–696.

58. **Sitia, R., A. Rubartelli, S. Deambrosio, D. Pozzi, and U. Hammerling.** 1985. Differentiation in the murine B cell lymphoma I.29: inductive capacities of lipopolysaccharide and *Mycoplasma fermentans* products. *Eur. J. Immunol.* **15:**570–575.

59. **Somerson, N. L., and M. K. Cook.** 1965. Suppression of Rous sarcoma virus growth in tissue cultures by *Mycoplasma orale. J. Bacteriol.* **90:**934–940.

60. **Stuart, P. M., G. H. Cassell, and J. G. Woodward.** 1989. Induction of class II MHC antigen expression in the macrophages by Mycoplasma species. *J. Immunol.* **142:**3392–3399.

61. **Stuart, P. M., G. H. Cassell, and J. G. Woodward.** 1990. Mycoplasma induction of class II MHC antigens, possible role in autoimmunity. *Zentralbl. Bakteriol. Suppl.* **20:**570–577.

62. **Teh, H. S., M. Ho, and W. R. McMaster.** 1985. Isolation and characterization of novel suppressor T cells from murine fetal thymus. *J. Immunol.* **135:**1582–1588.

63. **Teh, H. S., M. Ho, and L. D. Williams.** 1988. Suppression of cytotoxic responses by a supernatant factor derived from *Mycoplasma hyorhinis*-infected mammalian cell lines. *Infect. Immun.* **56:**197–203.

64. **Tumang, J. R., D. N. Posnett, B. C. Cole, M. K. Crow, and S. M. Friedman.** 1990. Helper T cell-dependent human B cell differentiation mediated by a mycoplasmal superantigen bridge. *J. Exp. Med.* **171:**2153–2158.

65. **Vasudevachari, M. B., T. C. Mast, and N. P. Salzman.** 1990. Suppression of HIV-1 reverse transcriptase activity by mycoplasma contamination of cell cultures. *AIDS Res. Hum. Retroviruses* **6:**411–416.

66. **Wayner, E. A., and C. G. Brooks.** 1984. Induction of NKCF-like activity in mixed lymphocyte tumor cell culture: direct involvement of mycoplasma infection of tumor cells. *J. Immunol.* **132:**2135–2142.

67. **Williamson, J. S. P., J. K. Davis, and G. H. Cassell.** 1986. Polyclonal activation of rat splenic lymphocytes after in vivo administration of *Mycoplasma pulmonis* and its relation to in vitro response. *Infect. Immun.* **52:**594–599.

68. **Wright, K.** 1990. Mycoplasmas in the AIDS spotlight. *Science* **248:**682–683.

69. **Yiu, S., and M. Yamazaki.** 1986. Induction of macrophage growth by lipids. *J. Immunol.* **136:**1334–1338.

VI. MOLECULAR BASIS OF MYCOPLASMA PATHOGENICITY

27. Pathogenic Determinants and Mechanisms

VICTOR V. TRYON and JOEL B. BASEMAN

INTRODUCTION

The virulence process of mycoplasma pathogens such as *Mycoplasma pneumoniae* is undeniably complex. The infected eucaryotic host will certainly be found to provide or compete for metabolic substrates such as lipid precursors and preformed purines and pyrimidines (see chapters 13 and 14), and the mycoplasmas are known to evade, as well as modulate, the accompanying host immune response (see chapters 28 and 29). However, our discussion of the determinants and mechanisms involved in the virulence process of the pathogenic mycoplasmas will emphasize the early events in the host-parasite interaction. These early events include adherence to host cells and elaboration of metabolic products that may injure or otherwise interfere with host metabolism. Our emphasis will be on the organisms and processes best known to us, that is, *M. pneumoniae* and *M. genitalium* and specific attachment to host cells. In addition, we intend to pay special attention to those areas that have not been well reviewed previously, such as the generation of oxygen radicals by mycoplasmas and developments in AIDS-related mycoplasmas.

Virulence of even these relatively simple organisms with limited genome size (on the order of one-sixth the size of the *Escherichia coli* genome) will probably be measured not through the effects of single peptides but rather through the summation of expression of a multitude of gene products such as adhesins, nutrient receptors, mitogens, polysaccharide polymers, and metabolic intermediates. The involvement of many individual virulence determinants prompts questions concerning the presence of integrated control mechanisms. However, even though coordinate control of the expression of protein adhesins in *M. pneumoniae* has been observed (102), little is known generally about global responses of mycoplasmas to changing host microenvironments. In fact, some of the long-lasting pathology following infection by mycoplasmas may be induced long after the organisms have been suppressed or cleared by the host response.

ADHERENCE TO HUMAN CELLS

Several flask-shaped mycoplasmas parasitic for the respiratory and urogenital tracts of humans and other animals have been reported (66, 98). The narrowed tip of these unique procaryotes appears to mediate attachment to human cells through the clustering of the mycoplasmal adhesins. The recent observation of significant DNA and protein similarities between the adhesins previously identified for *M. pneumoniae* and *M. genitalium* (55, 82, 139) and the potential adhesins of other mycoplasma species (53) suggests a family of putative adhesins whose continued study in *M. pneumoniae* and *M. genitalium* would be both instructive and illustrative for the mycoplasmas in general.

The extraordinary tip-oriented attachment of *M. pneumoniae* to tracheal epithelium was first described in 1973 (49, 50). Cytopathology was positively correlated with the number of adherent organisms and length of coincubation. Only recently has the molecu-

Victor V. Tryon and Joel B. Baseman • Department of Microbiology, University of Texas Health Science Center at San Antonio, 7703 Floyd Curl Drive, San Antonio, Texas 78284-7758.

lar basis for this polar attachment mechanism become even partially understood. Protein P1 (approximately 170 kDa) was implicated as a major adhesin in 1977, when studies revealed that mild trypsin treatment of *M. pneumoniae* resulted in the loss of P1 and the concomitant reduced adherence of mycoplasmas to eucaryotic cells (76, 81). When trypsin-treated mycoplasmas were transferred to new media and allowed to grow, adherence to host cells was restored along with the regeneration of mycoplasma proteins, including P1 (80, 81). Krause and Baseman first demonstrated selective binding of solubilized, radiolabeled P1 to glutaraldehyde-fixed host cells (101). Several groups independently localized P1 to the specialized tip of *M. pneumoniae* (14, 64, 79). Visual evidence for the clustering of P1 on the tip in virulent (i.e., adherent) *M. pneumoniae* and the failure of nonadherent organisms to cluster P1 was provided by immunoelectron microscopy by Baseman et al. (14). Further support for the functional role of P1 as an adhesin was obtained by using monoclonal and monospecific antibodies to P1 (and Fab fragments of these antibodies) to block adherence of *M. pneumoniae* to hamster respiratory epithelium and sheep erythrocytes (101). Antibodies randomly produced against other proteins from *M. pneumoniae* had no effect on attachment.

The expression of P1 alone, however, is not sufficient for adherence of *M. pneumoniae* to host cells. Comparative adherence assays and one- and two-dimensional protein profiles of wild-type *M. pneumoniae*, spontaneously arising nonadhering mutants, and the cognate revertants demonstrated four classes of noncytadhering mutants. Each mutant class varied in the expression of a small number of proteins (one to four peptides) (16, 100, 102). These experiments provided suggestive evidence for the involvement of multiple proteins, in addition to P1, in the adherence process.

One example of an additional protein involved in cytadherence is P30. As with P1, antibodies to P30 blocked adherence of *M. pneumoniae* to erythrocytes (16, 140). P30, like P1, is actively clustered at the tip of virulent, cytadhering *M. pneumoniae* (16). Later work showed that P30 shares considerable DNA and protein sequence similarities with P1 (54, 184).

Analogous adherence strategies were used to implicate a 140-kDa protein, P140, in the adherence of the then newly discovered *M. genitalium* (198). *M. genitalium* exhibited considerable serologic cross-reactivity with *M. pneumoniae* and adhered to human cells in a similar tip-mediated, sialic acid-dependent manner (55, 112, 114, 187, 198). As with adhesin P1, P140 was shown to be surface accessible and clustered at the tip of virulent organisms (82, 138, 139). Although not all monoclonal antibodies to P140 from *M. genitalium* recognized the P1 adhesin from *M. pneumoniae*, one class of anti-P140 monoclonal antibodies not only recognized P1 but also blocked cytadherence of *M. pneumoniae* (139). The structural basis for this finding will be discussed below.

Strong evidence exists to suggest that other proteins from *M. pneumoniae* and *M. genitalium* are involved in the cytadherence process. Other adhesin candidates are under investigation in several laboratories. As with our initial attempts in the molecular characterization of P1 (193), studies based on the expression of putative adhesins of these human pathogens in recombinant hosts continue to be hampered by the differences in the molecular biology of the mycoplasmas and *E. coli* (see chapter 19).

Several intriguing aspects about adhesins P1, P140, and P30 remain to be resolved. First, the cognate host ligands for the mycoplasmal adhesins have not been identified. Characterization of the eucaryotic side of this adhesin receptor question is under study by Loveless and Feizi (126) and others (73, 104, 115, 160). Although the host receptor for P1 has yet to be conclusively identified, the binding domain(s) within P1 has been characterized. Using monoclonal and monospecific antibodies to P1 that blocked attachment of *M. pneumoniae* to host cells and phage subclones expressing small fragments of the P1 structural gene, Dallo et al. (58) localized a receptor domain on P1 to 13 amino acids near the carboxy terminus of the mycoplasma adhesin. Involvement of other domains of the P1 protein has been suggested (74).

Still to be resolved is the molecular basis for the interaction between P1 and the Triton X-100-insoluble cytoskeletal shell observed in *M. pneumoniae* (88, 132, 135). The role that these interactions may play in clustering the adhesins at the tip of virulent mycoplasmas remains undetermined.

Other intriguing questions remain unresolved as well. Very shortly after the implication of P1 as an important adhesin, Krause and coworkers (103) reported the collection of spontaneously arising, noncytadhering mutants of *M. pneumoniae* at a high frequency (10^{-2} to 10^{-3} mutants per generation). Although these mutants showed variations in several peptides, fully virulent revertants expressing the entire complement of adherence-related peptides were obtained at a considerably lower frequency (102). The data suggest the possibility of coordinate expression of these adherence-related peptides, which is consistent with the observations of Inamine et al. (85) and Sperker et al. (179) for a P1 operon in *M. pneumoniae*.

Frequent mutations within the structural gene for P1 itself may occur. In our initial characterization of P1, we observed that as much as two-thirds of the structural gene for P1 could be found in multiple copies in the limited genome of *M. pneumoniae* (181, 184). The cell binding domain of P1 identified by Dallo et al. (58) was in a unique, or single-copy, region. Recent examination of P1 structural genes from different clinical isolates revealed major differences in the nucleotide sequences that resulted in significant changes in the amino acid compositions of cytadhesin P1 (57, 182, 183). As might be predicted, the single-copy regions remained conserved, while the multiple-copy regions of the P1 structural gene displayed considerable sequence divergency. Gerstenecker and Jacobs (74) have suggested that the assembled P1 adhesin-binding site not only consists of the 13-amino-acid region encoded by a single-copy segment of the gene (58, 101) but also includes additional peptide loops encoded by multicopy P1 structural fragments. This suggestion reinforces the postulate by Su et al. (181, 182) that sequence diversity generated by genetic recombination within the structural gene for P1 and P1-related sequences may affect not only immunogenicity of P1 but, more importantly, the cytadherence of *M. pneumoniae* and thus ultimately tissue tropism and pathobiology.

The genetic basis for the similarities between adhesins P1 of *M. pneumoniae* and P140 of *M. genitalium* was demonstrated by Dallo et al. (55, 56) and Inamine et al. (84). In addition to unique sequences, these two adhesins share stretches of substantial (>70%) DNA similarity. One such region of DNA similarity encodes the single-copy, 13-amino-acid host cell-binding domain of P1. This observed conservation of structure was important since it was shown earlier that monoclonal antibodies to P140 of *M. genitalium* could block attachment of *M. pneumoniae* to host eucaryotic cells (139).

If these two organisms have similar cell-binding domains, a common tissue tropism could then be expected. *M. genitalium* was first isolated in 1980 from the urethra of patients with nongonococcal urethritis (198), and it was generally assumed that the genitourinary tract was the principal site of colonization of this organism in humans. However, when Baseman and colleagues (15) examined mycoplasma isolates obtained years earlier from patients hospitalized with pneumonia, the isolates were found to be mixtures of both *M. pneumoniae* and *M. genitalium*. This discovery was made possible by the identification of DNA and amino acid sequences unique to P1 and P140 (55, 56). The coisolation of *M. pneumoniae* and *M. genitalium* supports the concept of similar structural properties of mycoplasma adhesins resulting in analogous biological functions such as tissue tropism. Recent work suggests that there may exist a family of P1-like adhesins among the pathogenic mycoplasmas, including *M. gallisepticum* and others (33, 53).

The adhesins of *M. pneumoniae* and *M. genitalium* share more than just a common cell-binding domain. In addition, and perhaps equally importantly, these mycoplasmal protein adhesins share striking similarities over short amino acid stretches with human and other mammalian proteins such as extracellular matrix peptides and major histocompatibility complex (MHC) polymers (184; unpublished data). These similarities may be responsible for triggering an anti-self immune response in the parasitized host. This immune response may account for the autoimmunelike manifestations reported with mycoplasma infections (22, 24, 113, 144, 209). The role that these similar epitopes may play in provoking a cross-reactive immune response remains to be tested experimentally, but it is interesting to note that a similar relationship between human immunodeficiency virus (HIV) and immune cell dysfunctions has recently been suggested (75, 77, 96).

MECHANISMS OF OXIDATIVE DAMAGE

Many biochemical processes, including general membrane toxicity (70, 71), phospholipases (165), and ATPase, have been suggested as the cause of epithelial membrane cytotoxicity induced by the pathogenic mycoplasmas. However, since the discovery that the hemolysin of *M. pneumoniae* and other mycoplasmas is hydrogen peroxide (178), it has been postulated that mycoplasma virulence may be due to reactive oxygen molecules secreted by these closely host cell associated organisms. The most immediate and visible consequences of the close approximation of the eucaryotic epithelial membrane by the pathogenic mycoplasmas

are localized tissue disruption and subsequent disorganization (28, 49, 50). It is these local cytotoxic effects which may best be explained by the production of highly reactive oxygen molecules.

Despite the demonstration that hemadsorption and virulence are separable events in *M. pneumoniae* (108, 116, 117, 210), it seems clear that cytadherence and virulence will remain proximal events for the major protean manifestations of respiratory disease. Consequently, the virulence properties of importance in addition to adherence (reviewed above) would appear to be those that act over a short distance and with cumulative rather than overwhelming effects, as has been observed for ciliary activity by Collier and Baseman (49) and Cherry and Taylor-Robinson (30). Although not considered here, these assumptions may have important relevance to extrapulmonary disease such as cerebral, myocardial, rheumatoid, and dermatological disorders reported in association with *M. pneumoniae* (29).

Lecce and Morton (107) suggested an oxygen-terminated respiratory chain and the presence of catalase in pleuropneumonialike organisms isolated from humans. Although an intact, full-length respiratory chain was confirmed for *M. hominis* 07 (now called *Mycoplasma arthritidis* 07) by VanDemark (200) and VanDemark and Smith (201), Pollack and coworkers (152, 154) later found no evidence for iron-containing cytochromes in *M. pneumoniae* or any other mycoplasma. Low and Zimkus (129) found H_2O_2 formation associated only with flavin mononucleotide-dependent $NADH_2$ oxidase partially purified from cell extracts of *M. pneumoniae*. It appears to be generally accepted now that the production of peroxide by mycoplasmas is an expected consequence of the characteristic, flavin-terminated electron transport chain.

Over 25 years ago, Somerson et al. (178) reported the identification of the *M. pneumoniae* and *Acholeplasma* (then called *Mycoplasma*) *laidlawii* hemolysins as hydrogen peroxide. Earlier work by the same group had demonstrated the oxygen-dependent production of a nonprotein, low-molecular-weight hemolysin (177). Their initial discovery included the suggestion that the toxicity of *M. pneumoniae* for erythrocytes, as well as respiratory tissues, was due to the production of peroxide. Identification of the hemolysin of *M. pneumoniae* as a peroxide was accompanied by the first visual confirmation of hemadsorption of guinea pig erythrocytes to colonies of *M. pneumoniae*. Hemadsorption by *M. pneumoniae* had been briefly reported a year earlier by Del Giudice and Pavia (59). Interestingly, in this abstract, the authors noted that hemadsorption was later followed by lysis of the erythrocytes.

Cohen and Somerson (41) discovered that the formation of hydrogen peroxide by *M. pneumoniae* was stimulated by glucose. On the basis of previous work of Cohen (36) and Cohen and Hochstein (37–40) with human erythrocyte enzymes, these investigators suggested that the rate of peroxide formation by *M. pneumoniae* was sufficient to result in oxidative damage to the erythrocytes. Observed cell damage included the loss of reduced glutathione, denaturation of hemoglobin, peroxidation of erythrocyte lipids, and eventually lysis of the erythrocytes.

Shortly after their initial discovery, Cohen and Somerson (42) reported the paradoxical presence of peroxidaselike activity in *M. pneumoniae*. This finding, however, explained the lack of accumulation of hydrogen peroxide in growth medium (42). No endogenous catalase activity was detected in *M. pneumoniae*. The loss of peroxide was instead attributed to a dynamic interplay between the secretion and destruction of hydrogen peroxide by mycoplasmas. This presumption foreshadowed the difficulties of studying the effects of highly reactive oxygen molecules in a complex environment rich in enzymes and lipids. In fact, the new catalase capture method proposed in that report was described by Cohen and Somerson as mimicking the situation in vivo, where H_2O_2 secreted by mycoplasmas impinged on and reacted with adjacent tissue (42).

In the same year as the report by Somerson et al. Low and colleagues briefly reported the production of hydrogen peroxide by *M. pneumoniae* (127, 128). Just after the original report by Somerson et al. (178), Thomas and Bitensky (191) independently reported the reduction of turkey and human hemoglobin by hydrogen peroxide formed by the avian respiratory pathogen *M. gallisepticum*. From these reports, it appeared as though peroxide formation might be a general characteristic as well as a specific virulence attribute of the mycoplasmas.

The first survey of peroxide activity of *Mycoplasma* species appeared 2 years later. Cole and colleagues (46) reported the catalase-inhibitable hemolytic activity of *M. pneumoniae*, *M. fermentans*, *M. salivarium*, *M. orale*, *M. arthritidis*, *M. pulmonis*, *M. neurolyticum*, and *M. gallisepticum*. In contrast, hemolytic activity that was not inhibited by catalase was reported for *M. hominis*, *M. mycoides* subsp. *capri*, and *M. bovigenitalium* (46). These studies revealed that guinea pig erythrocytes, which are low in endogenous catalase, were the most sensitive markers for hemolytic activity, while rabbit erythrocytes, which are high in catalase, were the least sensitive. Sobeslavsky and Chanock (176) reported similar findings in their survey of several mycoplasmas; however, they found that the characteristic narrow zone of hemolysis produced by *M. hominis* was inhibitable with catalase embedded in the agar overlay. Interestingly, all of the catalase-inhibitable hemolysins except the hemolysin of *M. salivarium* were also inhibited by peroxidase. Although sensitive to catalase, the hemolytic activity of *M. salivarium* was unaffected by 1,000 units of added peroxidase per ml.

The first test of the role of the peroxide hemolysins and host-produced catalase in virulence was reported by Brennan and Feinstein for *M. pulmonis* in normal, acatalasemic, and acatalic mice (26). In vitro studies showed that catalase in the culture medium stimulated the growth of *M. pulmonis* at 37°C and prolonged survival of the organism by up to 48 h at 25°C. Also, hydrogen peroxide production contributed to the overall virulence of this organism for mice. That is, more acatalic mice than normal or acatalasemic mice developed *M. pulmonis*-induced pneumonia at 3 days postinfection. The acatalic mice had more severe disease as well. In contrast and perhaps surprisingly, at day 5 after inoculation of *M. pulmonis*, fewer pneumonias occurred in the acatalic mice than in normal mice, which were more severely affected. Brennan and Feinstein suggested that H_2O_2 secretion by *M. pulmonis* in these catalase-deficient mice was overwhelmingly suicidal to the mycoplasma colonizers. In other words,

the lack of host catalase in the acatalic mice caused *M. pulmonis* to be overcome by its own production of hydrogen peroxide. According to these investigators, this unexpected difference was due to protection afforded to *M. pulmonis* by host catalase, which allowed the delayed elaboration of additional mycoplasma-generated toxic substances. Among other alternative explanations not explored at the time of this report is the possibility that the accumulated products of the catalase reaction (e.g., singlet oxygen) may have proven more harmful than the substrate hydrogen peroxide alone. The toxic effect of self-generated oxygen molecules on mycoplasmas will be considered later.

Chicken tracheal organ cultures were utilized by Cherry and Taylor-Robinson to confirm the role of hydrogen peroxide in the inactivation of ciliary activity caused by *M. mycoides* subsp. *capri* (30). The B3 strain of *M. mycoides* was compared with strains of *M. gallisepticum* in the same model system (31). Ciliostasis was inhibited by addition of catalase for *M. capri*, but not for the strains of *M. gallisepticum* tested. Cherry and Taylor-Robinson noted that chicken organ culture controls without organisms generated significant but varying levels of peroxide. Background activity thus obscured the effects that these organisms might have in this model system.

The ciliostatic activity could be induced by the addition of exogenous hydrogen peroxide in amounts similar to those generated by the mycoplasmas. Addition of catalase to the organ cultures resulted in delayed onset of ciliostasis. The presence of other unknown toxin or factors in the growth medium seemed unlikely to these investigators, since organism-free, conditioned organ culture media had no effect on ciliary activity. These results reinforce the importance of the proximity of cause-and-effect relationships, since organism-free, conditioned media that presumably contain mycoplasma-generated peroxides or other toxic factors had no effect on ciliary activity.

The bioavailability of the mycoplasma-produced hydrogen peroxide and the importance of the close approximation of the host and mycoplasmas are clearly illustrated by the report of "peroxide-independent" lactoperoxidase (LPO)-catalyzed iodination of cells in culture by Lanks and Chin (106). LPO-catalyzed iodination of surface-exposed membrane proteins is a biochemical tool which requires exogenously supplied enzyme (LPO) and hydrogen peroxide. Lanks and Chin described what appeared to be peroxide-independent iodination of murine L cells in culture (106). Later, these investigators determined that *M. hyorhinis* infecting the cell cultures supplied sufficient hydrogen peroxide for efficient iodination of several cell types in the presence of exogenous LPO. Therefore, iodination appeared independently of exogenously added hydrogen peroxide. Interestingly, iodinated peptides specific to *M. hyorhinis* were not detected. This was perhaps because the concentration of mycoplasma peptides was too low for detection, but it may also imply some endogenous protective system of the mycoplasmas. Surface proteins of other mycoplasmas are certainly accessible in vitro to LPO-catalyzed iodination, as demonstrated by us and many other research groups. Early work by Amar et al. (10) on the iodination of membrane proteins of *M. hominis* and *A. laidlawii* noted that exogenous H_2O_2 was not required when LPO was used to iodinate the membranes of these organisms. In contrast, hydrogen peroxide was required to iodinate the erythrocytes used as a control.

The effect of reactive oxygen species on the pathogenic mycoplasmas generating these molecules is also an important consideration. Jacobs and colleagues demonstrated the susceptibility of the mycoplasmas pathogenic for humans to the bacteriocidal peroxidase-H_2O_2-halide system of human polymorphoneutrophils (86). However, little consensus has been reached over time on the presence or absence in mycoplasmas of two potentially protective enzymatic activities, catalase (EC 1.11.1.6) and superoxide dismutase (SOD; EC 1.15.1.1). The tolerance of mycoplasmas to reactive oxygen molecules that occur inevitably as a result of aerobic respiration by mycoplasmas (even if truncated at site 1 of the respiratory chain) has been addressed primarily through the assay of the enzymatic activities of catalase, SOD, and peroxidase. Low et al. (127, 128) reported the lack of catalase in *M. pneumoniae* at about the time of the identification of the peroxide hemolysin by Somerson et al. (178). Somerson et al. (178) and Lipman et al. (117) also failed to detect catalase activity, and Lynch and Cole (130, 131) found no catalase activity in the *Mycoplasma* species tested, including *M. pneumoniae*, *M. gallisepticum*, *M. hominis*, and *M. pulmonis*. Low-level catalase activity was reported by Meier and Habermehl for *M. arthritidis*, *M. bovigenitalium*, and *M. pulmonis*. No activity was detected in *M. capricolum* (134).

SOD catalyzes the recombination of superoxide anions to H_2O_2 and O_2. The synthesis of SOD is generally induced in procaryotes under aerobic conditions. However, Lynch and Cole (130, 131) found no evidence for SOD activity in *M. pneumoniae* or other *Mycoplasma* species despite the presence of superoxide anions in measurable amounts and despite efforts to inhibit or inactivate media enzymes that might obscure mycoplasma enzyme activity. SOD activity was found in *A. laidlawii* (130, 131). Lynch and Cole suggested that the SOD-deficient *Mycoplasma* species might make use of the SOD and catalase activities of the eucaryotic host to protect mycoplasmas from the toxic effects of the superoxide anion and its reaction products. Kirby et al. confirmed the presence of SOD activity in *A. laidlawii* and the lack of activity in *M. pneumoniae* (97). Using crude cell extracts in a multiple isoenzyme expression assay, O'Brien and colleagues (146) generally confirmed the presence of SOD activity in *Acholeplasma* species and the absence of activity in *M. pneumoniae* and other *Mycoplasma* species. Trace SOD activity was found in *M. faucium*. Most recently, Meier and Habermehl (134) have demonstrated glucose-dependent production of both superoxide and H_2O_2 in several *Mycoplasma*, *Acholeplasma*, and *Ureaplasma* species. In contrast to most previous reports, SOD was detectable in several *Mycoplasma* species. This important disparity is difficult to reconcile but may be due to the level of enzyme purification performed prior to testing. Ultrafiltration studies showed the SOD activity to be associated with high-molecular-mass filtrates. Therefore, the measured SOD activity was not due simply to the enzyme-free transition metal complexes which are hypothesized to account for observed SOD activity in lactic acid bacteria (134).

If not SOD, what may protect mycoplasmas from the effects of superoxide? Other non-SOD strategies for dealing with superoxide anions and hydrogen peroxide generated in aerobic procaryotes include altered permeability to oxygen species, modification of enzymes to reduce sensitivity to hydrogen peroxide and oxygen radicals, and substitution of metal ions in the reaction centers.

Several model systems have been proposed to test the effect of mycoplasma-produced, reactive oxygen molecules on the eucaryotic host. The first such systems included tracheal ring organ cultures (30, 31, 49, 50, 80). More recently, ciliated epithelial cells and erythrocytes (6, 8), peripheral lymphocytes (11), human trisomy 21 fibroblasts (7, 87), and newborn mice (52) have been used to study mechanisms of cytotoxicity.

Almagor and colleagues found that virulent, metabolically active *M. pneumoniae* markedly decreased host catalase activity of erythrocytes, fibroblasts, and ciliated epithelial cells (6–8). Membranes isolated from skin fibroblasts had a fourfold increase in level of malonyldialdehyde, which was used as a marker for lipid peroxidation. Lipid peroxidation of eucaryotic membranes generally results in a "leaky" membrane. The combination of mycoplasma-produced hydrogen peroxide and unchecked endogenous production of hydrogen peroxide that was not properly detoxified was suggested as the cause of host cell damage.

Peroxidase was found by Arai and coworkers to block the induction of interferon in human peripheral lymphocytes cocultivated with *M. pneumoniae* FH (11). Peroxidase inhibition was successful only early in the cultivation period. Interferon was hypothesized to be induced by the production of cross-linked aldehydes on the lymphocyte surface as a result of *M. pneumoniae* metabolism in manner analogous to the inductive action of glucose oxidase.

Almagor et al. (7) used normal and trisomy 21 skin fibroblasts to test the hypothesis that the superoxide anion produced by *M. pneumoniae* is the reactive oxygen species responsible for the inhibition of host catalase. Trisomy 21 cells were used because the copper-zinc SOD activity is 50% greater than in normal cells. When infected with *M. pneumoniae*, these cells showed reduced levels of catalase inhibition. More dramatic effects were demonstrated in normal cells, in which the addition of exogenous SOD completely protected the host fibroblast catalase from the toxic effects of colonization by *M. pneumoniae*. The addition of exogenous catalase was not protective.

Continuing their studies in *M. pneumoniae*-infected skin fibroblasts, Almagor and colleagues (5) examined the protective role of the free radical scavenger vitamin E and cellular glutathione cycles in protection against oxidative challenge by *M. pneumoniae*-induced metabolites. Vitamin E-treated cells showed decreased inhibition of catalase activity and decreased lipid peroxidation, as measured by malonyldialdehyde accumulation. Fibroblasts with chemically reduced glutathione levels or increased levels of oxidized glutathione (glutathione disulfide) due to the elevated concentration of hydrogen peroxide as a consequence of *M. pneumoniae* infection showed increased levels of lipid peroxidation. These studies supported the suggestion that superoxide or other reactive oxygen species resulted in generalized oxidative damage to the host cell. Oxidative damage is a consequence of attack both by *M. pneumoniae*-synthesized oxidants and by unchecked, endogenously (host) produced toxic oxygen molecules such as hydrogen peroxide.

It seems clear that reactive oxygen molecules fit the a priori requirements necessary to explain the special type of cytotoxicity induced by *M. pneumoniae* and related human epithelial pathogens. That is, the action is generally over short distances, and the effects are cumulative rather than overwhelming. However, the question still remains as to whether hydrogen peroxide, superoxide anion, or other reactive oxygen molecules are responsible for the observed cytotoxicity.

We have reported the avid acquisition of host lactoferrin by *M. pneumoniae* (194). The possibility exists that binding of host lactoferrin by *M. pneumoniae* stably introduces reactive iron complexes in a microenvironment that also includes locally acidic concentrations (as a consequence of *M. pneumoniae* and host metabolism), hydrogen peroxide, and superoxide anion. The conditions could result in the generation of powerful and highly reactive hydroxy radicals through Haber-Weiss-type reactions. Similar mechanisms have been postulated to contribute to the microbicidal activity of phagocytes by Klebanoff and Waltersdorph (99). The impact of these hydroxy radical oxidants on both *Mycoplasma* species and their host cells has not been tested. However, as reported in the studies cited above, the pathogenic mycoplasmas seem resistant to the effects of oxidative molecules. These highly specialized pathogens may have evolved additional unique mechanisms to protect themselves from the consequence of their self-generated oxidative challenge.

CAPSULES, SLIME LAYERS, AND OTHER SURFACE STRUCTURES

Capsules, capsulelike galactans, floccular material, mats, naps, surface projections and fibrils, and electron-dense and fuzzy layers have all been described for many pathogenic mycoplasmas, from *M. mycoides* to, most recently, *M. genitalium*. These vague descriptions apply to observations of electron micrographs of mycoplasmas that are pathogens of humans and animals. Putative capsule staining with ruthenium red has been described for *M. synoviae* (1), *M. hyopneumoniae* (185), *M. dispar* (9, 78), *Ureaplasma urealyticum* (161), *M. gallisepticum* (186), and *M. pneumoniae* (207).

These amorphous structures extend some 20 to 30 nm outside the membrane and were suggested to be responsible for hemagglutination (1), adherence (207), and general virulence (9). The actual role in the virulence process, as well as the chemical composition of these fuzzy layers, remains almost as nebulous as the structures themselves. Examination of electron micrographs of fixed and stained mycoplasmas for extramembranous material was prompted by observations of two groups suggesting carbohydrates on the surface of mycoplasmas (89, 171) and the early observation of a galactan isolated from *M. mycoides* subsp. *mycoides* (150).

A galactose-furanose polymer slime layer has been isolated directly from *M. mycoides* subsp. *mycoides* from culture medium and the blood of infected cattle

(118, 199). When the polysaccharide was parenterally injected into cattle just prior to challenge with *M. mycoides*, a prolonged mycoplasmenia was observed (118). Anaphylactoid responses were observed earlier to subcomponents of the polymer, but the likely contamination with complex growth medium components makes interpretation of these experiments difficult (83).

Robertson and Smook (161) used ruthenium red and iron dextran linked to concanavalin A to identify an electron-dense mat outside of the membrane of two strains of *U. urealyticum*. The hexose α-methyl-D-mannoside was used to block the concanavalin A-iron attachment to the surface mat. Although the importance of this layer to cytadherence was speculated by the investigators, no experimental evidence for this role was provided.

Using ruthenium red and tannic acid, Wilson and Collier (207) provided suggestive visual evidence for a mucoprotein extracellular layer surrounding *M. pneumoniae* in fixed sections of *M. pneumoniae*-infected hamster tracheal ring cultures. No discrimination was made between a host or mycoplasmal origin for the extracellular layer.

As noted above, few experiments were directed toward examining the role that these extracellular layers may play in the pathogenesis of mycoplasmal disease. An essential understanding of the basic biochemistry of synthesis, attachment, and composition of the extracellular layers is lacking. Nonetheless, a few generalizations may be made. The layers described to date all appear anionic, as demonstrated by the use of ruthenium red to visualize the layer. In addition, the layers seem intimately associated with the membrane, since the capsulelike material survives centrifugation and other basic manipulations. One exception is *M. mycoides*, which appears to produce sufficient unattached material to interfere with the initial clearance by circulating antibody of the mycoplasmas. The polysaccharides described all appear to be immunogenic only when complexed to proteins. The issue of linkage of the polysaccharides to the cell membrane is unexamined but is discussed below. The issue of the biochemical structure of this anionic layer is not resolved. Wise and Watson (208) described densely distributed proteins on *M. hyorhinis*. These proteins were later identified as constituents of a variable lipoprotein system (164). These lipoproteins are a prominent, anionic surface layer likened by Rosengarten and Wise (164) to the crystalline surface layer of other bacteria (175). Whether these or related structures contribute to the anionic surface coating visualized by electron microscopy is unknown.

MYCOPLASMAL TOXINS AND GENERAL MEMBRANE TOXICITY

The evidence for the existence of mycoplasmal exotoxins and the role for these agents in the pathogenicity of mycoplasma infections were last reviewed by Tully in 1981 (197). Described as an enigma at the time of that review, the attribution of virulence properties to classic, exportable proteins produced by the mycoplasmas seems from the vantage point of time to be largely unfounded. Very little additional work on mycoplasmal exotoxins or endotoxinlike molecules was reported in the last decade. The two most enigmatic examples of mycoplasmal toxins include the neurotropic toxins associated with *M. gallisepticum* and *M. neurolyticum* (189, 195); these examples will be discussed briefly here.

The cerebral polyarteritis induced by *M. gallisepticum* S6 that results in a rapidly fatal encephalopathy in turkey poults has been postulated to result from some neurotoxic property (190, 192). In fact, the disease in poultry appears to be a complex disease syndrome that also includes chronic persistent arthritis and immune complex deposits in the glomeruli of the kidney (34, 35). Induction of the disease requires large numbers of organisms (10^8 to 10^9 CFU per bird) delivered intravenously. The cerebral polyarteritis is found only in the presence of foci of organisms (34, 35) and is rapidly resolved with antibiotic therapy. Although the antibiotics clear the necrotic, cerebral vascular lesions, the chronic inflammatory joint disease remains, suggesting an immunological etiology.

A neurotoxin produced by *M. neurolyticum* was suggested as the cause of the encephalopathy called rolling disease (195). The disease was originally described in mice used for the intracerebral transfer of toxoplasma (169) or yellow fever virus (65). The disease was later associated with a new mycoplasma, *M. neurolyticum*, that was thought to elaborate a potent extracellular neurotoxin (2, 195). Much of the early reports characterizing an elaborated exotoxin were in error because the small size of the mycoplasmas resulted in the failure of early investigators to fully remove whole organisms by centrifugation or filtration (196). Later work using more highly purified culture filtrates found little evidence for a protein-based, non-lipo-oligosaccharide toxin (196).

METABOLIC INTERRUPTION OF HOST METABOLISM

Nucleases

The elaboration of RNA and DNA exo- or endonucleases by pathogenic members of the mollicutes in general is just one way that these organisms may compete with the host for important metabolic precursors. The requirement for preformed metabolites such as purines and pyrimidines and ribose 1-phosphate is reviewed in part III of this volume, "Metabolism and Energy Utilization" (see especially chapters 11 and 13).

All mollicutes tested contain both RNA and DNA exonuclease activities (133, 149, 153, 159). These nuclease activities accounted for the original observations by Razin and Knight (158) that undegraded RNA and DNA fulfilled the requirement for nucleotide precursors for the mycoplasmas. Razin et al. (159) demonstrated that mycoplasmal nucleases were most active on native-conformation RNA and DNA. These activities appeared to be soluble and exported, since activity was tested by observing cleared zones around colonies grown on agar plates containing complex RNA or DNA.

Given the requirement for preformed nucleotide precursors and the elaboration of extracellular nucleases by pathogenic mycoplasmas, it seems probable that host DNA or RNA presents a potential nucleotide pool to the invading mycoplasmas and thus may be a target of these exported nuclease activities. Although this assumption has not been directly tested, mycoplasma infection of mammalian cells in culture is known to result in alterations in nucleic acid metabolism of host cells (167) and chromosomal aberrations (67, 148). One interesting observation yet to be followed up is the role that host purines may play in the pathogenesis of *M. pneumoniae* infections. Gabridge and Stahl (72) observed that added adenine spared the pathological effects on hamster tracheal ring cultures infected with *M. pneumoniae*.

Arginine Deiminase

Pollock et al. (92, 155) first reported the requirement of some mycoplasmas for arginine. Schimke and Barile (172) proposed a multienzyme arginine utilization pathway that resulted in the evolution of ammonia and carbon dioxide and the production of ATP. They showed that low-level arginine utilization of cells in culture was due to contamination with mycoplasmas and proposed low-level arginine utilization as an efficient method for detecting mycoplasma contamination of mammalian cells in culture.

While testing the hypothesis that mycoplasmas had an etiological role in rheumatoid arthritis, Copperman and Morton (51) discovered that *M. hominis*, an arginine-utilizing mycoplasma, inhibited rather than stimulated lymphocytes obtained from patients with rheumatoid arthritis. Further investigation revealed that progression in mitosis was reversibly inhibited by addition of whole or lysed *M. hominis*. Although mitosis was inhibited, no chromosomal abnormalities were observed. Inhibition was relieved by washing the lymphocytes and adding fresh medium and phytohemagglutinin without mycoplasmas.

The observation that *M. hominis* inhibited phytohemagglutinin-stimulated lymphocyte induction in vitro was extended to other arginine-requiring mycoplasmas by Barile and Leventhal (13). Inhibition induced by the arginine-requiring organisms could be relieved by the addition of excess arginine. Three glucose-fermenting mycoplasmas had no effect. Simberkoff et al. (174) reported similar findings with *M. arthritidis* and four other arginine-requiring mycoplasmas, including *M. hominis*. In this study, antisera raised to whole-cell *M. arthritidis* prevented the inhibitory effects of cell extracts of all five arginine-requiring mycoplasmas, suggesting that a closely related enzyme structure was responsible for inhibition in all of the organisms tested.

Effects of mycoplasma-derived arginine deiminase on mammalian cells in culture continue to be reported. Recently, Miyazaki et al. (136) reported that mycoplasma-derived arginine deiminase inhibited the growth of murine and human tumor cells in vitro and suggested the use of this enzyme for chemotherapy against human cancers.

Phospholipase

The finding that perinatal pathogens had high levels of phospholipase activity (19) and the discovery of phospholipase activity in *M. hominis* and *A. laidlawii* B (165, 202) led De Silva and Quinn (62) to postulate that phospholipase activity of *U. urealyticum* serovars could play a role in triggering premature labor (157). Phospholipase A_1, A_2, and C activities (reviewed in reference 61) were found in cell lysates of the three *U. urealyticum* serovars tested against target liposomes containing specifically radiolabeled phospholipids (62).

Membrane-bound lysophospholipase A activity was detected in *A. laidlawii* B by van Golde et al. (202). Sonication of the membrane preparations did not release significant amounts of enzyme activity. Fatty acid products of the lipase activity were recovered only as free acids and not incorporated into the acholeplasma lipids. Thus, the utility of this enzyme activity is unclear. Rottem et al. (165) reported a heat-labile, detergent-sensitive phospholipase A activity associated with the membrane of *M. hominis*. In contrast to the previous reports, an exported phospholipase A activity was detected in *A. laidlawii* and *M. mycoides* by Bhandari and Asnani (21). This activity was also heat labile and sensitive to detergent treatment but, unlike other phospholipase activities, was found to be hemolytic against mouse, rabbit, horse, sheep, cattle, and human erythrocytes.

All of the work discussed above was performed by using relatively crude enzyme preparations such as cell lysates or simple ammonium sulfate fractions. No test of the relevance of the phospholipase activity to virulence has been reported.

EVASION OF THE IMMUNE RESPONSE

Nonimmune Receptor-Ligand Interactions between Host Immunoglobulins and Mycoplasmas

M. arginini was found by Lemke et al. (110) to bind the Fc portion of immunoglobulin. The Fc receptor activity was discovered during an attempt to produce hybridomas secreting antibody with specificity for the Fc portion of immunoglobulin. Hybridomas contaminated with *M. arginini* exhibited this Fc-binding activity regardless of the antibody specificity. This lectin-like, Fc-binding activity was found with *M. arginini* but not *M. orale*. A similar agglutinating activity in *M. fermentans* was suggested earlier as having a role in the pathogenesis of rheumatoid arthritis (206). Nonimmune binding of immunoglobulin has been described for staphylococci (protein A), streptococci, *Neisseria* spp., *Haemophilus* spp. (205), and many other microorganisms.

All five *M. hominis* strains and the one *M. arginini* strain tested by Alexander et al. (4) expressed a 95- to 105-kDa protein that reacted with Fab fragments of immunoglobulin G from horses, humans, rabbits, and goats. The mycoplasma protein bound Fab, but not Fc, fragments of immunoglobulin, suggesting an interaction more like that of *Peptococcus magnus* (25, 143) than that of protein A from staphylococci (63).

Specific characterization of these immunoglobulin-binding activities of mycoplasmas has not been performed, and no studies designed to address the role in the virulence process have been reported.

Immunoglobulin A (IgA) protease activity for human subclass A1 has been reported for several genera of pathogenic procaryotes, including *Neisseria*, *Haemophilus*, *Streptococcus*, *Bacteroides*, and *Capnocytophaga* (95, 151). Given that *Ureaplasma* species colonize mucosal surfaces and are presumably exposed to IgA, Robertson and coworkers tested for IgA1 protease activity in 14 serotypes of *U. urealyticum* and in *M. pneumoniae*, *M. hominis*, and *A. laidlawii* (162). IgA protease activity was detected in most *Ureaplasma* strains tested, including all standard serotypes and 34 of 35 wild-type strains. No activity was found in *Mycoplasma*, *Acholeplasma*, and *Spiroplasma* species. Kilian et al. also found IgA protease activity to be exclusively associated with ureaplasmas (93, 94). Kapatais-Zoumbos et al. (91) confirmed these observations and further found that specificity of the protease was restricted to IgA from the cognate host. That is, IgA proteases found in human serovars of *U. urealyticum* were specific for human IgA, and IgA proteases from canine serovars were specific for canine immunoglobulin. To these investigators, this extraordinary host specificity was strong support for the suggestion that ureaplasmas from different hosts each represent distinct species and, further, that specificity of this potential virulence factor could play a role in the host specificity of pathogenic ureaplasmas.

Antigenic Variation

Antigenic variation in the mycoplasmas and the underlying gene rearrangements responsible for these differences are discussed in chapter 28. However, the potential importance to the virulence process suggests that a brief comment is appropriate here. Several pathogenic mycoplasmas, including *M. pneumoniae* (101, 103, 139, 182), *M. hominis* (3, 147), *M. pulmonis* (204), *M. fermentans* (180), and *M. hyorhinis* (145, 163, 164), have been shown to exhibit antigenic variation of surface accessible proteins or lipid-modified proteins. The in vivo expression of these variants in each organism has been documented. Although in vitro expression of the variable lipoproteins of *M. hyorhinis* appears to be random and independent, the coordinate regulation of major surface proteins from *M. pneumoniae*, including adhesins P1 and P30, has been observed (16, 103). Thus, in vivo variation in pathogenic mycoplasmas may have a role in evasion of the host immune response, but it is more likely to be responsible for necessarily variable interactions with host cells such as specific cytadherence.

Modulation of the Immune Response

One hallmark of mycoplasma infections is the induction of chronic disease states, suggesting an inability to efficiently clear invading organisms. Regulation of the host immune response by mycoplasmas is a complex and still evolving study.

Mycoplasmas have been shown to be potent polyclonal activators of both T and B cells in vitro and in vivo (168). These effects have been shown in mice and human lymphocytes (also other species) (47) and act through MHC-restricted or unrestricted pathways. B-cell proliferation, as well as immunoglobulin production, has been documented (23). Induction of T-cell proliferation may result in the formation of cytotoxic T cells (20, 211). Activation of lymphocytes may act directly through mycoplasma proteins or glycolipids or indirectly through activation of macrophages and monocytes and the subsequent release of cytokines such as interleukin-6 (156), interleukin-1 (44, 45), and interleukin-2 (111). The mitogenic, cytokine-inducing effects of *M. arthritidis* have been associated with inflammatory rheumatic disease in rats (27) and humans with histocompatibility antigen HLA-B1 (173).

Mycoplasma-derived macromolecules have also been shown to be immunosuppressive as well as proliferative and stimulatory (43, 68, 90, 105). These suppressive effects have been specifically characterized in *M. hyorhinis* (188) and *M. arthritidis* (48). Cole and Wells (48) suggested that the soluble T-cell mitogen of *M. arthritidis* contributed to disease by causing the host to be more susceptible to invasion by *M. arthritidis*. This effect was hypothesized to be mediated through the activation of host cells cytotoxic for allogeneic proliferating host lymphocytes and not due to previously suspected virulence processes such as a direct toxic effect of the small, basic protein T-cell mitogen or arginine depletion (12).

NEW VARIATIONS ON AN OLD THEME

Lo and coworkers recently reported that a new mycoplasma may be a significant cofactor or pathogen in patients with AIDS (122) and in individuals who die suddenly of overwhelming infection without any predisposing condition (120). Earlier reports by Lo had incorrectly concluded, on the basis of size, ability to transfect eucaryotic cells, and intracellular location (cytoplasmic and nuclear), that the new pathogen was a virus (or virus like) (119, 120, 123, 125). More recent reports identified the agent as a new mycoplasma species, *M. incognitus* (122). Most recently, Saillard et al. (170) used genetic and serological tests to demonstrate that *M. incognitus* is a strain of *M. fermentans*, a previously recognized mycoplasma infrequently isolated from the human urogenital tract (166) and bone marrow (141, 142).

Isolated strains of *M. fermentans* were previously shown to be pathogenic for mice, but not rabbits, rats, guinea pigs, or hamsters, by Gabridge et al. (69). However, the lethality in mice was dependent on the injection of very high numbers of organisms (10^{10}) intravenously and was similar to gram-negative endotoxic shock. Also noted was the observation that injection of fewer organisms ($<10^7$ CFU) resulted in a chronic disease that stunted growth of the mice (69). Lo and colleagues later attributed a wasting disease in silvered leaf monkeys to infection with *M. fermentans* strain incognitus (125).

The method of the initial isolation of the AIDS-associated mycoplasma remains one of the most controversial aspects of this recent discovery. Nucleic acids were extracted from spleen and Kaposi's sarcoma tissues from two patients with AIDS by using standard techniques that included proteinase K, sodium dodecyl sulfate, and phenol. The purified nucleic acid was then transfected by using calcium phosphate into murine NIH 3T3 cells in culture. After consecutive cycles of transfection, transformed cells that were persistently infected with what appeared to be large, enveloped complex virions were obtained (119). One transformant from the second cycle of transfection with Kaposi's sarcoma DNA was isolated and used to serially infect additional NIH 3T3 cells after passage through a 0.22-μm-pore-size filter (123). Cloned DNA fragments were obtained from this transformant and used to construct DNA probes and polymerase chain reaction primers. These reagents were used to identify mycoplasma-related sequences in DNA isolated from tissues in 7 of 10 patients with AIDS who were tested.

The viruslike infectious agent (VLIA) was pathogenic for silvered leaf monkeys (125). All four monkeys injected with pelleted particles of NIH 3T3 freeze-thaw cell lysates carrying VLIA showed wasting syndromes and died in 7 to 9 months. All four animals were positive for VLIA-specific DNA. Only one of the four animals developed a prominent antibody response to VLIA.

VLIA-specific DNA and VLIA-like particles were also detected in all six HIV antibody-negative patients examined who died suddenly after presenting originally with flulike illnesses (120). No humoral response to VLIA or inflammatory response in tissues with visible VLIA particles was detected.

Recently, Lo and coworkers (121) found 19 of 26 tissues from patients with AIDS to be positive by immunohistochemistry, using monoclonal antibodies produced against the VLIA particles obtained from transfected NIH 3T3 cells. Electron microscopy and in situ hybridization using single-stranded probes to DNA unique to *M. fermentans* strain incognitus were positive as well.

Using antibodies to *M. fermentans* strain incognitus generated previously by Lo's group, Bauer et al. (18) examined renal tissues from 203 patients with AIDS. Of the renal tissues from 20 patients with AIDS-associated nephropathy, 15 showed positive staining for mycoplasmas. The authors speculated that infection with *M. fermentans* may have contributed to the pathology that led to renal failure in their study population.

Testing the hypothesis that mycoplasmas might affect the progression of AIDS through the activation of HIV-infected cells, Chowdhury et al. (32) found that heat-killed *A. laidlawii* augmented HIV production and HIV-induced syncytium formation in several human T-cell lines. Virus production was measured by enzyme-linked immunosorbent assay (ELISA) with the HIV p24 protein as the antigen.

Lemaître and colleagues (109) reported that tetracycline analogs (principally monocycline and doxycline) protected a T-lymphoblastoid cell line from HIV-induced cell lysis and promoted the emergence of chronically HIV infected cells. Although protected from lysis, the cells continued to produce infectious virus for weeks, and other cytopathologies such as giant cell formation were still observed. These investigators suggested that tetracycline analogs eliminated a tetracycline-sensitive microorganism that acted synergistically with HIV to induce cell lysis. They speculated that the microorganism was introduced into their culture system by the HIV stock (cell culture supernatant) which had been passed through 0.45-μm-pore-size filters. Virus production was followed by measuring reverse transcriptase activity, using tritiated dTTP.

When *M. fermentans* strain incognitus was similarly coinfected with HIV in a different T-cell line, thereby introducing cell-dependent variables such as virus receptor densities, Lo and colleagues (124) found that HIV replication and production were unchanged when measured by ELISA for p24 and by electron microscopy. In contrast to the antibiotic-induced cell protection observed by Lemaître et al. (109), prominent cell death was observed, syncytium formation was completely prevented, and over 90% of the reverse transcriptase activity was inhibited when T cells were cocultivated with HIV and *M. fermentans* strain incognitus. Suppression or interference with reverse transcriptase activity by contamination of cells with *M. hyorhinis* had been reported previously (203).

The old theme in this still evolving investigation is that mycoplasmas are highly cell associated, are not reliably eliminated with even prolonged antibiotic treatment, and can confound the study of cell biology in as yet unpredictable ways. The new variation on the theme is the unequivocal demonstration of *M. fermentans* as an intracellular pathogen. This observation may be extended to other potentially AIDS associated mycoplasmas such as *M. pirum* and *M. genitalium* in the near future (60, 75).

Another old theme has a new variation. It has been suggested for decades that the mycoplasmas pathogenic for humans may provoke an immune response that is effectively anti-self (22, 24, 113). Several groups are investigating the still highly controversial hypothesis that AIDS is also an immunopathological progression that results not from a classical virulence process unique to HIV but rather from the induction of a deleterious host immune response provoked by HIV macromolecules that mimic self antigens (77). In support of this concept, Kion and Hoffman (96) demonstrated that alloimmune mice produced anti-self antibodies that were also reactive to gp120 and p24 of HIV even though these animals were never exposed to the virus.

In view of this hypothesis, it seems important to reiterate our observation that stretches of adhesins P1, P140, and P30 from *M. pneumoniae* and *M. genitalium* share amino acid similarities with mammalian proteins, including human matrix and MHC. In initial attempts to understand mycoplasmas as cofactors in AIDS, Montagnier et al. (137) generated rabbit polyclonal antisera to a synthetic peptide that replicated the predicted amino acid sequence in the binding site of P140 (53, 55). When HIV-infected donor peripheral lymphocytes or an HIV-infected T-cell blast cell line were treated with a relatively low dilution (1:50 or 1:200) of the polyclonal anti-P140-binding-site peptide, replication of HIV was reduced by up to 90%. Virus production was measured by p24-specific ELISA. The molecular basis for this effect might be due to a similarity of conformation between the peptide sequence of *M. genitalium* adhesin P140 and an undetermined surface protein of the virus or the cell. Alternatively, since we have shown that a family of adhesin-related molecules exists among pathogenic mycoplasmas, it may be that the effects of the antiadhesin sera are to inhibit undefined interactions between contaminating mycoplasmas and target cells. The effect of the antibody-antigen interaction was a

reduction in the triggering of viral replication. Reduced viral replication resulted in a concomitant sparing of host cells, which remained chronically infected with HIV but continued to produce virus at a substantially lower, sublethal level.

The actual role of any of these cofactor mechanisms in the development of immunodeficiency diseases (HIV associated or not) remains to be proven experimentally (17).

REFERENCES

1. **Ajufo, J. C., and K. G. Whithear.** 1978. Evidence for a ruthenium red-staining extracellular layer as the haemagglutinin of the WVU 1853 strain of *Mycoplasma synoviae. Aust. Vet. J.* **54:**502–504.

2. **Aleu, F., and L. Thomas.** 1966. Studies of PPLO infection. III. Electron microscopic study of brain lesions caused by *Mycoplasma neurolyticum* toxin. *J. Exp. Med.* **124:**1083–1088.

3. **Alexander, A. G.** 1987. Analysis of protein antigens of *Mycoplasma hominis*: detection of polypeptides involved in the human immune response. *Isr. J. Med. Sci.* **23:**608–612.

4. **Alexander, A. G., H. R. Lowes, and G. K. Kenny.** 1991. Identification of a mycoplasmal protein which binds immunoglobulins nonimmunologically. *Infect. Immun.* **59:**2147–2151.

5. **Almagor, M., I. Kahane, C. Gilon, and S. Yatziv.** 1986. Protective effects of the glutathione redox cycle and vitamin E on cultured fibroblasts infected by *Mycoplasma pneumoniae. Infect. Immun.* **52:**240–244.

6. **Almagor, M., I. Kahane, J. M. Wiesel, and S. Yatziv.** 1985. Human ciliated epithelial cells from nasal polyps as an experimental model for *Mycoplasma pneumoniae* infection. *Infect. Immun.* **48:**552–555.

7. **Almagor, M., I. Kahane, and S. Yatziv.** 1984. Role of superoxide anion in host cell injury induced by *Mycoplasma pneumoniae* infection. A study in normal and trisomy 21 cells. *J. Clin. Invest.* **73:**842–847.

8. **Almagor, M., S. Yatziv, and I. Kahane.** 1983. Inhibition of host cell catalase by *Mycoplasma pneumoniae*: a possible mechanism for cell injury. *Infect. Immun.* **41:**251–256.

9. **Almeida, R. A., and R. F. Rosenbusch.** 1991. Capsule-like surface material of *Mycoplasma dispar* induced by in vitro growth in culture with bovine cells is antigenically related to similar structures expressed in vivo. *Infect. Immun.* **59:**3119–3125.

10. **Amar, A., S. Rottem, and S. Razin.** 1974. Characterization of the mycoplasma membrane proteins. IV. Disposition of proteins in the membrane. *Biochim. Biophys. Acta* **352:**228–244.

11. **Arai, S., T. Munakata, and K. Kuwano.** 1983. Mycoplasma interaction with lymphocytes and phagocytes: role of hydrogen peroxide released from *M. pneumoniae. Yale J. Biol. Med.* **56:**631–638.

12. **Atkin, C. L., B. C. Cole, G. J. Sullivan, L. R. Washburn, and B. B. Wiley.** 1986. Stimulation of mouse lymphocytes by a mitogen derived from *Mycoplasma arthritidis.* V. A small basic protein from culture supernatants is a potent T cell mitogen. *J. Immunol.* **137:**1581–1589.

13. **Barile, M. F., and B. G. Leventhal.** 1968. Possible mechanism for mycoplasma inhibition of lymphocyte transformation induced by phytohaemagglutinin. *Nature* (London) **219:**751–752.

14. **Baseman, J. B., R. M. Cole, D. C. Krause, and D. K. Leith.** 1982. Molecular basis for cytadsorption of *Mycoplasma pneumoniae. J. Bacteriol.* **151:**1514–1522.

15. **Baseman, J. B., S. F. Dallo, J. G. Tully, and D. L. Rose.** 1988. Isolation and characterization of *Mycoplasma gen-*

italium strains from the human respiratory tract. *J. Clin. Microbiol.* **26:**2266–2269.

16. **Baseman, J. B., J. Morrison-Plummer, D. Drouillard, V. V. Tryon, and S. C. Holt.** 1987. Identification of a 32 kDa protein of *Mycoplasma pneumoniae* associated with hemadsorption. *Isr. J. Med. Sci.* **23:**474–479.

17. **Baseman, J. B., and R. Quackenbush.** 1990. Preliminary assessment of AIDS-associated mycoplasmas. *ASM News* **56:**5–9.

18. **Bauer, F. A., D. J. Wear, P. Angritt, and S.-C. Lo.** 1991. *Mycoplasma fermentans* (incognitus strain) infection in the kidneys of patients with acquired immunodeficiency syndrome and associated nephropathy: a light microscopic, immunohistochemical, and ultrastructural study. *Hum. Pathol.* **22:**63–69.

19. **Bejar, R., V. Curbelo, C. Davis, and L. Gluck.** 1981. Premature labour. II. Bacterial sources of phospholipase. *Obstet. Gynecol.* **57:**479–482.

20. **Bekoff, M. C., B. C. Cole, and H. M. Grey.** 1987. Studies on the mechanism of stimulation of T cells by the *Mycoplasma arthritidis*-derived mitogen. Role of class IIIE molecules. *J. Immunol.* **139:**3189–3194.

21. **Bhandari, S., and P. J. Asnani.** 1989. Characterization of phospholipase A_2 of *Mycoplasma* species. *Folia Microbiol.* **34:**294–301.

22. **Biberfeld, G.** 1971. Antibodies to brain and other tissues in cases of *Mycoplasma pneumoniae* infection. *Clin. Exp. Immunol.* **8:**319–333.

23. **Biberfeld, G., and E. Gronowicz.** 1976. *Mycoplasma pneumoniae* is a polyclonal B-cell activator. *Nature* (London) **261:**238–239.

24. **Biberfeld, G., and G. Sterner.** 1976. Smooth muscle antibodies in *Mycoplasma pneumoniae* infection. *Clin. Exp. Immunol.* **24:**287–291.

25. **Björck, L.** 1988. Protein L: a novel bacterial cell wall protein with affinity for Ig L chains. *J. Immunol.* **140:**1194–1197.

26. **Brennan, P. C., and R. N. Feinstein.** 1969. Relationship of hydrogen peroxide production by *Mycoplasma pulmonis* to virulence for catalase-deficient mice. *J. Bacteriol.* **98:**1036–1040.

27. **Cannon, G. W., B. C. Cole, J. R. Ward, J. L. Smith, and E. J. Eichwald.** 1988. Arthritogenic effects of *Mycoplasma arthritidis* T cell mitogen in rats. *J. Rheumatol.* **15:**735–741.

28. **Carson, J. L., A. M. Collier, and S.-C. S. Hu.** 1980. Ultrastructural observations on cellular and subcellular aspects of experimental *Mycoplasma pneumoniae* disease. *Infect. Immun.* **29:**1117–1124.

29. **Cassell, G. H., and B. C. Cole.** 1981. Mycoplasmas as agents of human disease. *N. Engl. J. Med.* **304:**80–89.

30. **Cherry, J. D., and D. Taylor-Robinson.** 1970. Growth and pathogenesis of *Mycoplasma mycoides* var. *capri* in chicken embryo tracheal organ cultures. *Infect. Immun.* **2:**431–438.

31. **Cherry, J. D., and D. Taylor-Robinson.** 1970. Peroxide production by mycoplasmas in chicken tracheal organ cultures. *Nature* (London) **228:**1099–1100.

32. **Chowdhury, M. I. H., T. Munakata, Y. Koyanagi, S. Kobayashi, S. Arai, and N. Yamamoto.** 1990. Mycoplasma can enhance HIV replication in vitro: a possible cofactor responsible for the progression of AIDS. *Biochem. Biophys. Res. Commun.* **170:**1365–1370.

33. **Clyde, W. A., Jr., and P. C. Hu.** 1986. Antigenic determinants of the attachment protein of *Mycoplasma pneumoniae* shared by other pathogenic *Mycoplasma* species. *Infect. Immun.* **51:**690–692.

34. **Clyde, W. A., and L. Thomas.** 1973. Pathogenesis studies in experimental mycoplasma disease: *M. gallisepticum* infections of turkeys. *Ann. N.Y. Acad. Sci.* **225:**413–424.

35. **Clyde, W. A., and L. Thomas.** 1973. Tropism of *Mycoplasma gallisepticum* for arterial walls. *Proc. Natl. Acad. Sci. USA* **70:**1545–1549.

36. **Cohen, G.** 1966. On the generation of hydrogen peroxide in erythrocytes by acetylphenylhydrazine. *Biochem. Pharmacol.* **15:**1775–1782.

37. **Cohen, G., and P. Hochstein.** 1961. Glucose-6-phosphate dehydrogenase and detoxication of hydrogen peroxide in human erythrocytes. *Science* **134:**1756–1757.

38. **Cohen, G., and P. Hochstein.** 1963. Glutathione peroxidase: the primary agent for the elimination of hydrogen peroxide in erythrocytes. *Biochemistry* **2:**1420–1428.

39. **Cohen, G., and P. Hochstein.** 1964. Generation of hydrogen peroxide in erythrocytes by hemolytic agents. *Biochemistry* **3:**895–900.

40. **Cohen, G., and P. Hochstein.** 1965. *In vivo* generation of H_2O_2 in mouse erythrocytes by hemolytic agents. *J. Pharmacol. Exp. Ther.* **147:**139–143.

41. **Cohen, G., and N. L. Somerson.** 1967. *Mycoplasma pneumoniae*: hydrogen peroxide secretion and its possible role in virulence. *Ann. N.Y. Acad. Sci.* **143:**85–87.

42. **Cohen, G., and N. L. Somerson.** 1969. Glucose-dependent secretion and destruction of hydrogen peroxide by *Mycoplasma pneumoniae*. *J. Bacteriol.* **98:**547–551.

43. **Cole, B. C., L. Golightly-Rowland, J. R. Ward, and B. B. Wiley.** 1970. Immunological response of rodents to murine mycoplasmas. *Infect. Immun.* **2:**419–425.

44. **Cole, B. C., and R. N. Thorpe.** 1983. Induction of human γ interferons by a mitogen derived from *Mycoplasma arthritidis* and by phytohemagglutinin: differential inhibition with monoclonal anti-HLA.DR antibodies. *J. Immunol.* **131:**2392–2396.

45. **Cole, B. C., and R. N. Thorpe.** 1984. I-E/I-C region-associated induction of murine gamma interferon by haplotype-restricted polyclonal T-cell mitogen derived from *Mycoplasma arthritidis*. *Infect. Immun.* **43:**302–307.

46. **Cole, B. C., J. R. Ward, and C. H. Martin.** 1968. Hemolysin and peroxide activity of *Mycoplasma* species. *J. Bacteriol.* **95:**2022–2030.

47. **Cole, B. C., L. R. Washburn, G. J. Sullivan, and J. R. Ward.** 1982. Specificity of a mycoplasma mitogen for lymphocytes from human and various animal hosts. *Infect. Immun.* **36:**662–666.

48. **Cole, B. C., and D. J. Wells.** 1990. Immunosuppressive properties of the *Mycoplasma arthritidis* T-cell mitogen in vivo: inhibition of proliferative responses to T-cell mitogens. *Infect. Immun.* **58:**228–236.

49. **Collier, A. M., and J. Baseman.** 1973. Organ culture techniques with mycoplasmas. *Ann. N.Y. Acad. Sci.* **225:**277–289.

50. **Collier, A. M., and W. A. Clyde, Jr.** 1969. *Mycoplasma pneumoniae* disease pathogenesis studied in tracheal organ culture. *Fed. Proc.* **28:**616.

51. **Copperman, R., and H. E. Morton.** 1966. Reversible inhibition of mitosis in lymphocyte cultures by non-viable mycoplasma. *Proc. Soc. Exp. Biol. Med.* **123:**790–795.

52. **Crouse, D. T., G. H. Cassell, K. B. Waites, J. M. Foster, and G. Cassady.** 1990. Hyperoxia potentiates *Ureaplasma urealyticum* pneumonia in newborn mice. *Infect. Immun.* **58:**3487–3493.

53. **Dallo, S. F., and J. B. Baseman.** 1990. Cross-hybridization between the cytadhesin genes of *Mycoplasma pneumoniae* and *Mycoplasma genitalium* and genomic DNA of *Mycoplasma gallisepticum*. *Microb. Pathog.* **8:**371–375.

54. **Dallo, S. F., A. Chavoya, and J. B. Baseman.** 1990. Characterization of the gene for a 30-kilodalton adhesin-related protein of *Mycoplasma pneumoniae*. *Infect. Immun.* **58:**4163–4165.

55. **Dallo, S. F., A. Chavoya, C. J. Su, and J. B. Baseman.** 1989. DNA and protein sequence homologies detected between the adhesins of *Mycoplasma genitalium* and *Mycoplasma pneumoniae*. *Infect. Immun.* **57:**1059–1065.

56. **Dallo, S. F., J. R. Horton, C. J. Su, and J. B. Baseman.** 1989. Homologous regions shared by adhesin genes of

Mycoplasma pneumoniae and *Mycoplasma genitalium*. *Microb. Pathog.* **6:**69–73.

57. **Dallo, S. F., J. R. Horton, C. J. Su, and J. B. Baseman.** 1990. Restriction fragment length polymorphism in the cytadhesin P1 gene of human clinical isolates of *Mycoplasma pneumoniae. Infect. Immun.* **58:**2017–2020.

58. **Dallo, S. F., C. J. Su, J. R. Horton, and J. B. Baseman.** 1988. Identification of P1 gene domain containing epitope(s) mediating *Mycoplasma pneumoniae* cytadherence. *J. Exp. Med.* **167:**718–723.

59. **Del Giudice, R. A., and R. Pavia.** 1964. Hemadsorption by *Mycoplasma pneumoniae* and its inhibition with sera from patients with primary atypical pneumonia. *Bacteriol. Proc. 1964,* p. 71.

60. **Del Giudice, R. A., J. G. Tully, D. L. Rose, and R. M. Cole.** 1985. *Mycoplasma pirum* sp. nov., a terminal structured Mollicute from cell cultures. *Int. J. Syst. Bacteriol.* **35:**285–291.

61. **Dennis, E. A.** 1983. Phospholipases, p. 307–353. *In* P. D. Boyer (ed.), *The Enzymes,* vol. 16. Academic Press, Inc., New York.

62. **De Silva, N. S., and P. A. Quinn.** 1986. Endogenous activity of phospholipases A and C in *Ureaplasma urealyticum. J. Clin. Microbiol.* **23:**354–359.

63. **Dossett, J. H., G. Kronvall, R. C. Williams, Jr., and P. G. Quie.** 1969. Antiphagocytic effects of staphylococcal protein A. *J. Immun.* **103:**1405–1410.

64. **Feldner, J., U. Göbel, and W. Bredt.** 1982. *Mycoplasma pneumoniae* adhesin localized to tip structure by monoclonal antibody. *Nature* (London) **298:**765–767.

65. **Findlay, G. M., E. Klieneberger, E. O. MacCallum, and R. D. Mackenzie.** 1938. Rolling disease—new syndrome in mice associated with a pleuropneumonia-like organism. *Lancet* **ii:**1511–1513.

66. **Fischer, M., and H. Kirchhoff.** 1987. Interaction of *Mycoplasma mobile* 163K with erythrocytes. *Zentralbl. Bakteriol. Hyg. Reihe* A **266:**497–505.

67. **Fogh, J., and H. Fogh.** 1965. Chromosome changes in PPLO-infected FL human amnion cells. *Proc. Soc. Exp. Biol. Med.* **119:**233–238.

68. **Foresman, M. D., K. C. F. Sheehan, and J. E. Swierkosz.** 1989. The regulation of murine B cell differentiation. I. Nonspecific suppression caused by *Mycoplasma arginini. Cell Immun.* **123:**354–372.

69. **Gabridge, M. G., G. D. Abrams, and W. H. Murphy.** 1972. Lethal toxicity of *Mycoplasma fermentans* for mice. *J. Infect. Dis.* **125:**153–160.

70. **Gabridge, M. G., C. K. Johnson, and A. M. Cameron.** 1974. Cytotoxicity of *Mycoplasma pneumoniae* membranes. *Infect. Immun.* **10:**1127–1134.

71. **Gabridge, M. G., and W. H. Murphy.** 1971. Toxic membrane fractions from *Mycoplasma fermentans. Infect. Immun.* **4:**678–682.

72. **Gabridge, M. G., and Y. D. Stahl.** 1978. Role of adenine in pathogenesis of *Mycoplasma pneumoniae* infections of tracheal epithelium. *Med. Microbiol. Immunol.* **165:**43–55.

73. **Geary, S. J., and M. G. Gabridge.** 1987. Characterization of a human lung fibroblast receptor site for *Mycoplasma pneumoniae. Isr. J. Med. Sci.* **23:**462–468.

74. **Gerstenecker, B., and E. Jacobs.** 1990. Topographical mapping of the P1-adhesin of *Mycoplasma pneumoniae* with adherence-inhibiting monoclonal antibodies. *J. Gen. Microbiol.* **136:**471–476.

75. **Goldsmith, M. F.** 1990. Science ponders whether HIV acts alone or has another microbe's aid. *JAMA* **264:**665–666.

76. **Gorski, F., and W. Bredt.** 1977. Studies on the adherence mechanism of *Mycoplasma pneumoniae. FEMS Microbiol. Lett.* **1:**265–267.

77. **Hoffmann, G. W., T. A. Kion, and M. D. Grant.** 1991. An idiotypic network model of AIDS immunopathogenesis. *Proc. Natl. Acad. Sci. USA* **88:**3060–3064.

78. **Howard, C. J., and R. N. Gourlay.** 1974. An electron microscopic examination of certain bovine mycoplasmas stained with ruthenium red and the demonstration of a capsule on *Mycoplasma dispar. J. Gen. Microbiol.* **83:**393–398.

79. **Hu, P. C., R. M. Cole, Y. S. Huang, J. A. Graham, D. E. Gardner, A. M. Collier, and W. A. Clyde, Jr.** 1982. *Mycoplasma pneumoniae* infection: role of a surface protein in the attachment organelle. *Science* **216:**313–315.

80. **Hu, P. C., A. M. Collier, and J. B. Baseman.** 1976. Interaction of virulent *Mycoplasma pneumoniae* with hamster tracheal organ cultures. *Infect. Immun.* **14:**217–224.

81. **Hu, P. C., A. M. Collier, and J. B. Baseman.** 1977. Surface parasitism by *Mycoplasma pneumoniae* of respiratory epithelium. *J. Exp. Med.* **145:**1328–1343.

82. **Hu, P. C., U. Schaper, A. M. Collier, W. A. Clyde, Jr., M. Horikawa, Y. S. Huang, and M. F. Barile.** 1987. A *Mycoplasma genitalium* protein resembling the *Mycoplasma pneumoniae* attachment protein. *Infect. Immun.* **55:**1126–1131.

83. **Hudson, J. R., S. Buttery, and G. S. Cottew.** 1967. Investigations into the influence of the galactan of *Mycoplasma mycoides* on experimental infection with that organism. *J. Pathol. Bacteriol.* **94:**257–273.

84. **Inamine, J. M., S. Loechel, A. M. Collier, M. F. Barile, and P. C. Hu.** 1989. Nucleotide sequence of the *MgPa* (*mgp*) operon of *Mycoplasma genitalium* and comparison to the *P1* (*mpp*) operon of *Mycoplasma pneumoniae. Gene* **82:**259–267.

85. **Inamine, J. M., S. Loechel, and P. C. Hu.** 1988. Analysis of the nucleotide sequence of the P1 operon of *Mycoplasma pneumoniae. Gene* **73:**175–183.

86. **Jacobs, A. A., I. E. Low, B. B. Paul, R. R. Strauss, and A. J. Sbarra.** 1972. Mycoplasmacidal activity of peroxidase-H_2O_2-halide systems. *Infect. Immun.* **5:**127–131.

87. **Kahane, I.** 1984. *In vitro* studies on the mechanism of adherence and pathogenicity of mycoplasmas. *Isr. J. Med. Sci.* **20:**874–877.

88. **Kahane, I., S. Tucker, D. K. Leith, J. Morrison-Plummer, and J. B. Baseman.** 1985. Detection of the major adhesin P1 in triton shells of virulent *Mycoplasma pneumoniae. Infect. Immun.* **50:**944–946.

89. **Kahane, I., and J. G. Tully.** 1975. Binding of plant lectins to mycoplasma cells and membranes. *J. Bacteriol.* **128:**1–7.

90. **Kaklamanis, E., and M. Pavlatos.** 1972. The immunosuppressive effect of mycoplasma infection. I. Effect on the humoral and cellular response. *Immunology* **22:**695–702.

91. **Kapatais-Zoumbos, K., D. K. F. Chandler, and M. F. Barile.** 1985. Survey of immunoglobulin A protease activity among selected species of *Ureaplasma* and *Mycoplasma*: specificity for host immunoglobulin A. *Infect. Immun.* **47:**704–709.

92. **Kenny, G. E., and M. E. Pollock.** 1973. Mammalian cell cultures contaminated with pleuropneumonia-like organisms. *J. Infect. Dis.* **112:**7–16.

93. **Kilian, M., M. B. Brown, T. A. Brown, E. A. Freundt, and G. H. Cassell.** 1984. Immunoglobulin A1 protease activity in strains of *Ureaplasma urealyticum. Acta Pathol. Microbiol. Immun. Scand. Sect. B* **92:**61–64.

94. **Kilian, M., and E. A. Freundt.** 1984. Exclusive occurrence of an extracellular protease capable of cleaving the hinge region of human immunoglobulin A1 in strains of *Ureaplasma urealyticum. Isr. J. Med. Sci.* **20:**938–941.

95. **Kilian, M., B. Thomsen, T. E. Petersen, and H. S. Bleeg.** 1983. Occurrence and nature of bacterial IgA protease. *Ann. N.Y. Acad. Sci.* **409:**612–624.

96. **Kion, T. A., and G. W. Hoffmann.** 1991. Anti-HIV and anti-anti-MHC antibodies in alloimmune and autoimmune mice. *Science* **253:**1138–1140.

97. **Kirby, T., J. Blum, I. Kahane, and I. Fridovich.** 1980. Distinguishing between Mn-containing and Fe-containing superoxide dismutases in crude extracts of cells. *Arch. Biochem. Biophys.* **201:**551–555.

98. **Kirchhoff, H., R. Rosengarten, W. Lotz, M. Fischer, and D. Lopatta.** 1984. Flask-shaped mycoplasmas: properties and pathogenicity for man and animals. *Isr. J. Med. Sci.* **20:**848–853.

99. **Klebanoff, S. J., and A. M. Waltersdorph.** 1990. Prooxidant activity of transferrin and lactoferrin. *J. Exp. Med.* **172:**1293–1303.

100. **Krause, D. C., and J. B. Baseman.** 1982. *Mycoplasma pneumoniae* proteins which selectively bind to host cells. *Infect. Immun.* **37:**382–386.

101. **Krause, D. C., and J. B. Baseman.** 1983. Inhibition of *Mycoplasma pneumoniae* hemadsorption and adherence to respiratory epithelium by antibodies to a membrane protein. *Infect. Immun.* **39:**1180–1186.

102. **Krause, D. C., D. K. Leith, and J. B. Baseman.** 1983. Reacquisition of specific proteins confers virulence in *Mycoplasma pneumoniae. Infect. Immun.* **39:**830–836.

103. **Krause, D. C., D. K. Leith, R. M. Wilson, and J. B. Baseman.** 1982. Identification of *Mycoplasma pneumoniae* proteins associated with hemadsorption and virulence. *Infect. Immun.* **35:**809–817.

104. **Krivan, H. C., L. D. Olson, M. F. Barile, V. Ginsburg, and D. D. Roberts.** 1989. Adhesion of Mycoplasma pneumoniae to sulfated glycolipids and inhibition by dextran sulfate. *J. Biol. Chem.* **264:**9282–9288.

105. **Lai, W. C., S. P. Pakes, I. Owusu, and S. Wang.** 1989. *Mycoplasma pulmonis* depresses humoral and cell-mediated responses in mice. *Lab. Anim. Sci.* **39:**11–15.

106. **Lanks, K. W., and N. W. Chin.** 1979. Lactoperoxidase-catalyzed iodination of cell cultures infected with mycoplasma. *In Vitro* **15:**503–506.

107. **Lecce, J. G., and H. E. Morton.** 1954. Metabolic studies on three strains of pleuropneumonia-like organisms isolated from man. *J. Bacteriol.* **67:**62–68.

108. **Leith, D. K., E. J. Hansen, R. M. Wilson, D. C. Krause, and J. B. Baseman.** 1983. Hemadsorption and virulence are separable properties of *Mycoplasma pneumoniae. Infect. Immun.* **39:**844–850.

109. **Lemaître, M., D. Guétard, Y. Hénin, L. Montagnier, and A. Zerial.** 1990. Protective activity of tetracycline analogs against the cytopathic effect of the human immunodeficiency viruses in CEM cells. *Res. Virol.* **141:**5–16.

110. **Lemke, H., R. Krausse, J. Lorenzen, and B. Havsteen.** 1985. Mycoplasma infection of cell lines can simulate the expression of Fc receptors by binding of the carbohydrate moiety of antibodies. *Eur. J. Immun.* **15:**442–447.

111. **Levin, D., H. Gershon, and Y. Naot.** 1985. Production of interleukin-2 by rat lymph node cells stimulated by *Mycoplasma pulmonis* membranes. *J. Infect. Dis.* **151:**541–544.

112. **Lind, K.** 1982. Serological cross-reactions between "*Mycoplasma genitalium*" and *M. pneumoniae. Lancet* **ii:**1158–1159.

113. **Lind, K., M. Hoier-Madsen, and A. Wiik.** 1988. Autoantibodies to the mitotic spindle apparatus in *Mycoplasma pneumoniae* disease. *Infect. Immun.* **56:**714–715.

114. **Lind, K., B. Ø. Lindhardt, H. J. Schütten, J. Blom, and C. Christiansen.** 1984. Serological cross-reactions between *Mycoplasma genitalium* and *Mycoplasma pneumoniae. J. Clin. Microbiol.* **20:**1036–1043.

115. **Lingwood, C. A., P. A. Quinn, S. Wilansky, A. Nutikka, H. L. Ruhnke, and R. B. Miller.** 1990. Common sulfoglycolipid receptor for mycoplasmas involved in animal and human infertility. *Biol. Reprod.* **43:**694–697.

116. **Lipman, R. P., and W. A. Clyde, Jr.** 1969. The interrelationship of virulence, cytadsorption, and peroxide formation in *Mycoplasma pneumoniae. Proc. Soc. Exp. Biol. Med.* **131:**1163–1167.

117. **Lipman, R. P., W. A. Clyde, Jr., and F. W. Denny.** 1969. Characteristics of virulent, attenuated, and avirulent *Mycoplasma pneumoniae* strains. *J. Bacteriol.* **100:**1037–1043.

118. **Lloyd, L. C., S. H. Buttery, and J. R. Hudson.** 1971. The effect of the galactan and other antigens of *Mycoplasma mycoides* var. *mycoides* on experimental infection with that organism in cattle. *Med. Microbiol.* **4:**425–439.

119. **Lo, S.-C.** 1986. Isolation and identification of a novel virus from patients with AIDS. *Am. J. Trop. Med. Hyg.* **35:**675–676.

120. **Lo, S.-C., M. S. Dawson, P. B. Newton III, M. A. Sonoda, J. W.-K. Shih, W. F. Engler, R. Y.-H. Wang, and D. J. Wear.** 1989. Association of the virus-like infectious agent originally reported in patients with AIDS with acute fatal disease in previously healthy non-AIDS patients. *Am. J. Trop. Med. Hyg.* **41:**364–376.

121. **Lo, S.-C., M. S. Dawson, D. M. Wong, P. B. Newton III, M. A. Sonoda, W. F. Engler, R. Y.-H. Wang, J. W.-K. Shih, H. J. Alter, and D. J. Wear.** 1989. Identification of *Mycoplasma incognitus* infection in patients with AIDS: an immunohistochemical, *in situ* hybridization and ultrastructural study. *Am. J. Trop. Med. Hyg.* **41:**601–616.

122. **Lo, S.-C., J. W.-K. Shih, P. B. Newton III, D. M. Wong, M. M. Hayes, J. R. Benish, D. J. Wear, and R. Y.-H. Wang.** 1989. Virus-like infectious agent (VLIA) is a novel pathogenic mycoplasma: *Mycoplasma incognitus. Am. J. Trop. Med. Hyg.* **41:**586–600.

123. **Lo, S.-C., J. W.-K. Shih, N.-Y. Yang, C.-Y. Ou, and R. Y.-H. Wang.** 1989. A novel virus-like infectious agent in patients with AIDS. *Am. J. Trop. Med. Hyg.* **40:**213–226.

124. **Lo, S.-C., S. Tsai, J. R. Benish, J. W.-K. Shih, D. J. Wear, and D. M. Wong.** 1991. Enhancement of HIV-1 cytocidal effects in CD4+ lymphocytes by the AIDS-associated mycoplasma. *Science* **251:**1074–1076.

125. **Lo, S.-C., R. Y.-H. Wang, P. B. Newton III, N.-Y. Yang, M. A. Sonoda, and J. W.-K. Shih.** 1989. Fatal infection of silvered leaf monkeys with a virus-like infectious agent (VLIA) derived from a patient with AIDS. *Am. J. Trop. Med. Hyg.* **40:**399–409.

126. **Loveless, R. W., and T. Feizi.** 1989. Sialo-oligosaccharide receptors for *Mycoplasma pneumoniae* and related oligosaccharides of poly-N-acetyllactosamine series are polarized at the cilia and apical-microvillar domains of the ciliated cells in human bronchial epithelium. *Infect. Immun.* **57:**1285–1289.

127. **Low, I. E., M. D. Eaton, and P. Proctor.** 1965. Relation of catalase to carbohydrate metabolism of *Mycoplasma pneumoniae. Bacteriol. Proc. 1965,* p. 77.

128. **Low, I. E., M. D. Eaton, and P. Proctor.** 1968. Relation of catalase to substrate utilization by *Mycoplasma pneumoniae. J. Bacteriol.* **95:**1425–1430.

129. **Low, I. E., and S. M. Zimkus.** 1973. Reduced nicotinamide adenine dinucleotide oxidase activity and H_2O_2 formation of *Mycoplasma pneumoniae. J. Bacteriol.* **116:**346–354.

130. **Lynch, R. E., and B. C. Cole.** 1980. *Mycoplasma pneumoniae:* a pathogen which manufactures superoxide but lacks superoxide dismutase. *Proc. Fed. Eur. Biochem. Soc. Symp.* **62:**49–56.

131. **Lynch, R. E., and B. C. Cole.** 1990. *Mycoplasma pneumoniae:* a prokaryote which consumes oxygen and generates superoxide but which lacks superoxide dismutase. *Biochem. Biophys. Res. Commun.* **96:**98–105.

132. **Maniloff, J.** 1981. Cytoskeletal elements in mycoplasmas and other prokaryotes. *BioSystems* **14:**305–312.

133. **Marcus, P. I., and I. Yoshida.** 1990. Mycoplasmas produce double-stranded ribonuclease. *J. Cell. Physiol.* **143:**416–419.

134. **Meier, B., and G. G. Habermehl.** 1990. Evidence for superoxide dismutase and catalase in Mollicutes and release of reactive oxygen species. *Arch. Biochem. Biophys.* **277:**74–79.

135. **Meng, K. E., and R. M. Pfister.** 1980. Intracellular struc-

tures of *Mycoplasma pneumoniae* revealed after membrane removal. *J. Bacteriol.* **144**:390–399.

136. **Miyazaki, K., H. Takaku, M. Umeda, T. Fujita, W. Huang, T. Kimura, J. Yamashita, and T. Horio.** 1990. Potent growth inhibition of human tumor cells in culture by arginine deiminase purified from a culture medium of a mycoplasma-infected cell line. *Cancer Res.* **50**:4522–4527.

137. **Montagnier, L., D. Berneman, D. Guétard, A. Blanchard, S. Chamaret, V. Rame, J. Vanrietschoten, K. Mabrouk, and E. Bahraoui.** 1990. Inhibition de l'infectiosité de souches prototypes du VIH par des anticorps dirigés contre une séquence peptidique de mycoplasme. *C.R. Acad. Sci.* **311**:425–430.

138. **Morrison-Plummer, J., D. H. Jones, K. Daly, J. G. Tully, D. Taylor-Robinson, and J. B. Baseman.** 1987. Molecular characterization of *Mycoplasma genitalium* species-specific and cross-reactive determinants: identification of an immunodominant protein of *M. genitalium*. *Isr. J. Med. Sci.* **23**:453–457.

139. **Morrison-Plummer, J., A. Lazzell, and J. B. Baseman.** 1987. Shared epitopes between *Mycoplasma pneumoniae* major adhesin protein P1 and a 140-kilodalton protein of *Mycoplasma genitalium*. *Infect. Immun.* **55**:49–56.

140. **Morrison-Plummer, J., D. K. Leith, and J. B. Baseman.** 1986. Biological effects of anti-lipid and anti-protein monoclonal antibodies on *Mycoplasma pneumoniae*. *Infect. Immun.* **53**:398–403.

141. **Murphy, W. H., C. Bullis, L. Dabich, R. Heyn, and C. J. D. Zarafonetis.** 1970. Isolation of mycoplasma from leukemic and nonleukemic patients. *J. Natl. Cancer Inst.* **45**:243–251.

142. **Murphy, W. H., I. J. Ertel, and C. J. D. Zarafonetis.** 1965. Virus studies of human leukemia. *Cancer* **18**:1329–1344.

143. **Myhre, E. B., and M. Erntell.** 1985. A non-immune interaction between the light chain of human immunoglobulin and a surface component of a *Peptococcus magnus* strain. *Mol. Immun.* **22**:879–885.

144. **Neimark, H.** 1983. Mycoplasma and bacterial proteins resembling contractile proteins: a review. *Yale J. Biol. Med.* **56**:419–423.

145. **Notarnicola, S. M., M. A. McIntosh, and K. S. Wise.** 1990. Multiple translational products from a *Mycoplasma hyorhinis* gene expressed in *Escherichia coli*. *J. Bacteriol.* **172**:2986–2995.

146. **O'Brien, S. J., J. M. Simonson, M. W. Grabowski, and M. F. Barile.** 1981. Analysis of multiple isoenzyme expression among twenty-two species of *Mycoplasma* and *Acholeplasma*. *J. Bacteriol.* **146**:222–232.

147. **Olson, L. D., C. A. Renshaw, S. W. Shane, and M. F. Barile.** 1991. Successive synovial *Mycoplasma hominis* isolates exhibit apparent antigenic variation. *Infect. Immun.* **59**:3327–3329.

148. **Paton, G. R., J. P. Jacobs, and F. T. Perkins.** 1965. Chromosome changes in human diploid-cell cultures infected with mycoplasma. *Nature* (London) **207**:43–45.

149. **Plackett, P.** 1957. Depolymerization of ribonucleic acid by extracts of *Asterococcus mycoides*. *Biochim. Biophys. Acta* **26**:664–665.

150. **Plackett, P., and S. H. Buttery.** 1958. A galactan from *Mycoplasma mycoides*. *Nature* (London) **182**:1236–1237.

151. **Plaut, A. G.** 1983. The IgA1 proteases of pathogenic bacteria. *Annu. Rev. Microbiol.* **37**:603–622.

152. **Pollack, J. D.** 1979. Respiratory pathways and energy-yielding mechanisms, p. 187–211. *In* M. F. Barile and S. Razin (ed.), *The Mycoplasmas*, vol. 1. Academic Press, New York.

153. **Pollack, J. D., and P. J. Hoffmann.** 1982. Properties of the nucleases of Mollicutes. *J. Bacteriol.* **152**:538–541.

154. **Pollack, J. D., A. J. Merola, M. Platz, and R. L. Booth, Jr.** 1981. Respiratory associated components of Mollicutes. *J. Bacteriol.* **145**:907–913.

155. **Pollock, M. E., P. E. Treadwell, and G. E. Kenny.** 1962. Effect of amino acid depletion by PPLO on morphology of cells in culture. *Fed. Proc.* **21**:161.

156. **Quentmeier, H., E. Schmitt, H. Kirchhoff, W. Grote, and P. F. Mühlradt.** 1990. *Mycoplasma fermentans*-derived high-molecular-weight material induces interleukin-6 release in cultures of murine macrophages and human monocytes. *Infect. Immun.* **58**:1273–1280.

157. **Quinn, P. A., J. Butany, M. Chipman, J. Taylor, and W. Hannah.** 1985. A prospective study of microbial infection in stillbirths and early neonatal death. *Am. J. Obstet. Gynecol.* **151**:238–249.

158. **Razin, S., and B. C. J. G. Knight.** 1960. The effects of ribonucleic acid, and deoxyribonucleic acid on the growth of Mycoplasma. *J. Gen. Microbiol.* **22**:504–519.

159. **Razin, S., A. Knyszynski, and Y. Lifshitz.** 1964. Nucleases of Mycoplasma. *J. Gen. Microbiol.* **36**:323–331.

160. **Roberts, D. D., L. D. Olson, M. F. Barile, V. Ginsburg, and H. C. Krivan.** 1989. Sialic acid-dependent adhesion of Mycoplasma pneumoniae to purified glycoproteins. *J. Biol. Chem.* **264**:9289–9293.

161. **Robertson, J., and E. Smook.** 1976. Cytochemical evidence of extramembranous carbohydrates on *Ureaplasma urealyticum* (T-strain mycoplasma). *J. Bacteriol.* **128**:658–660.

162. **Robertson, J. A., M. E. Stemler, and G. W. Stemke.** 1984. Immunoglobulin A protease activity of *Ureaplasma urealyticum*. *J. Clin. Microbiol.* **19**:255–258.

163. **Rosengarten, R., and K. S. Wise.** 1990. Phenotypic switching in mycoplasmas: phase variation of diverse surface lipoproteins. *Science* **247**:315–318.

164. **Rosengarten, R., and K. S. Wise.** 1991. The Vlp system of *Mycoplasma hyorhinis*: combinatorial expression of distinct size variant lipoproteins generating high-frequency surface antigenic variation. *J. Bacteriol.* **173**:4782–4793.

165. **Rottem, S., M. Hasin, and S. Razin.** 1973. Differences in susceptibility to phospholipase C of free and membrane-bound phospholipids of *Mycoplasma hominis*. *Biochim. Biophys. Acta* **323**:520–531.

166. **Ruiter, M., and H. M. M. Wentholt.** 1953. Isolation of a pleuropneumonia-like organism (G-strain) in a case of fusospirillary vulvovaginitis. *Acta Derm. Venereol.* **33**:123–129.

167. **Russell, W. C.** 1966. Alterations in the nucleic acid metabolism of tissue culture cells infected by mycoplasmas. *Nature* (London) **212**:1537–1540.

168. **Ruuth, E., and F. Praz.** 1989. Interactions between mycoplasmas and the immune system. *Immunol. Rev.* **112**:134–160.

169. **Sabin, A. B.** 1938. Identification of the filtrable, transmissible neurolytic agent isolated from toxoplasma-infected tissue as a new pleuropneumonia-like microbe. *Science* **88**:189–190.

170. **Saillard, C., P. Carle, J. M. Bové, C. Bébéar, S.-C. Lo, J. W.-K. Shih, R. Y.-H. Wang, D. L. Rose, and J. G. Tully.** 1990. Genetic and serologic relatedness between *Mycoplasma fermantans* strains and a mycoplasma recently identified in tissues of AIDS and non-AIDS patients. *Res. Virol.* **141**:385–395.

171. **Schiefer, H. G., U. Gerhardt, H. Brunner, and M. Krupe.** 1974. Studies with lectins on the surface carbohydrate structures of mycoplasma membranes. *J. Bacteriol.* **120**:81–88.

172. **Schimke, R. T., and M. F. Barile.** 1963. Arginine breakdown in mammalian cell culture contaminated with pleuroneumonia-like organisms (PPLO). *Exp. Cell Res.* **30**:593–596.

173. **Seitz, M., E.-M. Lemmel, J. Homfeld, and H. Kirchner.** 1989. Enhanced interferon-gamma production by lymphocytes induced by a mitogen from *Mycoplasma*

arthritidis in patients with ankylosing spondylitis. *Rheumatol. Int.* **9:**85–90.

174. **Simberkoff, M. S., G. J. Thorbecke, and L. Thomas.** 1969. Studies of PPLO infection. V. Inhibition of lymphocyte mitosis and antibody formation. *J. Exp. Med.* **129:**1163–1181.

175. **Smit, J.** 1986. Protein surface layers of bacteria, p. 343–376. *In* M. Inouye (ed.), *Bacterial Outer Membranes as Model Systems.* John Wiley & Sons, Inc., New York.

176. **Sobeslavsky, O., and R. M. Chanock.** 1968. Peroxide formation by mycoplasmas which infect man. *Proc. Soc. Exp. Biol. Med.* **129:**531–535.

177. **Somerson, N. L., R. H. Purcell, D. Taylor-Robinson, and R. M. Chanock.** 1965. Hemolysin of *Mycoplasma pneumoniae. J. Bacteriol.* **89:**813–818.

178. **Somerson, N. L., B. E. Walls, and R. M. Chanock.** 1965. Hemolysin of *Mycoplasma pneumoniae*: tentative identification as a peroxide. *Science* **150:**226–228.

179. **Sperker, B., P. C. Hu, and R. Herrmann.** 1991. Identification of gene proucts of the P1 operon of *Mycoplasma pneumoniae. Mol. Microbiol.* **5:**299–306.

180. **Städtlander, C. T. K.-H., C. Zuhua, H. L. Watson, and G. H. Cassell.** 1991. Protein and antigen heterogeneity among strains of *Mycoplasma fermentans. Infect. Immun.* **59:**3319–3322.

181. **Su, C. J., A. Chavoya, and J. B. Baseman.** 1988. Regions of *Mycoplasma pneumoniae* cytadhesin P1 structural gene exist as multiple copies. *Infect. Immun.* **56:**3157–3161.

182. **Su, C. J., A. Chavoya, S. F. Dallo, and J. B. Baseman.** 1990. Sequence divergency of the cytadhesin gene of *Mycoplasma pneumoniae. Infect. Immun.* **58:**2669–2674.

183. **Su, C. J., S. F. Dallo, and J. B. Baseman.** 1990. Molecular distinctions among clinical isolates of *Mycoplasma pneumoniae. J. Clin. Microbiol.* **28:**1538–1540.

184. **Su, C. J., V. V. Tryon, and J. B. Baseman.** 1987. Cloning and sequence analysis of cytadhesin gene (P1) from *Mycoplasma pneumoniae. Infect. Immun.* **55:**3023–3029.

185. **Tajima, M., and T. Yagihashi.** 1982. Interaction of *Mycoplasma hyopneumoniae* with the porcine respiratory epithelium as observed by electron microscopy. *Infect. Immun.* **37:**1162–1169.

186. **Tajima, M., T. Yagihashi, and Y. Miki.** 1982. Capsular material of *Mycoplasma gallisepticum* and its possible relevance to the pathogenic process. *Infect. Immun.* **36:**830–833.

187. **Taylor-Robinson, D., F. M. Furr, and J. G. Tully.** 1983. Serological cross-reaction between *Mycoplasma genitalium* and *M. pneumoniae. Lancet* **i:**527.

188. **Teh, H.-S., M. Ho, and L. D. Williams.** 1988. Suppression of cytotoxic responses by a supernatant factor derived from *Mycoplasma hyorhinis*-infected mammalian cell lines. *Infect. Immun.* **56:**197–203.

189. **Thomas, L.** 1967. The neurotoxins of *M. neurolyticum* and *M. gallisepticum. Ann. N.Y. Acad. Sci.* **143:**218–224.

190. **Thomas, L., and M. W. Bitensky.** 1966. Studies of PPLO infection. IV. The neurotoxicity of intact mycoplasmas, and their production of toxin *in vivo* and *in vitro. J. Exp. Med.* **124:**1089–1098.

191. **Thomas, L., and M. W. Bitensky.** 1966. Methaemoglobin formation by *Mycoplasma gallisepticum*: the role of hydrogen peroxide. *Nature* (London) **210:**963–964.

192. **Thomas, L., M. Davidson, and R. T. McCluskey.** 1966. Studies of PPLO infection. I. The production of cerebral polyarteritis by *Mycoplasma gallisepticum* in turkeys; the neurotoxic property of the mycoplasma. *J. Exp. Med.* **123:**897–912.

193. **Treviño, L. B., W. G. Haldenwang, and J. B. Baseman.** 1986. Expression of *Mycoplasma pneumoniae* antigens in *Escherichia coli. Infect. Immun.* **53:**129–134.

194. **Tryon, V. V., and J. B. Baseman.** 1987. The acquisition of human lactoferrin by *Mycoplasma pneumoniae. Microb. Pathog.* **3:**437–443.

195. **Tully, J. G.** 1964. Production and biological characteristics of an extracellular neurotoxin from *Mycoplasma neurolyticum. J. Bacteriol.* **88:**381–388.

196. **Tully, J. G.** 1974. Mycoplasma neurotoxins: partial purification of the toxin from *Mycoplasma neurolyticum. Colloq. INSERM* **33:**317–324.

197. **Tully, J. G.** 1981. Mycoplasmal toxins. *Isr. J. Med. Sci.* **17:**604–607.

198. **Tully, J. G., D. Taylor-Robinson, R. M. Cole, and J. M. Bové.** 1983. *Mycoplasma genitalium*, a new species from the human urogenital tract. *Int. J. Syst. Bacteriol.* **33:**387–396.

199. **Turner, A. W.** 1962. Circulating *M. mycoides* antigen as a cause of loss of agglutination and complement fixation reactivity during acute pleuropneumonia. *Aust. Vet. J.* **38:**401.

200. **VanDemark, P. J.** 1967. Respiratory pathways in the mycoplasma. *Ann. N.Y. Acad. Sci.* **143:**77–87.

201. **VanDemark, P. J., and P. F. Smith.** 1964. Respiratory pathways in the *Mycoplasma.* II. Pathway of electron transport during oxidation of reduced nicotinamide adenine dinucleotide by *Mycoplasma hominis. J. Bacteriol.* **88:**122–129.

202. **van Golde, L. M. G., R. N. McElhaney, and L. L. M. van Deenen.** 1971. A membrane-bound lysophospholipase from *Mycoplasma laidlawii* strain B. *Biochim. Biophys. Acta* **231:**245–249.

203. **Vasudevachari, M. B., T. C. Mast, and N. P. Salzman.** 1990. Suppression of HIV-1 reverse transcriptase activity by mycoplasma contamination of cell cultures. *AIDS Res. Hum. Retroviruses* **6:**411–416.

204. **Watson, H. L., L. S. McDaniel, D. K. Blalock, M. T. Fallon, and G. H. Cassell.** 1988. Heterogeneity among strains and a high rate of variation within strains of a major surface antigen of *Mycoplasma pulmonis. Infect. Immun.* **56:**1358–1365.

205. **Widders, P. R., J. W. Smith, M. Yarnall, T. C. McGuire, and L. B. Corbeil.** 1988. Non-immune immunoglobulin binding by "*Haemophilus somnus.*" *J. Med. Microbiol.* **26:**307–311.

206. **Williams, M. H., J. Brostoff, and I. M. Roitt.** 1970. Possible role of *Mycoplasma fermentans* in pathogenesis of rheumatoid arthritis. *Lancet* **ii:**277–280.

207. **Wilson, M. H., and A. M. Collier.** 1976. Ultrastructural study of *Mycoplasma pneumoniae* in organ culture. *J. Bacteriol.* **125:**332–339.

208. **Wise, K. S., and R. K. Watson.** 1983. *Mycoplasma hyorhinis* GDL surface protein antigen p120 defined by monoclonal antibody. *Infect. Immun.* **41:**1332–1339.

209. **Wise, K. S., and R. K. Watson.** 1985. Antigenic mimicry of mammalian intermediate filaments by mycoplasmas. *Infect. Immun.* **48:**587–591.

210. **Yayoshi, M.** 1983. Association between *M. pneumoniae* hemolysis, attachment and pulmonary pathogenicity. *Yale J. Biol. Med.* **56:**685–689.

211. **Yowell, R. L., B. C. Cole, and R. A. Daynes.** 1983. Utilization of T cell hybridomas to establish that a soluble factor derived from *Mycoplasma arthritidis* is truly a genetically restricted polyclonal T cell activator. *J. Immunol.* **131:**543–545.

28. Antigenic Variation

KIM S. WISE, DAVID YOGEV, and RENATE ROSENGARTEN

INTRODUCTION

Mycoplasmas occupy an extensive array of natural habitats which include but are not limited to several animal and plant hosts. Despite their minimal genomic capacity and metabolic limitations, these organisms have successfully adapted to conditions that may be considered quite challenging and which may vary rapidly. At a minimum, survival in a host requires the ability to acquire nutrients from diverse microenvironments encountered in assorted compartments, an ability to accommodate different physical conditions associated with these transient niches, and an effective means for transmission to similar or alternative host populations (24, 31, 59). In addition, highly evolved host defense mechanisms must be avoided to the extent that at least some organisms continue to propagate. A common strategy employed by microbial parasites to meet this demand is the generation of diversity (18, 24, 58, 84). In many biological systems, expenditure of energy is sacrificed to secure the flexibility to respond, or adapt by selection, to alternative and unpredictable environmental conditions. This tactic is used by several microbial species and is also effectively employed by multicellular host organisms, as perhaps best illustrated by the powerful diversity-generating systems underlying the adaptive immune system (113). Indeed, the interplay of competing cellular populations undergoing rapid diversification contributes fundamentally to the dynamic status of the host-microbe interaction.

The term "antigenic variation" is commonly used to describe the ability of microbial species to elaborate alternative forms of macromolecules recognized and distinguished by antibodies or other elements of immune recognition. Because of the importance of the vertebrate immune system in controlling unicellular microbes (both procaryotic and eucaryotic), a focus on molecular structures and genetic mechanisms creating epitopically distinct entities understandably dominates this subject when one is dealing with agents infecting immunocompetent individuals. In addition, the emergence of the monoclonal antibody (MAb) as a common tool for defining variant structures tends to emphasize the antigenic nature of microbial components, whether or not immune function plays a role in the recognition, selection, or ultimate fate of the agent bearing the structure. Structures on the microbial surface understandably receive special attention as likely targets of strong immunological selective pressure.

Kim S. Wise • Department of Molecular Microbiology and Immunology, M642 Medical Sciences Building, University of Missouri–Columbia, Columbia, Missouri 65212.   **David Yogev** • Department of Membrane and Ultrastructure Research, The Hebrew University–Hadassah Medical School, P.O. Box 1172, Jerusalem 91010, Israel.   **Renate Rosengarten** • Institut für Mikrobiologie und Tierseuchen, Tierärztliche Hochschule Hannover, Bischofsholer Damm 15, 3000 Hannover 1, Federal Republic of Germany.

The central role of antigenic variation notwithstanding, many adaptations at the microbial surface also involve critical systems mediating selective attachment to or penetration of host tissues, acquisition of metabolites, and transduction of sensory signals from the environment (24, 31, 57, 59). In this chapter, the antigenic aspects of mycoplasmal surface variation are addressed within the broader perspective of phenotypic variation encompassing additional parameters of diversity that may affect other, equally critical aspects of host adaptation.

Defining the molecular basis of mycoplasma adaptation is important to our understanding of the mycoplasma-host interaction and our ability to manipulate this interaction during deleterious infection and disease. More generally, molecular analysis has now begun to reveal novel strategies by which these evolutionarily unique organisms generate and maintain critical levels of population diversity. These include innovative structural adaptations of surface proteins particularly suited to wall-less procaryotes as well as genetic alterations exploiting apparently error-prone mechanisms to drive structural diversification. Thus, mycoplasmal solutions to the problem of maintaining diversity may be particularly instructive from a global perspective of genetic mechanisms, membrane protein structure, and population dynamics. From a practical standpoint, understanding specific principles underlying mycoplasma variation may identify general patterns and mechanisms that would improve our ability to predict how these agents adapt. Indeed, emerging evidence presented here, that intensive genetic and structural diversification operates in mycoplasma populations, is likely to change fundamental experimental premises and approaches to the analysis of mycoplasma pathogenicity. It is the intent of this chapter to (i) define newly identified structural and genetic aspects of mycoplasma variation recently derived from detailed analysis of one species, (ii) compare patterns of variation predicted by this system with variation observed in other mycoplasma species, and (iii) discuss the potential impact of mycoplasma variation both on the pathobiology of these organisms and on the design of future studies assessing mycoplasma interactions with their hosts.

DYNAMICS AND EVOLUTION OF MYCOPLASMA POPULATIONS

Defined Environments

Any study of variation in unicellular organisms requires definition of the population measured and definition of the parameter being monitored (85). Moreover, the nature and degree of variation occurring in one environment may or may not be reflected under different conditions. These constraints pose significant problems in defining any system of phenotypic or genotypic variation but are particularly severe in studies of fastidious organisms such as mycoplasmas. The issue of mycoplasma population variation is addressed in chapter 34, and only specific aspects are mentioned here. In a host, mycoplasmas not only may be exposed to physiologic fluctuations but also may

have to compete for or exploit niches with commensal microbial populations. Organisms may be subjected to external systems (e.g., phages, plasmids, or transformation-competent DNA) mediating exchange and mutation of exogenous genetic material (11, 58, 82). In contrast to life in a host habitat, a population monitored in vitro as a free-living culture may be subject to fewer environmental uncertainties, although variables such as genetic transfer systems and physiologic conditions in complex media may remain ill defined. Even in broth culture, phenotypic variation may differ from that occurring in an agar medium, and cocultivation of mycoplasmas with cultured cells in vitro creates yet another distinctive environment. In practice, most conventional protocols demand some transfer among such differing conditions in order to propagate organisms and to define and characterize phenotypic or genetic features. Despite such fundamental limitations, careful examination of populations in moderately consistent environments has yielded information on intrinsic properties of variation in many organisms, including mycoplasmas.

Population Sampling

Population sampling is also critical in understanding the dynamics of mycoplasma variation. An important distinction must be made between measurement of heterogeneity in a large population and documentation of altered properties that occur during sequential generations derived from individual organisms. For this reason, the analysis of clonal populations and the transference or change of phenotypic properties through clonal lineages may reveal features of variation inaccessible simply by analysis of bulk populations. In this context, clonality takes on an entirely operational definition, indicating only a population derived from a single organism, with the realization that sampling requires growth of the clone to a measurable population size, even though diversification may occur in the process.

Transient versus Heritable Variation

An additional, critical issue in assessing phenotypic variation and corresponding genetic alterations is the distinction between transient phenotypic changes that occur in individual organisms and heritable changes that are transmitted to the progeny of an organism. Mechanisms of gene regulation in response to environmental stimuli have been extensively documented for several microbial species (24, 31, 57, 59). In most of these cases, resulting phenotypic changes in individual organisms of a population are temporary and usually reversible and provide an important adaptive capability for responding to immediate changes in external conditions. In contrast, several mechanisms that generate random genetic alterations resulting in altered phenotypes have been documented (11, 24, 84). These changes may or may not be reversible and may occur in apparently programmed sequence, but they result ultimately in transmission of a mutation to immediate progeny populations which may subsequently undergo further mutational changes. The frequency and placement of mutations characterize the rate and complexity of diversification. Several microbial systems of phase variation or phenotypic switching that involve a wide variety of mutational mechanisms have been characterized (6, 11, 24, 42, 84). An inherent dividend of mutational processes is the potential incorporation of new phenotypic features into a population; however, the predominance of the new phenotype depends on the relative proportion of individuals bearing the marker at the time of population sampling. Random genetic processes inducing population diversity are critical elements in adaptation of microbes to new environments, especially in habitats such as the immunocompetent host, where mutational pathways that specifically recognize changes in microbial populations have likewise evolved.

Mycoplasmas may utilize transient regulatory mechanisms for phenotypic change as well as random mutational mechanisms for diversification. Indeed, these tactics for adaptation are by no means mutually exclusive. Molecular features of one mycoplasma system that identify several unique and superimposed mechanisms generating and maintaining population diversity have recently come to light. These are described below for the variable lipoprotein (Vlp) system of *Mycoplasma hyorhinis*, an organism showing antigenic variation with several aspects analogous to those found in other mycoplasma species.

THE Vlp SYSTEM OF *M. HYORHINIS*

Characteristics of *M. hyorhinis* Surface Antigens

Variable phenotypes and serogroups of *M. hyorhinis*

The presence of antigenic and other forms of phenotypic variation has been extensively examined in *M. hyorhinis*, one of over 70 species in the genus *Mycoplasma* (13, 74, 76, 77, 115). Like several members of this group, *M. hyorhinis* is an infectious agent and sometime pathogen, causing rhinitis, polyserositis, and chronic experimental arthritis in its natural swine host (79, 106). This agent is also a common and notorious contaminant of tissue cell cultures, in which it propagates as a cell surface parasite, and has been studied to define assorted aspects of mycoplasma-host cell interactions (17) (see chapter 26). Isolates of *M. hyorhinis* are known to differ with respect to their pathogenic potential, ability to adsorb to cells in vitro, and requirements for independent growth in agar medium.

In addition to these variant phenotypic features, antigenic heterogeneity was also identified in *M. hyorhinis* by earlier work defining and distinguishing intraspecies subgroups or serotypes by using polyspecific serologic reagents (34, 106). Interestingly, one early observation suggested that some organisms in a passaged strain of *M. hyorhinis* were resistant to growth-inhibiting antibodies and that these resistant populations could regenerate progeny, most of which regained susceptibility (39). More recently, a specific MAb mediating complement-dependent mycoplasmacidal killing of *M. hyorhinis* consistently spared a portion of the population treated (74). Thus, both antigenic heterogeneity in populations and instability of an antigenic phenotype in subsequent progeny populations have been documented, although the basis of these features has not been clear.

Distinct sets of size-variant and strain-variant surface proteins

More detailed examination of *M. hyorhinis* membrane surface components (13, 15, 74, 76, 77, 110) revealed distinct, antigenically defined sets of surface proteins on organisms of this species. Antigens within a set shared the MAb-defined epitope but showed variation in two parameters. First, when bulk populations propagated by standard passage in medium were assessed by sodium dodecyl sulfate-polyacrylamide gel electrophoresis (SDS-PAGE) and immunoblot analysis or by quantitative enzyme-linked immunosorbent assay (ELISA) inhibition tests, MAb-defined proteins were found to be either present or absent on particular strains; these differences were generally consistent after repeated broth passages. Moreover, some isolates displayed more than one set of antigens, and in other cases, quantitative differences in the average number of epitopes expressed per organism could be detected among strains by an ELISA inhibition test using whole organisms.

The second property to emerge from immunoblot analysis of SDS-PAGE-separated proteins was that of size variation. Proteins bearing the distinctive epitope of a set could occur in discrete sizes. Depending on the quantity of organisms sampled (10^6 to 10^8 per well), regularly spaced "ladders" composed of discrete steps with distinctive spacing were observed in some strains. Usually one size predominated in a strain, but this size varied widely among strains (13, 76).

Thus, at the level of bulk population analysis, *M. hyorhinis* displays (i) multiple sets of MAb-defined proteins, (ii) strain-variant expression of one or more of these antigen sets, and (iii) multiple size forms of antigens within each set, manifest either as distinctive ladders comprising discrete proteins in a particular strain or as variation among strains in the size of the epitope-bearing protein predominantly expressed.

Vlp surface membrane antigens containing repetitive protein structure

MAbs defining sets of size-variant and strain-variant antigens have been used in conjunction with biochemical procedures to determine the nature of the antigens recognized. Detergent phase partitioning of *M. hyorhinis* by using Triton X-114 delineated several amphiphilic proteins operationally defined as integral membrane proteins by their selective incorporation into detergent micelles (13, 74). In parallel studies, metabolic labeling of organisms with [³H]palmitate had revealed several lipid-associated proteins, all of which partitioned exclusively as integral membrane proteins (15). These proteins were subsequently shown by acid methanolysis to contain nonextractable, covalently bound lipid (13). Direct radioimmunoprecipitation with surface-binding MAbs defining variant antigens directly demonstrated that each set recognized was composed of size-variant lipoproteins that could be metabolically labeled with [³H]palmitate or with [³⁵S]cysteine (thus permitting easy identification of these translation products as strongly labeled Triton X-114-phase components) (13, 76, 77). Initial lipoprotein sets identified by MAbs could not be metabolically labeled with methionine, but selective incorporation of this amino acid was later used to define one additional set of size-variant lipoproteins (see below).

The surface location, orientation, and internal structure of Vlp antigens were determined by several strategies. Direct immunoelectron microscopy showed that specific antigens were densely packed on the external face of the mycoplasma's single limiting membrane (110), and trypsin treatment of intact cells further supported the surface accessibility of these proteins (74, 76, 110). The internal structure of these antigens was revealed by graded proteolytic digestion of SDS-PAGE gel-eluted antigens, which generated a periodic size-variant set of epitope-bearing partial tryptic fragments that mimicked the spontaneous ladders identified in cultures (13; unpublished observation). The analogous ladder could also be generated by graded trypsin treatment of intact cells expressing individual size-variant forms (76). Similar ladders could be generated from intact cells with carboxypeptidase Y, a protease that sequentially cleaves amino acids from the C-terminal end of proteins. Since the enzyme hydrolyses Arg and Lys residues at a much reduced efficiency, pauses at putative periodic trypsin sites are anticipated during hydrolysis. Generation of the predicted laddered set of partial carboxypeptidase products from intact cells argued for a periodic, repetitive polypeptide structure in these proteins and further indicated that the C terminus and most of the protein sequence were fully accessible outside the membrane, without interruption by transmembrane domains (76).

Thus, the external membrane face of *M. hyorhinis* displayed variable sets of lipid-modified surface membrane proteins defined by MAbs. Proteins in each set displayed size variation and were predicted to contain periodic structures in an exposed C-terminal region. All of these characteristics were later supported by protein features determined from sequence analysis of corresponding genes (see Fig. 4).

Analysis of Vlp and Other High-Frequency Phenotypic Switching in Isogenic Clonal Populations

The initial observations indicated that *M. hyorhinis* might create surface diversity through altered expression and structural variation of individual translation products exposed on the external surface of the membrane and suggested that diversification resided in the structure and expression of Vlps. To fully understand the capabilities of this system and to determine mechanisms regulating mycoplasma lipoprotein surface variation, several additional aspects needed to be determined: (i) the number, structural diversity, and antigenic relationships of alternative lipoprotein translation products, (ii) the possibility and parameters of phenotypic switching and the possible linkage or independence of Vlp switching to other phenotypic characteristics of the organism, and (iii) the possibility of combinatorial diversity arising from simultaneous expression of different products on single cells. Each of these issues is important in determining the nature

and limits of the diversity generated and is critical in comparing antigenic variation in mycoplasmas with known systems of bacterial surface variation and regulated expression of factors involved in infection and virulence (24, 59, 84). However, these questions could be addressed only by assessing precise changes occurring in individual cell lineages within a population. This was accomplished by using MAbs, differential metabolic labeling patterns, structural comparisons, and sequential patterns of expression in several clonal isogenic lineages of *M. hyorhinis* to rigorously define and document variation in the Vlp system of this organism. This analysis provided evidence for high-frequency phase variation in expression of Vlp proteins and established additional parameters of concomitant phenotypic switching involving colony opacity and morphology.

Phase variation in colony morphology and opacity

M. hyorhinis SK76, isolated as an arthritogenic agent and obtained as a multiply filter cloned isolate (78), was analyzed for its ability to diversify phenotypically during independent, cell-free growth in vitro (76, 77). Early- and late-passage broth cultures showed consistent heterogeneity in colony morphology when plated on standard agar medium. A stable proportion of three "morphotypes" (indicated as a percentage of the colonies plated from filtered broth culture) was independent from the number of passages: S (small-diameter; 98.6%), M (medium-diameter; 1.3%), and L (large-diameter; 0.1%) morphotypes. Filter cloning yielded purified cultures of each morphotype, but these populations showed switching to both of the alternative morphotypes. Lineages subsequently derived from these switched progeny either reverted to the original phenotype or again generated alternate phenotypes. Oscillating switches of L, S, and M morphotypes occurred at high frequencies (defined as the fraction of switched phenotype per cell per generation [93]), typically ranging from 10^{-4} to 10^{-2}. Extremely high switch frequencies ($\sim 3 \times 10^{-2}$, the maximum measurable) were apparent in some lineages; virtually every colony plated showed one morphotype spawning "sectors," subsequently shown to represent an alternative morphotype.

A second phenotype showing diversity in *M. hyorhinis* populations was colony opacity (76, 77). Subcloned lineages of each morphotype showed heterogeneity in this feature, which was therefore not linked to colony morphology. Lineages monitored for this trait generated oscillating transparent (tr) or opaque (op) populations at frequencies similar to those for morphotype switching, often with sectoring observed in all colonies plated. The ability to undergo reversible high-frequency, independent switching of colony morphotype and opacity was therefore a heritable feature of the organism.

Phase variation of Vlp expression

Marked phenotypic instability in Vlp expression was also identified in subcloned *M. hyorhinis* populations by immunostaining colonies with MAbs to assess expression of the corresponding epitope-bearing lipoproteins. Striking heterogeneity was observed both in populations derived from single colony isolates and within individual colonies, as demonstrated by extensive sectoring. Subcloned populations oscillating between expression (+) or absence (−) of a particular Vlp epitope showed extremely high switch frequencies. Sectored immunostaining was observed in all morphotypes and occurred in both op and tr colonies. Expression of specific Vlps therefore varied independently from other phenotypes. However, concomitant switches of two phenotypes (for example, op$^+$ → tr$^-$) were often observed. High-frequency phenotypic switching of colony morphology, opacity, and epitope expression occurred throughout this species, as documented in clonally purified strains (13) and in primary passages from filter-cloned American Type Culture Collection (Rockville, Md.) stocks of *M. hyorhinis*: ATCC 23839 (GDL); 25021, 25026, and 25077 (PG29); 17981 (BTS-7); and 27717 (a subcloned BTS-7 stock derived form 17981) (76).

Identification and characterization of distinct Vlps

The isolation of subcloned populations showing phase variation in surface epitope expression allowed SDS-PAGE and immunoblot confirmation of the corresponding Vlp expression state. Systematic analysis of phase variation in Vlp expression in *M. hyorhinis* SK76 revealed three distinct Vlps, each of which was shown to undergo high-frequency changes in size and expression (76, 77). The key to this strategy was to rigorously establish and analyze several clonally derived isogenic lineages representing specific, sequential phenotypic switches in successive generations. Selection of phenotypic variants was based on simultaneous scoring of colony opacity and Vlp epitope expression in sequential populations and on SDS-PAGE analysis of isolated clonal variants followed by immunoblotting of whole organism samples or fluorography of radiolabeled Triton X-114-phase protein samples. By expanding the range of MAb reagents used to identify specific Vlps and by comparing selective metabolic labeling profiles, three distinct surface lipoprotein antigens, VlpA, VlpB, and VlpC were identified (77).

Reversible variation in Vlp size and correlation with colony opacity

Initial studies using MAb to VlpC showed that strain SK76 expressed a heterogeneous ladder of amphiphilic, size-variant surface lipoproteins bearing the epitope, which differed from the more restricted, single-size variants expressed by other strains (76). This heterogeneous pattern was maintained in several subcloned lineages of the SK76 strain, even during transitions between morphotypes. In contrast, analysis of some derived lineages revealed marked variation in the size of VlpC. This was manifest as several discrete forms, each expressed separately on individual clones. Size-variant antigens were detected at a very high frequency in these subclones and collectively accounted for a large portion of the heterogeneous ladder in the original progenitor population. These spontaneously occurring size variants showed uniform spacing by SDS-PAGE (under reducing conditions) corresponding to a difference in apparent molecular mass of ~2.8

kDa. Analysis of clonal lineages therefore established that mechanisms also operate in these organisms to generate reversible antigen size variation at high frequency in isogenic populations.

In a lineage expressing only VlpC, a decrease in VlpC size had been observed during a switch from a tr to an op colony phenotype (76). The degree of opacity in plated populations actually varied widely, as did the range of Vlp sizes. To test the possibility that Vlp size correlated with opacity, clonal variants from different lineages expressing a single Vlp were assessed for both parameters. Extensive analysis of several such variants displaying a continuum from transparent to strongly opaque revealed an exact, inverse correlation between Vlp size and colony opacity (76, 77).

Colony opacity served as a convenient guide to establish extensive isogenic lineages of Vlp size variants and permitted characterization of several features of Vlp size variation. (i) Individual Vlp size variants could spontaneously increase or decrease by discrete, integral numbers of intervals; (ii) the size of any Vlp could increase or decrease in successive generations; (iii) although size variants of a particular Vlp were consistently associated with a characteristic degree of colony opacity, the absolute size of the different Vlps measured in SDS-PAGE did not determine this property; and (iv) in contrast to clonal variants expressing only one Vlp, for which colony opacity varied clearly as the size of the expressed Vlp, variants expressing more than one Vlp at a time (see below) appeared to have opacity phenotypes dictated by the largest Vlp expressed.

Structural and antigenic comparison of individual Vlps

Spontaneous isogenic size variants generated from clonally derived VlpC variants created a ladder with a highly characteristic, regular spacing of approximately 2.8 kDa. Analysis of VlpB revealed an analogous but distinguishable periodic structure with a closer spacing of approximately 2.3 kDa. Exceptions to the regularity of this pattern occasionally occurred; i.e., a spontaneous variant of a Vlp did not correspond to any rung of the ladder in the progenitor population (77).

The striking structural differences among Vlps suggested that the periodic structures of each protein were not identical. This variability was confirmed by showing that similarly sized variants of VlpB and VlpC yielded trypsin digestion products that were distinctive for each Vlp and indistinguishable from the spacing observed in spontaneous ladders in corresponding progenitor populations. Spacing of VlpA size variants appeared to be greater than that of either VlpB or VlpC.

Although Vlps were distinguishable by structural dissimilarity in their periodic structure, MAb-defined epitopes established additional means to characterize Vlp structures. Notably, while some MAbs were clearly able to distinguish Vlps, one MAb established the presence of a shared epitope on VlpB and VlpC. This finding suggested that structurally related portions of Vlps may exist. Thus, Vlps carried specific epitopes which were distinct for each translation product or which could be shared by multiple Vlps. Importantly, all Vlp-related MAbs were highly specific for *M. hyorhinis*, further indicating that the Vlp system was not dispersed outside the species (13).

The structural complexity and antigenic variation reflected in the Vlp system raised the question of whether this system of surface antigens was expressed or immunogenic in the natural swine host. That Vlps were targeted by the host immune system was shown by using serum antibody from swine with experimentally induced *M. hyorhinis* SK76-induced arthritis (78), which specifically recognized the prominent VlpA, VlpB, and VlpC size variants in immunoblots of Triton X-114-phase proteins of *M. hyorhinis* SK76 compared with control swine serum (77).

Independent phase variation and complex combinatorial expression of Vlps

In further studies, clonal lineages of Vlp expression variants were analyzed to document the parameters of phase variation involving multiple Vlps. Immunoscreening of colonies and subsequent SDS-PAGE analysis identified several phase variants representing oscillating states of Vlp expression (77). It was found that reciprocal states of expression involving two particular Vlps were not obligatorily linked; expression of one Vlp could eventually oscillate with expression of either of the other two Vlps. While the simplest case of phase variation involved expression of only one Vlp at a time, analysis of several clonal variants suggested that more than one Vlp could be expressed concomitantly. This was proven rigorously by screening replicate colony blots for double-expressing clones, using MAbs to distinct Vlps. Analysis of several cloned colonies and their progeny strongly argued that a single organism can express multiple Vlps. Supplemental studies using SDS-PAGE to monitor all Vlp products showed that clonal populations could express any one Vlp (VlpA, VlpB, or VlpC) or could simultaneously express any two or all Vlps in any combination. Notably, however, it appeared in all lineages examined that only a single size version of each Vlp could be expressed on a cell.

As anticipated from independent Vlp phase variation, switches involving concomitant phase variation

of multiple Vlps were generally observed at a lower frequency than documented for switches involving individual Vlps. Switches of multiple Vlps were not coordinately linked, since alternative combinations of Vlps occurred during subsequent phase transitions in several lineages studies. Finally, all attempts to detect clones lacking all Vlps were unsuccessful; metabolic labeling analysis of VlpB$^-$ VlpC$^-$ colonies (selected by negative immunoblot from assorted lineages) always yielded variants expressing VlpA (by the criteria defined above). In no case has a population been found that did not express at least one prominent [^{35}S]cysteine- and [^{3}H]palmitate-labeled Triton X-114-phase protein that could be categorized as VlpA, VlpB, or VlpC (77; unpublished observation).

Seven combinatorial classes of Vlp expression occur (Fig. 1). However, since each Vlp can vary in size within a population, the potential numbers of structural permutations per class is extremely high. For example, assuming at least 12 size variants of VlpA, approximately 25 of VlpB, and 30 of VlpC, the possible number of size-variant permutations in a cell expressing all three Vlps (the product of $12 \times 25 \times 30$) is about 9×10^3. Over 50 different individual size variants of VlpA, VlpB, or VlpC have been documented among clonal populations. Moreover, of the 42 possible phase transitions among the 7 combinatorial phenotypic classes shown in Fig. 1 (the permutations of seven items taken two at a time), 26 have been documented. Finally, it is noteworthy that the phenomenon of Vlp size variation is superimposed on Vlp phase variation. Changes in the size of each Vlp can occur either independently from or concomitantly with variation in Vlp expression.

Summary of features

Taken together, these results demonstrate that (i) a given Vlp phenotype, defined as a class comprising the combinatorial mosaic of Vlps expressed on a cell, can switch to any of six other Vlp combinatorial phenotypes, (ii) phase transitions involving multiple Vlp switches occur with each Vlp switching independently from the others, in a noncoordinate manner, (iii)

Class	Vlps Expressed	Size Variant Combinations		Phenotypic Transitions
		Possible No.	Documented No.	
1	VlpC	~30	25	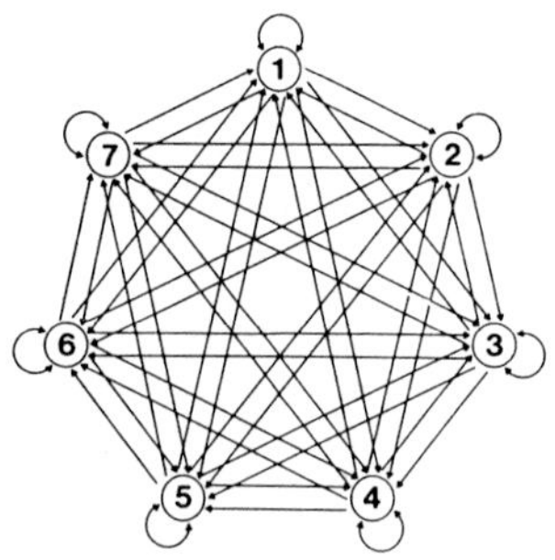
2	VlpB	~25	20	
3	VlpA	>12	5	
4	VlpC + VlpB	>750	15	
5	VlpC + VlpA	>360	13	
6	VlpB + VlpA	>300	12	
7	VlpC + VlpB + VlpA	>9,000	14	

Figure 1. Combinatorial repertoire and phase transitions of Vlp variants expressed in subcloned lineages of *M. hyorhinis* SK76. Data are derived from references 76 and 77.

phase variation of any Vlp may be (but is not necessarily) accompanied by concomitant size variation in that translation product, and (iv) only one size of a particular Vlp appears to occur per cell.

Organization and Structure of *vlp* Genes and Their Products

The *vlp* gene family cluster

A region of the *M. hyorhinis* SK76 chromosome containing genes encoding Vlp proteins has been identified by molecular cloning and mapping of specific genes corresponding to Vlp products (115). Regions encoding Vlp proteins were determined by analysis of subcloned DNA fragments placed under selective T7 RNA polymerase promoter control to express identifiable recombinant Vlp proteins in *Escherichia coli*. A map of the fully sequenced region containing *vlp* genes is shown in Fig. 2.

Two adjacent subcloned fragments generated distinct recombinant proteins with the unique epitope profiles of VlpB and VlpC, respectively. The subregion encoding VlpA was determined by an alternative strategy, based on the principle that Vlp size variation correlates with restriction fragment length polymorphism reflecting a periodic structure in the corresponding gene (see below). This was evaluated by using isogenic lineages of the SK76 strain expressing size variants of only VlpA. The three *vlp* genes are clustered within a 4-kb chromosomal segment. Three similarly oriented open reading frames (ORFs) predict features characteristic of the authentic corresponding Vlp products (see below). Each ORF is flanked 5' by a highly conserved 240-bp noncoding region containing *vlp* promoters (indicated as P in Fig. 2). A highly unusual feature of *vlp* genes is the presence of multiple, additional ORFs on both DNA strands overlapping the sequences encoding each *vlp* product (indicated by small solid arrows in Fig. 2). While none of these alternative ORFs predicts features consistent with authentic Vlp proteins, they may contribute in other ways to diversity in Vlp sequences (see below).

One of several chromosomal copies of a previously described insertion sequence (IS)-like element in *M. hyorhinis* (30) lies between the *vlpA* and *vlpB* genes, in an orientation aligning a translationally interrupted IS-encoded ORF in the same direction as *vlp* genes (see chapter 22). Synthetic oligonucleotides representing highly conserved or specific regions of *vlp* genes (see below) were used as probes in Southern blot hybridization of genomic DNA to determine that each gene existed as a single copy in the *M. hyorhinis* chromosome (115).

The organization of the *vlp* gene family depicted in Fig. 2 was consistently found in several clonal isolates within an extensive isogenic lineage developed from the SK76 strain and accounts for the expression of all known Vlp products detected in this lineage: the MAb-defined VlpB and VlpC products and the VlpA product selectively labeled with Met, an amino acid encoded exclusively in the *vlpA* coding sequence. No UGA (Trp) codons (69) were present in any of the *vlp* coding sequences.

Analysis of clonal variants within this lineage was particularly useful in determining several critical aspects of Vlp structure, variation, and phase-variant expression. Interestingly, however, this clonal lineage derived from SK76 failed to express one other MAb-defined Vlp (designated VlpE) which was known to be expressed in other *M. hyorhinis* strains (13, 75, 76, 77, 110). Further recent analysis of clonal isolates from these other strains has revealed up to three additional and distinct Vlp genes, one of which could be assigned to the authentic VlpE product (117). This finding indicated that *vlp* gene families may contain a variable number of individual members. Moreover, recent screening of a standard, passaged SK76 stock culture (derived originally from a multiply cloned isolate) revealed a very small variant population (<1% of the bulk culture) that expressed VlpE yet contained other characteristic antigenic and genomic signatures of the SK76 strain (75). Clonal isolates of these VlpE-expressing organisms indeed showed larger families of *vlp* genes (117). This unexpected result demonstrated that *vlp* gene families may be highly variable and that differences in Vlp expression within species or within strains may arise in some cases by dynamic loss or gain of genes or gene blocks, by currently unknown mechanisms. This is one of several features generating Vlp diversity in populations of *M. hyorhinis*.

Deduced structure of Vlp proteins

Conserved regions for membrane processing. Gene sequences *vlpA*, *vlpB*, and *vlpC* predict proteins with features characteristic of corresponding mycoplasma Vlp proteins. Several striking aspects of Vlp structural similarity, sequence divergence, and variability were associated with specific portions of these proteins (115). These regions are denoted I, II, and III and display features summarized in the prototype structure shown in Fig. 3. Region I represents a highly homologous N-terminal portion of Vlp proteins containing a typical procaryotic signal peptide sequence of 29 amino acids. This signal terminates with the tetrapeptide Ala-Ile-Ser-Cys, a motif consistent with a procaryotic prolipoprotein signal peptidase recognition sequence (112). The one Cys residue in each Vlp occurs within this sequence and is the predicted acylation

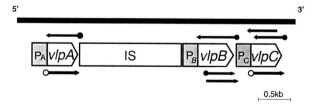

Figure 2. Organization of the *vlp* gene cluster in a subcloned lineage of *M. hyorhinis* SK76. The location and the orientation of Vlp ORFs are indicated by large open labeled arrows. Highly homologous regions 5' of each *vlp* gene are indicated by shaded boxes labeled P. The position of an IS-like element is shown by the large open box labeled IS. Solid arrows overlapping the Vlp ORFs indicate the location and orientation of additional ORFs in alternative reading frames. Open circles attached to arrows denote the presence of putative (NTG) initiation codons, and solid circles represent the additional presence of a putative ribosome binding site.

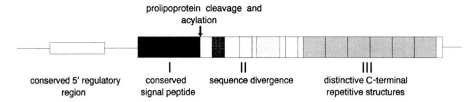

Figure 3. Schematic representation of Vlp structural features. The Vlp ORF is shown as a rectangle containing various regions (I, II, and III) bearing the features indicated. Distinctively shaded boxes in region II indicate reiterated sequences recurring within individual Vlps or among different Vlps. Shaded areas in region III represent tandemly repeated sequences distinctive for each Vlp that occur in variable numbers in Vlp size variants.

site, N terminus, and point of membrane anchorage of a mature, processed procaryotic lipoprotein (112). This single residue is also noteworthy in that the intense autoradiographic signal of Vlps in Triton X-114-phase proteins from [^{35}S]cysteine-labeled mycoplasmas (76, 77) argues further that Vlps are the most abundant membrane proteins in the organism. Indirect evidence that Vlp prolipoproteins are cleaved in mycoplasmas comes from the deduced sequence, placing all five Leu residues in VlpC within its signal peptide. Inability to metabolically label VlpC with [^{3}H]leucine, under conditions labeling several other amphiphilic *M. hyorhinis* proteins, suggested that the signal peptide of this Vlp is efficiently processed (unpublished observations). Further assessment of processing and lipid acylation is in progress.

Divergent mature Vlp surface proteins with a common charge motif. In contrast to region I, region II shows considerable sequence divergence among Vlps. For example, although VlpB and VlpC share an identical sequence for the first 20 residues of the predicted mature lipoproteins, comparison of all three mature Vlp proteins shows general sequence variation in region II. However, within these divergent regions are several short, sometimes overlapping blocks of homologous amino acid sequences (Fig. 3) that recur at variable locations within or among different Vlps. These are encoded by corresponding reiterated, oligomeric DNA sequences (115).

Region III also contains reiterated sequences; however, these occur in a striking array of tandem, in-frame units encoding 12 amino acids (in VlpB and VlpC) or 13 amino acids (in VlpA). These units create a periodic polypeptide structure extending nearly to the predicted C terminus of each Vlp. Amino acid and corresponding nucleotide sequences within periodic units are dissimilar among distinct Vlps. However, the overall composition and charge distribution within these proteins are remarkably consistent. Each mature Vlp protein (regions II and III) is predicted to be hydrophilic and to lack alpha-helix or beta structure (33). The N-terminal portions of mature Vlps (region II) contain few charged residues; over 95% of the sequence is composed of Ser, Thr, Asn, Gln, and Gly residues, with 46 to 51% representing Ser and Thr. In contrast, each region III periodic unit within any Vlp, while also rich in Ser and Thr (30%), contains a striking distribution of spaced charged residues creating a repeating motif $(+ \ - \ -)_n$ throughout the multiple tandem copies of these units. This feature is characteristic of Vlps and may significantly influence the physicochemical characteristics of the mycoplasma surface.

The orientation and placement of periodic sequences in *vlp* genes confirm earlier biochemical evidence (76, 77) predicting their presence in the surface exposed C-terminal region of these lipoproteins; indeed, single Lys residues in each unit provide precise cleavage sites predicting trypsin-generated ladders as well as the pause sites defined by graded carboxypeptidase Y proteolysis (77). In addition, the previously identified difference in spacing within the VlpC and VlpB size-variant ladders (77) now appears to reflect differences in structure rather than length of their periodic units, possibly influenced by multiple Pro residues in the VlpC sequence.

Spontaneous changes in repetitive sequences generating Vlp size variation

Examination of several phenotypic transitions in isogenic lineages of the SK76 strain showed that an incremental increase or decrease in the size of individual Vlp proteins was accompanied by concomitant expansion or contraction (by discrete increments) of restriction fragments bearing the corresponding *vlp* gene (115). That size variation at the DNA level occasionally occurred without expression of the corresponding protein further indicated that size variation was independent from phase variation. Since C-terminal periodic structure had been implicated in Vlp size variation, the precise changes occurring during size variation were determined by sequencing *vlpB* genes from two isolates predicted to vary in the number of periodic units. DNA sequences confirmed the presence in the longer gene of additional repetitive units in region III. Distinctive signatures downstream of the most 3′ periodic unit and upstream of the most 5′ periodic unit were preserved in both size-variant *vlpB* genes, indicating a precise deletion of four internal units that maintained the exact boundaries and reading frame throughout region III of the smaller spontaneous variant. These results (115) identify region III as the protein domain undergoing changes during Vlp size variation and suggest a precise insertion or deletion of periodic coding sequences as the underlying mechanism.

Possible mechanisms of size variation leading to precise deletion or insertion of sequences in region III include homologous recombination (2, 11, 71) and slipped-strand mispairing (51, 62). Similar mechanisms have been implicated in the generation of size-variant proteins in other bacteria (3, 32, 42). Some mycoplasmas have been shown to possess pathways of homologous recombination (53) and *recA* gene homologs (29). In addition, early evidence suggested that deficiencies in DNA polymerase editing may occur in *M. hyorhinis* (61). Thus, either sequence-specific recombination or error-prone replicative processes may contribute to *vlp* gene size variation as well as other features of *vlp* expression (see below). Notably, oligonucleotide probes specific for region III repetitive structures of each *vlp* gene failed to identify any other reservoirs of these units, suggesting that size variation involves only intragenic repetitive sequences. Interestingly, some *vlp* genes contain nonidentical repetitive structures that are grouped in various locations within region III (unpublished observations). This finding suggests a superimposed mechanism for sequence diversification in this region (see below).

Structural and antigenic consequences of Vlp expression at the cell surface

Characterization of the *vlp* gene complex revealed novel mechanisms for generating and maintaining structural surface variation, several features of which are depicted in the model proposed in Fig. 4. Vlps employ a common set of lipoprotein signal peptide sequences to process and anchor mature forms of the proteins in the single lipid bilayer membrane, presumably by lipid covalently linked to the N-terminal Cys residue and integrated into the outer leaflet of the membrane (112). These external surface products represent the major membrane-associated proteins of *M. hyorhinis*.

Epitope distribution. Mature Vlp proteins contain important sequence features allowing antigenic variation within a conserved structural framework. Sequence divergence in region II provides diversity that could create distinct epitopes on each Vlp, and region II sequences common to VlpB and VlpC could specify the shared epitopes distinguishing these products from VlpA. The epitopes currently defined on Vlps are likely to be determined by protein sequence, since it is highly improbable that the small recombinant fragments expressing Vlp products in *E. coli* would encode genes, with proper codon usage (69), sufficient to create multiple *M. hyorhinis* species-specific and Vlp-specific posttranslational modifications accounting for the four epitopes detected. The precise locations of key epitopes involved in antibody-mediated mycoplasma killing (74) or mycoplasma functional modulation of host cells (26, 77, 83) are being determined by mutational analysis of cloned *vlp* genes.

Surface properties. The preservation of region III periodic structure during size variation is striking, with the charge motif $(+ \; - \; -)_n$ maintained throughout this region of all Vlps during high-frequency size variation. This feature is consistent with the low isoelectric point observed for some Vlps (15) and predicts a strong dependence of this property on Vlp size (determined by the number of region III periodic units present). Conservation of this distinctive structure among Vlps, its maintenance during combinatorial Vlp expression, and the inability as yet to identify mycoplasma variants lacking Vlps all suggest a possible function for these abundant proteins beyond antigenic variation for immune avoidance. Vlp proteins are perhaps the fundamental cellular coat structure of these wall-less procaryotes. The capacity to elaborate a layer varying in thickness or charge density (depending on Vlp size) suggests a possible function of Vlp expression and size variation in modulating surface properties that could affect ion and macromolecular permeability, cell shape, or cell-cell interactions (possibly reflected in the observed inverse correlation of colony opacity with Vlp size). In this sense, Vlps may be similar to paracrystalline S-layer proteins of several eubacteria and archaebacteria (87, 88), which are

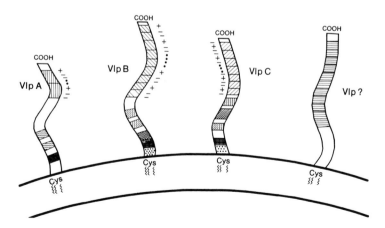

Figure 4. Schematic representation showing proposed features of Vlp expressed at the mycoplasma membrane surface. Key features include (i) membrane anchorage by lipid covalently bound to the N-terminal Cys residue of mature Vlp proteins, (ii) uncharged regions and the repetitive, size-variant C-terminal region carrying the charge motif $(+ \; - \; -)_n$, and (iii) different regions of sequence homology (similarly shaded) that are shared by or reiterated within individual Vlps. Features indicated are based on *vlpA*, *vlpB*, and *vlpC* gene sequences reported in reference 115. The undesignated Vlp indicates the probable combinatorial expression of several additional Vlp products in organisms containing expanded *vlp* gene families. The exact spatial orientation of Vlp polypeptide chains is not known. They are indicated in extended form for purposes of illustration.

hypothesized to mediate similar functions in lieu of conventional eubacterial cell walls.

Host interactions. Clearly, variation in such a layer could also profoundly affect the interaction of *M. hyorhinis* with host cell surfaces and could determine important parameters of self-recognition and contact between mycoplasmas themselves, including their striking aggregation and lateral mobility during surface colonization of some lymphoid cells (17). The virtual continuum of potential surface properties provided by Vlp combinatorial expression and size-variant permutations could provide an inherent plasticity and extreme sensitivity for responding to environmental conditions or could play a role in recognition of several host cells adhesin molecules implicated in pathogenic pathways (31, 107).

Perhaps the most intriguing aspect of the Vlp system is its potential role in modulating the characteristics of host cells with which the mycoplasma interacts. MAbs used to define Vlps indeed mediate interesting effects in cell cultures contaminated with *M. hyorhinis*. A MAb recognizing a common epitope shared by VlpB and VlpC has been shown to inhibit propagation of mycoplasma infections in cell culture, implying that it interferes directly with the organism's ability to replicate or to adhere and colonize the lymphoid cells in that study (40). Perhaps more striking is the effect of the MAb to VlpB. The target of this MAb (DD9) was originally described as a surface component of an invasive sarcoma cell line (91), but was later ascribed to a surface antigen of *M. hyorhinis* that contaminated that line (26). Interestingly, these and later reports (83) documented that the invasiveness of the cell line in vitro was dependent on infection with *M. hyorhinis* and could be completely reversed by treating the cultures with Fab fragments of the DD9 MAb. This finding strongly implicates the mycoplasma in dictating host cell properties and implicates VlpB as a surface molecule that may mediate this effect (77). These MAb-mediated effects might reflect alteration of attachment, surface distribution, or metabolic states of the mycoplasma, or they could engender more direct interactions of the Vlp with host cells through specific modulation of cellular function. Finally, the well-documented role of the lipopeptide portions of lipoproteins as mitogens and modulators of cellular signaling pathways (38) may be an important additional feature to consider in examining possible immunomodulatory roles for Vlps.

Mechanism of Vlp Phase Variation

Lack of chromosomal rearrangement or frameshift mutations during Vlp phase variation

Surface diversity generated by structural variation of individual *vlp* gene products is further potentiated by apparently random phase variation in expression of Vlp proteins (77). Mechanisms regulating the high-frequency phase variation of *vlp* gene products were therefore investigated. A variety of DNA sequences alterations are known to mediate bacterial phase variation, including duplicative (nonreciprocal) transposition of genes to or from expression sites as well as sequence inversions, insertions, or frameshift muta-

tions affecting gene transcription or translation (1, 6, 11, 24, 45–47, 54, 58, 82, 92). Having established that each *vlp* gene occurs as a single chromosomal copy, the possibility was examined that changes in the location or multiplicity of *vlp* genes might be associated with phenotypic switches involving phase transitions between on or off expression states of Vlp products. In an extensive subcloned lineage, switches in expression of several individual or combinatorial Vlp transitions were found to be unaccompanied by detectable changes in characteristic genomic restriction fragments. Lack of polymorphism at the DNA level argued against long-range transpositions or duplication of *vlp* genes during Vlp phase variation.

In the absence of data indicating genomic rearrangements associated with Vlp phase variation, the possibility of phase-associated frameshift mutations in *vlp* coding sequences was similarly examined in this lineage. No changes in individual *vlp* coding sequences were observed during on/off phase transitions, thereby ruling out frameshift mutations as a means of controlling phase variation. Moreover, sequences of the *vlp* genes in the off state directed expression of authentic recombinant Vlp products in *E. coli*.

Association of Vlp phase variation with frequent mutations in a homopolymeric poly(A) tract in *vlp* promoter regions

Lack of DNA sequence alteration in *vlp* structural genes during phase variation raised the possibility that this process is controlled at the transcriptional level. Several features of *vlp* genes are indeed consistent with their possible independent, transcriptional regulation (115). Highly homologous 5′ regions flanking each *vlp* structural gene (Fig. 2) contain several features potentially involved in *vlp* gene expression (depicted in more detail in Fig. 5). Primer extension studies using isolates expressing individual Vlps identified similar transcription initiation sites for each *vlp* gene, 116 to 118 bp upstream of the proposed translation initiation codons. A potential −10 hexamer is present 5 bp upstream of the +1 transcription start site for each *vlp* gene. Two directly repeated 25- to 27-bp sequences (DR1-a and -b), separated by 15 to 16 bp, predict sites on the same side of a B-DNA helix that resemble other procaryotic sequences that accommodate DNA-binding regulator proteins (35, 56, 70, 73, 108). The DR1 structure is in a position typical of positive-regulating activator protein binding sites in procaryotic systems (73), upstream of the transcription initiation site and accessible for possible interaction with RNA polymerase. A striking region of contiguous adenine residues [poly(A)] occurs between the DR1 structure and the transcriptional start site. A second set of distinct, directly repeating 16-bp sequences (DR2-a and -b) and a palindromic stem-loop structure with small direct repeats in the loop (not shown) occur downstream of the transcriptional start and preceding the proposed ribosome binding site. In addition to transcriptional features 5′ of each *vlp* gene, inverted repeat sequences capable of forming stem-loop structures typical of rho-independent transcriptional terminators occur 3′ of *vlpA* ($\Delta G = -14.9$ kcal [1 cal = 4.184 J]), *vlpB* ($\Delta G = -9.6$ kcal), and *vlpC* ($\Delta G = -16.5$ kcal).

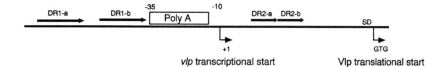

Figure 5. Characteristic features of promoter regions flanking *vlp* genes. Direct repeats DR1 and DR2 represent putative sites binding cell regulatory factors. The homopolymeric poly(A) tract undergoing high-frequency mutations affecting Vlp phase variation is shown, located between the DR1 site and the transcriptional start. A putative Shine-Dalgarno ribosome binding site (SD) and GTG initiation codon are also indicated.

To monitor possible changes upstream of *vlp* genes that might affect expression and phase variation, DNA sequences of 5′ flanking regions were determined in several isolates in different phase states of Vlp expression. The only sequence difference observed within a region 250 bp upstream of the *vlpA* or *vlpB* gene during phase switches was a change in the length of the poly(A) region. The on and off expression states corresponded exactly to lengths of 17 and 18 residues, respectively, in the poly(A) tract. Longer stretches of up to 20 A residues have been identified in poly(A) regions of two *vlpC* genes from isolates in the off state. Since a mutation affecting the length of the poly(A) tract is the only sequence change detected during phase transitions, is highly correlated with the independent expression state of multiple *vlp* genes, and occurs at a location that could affect transcription initiation, this mechanism is strongly implicated as an element controlling Vlp phase variation.

It is interesting to speculate that transcriptional control of phase variation occurs by critical changes within the poly(A) region affecting the spacing or secondary structure between the −10 site and −35 or DR1-b structures. A similar mechanism has recently been proposed by Willems et al. (108) to regulate phase variation of the *Bordetella pertussis fim* gene, whereby transcription may be controlled by critical changes in the length of a poly(C) tract lying between a putative activator binding sequence and polymerase binding site. *vlp* promoters contain both a putative −35 region (TTGCAA in *vlpA* or TTCAAA in *vlpB* and *vlpC*) contiguous with and partially overlapping the poly(A) tract and the adjacent DR1 repeat structures. Whether these or other structures (Fig. 5) are involved in positive or negative regulation of *vlp* genes (56) is yet to be determined. In recent studies, gel shift assays suggest that a cell factor may specifically bind to the *vlp* promoter regions, although the precise target sequences have not been delineated (unpublished observation). The possibility that *vlp* gene transcription may require or be controlled by other gene products supports the idea that expression of genes in the *vlp* family may be influenced by more global regulatory systems (57, 59) possibly present in the organism. This is not known at the present.

As to the mechanism underlying the mutations within the poly(A) region, it has been shown that regions with reiterated bases are hot spots for small insertions or deletions due to transient misalignment during replication (51, 62, 94). Such a stochastic mechanism might statistically favor insertion or deletion of a single base, which may be sufficient for the regulation of *vlp* genes. It might indeed be expected that mutations resulting in insertion or deletion of several A residues could generate progeny with a decreased probability of subsequent switching in that *vlp* gene. This could explain the imbalance in off versus on switch frequencies observed in some lineages. Overall, the structures of regions flanking *vlp* genes suggest that Vlp expression and phase variation may be determined by complex regulation of gene expression, including several mechanisms affecting transcriptional processes (10, 14, 25, 56, 73, 86, 108).

Origin, Sequence Divergence, and Rearrangement of *vlp* Genes

Possible origins of *vlp* genes

G + C composition of *vlp* genes. An unusual characteristic of *vlp* structural genes is their disproportionately high G + C content. The average genomic base composition of *M. hyorhinis* is ~27% G + C (8). This low G + C content is also reflected in five structural genes in this organism (26, 63, 116), in additional ORFs flanking the *vlp* gene family (unpublished observations), and in ORFs associated with IS-like elements probably transmitted among mycoplasma species of swine (see chapter 22). In contrast, the ORFs encoding Vlp proteins show a composition of 39 to 41% G + C. Moreover, the boundary of this feature is abrupt; the highly conserved 5′ regions flanking *vlp* genes (Fig. 2) contain only 17% G + C. This localized bias in base composition might argue that sequences encoding Vlps were acquired from an exogenous source, since emergence of specific G + C-rich regions in an organism subjected to strong AT-biased mutational pressure (69) seems quite unlikely.

Selection involving overlapping ORFs. Maintenance of this compositional bias might be further explained by the unusual presence of multiple ORFs, on both strands, overlapping the sequences encoding each Vlp protein (indicated by small solid arrows in Fig. 2). It is not yet known whether products encoded by alternative ORFs are expressed in *M. hyorhinis*. Nevertheless, the elevated G + C content might reflect constraints imposed by selection against nonsense mutations in the several ORFs overlapping *vlp* gene regions, particularly if these coding regions provide a specific advantage to the organism. It is noteworthy that ORFs encoding Vlp sequences contain no UGA codons, whereas some alternative ORFs do. The use of the UGA (Trp) codon by mycoplasmas (69) thus enhances the potential use of such alternative coding regions.

Sequence divergence in overlapping ORFs

Reiterated sequences and alternative reading frames within *vlp* genes may also play a key role in their evolution as diversity-generating sequences. Frameshift mutations in any *vlp* gene downstream of the Cys residue could, in principle, create an entirely new lipoprotein or, with multiple mutations, a hybrid protein containing variable portions of divergent sequence. Although alternate ORFs predict sequence features quite incompatible with authentic Vlps, they may be a critical source for mutational divergence of Vlp sequences. Repetitive oligomeric sequences with overlapping ORFs have indeed been proposed as important primitive coding elements (66, 89, 114) on the basis of their ability to encode products of substantial length, their resistance to insertions or substitutions that might create termination codons, and their ability to rapidly create divergent sequences by frameshift mutations (66). Duplication or exchange of small segments of sequence through ectopic recombination among extensive reiterated sequences throughout *vlp* genes (2, 71) and the likelihood of error-prone DNA replication in these organisms (51, 61) would further facilitate the use of such sequences in *vlp* gene diversification.

vlp gene rearrangements

It is not clear whether *vlp* coding regions and their 5′ flanking sequences have been acquired as blocks of multiple genes or evolved from a single copy introduced into the organism. Although originally undetected in immunoblot searches of SK76 clonal isolates, recently discovered clones with greatly enlarged *vlp* gene families have been discovered in passaged SK76 populations. This finding indicates a powerful population dynamic of chromosomal rearrangements involving sets of *vlp* genes. It is possible that any small repetitive regions could serve as sites for deletions or insertions of genes by a variety of mechanisms (2, 37, 71). Indeed, partial examination of regions flanking different-sized *vlp* clusters in two clonal isolates revealed identical boundaries near the homologous and repetitive DR1 structures (Fig. 5) of the distinct 5′ *vlp* genes in each family (117). Lysogenic phage (36) and apparently transmissible IS-like sequences (see chapter 22) reported for *M. hyorhinis* offer additional elements potentially capable of introducing or rearranging *vlp* genes. In this sense, the *vlp* gene family might resemble some phage-encoded or IS-associated virulence factors recently reported in other eubacteria (9, 45, 60, 72).

Summary of *vlp* Attributes Generating Diversity in *M. hyorhinis*

Viewed from the perspective of population dynamics, the *vlp* gene system contributes to phenotypic fluctuations by several mechanisms, including (i) gain or loss of multiple, homologous yet divergent genes, (ii) several potential intragenic mutations affecting sequence divergence, (iii) high-frequency reiteration or deletion of periodic coding regions, (iv) random mutational pathways affecting the transcription of *vlp* genes, which generates a combinatorial repertoire of Vlp surface mosaics, and (v) possible control by putative global regulatory systems in this organism.

The Vlp system of *M. hyorhinis* represents an unprecedented combination of genetic and structural attributes providing a highly plastic set of variant proteins at the surface membrane of this microbe. Use of conserved as well as uniquely variant procaryotic lipoprotein domains as a structural basis for antigenic and possibly functional variation is an adaptation perhaps ideally suited to the wall-less mycoplasmas. Provision of a system for combinatorial expression of multiple Vlp products further enhances the potential response of the system to environmental changes, either by selection of specific mycoplasma populations in the host or through signals modulating functionally distinct mosaics of Vlp products (24, 31, 107). From an evolutionary standpoint, the apparently exogenous origin of the Vlp system also emphasizes a possibly critical role for epigenetic factors during reduction evolution and perhaps concomitant host adaptation of this genomically limited group of organisms.

ANTIGENIC VARIATION AND HETEROGENEITY IN OTHER MYCOPLASMAS AND PROCARYOTES

Variation Involving Lipoproteins or Repetitive Protein Structure

Extensive literature documents the widespread presence throughout the eubacterial kingdom of diverse systems and genetic mechanisms that maintain heterogeneity in a variety of proteins and other macromolecules. Excellent reviews of this subject are available (24, 55, 58, 84). However, some specific examples that resemble molecular motifs described in the Vlp system are noteworthy. First, lipoproteins are becoming increasingly appreciated as important membrane surface constituents of mycoplasmas and may represent an adaptation for several functions, including transport proteins (26) and other surface molecules (19, 20, 64, 109). Specific examples of variable lipoproteins in mycoplasmas are discussed below. Some variable lipoproteins also occur in other bacteria. The *Neisseria* H.8 antigen contains repetitive primary sequence structure and can occur in multiple contexts with alternative domains appended to the lipoprotein sequence (111). Lipoproteins also constitute major variant proteins in *Borrelia* species, including OspA and OspB products in *Borrelia burgdorferi* (12) and a large repertoire of alternative products encoded in an extensive family of mobile, plasmid-encoded genes in *B. hermsii* (6, 16, 41). Additional examples of variation based on the procaryotic lipoprotein structure are likely to emerge in the future.

The other striking feature of Vlp proteins, found also in assorted bacteria, is the use of tandemly repetitive protein structure. Pertinent examples include the M proteins of streptococci (32) and surface proteins of *Rickettsia rickettsiae* (4) and *Anaplasma marginale* (3). All of these are known or proposed to participate in spontaneous size variations. Mycoplasma proteins with internally reiterated structures have been reported to be present in *M. pneumoniae* and *M. genitalium* (see chapters 22 and 27).

Systems of Variation and Heterogeneity in Other Mycoplasma Species

Genomic and structural diversity occur in many mycoplasma species (see chapter 34). Features of selected mycoplasma species closely resemble and may be mechanistically analogous to the characteristics found in the Vlp system. These are described below. It should be noted that the molecular basis of variation detailed for the Vlp system predicts several characteristics that, when measured in bulk culture, superficially resemble several of the examples cited. These include (i) strain variability, (ii) possible expression of epitopes defining serovarlike sets of proteins shared among or unique to subsets of organisms, (iii) size variation, (iv) amphiphilic membrane lipoproteins, (v) variation in colony opacity and morphology, and (vi) extensive genomic variation, based on insertion, deletion, or rearrangements of gene blocks or on high-frequency random mutations generating restriction fragment length polymorphisms. Several mechanisms other than those defined in the Vlp system may also create any of these phenotypic characteristics. Therefore, while it may be useful to use the Vlp system as a paradigm of variation in mycoplasmas, other models and possibilities should not be ruled out in particular systems, especially those for which genetic mechanisms have not been established. Some examples are given below.

M. hominis

Extensive variability has been observed with respect to genetic restriction patterns, protein profiles, and serologically or MAb-defined surface antigens (see chapter 34). Recent work particularly emphasizing features resembling Vlp proteins describes amphiphilic, lipid-labeled proteins that vary in size and expression among several human isolates, including several derived longitudinally from a single patient with inflammatory arthritis (67, 68). These authors raise the possibility that variation could occur in the human host.

U. urealyticum

In *Ureaplasma urealyticum*, size-variant and strain-variant patterns of surface proteins have been documented that generate characteristic ladders and express epitopes defining marked strain heterogeneity (98, 103). In one case, serovar-specific proteins have been shown to be lipid modified and amphiphilic (98).

M. pulmonis

A system of variable protein (V-1) antigens closely resembling the Vlp system has been extensively documented (see chapter 24). In particular, variant surface antigens are hydrophobic, express shared as well as specific epitopes, and show size-dependent isoelectric variation (43, 104, 105). Variation in colony opacity, long observed in this species (21–23, 52), has been argued to vary with selective patterns of V-1 expression (104), as has colony morphology (28). Size and expression of V-1 antigens undergo high-frequency phase switching (27, 105). Isoelectric variants of V-1 have been proposed to correlate with the ability of cells to adsorb the P1 virus of this species (27), and complex V-1 patterns have been proposed to be associated with disease characteristics in rodents (96). In contrast to the repetitive structures generating size variation in the Vlp system, size variation in V-1 antigen was proposed to arise from assembly of subunit structures (104). In recent studies by another group, clinical isolates of *M. pulmonis* have been shown to express variable patterns, sizes, and combinations of proteins resembling some features of the V-1 antigen (49), further suggesting that systems creating variable antigens may be operating in natural populations of this species.

M. fermentans

Recent analysis of this species has shown restriction fragment length polymorphism differences among strains, using probes recognizing an IS-like element (44). Strain differences in size and expression of some proteins have also been noted within this species (80, 90). Recently, a family of variant membrane surface lipoproteins has been shown to undergo high-frequency, noncoordinate phase variation, and the gene corresponding to one variant protein displays a typical procaryotic lipoprotein signal peptide (97). Thus, a system quite analogous to the Vlp system of *M. hyorhinis* may occur in this species.

M. gallisepticum

M. gallisepticum has been shown to display both genotypic (81) and extensive antigenic (5, 7) diversity among several isolates, involving amphiphilic membrane proteins recognized by host antibodies. This extends the observation of antigenic diversification to mycoplasma species of avian hosts.

M. pneumoniae

Variation in *M. pneumoniae* is reviewed in chapters 24 and 27. Heterogeneity among clinical isolates (95) and reversible, high-frequency mutations affecting cytadhesion (48) and structural analysis of other phase-variable proteins (65) have been documented in this species.

Other species

Heterogeneity that could be based on variant antigen systems has also been observed in *M. arthritidis* (101, 102) and in amphiphilic proteins of *M. ovipneumoniae* (99). Variation in colony morphology has been noted in *M. mycoides* (50, 100). The species listed here may not be inclusive, but they clearly indicate the wide occurrence of genomic and phenotypic heterogeneity among mycoplasmas.

FUTURE CONSIDERATIONS OF ANTIGENIC VARIATION IN MYCOPLASMAS

The detailed molecular description of one system of antigenic variation and the literature describing the extent of diversity-generating systems among species strongly suggest that such systems may be extremely widespread among mycoplasmas. In addition, these systems are complex at the genetic level and yield complex patterns when assessed in populations. Several considerations and issues will need to be addressed in future studies of such organisms, in terms of experimental approaches and interpretations.

(i) It is important to realize that mycoplasmas occur as rapidly mutating populations.

(ii) Diversification may occur in very short periods, even during growth from a single organism to a colony.

(iii) Host environments as well as those used for in vitro cultivation may be quite selective for populations. Sampling the host population by cultivation may select particular phenotypes; reintroduction of populations into the host after in vitro cultivation may similarly select subpopulations. Classic techniques generally fail to address the distribution of phenotypes in the host or in cultured populations.

(iv) Attempts to correlate phenotypes determined in vitro with properties of the organism in vivo are inherently limited by lack of knowledge about the selection or dynamics of populations in either environment.

(v) Since differences in the capacity to diversify may be as important for infection or disease as the elaboration of specific gene products, efforts using new technologies to assess the distribution and phenotypes of populations within the host will be increasingly needed. An understanding of the molecular genetic basis for antigenic structure and variation is critical in this regard, since the expression state of genes must be determined either by detecting a gene product (transcript or protein) or by defining mutations that specify the expression state and nature of the product, as has been accomplished with *vlp* genes. This strategy will be especially critical in the absence of versatile systems for classic mutational analysis of mycoplasmas.

Acknowledgments. Work by the authors discussed in this chapter was supported in part by Public Health Service grant AI31656 from the National Institutes of Health (K.S.W.) and a grant from the University of Missouri Weldon Spring Fund (K.S.W.). D.Y. was the recipient of fellowships from the Rothschild Foundation and the University of Missouri–Columbia Molecular Biology Program. R.R. was the recipient of a fellowship (Ro 739/1-1) from the Deutsche Forschungsgemeinschaft.

REFERENCES

1. **Abraham, J. M., C. S. Freitag, J. R. Clements, and B. I. Eisenstein.** 1985. An invertible element of DNA controls phase variation of type 1 fimbriae of *Escherichia coli*. *Proc. Natl. Acad. Sci. USA* **82**:5724–5727.
2. **Albertini, A. M., M. Hofer, M. P. Calos, and J. H. Miller.** 1982. On the formation of spontaneous deletions: the importance of short sequence homologies in the generation of large deletions. *Cell* **29**:319–328.
3. **Allred, D. R., T. C. McGuire, G. H. Palmer, S. R. Leib, T. M. Harkins, T. F. McElwain, and A. F. Barbet.** 1990. Molecular basis for surface antigen size polymorphisms and conservation of a neutralization-sensitive epitope in *Anaplasma marginale*. *Proc. Natl. Acad. Sci. USA* **87**:3220–3224.
4. **Anderson, B. E., G. A. McDonald, D. C. Jones, and R. L. Regnery.** 1990. A protective protein antigen of *Rickettsia rickettsii* has tandemly repeated, near-identical sequences. *Infect. Immun.* **58**:2760–2769.
5. **Avakian, A. P., S. H. Kleven, and D. H. Ley.** 1991. Comparison of *Mycoplasma gallisepticum* strains and identification of immunogenic integral membrane proteins with Triton X-114 by immunoblotting. *Vet. Microbiol.* **29**:319–328.
6. **Barbour, A. G.** 1990. Antigenic variation of a relapsing fever *Borrelia* species. *Annu. Rev. Microbiol.* **44**:155–171.
7. **Barbour, E. K., J. A. Newman, J. Sasipreeyajan, A. C. Caputa, and M. A. Muneer.** 1989. Identification of the antigenic components of the virulent *Mycoplasma gallisepticum* (R) in chickens: their role in differentiation from the vaccine strain (F). *Vet. Immunol. Immunopathol.* **21**:197–206.
8. **Barile, M. F., and S. Razin (ed.).** 1979. *The Mycoplasmas*, vol. 1. Academic Press, Inc., New York.
9. **Barondess, J. J., and J. Beckwith.** 1990. A bacterial virulence determinant encoded by lysogenic coliphage λ. *Nature* (London) **346**:871–874.
10. **Belland, R. J.** 1991. H-DNA formation by the coding repeat elements of neisserial *opa* genes. *Mol. Microbiol.* **5**:2351–2360.
11. **Berg, D. E., and M. M. Howe (ed.).** 1989. *Mobile DNA.* American Society for Microbiology, Washington, D.C.
12. **Bergström, S., V. G. Bundoc, and A. G. Barbour.** 1989. Molecular analysis of linear plasmid-encoded major surface proteins, OspA and OspB, of the Lyme disease spirochaete *Borrelia burgdorferi*. *Mol. Microbiol.* **3**:479–486.
13. **Boyer, M. J., and K. S. Wise.** 1989. Lipid-modified surface protein antigens expressing size variation within the species *Mycoplasma hyorhinis*. *Infect. Immun.* **57**:245–254.
14. **Braaten, B. A., L. B. Blyn, B. S. Skinner, and D. A. Low.** 1991. Evidence for a methylation-blocking factor (*mbf*) locus involved in *pap* pilus expression and phase variation in *Escherichia coli*. *J. Bacteriol.* **173**:1789–1800.
15. **Bricker, T. M., M. J. Boyer, J. Keith, R. Watson-McKown, and K. S. Wise.** 1988. Association of lipids with integral membrane surface proteins of *Mycoplasma hyorhinis*. *Infect. Immun.* **56**:295–301.
16. **Burman, N., S. Bergström, B. I. Restrepo, and A. G. Barbour.** 1990. The variable antigens Vmp7 and Vmp21 of the relapsing fever bacterium *Borrelia hermsii* are structurally analogous to the VSG proteins of the African trypanosome. *Mol. Microbiol.* **4**:1715–1726.
17. **Cole, B. C., Y. Naot, E. J. Stanbridge, and K. S. Wise.** 1985. Interactions of mycoplasmas and their products with lymphoid cells in vitro, p. 203–257. *In* S. Razin and M. F. Barile (ed.), *The Mycoplasmas*, vol. 4. *Mycoplasma Pathogenicity*. Academic Press, Inc., New York.
18. **Coote, J. G.** 1991. Antigenic switching and pathogenicity: environmental effects on virulence gene expression in *Bordetella pertussis*. *J. Gen. Microbiol.* **137**:2493–2503.
19. **Dahl, C. E., J. S. Dahl, and K. Bloch.** 1983. Proteolipid formation in *Mycoplasma capricolum*. *J. Biol. Chem.* **258**:11814–11818.
20. **Dahl, C. E., N. C. Sacktor, and J. S. Dahl.** 1985. Acylated proteins in *Acholeplasma laidlawii*. *J. Bacteriol.* **162**:445–447.
21. **Davidson, M. K., S. E. Ross, J. R. Lindsey, and G. H. Cassell.** 1988. Colony opacity, hemadsorption, hemolysis, and mitogenicity are not associated with virulence of *Mycoplasma pulmonis*. *Infect. Immun.* **56**:2169–2173.
22. **Deeb, B. J., and G. E. Kenny.** 1967. Characterization of *Mycoplasma pulmonis* variants isolated from rabbits. I. Identification and properties of isolates. *J. Bacteriol.* **93**:1416–1424.

23. **Deeb, B. J., and G. E. Kenny.** 1967. Characterization of *Mycoplasma pulmonis* variants isolated from rabbits. II. Basis for differentiation of antigenic subtypes. *J. Bacteriol.* **93:**1425–1429.

24. **DiRita, V. J., and J. J. Mekalanos.** 1989. Genetic regulation of bacterial virulence. *Annu. Rev. Genet.* **23:**455–482.

25. **Dorman, C. J., N. N. Bhriain, and C. F. Higgins.** 1990. DNA supercoiling and environmental regulation of virulence gene expression in *Shigella flexneri*. *Nature* (London) **344:**789–792.

26. **Dudler, R., C. Schmidhauser, R. W. Parish, R. E. H. Wettenhall, and T. Schmidt.** 1988. A mycoplasma high-affinity transport system and the *in vitro* invasiveness of mouse sarcoma cells. *EMBO J.* **7:**3963–3970.

27. **Dybvig, K., J. Alderete, H. L. Watson, and G. H. Cassell.** 1988. Adsorption of mycoplasma virus P1 to host cells. *J. Bacteriol.* **170:**4373–4375.

28. **Dybvig, K., J. Simecka, H. Watson, and G. Cassell.** 1989. High-frequency variation in *Mycoplasma pulmonis* colony size. *J. Bacteriol.* **171:**5165–5168.

29. **Dybvig, K., and A. Woodard.** 1992. Cloning and DNA sequencing of a *Mycoplasma recA* gene. *J. Bacteriol.* **174:**778–784.

30. **Ferrell, R. V., M. B. Heidari, K. S. Wise, and M. A. McIntosh.** 1989. A mycoplasma genetic element resembling prokaryotic insertion sequences. *Mol. Microbiol.* **3:**957–967.

31. **Finlay, B. B., and S. Falkow.** 1989. Common themes in microbial pathogenicity. *Microbiol. Rev.* **53:**210–230.

32. **Fischetti, V. A.** 1991. Streptococcal M protein. *Sci. Am.* **264:**32–39.

33. **Garnier, J., D. J. Ogusthorpe, and B. J. Robson.** 1978. Analysis of the accuracy and implications of simple methods for predicting the secondary structure of globular proteins. *Mol. Biol.* **120:**97–120.

34. **Goiš, M., F. Kuksa, J. Franz, and D. Taylor-Robinson.** 1974. The antigenic differentiation of seven strains of *Mycoplasma hyorhinis* by growth-inhibition, metabolism-inhibition, latex-agglutination, and polyacrylamide-gel-electrophoresis tests. *J. Med. Microbiol.* **7:**105–115.

35. **Gottesman. S.** 1984. Bacterial regulation: global regulatory networks. *Annu. Rev. Genet.* **18:**415–441.

36. **Gourlay, R. N., S. G. Wyld, and M. E. Poulton.** 1983. Some characteristics of mycoplasma virus Hr1, isolated from and infecting *Mycoplasma hyorhinis*. *Arch. Virol.* **77:**81–85.

37. **Haas, R., and T. F. Meyer.** 1986. The repertoire of silent pilus genes in *Neisseria gonorrhoeae*: evidence for gene conversion. *Cell* **44:**107–115.

38. **Hauschildt, S., U. Steffens, L. Wagner-Roos, and W. G. Bessler.** 1988. Role of proteinkinase C and phosphatidylinositol metabolism in lipopeptide-induced leukocyte activation as signal transducing mechanism. *Mol. Immunol.* **25:**1081–1086.

39. **Hayflick, L., and E. Stanbridge.** 1967. Isolation and identification of mycoplasma from human clinical materials. *Ann. N.Y. Acad. Sci.* **143:**608–621.

40. **Hemler, M. E., and J. Strominger.** 1982. Monoclonal antibodies reacting with immunogenic mycoplasma proteins present in human hematopoietic cell lines. *J. Immunol.* **129:**2734–2738.

41. **Hinnebusch, J., S. Bergström, and A. G. Barbour.** 1990. Cloning and sequence analysis of linear plasmid telomeres of the bacterium *Borrelia burgdorferi*. *Mol. Microbiol.* **4:**811–820.

42. **Hollingshead, S. K., V. A. Fischetti, and J. R. Scott.** 1987. Size variation in group A streptococcal M protein is generated by homologous recombination between intragenic repeats. *Mol. Gen. Genet.* **207:**196–203.

43. **Horowitz, S. A., B. Garrett, J. K. Davis, and G. H. Cassell.** 1987. Isolation of *Mycoplasma pulmonis* membranes and identification of surface antigens. *Infect. Immun.* **55:**1314–1320.

44. **Hu, W. S., R. Y.-H, Wang, R.-S. Liou, J. W.-K. Shih, and S.-C. Lo.** 1990. Identification of an insertion-sequence-like genetic element in the newly recognized human pathogen *Mycoplasma incognitus*. *Gene* **93:**67–72.

45. **Jalajakumari, M. B., C. J. Thomas, R. Halter, and P. A. Manning.** 1989. Genes for biosynthesis and assembly of CS3 pili of CFA/II enterotoxigenic *Escherichia coli*: novel regulation of pilus production by bypassing an amber codon. *Mol. Microbiol.* **3:**1685–1695.

46. **Jonsson, A.-B., G. Nyberg, and S. Normark.** 1991. Phase variation of gonococcal pili by frameshift mutation in pilC, a novel gene for pilus assembly. *EMBO J.* **10:**477–488.

47. **Kitten, T., and A. G. Barbour.** 1990. Juxtaposition of expressed variable antigen genes with a conserved telomere in the bacterium *Borrelia hermsii*. *Proc. Natl. Acad. Sci. USA* **87:**6077–6081.

48. **Krause, D. C., D. K. Leith, and J. B. Baseman.** 1983. Reacquisition of specific proteins confers virulence in *Mycoplasma pneumoniae*. *Infect. Immun.* **39:**830–836.

49. **Lai, W. C., M. Bennett, S. P. Pakes, and S. S. Murphree.** 1991. Potential subunit vaccine against *Mycoplasma pulmonis* purified by a protective monoclonal antibody. *Vaccine* **9:**177–184.

50. **Leach, R. H., M. Costas, and D. L. Mitchelmore.** 1989. Relationship between *Mycoplasma mycoides* subsp. *mycoides* ('large-colony' strains) and *M. mycoides* subsp. *capri*, as indicated by numerical analysis of one-dimensional SDS-PAGE protein patterns. *J. Gen. Microbiol.* **135:**2993–3000.

51. **Levinson, G., and G. A. Gutman.** 1987. Slipped-strand mispairing: a major mechanism for DNA sequence evoluation. *Mol. Biol. Evol.* **4:**203–221.

52. **Liss, A., and R. A. Heiland.** 1983. Colonial opacity variation in *Mycoplasma pulmonis*. *Infect. Immun.* **41:**1245–1251.

53. **Mahairas, G., and F. C. Minion.** 1989. Transformation of *Mycoplasma pulmonis*: demonstration of homologous recombination, introduction of cloned genes, and preliminary description of an integrating shuttle system. *J. Bacteriol.* **171:**1775–1780.

54. **Marrs, C. F., W. W. Ruehl, G. K. Schoolnik, and S. Falkow.** 1988. Pili gene phase variation of *Moraxella bovis* is due to an inversion of the pilin genes. *J. Bacteriol.* **170:**3032–3039.

55. **Maskell, D. J., M. J. Szabo, P. D. Butler, A. E. Williams, and E. R. Moxon.** 1991. Molecular analysis of a complex locus from *Haemophilus influenzae* involved in phase-variable lipopolysaccharide biosynthesis. *Mol. Microbiol.* **5:**1013–1022.

56. **Matthews, K. S.** 1992. DNA looping. *Microbiol. Rev.* **56:**123–136.

57. **Mekalanos, J. J.** 1992. Environmental signals controlling expression of virulence determinants in bacteria. *J. Bacteriol.* **174:**1–7.

58. **Meyer, T. F.** 1987. Molecular basis of surface antigen variation in *Neisseria*. *Trends Genet.* **3:**319–324.

59. **Miller, J. F., J. J. Mekalanos, and S. Falkow.** 1989. Coordinate regulation and sensory transduction in the control of bacterial virulence. *Science* **243:**916–922.

60. **Miller, V. L., J. B. Biliska, and S. Falkow.** 1990. Nucleotide sequence of the *Yersinia enterocolitica ail* gene and characterization of the Ail protein product. *J. Bacteriol.* **172:**1062–1069.

61. **Mills, B. L., E. J. Stanbridge, W. D. Sedwick, and D. Korn.** 1979. Purification and partial characterization of the principal deoxyribonucleic acid polymerase from *Mycoplasmatales*. *J. Bacteriol.* **132:**641–649.

62. **Murphy, G. L., T. D. Connell, D. S. Barritt, M. Koomey, and J. G. Cannon.** 1989. Phase variation of gonococcal protein. II. Regulation of gene expression by slipped-

strand mispairing of a repetitive DNA sequence. *Cell* **56**:539–547.

63. **Notarnicola, S. M., M. A. McIntosh, and K. S. Wise.** 1991. A *Mycoplasma hyorhinis* protein with sequence similarities to nucleotide-binding enzymes. *Gene* **97**:77–85.

64. **Nyström, S., K.-E. Johansson, and A. Wieslander.** 1986. Selective acylation of membrane proteins in *Acholeplasma laidlawii*. *Eur. J. Biochem.* **156**:85–94.

65. **Ogle, K. F., K. K. Lee, and D. C. Krause.** 1991. Cloning and analysis of the gene encoding the cytadherence phase-variable protein HMW3 from *Mycoplasma pneumoniae*. *Gene* **97**:69–75.

66. **Ohno, U.** 1984. Birth of a unique enzyme from an alternative reading frame of the preexisted, internally repetitious coding sequence. *Proc. Natl. Acad. Sci. USA* **81**:2421–2425.

67. **Olson, L. D., C. A. Renshaw, S. W. Shane, and M. F. Barile.** 1991. Successive synovial *Mycoplasma hominis* isolates exhibit apparent antigenic variation. *Infect. Immun.* **59**:3327–3329.

68. **Olson, L. D., S. W. Shane, A. A. Karpas, T. M. Cunningham, P. S. Probst, and M. F. Barile.** 1991. Monoclonal antibodies to surface antigens of a pathogenic *Mycoplasma hominis* strain. *Infect. Immun.* **59**:1683–1689.

69. **Osawa, S., T. H. Jukes, K. Watanabe, and A. Muto.** 1992. Recent evidence for evolution of the genetic code. *Microbiol. Rev.* **56**:229–264.

70. **Pabo, C. O., and R. T. Sauer.** 1984. Protein-DNA recognition. *Annu. Rev. Biochem.* **53**:293–321.

71. **Petes, D. T., and C. W. Hill.** 1988. Recombination between repeated genes in microorganisms. *Annu. Rev. Genet.* **22**:147–168.

72. **Pulkkinen, W. S., and S. I. Miller.** 1991. A *Salmonella typhimurium* virulence protein is similar to a *Yersinia enterocolitica* invasion protein and a bacteriophage lambda outer membrane protein. *J. Bacteriol.* **173**:86–93.

73. **Raibaud, O., and M. Schwartz.** 1984. Positive control of transcription initiation in bacteria. *Annu. Rev. Genet.* **18**:173–206.

74. **Riethmann, H. C., M. J. Boyer, and K. S. Wise.** 1987. Triton X-114 phase fractionation of an integral membrane surface protein mediating monoclonal antibody killing of *Mycoplasma hyorhinis*. *Infect. Immun.* **55**:1094–1100.

75. **Rosengarten, R., P. Theiss, D. Yogev, and K. S. Wise.** Unpublished data.

76. **Rosengarten, R., and K. S. Wise.** 1990. Phenotypic switching in mycoplasmas: phase varition of diverse surface lipoproteins. *Science* **247**:315–318.

77. **Rosengarten, R., and K. S. Wise.** 1991. The Vlp system of *Mycoplasma hyorhinis*: combinatorial expression of distinct size variant lipoproteins generating high-frequency surface antigenic variation. *J. Bacteriol.* **173**:4782–4793.

78. **Ross, R., S. Dale, and J. Duncan.** 1973. Experimentally induced *Mycoplasma hyorhinis* arthritis of swine: immune response to 26th postinoculation week. *Am. J. Vet. Res.* **34**:367–373.

79. **Ross, R. F.** 1973. Pathogenicity of swine mycoplasmas. *Ann. N.Y. Acad. Sci.* **225**:347–368.

80. **Saillard, C., P. Carle, J. M. Bové, C. Bébéar, S.-C. Lo, J. W.-K. Shin, R. Y.-H. Wang, D. L. Rose, and J. G. Tully.** 1990. Genetic and serologic relatedness between *Mycoplasma fermentans* strains and a mycoplasma recently identified in tissues of AIDS and non-AIDS patients. *Res. Virol.* **141**:385–395.

81. **Santha, M., K. Lukacs, K. Burg, S. Bernath, I. Rasko, and L. Stipkovits.** 1988. Intraspecies genotypic heterogeneity among *Mycoplasma gallisepticum* strains. *Appl. Environ. Microbiol.* **54**:607–609.

82. **Saunders, J. R.** 1989. Modulating bacterial virulence. *Nature* (London) **338**:622–623.

83. **Schmidhauser, C., R. Dudler, T. Schmidt, and R. W. Parish.** 1990. A mycoplasmal protein influences tumour cell invasiveness and contact inhibition *in vitro*. *J. Cell Sci.* **95**:499–506.

84. **Seifert, H. S., and M. So.** 1988. Genetic mechanisms of bacterial antigenic variation. *Microbiol. Rev.* **52**:327–336.

85. **Selander, R. K., D. A. Caugant, and T. S. Whittam.** 1987. Genetic structure and variation in natural populations of *Escherichia coli*, p. 1625–1648. *In* F. C. Neidhardt, J. L. Ingraham, K. B. Low, B. Magasanik, M. Schaechter, and H. E. Umbarger (ed.), *Escherichia coli and Salmonella typhimurium: Cellular and Molecular Biology*, vol. 2. American Society for Microbiology, Washington, D.C.

86. **Simons, R. W., and N. Kleckner.** 1988. Biological regulation by antisense RNA in prokaryotes. *Annu. Rev. Genet.* **22**:567–600.

87. **Sleytr, U. B., and P. Messner.** 1988. Crystalline surface layers in procaryotes. *J. Bacteriol.* **170**:2891–2897.

88. **Smit, J.** 1986. Protein surface layers of bacteria, p. 343–376. *In* M. Inouye (ed.), *Bacterial Outer Membranes as Model Systems*. John Wiley & Sons, Inc., New York.

89. **Smith, G. P.** 1976. Evolution of repeated DNA sequences by unequal crossover. *Science* **191**:528–535.

90. **Stadtländer, C. T. K.-H., C. Zuhua, H. L. Watson, and G. H. Cassell.** 1991. Protein and antigen heterogeneity among strains of *Mycoplasma fermentans*. *Infect. Immun.* **59**:3319–3322.

91. **Steinemann, C., M. Fenner, H. Binz, and R. W. Parish.** 1984. Invasive behavior of mouse sarcoma cells is inhibited by blocking a 37,000-dalton plasma membrane glycoprotein with Fab fragments. *Proc. Natl. Acad. Sci. USA* **81**:3747–3750.

92. **Stibitz, S., W. Aaronson, D. Monack, and S. Falkow.** 1989. Phase variation in *Bordetella pertussis* by frameshift mutation in a gene for a novel two-component system. *Nature* (London) **338**:266–269.

93. **Stocker, B. A. D.** 1949. Measurements of rate of mutation of flagellar antigenic phase in *Salmonella typhimurium*. *J. Hyg.* **47**:398–413.

94. **Streisinger, G., and J. E. Owen.** 1985. Mechanisms of spontaneous and induced frameshift mutation in bacteriophage T4. *Genetics* **109**:633–659.

95. **Su, C. J., S. F. Dallo, and J. B. Baseman.** 1990. Molecular distinctions among clinical isolates of *Mycoplasma pneumoniae*. *J. Clin Microbiol.* **28**:1538–1540.

96. **Talkington, D. F., M. T. Fallon, H. L. Watson, R. K. Thorp, and G. H. Cassell.** 1989. *Mycoplasma pulmonis* V-1 surface protein variation: occurrence *in vivo* and association with lung lesions. *Microb. Pathog.* **7**:429–436.

97. **Theiss, P., M. F. Kim, and K. S. Wise.** 1992. High frequency antigenic and phase variation of *Mycoplasma fermentans* membrane lipoproteins generating diverse surface mosaics for host interactions, abstr. G-32, p. 164. *Abstr. 92nd Gen. Meet. Am. Soc. Microbiol. 1992.* American Society for Microbiology, Washington, D.C.

98. **Thirkell, D., A. D. Myles, and W. C. Russell.** 1991. Palmitoylated proteins in *Ureaplasma urealyticum*. *Infect. Immun.* **59**:781–784.

99. **Thirkell, D., R. K. Spooner, G. E. Jones, and W. C. Russell.** 1990. Polypeptide and antigenic variability among strains of *Mycoplasma ovipneumoniae* demonstrated by SDS-PAGE and immunoblotting. *Vet. Microbiol.* **21**:241–254.

100. **Valdivieso-Garcia, A., and S. Rosendal.** 1982. Variation in colony size of *Mycoplasma mycoides* subspecies *mycoides* isolated from goats. *Vet. Rec.* **110**:470.

101. **Washburn, L. R., and S. Hirsch.** 1990. Comparison of four *Mycoplasma arthritidis* strains by enzyme immunoassay, metabolism inhibition, one- and two-dimen-

sional electrophoresis, and immunoblotting. *J. Clin. Microbiol.* **28:**1974–1981.

102. **Washburn, L. R., J. R. Ramsay, and L. K. Roberts.** 1985. Characterization of the metabolism inhibition antigen of *Mycoplasma arthritidis. Infect. Immun.* **49:**357–364.

103. **Watson, H. L., D. K. Blalock, and G. H. Cassell.** 1990. Variable antigens of *Ureaplasma urealyticum* containing both serovar-specific and serovar-cross-reactive epitopes. *Infect. Immun.* **58:**3679–3688.

104. **Watson, H. L., K. Dybvig, D. K. Blalock, and G. H. Cassell.** 1989. Subunit structure of the variable V-1 antigen of *Mycoplasma pulmonis. Infect. Immun.* **57:**1684–1690.

105. **Watson, H. L., L. S. McDaniel, D. K. Blalock, M. T. Fallon, and G. H. Cassell.** 1988. Heterogeneity among strains and a high rate of variation within strains of a major surface antigen of *Mycoplasma pulmonis. Infect. Immun.* **56:**1358–1363.

106. **Whittlestone, P.** 1979. Porcine mycoplasmas, p. 133–176. *In* J. G. Tully and R. F. Whitcomb (ed.), *The Mycoplasmas,* vol. 2. Academic Press, Inc., New York.

107. **Wick, M. J., J. L. Madara, B. N. Fields, and S. J. Normark.** 1991. Molecular cross talk between epithelial cells and pathogenic microorganisms. *Cell* **67:**651–659.

108. **Willems, R., A. Paul, H. G. J. van der Heide, A. R. ter Avest, and F. R. Mooi.** 1990. Fimbrial phase variation in *Bordetella pertussis:* a novel mechanism for transcriptional regulation. *EMBO J.* **9:**2803–2809.

109. **Wise, K. S., and M. F. Kim.** 1987. Major membrane surface proteins of *Mycoplasma hyopneumoniae* selectively modified by covalently bound lipid. *J. Bacteriol.* **169:**5546–5555.

110. **Wise, K. S., and R. K. Watson.** 1983. *Mycoplasma hyorhinis* GDL surface protein antigen p120 defined by monoclonal antibody. *Infect. Immun.* **41:**1332–1339.

111. **Woods, J. P., J. F. Dempsey, T. H. Kawula, D. S. Barritt, and J. G. Cannon.** 1989. Characterization of the neisserial lipid-modified azurin bearing the H.8 epitope. *Mol. Microbiol.* **3:**583–591.

112. **Wu, H.** 1987. Post-translational modification and processing of membrane proteins in bacteria, p. 37–71. *In* M. Inouye (ed.), *Bacterial Outer Membranes as Model Systems.* John Wiley & Sons, Inc., New York.

113. **Yanocopoulos, G. D., and F. W. Alt.** 1986. Regulation of the assembly and expression of variable-region genes. *Annu. Rev. Immunol.* **4:**339–368.

114. **Yčas, M.** 1972. *De novo* origin of periodic proteins. *J. Mol. Evol.* **2:**17–27.

115. **Yogev, D., R. Rosengarten, R. Watson-McKown, and K. Wise.** 1991. Molecular basis of *Mycoplasma* surface antigenic variation: a novel set of divergent genes undergo spontaneous mutation of periodic coding regions and 5′ regulatory sequences. *EMBO J.* **10:**4069–4079.

116. **Yogev, D., R. Watson-McKown, M. A. McIntosh, and K. S. Wise.** 1991. Sequence and Tn*phoA* analysis of a *Mycoplasma hyorhinis* protein with membrane export function. *J. Bacteriol.* **173:**2035–2044.

117. **Yogev, D., R. Watson-McKown, R. Rosengarten, and K. S. Wise.** Unpublished data.

29. Immunity and Vaccine Development

JANE S. ELLISON, LYN D. OLSON, and MICHAEL F. BARILE

INTRODUCTION

Mycoplasmas cause severe respiratory, arthritic, and urogenital diseases of humans which result in considerable economic labor hours lost. The incidence of respiratory tract infections due to *Mycoplasma pneumoniae* in the United States during an epidemic year has been estimated to be 8 to 15 million cases (60, 61). The incidence and pathogenesis of the recognized human mycoplasma pathogens are covered elsewhere in this volume (see chapters 25 and 27). Mycoplasmas also cause severe diseases in virtually all mammalian species studied, and animal mycoplasmoses are of major economic importance because their high morbidity and mortality rates result in reduced food production from cattle, sheep, goats, swine, and poultry (see chapter 24). The high frequency of respiratory mycoplasma diseases among laboratory mice and rats jeopardizes the usefulness of these animals as models for biomedical research (29, 116). Vaccine development for animal mycoplasma diseases has been reviewed elsewhere (5, 7). This chapter will concentrate on development of vaccines against human diseases.

Although antibiotic therapy is helpful and can reduce the severity of mycoplasma diseases, treatment does not eliminate colonization or abort infection, and antibiotic resistance can develop (see chapter 31). Thus, vaccines are the most promising approach to the control of mycoplasma infections in humans and animals. Support for the development of an *M. pneumoniae* vaccine is provided by the fact that recovery from disease provides individuals some protection against reinfection (43, 56–59). Experimentally infected hamsters (9, 10) and chimpanzees (12, 14) are fully protected against rechallenge. Also, strains of *M. pneumoniae* isolated from different epidemics show very little variation and have marked antigenic and genotypic homogeneity (37, 176, 186).

Whereas humoral immune mechanisms play a major role in protection against systemic infections, protection against mycoplasma diseases of the mucosal surface appears to be accomplished via complex local and cell-mediated immune mechanisms which are as yet not completely understood. A comprehensive discussion of host defense mechanisms against mucosal surface disease may be found elsewhere (59, 68, 76, 128). The following summary outlines key features of the immune process as they relate to vaccine development.

PATHOGENIC HUMAN MYCOPLASMAS

M. pneumoniae

Protective antigens

Because the host must defend itself from noxious tissue-damaging substances to avoid or abort disease, the toxic and virulence components of a pathogen are generally the most effective protective antigens. A protein-rich cell extract prepared from virulent *M. pneumoniae* 1428 and given intratracheally (i.t.) to hamsters induced histopathological lung changes remarkably similar to those produced during infection (36). Hamsters immunized with the extract were protected from developing disease when challenged with virulent organisms (8–10, 15). The extract contained hemagglutination, attachment inhibition, ciliostatic, chemotactic, and proteolytic activities (31, 32, 36). The ciliostatic activity was heat and protease resistant and induced ciliary damage and ciliocytophoria in tracheal organ cultures in vitro or when inoculated i.t. in hamsters. The chemotactic activity induced an intense peribronchial and perivascular infiltration of cells similar to that induced by infection with virulent *M. pneumoniae* (36). The components responsible for the ciliotoxic and cell recruitment activities have not been

Jane S. Ellison, Lyn D. Olson, and Michael F. Barile • Laboratory of Mycoplasma, Division of Bacterial Products, Center for Biologics Evaluation and Research, Food and Drug Administration, Bethesda, Maryland 20892.

isolated or characterized. Another virulence factor, the ability to inhibit host cell catalase activity, provides *M. pneumoniae* with an additional mechanism for causing injury to host cells (3). The virulence components responsible for each of these toxic activities are potential immunogens.

Attachment initiates infection, and the ability to attach correlates with virulence and pathogenicity in a given strain (35). *M. pneumoniae* attaches via a specialized tip structure (80, 82), and a 169-kDa membrane protein (designated P1), which is found concentrated on the tip structure (16, 80), mediates attachment. Hemadsorption-defective (HA⁻) mutants either lack the P1 cytadhesin or are unable to cap P1 on the attachment organelle and thus are unable to attach and produce disease (16, 80, 55, 100). Monoclonal antibodies (MAbs) to P1 block hemadsorption or the gliding motility of *M. pneumoniae* and reduce its ability to produce lung lesions in infected hamsters without affecting viability of the organism (24). Purified anti-P1 immunoglobulin blocks adsorption to erythrocytes and hamster tracheal rings in vitro without reducing viability or inhibiting glucose metabolism of the mycoplasma (105). The consistent presence of antibodies to P1 in patient sera (91, 93, 176) and respiratory secretions (83) confirms the significance of P1 as a major immunogen.

Recently, a 90- and a 40-kDa protein were shown to be immunodominant, surface exposed, localized on the terminal tip attachment apparatus, present in pathogenic strains, absent in the nonpathogenic strain, and probably involved in attachment. These proteins should also be considered as potential candidate immunogens for inclusion in an acellular *M. pneumoniae* vaccine (62a).

Cytadsorption may be a complex process involving surface proteins other than the P1 cytadhesin, and each of these accessory adhesins may be a potential immunogen. A study of 22 HA⁻ mutants identified seven non-P1 proteins as possible accessories in attachment. Spontaneous HA⁺ revertants, which had regenerated the missing proteins, also regained the ability to attach to hamster tracheal rings in vitro and to produce pneumonia in hamsters (106). Protease treatment of virulent strains resulted in the loss of P1 and a smaller protein (P2) as well as in the loss of attachment capability and virulence. Regeneration of both of these proteins was accompanied by restoration of the ability to attach and to produce disease (82). In a separate study, a 32-kDa protein was also found to be clustered on the tip organelle (17) and may play a role in attachment to nonsialylated receptors (72, 108, 134). Pathogenic strain M129-B7 and isogenic avirulent strain M129-B169 have identical protein profiles except that the avirulent strain has lost a 45-kDa protein and two other protein bands are nonreactive with MAbs against analogous proteins in the pathogenic strain (82), suggesting that these proteins may also play a role in the attachment process. Thus, loss of attachment and virulence can result from either a loss or an alteration in the adhesins or from the fact that the adhesins are not exposed on the membrane surface as a result of structural changes. In most patients, immunoglobulin G (IgG) antibody from sera and respiratory secretions bind most strongly to P1 and an 88- to 90-kDa protein on immunoblots (83, 176), but patient sera

and respiratory secretions also react with numerous other protein bands ranging in size from 193 to 33 kDa. Sera from convalescent patients have consistently higher levels of antibody reactive with these proteins than do sera from patients in the acute stage of disease (176).

The principal protein antigens of *M. pneumoniae* appear to be stable in clinical isolates collected and preserved over a considerable period of time (176). Conversely, most other mycoplasma species, including *M. hominis* and *Ureaplasma urealyticum* (discussed later), exhibit extensive antigenic variability (also see chapters 28 and 33). Many DNA sequences, including one which exceeds 400 bp in length, are repeated 8 to 10 times within the *M. pneumoniae* genome (47, 164, 181); at least one representative of each repetitive element resides within or adjacent to the P1 operon (47). This finding has led to speculation that the P1 region of the *M. pneumoniae* genome may be subject to frequent recombination events causing antigenic variation within the P1 protein. Several recent studies indicate that variation does occur within the P1 adhesin gene. Premature truncation of P1 due to a frameshift mutation results in loss of cytadsorption (165), and restriction fragment length polymorphisms within the P1 gene have been demonstrated also (52).

The antigens that elicit growth-inhibiting, metabolism-inhibiting (MI), and complement-fixing (CF) antibodies to *M. pneumoniae* have been shown to be membrane glycolipids (28, 146). Glycolipid antibodies probably play a major role in clearance of organisms and recovery from disease; however, they do not appear to be directly involved in protection against disease. Immunization with reaggregates of *M. pneumoniae* glycolipids and *Acholeplasma laidlawii* membrane proteins provided hamsters with no significant protection against challenge with virulent organisms, even though CF and MI serum antibodies were induced (27, 147). Other studies have found no correlation between protection and the level of MI antibody (8–10, 15, 77). Conversely, a membrane polysaccharide fraction was immunogenic and provided some protection against challenge in hamsters (27).

Two classes of host tissue receptors for *M. pneumoniae* adhesins have been identified: sialic acid-containing glycoproteins (35, 148) and sulfated glycolipids (108). Although the interactions between the sialic acid-containing glycoconjugate receptors and the binding domains of P1 are well documented, these interactions remain to be completely elucidated. For example, recent studies have identified three regions of P1 that appear to be involved in adherence, although they may not be the immunodominant regions (53, 95, 96).

Protective immune mechanisms

Hamsters (8–11) or chimpanzees (15) recovering from experimentally induced *M. pneumoniae* pneumonia are fully protected against challenge. However, the amount and duration of protection from natural infection in patients to subsequent reinfection are less clear (43–45, 56–62). The general consensus from the available literature indicates that infection early in life confers short-lived protection, but as the population grows older, protection is maintained for longer periods. Also, the severity of infection in parents is generally less severe than that in young adults. The attack rate also varies; there is a lower attack rate in young adults over 15 years of age than in those under 15 and still fewer cases in the middle-age population. Cases of reinfection have been reported (18, 60, 62), but this is a rare event in older adults. Because infection occurs infrequently in older patients, exposure early in life may protect against reinfection in later life (113). Thus, the overall findings would indicate that immunization should provide a useful approach to prevention of infection and disease, especially among children and young adults. It has been speculated that protection in older adults may be due to the accumulation of cross-reactive antibodies to other bacterial infections, which would be similar to findings seen in adults immunized against *Haemophilus influenzae* infections (90a). However, this possibility is speculative and remains to be determined.

The mechanisms responsible for protection against respiratory mucosal infections, including *M. pneumoniae* pneumonia, are not well understood. The available literature suggests that the secretory IgA (sIgA) class of antibodies is the predominant isotype involved in protection against mucosal surface infections (68, 76, 128), and most of the IgA found in secretions is locally produced (86). Repeated subcutaneous (s.c.) or intramuscular (i.m.) administration of antigens has generally been ineffective in evoking specific local mucosal immunity, presumably because of an inadequate sIgA response (98, 109). However, antigen administered by the intraperitoneal (i.p.) route can induce a primary reaction (also referred to as priming) whereby a relatively long-lasting immunological memory of the antigen is created in the form of antigen-specific IgA memory cells (30, 98, 142). Depending on the type of antigen, and the route and schedule by which it is administered, these IgA memory cells can migrate throughout the lymphoid system, reaching distant unstimulated mucosal sites far from the priming site, or they can settle in lymphoid tissues near the site of priming (98). In either case, subsequent contact with the same antigen can trigger the IgA memory cells to become IgA-secreting plasma cells. Since parenteral immunization can suppress or interfere with the secondary mucosal immune response in some cases (142), it is advisable to determine early in the development of a particular vaccine those conditions which induce the optimal mucosal immune response for the particular immunogen and mucosal surface to be protected.

Pulmonary disease induced with virulent *M. pneumoniae* i.t. protects hamsters from subsequent challenge, whereas hamsters given the agent parenterally are not protected, suggesting that local and cell-mediated immune mechanisms are involved in the protective response (8–10, 15). In addition, IgA-bearing cells and IgA antibodies present in the lumen of the lung correlate better with protection than do serum antibody titers (25, 26), and factors present in lung washings of immune hamsters protect against ciliary tissue damage and dysfunction (166). Since IgA does not bind complement, it cannot be involved in complement-mediated phagocytosis or mycoplasmacidal activities. Whether IgA prevents attachment, and thereby prevents disease, remains to be determined

(45). Although preventing attachment is crucial, the vaccine must also prevent ciliotoxicity and the development of pulmonary histopathological lesions. Development of pulmonary lesions appears to be T cell dependent. However, it is not known whether the histopathological lesions are immunologically mediated or a result of a toxic component of the pathogen and infection (44). Perhaps both are involved. In any case, presentation of the antigen is very important. In hamster studies, the most effective route and schedule of antigen presentation which induced protection to *M. pneumoniae* diseases against challenge was the i.p.-i.t. priming-booster immunization schedule (8–10, 15). Other investigators have found a priming i.p. dose followed by local administration of inactivated microbial cells or antigens to be effective in inducing mucosal surface protection (137, 142). A similar immunization strategy has been successful in inducing resistance to *M. pulmonis* in mice, to *M. gallisepticum* in chickens, and to *M. bovis* in cattle; however, it has failed to induce protection against *M. pulmonis* infection in rats and to *M. hyopneumoniae* infection in swine (5, 7).

Vaccine strategies

The current working concept for successful immunization can be stated simply as follows: preventing attachment prevents initiation of disease, and preventing tissue damage prevents or reduces the severity of disease (5, 7). Several conditions must be met for immunization to be successful: (i) a vaccine must contain a protective immunogen(s), (ii) the antigens must be genetically and phenotypically stable, (iii) the route and presentation must elicit a protective respiratory mucosal immune response, and (iv) the vaccine must protect without inducing untoward toxic reactions or adverse immune abnormalities, including potentiation of disease (49, 64, 102). Because certain vaccines can potentiate disease, vaccinees must be carefully monitored. Patients immunized with various formalin-inactivated viral, chlamydial, or mycoplasmal vaccines have developed accelerated, potentiated disease upon subsequent infection (49, 64, 102). Patient volunteers (159, 160) and hamsters (8–10, 15, 43) immunized with formalin-inactivated *M. pneumoniae* vaccine developed a more severe pneumonia following challenge than did nonimmunized subjects. Potentiation of mycoplasmal diseases has also been reported for chickens immunized with inactivated *M. gallisepticum* (1) and for pigs immunized with either *M. hyopneumoniae* antigens (151) or a whole-cell formalin-inactivated vaccine (107). This apparent sensitization following immunization dictates caution in the evaluation of experimental vaccines and careful, methodical follow-up and surveillance of immunized subjects.

Inactivated vaccines. Shortly after Chanock et al. (38) reported that *M. pneumoniae* was the cause of primary atypical pneumonia, a series of seven different formalin-inactivated vaccine formulations was developed and used in 11 separate field trial studies. These vaccines were given to more than 40,000 military recruits, university students, or children confined to institutions over a 15-year period. Small numbers of immunized human volunteers were hospitalized and challenged with virulent organisms (see references 5,

8, 11, and 15 for references). Seroconversion rates ranged form 0 to 90%, but reduction in naturally occurring disease ranged from only 28 to 67%. A commercially prepared, formalin-inactivated vaccine with an alum adjuvant, used to immunize approximately 24,000 military recruits, was reported to cause a 48 to 60% reduction in all types of nonbacterial pneumonias (129–131); however, these studies did not provide isolation and seroconversion data specific for diagnosis of *M. pneumoniae* disease, making evaluation of these findings difficult. One of the better formalin-inactivated vaccines, lot OSU-1A, provided about 67% protection against naturally occurring disease (180). In other studies, some of the immunized volunteers, who failed to seroconvert, developed a more severe, potentiated form of pneumonia upon challenge than did nonimmunized control patients (159, 160).

The poor correlation between seroconversion rates and protection in immunized human subjects and in hamsters led to the development of a hamster immunization-challenge potency assay (8–10, 15). Two human doses of lot OSU-1A vaccine, given to hamsters by either the i.t., s.c., i.m., or i.p. route, provided very little protection against challenge. Hamsters immunized i.m. or s.c. with only one dose of lot OSU-1A developed more severe histopathological lung lesion scores than did nonimmunized hamsters when challenged (5, 7–10, 15). Good protection was achieved in hamsters given six doses of the OSU-1A vaccine or three doses of OSU-1A in alum adjuvant, but this schedule was considered impractical for general use in humans. In an earlier study, another formalin-inactivated vaccine containing complete Freund's adjuvant did not protect hamsters from challenge (57).

Overall, data obtained from both human field trial and animal studies indicate that formalin-inactivated *M. pneumoniae* vaccines were not very effective in preventing naturally occurring *M. pneumoniae* disease. The relatively low rate of protection may be due to insufficient amounts of protective immunogens, poor immunological responses, suboptimal routes of immunization, inability to stimulate a primary immunological response, failure to stimulate migration of immune cells to the mucosal site of infection, or failure to stimulate local immune mechanisms required for protection against mucosal surface diseases. Suppression of humoral antibody or cell-mediated immune responses (58) could also be involved, but this possibility remain to be determined. Presently, all attempts to produce a formalin-inactivated vaccine commercially have been discontinued.

Live vaccines. Development of live attenuated vaccines by repeated subculture in artificial media resulted in decreased virulence and a corresponding decrease in the protective immunological response (48). A live, attenuated, high-broth-passage vaccine provided maximum protection in hamsters when it was given by the intranasal route, supporting the contention that live vaccines induce protection by stimulating local mucosal defense mechanisms (57). Serum antibody levels did not correlate with protection, but bronchial washings contained growth-inhibiting antibodies, indicating that a local immune response had occurred. Although this live attenuated vaccine showed promise in animal studies, it was unsuitable for human use because it retained some of its virulence in hamsters.

Another approach involved development of temperature-sensitive mutant vaccines, which could grow at 30 to 32°C but not at 37 to 38°C, the core temperature of the lung. These temperature-sensitive mutant strains were expected to colonize and infect upper respiratory oropharyngeal tissues and stimulate an immune response, but they were not expected to produce pneumonia because of their inability to grow at pulmonary core temperatures. In the hamster model, temperature-sensitive mutant vaccines behaved as expected and provided significant protection against challenge (25, 162, 163). However, they caused moderately severe bronchitis or pneumonia in human volunteers (25, 75) and were unacceptable for general human use. Attempts to produce temperature-sensitive mutant vaccines against *M. pneumoniae* were discontinued.

Live HA$^-$ mutant strain P24-S1, derived from virulent strain FH-P24 and identical to its virulent parent in protein profile and antibody staining patterns with patient sera, retains the ability to attach to cultured hamster lung cells and to colonize hamster lung and tracheal tissues (184). Immunization of hamsters by aerosol inhalation of P24-S1 induced IgG with CF activity in serum and bronchial washings and macrophage migration inhibition activity; 50% of hamsters immunized with P24-S1 were protected from challenge with the virulent parent strain. In another study, 70% of the mice immunized with P24-S1 were protected, compared with 20% protected by passive immunization with guinea pig hyperimmune serum (185).

Whereas live vaccines remain a conceptually viable approach for protection against *M. pneumoniae*, all previous efforts have been disappointing, and these vaccines have not been approved for general use for various reasons. They have either not been genetically stable, reverted to the virulent phenotype, or failed to stimulate a protective mucosal immune response.

Cell-free component vaccines. Studies with the protein-rich *M. pneumoniae* cell extract described above have demonstrated that an acellular vaccine is feasible when the immunogen is presented by an optimal route (8–10, 15, 31–34, 36, 37). In addition, an acellular membrane polysaccharide vaccine induced some protection against challenge in guinea pigs (23, 27).

Because the P1 cytadhesin of *M. pneumoniae* is essential for attachment, it has long been regarded as an excellent candidate component of a purified vaccine. The P1 protein isolated by preparative sodium dodecyl sulfate-polyacrylamide gel electrophoresis (SDS-PAGE) was used to immunize guinea pigs in two studies. In one study, two doses were given intranasally 4 weeks apart (92), and in another study, a single dose in Freund's adjuvant was given i.p. (97). Animals were challenged 4 weeks postimmunization. In both studies, immunized animals developed significant systemic and local IgA immune responses. Unfortunately, plate counts of viable organisms from the lung tissues were not performed in either study (92, 97), making it impossible to determine whether the elevated antibody response prevents colonization of *M. pneumoniae* in the lung. However, in the second study, P1 antigen was detected by enzyme-linked immunosorbent assay in the bronchial washings of only one of the three P1-

immunized animals following challenge with *M. pneumoniae*, while positive P1 antigen was detected in all three infected animals (97). These findings suggest that the local immunity of animals immunized with P1 protein by the i.p. route is able to prevent or diminish colonization of the lung upon subsequent *M. pneumoniae* infection. On the other hand, histopathological examination revealed intense peribronchiolar and perivascular infiltration of lung tissue with lymphocytes in both immunized and nonimmunized animals upon challenge with the virulent organism. Hilar lymph nodes from immunized and subsequently challenged animals, as well as from twice-infected animals, appeared to be depleted of specific stimulable lymphocytes, suggesting transfer of immunocompetent lymphocytes to inflammation sites. Similarities between these lung lesions and lung hypersensitivity reactions produced by other means have been noted by several investigators (9, 56, 97). It is possible that the epitope(s) responsible for this peribronchial cell recruitment activity differs from the P1 epitope(s) that reacts with attachment-blocking antibodies (73, 94, 95, 96), and an engineered P1 fragment in which the cell recruitment activity has been reduced or eliminated could be an excellent component candidate for an acellular vaccine (73, 95, 96). However, it is most likely that components other than P1 are responsible for ciliotoxicity as well as peribronchial cell recruitment and that these are also important immunogens (8–10, 15, 31–34, 36, 37).

Recombinant DNA vaccine candidates. The P1 gene is part of a three-gene operon which encodes 28- and 130-kDa proteins in addition to P1 (169 kDa). The entire operon has been sequenced and is believed to be transcribed as a single polycistronic message (87). Only portions of the P1 protein have been expressed in *Escherichia coli* (53, 63, 156, 173), primarily because the UGA codon that codes for tryptophan in *M. pneumoniae* terminates translation in *E. coli* (88, 156).

As mentioned previously, the mature P1 adhesin contains multiple antigenic determinants (84), and several laboratories have sought to map the immunodominant and biofunctional domains by examining the reactivity of contiguous or overlapping peptide segments with specific MAbs against P1 or with sera from convalescent patients (53, 73, 95). A 13-amino-acid sequence located near the C terminus was identified as a mediator of adherence with attachment-inhibiting anti-P1 MAbs; the same sequence was reactive with patient sera as well (53). Two other adherence sites were identified, one near the N terminus of the protein and the other located in the middle of the protein. Both of these epitopes were recognized by patient sera also (94). Close contact among the three functional domains appears to be necessary for adherence and is probably achieved by folding of the protein. Recently, Jacobs and coworkers (96) identified a T-cell epitope that overlaps the C-terminal end of a B-cell epitope; both lie within one of the three immunodominant domains. The ability to stimulate both humoral and cellular immune responses would explain the relatively high antibody levels against P1 observed in patients. If peptides containing amino acid sequences corresponding to the three P1 immunodominant regions are capable of eliciting attachment-blocking antibodies, such synthetic peptides could be excellent candidates for use as chemically defined immunogens that could be produced in large quantities by using recombinant DNA techniques.

As indicated previously, the route of antigen presentation is very important in attempts to induce protection against respiratory mucosal infections. Because the i.p.-i.t. priming-immunization schedule used successfully with animals is not suitable for human use, other routes of antigen presentation are being explored. A live adenovirus recombinant vaccine has been developed by cloning a three-fragment component of the *M. pneumoniae* P1 gene into an adenovirus vector (114). The *M. pneumoniae* DNA insert consists of a leader signal sequence, a sequence that encodes an epitope recognized by a specific MAb (M-328), and a transfer-stop sequence. In principle, orally administered recombinant adenovirus vaccine would be expected to induce an asymptomatic infection of the lower intestinal tract. It is hoped that the virus will replicate in the gut mucosa and then produce and excrete the P1 fragment, which, in turn, will stimulate a disseminated mucosal immune response that will result in respiratory IgA secretion. Specific antigen-activated lymphocytes from gut-associated lymphoid follicles could migrate to bronchus-associated lymphoid tissue through the common mucosal immunity system, from which they could be recruited to initiate a protective sIgA response following respiratory exposure to P1. Expression of the P1 peptide by human 293 cell cultures infected with the recombinant adenovirus was demonstrated by using immunofluorescent staining and Western immunoblot analyses. Preliminary studies in cotton rats, which are susceptible to both *M. pneumoniae* and adenovirus, indicate that anti-P1 antibodies were produced following immunization with the recombinant adenovirus vaccine (79a).

M. hominis

Potential virulence/immunogenic components

Pathogenic strains of *M. hominis* isolated from different tissues of patients with a variety of disease processes and from contaminated or infected cell culture substrates are very heterogeneous, having markedly different antigens and immunogens (78), attachment protein adhesins (90), isozymes (140), polypeptide compositions (39, 40, 110), DNA homology (13), and DNA restriction enzyme patterns (40). Antigenic and genetic variation in *M. hominis* are discussed in chapters 28 and 34.

The ability to metabolize arginine for the production of ATP is an important property of *M. hominis*. Arginine-utilizing mycoplasmas can rapidly deplete the medium of arginine, an essential amino acid, in infected or contaminated cell cultures. This, in turn, can alter the metabolism and function of infected fibroblastic cell cultures, lymphocyte cultures, and other such tissue cells grown in vitro. Alterations in protein and nucleic acid synthesis, cell division and growth, karyology, lymphocyte blast formation, and virus propagation have been observed in infected cell cultures depleted of arginine (see reference 4 for references). Arginine deiminase, the initial enzyme involved in the three-enzyme arginine dihydrolase pathway, has been suggested, although not proven, to correlate with virulence (179). Another potential virulence factor/immunogen among arthritogenic strains, such as strain 1620 (isolated from a patient with septic arthritis), consists of those components responsible for the severe inflammatory and lymphocyte recruitment activity demonstrated in experimentally induced *M. hominis* arthritis in chimpanzees (14).

Because attachment correlates with pathogenicity in *M. hominis* (90), the components that mediate attachment are potentially important immunogens. Recent studies have focused on identifying adhesins and surface antigens in pathogenic strains. Alexander (2) identified eight proteins from *M. hominis* 49L, ranging from 135 to 37 kDa, as candidate surface antigens by examining antibody staining patterns with sera of patients with invasive *M. hominis* diseases; paired sera taken during acute and convalescent stages of disease were compared on immunoblots in this study. Two proteins identified in this manner (115 and 98 kDa) were common to six other clinical isolates. In a prospective study of *M. hominis* in relation to pregnancy complications, paired prenatal and postpartum sera were used to identify two proteins (50 and 58 kDa) from strain PG21 that were recognized only by sera of patients with culture-positive *M. hominis* infections (155). Culture-positive women, whose prenatal serum contained antibodies against the same two proteins, appeared to have fewer pregnancy and postpartum complications (postpartum fever or endometritis). This finding suggests that antibodies against these two proteins, when present prior to pregnancy, may provide some protection against these complications in women who are colonized with *M. hominis*. If so, these proteins could be potential protective immunogens. In another recent comprehensive study, three species-specific MAbs, generated against arthritogenic strain 1620, were used to probe 17 clinical isolates from diverse clinical sources (141). A surface protein of approximately 94 kDa was observed to be reactive in most of these strains, suggesting that this protein may be an important immunogenic component.

Immunological aspects

The severity of disease and failure to treat or adequately control *M. hominis* infections with antibiotics (see chapter 31) supports vaccine development as a highly desirable goal. An acute, severe, septic arthritis was experimentally induced in chimpanzees by intraarticular inoculation of 10^5 color-changing units of strain 1620 (12, 14). Following convalescence, the recovered chimpanzees were resistant to reinfection upon challenge with 10^8 color-changing units of strain 1620. Thus, a previous infection protected against subsequent exposure, suggesting that immunization should provide a meaningful approach to protection (14). Since laboratory reference type strain PG21 produced no overt clinical disease, studies are under way in our laboratory to compare the protein profiles of arthritogenic and nonarthritogenic strains.

Presently, no vaccines have been prepared from *M. hominis* for use in humans. Development of a vaccine against all *M. hominis* infections may pose difficult technical challenges because the virulence/immuno-

genic components may differ according to the particular strain(s) and the disease(s) they produce. Thus, different vaccine components specific for each different disease entity may be needed. Additional study is needed to further define the mechanisms of pathogenesis and to identify the virulent and pathogenic components and the protective immunogens for each of the strains which cause these diverse clinical diseases. Studies on the genomic and phenotypic properties and molecular biology of these pathogenic strains would help in the characterization of the protective immunogens.

U. urealyticum

Immunological aspects

Because of the frequency and severity of disease and the failure of antibiotic therapy to eliminate or adequately control some *U. urealyticum* infections (167), vaccine development would provide a feasible approach for prevention of these diseases. In fact, we have shown that chimpanzees recovering from experimentally induced *U. urealyticum* septic arthritis are fully protected against challenge (14). However, there are at least 14 distinct serological groups (serovars) within the species, and these fall into two genomic clusters based on DNA-DNA homology, DNA restriction patterns, SDS-PAGE protein profiles, and sensitivity to magnesium salts (6, 20, 21). Because these 14 serovars are antigenically distinct, each with potentially different virulence/immunogenic protein components, vaccine development for prevention of all ureaplasmal diseases would present challenging technical problems. Moreover, only a limited amount of information is available on the virulence/immunogenic protein components among each of these 14 serovars. Some antigenic diversity has been observed within each serovar of human origin, and these serovars differ from strains isolated from nonhuman primates. For example, human *U. urealyticum* serovar VIII strains have a 96-kDa surface-exposed protein which contains at least four distinct epitopes (171, 172). Strains isolated from chimpanzees lacked the 96-kDa protein but were otherwise similar to the human isolates on immunoblots. The 96-kDa component has not been detected in any of the other nonhuman *Ureaplasma* species or serovars examined.

It has been well established that all *U. urealyticum* serovars tested possess an IgA1-specific protease, which degrades human IgA1 (but not human IgA2 or IgA of animal origin) into the two Fab and Fc fragments (101, 149). Because IgA antibodies are believed to be a major defense mechanism in protecting against surface mucosal infection, IgA protease activity has been associated with pathogenicity. Many human bacterial pathogens that produce mucosal infections also possess a specific IgA protease, whereas nonpathogenic species or strains of the same genus do not (103, 150). Because these pathogens can degrade IgA1, they may overcome local immune defenses and gain entry into the respiratory tract and cause mucosal infection. Thus, IgA1 protease(s) may be an important virulence/immunogenic component.

The genus *Ureaplasma* is unique among organisms

belonging to the class *Mollicutes* because it requires urea for energy. The breakdown of urea results in the production of ATP and the release of ammonia. As with other procaryotes that exhibit urease activity, ureaplasmas are capable of inducing urinary calculi (stones) in patients infected with ureaplasmas and in experimentally infected animals. Thus, urease may be another virulence factor and a potential immunogen. Five distinct urease epitopes have been identified by using anti-urease MAbs (172). Only the human and chimpanzee isolates examined contained all five of these epitopes. The distribution of the five epitopes appeared to vary among isolates obtained from different animal *Ureaplasma* species. Because the chimpanzee strains were similar to the human *U. urealyticum* strains, the chimpanzee may be an appropriate animal model for the study of *U. urealyticum* infection.

The lipoglycan (formerly called lipopolysaccharide) layer surrounding *Ureaplasma* cells is another potentially important immunogen. Lipoglycans, which make up about 5% of cell dry weight, have endotoxin-like properties. They cause febrile responses in rabbits and produce a positive *Limulus* amoebocyte lysate test (157). Similar lipoglycans in *Acholeplasma* species modulate immune responsiveness of the host to certain antigens and are mitogenic to lymphocyte cultures in vitro (161).

Other potential virulence/immunogenic components of *U. urealyticum* include those factors responsible for the severe inflammatory and lymphocyte recruitment activity in synovial exudates of chimpanzees with septic arthritis experimentally induced with *U. urealyticum* (14). No vaccines have been prepared from *U. urealyticum* for use in humans.

Clearly, additional studies are required to better define the mechanisms and components of virulence and pathogenicity among the various serovars of *U. urealyticum*. We must also identify the critical immunogenic components capable of inducing protection against the various diseases caused by this diverse serological group of organisms. Study of the molecular biology of these pathogens would also be useful in the characterization of the immunogens.

M. genitalium

Potential virulence/immunogenic components

M. genitalium has been implicated in nongonococcal urethritis and other urogenital diseases, including pelvic inflammatory disease (see chapter 25). Initially believed to inhabit the urogenital tract, its isolation from homosexual males with nongonococcal urethritis with greater frequency than from heterosexuals has recently led to speculation that it may be a component of the gastrointestinal flora. Evidence suggesting a role for *M. genitalium* in arthritic and respiratory diseases, either alone or acting synergistically with other agents, has also been amassed (16a). *M. genitalium* caused experimentally induced urogenital infections in male and female chimpanzees, monkeys, tamarins, and marmosets. The disease was characterized by colonization of the urethral or vaginal tissues, overt signs of clinical disease, and a pronounced serum antibody response (169, 170, 175).

Attachment of *M. genitalium* to ciliated epithelial cells is mediated by an adhesin designated MgPa that appears to be analogous to the P1 protein of *M. pneumoniae* (50, 89). Like P1, MgPa is the immunodominant surface antigen recognized by sera from infected mice, guinea pigs, hamsters, and chimpanzees (85, 133, 168); it also is located on the attachment tip (85). Furthermore, MgPa is encoded by a three-gene operon analogous to the P1 operon of *M. pneumoniae* (89). The MgPa operon has been cloned, sequenced, and found to share extensive homology with the P1 operon of *M. pneumoniae*. These observations are consistent with reports of serological cross-reactivity between MgPa and P1 proteins (22, 115) as well as between other common protein epitopes shared by the two organisms (42, 154).

Immunological aspects

Although *M. pneumoniae* and *M. genitalium* are genomically distinct species, they have many characteristics, properties, and activities in common. These include morphological and ultrastructural similarities and marked antigenic cross-reactivity (50, 51, 115, 133, 174) in addition to the similarities in their major adhesin proteins. Because of their extensive immunological and serological similarities, it is difficult or impossible to distinguish the serological response to infection between these two species by using the conventional MI or CF test procedures currently used for the diagnoses of *M. pneumoniae* disease. These similarities in serological response have important ramifications for the differential diagnosis of *M. pneumoniae* and *M. genitalium* disease. Similarities in serological responses and the clinical features of pneumonia produced by the two organisms (175) would also pose difficulties in evaluating vaccine efficacy for the prevention of either *M. pneumoniae* or *M. genitalium* disease, assuming that the immunogens for these two genomically distinct species are not identical or equally protective. There is no information available on the development of vaccines directed against *M. genitalium* disease.

M. fermentans

The significance of *M. fermentans* as a human pathogen remains to be established. However, this agent has been implicated recently in the pathogeneses of AIDS and in non-AIDS fatal pulmonary illness with systemic complications (112,121–124). These reports have stimulated interest among various laboratories in investigating the basic molecular biology and genomic properties and in identifying the pathogenic, virulence, and immunogenic components of this species.

Incidence and pathogenesis

M. fermentans was first isolated by Ruiter and Wentholt in 1953 (152) from the urogenital tract of two patients with genital infections. These findings were confirmed by Nicol and Edwards (139). *M. fermentans* has been recovered with low frequency (about 1% of specimens) from the human urogenital tract of asymptomatic patients and even less frequently from the human oral cavity (111, 126, 127). *M. fermentans* has also been found on rare occasions in the urogenital tract of nonhuman primates (54).

M. fermentans was isolated from bone marrow of leukemic and nonleukemic patients by using cell culture procedures (135, 136). Some critics believed that these isolates were cell culture contaminants. Mice experimentally infected with these leukemic *M. fermentans* strains produced several distinct disease entities (65, 66, 143). The i.p. injection of 10^{10} CFU in germ-free mice produced a lethal toxicity similar to endotoxic shock caused by gram-negative organisms and led to death within 24 to 48 h. On examination, the histopathological changes indicated that an overwhelming systemic infection with necrosis had occurred, but there was no neurological involvement. A lesser inoculum of 10^9 to 10^8 CFU resulted in an acute or chronic leukemoid disease, whereas a dose of less than 10^7 CFU resulted in a lifelong low-grade, growth-stunting infection. Experimental infection of rats resulted in a prolonged persistent colonization of *M. fermentans* in various tissues but particularly in lymphoid tissue, bone marrow, articular cartilage, and blood (177). Nonviable cell membranes from *M. fermentans* were also toxic for mice (66, 143). Both viable cells and nonviable membrane preparations from *M. fermentans* were toxic for mouse thymocytes (67), and membranes and globular proteins from *M. fermentans* were cytotoxic for rat lymphocytes (74).

M. fermentans has profound mitogenic activity for human B and T lymphocytes (19) and also for murine B-lymphoma cells (158). A high-molecular-weight material (MDHM) derived from *M. fermentans* caused differentiation of concanavalin A-stimulated mouse thymocytes to cytolytic effector T cells (145). Although it was not mitogenic for murine spleen cells, MDHM induced the release of high titers of interleukin-6 (IL-6) from peritoneal macrophages and human monocytes. The effect of MDHM was inhibited by monoclonal anti-IL-6 antibody. These findings may have clinical significance, since excessive production of IL-6 in the synovial fluid, resulting in T- and B-cell activation, has been a phenomenon observed in chronically inflamed arthritic joints (79, 178).

M. fermentans has been isolated from synovial fluids of several patients with rheumatoid arthritis (182, 183) and was reputed to play a role in the pathogenesis of this disease (46). An experimental polyarthritis was induced by the i.p. inoculation of *M. fermentans* in rabbits. Synovial tissues and fluids from these animals contained *M. fermentans*-specific IgG, rheumatoid factor, phagocytic cells, and deposited immune complexes (99). In female grivet monkeys, an acute salpingitis and parametritis with significant rises in serum antibody titers developed after the experimental inoculation of this agent into the uterine tubes (132).

Most recently, Lo and colleagues (120–124) reported the isolation of a novel virus from a mouse cell culture line transfected with the DNA from human Kaposi's sarcoma tissue. The agent was initially described as a viruslike infectious agent (VLIA) and was detected intracellularly, using MAbs and DNA probes, in various tissues from AIDS patients and non-AIDS patients who died of a fatal necrotic pulmonary disease (121-124). The six non-AIDS patients were diagnosed initially as having a mycoplasma pneumonia, but the

illness rapidly developed into a fulminating necrotizing disease, a condition which is quite uncharacteristic of known mycoplasma diseases. Subsequently, each of the patients died abruptly within a 7-week period from onset of symptoms. VLIA-specific DNA was detected in various organs, including the liver, spleen, kidney, lymph nodes, and brain, yet these patients had no appreciable serum antibody responses. The VLIA agent was subsequently shown to be a mycoplasma and was designated *M. incognitus* (123). However, extensive DNA, protein, and serological analyses demonstrated clearly that the VLIA agent is a strain of *M. fermentans* (153).

The initial report generated much controversy, because mycoplasmas are common and notorious contaminants of cell culture lines and because it seemed quite unlikely that a eucaryotic tissue cell was capable of transfection with mycoplasma DNA. Moreover, *M. fermentans* has been isolated from contaminated cell cultures with high frequency in recent years. Prior to 1980, only about 1% of the cell culture contaminants were identified as *M. fermentans* (4, 144), but between 1981 and 1987, 690 (21%) of the 3,296 cell culture contaminants isolated were shown to be *M. fermentans* (53a). Yoshida et al. (187) also reported that 13 (24%) of their 57 positive isolations were *M. fermentans*. In addition, some strains of *M. fermentans*, such as strain IM1, a cell culture contaminant, were just as fastidious as the VLIA strain (123). Both grew well in cell culture systems but poorly in broth or on agar, and both had special nutritional requirements for growth on agar; they preferred an anaerobic environment (5% CO_2 in N_2) and grew best in either Herderschee's medium (strain IM1), which contains 7% sucrose (144), or the SP-4 medium for VLIA.

In other studies, Lemaître et al. (112) reported that the in vitro cytopathogenicity in cell cultures infected with human immunodeficiency virus was due to a mycoplasma contaminant, which was recently identified as *M. fermentans* (132a). The significance of these findings as they relate to pathogenesis of human immunodeficiency virus-related disease remains to be determined.

Potential virulence/immunogenic components

There is very little information available regarding the virulence/immunogenic components of *M. fermentans*. Some strains are known to exhibit marked antigenic or serological variation. *M. fermentans* is somewhat unusual in having both arginine dihydrolase and glucose fermentation activities, but different strains vary widely with respect to arginine deiminase activity (138). Clearly, additional studies are required to define the mechanisms and components of virulence and pathogenicity and to determine, in fact, whether these organisms are bona fide human pathogens. Further work is also needed to identify immunogenic components of these agents and to elucidate their molecular biology.

FUTURE OUTLOOK

There are urgent needs for effective mycoplasma vaccines for humans and animals because of (i) the high prevalence of disease in humans and severity of mycoplasma diseases in animals, frequently resulting in death (61), (ii) the prolonged, protracted course of infection, and (iii) the failure of antibiotics and other therapeutic approaches to eradicate the mycoplasmas and abort the infectious disease process. Even though humans and animals that have recovered from naturally acquired mycoplasma diseases are resistant to rechallenge, the efforts to develop effective and safe vaccines have been only partially successful (5, 7). The overall success obtained with formalin-inactivated vaccines in humans has been extremely disappointing, even though successful inactivated vaccines have been developed for prevention of contagious bovine pleuropneumonia (69–71), contagious caprine pleuropneumonia (117), and *M. gallisepticum* disease in chickens (104). Live, attenuated vaccines are also being used to control these same animal diseases (104, 118, 119, 125), but no acceptable live vaccine has been developed for human use.

Prevention of mycoplasmal diseases poses challenging technical problems because basic information regarding disease pathogenesis is incomplete in many critical areas, including (i) the basic immune mechanisms that protect against mucosal surface infections of the respiratory, urogenital, and synovial systems, (ii) the infectious process induced by mycoplasma pathogens of humans and animals, and (iii) the disease-related antigens and the protective immunogens required to induce protection against each mycoplasma disease. Much has been learned about the mechanism of pathogenesis, the virulence and immunogenic components, and the immune response to *M. pneumoniae* in recent years, and some of this knowledge may be applicable to other mycoplasma pathogens as well. Thus, continued studies are needed to define mechanisms of pathogenesis and to identify potential immunogens capable of inducing protective immunological responses to mycoplasma pathogens. In addition, the optimal protective immune response must be established for each mycoplasma disease, and the relative contribution of humoral, local, and cell-mediated mechanisms in development of resistance must be determined. The best immunization route and schedule for stimulating the protective immune mechanisms responsible for resistance must be defined. The immune response to mycoplasma infections may play a critical role in the pathogenesis of disease and may be responsible for the histopathological lesions and the autoimmune manifestations seen with mycoplasma diseases. For this reason, it may be necessary to use engineered immunogens capable of eliciting a protective response but lacking the components that induce the intense cell recruitment that contributes to lesions in lungs and joints. A number of inactivated vaccines have also induced potentiated disease. Thus, a vaccine must protect without inducing adverse toxic effects or untoward immunological reactions. The investigator must be cognizant of the possibility of undesirable reactions that can develop and must rule out undesirable reactivity before vaccines are made available for general use.

REFERENCES

1. **Adler, H. E., and J. M. Lamas da Silva.** 1970. Immunization against *Mycoplasma gallisepticum*. *Avian Dis.* **14**:763–769.

2. **Alexander, A. G.** 1987. Analysis of protein antigens of *Mycoplasma hominis*: detection of polypeptides involved in the human immune response. *Isr. J. Med. Sci.* **23**:608–612.

3. **Almagor, M., S. Yatziv, and I. Kahane.** 1983. Inhibition of host cell catalase by *Mycoplasma pneumoniae* infection: a possible mechanism for cell injury. *Infect. Immun.* **41**:251–256.

4. **Barile, M. F.** 1979. Mycoplasma-tissue cell interactions, p. 425–474. *In* J. G. Tully and R. F. Whitcomb (ed.), *The Mycoplasmas*, vol. 2. *Human and Animal Mycoplasmas*. Academic Press, Inc., New York.

5. **Barile, M. F.** 1985. Immunization against mycoplasma infections, p. 451–492. *In* S. Razin and M. F. Barile (ed.), *The Mycoplasmas*, vol. 4. *Mycoplasma Pathogenicity*. Academic Press, Inc., Orlando, Fla.

6. **Barile, M. F.** 1986. DNA homologies and serologic relationships among ureaplasmas from various hosts. *Pediatr. Infect. Dis.* **5**(Suppl.):296–299.

7. **Barile, M. F., J. M. Bové, J. M. Bradbury, G. H. Cassell, W. A. Clyde, Jr., G. S. Cottew, and P. Whittlestone.** 1985. Current status on the control of mycoplasmal diseases of man, animals, plants and insects. *Bull. Inst. Pasteur* **83**:339–373.

8. **Barile, M. F., D. K. F. Chandler, H. Yoshida, M. W. Grabowski, R. Harasawa, and O. A. Ahmed.** 1981. Hamster challenge potency assay for evaluation of *Mycoplasma pneumoniae* vaccines. *Isr. J. Med. Sci.* **17**:682–686.

9. **Barile, M. F., D. K. F. Chandler, H. Yoshida, M. W. Grabowski, R. Harasawa, and S. Razin.** 1988. Parameters of *Mycoplasma pneumoniae* infection in Syrian hamsters. *Infect. Immun.* **56**:2443–2449.

10. **Barile, M. F., D. K. F. Chandler, H. Yoshida, M. W. Grabowski, and S. Razin.** 1988. Hamster challenge potency assay for evaluation of *Mycoplasma pneumoniae* vaccines. *Infect. Immun.* **56**:2450–2457.

11. **Barile, M. F., M. W. Grabowski, D. K. F. Chandler, K. Izumikawa, and K. Zoumbos.** 1983. Current approaches in the development of *Mycoplasma pneumoniae* vaccines for the prevention of primary atypical pneumonia. *Chemoterapia* **2**:80–81.

12. **Barile, M. F., M. W. Grabowski, P. J. Snoy, D. K. F. Chandler.** 1987. The superiority of the chimpanzee animal model to study the pathogenicity of known *Mycoplasma pneumoniae* and reputed mycoplasma pathogens. *Isr. J. Med. Sci.* **23**:556–560.

13. **Barile, M. F., M. W. Grabowski, E. B. Stephens, S. J. O'Brien, J. M. Simonson, K. Izumikawa, D. K. F. Chandler, D. Taylor-Robinson, and J. G. Tully.** 1983. *Mycoplasma hominis*-tissue cell interactions: a review with new observations on phenotypic and genotypic properties. *Sex. Transm. Dis.* **10**(Suppl.):345–354.

14. **Barile, M. F., P. J. Snoy, L. M. Miller, M. W. Grabowski, D. K. F. Chandler, A. Blanchard, T. M. Cunningham, L. D. Olson, and A. P. Guruswamy.** 1990. Mycoplasma-induced septic arthritis in chimpanzees, p. 389–393. *In* G. Stanek, G. H. Cassell, J. G. Tully, and R. F. Whitcomb (ed.), *Recent Advances in Mycoplasmology*. Gustav Fischer Verlag, New York.

15. **Barile, M. F., H. Yoshida, D. K. F. Chandler, M. W. Grabowski, and R. Hawasawa.** 1982. The hamster-immunization-protection-challenge-potency assay for evaluation of mycoplasma pneumoniae vaccines, p. 202–211. *In* J. B. Robbins, J. C. Hill, and J. C. Sadoff (ed.), *Seminars in Infectious Diseases*, vol. 4. *Bacterial Vaccines*. Thieme-Stratton, Inc., New York.

16. **Baseman, J. B., R. M. Cole, D. C. Krause, and D. K. Leith.** 1982. Molecular basis for cytadsorption of *Mycoplasma pneumoniae*. *J. Bacteriol.* **151**:1514–1522.

16a. **Baseman, J. B., S. F. Dallo, J. G. Tully, and D. L. Rose.** 1988. Isolation and characterization of *Mycoplasma gen-*

500   ELLISON ET AL.

italium strains from the human respiratory tract. *J. Clin. Microbiol.* **26:**2266–2269.

17. **Baseman, J. B., J. Morrison-Plummer, D. Drouillard, B. Puleo-Scheppke, V. V. Tryon, and S. C. Holt.** 1987. Identification of a 32-kilodalton protein of *Mycoplasma pneumoniae* associated with hemadsorption. *Isr. J. Med. Sci.* **23:**474–479.

18. **Biberfeld, G.** 1974. Cell-mediated immune response following *Mycoplasma pneumoniae* infection in man. II. Leukotyce migration inhibition. *Clin. Exp. Immunol.* **17:**43–49.

19. **Biberfeld, G., and E. Nilsson.** 1978. Mitogenicity of *Mycoplasma fermentans* for human lymphocytes. *Infect. Immun.* **21:**48–54.

20. **Blanchard, A.** 1990. *Ureaplasma urealyticum* urease genes: use of a UGA tryptophan codon. *Mol. Microbiol.* **4:**669–676.

21. **Blanchard, A., S. Razin, G. E. Kenny, and M. F. Barile.** 1988. Characteristics of *Ureaplasma urealyticum* urease. *J. Bacteriol.* **170:**2692–2697.

22. **Bredt, W., B. Kleinman, and E. Jacobs.** 1987. Antibodies in the sera of *Mycoplasma pneumoniae*-infected patients against proteins of *Mycoplasma genitalium* and other mycoplasmas of man. *Zentralbl. Bakteriol. Hyg. Reihe A* **266:**32–42.

23. **Brunner, H.** 1981. Protective efficacy of *Mycoplasma pneumoniae* polysaccharides. *Isr. J. Med. Sci.* **17:**678–681.

24. **Brunner, H., J. Feldner, and W. Bredt.** 1984. Effect of monoclonal antibodies to the attachment-tip on experimental *Mycoplasma pneumoniae* infection of hamsters: a preliminary report. *Isr. J. Med. Sci.* **20:**878–881.

25. **Brunner, H., H. Greenberg, W. D. James, R. L. Horswood, and R. M. Chanock.** 1973. Decreased virulence and protective effect of genetically stable temperature-sensitive mutants of *Mycoplasma pneumoniae. Ann. N.Y. Acad. Sci.* **225:**436–452.

26. **Brunner, H., H. B. Greenberg, W. D. James, R. L. Horswood, R. B. Couch, and R. M. Chanock.** 1973. Antibody to *Mycoplasma pneumoniae* in nasal secretions and sputa of experimentally infected human volunteers. *Infect. Immun.* **8:**612–620.

27. **Brunner, H., and B. Prescott.** 1982. Effect of *Mycoplasma pneumoniae* polysaccharides and glycolipids on prophylaxis of experimental disease, p. 190–197. *In* J. B. Robbins, J. C. Hill, and J. C. Sadoff (ed.), *Seminars in Infectious Diseases*, vol. 4. *Bacterial Vaccines.* Thieme-Stratton, Inc., New York.

28. **Brunner, H., S. Razin, A. R. Kalica, and R. M. Chanock.** 1971. Lysis and death of *Mycoplasma pneumoniae* by antibody and complement. *J. Immunol.* **106:**907–916.

29. **Cassell, G. H., J. R. Lindsey, and J. K. Davis.** 1981. Respiratory and genital mycoplasmas of laboratory rodents: implications for biomedical research. *Isr. J. Med. Sci.* **17:**548–554.

30. **Cebra, J. L., J. A. Fuhrman, D. A. Horsfall, and R. D. Shahin.** 1982. Natural and deliberate priming of IgA responses to bacterial antigens by the mucosal route, p. 6–12. *In* J. B. Robbins, J. C. Hill, and J. C. Sadoff (ed.), *Seminars in Infectious Diseases*, vol. 4. *Bacterial Vaccines.* Thieme-Stratton, Inc., New York.

31. **Chandler, D. K. F., and M. F. Barile.** 1980. Ciliostatic, hemagglutinating and proteolytic activities in a cell extract of *Mycoplasma pneumoniae. Infect. Immun.* **29:**1111–1116.

32. **Chandler, D. K. F., and M. F. Barile.** 1982. *In vitro* activities of *Mycoplasma pneumoniae* extract, p. 186–189. *In* J. B. Robbins, J. C. Hill, and J. C. Sadoff (ed.), *Seminars in Infectious Diseases*, vol. 4. *Bacterial Vaccines.* Thieme-Stratton, Inc., New York.

33. **Chandler, D. K. F., and M. F. Barile.** 1983. *Mycoplasma pneumoniae* attachment to WiDr cell cultures: competitive inhibition assays. *Yale J. Biol. Med.* **56:**679–683.

34. **Chandler, D. K. F., A. M. Collier, and M. F. Barile.** 1982. Attachment of *Mycoplasma pneumoniae* to hamster tracheal organ cultures, tracheal outgrowth monolayers, human erythrocytes, and WiDr human tissue culture cells. *Infect. Immun.* **35:**937–942.

35. **Chandler, D. K. F., M. W. Grabowski, and M. F. Barile.** 1982. *Mycoplasma pneumoniae* attachment: competitive inhibition by mycoplasmal binding component and sialic acid-containing glycoconjugates. *Infect. Immun.* **38:**598–603.

36. **Chandler, D. K. F., M. W. Grabowski, A. S. Rabson, and M. F. Barile.** 1987. Further studies on the *Mycoplasma pneumoniae* extract: ciliostatic and cell recruitment activities. *Isr. J. Med. Sci.* **23:**580–584.

37. **Chandler, D. K. F., S. Razin, E. B. Stephens, R. Harasawa, and M. F. Barile.** 1982. Genomic and phenotypic analyses of *Mycoplasma pneumoniae* strains. *Infect. Immun.* **38:**604–609.

38. **Chanock, R. M., L. Hayflick, and M. F. Barile.** 1962. Growth on artificial medium of an agent associated with atypical pneumonia and its identification as a PPLO. *Proc. Natl. Acad. Sci. USA* **48:**41–49.

39. **Christiansen, C., G. Christiansen, and O. F. Rasmussen.** 1987. Heterogeneity of *Mycoplasma hominis* as detected by a probe for *atp* genes. *Isr. J. Med. Sci.* **23:**591–594.

40. **Christiansen, G., and H. Anderson.** 1988. Heterogeneity among *Mycoplasma hominis* strains as detected by probes containing parts of ribosomal ribonucleic acid genes. *Int. J. Syst. Bacteriol.* **38:**108–115.

41. **Christiansen, G., H. Anderson, S. Birkelund, and E. A. Freundt.** 1987. Genomic and gene variation in *Mycoplasma hominis. Isr. J. Med. Sci.* **23:**595–602.

42. **Cimolai, N., L. E. Bryan, M. To, and D. E. Woods.** 1987. Immunological cross-reactivity of a *Mycoplasma pneumoniae* membrane-associated protein antigen with *Mycoplasma genitalium* and *Acholeplasma laidlawii. J. Clin. Microbiol.* **25:**2136–2139.

43. **Clyde, W. A., Jr.** 1971. Immunopathology of experimental *Mycoplasma pneumoniae* disease. *Infect. Immun.* **4:**757–763.

44. **Clyde, W. A., Jr.** 1983. *Mycoplasma pneumoniae* respiratory disease symposium: summation and significance. *Yale J. Biol. Med.* **56:**523–527.

45. **Clyde, W. A., Jr., and G. W. Fernald.** 1983. Mycoplasmas: the pathogens' pathogen. *Cell. Immunol.* **82:**88–97.

46. **Cole, B. C., L. R. Washburn, and D. Taylor-Robinson.** 1985. Mycoplasma-induced arthritis, p. 107–160. *In* S. Razin and M. F. Barile (ed.), *The Mycoplasmas*, vol. 4. *Mycoplasma Pathogenicity.* Academic Press, Inc., Orlando, Fla.

47. **Colman, S. D., P. C. Hu, and K. F. Bott.** 1990. Prevalence of novel repeat sequences in and around the *P1* operon in the genome of *Mycoplasma pneumoniae. Gene* **87:**91–96.

48. **Couch, R. B., T. R. Cate, and R. M. Chanock.** 1964. Infection with artificially propagated Eaton agent (*Mycoplasma pneumoniae*): implications for development of attenuated vaccine for cold agglutinin-positive pneumonia. *JAMA* **187:**442–447.

49. **Craighead, J. E.** 1975. Report of a workshop: disease accentuation after immunization with inactivated microbial vaccines. *J. Infect. Dis.* **131:**749–754.

50. **Dallo, S. F., A. Chavoya, C. J. Su, and J. B. Baseman.** 1989. DNA and protein sequence homologies between the adhesins of *Mycoplasma genitalium* and *Mycoplasma pneumoniae. Infect. Immun.* **57:**1059–1065.

51. **Dallo, S. F., J. R. Horton, C. J. Su, and J. B. Baseman.** 1989. Homologous regions shared by adhesin genes of *Mycoplasma pneumoniae* and *Mycoplasma genitalium. Microb. Pathog.* **6:**69–73.

52. **Dallo, S. F., J. R. Horton, C. J. Su, and J. B. Baseman.** 1990. Restriction fragment length polymorphism in the

cytadhesin P1 gene of human clinical isolates of *Mycoplasma pneumoniae*. *Infect. Immun.* **58:**2017–2020.

53. **Dallo, S. F., C. J. Su, J. R. Horton, and J. B. Baseman.** 1988. Identification of P1 gene domain containing epitope(s) mediating *Mycoplasma pneumoniae* cytadherence. *J. Exp. Med.* **167:**718–723.

53a. **Del Giudice, R. A.** Personal communication.

54. **Del Giudice, R. A., and T. R. Carski.** 1969. Recovery of human mycoplasmas from simian tissues. *Nature* (London) **222:**1088–1089.

55. **Feldner, J., U. Göbel, and W. Bredt.** 1982. *Mycoplasma pneumoniae* adhesin localized to tip structure by monoclonal antibody. *Nature* (London) **298:**765–767.

56. **Fernald, G. W.** 1979. Humoral and cellular immune responses to mycoplasmas, p. 399–423. *In* J. G. Tully and R. F. Whitcomb (ed.), *The Mycoplasmas*, vol. 2. *Human and Animal Mycoplasmas.* Academic Press, Inc., New York.

57. **Fernald, G. W., and W. A. Clyde, Jr.** 1970. Protective effect of vaccines in experimental *Mycoplasma pneumoniae* disease. *Infect. Immun.* **1:**559–565.

58. **Fernald, G. W., and W. A. Clyde, Jr.** 1983. Immune responses to *Mycoplasma pneumoniae* infections, p. 270–288. *In* J. Bienenstock (ed.), *Immunology of the Lung.* McGraw-Hill Book Co., Hamburg, Germany.

59. **Fernald, G. W., W. A. Clyde, Jr., and F. W. Denny.** 1981. p. 415–439. *In* A. J. Nahmias and R. J. O'Reilly (ed.), *Immunology of Human Infections.* Plenum Medical Book Co., New York.

60. **Fernald, G. W., A. M. Collier, and W. A. Clyde, Jr.** 1975. Respiratory infections due to *Mycoplasma pneumoniae* in infants and children. *Pediatrics* **55:**327–335.

61. **Foy, H. M., and I. D. Allan.** 1982. Frequency of *Mycoplasma pneumoniae* pneumonia. *Lancet* **i:**392.

62. **Foy, H. M., H. Ochs, S. D. Davis, G. E. Kenny, and R. R. Luce.** 1973. *Mycoplasma pneumoniae* infections in patients with immunodeficiency syndromes: report of four cases. *J. Infect. Dis.* **127:**388–393.

62a. **Franzoso, G., P.-C. Hu, G. Meloni, and M. F. Barile.** 1992. Abstr. 9th Int. Congr. Organ. Mycoplasmology, Ames, Iowa.

63. **Frydenberg, J., K. Lind, and P. C. Hu.** 1987. Cloning of *Mycoplasma pneumoniae* DNA and expression of P1-epitopes in *Escherichia coli. Isr. J. Med. Sci.* **23:**759–762.

64. **Fulginiti, V. A., J. J. Eller, A. W. Downie, and C. H. Kempe.** 1967. Altered reactivity to measles virus: atypical measles in children previously immunized with inactivated measles virus vaccines. *JAMA* **202:**1075–1080.

65. **Gabridge, M. G.** 1974. Role of gram negative sepsis in lethal toxicity induced by *Mycoplasma. J. Infect. Dis.* **130:**529–533.

66. **Gabridge, M. G., G. D. Abrams, and W. H. Murphy.** 1972. Lethal toxicity of *Mycoplasma fermentans* for mice. *J. Infect. Dis.* **125:**153–160.

67. **Gabridge, M. G., D.-M. Yip, and K. Hedges.** 1975. Levels of lysosomal enzymes in tissues of mice infected with *Mycoplasma fermentans. Infect. Immun.* **12:**233–239.

68. **Gallin, J. I., and A. S. Fauci (ed.).** 1985. *Advances in Host Defense Mechanisms*, vol. 4. *Mucosal Immunity*, p. 1–196. Raven Press, New York.

69. **Garba, S. A., A. Ajayi, L. D. Challa, M. K. Bello, J. N. Z. Gazama, H. Gimba, J. Ngbede, B. Bitrus, and A. O. Adeoye.** 1986. Field trial of inactivated oil-adjuvant Gladysdale strain vaccine for contagious bovine pleuropneumonia. *Vet. Rec.* **119:**376–377.

70. **Garba, S. A., and R. J. Terry.** 1986. Immunogenicity of oil-based contagious bovine pleuropneumonia vaccine in cattle. *Vaccine* **4:**266–270.

71. **Garba, S. A., R. J. Terry, D. S. Adegboye, A. G. Lamorde, and J. A. Abalaka.** 1989. The choice of adjuvants in mycoplasma vaccines. *Microbios* **57:**15–19.

72. **Geary, S. J., and M. G. Gabridge.** 1987. Characterization

73. **Gerstenecker, B., and E. Jacobs.** 1989. Topological mapping of the P1-adhesin of *Mycoplasma pneumoniae* with adherence-inhibiting monoclonal antibodies. *J. Gen. Microbiol.* **136:**471–476.

74. **Gorina, L. G., A. V. Zilfian, K. S. Saiadian, S. A. Goncharova, and A. V. Vartanian.** 1988. Cytotoxic action of the individual membrane components of *Mycoplasma arthritidis* and *M. fermentans* in rat lymphocytes. *Zh. Mikrobiol. Epidemiol. Immunobiol.* **2:**82–87.

75. **Greenberg, H., C. M. Helms, H. Brunner, and R. M. Chanock.** 1974. Asymptomatic infection of adult volunteers with a temperature-sensitive mutant of *Mycoplasma pneumoniae. Proc. Natl. Acad. Sci. USA* **71:**4015–4019.

76. **Hanson, L. A., and C. Svanborg Eden (ed.).** 1987. Mucosal immunobiology: cellular molecular intractions in the mucosal immune system, p. 1–330. Karger, Basel.

77. **Hayatsu, E.** 1978. Acquired immunity to *Mycoplasma pneumoniae* in hamsters. *Microbiol. Immunol.* **22:**181–195.

78. **Hollingdale, M. R., and R. M. Lemcke.** 1970. The antigens of *Mycoplasma hominis. J. Hyg.* **67:**585–602.

79. **Hossiau, F. A., J.-P. Devogelaer, J. van Damme, C. Nagant de Deuxchaisnes, and J. van Snick.** 1988. Interleukin-6 in synovial fluid and serum of patients with rheumatoid arthritis and other inflammatory arthritides. *Arthritis Rheum.* **31:**784–788.

79a. **Hu, P.-C.** Personal communication.

80. **Hu, P.-C, R. M. Cole, Y.-S. Huang, J. A. Graham, D. E. Gardner, A. M. Collier, and W. A. Clyde, Jr.** 1982. *Mycoplasma pneumoniae* infection: role of a surface protein in the attachment organelle. *Science* **216:**313–315.

81. **Hu, P.-C., A. M. Collier, and J. B. Baseman.** 1977. Surface parasitism by *Mycoplasma pneumoniae* of respiratory epithelium. *J. Exp. Med.* **145:**1328–1343.

82. **Hu, P.-C., A. M. Collier, and W. A. Clyde.** 1984. Serological comparison of virulent and avirulent *Mycoplasma pneumoniae* by monoclonal antibodies. *Isr. J. Med. Sci.* **20:**870–873.

83. **Hu, P.-C, C.-H, Huang, A. M. Collier, and W. A. Clyde, Jr.** 1983. Demonstration of antibodies to *Mycoplasma pneumoniae* attachment protein in human sera and respiratory secretions. *Infect. Immun.* **41:**437–439.

84. **Hu, P.-C, C.-H. Huang, Y.-S. Huang, A. M. Collier, and W. A. Clyde, Jr.** 1985. Demonstration of multiple antigenic determinants on *Mycoplasma pneumoniae* attachment protein by monoclonal antibodies. *Infect. Immun.* **50:**292–296.

85. **Hu, P.-C, U. Schaper, A. M. Collier, W. A. Clyde, Jr., M. Horikawa, Y.-S. Huang, and M. F. Barile.** 1987. A *Mycoplasma genitalium* protein resembling the *Mycoplasma pneumoniae* attachment protein. *Infect. Immun.* **55:**1126–1131.

86. **Husband, A. J., R. Scicchitano, and R. F. Sheldrake.** 1986. Origin of IgA at mucosal sites, p. 1157–1162. *In* J. R. McGhee, J. Mestecky, P. L. Ogra, and J. Bienenstock (ed.), *Recent Advances in Mucosal Immunology. Part B: Effector Functions.* Plenum Press, New York.

87. **Inamine, J. M., T. P. Denny, S. Loechel, U. Schaper, C.-H. Huang, K. F. Bott, and P.-C. Hu.** 1988. Nucleotide sequence of the P1 attachment-protein gene of *Mycoplasma pneumoniae. Gene* **64:**217–229.

88. **Inamine, J. M., K. C. Ho, S. Loechel, and P.-C. Hu.** 1990. Evidence that UGA is read as a tryptophan codon rather than as a stop codon by *Mycoplasma pneumoniae, Mycoplasma genitalium,* and *Mycoplasma gallisepticum. J. Bacteriol.* **172:**504–506.

89. **Inamine, J. M., S. Loechel, A. M. Collier, M. F. Barile, and P.-C. Hu.** 1989. Nucleotide sequence of the MgPa (*mgp*) operon of *Mycoplasma genitalium* and compari-

son to the P1 (*mpp*) operon of *Mycoplasma pneumoniae.* *Gene* **82:**259–267.

90. **Izumikawa, K., D. K. F. Chandler, M. W. Grabowski, and M. F. Barile.** 1987. Attachment of *Mycoplasma hominis* to human cell cultures. *Isr. J. Med. Sci.* **23:**603–607.

90a. **Jacobs, E.** Personal communication.

91. **Jacobs, E., A. Bennewitz, and W. Bredt.** 1986. Reaction pattern of human anti-*Mycoplasma pneumoniae* antibodies in enzyme-linked immunosorbent assays and immunoblotting. *J. Clin. Microbiol.* **23:**517–522.

92. **Jacobs, E., M. Drews, A. Stuhlert, C. Buttner, P. J. Klein, M. Kist, and W. Bredt.** 1988. Immunological reaction of guinea-pigs following intranasal *Mycoplasma pneumoniae* infection and immunization with the 168 kDa adherence protein. *J. Gen. Microbiol.* **134:**473–479.

93. **Jacobs, E., K. Fuchte, and W. Bredt.** 1986. A 168-kilodalton protein of *Mycoplasma pneumoniae* used as antigen in a dot enzyme-linked immunosorbent assay. *Eur. J. Clin. Microbiol.* **5:**435–440.

94. **Jacobs, E., B. Gerstenecker, B. Mader, C.-H. Huang, P.-C. Hu, R. Halter, and W. Bredt.** 1989. Binding sites of attachment-inhibiting monoclonal antibodies and antibodies from patients on peptide fragments of the *Mycoplasma pneumoniae* adhesin. *Infect. Immun.* **57:**685–688.

95. **Jacobs, E., A. Pilatschek, B. Gerstenecker, K. Oberle, and W. Bredt.** 1990. Immunodominant epitopes of the adhesin of *Mycoplasma pneumoniae.* *J. Clin. Microbiol.* **28:**1194–1197.

96. **Jacobs, E., R. Rock, and L. Dalehite.** 1990. A B cell-, T cell-linked epitope located on the adhesin of *Mycoplasma pneumoniae.* *Infect. Immun.* **58:**2464–2469.

97. **Jacobs, E., A. Stuhlert, M. Drews, K. Pumpe, H. E. Schafer, M. Kist, and W. Bredt.** 1988. Host reactions to *Mycoplasma pneumoniae* infections in guinea-pigs preimmunized systemically with the adhesin of this pathogen. *Microb. Pathog.* **5:**259–265.

98. **Jeurissen, S. H. M., E. Claassen, N. Van Rooijen, and G. Kraal.** 1985. Intra-intestinal priming leads to antigen-specific IgA memory cells in peripheral lymphoid organs. *Immunology* **56:**417–423.

99. **Kagan, G. Y., Y. V. Vulfovich, A. V. Zilfyan, I. V. Zheverzh, and N. A. Gamova.** 1982. Experimental polyarthritis induced by *Mycoplasma fermentans* in rabbits. *Zh. Mikrobiol. Epidemiol. Immunobiol.* **3:**107–110.

100. **Kahane, I., S. Tucker, and J. B. Baseman.** 1985. Detection of *Mycoplasma pneumoniae* adhesin (P1) in the nonhemadsorbing population of virulent *Mycoplasma pneumoniae.* *Infect. Immun.* **49:**457–458.

101. **Kapatais-Zoumbos, K., D. K. F. Chandler, and M. F. Barile.** 1985. Survey of immunoglobulin A protease activity among selected species of *Ureaplasma* and *Mycoplasma*: specificity for host immunoglobulin A. *Infect. Immun.* **47:**704–709.

102. **Kapikian, A. Z., R. H. Mitchell, R. M. Chanock, R. A. Shvedoff, and C. E. Stewart.** 1969. An epidemiologic study of altered clinical reactivity to respiratory syncytial (RS) virus infection in children previously vaccinated with an inactivated RS virus vaccine. *Am. Epidemiol.* **89:**405–421.

103. **Kilian, M., B. Thomsen, T. E. Peterson, and T. E. Bleeg.** 1983. Occurrence and nature of bacterial IgA proteases. *Ann. N.Y. Acad. Sci.* **409:**612–624.

104. **Kleven, S. H., J. R. Glisson, M. Y. Lin, and F. D. Talkington.** 1984. Bacterins and vaccines for the control of *Mycoplasma gallisepticum.* *Isr. J. Med. Sci.* **20:**989–991.

105. **Krause, D. C., and J. B. Baseman.** 1983. Inhibition of *Mycoplasma pneumoniae* hemadsorption and adherence to respiratory epithelium by antibodies to a membrane protein. *Infect. Immun.* **39:**1180–1186.

106. **Krause, D. C., D. K. Leith, and J. B. Baseman.** 1983. Reacquisition of specific proteins confers virulence in *Mycoplasma pneumoniae.* *Infect. Immun.* **39:**830–836.

107. **Kristensen, B., P. Paroz, J. Nicolet, M. Wanner, and A. L. de Weck.** 1981. Cell-mediated and humoral immune response in swine after vaccination and natural infection with *Mycoplasma hyopneumoniae.* *Am. J. Vet. Res.* **42:**784–788.

108. **Krivan, H. C., L. D. Olson, M. F. Barile, V. Ginsberg, and D. D. Roberts.** 1989. Adhesion of *Mycoplasma pneumoniae* to sulfated glycolipids and inhibition by dextran sulfate. *J. Biol. Chem.* **264:**9283–9288.

109. **Lange, S., and J. Holmgren.** 1978. Protective antitoxic cholera immunity in mice: influence of route and number of immunizations and mode of action of protective antibodies. *Acta Pathol. Microbiol. Scand.* **86:**145.

110. **Lee, G. Y., and G. B. Kenny.** 1987. Humoral immune response to polypeptides of *Ureaplasma urealyticum* in women with postpartum fever. *J. Clin. Microbiol.* **25:**1841–1844.

111. **Lelijveld, J. L. M., A. Leentvaar-Kuijpers, A. C. Hekker, A. A. Polak-Vogelzang, and R. F. E. De Wit.** 1981. Some sexually transmitted diseases in female visitors of an out-patient department for venereal diseases in Utrecht, Netherlands. *Ned. Tijdschr. Geneeskd.* **125:**463–466.

112. **Lemaître, M., D. Guétard, Y. Hénin, L. Montagnier, and A. Zerial.** 1990. Protective activity of tetracycline analogues against the cytopathic effect of the human immunodeficiency viruses in CEM cells. *Res. Virol.* **141:**5–16.

113. **Lemcke, R. M.** 1973. Summary of discussion. Workshop on the mycoplasmatales as agents of disease. Session II: Immunology. *J. Infect. Dis.* **127**(Suppl.):66–68.

114. **Li, C.-M., S. Loechel, and P.-C. Hu.** 1990. Development of a *Mycoplasma pneumoniae*-adenovirus recombinant vaccine. *IOM Lett.* **1:**119–120.

115. **Lind, K., B. O. Lindhardt, J. H. Schutten, J. Blom, and C. Christiansen.** 1984. Serological cross-reactions between *Mycoplasma genitalium* and *Mycoplasma pneumoniae.* *J. Clin. Microbiol.* **20:**1036–1042.

116. **Lindsey, J. R.** 1986. Prevalence of viral and mycoplasmal infections in laboratory rodents, p. 801–808. *In* P. N. Bhatt, R. O. Jacoby, H. C. Morse, and A. E. New (ed.), *Viral and Mycoplasmal Infections of Laboratory Rodents: Effects on Biomedical Research.* Academic Press, Inc., Orlando, Fla.

117. **Litamoi, J. K., F. K. Lijodi, and E. Nandokha.** 1989. Contagious caprine pleuropneumonia: some observations in a field vaccination trial using inactivated *Mycoplasma* strain F38. *Trop. Anim. Health Prod.* **21:**146–150.

118. **Lloyd, L. C.** 1969. Contagious bovine pleuropneumonia. Aspects of eradication in Australia. *Bull. Off. Int. Epizoot.* **71:**1329–1334.

119. **Lloyd, L. C., and E. R. Trethewie.** 1970. Contagious bovine pleuropneumonia, p. 172–197. *In* J. T. Sharp (ed.), *The Role of Mycoplasmas and L-Forms of Bacteria in Disease.* Charles C Thomas, Springfield, Ill.

120. **Lo, S.-C.** 1986. Isolation and identification of a novel virus from patients with AIDS. *Am. J. Trop. Med. Hyg.* **35:**675–676.

121. **Lo, S.-C., M. S. Dawson, P. B. Newton III, M. A. Sonoda, J. W.-K. Shih, W. F. Engler, R. Y.-H. Wang, and D. J. Wear.** 1989. Association of the virus-like infectious agent originally reported in patients with AIDS with acute fatal disease in previously healthy non-AIDS patients. *Am. J. Trop. Med. Hyg.* **41:**364–376.

122. **Lo, S.-C., M. S. Dawson, D.-M. Wong, P. B. Newton III, M. A. Sonoda, W. F. Engler, R. Y.-H. Wang, J. W.-K. Shih, H. J. Alter, and D. J. Wear.** 1989. Identification of *Mycoplasma incognitus* infection in patients with AIDS: an immunohistochemical, in situ hybridization and ultrastructural study. *Am. J. Trop. Med. Hyg.* **41:**601–616.

123. **Lo, S.-C., J. W.-K. Shih, P. B. Newton III, D.-M. Wong, M. M. Hayes, J. R. Benish, D. J. Wear, and R. Y.-H. Wang.** 1989. Virus-like infectious agent (VLIA) is a novel pathogenic mycoplasma: *Mycoplasma incognitus.* *Am. J. Trop. Med. Hyg.* **41:**586–600.

124. **Lo, S.-C., J. W.-K. Shih, N.-Y. Yang, C. Y. Ou, and R. Y.-H. Wang.** 1989. A novel virus-like infectious agent in patients with AIDS. *Am. J. Trop. Med. Hyg.* **41:**213–226.

125. **MacOwan, K. J., and J. E. Minette.** 1978. The effect of high passage *Mycoplasma* strain F38 on the course of contagious carpine pleuropneumonia (CCPP). *Trop. Anim. Health. Prod.* **10:**31–35.

126. **Mårdh, P. A., and L. Westrom.** 1970. T-mycoplasma in the genito-urinary tract of the female. *Acta Pathol. Microbiol. Scand. Sect. B* **78:**374–376.

127. **Mårdh, P. A., and L. Westrom.** 1970. Tubal and cervical cultures in acute salpingitis with special reference to *Mycoplasma hominis* and T-strain mycoplasmas. *Br. J. Vener. Dis.* **46:**179–186.

128. **McGhee, J. R., J. Mestecky, P. L. Ogra, and J. Bienenstock (ed.).** 1986. *Recent Advances in Mucosal Immunology. Part B: Effector Functions*, p. 877–1897. Plenum Press, New York.

129. **Mogabgab, W. J.** 1973. Efficacy of inactivated *Mycoplasma pneumoniae* vaccine demonstrated by protection in large field trials. *Ann. N.Y. Acad. Sci.* **225:**453–461.

130. **Mogabgab, W. J.** 1973. Protective efficacy of killed *Mycoplasma pneumoniae* vaccine measured in large-scale studies in a military population. *Am. Rev. Respir. Dis.* **108:**899–908.

131. **Mogabgab, W. J., S. Marchand, G. Mills, and R. Beville.** 1975. Efficacy of inactivated *Mycoplasma pneumoniae* vaccine in man. *Dev. Biol. Stand.* **28:**597–608.

132. **Moller, B. R., E. A. Freundt, and P. A. Mårdh.** 1980. Experimental pelvic inflammatory disease provoked by *Chlamydia trachomatis* and *Mycoplasma hominis* in grivet monkeys. *Am. J. Obstet. Gynecol.* **138:**990–995.

132a.**Montagnier, L.** Personal communication.

133. **Morrison-Plummer, J., D. H. Jones, K. Daly, J. G. Tully, D. Taylor-Robinson, and J. B. Baseman.** 1987. Molecular characterization of *Mycoplasma genitalium* species-specific and cross-reactive determinants: identification of an immunodominant protein of *M. genitalium. Isr. J. Med. Sci.* **23:**453–457.

134. **Morrison-Plummer, J., D. K. Leith, and J. B. Baseman.** 1986. Biological effects of anti-lipid and anti-protein monoclonal antibodies on *Mycoplasma pneumoniae. Infect. Immun.* **53:**398–403.

135. **Murphy, W. H., C. Bullis, L. Dabich, R. Heyn, and C. J. D. Zarafonetis.** 1970. Isolation of *Mycoplasma* from leukemic and nonleukemic patients. *J. Natl. Cancer Inst.* **45:**243–351.

136. **Murphy, W. H., C. Bullis, E. J. Ertel, and C. J. D. Zarafonetis.** 1967. Mycoplasma studies of human leukemia. *Ann. N.Y. Acad. Sci.* **143:**544–556.

137. **Murray, M.** 1973. Local immunity and its role in vaccination. *Vet. Rec.* **93:**500–504.

138. **Nakashima, T.** 1984. Isolation and biological characteristics of phenotypic variants of *Mycoplasma fermentans. J. Karume Med. Assoc.* **47:**765–779.

139. **Nicol, C. S., and D. G. Edwards.** 1983. Role of organisms of the pleuropneumonia group in human genital infections. *Br. J. Vener. Dis.* **29:**141–150.

140. **O'Brien, S. J., J. M. Simonson, M. W. Grabowski, and M. F. Barile.** 1981. Analysis of multiple isozyme expression among twenty-two species of *Mycoplasma* and *Acholeplasma. J. Bacteriol.* **146:**222–232.

141. **Olson, L. D., S. W. Shane, A. A. Karpas, T. M. Cunningham, P. G. Probst, and M. F. Barile.** Monoclonal antibodies to pathogenic *Mycoplasma hominis* surface antigens. Submitted for publication.

142. **Pierce, N. F., and F. T. Koster.** 1980. Priming and suppression of the intestinal immune response to cholera toxoid/toxin by parenteral toxoid in rats. *J. Immunol.* **124:**307–311.

143. **Plata, E. J., M. R. Abell, and W. H. Murphy.** 1973. Induction of leukemoid disease in mice by *Mycoplasma fermentans. J. Infect. Dis.* **128:**588–597.

144. **Polak-Vogelzang, A. A., J. Brugman, and R. Reijgers.** 1987. Comparison of two methods for detection of Mollicutes (Mycoplasmatales and Acholeplasmatales) in cell cultures in The Netherlands. *Antonie van Leeuwenhoek J. Microbiol. Serol.* **53:**107–118.

145. **Quintmeier, H., E. Schmitt, H. Kirchhoff, W. Grote, and P. F. Muhlradt.** 1990. *Mycoplasma fermentans*-derived high-molecular-weight material induces interleukin-6 release in cultures of murine macrophages and human monocytes. *Infect Immun.* **58:**1273–1280.

146. **Razin, S., B. Prescott, G. Caldes, W. D. James, and R. M. Chanock.** 1970. Role of glycolipids and phosphatidylglycerol in the serological activity of *Mycoplasma pneumoniae. Infect. Immun.* **1:**408–416.

147. **Razin, S., B. Prescott, W. D. James, G. Caldes, J. Valdesuso, and R. M. Chanock.** 1971. Production and properties of antisera to membrane glycolipids of *Mycoplasma pneumoniae. Infect. Immun.* **3:**420–423.

148. **Roberts, D. D., L. D. Olson, M. F. Barile, V. Ginsburg, and H. C. Krivan.** 1989. Sialic acid-dependent adhesion of *Mycoplasma pneumoniae* to purified glycoproteins. *J. Biol. Chem.* **264:**9289–9293.

149. **Robertson, J. A.** 1986. Potential virulence factors of *Ureaplasma urealyticum. Pediatr. Infect. Dis.* **5** (Suppl.):322–324.

150. **Robertson, J. A., M. E. Stemler, and G. W. Stemke.** 1984. Immunoglobulin A protease activity of *Ureaplasma urealyticum. J. Clin. Microbiol.* **19:**255–258.

151. **Ross, R. F., B. J. Zimmerman-Erickson, and T. F. Young.** 1984. Characteristics of protective activity of *Mycoplasma hyopneumoniae* vaccine. *Am. J. Vet. Res.* **45:**1899–1905.

152. **Ruiter, M, and H. M. M. Wentholt.** 1953. Isolation of a pleuropneumonia-like organism (G-strain) in a case of fusospirillary vulvovaginitis. *Acta Dermat. Venereol.* **33:**123–129.

153. **Saillard, C., P. Carle, J. M. Bové, C. Bébéar, S.-C. Lo, J. W.-K. Shih, R. Y.-H. Wang, D. L. Rose, and J. G. Tully.** 1990. Genetic and serological relatedness between *Mycoplasma fermentans* strains and a mycoplasma recently identified in tissues of AIDS and non-AIDS patients. *Res. Virol.* **141:**385–395.

154. **Sasaki, Y., M. Shintani, H. Watanabe, and T. Sasaki.** 1989. *Mycoplasma genitalium* and *Mycoplasma pneumoniae* share a 67 kilodalton protein as a main cross-reactive antigen. *Microbiol. Immunol.* **33:**1059–1062.

155. **Schalla, W. O., and H. R. Harrison.** 1987. Western blot analysis of the human serum response to *Mycoplasma hominis. Isr. J. Med. Sci.* **23:**613–617.

156. **Schaper, U., J. S. Chapman, and P.-C. Hu.** 1987. Preliminary indication of unusual codon usage in the DNA sequence of the attachment protein of *Mycoplasma pneumoniae. Isr. J. Med. Sci.* **23:**361–367.

157. **Seid, R. C., Jr., P. F. Smith, G. Guevarra, H. D. Hochstein, and M. F. Barile.** 1980. Endotoxin-like activities of mycoplasmal lipopolysaccharides (lipoglycans). *Infect. Immun.* **29:**990–994.

158. **Sitia, R., A. Rubartelli, S. Deambrosis, D. Pozzi, and U. Hammerling.** 1985. Differentiation in the murine B cell lymphoma 129: inductive capacities of lipopolysaccharide and *Mycoplasma fermentans* products. *Eur. J. Immunol.* **15:**570–575.

159. **Smith, C. B., R. M. Chanock, W. T. Friedewald, and R. H. Alford.** 1967. *Mycoplasma pneumoniae* infections in volunteers. *Ann. N.Y. Acad. Sci.* **143:**471–483.

160. **Smith, C. B., W. T. Friedewald, and R. M. Chanock.** 1967. Inactivated *Mycoplasma pneumoniae* vaccine: evaluation in volunteers. *JAMA* **199:**353–358.

161. **Smith, P. F.** 1987. Antigenic character of membrane lipoglycans from mollicutes—a review. *Isr. J. Med. Sci.* **23:**448–452.

162. **Steinberg, P., R. L. Horswood, H. Brunner, and R. M. Chanock.** 1971. Temperature-sensitive mutants of *My-*

coplasma pneumoniae. II. Response of hamsters. *J. Infect. Dis.* **124:**179–187.

163. **Steinberg, P., R. L. Horswood, and R. M. Chanock.** 1969. Temperature-sensitive mutants of *Mycoplasma pneumoniae*. I. *In vitro* biologic properties. *J. Infect. Dis.* **120:**217–224.

164. **Su, C.-J., A. Chavoya, and J. B. Baseman.** 1988. Regions of *Mycoplasma pneumoniae* cytadhesin P1 structural gene exist as multiple copies. *Infect. Immun.* **56:**3157–3161.

165. **Su, C.-J., A. Chavoya, and J. B. Baseman.** 1989. Spontaneous mutation results in loss of the cytadhesin (P1) of *Mycoplasma pneumoniae*. *Infect. Immun.* **57:**3237–3239.

166. **Taylor, G., and D. Taylor-Robinson.** 1974. The part played by cell-mediated immunity in mycoplasma respiratory infections. *Dev. Biol. Stand.* **28:**195–210.

167. **Taylor-Robinson, D., and P. M. Furr.** 1986. Clinical antibiotic resistance of *Ureaplasma urealyticum*. *Pediatr. Infect. Dis.* **5:**S335–S337.

168. **Taylor-Robinson, D., P. M. Furr, and N. F. Hanna.** 1985. Microbiological and serological study of non-gonococcal urethritis with special reference to *Mycoplasma genitalium*. *Genitourin. Med.* **61:**319–324.

169. **Taylor-Robinson, D., P. M. Furr, J. G. Tully, M. F. Barile, and B. R. Moller.** 1987. Animal models of *Mycoplasma genitalium* urogenital infections. *Isr. J. Med. Sci.* **23:**561–564.

170. **Taylor-Robinson, D., J. G. Tully, and M. F. Barile.** 1985. Urethral infection in male chimpanzees produced experimentally by *Mycoplasma genitalium*. *Br. J. Exp. Pathol.* **66:**95–101.

171. **Thirkell, D., A. D. Myles, and W. C. Russell.** 1989. Serotype 8- and serocluster-specific surface expressed antigens of *Ureaplasma urealyticum*. *Infect. Immun.* **57:**1697–1701.

172. **Thirkell, D., A. D. Myles, and D. Taylor-Robinson.** 1990. A comparison of four major antigens in five human and several animal strains of ureaplasmas. *J. Med. Microbiol.* **32:**163–168.

173. **Trevino, L. B., W. G. Haldenwang, and J. B. Baseman.** 1986. Expression of *Mycoplasma pneumoniae* antigens in *Escherichia coli*. *Infect. Immun.* **53:**129–134.

174. **Tully, J. G., D. Taylor-Robinson, R. M. Cole, and D. L. Rose.** 1981. A newly discovered mycoplasma in the human urogenital tract. *Lancet* **i:**1288–1291.

175. **Tully, J. G., D. Taylor-Robinson, D. L. Rose, P. Furr, C. E. Graham, and M. F. Barile.** 1986. Urogenital challenge of primate species with *Mycoplasma genitalium* and

characteristics of infection induced in chimpanzees. *J. Infect. Dis.* **153:**1046–1054.

176. **Vu, A. C., H. M. Foy, F. D. Cartwright, and G. E. Kenny.** 1987. The principal protein antigens of isolates of *Mycoplasma pneumonia* as measured by levels of immunoglobulin G in human serum are stable in strains collected over a 10-year period. *Infect. Immun.* **55:**1830–1836.

177. **Vulfovich, Y. V., A. V. Zilfian, I. V. Zheverzheeva, N. A. Gamova, and G. Y. Kagan.** 1981. Prolonged persistence of *Mycoplasma arthritidis* and *Mycoplasma fermentans* in the body of experimentally-infected rats. *Zh. Mikrobiol. Epidemiol. Immunobiol.* **1:**14–17.

178. **Waage, A., C. Kaufmann, T. Espevik, and G. Husby.** 1989. Interleukin-6 in synovial fluid from patients with arthritis. *Clin. Immunol. Immunopathol.* **50:**394–398.

179. **Weickmann, J. L., and D. E. Farhney.** 1977. Arginine deiminase from *Mycoplasma arthritidis*: evidence for multiple forms. *J. Biol. Chem.* **252:**2615–2620.

180. **Wenzel, R. P., R. B. Craven, J. A. Davies, J. O. Hendley, B. H. Hamory, and J. M. Gwaltney, Jr.** 1977. Protective efficacy of an inactivated *Mycoplasma pneumoniae* vaccine. *J. Infect. Dis.* **136:**S204–S207.

181. **Wenzel, R., and R. Herrmann.** 1988. Repetitive DNA sequences in *Mycoplasma pneumoniae*. *Nucleic Acids Res.* **16:**8337–8350.

182. **Williams, M. H., J. Brostoff, and I. M. Roitt.** 1970. Possible role of *Mycoplasma fermentans* in pathogenesis of rheumatoid arthritis. *Lancet* **ii:**277–280.

183. **Williams, M. H., and F. E. Bruckner.** 1971. Immunological reactivity of *Mycoplasma fermentans* in patients with rheumatoid arthritis. *Ann. Rheum. Dis.* **30:**271–273.

184. **Yayoshi, M., M. Araake, E. Hayatsu, T. Takezawa, and M. Yoskioka.** 1985. Immunogenicity and protective effect of hemolysis mutants of *Mycoplasma pneumoniae*. *Microbiol. Immunol.* **29:**1029–1037.

185. **Yayoshi, M., U. Gakuin, E. Hayatsu, and M. Yoskioka.** 1989. Protective effects of *Mycoplasma pneumoniae* live vaccine or its hyperimmune serum on the experimental infection in mice. *Kansenshogaku Zasshi* **63:**684–691.

186. **Yogev, D., D. Halachmi, G. E. Kenny, and S. Razin.** 1988. Distinction of species and strains of mycoplasmas (Mollicutes) by genomic DNA fingerprints with an rRNA gene probe. *J. Clin. Microbiol.* **26:**1198–1201.

187. **Yoshida, T., N. Yanai, M. Kawase, H. Mizzusawa, K. Yakamoto, and M. Takeuchi.** 1989. Identification of mycoplasmas contaminating animal cell lines. *Inst. Ferment. Res. Commun.* (Osaka) **4:**13–19.

30. Serodiagnosis

GEORGE E. KENNY

INTRODUCTION

Diagnosis of mycoplasmal infections by isolation of the organism is difficult because mycoplasmas grow slowly and require complex media for isolation, whereas most bacterial pathogens may be readily cultivated in the clinical microbiological laboratory relatively quickly. As a consequence, few laboratories offer culturing services. Therefore, serodiagnostic methods could be as important for diagnosis of mycoplasmal infections as they are for diagnosis of viral infections, the agents of which also may be difficult to cultivate. However, serodiagnostic methods for diagnosis of mycoplasmal infections are much less advanced because of the much greater antigenic complexity of mycoplasmas than of viruses. This chapter summarizes the methods and approaches that have been used for my-

coplasmas and provides concepts for the development and evaluation of new serodiagnostic tests.

Serodiagnosis has two important epidemiological and clinical uses: (i) to determine the incidence of new infections by using serology to detect antibodies produced during infection and disease, and (ii) to determine the prevalence of past infections in a population by testing individuals for any antibodies at all, the inference being that those who have antibodies have been infected sometime in the past.

The classic antibody response in an infectious disease shows three phases: (i) a rapid production of antibodies during weeks 1 to 3 of disease, (ii) a peak in antibody levels some 2 to 4 weeks after infection, and (iii) a gradual decrease in antibody levels in months to years following recovery from the illness. The demonstration of a significant antibody increase between

George E. Kenny • Department of Pathobiology, SC-38, School of Public Health and Community Medicine, University of Washington, Seattle, Washington 98195.

convalescent- and acute-phase sera from an ill individual suggests that infection with the particular agent has occurred recently. Thus, if the symptoms are compatible with those usually produced by the agent, a serological diagnosis is possible if an antibody increase can be documented. Operationally, the accepted criterion for a positive test has been the demonstration of a fourfold titer increase between acute- and convalescent-phase sera taken at onset and several weeks later when sera are tested by using twofold serial dilutions. The criterion of a fourfold rise has been accepted because twofold dilution tests are considered to have an intrinsic error of plus or minus one twofold dilution. The performance of a serodiagnostic test by using the criterion of a fourfold antibody rise can be evaluated by plotting the distribution of titer rises and falls in a population of persons with the disease (Fig. 1 shows an example for *Mycoplasma pneumoniae* pneumonia and the lipid complement fixation [CF] test). A large number of persons showed no titer rise (0 titer in Fig. 1) because the symptoms of *M. pneumoniae* pneumonia are so insidious and mild that many patients do not initially seek medical care but wait until the disease fails to improve. Thus, their acute-phase sera are collected well into the disease and possess antibody. Of the 353 persons who had fourfold rises, the geometric mean rise was 20.8-fold. In comparison with the 353 fourfold rises, only 83 persons showed a fall in titer. An excess of rises over falls should be seen in any test that is really measuring antibody increases to recent infections. If the test were to show an equal number of rises and falls, the concern would be that the rises and falls result from the statistical error inherent in the test. If titer rises were small (maximum of four- to eightfold), repetition of the results would show whether the rises and falls are due to the inherent error of the test.

The demonstration of antibodies in healthy individuals is taken to mean that these individuals have been infected with the agent in the past. Determination of cutoff values is difficult when serum titers are low. Cutoff values can best be established by measuring the long-term persistence of antibody in individuals known to be infected in the past.

Although demonstration of an antibody rise in acute- and convalescent-phase sera is the most stringent serodiagnostic method of determining the mycoplasmal etiology of a recent infection, a second method of diagnosis is to demonstrate the appearance of immunoglobulin M (IgM) class antibodies, since these antibodies usually but not always peak quickly and decline to low levels within months. Demonstration of IgM antibodies has the advantage that only a single serum needs to be tested, and this sample can be obtained quite early in infection in some infections. The IgM criterion has disadvantages in that the IgM response to some antigens, particularly carbohydrate or glycolipid antigens, may be prolonged, and adults may produce only IgG antibodies (a problem more marked with protein antigens).

A third method for serodiagnosis of recent infections is to determine a diagnostic antibody titer, since peak titers are frequently seen during or shortly after disease. Sera that show values equal to or greater than this value are considered positive. This criterion will not yield as accurate a timing of infection as will the antibody increase criterion because peak antibody levels may be observed for months after recovery.

TYPES OF SEROLOGICAL TESTS

The serodiagnostic tests can be divided into four methods. In the first method, the ability of antiserum to prevent growth or prevent the production of a metabolic product is used as an indicator. This procedure is highly species specific because it is a major method for distinguishing species. In the second method, the antigen is an extract of whole mycoplasmas, and antibodies are detected by CF tests, dot blot tests, and enzyme-linked immunosorbent assays (ELISAs). A third procedure is the use of a partially purified or purified antigen in an ELISA or similar test. Such tests include the use of lipid extracts in the CF tests for infections. The fourth category of test is the use of Western immunoblotting to determine and analyze polypeptides involved in the immune response.

Metabolic Inhibition Test

The simplest test is the metabolic inhibition test, which measures the growth of organisms by their ability to produce a metabolic product such as acid from glucose or failure to reduce tetrazolium or produce ammonia from either arginine or urea, depending on whether the particular species utilizes these substrates. Fixed amounts of organisms, diluted in medium, are mixed with serum in doubling twofold dilutions. The resulting mixtures are incubated in tubes or on microtiter plates for a period of time sufficient to

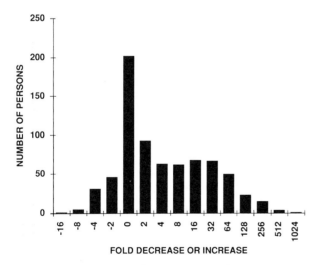

Figure 1. Distribution of fold increases or decreases in antibody between acute- and convalescent-phase sera from 731 persons with pneumonia and isolates of *M. pneumoniae*. Antibodies were measured by the lipid CF test from sera tested in a previous study (22). A total of 202 persons showed no antibody increase, indicated by the 0, and 353 showed a fourfold or greater rise. Fold increases are positive values for serum pairs with higher titers in convalescent phase and negative values for serum pairs which show decreases in titer.

produce a color reaction in the control wells without organisms. The serum titer is reported as the highest dilution of serum that prevents formation of the metabolic product. Prolonged incubation of the test usually leads to an apparent decrease in serum titer; consequently, the incubation time must be constant and paired sera must be tested in the same test run.

CF Test

The CF test relies on the ability of antigen-antibody complexes (mycoplasmas and their respective antibodies) to fix complement. The reaction is visualized by the failure of sheep erythrocytes sensitized with antibodies to sheep erythrocytes (hemolysin) to lyse in the presence of the test serum, which in reacting with the antigen removes complement from the system. The amount of complement consumed in the test is defined by the concentration of erythrocytes used. Since the erythrocyte concentration is standardized between laboratories, titers can be compared between studies. The end point is usually defined as the least amount of serum that completely prevents lysis of the erythrocytes in a test using 4 U of antigen, 2 U of complement, and serial twofold dilutions of serum. Since the test results may vary twofold from run to run, paired sera must be tested in the same run.

Fluorescent Antibody Test

The indirect immunofluorescence test is used to detect antibodies in patient sera (14). Organisms are fixed to tissue culture cells, or infected lung sections from embryonated hen eggs are used as the antigen (14) and fixed to glass slides. The slides or wells are incubated with dilutions of patient serum, and the binding of these antibodies is detected with a fluorescein-conjugated antiserum against the bound immunoglobulins. This procedure has advantages in that very small amounts of antigen are necessary and specific immunoglobulin classes can be detected. The difficulty of the procedure has discouraged its use. The label for the test also can be an enzyme that can be visualized with a histochemical stain used for detection of the enzyme activity localized in the vicinity of the antigen on the tissue. This procedure provides for permanent slides and permits the use of an ordinary microscope rather than a UV microscope. The use of electron-dense labels permits electron microscopy to be done for identification of antigens at the ultrastructural level.

ELISA

ELISA is very closely related in concept to the fluorescent antibody test with the exceptions that an enzyme-linked conjugated antiglobulin is used to detect the antibody and detection of the reaction is spectrophotometric rather than visual (10). The usual format is an indirect test with the antigen immobilized on a plastic surface. The antigen is reacted with dilutions of patient sera, and the resultant binding of patient serum antibodies is detected with a labeled antibody against the immunoglobulin. The most common enzymes used are horseradish peroxidase and alkaline phosphatase. As in the immunofluorescence test, antibodies that are specific to the heavy chains and thus specific to the major immunoglobulin classes can be used. The ease of use and sensitivity of ELISA had led to its widespread adaptation, particularly in view of the extensive technology available to facilitate testing of many sera. One major drawback is the fact that titers cannot be compared between laboratories because of difficulties in standardizing both the antigen and the conjugate.

Western Immunoblotting

The Western blot (38) is the only analytical method commonly used to define specific target antigens in an organism. Proteins separated by polyacrylamide gel electrophoresis are transferred electrophoretically to nitrocellulose. Strips are cut from nitrocellulose imprints from slab gels and used to assay patient sera for antibodies by immersing the nitrocellulose into dilutions of the serum. After washing, bound antibodies are detected with a enzyme-conjugated antibody to the target immunoglobulin. The enzyme label is detected with a histochemical stain that precipitates in the nitrocellulose and identifies the molecular weights of reactive polypeptides.

EVALUATION OF SERODIAGNOSTIC TESTS

The clinical usefulness of a serodiagnostic test is dependent on the ability of the test to distinguish healthy individuals (or animals) from individuals with the disease; the reliability of this distinction is defined by the sensitivity and specificity of the assay (22, 40). The terms "sensitivity" and "specificity" have epidemiological meanings that are distinct from common biological meanings.

Sensitivity and Specificity

The sensitivity of an assay is defined as the ability of the test to identify individuals with the disease in the group of diseased individuals and is defined in percentage terms as (diseased individuals with a positive test/all diseased individuals tested) × 100. The specificity of the test is the ability of the test to identify individuals without disease in a healthy population and is defined in percentage terms as (nondiseased individuals with negative test/all nondiseased individuals tested) × 100.

Note that these definitions are entirely different from and should not be confused with the common biological definitions of these terms. Sensitivity is commonly considered to be the ability of a test to measure small quantities of material; in contrast, epidemiological usage defines sensitivity as the ability of a test to detect disease. Similarly, specificity in the epidemiological sense does not imply the ability to distinguish between diseases or organisms but instead indicates the ability to successfully identify well individuals in a population of healthy individuals.

Determination of Predictive Values

The positive predictive value of a serological test measures the ability of a test to quantify true infections in a population of individuals with a positive test. The negative predictive value is the reverse, distinguishing the true negative individuals from individuals with a negative test who have the disease: positive predictive value = (individuals with disease with a positive test/total individuals with a positive test) × 100; negative predictive value = (healthy individuals with a negative test/total individuals with negative test) × 100.

Table 1 is a two-way table that defines how the data can be presented in order to calculate sensitivity, specificity, and positive and negative predictive values.

DEFINING REFERENCE POPULATIONS FOR EVALUATION OF SERODIAGNOSTIC TESTS

It is necessary to define a reference standard for diagnosis of disease that is independent of the serodiagnostic test being evaluated. Culture positivity is an important means of defining ill persons if the presence of the organism correlates with disease. Such a correlation is apparent in both *M. pneumoniae* and *M. pulmonis* infections, and serodiagnostic tests have been evaluated by using culture-positive individuals as the reference.

Serological Detection of *M. pneumoniae* Pneumonia

Clinical diagnosis of pneumonia due to *M. pneumoniae* is difficult because the disease cannot be distinguished clinically from pneumonias of other etiology (12). We evaluated the CF test with the lipid antigen (21) in a population of individuals who had pneumonia and from whom *M. pneumoniae* was isolated (Table 2 [22]). The sensitivity of serology, using as a criterion of positivity the fourfold antibody rise, was 53% (360 of 674 culture-positive persons; Table 2). However, when individuals with no titer rise but with titers of ≥32

Table 2. Sensitivity and specificity of serology with lipid antigen for the diagnosis of *M. pneumoniae* pneumonia in patients with and without isolates of *M. pneumoniae*[a]

Isolation result	Fourfold antibody increase	No fourfold antibody increase		Total
		≥32	≤16	
Positive	360	247	67	674
Negative	165	180	2,527	2,872
Total	525	427	2,594	3,546

[a] From reference 22.

were added to the 360 persons with a fourfold rise in antibody, the sensitivity increased to 90% (607 of 674). Fifty-eight percent of the persons who showed no fourfold rises in antibodies as measured by the lipid CF test (Fig. 1) showed titers of 1:64 or 1:128 and would have been counted as positive by using the ≥32 titer criterion. The specificity of the lipid CF test was 89% (2,527 of 2,872; Table 2).

The positive predictive value of the CF test was 64% (of 952 persons with positive serology, 607 had isolates; Table 2). The negative predictive value is 2,527/2,594, or 97%, for the population of pneumonia patients in Table 2. The positive predictive value is low for *M. pneumoniae* pneumonia because of the large number of individuals who have negative cultures but positive serology.

Serological Detection of *M. pulmonis* Infections

Cassell et al. (8) compared serology and culture for determining the prevalence of *M. pulmonis* infections in mice and rats. They used an ELISA with a lysate of whole organisms as the antigen and compared the serological data with isolation of the organism. For rats, they found that ELISA antibodies were found in all of 336 animals that were positive by culture (Table 3A), for a sensitivity of 100%. The specificity of the ELISA versus culture for rats was 83% (176 of 213 culture-negative rats also were ELISA negative). The ELISA test was both less sensitive and less specific for detection of infection in mice, with a sensitivity of 64% and specificity of 76% (Table 3B). These results suggest

Table 1. Calculation of sensitivity, specificity, positive predictive value, and negative predictive value for serological tests[a]

	Serological test	
	Positive	Negative
Disease positive	A	B
Disease negative	C	D

$$\text{Sensitivity} = \frac{A}{A + B} \times 100$$

$$\text{Specificity} = \frac{D}{C + D} \times 100$$

$$\text{Positive predictive value} = \frac{A}{A + C} \times 100$$

$$\text{Negative predictive value} = \frac{D}{B + D} \times 100$$

[a] A through D represent number of persons or animals.

Table 3. Sensitivity and specificity of ELISA for detection of *M. pulmonis* infections in rats and mice

Culture	ELISA		Total
	No. positive	No. negative	
A. Rats[a]			
Positive	336	0	336
Negative	37	176	213
Total	373	176	549
B. Mice[b]			
Positive	53	30	83
Negative	122	385	507
Total	175	415	590

[a] Data adapted from Table 2 of reference 8.
[b] Data adapted from Table 3 of reference 8.

that culture of mice was less effective than culture of rats. In another study with rats, using a higher test serum concentration in a microELISA test, the sensitivity and specificity of ELISA versus culture were both 98% (31). Serodiagnosis is greatly aided in other animal systems in which experimentally infected animals can easily be differentiated from control uninfected animals (if such can be obtained).

Antibody Responses upon Colonization with Mycoplasmas

In contrast to the cases (*M. pneumoniae* and *M. pulmonis*) in which infection with mycoplasmas leads to growth in deeper tissues and the appearance of antibody, mycoplasmas frequently colonize surface sites of the host without demonstrable disease. This poses a problem, since disease cannot be used to define the ill population. Furthermore, we need to know whether the host makes antibodies in response to such surface infections. It is well recognized that *Ureaplasma urealyticum* and *M. hominis* are common colonizers of humans and that they are opportunists, particularly in the immediate postpartum period. Lin et al. (28) found significant changes in antibody titers to *M. hominis* around the time of delivery in most pregnant women (88%) infected with *M. hominis* and fewer but still significant changes in titers to *U. urealyticum* (40%) of women colonized with *U. urealyticum*. Gibbs et al. (13) found a greater increase in *U. urealyticum* antibodies in women with intra-amniotic infections than in women who were colonized with *U. urealyticum* without intra-amniotic infection. These results establish that persons do make antibody to these agents when the organisms penetrate to deeper sites, but they do not give evidence for the production of antibodies upon colonization of the vagina.

DEVELOPMENT AND REFINEMENT OF SERODIAGNOSTIC TESTS FOR *M. PNEUMONIAE*

The efforts ongoing to provide serodiagnosis of *M. pneumoniae* pneumonia provide a good example for strategies being applied to the development of new tests for serodiagnosis of mycoplasmal infections.

CF and Metabolic Inhibition Tests

Although the fluorescent antibody test (14) was important in the initial definition of the role that *M. pneumoniae* played in atypical pneumonia, two tests, the CF test with lipid antigen (21) and the metabolic inhibition test (35), came into general usage. The results of the two tests correlated well (36). The CF antibodies were of both IgG and IgM classes, as might be expected (11, 34). As discussed above, the CF test using the criterion of a fourfold rise or a titer of ≥32 in the sera detected 90% of pneumonias caused by *M. pneumoniae* isolates (22). Since the principal antigens were found to be relatively simple glycolipids (4, 33) and serologically related lipids have been found in spinach (23), it was not surprising that false-positive reactions have

been found. The most notable example is the antibody increase by lipid CF seen in persons with meningitis caused by ordinary bacteria (24, 25). The reason for this cross-reaction is unknown, but its existence warrants caution in interpreting data from unusual syndromes in persons from whom *M. pneumoniae* has not been isolated. In addition, *M. pneumoniae* shares lipid antigens with *M. genitalium* (29), an organism that has proven most difficult to isolate. Despite these reservations, the lipid CF test has good sensitivity and specificity in populations of persons with pneumonia.

Development of ELISA for *M. pneumoniae* Pneumonia

The difficulties with CF assays using partially purified or crude antigens derived from whole organisms have led to use of the highly sensitive ELISA (10) for diagnosis of *M. pneumoniae* pneumonia. The initial assays used solubilized whole organisms, with the expectation that the tests might measure antibodies to most of the antigens in the mixture. This is not the case, since antibodies can be detected only to antigens which compose at least 1% of the total protein (20), a situation which poses problems for an organism composed of several hundred proteins as well as contaminants from the medium in which the organism was grown. In addition, the relatively small amount of antigen coated in the mixture yields a test which has a shallow slope when optical density is plotted against the log of the serum dilution (20).

Detection of IgM in *M. pneumoniae* Infections

Interest in the fluorescent antibody test has revived because of the ability of the test to measure antibody classes without extensive fractionation of the sera. Sillis showed that detection of IgM by immunofluorescence identified fewer infections than did either the CF test or IgA and IgG immunofluorescence tests (37) in persons who were culture positive. In assays by μ-capture ELISA (43), Wreghitt and Sillis showed that IgM antibodies persisted for 4 to 5 weeks after infection and even longer when measured by indirect ELISA. Vikerfors et al. (41) found IgM antibodies in 80% of infections and then only 9 days after onset. By indirect ELISA for IgM, van Griethuysen et al. (39) showed that IgM antibodies could be detected in paired sera of 32 of 47 patients with a fourfold CF antibody rise, and convalescent-phase sera of 6 of the 47 patients were also negative. Thus, detection of IgM does not provide for rapid diagnosis, since sera would optimally need to be collected at least a week after onset. In addition, the persistence of IgM against *M. pneumoniae* after infection would hinder determination of the timing of infections by using a single serum specimen.

Western Immunoblotting

Western blotting has proved to be a most important serodiagnostic method since it not only detects antibodies but also enables the molecular weights of the antigens involved to be directly determined. A number of studies have been carried out by immunoblotting human sera from persons with *M. pneumoniae* pneumonia (16, 17, 27, 42) and have shown overall that convalescent-phase sera from patients consistently recognize five peptides ranging in molecular mass from 35 to 170 kDa (16, 17, 42). The specific pattern formed confirms the data obtained from ELISA or other serodiagnostic tests. Western blotting was important in demonstrating that the antibody responses seen in purulent meningitis against the lipid CF antigen were not true responses to *M. pneumoniae* (24, 25). Western blotting has also served as an important guide for the selection of candidate peptides for prospective ELISAs.

Development of ELISAs for Diagnosis of *M. pneumoniae* Pneumonia with Defined Protein Antigens

The recognition that the P1 protein (165 to 170 kDa) is a major proteinaceous immunogen of *M. pneumoniae* (15, 27), and the fact that this protein has been sequenced, has led to the development of assays with purified proteins. Jacobs et al. (18) used a purified P1 protein fraction in an ELISA and found immune responses in persons with *M. pneumoniae* pneumonia. Papierok et al. (32) used the high-molecular-weight proteins also in an ELISA format. Both tests showed antibody increases between acute- and convalescent-phase sera, but the magnitudes of the titer changes were no greater than those seen in the CF test. These studies have been carried further: Jacobs et al. (19) have shown that two regions of the P1 peptide between leucine 801 and leucine 1139 contain reactive epitopes. Both regions show some homology with the sequence known for the cross-reacting 140-kDa antigen from *M. genitalium* (19). Not only does the 140-kDa protein of *M. genitalium* show homology with the P1 protein of *M. pneumoniae* (9), but *M. genitalium* also may be present in the respiratory tract (3). Despite these reservations, the developments indicate that serological assays using defined antigens are possible in diagnosis of *M. pneumoniae*. Purification of antigens will be required because *M. pneumoniae* shows a 62-kDa protein which binds the conjugate (42) and might be an immunoglobulin-binding protein, as appears to be the case for a 95- to 105-kDa protein in *M. hominis* (1).

Perspectives on the Serodiagnosis of *M. pneumoniae* Pneumonia

My current recommendation for serodiagnosis of *M. pneumoniae* pneumonia is the lipid CF test, since antigen is commercially available and the test has been well established. However, when antibody increases are seen in patients without pneumonia, the Western blot should be used as the confirmatory test. Regrettably, there is no commercial source for prepared strips. This solution is temporary because we should have better and more specific tests than the lipid CF test in the future. Such tests need to be evaluated against sera from patients from whom the organism has been isolated or detected by noncultural means in order to determine the sensitivities and specificities of these new assays, using a standard which is based on a different principle. The present practice of comparing new tests with the CF test as the only reference standard defeats the purpose of attempting to develop newer more specific tests, since the new test can be no better than the reference system. It must be remembered that the CF test does not show 100% sensitivity (22) (see above).

STATUS OF SEROLOGICAL TESTS FOR OTHER MYCOPLASMAS

The information concerning the other mycoplasmas is much less detailed than that for *M. pneumoniae* and *M. pulmonis* and is presented in summary form. A number of ELISAs using solubilized whole-organism antigens have been developed.

Human Genital Mycoplasmas

ELISAs for detection of human serum antibodies have been developed for both *M. hominis* and *U. urealyticum* (6, 7), using lysed whole organisms for the antigen. Persons positive by culture for *M. hominis* had a significantly greater positivity by ELISA, and 6 of 10 patients with postpartum fever of *M. hominis* etiology showed antibody increases (6). The ELISA for *U. urealyticum* showed small antibody changes with sera from males with nongonococcal urethritis of possible ureaplasmal etiology (7). The response appeared to be independent of serovar and similar to that seen by immunoblotting of sera from women with postpartum fever of ureaplasmal etiology (26).

Animal Mycoplasmas

Veterinary diagnostic problems differ from those related to diagnosis of humans in that the interest is in detection of infected animals and not in treatment, except for valuable animals. Consequently, low-cost serodiagnostic tests are needed to measure the prevalence of antibodies to veterinary pathogens. Evaluation of serodiagnostic tests for *M. hyopneumoniae* is complicated by the difficulties in isolation of the organism and by the finding that infected animals do not necessarily show lesions (30). Serology by the CF test correlated well by herd with disease in that herds which had animals with lesions also had the highest prevalence of antibody. In a comparison of tests for animals experimentally infected with *M. hyopneumoniae* (5), antibodies were found to persist longer when measured by ELISA than when measured by the CF test, which would be important in identifying infected herds. Western blotting showed that pigs respond as well to *M. hyopneumoniae* as humans do to *M. pneumoniae*. Western blotting also showed distinctive patterns in infected chickens for both *M. synoviae* and *M. gallisepticum* (2). Chickens consistently responded to six proteins of *M. gallisepticum* and two proteins of *M. synoviae* when infected with the homologous organism.

CONCLUSIONS

Serodiagnosis of mycoplasmal infections can be accomplished when colonization results in infection with resultant stimulation of the immune response, as is the case for *M. pneumoniae, M. pulmonis, M. gallisepticum,* and other invasive mycoplasmas. We presently do not know whether colonization of surface sites, such as the vagina, urethra, and oropharynx, with the opportunistic mycoplasmas gives rise to measurable antibody. When antibody is present, the most definitive serodiagnostic test is the Western immunoblot, which yields a specific pattern of protein antigen recognition.

In the evaluation of tests, the most important determination is the sensitivity and specificity of a serological test relative to a test or diagnostic method which is unrelated to the immune response. Such "gold standards" could include (i) individuals who are culture or probe positive and ill, (ii) experimentally infected animals, or (iii) animals with specific clinical or pathological evidence of disease.

Acknowledgments. I thank H. M. Foy for helpful criticism and F. D. Cartwright for preparation of data.

REFERENCES

1. **Alexander, A. G., H. R. Lowes, and G. E. Kenny.** 1991. Identification of a mycoplasmal protein which binds immunoglobulins nonimmunologically. *Infect. Immun.* **59:**2147–2151.
2. **Avakian, A. P., and S. H. Kleven.** 1990. The humoral immune response of chickens to *Mycoplasma gallisepticum* and *Mycoplasma synoviae* studied by immunoblotting. *Vet. Microbiol.* **24:**155–169.
3. **Baseman, J. B., S. F. Dallo, J. G. Tully, and D. L. Rose.** 1988. Isolation and characterization of *Mycoplasma genitalium* from the human respiratory tract. *J. Clin. Microbiol.* **26:**2266–2269.
4. **Beckman, B. L., and G. E. Kenny.** 1968. Immunochemical analysis of serologically active lipids of *Mycoplasma pneumoniae. J. Bacteriol.* **96:**1171–1180.
5. **Bereiter, M., T. F. Young, H. S. Joo, and R. F. Ross.** 1990. Evaluation of the ELISA and comparison to the complement fixation test and radial immunodiffusion enzyme assay for detection of antibodies against *Mycoplasma hyopneumoniae* in swine serum. *Vet. Microbiol.* **25:**177–192.
6. **Brown, M. B., G. H. Cassell, W. M. McCormack, and J. K. Davis.** 1987. Measurement of antibody to *Mycoplasma hominis* by an enzyme-linked immunoassay and detection of class-specific antibody response in women with postpartum fever. *Am. J. Obstet. Gynecol.* **156:**701–708.
7. **Brown, M. B., G. H. Cassell, D. Taylor-Robinson, and M. C. Shepard.** 1983. Measurement of antibody to *Ureaplasma urealyticum* by an enzyme-linked immunosorbent assay and detection of antibody responses in patients with nongonococcal urethritis. *J. Clin. Microbiol.* **17:**288–295.
8. **Cassell, G. H., J. R. Lindsey, J. K. Davis, M. K. Davidson, M. B. Brown, and J. G. Mayo.** 1981. Detection of natural *Mycoplasma pulmonis* infection in rats and mice by an enzyme linked immunosorbent assay (ELISA). *Lab. Anim. Sci.* **31:**676–682.
9. **Dallo, S. F., A. Chavoya, C.-J. Su, and J. B. Baseman.** 1989. DNA and protein sequence homology between the adhesins of *Mycoplasma genitalium* and *Mycoplasma pneumoniae. Infect. Immun.* **57:**1059–1065.
10. **Engvall, E., and P. Perlman.** 1972. Enzyme-linked immunosorbent assay, ELISA. III. Quantitation of specific antibodies by enzyme-linked anti-immunoglobulin in antigen-coated tubes. *J. Immunol.* **109:**129–135.
11. **Fernald, G. W., W. A. Clyde, and F. W. Denny.** 1967. Nature of the immune response to *Mycoplasma pneumoniae. J. Immunol.* **98:**1028–1038.
12. **Foy, H. M., G. E. Kenny, M. K. Cooney, and I. D. Allen.** 1979. Long-term epidemiology of infections with *Mycoplasma pneumoniae. J. Infect. Dis.* **139:**681–687.
13. **Gibbs, R. S., G. H. Cassell, J. K. Davis, and P. J. St. Clair.** 1986. Further studies on genital mycoplasma in intra-amniotic infection: blood cultures and serological response. *Am. J. Obstet. Gynecol.* **154:**717–724.
14. **Hers, J. F. P.** 1963. Fluorescent antibody technique in respiratory viral diseases. *Am. Rev. Respir. Dis.* **88:**316–338.
15. **Hu, P. C., R. M. Cole, Y. S. Huang, J. A. Graham, D. D. Gardner, A. M. Collier, and W. A. Clyde, Jr.** 1982. *Mycoplasma pneumoniae* infection: role of a surface protein in the attachment organelle. *Science* **216:**313–315.
16. **Hu, P. C., C. H. Huang, A. M. Collier, and W. A. Clyde, Jr.** 1982. Demonstration of antibodies to *Mycoplasma pneumoniae* attachment protein in human sera and respiratory secretions. *Infect. Immun.* **41:**437–439.
17. **Jacobs, E., A. Bennewitz, and W. Bredt.** 1986. Reaction pattern of human anti-*Mycoplasma pneumoniae* antibodies in enzyme-linked immunosorbent assays and immunoblotting. *J. Clin. Microbiol.* **23:**517–522.
18. **Jacobs, E., K. Fuchte, and W. Bredt.** 1986. A 168-kilodalton protein of *Mycoplasma pneumoniae* used as antigen in a dot enzyme-linked immunosorbent assay. *Eur. J. Clin. Microbiol.* **5:**435–440.
19. **Jacobs, E., A. Pilatschek, G. Gerstenecker, K. Oberle, and W. Bredt.** 1990. Immunodominant epitopes of the adhesin of *Mycoplasma pneumoniae. J. Clin. Microbiol.* **28:**1194–1197.
20. **Kenny, G. E., and C. L. Dunsmoor.** 1983. Principles, problems, and strategies in the use of antigenic mixtures for the enzyme-linked immunosorbent assay. *J. Clin. Microbiol.* **17:**655–665.
21. **Kenny, G. E., and J. T. Grayston.** 1965. Eaton pleuropneumonia-like organism (*Mycoplasma pneumoniae*) complement-fixing antigen: extraction with organic solvents. *J. Immunol.* **95:**19–25.
22. **Kenny, G. E., G. G. Kaiser, M. K. Cooney, and H. M. Foy.** 1990. Diagnosis of *Mycoplasma pneumoniae* pneumonia: sensitivities and specificities of serology with lipid antigen and isolation of the organism on soy peptone medium for identification of infections. *J. Clin. Microbiol.* **28:**2087–2093.
23. **Kenny, G. E., and R. M. Newton.** 1973. Close serological relationship between glycolipids of *Mycoplasma pneumoniae* and glycolipids of spinach. *Ann. N.Y. Acad. Sci.* **225:**54–61.
24. **Kleemola, M., and H. Kayhty.** 1982. Increase in titers of antibodies to *Mycoplasma pneumoniae* in patients with purulent meningitis. *J. Infect. Dis.* **146:**284–288.
25. **Kleemola, M., H. Kayhty, and R. Raty.** 1983. Reply. Presence of antibodies to *Mycoplasma pneumoniae* in patients with bacterial meningitis. *J. Infect. Dis.* **148:**363–365.
26. **Lee, G. Y., and G. E. Kenny.** 1987. Humoral immune response to polypeptides of *Ureaplasma urealyticum* in women with postpartum fever. *J. Clin. Microbiol.* **25:**1841–1844.
27. **Leith, D. K., L. B. Trevino, J. G. Tully, and J. B. Baseman.** 1983. Host discrimination of *Mycoplasma pneumoniae* proteinaceous immunogens. *J. Exp. Med.* **157:**502–514.
28. **Lin, J.-S., K. Radnay, M. I. Kendrick, B. Rosner, and E. H. Kass.** 1978. Serologic studies of human genital mycoplasmas: distribution of titers of mycoplasmacidal antibody to *Ureaplasma urealyticum* and *Mycoplasma hominis* in pregnant women. *J. Infect. Dis.* **137:**266–273.
29. **Lind, K., B. O. Lindhardt, H. J. Schutten, J. Blom, and C.**

Christiansen. 1984. Serological cross-reactions between *Mycoplasma genitalium* and *Mycoplasma pneumoniae*. *J. Clin. Microbiol.* **20:**1036–1043.

30. **McKean, J. D., J. J. Andrews, and D. O. Farrington.** 1979. Evaluation of diagnostic procedures for detection of mycoplasmal pneumonia of swine. *J. Am. Vet. Med. Assoc.* **174:**177–180.

31. **Mia, A. S., D. M. Kravcak, and G. H. Cassell.** 1981. Detection of *Mycoplasma pulmonis* antibody in rats and mice by a rapid micro enzyme linked immunosorbent assay. *Lab. Anim. Sci.* **31:**356–359.

32. **Papierok, G., C. Defives, A. Daunizeau, P. Wattré, and J.-C. Derieux.** 1988. Preparative electroelution of specific protein antigens from *Mycoplasma pneumoniae*: use in an enzyme-linked immunosorbent assay (ELISA). *Ann. Inst. Pasteur Microbiol.* **139:**589–603.

33. **Plackett, P., B. P. Marmion, E. J. Shaw, and R. M. Lemcke.** 1969. Immunochemical analysis of *Mycoplasma pneumoniae*. 3. Separation and chemical identification of serologically active lipids. *Aust. J. Exp. Biol. Med. Sci.* **47:**171–195.

34. **Schmidt, N. J., E. J. Lennette, J. Dennis, and P. S. Gee.** 1966. On the nature of complement-fixing antibodies to *Mycoplasma pneumoniae*. *J. Immunol.* **97:**95–99.

35. **Senterfit, L. B., and K. E. Jensen.** 1966. Antimetabolic antibodies to *Mycoplasma pneumoniae* measured by tetrazolium reduction inhibition. *Proc. Soc. Exp. Biol. Med.* **122:**786–790.

36. **Senterfit, L. B., J. D. Pollack, and N. L. Somerson.** 1972. Antibodies to *Mycoplasma pneumoniae*: correlation of complement fixation and tetrazolium reduction inhibition tests. *Proc. Soc. Exp. Biol. Med.* **140:**1294–1297.

37. **Sillis, M.** 1990. The limitation of IgM assays in the serological diagnosis of *Mycoplasma pneumoniae* infection. *J. Med. Microbiol.* **33:**253–258.

38. **Towbin, H., T. Staehelin, and J. Gordon.** 1989. Immunoblotting in the clinical laboratory. *J. Clin. Chem. Clin. Biochem.* **27:**495–501.

39. **van Griethuysen, A. J. A., R. de Graaf, J. A. M. van Druten, F. W. A. Heessen, J. T. M. van der Logt, and A. M. van Loon.** 1984. Use of the enzyme-linked immunosorbent assay for the early diagnosis of *Mycoplasma pneumoniae* infection. *Eur. J. Clin. Microbiol.* **3:**116–121.

40. **Vecchio, T. J.** 1966. Predictive value of a single diagnostic test in unselected populations. *N. Engl. J. Med.* **274:**1171–1173.

41. **Vikerfors, T., G. Brodin, M. Grandien, L. Hirschberg, A. Krook and C.-A. Petterson.** 1988. Detection of specific IgM antibodies for the diagnosis of *Mycoplasma pneumoniae*: a clinical evaluation. *Scand. J. Infect. Dis.* **20:**601–610.

42. **Vu, A. C., H. M. Foy, F. D. Cartwright, and G. E. Kenny.** 1987. The principal protein antigens of isolates of *Mycoplasma pneumoniae* as measured by levels of immunoglobulin G in human serum are stable in strains collected over a 10-year period. *Infect. Immun.* **55:**1830–1836.

43. **Wreghitt, T. G., and M. Sillis.** 1985. A μ-capture ELISA for detecting *Mycoplasma pneumoniae* IgM: comparison with indirect immunofluorescence and indirect ELISA. *J. Hyg.* (Cambridge) **94:**217–227.

31. Antibiotic Resistance

MARILYN C. ROBERTS

INTRODUCTION

Antibiotics are among the most valuable and most utilized therapeutic agents in medical practice and account for over 30% of the budgets of hospital pharmacies. The introduction of antibiotics into human medicine as well as for agricultural uses has led to the recognition of antibiotic-resistant bacteria (30, 43). Antibiotic resistance can arise as a result of gene mutation or the acquisition of new genetic material, or it can be innate to the species, genus, or family (30). All three types of antibiotic resistance have been found in mycoplasmas (8, 12, 37–39, 44, 45, 54, 56, 60, 61).

Mutation is the occurrence of a heritable change in the DNA of an organism, which can be transferred to daughter cells during active growth (30). Chromosomal mutation to antibiotic resistance has been recognized for over 40 years in bacteria and has also been documented in mycoplasmas (22, 30, 37, 38). The frequency with which chromosomal mutations occur varies over a wide range and differs from one antibiotic to another and from one species to another (30). However, it is only rarely transferred from one cell to another or from one species to another in nature (44). The level of drug resistance as a result of mutation is variable and depends on the kind of gene affected and the nature of the mutation (30). It is most often due to a DNA base substitution, although deletions or insertions can also cause mutations, and is generally rare under natural conditions.

Chromosomal drug resistance usually causes changes in existing cellular structures that either make the bacterial cell impermeable to one or more antibiotics or render specific target sites within the microorganism indifferent to the presence of the antibiotic (30). For most antibiotics, single mutations raise the level of resistance only moderately (two- to three-fold), although exceptions do exist. Selection for multiple mutations can be done in the laboratory by a stepwise process. The mutants obtained usually have higher antibiotic resistance to the antibiotic than do single-step mutants (22, 30).

In one study, mutation frequencies to streptomycin resistance were 10^{-4} for the arginine-utilizing mycoplasmas *Mycoplasma hominis* and *M. arginini* and 10^{-7} for *M. pneumoniae*, *M. gallisepticum*, and *Acholeplasma laidlawii* (22). Streptomycin resistance was found to be a single-step mutation which conferred high-level resistance. In contrast, resistance to aminoglycosides was found to be stepwise, with a frequency of 10^{-4} to 10^{-7} for each step. With stepwise selection, resistance to 10 mg/ml could be achieved for aminoglycosides. Similar findings have been reported for *M. mycoides* subsp. *mycoides*; single-step mutation rates of 10^{-8} to 10^{-9} were reported for streptomycin, spectinomycin, tylosin, erythromycin, and novobiocin (28). Single-step, high-level resistance (>100 µg/ml) to novobiocin, spectinomycin, or streptomycin was achieved in this strain, although high-level tetracycline mutants were not obtained even with multiple-step selection. In contrast, high-level tetracycline-resistant mutants could be produced in a stepwise fashion for *M. arginini* (22) and for bovine strains of mycoplasma (37, 38). Domeruth (8) reported mutation frequencies of 10^{-8} for high-level resistance to streptomycin and erythromycin in avian mycoplasmas, and Koostra et al. (27) found mutation frequencies of 10^{-7} to 10^{-9} for resistance to chloramphenicol, chlortetra-

Marilyn C. Roberts • Department of Pathobiology, SC-38, School of Public Health and Community Medicine, University of Washington, Seattle, Washington 98195.

513

cycline, and erythromycin in a number of mycoplasmas. Thus, the mollicutes have frequencies of mutation to resistance to a variety of antibiotics which are similar to those described for gram-negative and gram-positive bacteria for both one-step high-level resistance and stepwise resistance (30).

Acquisition of new genetic material, by either a plasmid or a transposon, has been recognized only recently in the mycoplasmas (5, 47, 49, 51), although it was first identified in bacteria in 1960 (30, 44). Plasmids are extrachromosomal elements that represent a reasonably stable but dispensable gene pool in bacteria. Many carry antibiotic resistance genes (30). Plasmids have been found in various mycoplasma and spiroplasma species (41); however, none have been shown to normally carry antibiotic resistance genes. Transposons are transposable elements which are defined genetic entities that are capable of inserting at many different sites in the chromosome or on plasmids. They often carry antibiotic resistance genes and carry one or more specific functions that act to mediate and regulate the transposition activity. Conjugative transposons have the additional ability to mediate their own transfer between cells and species by a conjugationlike process (7). Antibiotic resistance genes found on plasmids and transposons, in general, code for proteins that may enzymatically destroy the antibiotic, modify the antibiotic to an innocuous form, or interact with the cell envelope to make the cell envelope impermeable to the antibiotic (30, 44). There are exceptions, such as the Tet M determinant, which is the only naturally occurring antibiotic-resistant transposon that has been found in mycoplasmas. The *tetM* gene codes for a protein which binds to the ribosomes, protecting them from the action of tetracycline (34).

Innate antibiotic resistance is defined as resistance which is found in all members of a group (30). The mechanism of resistance in various mycoplasma species has not been well studied. However, innate resistance is usually due to the species' or group's basic physiological and biochemical makeup, which might either eliminate the target, reduce access to the target, or modify the target so that the antibiotic is no longer effective. Examples of some of these types of mechanisms have been found in various mycoplasmas. Differences in innate antibiotic susceptibility (Tables 1 to 3) have been used to isolate mycoplasmas from specimens and to separate different species from each other in the same sample (23, 41). The mollicutes, as a group, have been considered innately resistant to penicillins and cephalosporins because they lack cell walls and the peptidoglycans which are major structural components of the cell wall. Since these structures and corresponding enzymes (the penicillin-binding proteins) are missing in the mollicutes, there is no target for either the penicillins or cephalosporins to bind (42). Thus, since they lack the target, mycoplasmas are generally immune to the action of these agents. This is one of the unique characteristics found in the mollicutes. The resistance to β-lactams has been exploited for isolation of mycoplasmas from specimens which are contaminated with other bacteria (23).

More recently, Gadeau et al. (12) have examined rifampin susceptibility of *Spiroplasma* spp., *A. laidlawii*, and *M. mycoides* and found that they were 10- to 100-

Table 1. MICs of tetracycline for human mycoplasmas

	MIC (µg/ml) for:		
M. hominis	*M. pneumoniae*	*U. urealyticum*	Reference
>256	≤0.004–0.063	0.063–>256[a]	63
0.25–1	ND[b]	0.25–≥16[a]	62
0.2–0.8	1.6–3.2	0.2–0.8	32
0.2–3.1	ND	0.4–1.6	2
0.1–0.4	ND	0.1–1.6	6
ND	0.1–0.8	ND	61
ND	0.06–0.4	ND	19
0.5–>128	0.25–1	0.5–>128[a]	67
ND	0.1–12.8	ND	36
0.25–>32[a]	ND	0.25–1	51

[a] The large spread of tetracycline resistances in these studies is most likely due to a bimodal distribution of sensitive and resistant strains for *M. hominis* and *U. urealyticum*. All strains in our laboratory with MICs of >10 µg/ml carry the Tet M determinant (44, 47, 48).
[b] ND, not determined.

fold more resistant to rifampin than was an *Escherichia coli* control. Rifampin inhibits eubacteria by combining with RNA polymerase and preventing initiation of RNA synthesis. The authors demonstrated that spiroplasmal RNA polymerases were nonsusceptible to concentrations of rifampin 1,000 times higher than those inhibiting the *E. coli* RNA polymerase and suggested that the β subunit of the spiroplasmal enzyme has a low affinity for binding rifampin. Others have shown that ureaplasmas are also nonsusceptible to rifampin, which suggests that this characteristic is widely distributed among the mycoplasmas and may be a general property of the mollicutes, similar to the nonsusceptibility seen with penicillins and cephalosporins.

Erythromycin is another antibiotic to which many mycoplasma species are uniquely resistant (52). Exceptions include *M. pneumoniae* and *Ureaplasma urealyticum* (31, 51, 55, 59, 61, 67). In contrast, many mycoplasma species are susceptible to lincomycin, whereas *U. urealyticum* is innately resistant to 20 to 30 µg/ml (2, 31, 67, 68). Other examples of innate resistance are discussed below.

CLASSES OF ANTIBIOTICS

Tetracyclines

Tetracycline and the related compounds minocycline and doxycycline bind to ribosomes, preventing their proper function (30). Antibiotics in this group are among the few that are effective against virtually all species of mollicutes. Tetracycline is a broad-spectrum antibiotic with relatively low toxicity and few side effects. However, it is not used in young children or during pregnancy. Recent evidence indicates that tetracycline binds to the S7 protein of the 30S subunit of the ribosome and prevents the binding of the aminoacyl-tRNA to the ribosome acceptor site (54), resulting in blocking of protein production. In general, tetracyclines are considered bacteristatic, and this property seems to apply for the mollicutes as well.

In nature, high-level resistance to tetracycline is rarely due to chromosomal mutations. However, as

Table 2. MICs of other antibiotics[a]

Antibiotic	MIC (µg/ml) for:			Reference
	M. hominis	M. pneumoniae	U. urealyticum	
Erythromycin	>100	0.8–1.6	0.4–0.8	32
	>128	≤0.06–8	8->128	67
	500–1,000	ND[b]	6.2–25	2
	ND	0.002–400	ND	36
	>64	ND	0.25–1	51
	ND	0.6–4.8	ND	55
Chloramphenicol	12.8–25.6	ND	12.8–25.6	32
	0.5–0.8	ND	0.4–3.1	1
	<0.2–0.8	ND	0.4–3.1	6
	ND	0.8–4.8	ND	19
	ND	1.6–6.4	ND	61
	ND	1.6–12.8	ND	36
Streptomycin	12.5–200	ND	0.8–3.1	2
	ND	0.2–0.4	ND	19
	ND	0.1–1.2	ND	61
	12.5–50	ND	0.8–12.5	6
	ND	1->100	ND	36
Spectinomycin	<0.3–10	ND	<0.3–10	14
	1->128	0.25–2	4–128	67
	ND	ND	2->16	25
	ND	0.6–4.8	ND	55
Lincomycin	0.2–0.4	40	20–80	32
	0.5–16	2–32	64->128	67
	1.6–6.2	ND	100->1,000	2
	0.5–16	2–32	64->128	67
Clindamycin	0.06–0.25	ND	1–32	18
	≤0.06–2	0.5–4	2->128	67
	0.2–3.1	ND	25–50	2
Gentamicin	3.2–6.4	3.2–6.4	ND	32
	6.2–25	ND	3.1–25	2
	0.8–3.1	ND	0.4–12.5	6
	ND	0.4–0.8	ND	19
Ciprofloxacin	0.5–1.0	ND	2–64	26
	0.25–0	ND	0.5–2.0	41
	0.5–1	ND	1–4	62
	0.5–8	2–8	2–16	67
Difloxacin	2–32	1–8	4->256	63
	0.25–1	ND	0.5–2.0	26
	0.25–1	ND	0.5–1	62
Nalidixic acid	≥256	ND	64–256	26
	>128	32–128	ND	67
	ND	ND	2–128	2

[a] The large spread of MICs between laboratories can best be explained as lack of standard antibiotic susceptibility testing conditions. The large spread of MICs within one study may be due to some resistant organisms in the study but is more likely due to nonreproducibility under the assay conditions used.
[b] ND, not determined.

stated above, in some species of mycoplasmas, stepwise mutations to high-level tetracycline resistance can be selected under laboratory conditions (22). These mutations may either reduce the ability of the tetracycline to enter the cell or modify the ribosomes so they have a reduced binding affinity for tetracycline. Both types of mechanisms have been identified in other bacterial species, although the specific changes in the stepwise tetracycline resistance of mycoplasmas have not been characterized.

More recently, high-level tetracycline resistance (MICs of ≥10 µg/ml) in strains of M. hominis and U. urealyticum has been associated with the presence of the Tet M determinant (4, 5, 10, 43, 46, 47, 49). This determinant is often associated with a conjugative

transposon and has a wide host range among urogenital bacteria of human origin (44, 46). The Tet M determinant codes for production of a protein which binds to ribosomes, making them resistant to tetracycline both in vivo and in vitro. This determinant has been cloned and sequenced from a U. urealyticum strain and shown to be 95% related, at both the DNA and the predicted amino acid sequence levels, to previously characterized determinants isolated from the genus Streptococcus (53). The amino acid sequence of the Tet M determinant has been shown to be related to various characterized elongation factors, and two proposed mechanisms of resistance have been proposed (54). The tetM gene product could bind to the ribosome, preventing tetracycline binding to the S7 pro-

Table 3. MICs for animal mycoplasmas

Antibiotic	MIC (µg/ml) for:			Reference
	M. hyopneumoniae	*M. hyosynoviae*	*M. gallisepticum*	
Tetracycline	ND[a]	ND	0.8–0.16	64
	1.0–8.2	ND	ND	65
	4–16	0.25–4	0.13–1	67
Erythromycin	ND	ND	0.02–80[b]	64
	1.2–9.2	ND	ND	65
	ND	>128	≥0.06	67
Spectinomycin	ND	ND	1–20	16
	ND	ND	1.25–2.5	64
	ND	ND	1.56–6.25	68
	16	16	8–16	67
Lincomycin	ND	ND	1–10	16
	ND	ND	1.25–40	64
	0.06–0.1	ND	ND	65
	ND	0.39–1.56	ND	68
	8	8	32	67
Tylosin	0.05–0.1	0.05–5	ND	17
	ND	ND	0.02–>2.5	64
	ND	0.045–6.25	ND	68
	4	≤0.06	0.06–0.13	67
Tiamulin	0.025–0.05	0.05–0.01	ND	17
	ND	ND	0.005–0.8	64
Gentamicin	0.25–0.5	0.25–0.5	ND	17
	>50	ND	ND	65
	ND	0.78–6.25	ND	68
Ciprofloxacin	0.005–0.01	0.5–1	ND	17
	ND	1	1	67
Rifampin	1.6–3.1	ND	ND	65
	32	128	ND	67

[a] ND, not determined.
[b] Represents both susceptible and resistant strains showing a bimodal distribution of resistance to erythromycin (64).

tein but permitting productive binding of the aminoacyl-tRNA, or it could act as a tetracycline-resistant elongation factor.

The Tet M determinant has been transferred by conjugation and transformation to various species of mycoplasmas and acholeplasmas, in which it is found integrated into the chromosome and confers tetracycline resistance to the transformants and transconjugants (9, 31, 48). This determinant has been found in *M. hominis* and *U. urealyticum* strains from North America, Africa, Europe, and more recently Asia, suggesting that it is widely distributed among these populations. It is the only naturally acquired antibiotic resistance determinant that has been found in clinical strains of the mollicutes. The Tet M determinant has recently been used as part of cloning vectors to transform DNA back into mycoplasmas (31).

MLS Group

The most commonly used members of the macrolide-lincosamide-streptogramin B (MLS) family of antibiotics are clindamycin, erythromycin, lincosamides, spiramycin, streptogramin B, and tylosin (11, 30). They are most active on gram-positive bacteria and mycoplasmas and are generally bacteristatic, although some may be bactericidal at very high concentrations. Resistance to one antibiotic does not always

mean resistance to all antibiotics within the MLS group (33, 40). This is especially true for the mollicutes. It is known that *M. hominis* as well as many other mycoplasmas are resistant to erythromycin but susceptible to lincomycin, whereas the reverse is true of *U. urealyticum* (61).

The antibiotics are closely related in their modes of action and appear to share a common or overlapping binding site in the ribosomes (3, 15). The antimicrobial action of this group is not entirely clear but is believed to be linked to the ability of the MLS antibiotics to inhibit protein synthesis at the ribosomal level by binding to the 50S subunit. After an antibiotic binds, it appears to prevent the shift of the peptidyl-tRNA from the acceptor site back to the donor site on the ribosome during peptide synthesis, blocking protein production (15). Other data suggest that the macrolides act to break up the mRNA-bound 70S ribosomal complex and allow degradation of the 50S subunit.

Naturally occurring MLS-resistant strains of mycoplasmas have been described for a variety of species, including *M. pneumoniae* and *U. urealyticum* (2, 35, 37, 67). Four different mechanisms of resistance have been suggested for bacteria: (i) lack of entrance into the cell, (ii) chemical inactivation of the MLS antibiotic, (iii) lack of binding to the ribosomal target, and (iv) lack of an inhibitory response upon binding to the ribosome target. There is controversy over whether lack of drug accumulation is a viable option; some studies support this view, while others do not (15). There is well-documented evidence that degradation of macrolides by plasmid-coded esterases or enzymes which phosphorylate the drug renders the drug inactive and causes drug resistance (mechanism ii) (15). Lack of an inhibitory response to binding has also been documented for some gram-negative species (mechanism iv). The best-characterized resistance mechanism to MLS antibiotics is due to the dimethylation of the 23S rRNA by a specific methylase, making the binding site on the altered 50S ribosomal subunit no longer accessible (mechanism iii). This class of enzyme is widely distributed among gram-positive bacteria and has recently been found in strains of enteric bacteria as well. The mechanism of resistance in the MLS-resistant mycoplasmas has not been extensively studied. Nevertheless, macrolide-resistant *U. urealyticum* isolates have been shown to have a sixfold reduction in intracellular macrolide influx and accumulation and a reduction in antibiotic binding to the ribosomes compared with a susceptible strain (37). In addition, the most widespread MLS resistance mechanism described for bacteria is due to the acquisition of new genes which are often associated with conjugative transposons and can be found with the Tet M determinant (7). The possibility that these genes exist in the mollicutes or could be introduced into the group should be examined.

Quinolones

Fluoroquinolones are potent synthetic agents. Intense development has produced a large family of newer compounds that are active against a broad range of bacteria, including mycoplasmas. These drugs may be the treatment of choice for many mycoplasma diseases, in both humans and animals, in the future. Derivatives of these antibiotics may also be useful for treating tissue cultures (35). The primary target of nalidixic acid, as well as the newer fluoroquinolones, is DNA gyrase (67). These drugs appear to antagonize the A subunit of the gyrase and thus block DNA replication. Purified DNA gyrase has a variety of activities and is required for DNA replication and certain aspects of transcription, DNA repair, recombination, and transposition (67). The quinolones characteristically kill bacteria rapidly. However, at high concentrations, decreased killing is seen with some bacterial species, including mycoplasmas. Spontaneous mutations to high-level nalidixic acid resistance are relatively common in many bacterial species and are due to changes in the DNA gyrase subunit at a frequency of 10^{-6} to 10^{-8} (67). However, many mycoplasma species are innately resistant to nalidixic acid (26). Mutations can produce cross-resistance to a variety of fluoroquinolones, although, as with the MLS antibiotics, not all mutations confer resistance to all members of the fluoroquinolone family (67). High-level single-step mutations conferring resistance to some of the fluoroquinolones do occur (67), but for most species, selection of high-level resistance requires serial passage in the presence of increasing drug concentrations (24, 67). All resistance found to date has been located on the bacterial chromosome, and neither plasmid-encoded resistance nor transferable resistance in clinical strains has been described (67).

Various mycoplasma species differ in susceptibility to different members of the fluoroquinolone family, with nalidixic acid and cinoxacin MICs ranging from 64 to 256 µg/ml for all *M. hominis* and *U. urealyticum* strains examined (26), suggesting innate resistance to these compounds at least in these two species.

The susceptibilities of *M. hominis* and *U. urealyticum* to the newer quinolones are similar to the susceptibilities of gram-positive organisms such as streptococci (26, 67). Both the streptococci and mycoplasmas are 5- to 10-fold less susceptible than gram-negative enteric organisms to the fluoroquinolones, but the level of susceptibility depends on the species and the quinolone tested. The data that are accumulating suggest that not all species of mycoplasmas react to quinolones in the same way, nor do all quinolones have identical biochemical properties (24a, 26, 67). Thus, as new quinolones are produced, each will have to be tested on a bank of organisms to determine its MIC for each species.

Aminoglycosides

The aminoglycoside antibiotics constitute a large group of compounds, the majority of which are produced by actinomycetes of the genus *Streptomyces* (30). The most commonly used members of the group for treatment of disease include kanamycin, gentamicin, tobramycin, and amikacin. The aminoglycosides are relatively stable over a wide pH and temperature range; because of their potential toxicity, they are primarily used to treat serious infections caused by gram-negative organisms. Although these drugs are not routinely used for treatment of human mycoplasma disease, they have been used to prevent and eliminate mycoplasma contamination in tissue cultures (13, 22).

Ribosomes have been identified as the primary targets for the action of aminoglycosides; some antibiotics bind to the 30S subunit, and others bind to both the 30S and 50S subunits (30). In addition, a number of different and apparently unrelated physiological effects are seen with these drugs (30). Mutational resistance to aminoglycosides has been described for various mycoplasma species and can be a multistep or high-level single-step type of resistance (22, 28). Resistant mutations in the ribosomes are found in other bacterial species, and presumably occur in mycoplasmas as well, and account for the resistance seen.

The most common type of aminoglycoside resistance in other bacterial species is due to the presence of new genes which enzymatically modify the antibiotics (30). Three types of enzymes have been found in both gram-positive and gram-negative bacteria: acetyltransferases, phosphotransferases, and nucleotidyltransferases (30). Some of the gram-positive enzymes are associated with conjugative transposons and thus are able to be transferred by conjugation to other species (7, 44). To date, none of these enzymes has been found to occur naturally in mycoplasmas, but one transposon encoding gentamicin resistance has been introduced by transformation into mycoplasma strains, in which it is expressed (31). Some of these genes are found in large conjugative transposons which usually include the Tet M determinant, and thus the potential exists for transfer by conjugation. Thus, if these genes can be introduced into mycoplasmas, they probably would be stable and confer antibiotic resistance to aminoglycosides. Therefore, one could hypothesize that at some time in the future, it is likely that these enzymes will become established in various mycoplasma species.

Chloramphenicol

Chloramphenicol is not generally used for treatment of mycoplasma disease because of its potential toxicity, but it has been used to treat tissue cultures (22). This antibiotic inhibits bacterial protein synthesis by binding to the 50S subunit of the ribosome and inhibiting the peptidyltransferase step (30). Some strains have been found to have nonenzymatic resistance to chloramphenicol due to prevention of antibiotic entry into the cell, but most resistance in both gram-positive and gram-negative species is due to the acquisition of chloramphenicol acetyltransferases, which modify the drug to an inactive form (44).

In general, mycoplasmas are more resistant to chloramphenicol than are gram-negative bacteria but have resistance levels similar to those found in some gram-positive cocci such as *Staphylococcus aureus* and *Enterococcus faecalis*. Selection for stepwise resistance can be done in mycoplasmas and most likely represents changes in the ribosomes or permeability, similar to that found for mutations in other bacterial species (30).

ANTIBIOTIC SUSCEPTIBILITY TESTING

As antibiotic-resistant strains of mycoplasma have appeared and become more common, antibiotic susceptibility testing of mycoplasmas has become more important. In addition, a number of new antibiotics have appeared in the last few years, and their action against mycoplasmas can be assayed only by antibiotic susceptibility testing. As a result, the need for testing mycoplasmas has increased. A number of factors influence the results of antibiotic testing: the culture medium and its components, incubation conditions, and the inocula (30, 67). Standard conditions should be defined and used so that susceptibility test results are reproducible from one experiment to another and from one laboratory to another. Unfortunately, standard conditions for antibiotic susceptibility testing of mycoplasmas do not exist, and it is apparent that the media, number of organisms used in the inocula, and length of incubation time vary among laboratories (1, 6, 18, 19, 25, 26, 29, 32, 36, 43, 50, 56, 57). As a result, comparison of data from different laboratories is often difficult or impossible, as Tables 1 to 3 indicate. Two major types of testing have been done for both bacteria and mycoplasmas: the agar dilution and broth dilution tests (30). Agar dilution testing is more commonly used for bacteria, while broth testing has generally been used for mycoplasmas (50, 57). The mollicutes tend to grow more slowly than bacteria, and this property can complicate interpretation of the end point of the susceptibility test due to inactivation of labile antibiotics. This can be a problem with both agar and broth tests. The agar dilution test

should be used whenever possible, and a standard format should be adopted by all laboratories interested in doing antibiotic susceptibility testing.

Agar Dilution Test

The agar dilution test is the standard bacteriologic test used to determine the MIC of an antibiotic (30). The basic method involves incorporation of the antibiotic into liquefied agar or agarose medium, which is then mixed, poured into petri plates, and allowed to solidify. A series of plates containing increasing concentrations of the antibiotic is prepared. A standardized inoculum is used; with the aid of a multiple-inoculum replicator, different strains are spotted onto each plate. After incubation, the MIC end point is read as the lowest concentration which completely inhibits growth. A single colony or a faint haze of growth is disregarded (30). Standard agar dilution methods have four major advantages over broth dilution methods for bacteria. The use of an inoculum replicating apparatus allows for large numbers of strains to be tested at the same time. Microbial heterogeneity, including a mixture of susceptible and resistant organisms, or a spontaneous resistant mutant can be readily detected by observing the bacterial growth on the agar surface. This is not possible in a broth test. The medium may be supplemented with a variety of products to permit testing of nutritionally fastidious microorganisms that cannot be tested satisfactorily in a clear broth medium. The standard procedure may be modified in a number of ways to permit testing of particular microorganisms and is quite acceptable as long as appropriate controls are included to demonstrate that the modification does not affect the end result. Agar dilution MICs tend to be lower than broth dilution MICs because in broth dilution tests, a single surviving CFU can grow to produce visible turbidity. This single CFU may be resistant as a result of acquisition of new genetic material, by a mutation, or may represent a true mixture of resistant and susceptible cells (30), although growth also depends on the antibiotic being tested (66). Differences between the agar and broth dilution tests may vary with different microorganisms and antibiotic combinations (30).

Because of the advantages of the agar dilution test, we have adapted this test for mycoplasma antibiotic susceptibility testing (24–26). *M. hominis* was used as the model system for mycoplasmas. As a result, when other species of mycoplasmas are used, the medium, agar plates, and incubation times need to be varied to accommodate the different physiological characteristics of the organisms.

The basic method for mycoplasmas and ureaplasmas is as follows. The broth medium used for growth is soy peptone fresh yeast dialysate broth (20) supplemented with 20% agamma horse serum, 0.001% phenol red, and 200 U of penicillin per ml. For *U. urealyticum*, the dialysate broth is supplemented with 5 mM urea, 10 mM MES [2-(N-morpholino)-ethanesulfonic acid], 10% agamma horse serum, 1 mM Na_2SO_3 (freshly prepared), 0.001% phenol red, and 200 U of penicillin per ml. The final pH of the broth medium is 7.0 to 7.3 for *M. hominis* and 6.0 to 6.3 for *U. urealyticum* (23, 25, 26). The agar medium used for antibiotic susceptibility testing for *M. hominis* is H agar. The H-agar base contains (per liter of water) 20 g of soy peptone (HySoy, Sheffield Chemical Co., Norwich, N.Y.), 5 g of NaCl, 10 g of agarose, and 2 ml of a 1% phenol red solution. The pH is adjusted to 7.3. The complete H-agar medium contains 70 ml of agar base, 10 ml of fresh yeast dialysate, 20 ml of horse serum, and 200 μg of penicillin per ml. The final pH of the agar medium, incubated in 5% CO_2 in air at 37°C, is 6.8 to 7.0; however, no significant difference in end points is seen when the pH varies between 6.8 and 7.3. For testing susceptibilities of ureaplasmas, U agar is used. U-agar base contains 4.25 g of MES (acid form), 12 g of agarose, and 2 ml of 1% phenol red (21). The pH is adjusted to between 5.8 and 6.0. The complete medium contains 70 ml of U-agar base, 10 ml of fresh yeast extract dialysate, 3 mM urea (0.3 ml of filter-sterilized 1 M urea per 100 ml of agar medium), 200 U of penicillin per ml, and 20% whole horse serum. The final pH of the U agar is 6.0 to 6.1 when incubated at 37°C in an atmosphere of 5% CO_2 in air. Complete agar medium (25 ml) is poured into 100-mm^2 plastic petri dishes, which results in an agar thickness of 2.5 mm. Plates are held in the dark at room temperature for 48 h to allow evaporation of excess surface moisture so that inocula are readily imbibed by the agar (25, 26).

Preparation of the inocula is the most difficult part of the procedure. The use of patient material such as urine is not suitable for antibiotic susceptibility testing inocula because the concentration of mycoplasmas in urine can range from 10^1 to 10^8 CFU. It is also important that the organisms to be tested are in the logarithmic growth phase. To achieve this, we have found that the following procedure works well. For mycoplasmas, stock frozen cultures (known to be viable at high plate counts) are thawed at room temperature, diluted 1:100 in fresh medium, and incubated for 24 h at 37°C. The tube is then subcultured at a 1:100 dilution into a new broth tube. The two tubes are incubated for an additional 24 h. If the initial tube shows a haze or a slight alkaline pH shift after 24 h, the subculture is used for the inocula. If no reaction is observed, samples from both tubes are mixed and used (26). For ureaplasmas, the frozen stock culture is inoculated into ureaplasmal broth at 1:100 dilution. Eighteen hours later, a sample from the culture is serially diluted 1:100 and 1:10,000 into two new tubes of medium. These three tubes are incubated for 24 h, and the highest dilution which has a color change from yellow to pink is used for the inocula (25, 26). For testing of susceptibilities, serial 10-fold dilutions of the organisms are prepared in dialysate broth supplemented with 2% horse serum. For mycoplasmas, samples of the 10^{-2} and 10^{-3} dilutions are placed into the wells of a Steers replicator and plated onto the H-agar surface (0.025 ml per spot). Cultures are incubated in 5% CO_2 in air. On days 3, 4, and 5, the colonies are counted. For ureaplasmas, serial 10-fold dilutions are plated onto U agar. Colonies are stained on days 3 and 4 by spraying the plates with a calcium chloride-urea stain. For *M. pneumoniae*, plates are sealed with Parafilm and examined weekly for 3 weeks. All plates are viewed with a stereoscopic dissecting microscope at a magnification of ×40. The MIC is the concentration of antibiotic which completely prevents colony formation in spots known to contain 30 to 300 CFU, as judged by control plates which have no antibiotic. The MIC_{50} is the concentration of antibiotic which prevents colony formation of 50% of the strains tested, and the MIC_{90} is the concentration which prevents growth of 90% of the strains tested (30).

The agar dilution test eliminates the carryover effect whereby large inocula of ureaplasmas cause a color change in the broth medium whether or not the organisms are alive (25, 26). The only way to control for this effect is by using small inocula. Considerable care in determining the inoculum size is required because the minute colonies which form at high concentrations of ureaplasmas are nearly invisible and stain poorly with the calcium chloride-urea stain. In addition to the crowding effect, ureaplasmal colonies decrease in size and stainability as the amount of antibiotic increases, even though the MIC has not been reached.

The agarose medium recommended for the ureaplasmas is designed to give maximal colony size by virtue of its optimal concentration of 3 mM urea and high buffer capacity. This medium will also support growth of *M. hominis*. Thus, one medium can be used for susceptibility testing of both species, and the susceptibility of mixed cultures of ureaplasmas and mycoplasmas can also be assessed provided that sufficient ureaplasmas are present in the mixture and the mycoplasmas make colonies within 4 days. Therefore, unless it is known that the isolate is a pure culture of ureaplasmas, the agar plates should be stained to identify ureaplasmas specifically, since colonies of *M. hominis* under partial inhibition by antibiotics may appear to be as small as ureaplasmal colonies. The inclusion of phenol red in the medium permits colorimetric determination of the urease activity, which is particularly important when colonies are small and not stainable with the calcium chloride-urea stain. The pink color of the stain develops 2 to 24 h after the stain has been added. In contrast, without additional urea, only a faint pH change is seen. With most antibiotics, the shelf life of the medium is about 7 days at 4°C.

An alternative agar dilution technique has been developed for *M. pneumoniae* and *M. hominis* (1). In this assay, Hayflick's modified agar medium supplemented with 20% horse serum, pH 7.6, and containing serial dilutions of the antibiotics was used. These media were inoculated with 10^4 to 10^5 color-changing units and incubated in the presence of 5% CO_2 for 1 to 2 days for *M. hominis* and 4 days for *M. pneumoniae*. The end point was read as the lowest antibiotic concentration for which no colonies could be detected on that agar at the time when visible growth could be seen on the control plate containing no antibiotic.

Broth Dilution Tests

Broth dilution tests are usually preferred for studying the bactericidal activity of antimicrobial agents because subcultures can be made easily at different time intervals (30). In broth dilution tests, the lowest concentration of antibiotic which prevents visible growth after 18 to 24 h of incubation is defined as the MIC for bacteria. For mycoplasmas, this definition has been modified to the lowest dilution which prevents a color change in the media (1, 50, 57). For ureaplasmas, the broth dilution method determines an alkaline shift in pH due to hydrolysis of urea and is thus a metabolic inhibition test. If a mixture of susceptible and resistant cells is tested, the sample will appear resistant. Therefore, for the broth dilution test, clones of the isolates need to be prepared for broth testing, whereas uncloned isolates can be tested by agar dilution. In addition, the presence of resistant mutants in the inoculum will be read as resistant. Both macro- and microdilution tests have been used.

The standard macrodilution test for bacteria as described by Lorian (30) is as follows. The test is done in sterile capped tubes (13 by 100 mm). Twofold dilutions of the antibiotic are prepared, using separate pipettes to make the antibiotic dilutions. One tube has no antibiotics and is the control. The standard inoculum is a log-phase culture which has approximately 5×10^5 CFU/ml. All tubes are inoculated with equal volumes of the bacterial suspension, mixed, and incubated for 16 to 18 h at 36°C in an aerobic incubator. The broth used for the test depends on the organisms to be tested, and cation supplementation to 50 mg of Ca^{2+} per liter and 25 mg of Mg^{2+} per liter is indicated, especially for aminoglycoside testing. To modify this protocol for mycoplasmas, the broth medium needs to support the growth of mycoplasmas and provide a color end point rather than a measure of turbidity, and the time of incubation needs to be adjusted for the particular species to be tested. The inoculum can be prepared as described above for the agar dilution test, since this procedure will produce at least some cells in log phase.

The standard microtiter broth dilution antibiotic susceptibility test as described by Lorian (30) is as follows. Broth medium supplemented with Ca^{2+} and Mg^{2+} is used. Each antibiotic solution is made and dispensed into a 96-well tray, which can then be sealed and stored at $-20°C$ or below for up to 2 weeks. Log-phase cells are grown, and an inoculum of 1×10^4 to 5×10^4 CFU is added to each well. The trays are sealed and incubated as described above for the macrodilution test.

Senterfit has modified the microdilution test for mycoplasmas by using between 10^3 and 10^4 CFU (57). However, the organisms are grown for just a few hours, which for most species of mycoplasma is not long enough to put them in log phase. Therefore, the inoculum should be prepared as described for the agar dilution test. The same broth media can be used both for the broth dilution test and for growth of the inoculum for the agar and broth dilution tests. Both the macro- and microdilution tests can be incubated at 35°C and read after 24 h for many mycoplasma and ureaplasma strains, while 5 to 7 days is needed for *M. pneumoniae*. Larger numbers of organisms seem to be required for testing mycoplasmas and spiroplasmas isolated from plant sources. Liao and Chen (29) found that 10^6 CFU was useful for testing these organisms.

Bébéar et al. have developed a broth microdilution technique for use with *U. urealyticum* (1). The method uses Shepard liquid medium (58) containing antibiotic dilutions, which are inoculated with ureaplasmas to yield approximately 5×10^3 to 5×10^4 color-changing units in 0.2 ml and incubated in the presence of 5% CO_2. The inoculum is prepared by growing the strains for 18 h in Shepard medium without antibiotics to a final density of 10^6 to 10^7 color-changing units

per ml. Shepard medium includes tryptic soy broth (2.4%), horse serum (20%), urea (0.08%), cysteine HCl (0.01%), yeast extract (2%), and phenol red (0.002%), pH 6 (59). The initial MIC is read as the lowest antibiotic concentration inhibiting color change at the time when the indicator in the control well, without antibiotic, just changes color, usually after 1 day. Final MIC is the lowest concentration without color change that remains stable after 48 h of incubation.

Mycoplasmacidal Tests (Killing Curves)

Killing curve techniques measure the bactericidal activity of the antibiotic being tested, thus providing a dynamic picture of antimicrobial action and interaction over time, based on serial colony counts. However, the repetitive colony counts that are required are tedious to perform and limit the number of antimicrobial concentrations that can be tested with any isolate (30). As a result, the concentrations to be tested must represent concentrations which are achievable at the presumed site of the infection. With many antibiotics and organisms, an increasing proportion of the inoculum is killed as the concentration is increased. However, subpopulations surviving are a problem, because a portion of the inoculum may remain viable and survive to grow out if the cells are subcultured by removal from the antibiotic-containing media. Thus, the definition of MBC for bacteria according to Lorian (30) is the minimum concentration of antibiotic which allows survival of no more than a statistically arbitrary minimum proportion of a defined inoculum with incubation under defined conditions. Most laboratories have used a standard end point for assay as the achievement of 3 log_{10} units or 99.9% killing of the original inoculum. However, end points of 99.9% killing are dependent on the inoculum density plus the statistical variability of the procedures (30).

For bacteria, most methods use a final inoculum of 10^5 to 10^6 CFU/ml, which is produced by diluting an overnight culture. This protocol needs some modification for mycoplasmas (58). The initial sampling for colony counts should take place as soon as the inoculum is added. A control tube with the strain but no antibiotic is prepared at the same time for comparison.

It may be necessary to inactivate or greatly dilute the broth with the antibiotic in it to obtain accurate colony counts for particularly susceptible organisms. After incubation at 35 to 37°C, colony counts can be determined. This technique can be used to examine the interaction of two different antimicrobial agents combined in a single plate (30). For adaptation to mycoplasmas, the broth and solid media described for the agar dilution test can be used, and the inocula are handled as described above. When mycoplasmas and especially ureaplasmas are used, the rapid rate of loss of viability under nonantibiotic conditions must be taken into account, since a culture of ureaplasmas becomes nonviable after 24 h of growth in normal broth media (25, 26). The loss of viability may be delayed in the presence of antibiotics, which makes the time course of the experiment important to the interpretation of the results. The length of time for which killing experiments need to be run has not been well characterized and will differ for different species and antibiotic combinations. Relatively few killing curves for mycoplasmas have been reported, and a systematic examination of this technique with a number of species and antibiotics is required. If very long experiments are done, the colony count may fall below detectable limits and regrowth may be seen (67). Regrowth of the culture may be due to survival of a single antibiotic-resistant mutant cell, which over time will grow to detectable levels. This phenomenon is commonly found at high concentrations of quinolones, and the surviving bacteria are not resistant to the drug (67), suggesting that the observation is a characteristic of the antibiotic (30).

With the use of killing curves, antibiotics can be evaluated and the tentative cidal nature of the drug with different species of mycoplasmas can be determined. This information can then be used to evaluate new antibiotics or combinations of drugs.

MIC

A large number of susceptibility studies have been done with the human mycoplasmas *M. hominis*, *M. pneumoniae*, and *U. urealyticum*. To illustrate the problem in comparing susceptibility testing from different laboratories, MIC values for these three organisms have been compiled from some of the published studies (Table 1 and 2). The studies used either agar or broth dilution. In Table 1, the wide range of tetracycline MICs seen with many of the *M. hominis* and *U. urealyticum* isolates can be explained as attributable to a bimodal distribution of MICs due to populations of susceptible organisms (MIC of <10 μg/ml) and resistant strains (MIC of >10 μg/ml) (45, 48). All resistant strains that we and others have tested owe their resistance to the presence of the Tet M determinant (5, 47, 49, 51). Therefore, the strains listed in Table 1 with a wide range of tetracycline MICs probably represent the testing of a mixture of susceptible and resistant strains.

Similarly, the wide range of MICs found for erythromycin resistance may also be due to a mixture of susceptible and resistant strains, since resistant strains have been described for both *M. pneumoniae* and *U. urealyticum* (25, 37). This may also be true for lincomycin and *M. hominis*, since lincomycin resistance has been found in clinical gram-positive isolates (40).

In contrast, the wide range of MICs found with chloramphenicol, spectinomycin, and gentamicin is not so easily explained and is most likely due to variations from one laboratory to another in how the test was performed, the media that were used, and when the test was read. Tables 2 and 3 illustrate the need for a uniform assay to allow easy comparisons between different studies. The large spread of MICs within one study may be due to testing of a mixture of resistant and susceptible organisms. This is more likely for antibiotics for which resistant mutants arise easily in the laboratory, such as streptomycin (22), or with antibiotics for which resistant strains have been isolated. Nevertheless, it is also possible that the large MIC range is due to nonreproducibility under the assay conditions used or to the difficulties with particular antibiotics, such as spectinomycin (25), under the test conditions needed for these slowly growing organisms.

An analogous situation exists with the animal mycoplasmas, three species of which are listed in Table 3. Many of the antibiotics that are tested against animal mycoplasmas differ from those tested for human isolates, because human and animal diseases are often treated with different antibiotics (69).

Data for antibiotic resistance in bacterial species suggest that over the past 10 years, the actual number of species and genera that are resistant to antibiotics has increased (30, 44). This same situation has been documented for tetracycline resistance in *M. hominis* and *U. urealyticum* (46, 47, 49). Therefore, it is very likely that over time, antibiotic resistances will continue to increase in the mollicutes, both by mutation and by acquisition of new genetic material. As a result, continual surveillance is needed to monitor the spread of antibiotic resistance and to determine the potential impact on antibiotic therapy.

In response to this increase in antibiotic resistance, there are now several commercial systems available for susceptibility testing of mycoplasmas to antibiotics (41). The limit of the current systems is that only one or two concentrations of each antibiotic can be tested, which makes interpretation more difficult than for the classical MIC assay. Renaudin and Bébéar (42) compared a commercial system with the standard MIC determination and found the commercial system to be generally suitable for clinical laboratory use. However, more comparisons need to be done, and one must be careful in the interpretation of these tests since only one or two concentrations of antibiotics are used. It is likely that over time, other commercial systems will become available for susceptibility testing; as each becomes available, it must be tested and compared against other systems. If a commercial system is found to be reproducible, to give accurate values, and to be flexible and inexpensive, such a kit would greatly help in standardization of the mycoplasma antibiotic susceptibility testing and allow direct comparison of data between laboratories.

Acknowledgment. My work was supported by Public Health Service grant AI24136.

REFERENCES

1. **Bébéar, C., P. Cantet, H. Renaudin, and C. Quentin.** 1985. Activité comparée de la minocycline et doxycycline sur les mycoplasmes pathogènes pour l'homme. *Pathol. Biol.* **33**:577–580.

2. **Braun, P., J. O. Klein, and E. H. Kass.** 1970. Susceptibility of genital mycoplasmas to antimicrobial agents. *Appl. Microbiol.* **19**:62–70.

3. **Brisson-Noel, A., P. Trieu-Cuot, and P. Courvalin.** 1988. Mechanism of action of spiramycin and other macrolides. *J. Antimicrob. Chemother.* **22**(Suppl. B):13–23.

4. **Brown, J. T., and M. C. Roberts.** 1987. Cloning and characterization of *tet* M from a *Ureaplasma urealyticum* strain. *Antimicrob. Agents Chemother.* **31**:1852–1854.

5. **Brunet, B. B. de Barbeyrac, H. Renaudin, and C. Bebear.** 1989. Detection of tetracycline-resistant strains of *Ureaplasma urealyticum* by hybridization assays. *Eur. J. Clin. Microbiol. Infect. Dis.* **8**:636–638.

6. **Campello, C., E. Crevatin, G. Nedoclan, and L. Magori.**

1980. Antibiosensibilita de stipiti di Micoplasma isolatei dalle vie respiratorie e genitali di sogetti san. *Friuli Med.* **35**:247–258.

7. **Clewell, D. B., and C. Gawron-Burke.** 1986. Conjugative transposons and the dissemination of antibiotic resistance in *Streptococci*. *Annu. Rev. Microbiol.* **40**:635–659.

8. **Domeruth, C. H.** 1960. Antibiotic resistance and mutation rates of mycoplasma. *Avian Dis.* **4**:456–466.

9. **Dybvig, K., and J. Alderete.** 1988. Transformation of *M. pulmonis* and *Mycoplasma hyorhinis*: transposition of Tn*916* and formation of cointegrate structures. *Plasmid* **20**:33–41.

10. **Evans, R. T., and D. Taylor-Robinson.** 1978. The incidence of tetracycline-resistant strains of *Ureaplasma urealyticum. J. Antimicrob. Chemother.* **4**:57–63.

11. **Fishman, S. E., K. Cox, J. L. Larson, P. A. Reynolds, E. T. Seno, W.-K. Yeh, R. Van Frank, and C. L. Hershberger.** 1987. Cloning genes for the biosynthesis of a macrolide antibiotic. *Proc. Natl. Acad. Sci. USA* **84**:8248–8252.

12. **Gadeau, A.-P., C. Mouches, and J. M. Bové.** 1986. Probable insensitivity of *Mollicutes* to rifampin and characterization of spiroplasma DNA-dependent RNA polymerase. *J. Bacteriol.* **166**:824–828.

13. **Gardella, R. S., and R. A. Del Giudice.** 1984. Antibiotic sensitivities and elimination of mycoplasmas from infected cell cultures. *Isr. J. Med. Sci.* **20**:931–934.

14. **Gnarpe, H.** 1974. Spectinomycin and doxycycline in treatment of acute venereal disease: their influence on genital mycoplasmas and on the serum bactericidal effect. *Microbios* **10**:247–252.

15. **Goldman, R. C., and S. K. Kadam.** 1989. Binding of novel macrolide structures to macrolides-lincosamides-streptogramin B-resistant ribosomes inhibits protein synthesis and bacterial growth. *Antimicrob. Agents Chemother.* **33**:1058–1066.

16. **Hamdy, A. H.** 1970. Efficacy of lincomycin and spectinomycin against avian mycoplasmas. *Antimicrob. Agents Chemother.* **1**:522–530.

17. **Hannan, P. C. T., P. J. O'Hanlon, and N. H. Rogers.** 1989. In vitro evaluation of various quinolone antibacterial agents against veterinary mycoplasmas and porcine respiratory bacterial pathogens. *Res. Vet. Sci.* **46**:202–211.

18. **Harrison, H. R., R. M. Riggin, E. R. Alexander, and L. Weinstein.** In vitro activity of clindamycin against strains of *Chlamydia trachomatis, Mycoplasma hominis* and *Ureaplasma urealyticum* isolated from pregnant women. *Am. J. Obstet. Gynecol.* **149**:477–480.

19. **Jao, R. L., and M. Finland.** 1967. Susceptibility of *Mycoplasma pneumoniae* to 21 antibiotics in vitro. *Am. J. Med. Sci.* **253**:639–650.

20. **Kenny, G. E.** 1967. Heat lability and organic solvent solubility of *Mycoplasma* antigens. *Ann. N.Y. Acad. Sci.* **143**:676–681.

21. **Kenny, G. E.** 1983. Inhibition of the growth of *Ureaplasma urealyticum* by a new urease inhibitor, flurofamide. *Yale J. Biol. Med.* **56**:717–722.

22. **Kenny, G. E.** 1985. Mycoplasma contamination of cell cultures, p. 210–227. *In* I. Gylstorff (ed.), *Infectionen durch Mycoplasmatales.* VEB Gustav Fischer, Jena, Germany.

23. **Kenny, G. E.** 1985. Mycoplasmas, p. 407–411. *In* E. H. Lennette, A. Balows, W. J. Hausler, Jr., and H. J. Shadomy (ed.), *Manual of Clinical Microbiology*, 4th ed. American Society for Microbiology, Washington, D.C.

24. **Kenny, G. E., and F. D. Cartwright.** 1990. Selection of mutants of *Mycoplasma hominis* resistant to sparfloxacin. *Program Abstr. 30th Intersci. Conf. Antimicrobial Agents Chemother.*, abstr. 14.

24a.**Kenny, G. E., and F. D. Cartwright.** 1991. Susceptibility of *Mycoplasma pneumoniae* to several new quinolones, tetracycline, and erythromycin. *Antimicrob. Agents Chemother.* **35**:587–589.

25. **Kenny, G. E., F. D. Cartwright, and M. Roberts.** 1986. Agar dilution method for determination of antibiotic susceptibility of *Ureaplasma urealyticum. Pediatr. Infect. Dis.* **5**:S332–S334.

26. **Kenny, G. E., T. M. Hooton, M. C. Roberts, F. D. Cartwright, and J. Hoyt.** 1989. Susceptibilities of genital mycoplasmas to the newer quinolones as determined by the agar dilution method. *Antimicrob. Agents Chemother.* **33**:103–107.

27. **Koostra, W. L., J. N. Adams, and P. F. Smith.** 1966. In vitro selection and identification antibiotic-resistant mycoplasma mutants. *J. Bacteriol.* **91**:2386–2387.

28. **Lee, D. H., R. J. Miles, and J. R. M. Inal.** 1987. Antibiotic sensitivity and mutation rates to antibiotic resistance in *Mycoplasma mycoides* ssp. *mycoides. Epidemiol. Infect.* **98**:361–368.

29. **Liao, C. H., and T. A. Chen.** 1981. In vitro susceptibility and resistance to two spiroplasmas to antibiotics. *Phytopathology* **71**:442–445.

30. **Lorian, V.** 1986. *Antibiotics in Laboratory Medicine.* Williams & Wilkins, Baltimore.

31. **Mahairas, G. G., and F. C. Minion.** 1989. Transformation of *Mycoplasma pulmonis*: demonstration of homologous recombination, introduction of cloned genes, and preliminary description of an integrating shuttle system. *J. Bacteriol.* **171**:1775–1780.

32. **Mårdh, P.-A.** 1975. Human respiratory tract infections with *Mycoplasmas* and their in vitro susceptibility to tetracyclines and some other antibiotics. *Chemotherapy* **21**:47–57.

33. **Mathisen, G. E.** 1989. Antibiotic pharmacology erythromycin (part 1). *APUA Newsl.* **7**:4–5.

34. **McMurry, L. M., B. H. Park, V. Burdett, and S. B. Levy.** 1987. Energy-dependent efflux mediated by class L (TetL) tetracycline resistance determinant from streptococci. *Antimicrob. Agents Chemother.* **31**:1648–1650.

35. **Mowles, J. M.** 1988. The use of ciprofloxacin for the elimination of mycoplasma from naturally infected cell lines. *Cytotechnology* **1**:355–358.

36. **Nitu, Y., H. Kubota, S. Hasegawa, S. Komatsu, M. Horikawa, and T. Suetake.** 1974. Susceptibility of *Mycoplasma pneumoniae* to antibiotics in vitro. *Jpn. J. Microbiol.* **18**:149–155.

37. **Palu, G., S. Valisena, M. F. Barile, and G. A. Meoni.** 1989. Mechanism of macrolide resistance in *Ureaplasma urealyticum*: a study on collection and clinical strains. *Eur. J. Epidemiol.* **5**:146–153.

38. **Pilaszek, J., and M. Truszczynski.** 1980. A possibility of acquiring and losing resistance to antibiotics in bovine mycoplasma strains. I. Acquiring and losing resistance to tylosin. *Bull. Vet. Inst. Pulawy* **24**:25–41.

39. **Pilaszek, J., and M. Truszczynski.** 1980. A possibility of acquiring and losing resistance to antibiotics in bovine mycoplasma strains. II. Acquiring and losing resistance to chloramphenicol, oxytetracycline, neomycin and streptomycin. *Bull. Vet. Inst. Pulawy* **24**:25–41.

40. **Quiros, L. M., S. Fidalgo, F. J., Mendez, C. Hardisson, and J. A. Salas.** 1988. Novel mechanisms of resistance to lincosamides in *Staphylococcus* and *Arthrobacter* spp. *Antimicrob. Agents Chemother.* **32**:420–425.

41. **Razin, S.** 1985. Molecular biology and genetics of mycoplasmas (*Mollicutes*). *Microbiol. Rev.* **49**:419–455.

42. **Renaudin, H., and C. Bébéar.** 1990. Evaluation des systèmes *Mycoplasma* PLUS et SIR *Mycoplasma* pour la détection quantitative et l'étude de la sensibilité aux antibiotiques des mycoplasmes genitaux. *Pathol. Biol.* **38**:431–435.

43. **Ridgway, G. L., B. Mumtaz, F. G. Gabriel, and J. D. Oriel.** 1984. The activity of ciprofloxacin and other 4-quinolones against *Chlamydia trachomatis* and *Mycoplasmas* in vitro. *Eur. J. Clin. Microbiol.* **3**:344–346.

44. **Roberts, M. C.** 1989. Gene transfer in the urogenital and respiratory tract, p. 347–375. *In* S. B. Levy and R. V.

Miller (ed.), *Gene Transfer in the Environment*. McGraw-Hill Publishing Co., New York.

45. **Roberts, M. C., and S. L. Hillier.** 1990. Genetic basis of tetracycline resistance in urogenital bacteria. *Antimicrob. Agents Chemother.* **34:**261–264.

46. **Roberts, M. C., and G. E. Kenny.** 1986. Dissemination of the *tet M* tetracycline resistance determinant to *Ureaplasma urealyticum. Antimicrob. Agents Chemother.* **29:**350–352.

47. **Roberts, M. C., and G. E. Kenny.** 1986. Tetracycline resistant *Ureaplasma urealyticum. Pediatr. Infect. Dis.* **5:**S338–S340.

48. **Roberts, M. C., and G. E. Kenny.** 1987. Conjugal transfer of transposon Tn*916* from *Streptococcus faecalis* to *Mycoplasma hominis. J. Bacteriol.* **169:**3836–3839.

49. **Roberts, M. C., L. A. Koutsky, D. LeBlanc, K. K. Holmes, and G. E. Kenny.** 1985. Tetracycline resistant *Mycoplasma hominis* strains containing streptococcal *tet M* sequences. *Antimicrob. Agents Chemother.* **28:**141–143.

50. **Robertson, J. A., J. E. Coppola, and O. R. Heisler.** 1981. Standardized method for determining antimicrobial susceptibility of strains of *Ureaplasma urealyticum* and their response to tetracycline, erythromycin, and rosaramicin. *Antimicrob. Agents Chemother.* **28:**53–58.

51. **Robertson, J. A., G. W. Stemke, S. G. MacLellan, and D. Taylor.** 1988. Characterisation of tetracycline-resistant strains of *Ureaplasma urealyticum. J. Antimicrob. Chemother.* **21:**319–332.

52. **Rylander, M., and H. O. Hallander.** 1988. In vitro comparison of the activity of doxycycline, tetracycline, erythromycin and a new macrolide, CP 62993, against *Mycoplasma pneumoniae, Mycoplasma hominis,* and *Ureaplasma urealyticum. Scand. J. Infect. Dis.* **53:**12–17.

53. **Sanchez-Pescador, R., J. T. Brown, M. Roberts, and M. S. Urdea.** 1988. The nucleotide sequence of the tetracycline resistance determinant tet M from *Ureaplasma urealyticum. Nucleic Acids Res.* **16:**1216–1217.

54. **Sanchez-Pescador, R., J. T. Brown, M. Roberts, and M. S. Urdea.** 1988. Homology of the TetM with translocational elongation factors: implications for potential modes of tet M conferred tetracycline resistance. *Nucleic Acids Res.* **16:**1218.

55. **Schwartz, J. L., and D. Perlman.** 1971. Antibiotic resistance mechanisms in *Mycoplasmas* species. *J. Antibiot.* **24:**574–576.

56. **Senterfit, L. B.** 1981. Comparative in vitro sensitivity of *Mycoplasma pneumoniae* to rosaramicin, erythromycin, tetracycline and spectinomycin. *Drugs Exp. Clin. Res.* **3:**317–319.

57. **Senterfit, L. B.** 1983. Antibiotic sensitivity testing of mycoplasmas. *Methods Mycoplasmol.* **2:**397–401.

58. **Shepard, M. C., and C. D. Lunceford.** 1976. Differential agar medium (A7) for identification of *Ureaplasma urealyticum* (human T mycoplasmas) in primary cultures of clinical material. *J. Clin. Microbiol.* **3:**613–625.

59. **Shepard, M. C., C. D. Lunceford, and R. L. Baker.** 1966. T-strain mycoplasma selective inhibition by erythromycin *in vitro. Br. J. Vener. Dis.* **42:**21–24.

60. **Steers, E., E. L. Foltz, and B. S. Graves.** 1959. An inocula replicating apparatus for routine testing of bacterial susceptibility to antibiotics. *Antibiot. Chemother.* **9:**307–311.

61. **Stopler, T., and D. Branski.** 1986. Resistance of *Mycoplasma pneumoniae* to macrolides, lincomycin and streptogramin B. *J. Antimicrob. Chem.* **18:**359–364.

62. **Stopler, T., C. B. Gerichter, and D. Branski.** 1980. Antibiotic-resistant mutants of *Mycoplasma pneumoniae. Isr. J. Med. Sci.* **16:**169–173.

63. **Tjiam, K. H., J. H. T. Wagenvoort, B. van Klingeren, P. Piot, E. Stolz, and M. F. Michel.** 1986. In vitro activity of the two new 4-quinolones A56619 and A56620 against *Neisseria gonorrhoeae, Chlamydia trachomatis, Mycoplasma hominis, Ureaplasma urealyticum* and *Gardnerella vaginalis. Eur. J. Clin. Microbiol.* **5:**498–501.

64. **Waites, K. B., G. H. Cassell, K. C. Canupp, and P. B. Fernandes.** 1988. In vitro susceptibilities of mycoplasmas and ureaplasmas to new macrolides and arylfluoroquinolones. *Antimicrob. Agents Chemother.* **32:**1500–1502.

65. **Whitear, K. G., D. D. Bowtell, E. Ghiocas, and K. L. Hughes.** 1983. Evaluation and use of a micro-broth dilution procedure for testing sensitivity of fermentative avian mycoplasmas to antibiotics. *Avian Dis.* **27:**937–949.

66. **Williams, P. P.** 1978. In vitro susceptibility of *Mycoplasma hyopneumoniae* and *Mycoplasma hyorhinis* to fifty-one antimicrobial agents. *Antimicrob. Agents Chemother.* **14:**210–213.

67. **Wolfson, J. S., and D. C. Hooper.** 1989. Fluoroquinolone antimicrobial agents. *Clin. Microbiol. Rev.* **2:**378–424.

68. **Yancey, R. J., Jr., and L. K. Klein.** 1988. In-vitro activity of trospectomycin sulfate against *Mycoplasma* and *Ureaplasma* species isolated from humans. *J. Antimicrob. Chemother.* **21:**731–736.

69. **Zimmerman, B. J., and R. F. Ross.** 1975. Determination of sensitivity of *Mycoplasma hyosynoviae* to tylosin and selected antibacterial drugs by a microtiter technique. *Can. J. Comp. Med.* **39:**17–21.

32. Mycoplasmas and AIDS

SHYH-CHING LO

INTRODUCTION

The acquired immune deficiency syndrome (AIDS) is characterized by profound immunoincompetence and development of various opportunistic infections (8, 34, 61). Patients with progressive AIDS lose a specific subset of CD4$^+$ lymphocytes (immunodeficiency) and also suffer dysfunction of multiple organ systems, such as central nervous system function (AIDS dementia), cardiac function (AIDS cardiomyopathy), liver functions (AIDS hepatitis), and renal function (AIDS-associated nephropathy) (9, 16, 56, 57, 72). In addition, many AIDS patients develop uncommon tumors such as Kaposi's sarcoma, B-cell lymphoma, and Hodgkin's disease (8, 34, 61). Failure of immune function often leads to opportunistic infections with *Pneumocystis carinii*, *Toxoplasma gondii*, *Mycobacterium avium-intracellulare*, *Mycobacterium tuberculosis*, *Histoplasma capsulatum*, *Candida* sp., *Cryptococcus neoformans*, *Cryptosporidium* sp., and cytomegalovirus, which cause death in most patients with AIDS.

A human retrovirus, human immunodeficiency virus type 1 (HIV-1), is accepted by scientists and clinicians as the primary etiologic agent causing AIDS (1, 27, 65, 72). This virus can be recovered from cultured peripheral blood mononuclear cells of individuals with AIDS or AIDS-related complex and many asymptomatic individuals in the known risk groups (65). HIV-1 infection of human CD4$^+$ lymphocytes in cultures can produce cytopathic effects (1), which explains the depletion of CD4$^+$ lymphocytes in patients with AIDS. For many years, most investigators have believed that HIV-1 by itself is sufficient to cause profound immunodeficiency, to destroy parenchymal cells in different organs, to cause functional failure in a variety of organ systems, and also to lead to development of various tumors. However, there are still many unanswered questions as to how HIV-1 actually causes the complex disease described as AIDS. It is particularly difficult to explain the wide variation in the time of disease incubation, ranging from months to more than 10 years, and in the speed of disease progression among HIV-1-infected patients. The questions also focus on why so few cells are infected with HIV-1 but so many are destroyed (20). And, if it is direct cell killing of CD4$^+$ lymphocytes by HIV-1 that results in immunodeficiency, why does the clinical disease take more than 10 years to occur? Most infected patients apparently have a high titer of antibodies to HIV-1 in the long latency phase following HIV-1 infection. Why, in contrast to other viral infections, do antibodies to HIV-1 fail to protect patients from developing AIDS disease?

When patients begin to develop the devastating disease, only a few cells are found to be infected with the virus, and little viral burden is identified in diseased tissues. Furthermore, HIV-1 infection of experimental animals, including chimpanzees, has not produced any specific illness other than transient lymphadenopathy despite evidence of persistent HIV-1 viremia for nearly 9 years. All the findings suggest that HIV-1 may be a necessary but not a sufficient cause of AIDS dis-

Shyh-Ching Lo • Division of Molecular Pathobiology, Department of Infectious and Parasitic Disease Pathology, Armed Forces Institute of Pathology, Washington, D.C. 20306-6000.

ease. Two major theories on the pathogenesis of AIDS have recently been advanced in an attempt to answer some of these questions. First, an infectious agent(s) other than HIV-1 may play an important role in promoting the disease progression of AIDS (11). Second, there are many prominent autoimmune manifestations in patients with AIDS. Autoimmune disorders secondary to unknown mechanisms are likely to be responsible for the gradual immune decay, including the characteristic hallmark of CD4$^+$ lymphocyte depletion (50).

A class of organisms, termed *Mollicutes*, are the smallest organisms capable of self replication and cause many different forms of disease in animals (see chapters 24 and 25), in plants, and in insects (see chapter 23). The mycoplasma-associated diseases in animals can be severe and even fatal (28). Infections with mycoplasmas in humans, on the other hand, are usually considered self-limiting and clinically nonimportant. Other than atypical pneumonia (*Mycoplasma pneumoniae* pneumonia) (49, 55), some infections of the genitourinary system by the ureaplasmas or *Mycoplasma hominis* (67, 69), and occasional reports of hematogenous invasion or dissemination (51), mycoplasmas have not been previously associated with any significant human diseases (see chapter 25). The negative evidence is mainly due to the fact that mycoplasmas are difficult to culture from diseased tissues and serological evidence of mycoplasmal infections is not convincing. However, mycoplasmas are a heterogeneous group of microorganisms. Many of these extraordinary organisms are capable of producing systemic, debilitating disease as well as profoundly altering immune functions of the infected animal hosts. Prominent manifestations of immune dysfunction and autoimmune disorders in mycoplasmal infections have been well documented both in animals (7, 13, 23) and in humans (6, 12, 38, 60) (see chapters 27 and 29).

In the search for another infectious agent(s) which might play a key role in the complex pathogenesis of AIDS, recent attention has focused on several species of mycoplasma (22, 73). The finding of systemic mycoplasmal infections in many patients with AIDS (41, 45) may be highly significant. Infections with a hidden agent(s) like mycoplasma(s) in patients with AIDS may explain a number of unusual disease processes, including multiple organ failure and autoimmune disorders, commonly found in AIDS. Our studies and others (11, 37, 46, 73) have shown that mycoplasma(s) is indeed a reasonable candidate whose coinfection may greatly increase the frequency of development of clinical AIDS in patients infected with HIV-1. This brief review will attempt to give a general outline of the current understanding on the mycoplasmas associated with AIDS and their potential role in the disease process.

THE AIDS-ASSOCIATED MYCOPLASMAS

Infections with some specific species of mycoplasmas have been identified much more frequently in patients with AIDS and/or infected with HIV-1 than in non-HIV-infected control subjects. The organisms can be either directly identified in the diseased tissues by molecular and immunohistological techniques, or isolated from the body fluids of HIV-1-infected patients. These mycoplasmas include *Mycoplasma fermentans*, *Mycoplasma pirum*, *Mycoplasma genitalium*, and *Mycoplasma penetrans*. Biochemically, all of these organisms are glucose-fermenting mycoplasmas. It is interesting that *M. fermentans*, *M. pirum*, and *M. penetrans* can hydrolyze arginine as well. Presently, among these four species of AIDS-associated mycoplasmas, we have more information about *M. fermentans* and its association with disease processes in the infected tissues. The association between this particular species of mycoplasma and AIDS is apparently world wide and not limited to patients in North America and Europe. Interaction between *M. fermentans* and HIV-1 has also been examined more closely in vitro.

M. penetrans is a previously unknown mycoplasma recently isolated from HIV-1-infected patients with AIDS (42, 43). The significance of its infection in AIDS or in any human disease awaits the findings of future studies.

Mycoplasma fermentans

M. fermentans was initially isolated from the human urogenital tract in the early 1950s (63, 64). However, the mycoplasma was rarely identified. It was not known whether the organism was rare or was too fastidious to grow in cultures with present media (33). Little evidence was presented to correlate the organism with human urogenital disease. *M. fermentans* was later reported to be isolated from bone marrow of leukemic and nonleukemic patients in the 1970s (54). The organisms induced leukemoid disease with lymphadenopathy in experimentally infected animals (59). In that study, leukemoid disease was not induced in animals with parallel infections by *Mycoplasma hominis*, *Mycoplasma orale*, or *Mycoplasma salivarium*. Inoculation of *M. fermentans* in higher doses could induce fulminant syndromes resembling endotoxin shock, disseminated intravascular coagulation, or gramnegative-like sepsis in experimental animals (24, 25). Other studies reported cytotoxic effects of *M. fermentans* on mouse thymocytes (26) and prominent mitogenic effects on human peripheral lymphocytes (5). However, whether *M. fermentans* is truly pathogenic in humans has not been further investigated until recently.

Findings of systemic *M. fermentans* infections in many patients with AIDS (41, 45) have drawn widespread attention to the possible role of this organism in human diseases, including AIDS. However, identification of mycoplasmal infections has always been a challenge. Culture isolation of mycoplasmas directly from infected tissues is extremely difficult. Infection with these procaryotes may not produce a high titer of antibody response in the hosts. The cell wall-free, pleomorphic organisms cannot be demonstrated in infected tissues by special stains developed to reveal fungi, bacteria, or parasites. Even with the help of electron microscopy, the small, pleomorphic mycoplasmal particles are difficult to distinguish from fragments of cellular cytoplasm or organelles released from degenerating cells. Ultrastructural identification and interpretation can be highly complicated and controversial. Thus demonstration of mycoplasmal infection in the diseased tissues of immune-compromised AIDS patients often depends on the use of several techniques based on more than one diagnostic principle. The evidence of a high prevalence of *M. fermentans* infections in patients with AIDS is summarized below according to immunohistochemistry, electron microscopy, polymerase chain reaction (PCR), in situ hybridization, and culture isolation.

Histopathological identification of *M. fermentans* infections

We reported that many patients with AIDS had systemic infection with *M. fermentans*. In an early study (41) using Formalin-fixed, paraffin-embedded tissue from AIDS patients, rabbit antiserum raised specifically against *M. fermentans* (incognitus strain) stained reticuloendothelial cells or macrophages in the subcapsular sinus of AIDS patients' lymph nodes. Also stained were degenerating cells within lesions containing mononuclear lymphohistiocytes in brain tissues from patients with clinical encephalopathy and histopathological evidence of idiopathic subacute encephalitis, as well as in neuroglial cells in periventricular and perivascular areas in three other patients who had clinical encephalopathy but no histopathological evidence of encephalitis. To further facilitate the technique of direct identification of *M. fermentans* infection in tissues from patients with AIDS, we developed a series of monoclonal antibodies (MAbs) for immunohistochemistry. The incognitus strain of *M. fermentans*, grown in cell-free modified SP-4 medium, was used to prepare the MAbs (44). In immunoblot analyses, many of the MAbs reacted only with the incognitus strain and not with other species of human mycoplasmas, including the closely related type strain of *M. fermentans* (PG-18).

We focused our histopathological study on tissues from 34 patients who had clinical manifestations of functional deficit, or who displayed abnormalities of certain organ systems and tissues with histopathological lesions of necrosis or inflammation without an etiological agent being identified (41). Using immunohistochemistry and MAbs, we presented evidence of *M. fermentans* infection in thymus, liver, spleen, lymph node, or brain tissue from 22 of 32 homosexuals, intravenous drug abusers, or transfusion-associated pediatric patients with AIDS. *M. fermentans*-specific antigens were found in these infected tissues (Fig. 1) with only mild histopathological changes. Although occasional degenerating cells with disruption or even patchy necrosis were noted, there was no significant tissue reactive process or acute inflammatory reaction. We also identified *M. fermentans* infection in two placentas delivered by two patients with AIDS. In the study, areas of tissues with positive immunostaining for *M. fermentans*-specific antigens were retrieved and examined by electron microscopy. We observed characteristic ultrastructures with morphologic features typical of mycoplasmas in the tissues positive for incognitus strain-specific antigens (Fig. 2). *M. fermentans*-specific genetic material was also detected in these tissues (see the following section).

As mentioned earlier, patients with AIDS often develop significant dysfunction in multiple organ systems including the immune system, hematopoietic system, brain, heart, liver, joints, gastrointestinal tract, and kidney. In our studies, the functional deficit

of various organ systems which showed no other etiological agent appeared to be directly associated with a hidden mycoplasmal infection (41, 45). As a typical example, infection with *M. fermentans* in kidneys was shown to be associated with development of the kidney failure commonly termed AIDS-associated nephropathy in HIV-1-infected patients with AIDS (3). Other than the functional abnormality, the major morphologic characteristics that emerged in AIDS-associated nephropathy were: (i) focal segmental and global glomerulosclerosis, frequently characterized by visceral epithelial cell hypertrophy and vacuolization; (ii) microcystic dilatation of tubules which contain large proteinaceous casts; (iii) tubular cell degeneration and necrosis; and (iv) variable degrees of interstitial edema and inflammation (3, 16). We studied renal tissues from 203 HIV-1-infected patients with AIDS. Of the 203, 20 showed light-microscopic changes characteristic of AIDS-associated nephropathy. Fifteen of the 20 (group A) were examined by immunohistochemistry using *M. fermentans* (incognitus strain)-specific MAbs and electron microscopy. Renal tissues from all 15 patients showed positive staining for the incognitus strain mycoplasmal antigens within glomerular endothelial and epithelial cells, glomerular basement membrane, tubular epithelial cells and casts, and mononuclear interstitial cells. Ultrastructural study of these 15 cases revealed mycoplasmalike structures in these locations and others. In a parallel study, renal tissues from 15 patients with AIDS who had essentially normal renal histology or mild interstitial mononuclear cell infiltration (group B) were also examined. These tissues showed no evidence of *M. fermentans* infection in renal parenchymal cells.

Molecular genetic evidence of *M. fermentans* infection

To verify the immunohistochemistry results, our laboratory has also developed molecular techniques for identification of *M. fermentans*-specific genetic materials in infected tissues. DNA from *M. fermentans* (incognitus strain) was extracted, digested, and cloned into λ Charon 28. A clone was subcloned into phage M13, and two specific DNA probes (2.2 and 8.6 kb) were obtained. The first 200 bp at one of the terminal ends of the 2.2-kb fragment were sequenced (45). By PCR, using pairs of synthetic primers identical to specific sequences, the presence of *M. fermentans* was detected in DNA isolated from spleen, liver, brain, or lymph node tissues, Kaposi's sarcoma, or peripheral blood mononuclear cells from 7 of 10 patients with AIDS, but not in five different tissues and one tumor derived from five control subjects without AIDS (45).

An in situ hybridization technique using ^{35}S-labeled cloned *M. fermentans* (incognitus strain) DNA inserted into M13mp19 vector as a probe was also developed (40) to directly identify *M. fermentans* DNA in infected lymphocyte cultures (Fig. 3). The technique identified *M. fermentans* DNA in thymus, liver, and spleen tissues from patients with AIDS and in placentas delivered by two women with AIDS (41). Kupffer cells and occasional hepatocytes in the liver, infiltrating lymphoid cells and histiocytes in portal tracts of another liver, and lymphocytes in white pulp of the spleen were found to be positive by hybridization. These tissues were those previously found to be positive for *M. fer-*

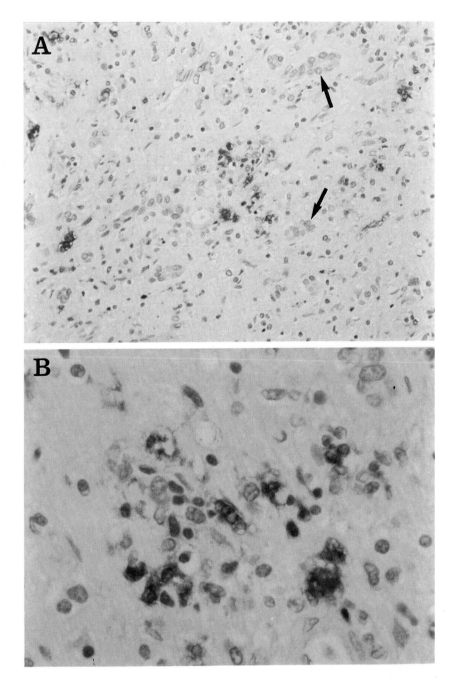

Figure 1. (A) Photomicrograph of a portal area in liver from an AIDS patient, showing patchy areas of necrosis. Prominent infiltrates of chronic inflammatory cells and proliferation of bile ducts (arrows) are identified. Many lymphohistiocytes stain intensely positive for *M. fermentans*-specific antigens. (×390.) (B) Higher magnification of the positively immunostained cells in panel A. Some positive cells show prominent cytopathological changes and cell disruption. (×780.) The same portal area shown in panel A, in a subsequent tissue section immunostained by a nonspecific MAb with the same isotype (IgGl/k), revealed no positive immunochemical reaction (not shown). (Modified from reference 41.)

mentans infection by immunohistochemistry using MAbs specific to *M. fermentans* (previous section). Parallel sections from the same tissues did not hybridize with vector DNA without the insert of incognitus DNA. Nor were positive signals found in five spleen and liver tissues from three patients who died of non-AIDS conditions, when these tissues were hybridized with the *M. fermentans*-specific DNA probe.

However, in situ hybridization using ^{35}S-labeled DNA probes is a very time-consuming and highly delicate procedure. We have therefore focused on applying newly available molecular genetic information to develop another assay, highly sensitive and specific, but much less labor intensive, for rapid diagnosis of *M. fermentans* infection. We recently used a new PCR assay system to amplify a 206-nucleotide specific gene

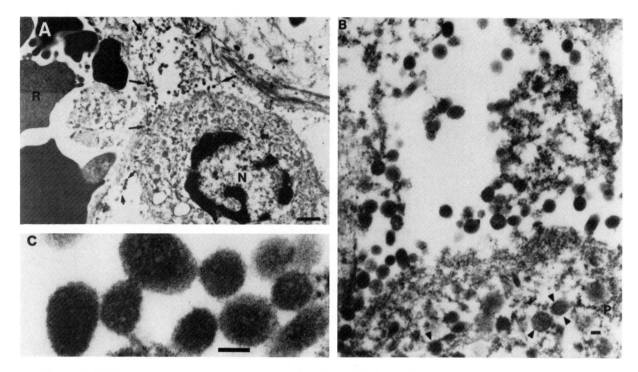

Figure 2. (A) Electron microscopy of a periportal area of an AIDS patient's liver immunostained positive for *M. fermentans*-specific antigens. Electron-dense mycoplasmalike particles are seen extracellularly in an area surrounding a small vessel (arrows). Nucleus (N) of a mononuclear lymphohistiocyte, and erythrocytes (R) in the small vessel, are shown. Bar, 900 nm. (B) Higher magnification of the mycoplasmalike microorganisms found in the empty extracellular space and along the outer surface of the lymphohistiocyte shown in panel A. Many intracellular particles (arrowheads) can also be identified and are difficult to differentiate from the extracellular particles. Polysomal structure (P) is shown. Bar, 100 nm. (C) Higher magnification of the mycoplasmalike microorganisms lining the outer surface of the lymphohistiocyte. Typical electron-dense structure of internal matrix with fine granular configuration is shown. Bar, 100 nm. (Modified from reference 41.)

sequence within the insertion sequence (IS)-like element of *M. fermentans* (70, 71). The IS-like genetic element was found only in *M. fermentans* and not in other human or animal mycoplasmas (32). The potentially transposable IS-like element exists in multiple copies in the *M. fermentans* genome (32). The PCR assay selectively amplified DNA from all strains of *M. fermentans* tested, but not DNA from other human or animal mycoplasmas, bacteria, fungi, monkeys, or humans (70). The *M. fermentans*-specific PCR has provided a much-needed detection assay for the study of this AIDS-associated mycoplasma in patients with AIDS.

Using the newly developed PCR, both our laboratory and R. Hawkins and his associates have detected a high prevalence of *M. fermentans* infection in urine (18) and blood (29) from HIV-1-infected patients but not in HIV-1-negative control subjects. Figure 4 reveals the PCR amplification of the 206-nucleotide specific gene sequence within the *M. fermentans* IS-like element from urine sediments of HIV-1-infected patients. Approximately 23% of urine samples (18) and 9% of blood samples (29) from the HIV-1-infected patients in the studies were found to be positive for this organism by PCR. None of the urine and blood samples from HIV-1-negative, non-AIDS controls tested positive. We believe this highly sensitive and specific assay will facilitate a rapid and reliable diagnosis of *M. fermentans*

infection in clinical samples for other investigators who are studying AIDS disease.

Isolation of *M. fermentans* by culture techniques

M. fermentans is known to be fastidious and difficult to isolate. From our own experience, attempts to isolate *M. fermentans* from infected tissues are frustrating. Many blood and tissue components have been found to be inhibitory to mycoplasma in culture. Prompted by our finding of prominent *M. fermentans* infection in AIDS-associated nephropathy (3), we anticipated that the urine from HIV-positive AIDS patients might have *M. fermentans* present. Our laboratory has specifically examined urine samples from patients with AIDS. We isolated *M. fermentans* from 3 of 43 urine samples from HIV-1-infected patients (18). These three urine samples tested strongly positive for this mycoplasma by PCR. *M. fermentans* could not be isolated by culture from another seven urine samples in this group which also tested positive by PCR. None of the 50 urines from HIV-1-uninfected controls tested positive by PCR or produced a positive culture for *M. fermentans*.

Luc Montagnier and his associates reported *M. fermentans* isolation from blood samples of HIV-1-infected patients (37, 53). The organism was isolated

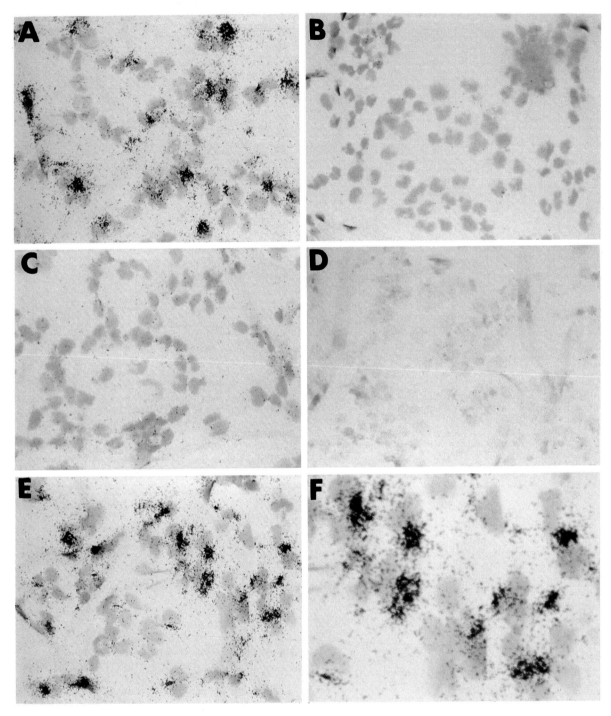

Figure 3. Detection of *M. fermentans* infection by in situ hybridization in CEM human lymphocyte cell line cultures. About 10^3 color-changing units of *M. fermentans* was inoculated into 10^6 CEM lymphocytes, incubated for 2 h at 37°C, washed once with RPMI 1640, and resuspended in RPMI 1640 with 10% fetal bovine serum. A separate set of cultures were treated without *M. fermentans* and served as control. All the cultures were refed (50% replacement) with fresh medium every other day. On day 14, 10^5 cells from either *M. fermentans*-infected or control cultures were washed once with phosphate-buffered saline and cytospun onto a glass slide. (A) CEM cells from the infected cultures were probed with ^{35}S-labeled cloned *M. fermentans* DNA (psb-2.2) inserted into M13mp19 cloning vector (38). Strong labeling is seen associated with infected cells. (×200.) (B) CEM cells from the noninfected control culture show no positive signal of hybridization. (×200.) (C) CEM cells from an infected culture, hybridized with ^{35}S-labeled M13mp19 cloning vector DNA not containing the 2.2-kb insert of *M. fermentans* DNA, also show no hybridization labeling. (×200.) (D) The positive labeling shown in panel A is highly sensitive to pretreatment of these infected cells with DNase (100 μg/ml in 50 mM Tris–7 mM MgCl$_2$, 37°C, 30 min) before hybridization. (×200.) (E) The positive labeling associated with the infected CEM cells, on the other hand, is apparently resistant to pretreatment with RNase (100 μg/ml in phosphate-buffered saline, 37°C, 30 min) before hybridization of these cells. (×200.) (F) Higher magnification of panel A. (×400.)

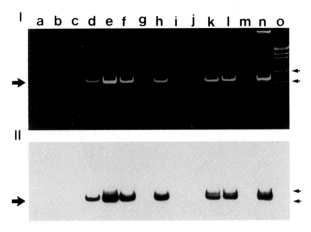

Figure 4. Analysis of PCR-amplified products from representative urine sediment samples from HIV-1-infected patients with AIDS and from HIV-negative non-AIDS donors. RW004 (5'-GGACTATTGTCTAAACAATTTCCC-3') and RW005 (5'-GGTTATTCGATTTCTAAATCGCCT-3') were the primer pair used in PCR amplification. RW006 (5'-GCTGTGGCCATTCT-CTTCTACGTT-3') with the internal nucleotide sequence was used as a probe to verify the fidelity of amplification. PCR products were analyzed both by electrophoresis in a polyacrylamide gel stained with ethidium bromide (I) and by hybridization with a ^{32}P-labeled RW006 probe (II), following electrophoretic transfer of DNA to a nylon membrane. Lane a, PCR reaction cocktail without DNA; lanes b and c, urine sediment samples from HIV-negative control donors; lanes d through m, urine sediment samples from HIV-positive AIDS patients; lane n, 1 fg of *M. fermentans* (incognitus strain) DNA diluted into 1 μg of human placental DNA; lane o, plasmid pUC18 DNA digested with *Msp*I, serving as size markers. Large arrows on the left indicate the positions of the 206-bp diagnostic band for *M. fermentans*. Small arrows on the right indicate the positions of the two bands of *Msp*I-digested pUC18 DNA of 242 bp (top arrow) and 190 bp (bottom arrow).

from peripheral blood mononuclear cell cultures. More recently, W. M. McCormack and his associates also reported isolation of *M. fermentans* from 14 of 180 urine samples from HIV-1-infected patients with AIDS (10). Some additional isolates were apparently glucose fermenters but have not been fully characterized yet (also see *M. pirum*, below). The findings are consistent with our earlier contention that patients with HIV-1 infection or AIDS have a high prevalence of infection by *M. fermentans*. Investigators should continue to modify and improve culture techniques as well as media to develop a more effective culture system.

Mycoplasma pirum

All isolates of the species *M. pirum* were previously from human cell cultures (19, 35). The true origin or natural host for this species has not been documented. The organisms have an organized terminal structure and metabolize both glucose and arginine for growth. Both morphological and biochemical properties are unusual in comparison with other human mycoplasmas (19). Recent reports by Montagnier and his associates of the isolation of *M. pirum* from primary cultures of peripheral mononuclear cells prepared from blood of AIDS patients (37, 53) suggest that the mycoplasma

is from humans. The mycoplasma apparently has been isolated on two occasions from the blood of patients with AIDS. In this context, four mycoplasmas isolated by Chirgwin et al. from 180 urine samples from HIV-1-infected patients with AIDS were recently reported as *M. pirum* (10). If the true identity of these isolates is confirmed, the uncertainty of the origin of *M. pirum* can finally be solved. However, further studies are still needed before the possible role of this organism in AIDS can be determined.

Mycoplasma genitalium

M. genitalium was originally isolated from the urethra of two male homosexuals with nongonococcal urethritis more than 10 years ago (68). The organism possesses a specialized terminal structure for attachment and metabolizes glucose for growth (31). However, the isolation has been difficult to repeat. An extensive number of samples from patients with urogenital diseases have been examined without any positive result. More recently, some strains of this organism were identified in the human respiratory tract, along with *Mycoplasma pneumoniae* (2). This finding suggests that *M. genitalium* may be a respiratory tract mycoplasma. Thus, the true location or the primary site for this organism in humans is still uncertain. Despite their distinct genetic make-up, there are prominent serological and antigenic cross-reactions between *M. genitalium* and *M. pneumoniae* (31). To assess the role of *M. genitalium* in human diseases more accurately, it becomes crucial to have an effective diagnostic procedure which can clearly distinguish infections with these two organisms in patients.

Montagnier and associates detected *M. genitalium* in blood samples of one patient with AIDS by a PCR system which could presumably amplify only *M. genitalium* DNA and not DNA from other mycoplasma species, including *M. pneumoniae* (53). So far *M. genitalium* has not been isolated from patients infected with HIV-1 or with AIDS. However, this is most likely due to the fact that the organism is too fastidious to grow in present culture systems. To elicit antibodies, Montagnier et al. (52) used two synthetic peptides derived from the adhesion protein of *M. genitalium* (17), which enables the organism to adhere to culture dish surfaces and attach to cells. One of the peptides was derived from a highly conserved region of the attachment protein which mediates binding. The resulting antibody to this particular peptide also recognized a similar region of adhesion protein from *M. pneumoniae* but did not recognize any HIV-1 protein. The antibody was shown to prevent HIV-1 infection and replication in human lymphocyte cultures. The second peptide, from the carboxy terminus of the adhesion protein, is not involved in attachment. The antibody to the second peptide had no effect on HIV-1 infection and replication. There are many possible interpretations of this observation. Montagnier et al. suggested that mycoplasmas such as *M. genitalium* could modulate infection and proliferation of HIV-1 in human lymphocytes (52). Root-Bernstein and Hobbs (62) proposed an alternative mechanism to explain the observed inhibition, based upon homologies or cross-reactivities identified between the adhesion peptide and the CD4 class II major histocompatibility complex proteins of human T lymphocytes.

At present, it is still too early to speculate on any possible role of *M. genitalium* in AIDS. However, many studies are in progress to determine the interaction between *M. genitalium* and HIV-1, the pathogenesis of this organism in chimpanzees with or without HIV-1 infection, and the scope of *M. genitalium* infection in different high-risk groups of AIDS patients.

Mycoplasma penetrans

A previously unknown mycoplasma was recently isolated in our laboratory from urine sediments of six HIV-1-infected patients with AIDS (43). The cell wall-free organism formed "fried-egg" colonies on SP-4 agar plates and could be repeatedly isolated from these patients in subsequent attempts. The organism requires cholesterol to grow and metabolizes both glucose and arginine. It possesses a unique terminal structure for attachment to eucaryotic cells (42, 43). There are two sharply divided compartments, a densely packed terminal structure and the body (Fig. 5). In addition to having the properties of adhesion, hemadsorption, and cytadsorption, the organism is highly invasive and capable of penetrating into the cytoplasm of mammalian cells through its unusual tiplike structure (Fig. 6). Detailed serological and DNA analyses have revealed that this mycoplasma is indeed a new species. Thus, a new name of *Mycoplasma penetrans* has been assigned, pertinent to its unusual properties (42).

Invading *M. penetrans* cells often had their tiplike structure deeply buried in the cytoplasm of infected mammalian cells (42, 43). Extensive invasion of *M. penetrans* into infected cells produced cytopathic effects and led to cell death. Using electron microscopy, we have examined directly the urine sediments which grew *M. penetrans* in high titer without other identifiable infectious agent. Organisms with the characteristic features of *M. penetrans* could be seen adhering to the surface as well as invading into the cytoplasm of urothelial cells (Fig. 7). Therefore, *M. penetrans* with its specialized tip structure apparently uses the same process documented in a variety of cell cultures to adhere to the surface and to invade the cytoplasm of urothelial cells in the patient's urogenital tract.

We believe that the finding of a previously unknown organism with many properties closely associated with virulence in pathogenic mollicutes is significant. Our laboratory is examining the scope of infection with the novel mycoplasma in various human diseases, especially in AIDS. Our preliminary serological study using enzyme-linked immunosorbent assay and Western blot (immunoblot) analysis reveals a high prevalence (40%) of antibodies to *M. penetrans* in AIDS patients infected with HIV-1. In comparison, a low incidence (0.3%) of antibody titer is found in sera from non-HIV-infected control subjects. There is also a low prevalence (0.9%) of the antibodies in patients attending sexually transmitted disease clinics. In addition, of more than 150 HIV-negative patients with different non-AIDS disease states, many associated with immune dysfunction and/or low leukocyte counts, none tested positive for the antibodies. The newly discovered mycoplasma, apparently not a commensal organism in humans and not a simple opportunistic infection commonly occurring in immune-compromised hosts, is uniquely associated with HIV-1 infection and AIDS disease. Prompted by these findings, our laboratory is now actively engaged in the development of a PCR assay for sensitive and rapid diagnosis of *M. penetrans* infection in various clinical specimens. MAbs will also be prepared to detect *M. penetrans* in infected tissues by immunohistochemistry. The significance of *M. penetrans* infection in AIDS will continue to be assessed in future studies.

INTERACTION BETWEEN AIDS-ASSOCIATED MYCOPLASMAS AND HIV-1

Findings of a high prevalence of *M. fermentans* infection in patients infected with HIV-1 have raised the possibility that the two infectious agents may interact synergistically and that mycoplasmas could play a significant disease-promoting role in HIV-infected patients. We have examined the effects of *M. fermentans* (incognitus strain) on HIV-1 infection of CD4$^+$ human lymphocytic CEM cells in culture (46). Coinfection with the incognitus strain significantly enhanced the ability of HIV-1 to induce cytopathic effects on human T-lymphocytes in vitro. Syncytium formation of HIV-infected T cells was essentially eliminated in the presence of *M. fermentans* (incognitus strain), despite prominent cell death. In addition, *M. fermentans* apparently produced a factor that inhibited the standard reverse transcriptase enzyme assay. However, replication and production of infectious HIV-1 particles continued during the coinfection. The modification of the biological properties and the up-regulation of HIV-1 cytopathogenicity by coinfection with *M. fermentans* may have clinical implications in the pathogenesis of AIDS.

Montagnier and associates reported earlier that the cell killing effect of HIV-1 in cultures could be significantly reduced by tetracycline antibiotics (36). The tetracycline-treated cultures continued to produce a high titer of HIV-1 in the absence of any cytocidal effect. The authors suggested that a tetracycline-sensitive procaryotic agent, most likely a mycoplasma, was involved with the cytocidal effect observed in the HIV-infected cultures. Indeed, in additional studies they confirmed mycoplasma as the hidden agent in the cultures (37). The contaminating mycoplasma was later isolated from CEM U13 cells and identified as a strain of *M. fermentans* (37). In this study, Montagnier et al. showed that, following infection of lymphoblastoid (CEM) or promonocytic (U937 and THP$_1$) cell lines with HIV-1, cytopathic effect on these cells was observed only in association with mycoplasma contamination. HIV-1 alone failed to kill human T-lymphocytes effectively. The authors concluded that the HIV-1 cytopathogenicity in human lymphocytes and monocytic cells appeared to be a mycoplasma-dependent process. These results also confirmed our earlier report that *M. fermentans* was able to markedly enhance the ability of HIV-1 to kill infected human lymphocytes in vitro (46).

The interaction between mycoplasms and HIV-1 is complex. Depending on the species of mycoplasma,

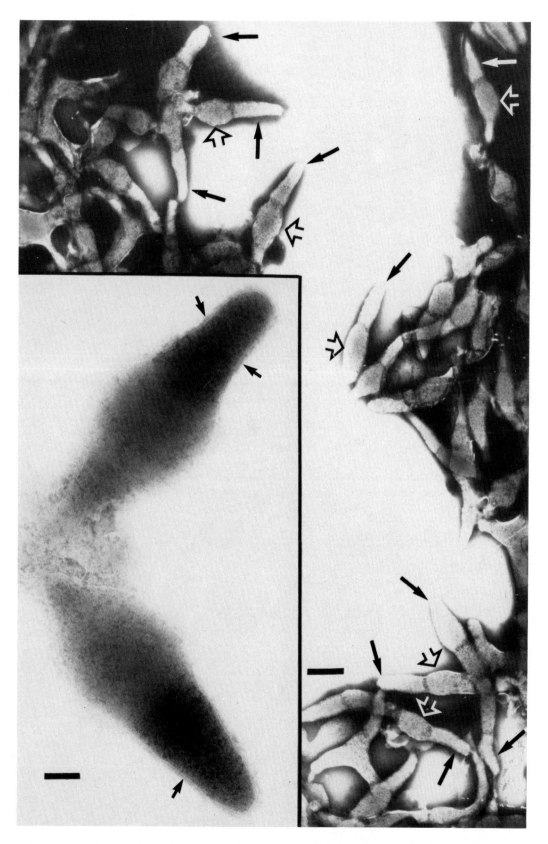

Figure 5. Electron micrographs of *M. penetrans*. Mycoplasma from a 5-day culture in SP-4 broth, negatively stained by phosphotungstic acid. Most organisms are rodlike with an elongated flask shape. There are two distinct compartments: a densely packed tiplike structure (arrows) and a broader body compartment (broad arrows). Bar, 400 nm. Insert reveals two organisms with "positive" staining. Phosphotungstic acid has entered the organisms, presumably due to leakage of the membrane, during preparation of negative staining. The densely packed tiplike structure of *M. penetrans* is highly evident. A surface layer (arrows) external to the cell membrane on the tiplike structure is noted. Bar, 100 nm. (Modified from reference 43.)

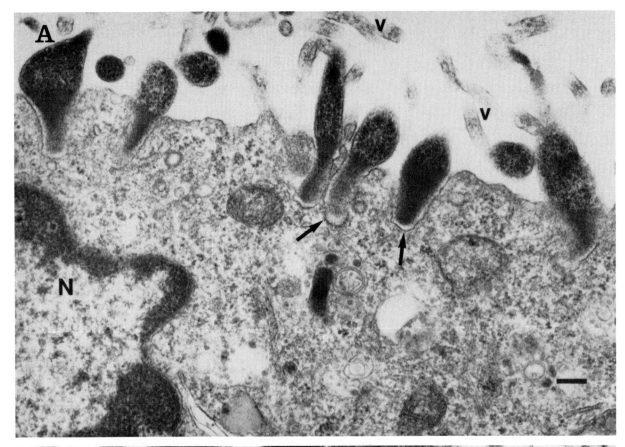

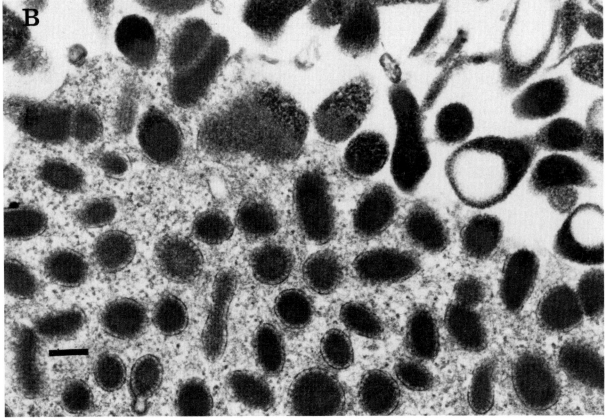

the effect on HIV-1 cytopathic activity in infected human lymphocyte cultures can be quite variable and even completely opposite. Current studies show that *M. fermentans* is highly effective in up-regulation of HIV-1 pathogenicity in human lymphocytes in vitro. The actual mechanisms responsible for the synergistic effects on cell killing are not clear. Since the cultures are normally replenished with fresh medium every other day, the cytopathic effect is not likely to be due to simple nutritional depletion in the mycoplasma-infected cultures. Many other mycoplasmas, including arginine-hydrolyzing *M. orale*, glucose-fermenting *M. genitalium*, and *M. pirum*, which hydrolyzes both glucose and arginine for growth, are found to have little or no effect on HIV-1 cytopathogenicity in coinfected human lymphocyte cultures (unpublished data). In one previous report, *M. hyorhinis*, a swine mycoplasma, even had a down-regulatory effect on the HIV-1 pathogenicity in cultures coinfected with both agents (58). In this context, our preliminary study reveals that *M. penetrans*, the newly isolated mycoplasma from patients with AIDS, has a profound synergistic effect on HIV-1 cytopathogenic activities in infected human lymphocyte cultures. Therefore, among mycoplasmas that are presently associated with AIDS, it appears that only *M. fermentans* and *M. penetrans* have prominent effects on enhancing HIV-1 cytopathogenicity in vitro.

EXPERIMENTAL INFECTION OF *M. FERMENTANS* IN NONHUMAN PRIMATES

In earlier studies (40, 45, 47), before the incognitus strain of *M. fermentans* was fully characterized, the organism was called a viruslike infectious agent (VLIA) and was thought to be most likely a large DNA virus. To examine whether the VLIA/incognitus strain was pathogenic, we inoculated VLIA/incognitus strain grown and isolated from a transformed NIH 3T3 cell culture into four silvered leaf monkeys (SL2 through 5) intraperitoneally (47). One additional monkey (SL1) was inoculated with supernatants prepared from control cultures of NIH 3T3 cells and served as the control.

All four monkeys inoculated with VLIA/incognitus strain exhibited a wasting syndrome and died in 7 to 9 months (47). The progressive weight loss lacks a good explanation. No diarrhea was observed during infection. The monkeys appeared to have a normal food intake. No febrile response could be detected in the moribund animals which showed the most prominent weight loss. On the contrary, these moribund animals were often hypothermic. Examination of thyroids at necropsy was normal and unremarkable. Two monkeys had a transient lymphadenopathy in earlier stages. Two moribund animals showed lymphopenia. Unfortunately, the MAb which stains CD4$^+$ cells representing the helper subset of lymphocytes in humans does not stain the lymphocytes of silvered leaf monkeys. Consequently, it was not possible to determine changes in lymphocyte subpopulations. Although three of the mycoplasma-infected monkeys had persistent low-grade fever early in the infection, the animals became afebrile in the later stages.

Development of specific antibody to the mycoplasma could best be documented by the changes of overall serological immunoreaction patterns in Western blot analysis of serial bleeding samples, including sera obtained before mycoplasma inoculation. One infected monkey had a more prominent antibody response which occurred 7 months after mycoplasma inoculation. The other two monkeys had only a transient or poor antibody response in the later stages. One infected monkey (SL4) failed to produce any significant antibody response. Radioimmunoassay revealed periodic mycoplasma antigenemia in these infected animals during the course of the experiment. The monkey (SL4) which showed no detectable antibody response had the most persistent mycoplasma antigenemia and was the first animal to succumb to the infection. The control monkey was sacrificed 8 months after the last mycoplasma-inoculated monkey succumbed and showed neither an antibody response nor evidence of antigenemia.

Mycoplasma-specific DNA could be directly detected by PCR in necropsy tissues of all four infected monkeys. Mycoplasma infection was identified in all four spleens, in two of four livers, in one of two kidneys, and in all three brains tested from these four animals, but not in the tissues from the control monkey. One monkey which exhibited neurological symptoms in the terminal stage was found by PCR to have mycoplasmal DNA in the brain. The necropsy tissues of the livers of two monkeys and the spleen of a third, which appeared to contain the most abundant amount of mycoplasma-specific DNA, also stained positively with *M. fermentans*-specific polyclonal antiserum and MAbs. Many positively stained hepatocytes and Kupffer cells showed profound cytopathic changes with degeneration, disruption, and necrosis (Fig. 8). Direct electron microscopy of these tissues revealed many areas with numerous particles having characteristic mycoplasma ultrastructure (Fig. 9). Most of the mycoplasmalike particles were found in the extracellular tissue matrix and sinusoidal spaces. However, many typical particles could also be identified in the cytoplasm of hepatocytes and degenerating Kupffer cells.

At necropsy, no malignant tumor, bacterial or fungal opportunistic infection, or viral inclusion body could be identified in any of the tissues examined. In

Figure 6. Adhesion and invasion of *M. penetrans* into mammalian cells. (A) Tiplike structures of densely packed fine granules deeply penetrate into the cytoplasm of a human endothelial cell in an infected culture, and the broader body compartments remain outside. The deeply invaginated membrane (arrows), nucleus (N), and microvilli (V) of the endothelial cell are shown. Bar, 200 nm. (B) Numerous *M. penetrans* cells adhering to the cell surface and invading the cytoplasm of a human embryo kidney cell in a 4-day culture. We assume that most of the organisms inside the cytoplasm are visible as cross-sections of their inserted tiplike structures. This section also shows some organisms lining up on the cell surface, with their tiplike structures (arrows) beginning to invade the cytoplasm. Extracellular organisms with vacuoles are also seen. Bar, 125 nm. (Modified from references 42 and 43.)

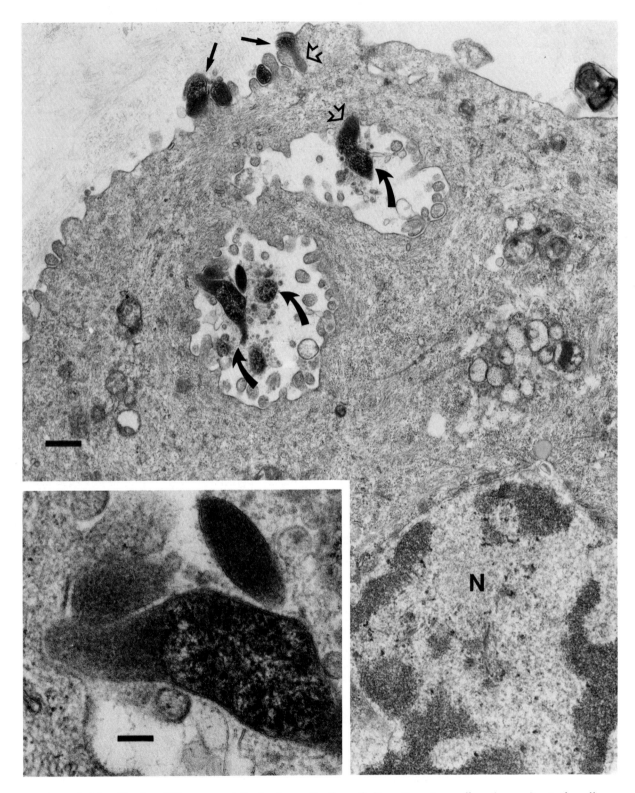

Figure 7. Identification of *M. penetrans* infection in a patient's urothelium. Organisms adhere (arrows) onto the cell surface and pierce their tip compartments (broad arrows) into the cytoplasm of a urogenital epithelial cell. Many organisms (curved arrows), with their tiplike structure with densely packed fine granules inserted into the cytoplasm, are found in either intracellular membrane-bound vesicles or a deeply invaginated cell process. Insert shows the adhesion and invasion processes in the intracellular vesicle at higher magnification. N, nucleus.

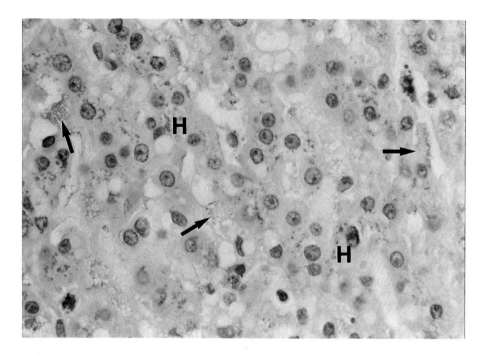

Figure 8. Immunohistochemistry detection of *M. fermentans* (incognitus strain) antigens using MAb (G2 9H8) in the liver of a monkey (SL2) experimentally infected with incognitus strain. Positive staining is found on linings of sinusoidal space, Kupffer cells, and some hepatocytes in the liver of monkey SL2. Many positively stained cells (arrows) show significant cytopathological changes with degeneration and disruption. Hemosiderin (H) pigments are identified in many hepatocytes. No tissue inflammatory reaction is found. (×880.)

an attempt to reisolate the VLIA/incognitus strain from the infected monkey, we cocultivated peripheral blood mononuclear cells from the moribund monkeys with normal human peripheral mononuclear cells, NIH 3T3 cells, and monkey BSC cells. No VLIA/incognitus strain was recovered. We also did not detect any evidence of retroviruses in these cultures.

It is remarkable that although all the VLIA/incognitus strain-inoculated monkeys suffered a systemic mycoplasmal infection, there was no acute inflammatory lesion or prominent reactive process, other than the atypical antibody responses, in any of the tissues examined at necropsy. The mycoplasma might have infected a key component(s) of the host immune system, resulting in a defective immune response, or might have special biological properties and mechanisms which either block or elude the immune surveillance of the infected host.

RESPIRATORY DISTRESS SYNDROME AND SYSTEMIC DISEASE ASSOCIATED WITH *M. FERMENTANS* INFECTION

Our laboratory reported a previously unrecognized fulminant disease apparently associated with systemic *M. fermentans* infection (40). Previously healthy HIV-negative patients, without any known risk of AIDS disease, presented with flulike illness, deteriorated rapidly, and developed adult respiratory distress syndrome and/or systemic disease with multiple organ failure (40). The clinical laboratory studies in these

patients included exhaustive pre- and postmortem blood and biopsy tissue cultures for bacterial, fungal, and viral agents and complete serological screening for a spectrum of likely infectious agents, including bacteria, viruses, rickettsia, chlamydia, and *M. pneumoniae*. As the disease rapidly progressed, some patients presented clinical pictures of disseminated intravascular coagulation. Clinicians taking care of these patients and pathologists studying the cases believed the patients were dying of a fulminant infectious process. However, no etiological agent could be identified. More remarkably, postmortem examinations showed histopathological lesions of extensive necrosis involving lung, liver, spleen, lymph nodes, adrenal glands, heart, and brain in these patients. Again, no viral, bacterial, fungal, or parasitic agent could be identified in the lesions or in the diseased tissues by routine histopathological workups for various infectious agents.

In this study, *M. fermentans* was identified and found to be concentrated in the advancing margins of necrosis in the diseased tissues by immunohistochemistry using specific antibodies raised against the incognitus strain of *M. fermentans* (38). In situ hybridization assays using cloned incognitus strain DNA (psb-2.2) as a probe, as described in the earlier section, also detected *M. fermentans* DNA in the advancing margins of the necrotizing lesions (Fig. 10). Furthermore, mycoplasmalike particles were also found intracellularly and extracellularly in the histopathological lesions by electron microscopy. Therefore, we believe there is a previously unrecognized human mycoplasma disease asso-

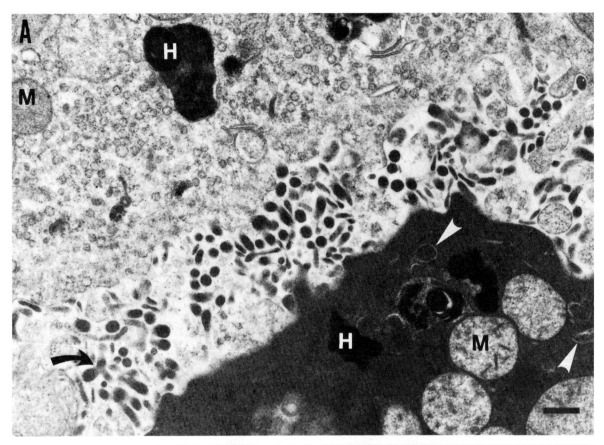

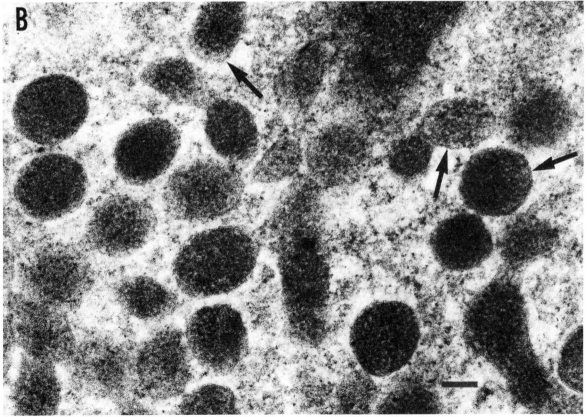

ciated with systemic *M. fermentans* infections which might lead to a fatal outcome in apparently non-immunocompromised, previously healthy patients.

Two similar cases of previously healthy, non-HIV-infected patients found to have systemic infection with *M. fermentans* were also recently reported (4, 39). One patient recovered after a nearly fatal course of adult respiratory distress syndrome as well as multiple organ failure (4). The other patient had extensive necrotizing lesions in spleen and liver associated with *M. fermentans* infection (Fig. 11). This young man also developed pulmonary symptoms. Fortunately, following splenectomy and liver wedge biopsy, he was diagnosed in time and treated successfully with doxycycline (39). His liver function returned to normal and he regained 40 lb of previously lost weight. He has been followed closely for more than 20 months without any sign of relapse.

After the unusual cases were reported to have a hidden systemic infection with *M. fermentans*, we started to receive some potential cases with similar clinico-pathological presentations submitted from outside pathologists and infectious disease experts. Some of these cases have been confirmed by immunohistochemistry, PCR assay, and electron microscopy to have fulminant pulmonary as well as systemic infection with *M. fermentans*. The infected lungs revealed histopathological changes closely resembling those commonly seen in pneumonitis of patients with AIDS. The typical cases will be presented in the future. Recently, R. Dular of Ottawa, Ontario, Canada, reported approximately 30 isolations of *M. fermentans* from previously healthy non-AIDS patients who had a sudden onset of a severe and often fatal form of respiratory distress syndrome (21). These isolations were made among approximately 150 clinical pulmonary specimens submitted to the Ontario Laboratory of Hygiene in a period of 8 to 9 months. *M. fermentans* was often isolated without any other etiological agent. The finding supports our earlier contention that there is a fulminant form of human disease with adult respiratory distress syndrome and/or multiple organ failure which is associated with pulmonary and systemic *M. fermentans* infection.

POSSIBLE ROLE OF MYCOPLASMAS IN AIDS DISEASE

We find that the pathogenesis of mycoplasmal infection per se is complicated and atypical. In *M. fer-*

mentans infection, the histopathology of infected tissues from experimental animals and patients ranged from no pathological change to fulminant necrosis with or without an associated inflammatory tissue reaction. We believe this unusual form of pathogenesis is likely due to one of two mechanisms: either the mycoplasmal infection concomitantly causes damage to key components of the hosts' immune system, or the pathogen has special biological properties to elude the immunosurveillance of the infected hosts. Although the role of *M. fermentans* infection and its actual relationship with AIDS disease or HIV-1 infection is not clear, the findings of systemic infection by direct identification of the pathogen in brain, liver, spleen, or thymus of these patients should be clinically important.

There are three general possibilities for the potential significance of infections with the AIDS-associated mycoplasmas. First, the mycoplasmas could simply represent opportunistic infections found in immunocompromised patients with AIDS. Second, infections with mycoplasmas such as *M. fermentans* and *M. penetrans* markedly enhance the pathogenicity of other human viruses including HIV-1, a phenomenon demonstrated in in vitro studies. Therefore, infections with some species of mycoplasma may promote the disease progression of AIDS. Finally, it is possible that the microbe itself is pathogenic in humans. This final consideration is supported by our findings in the animal experiment using nonhuman primates and by the association between *M. fermentans* infection and those previously healthy non-AIDS patients dying of an acute disease. The newly found *M. penetrans*, which has all the properties associated with virulence in pathogenic mollicutes, may also be pathogenic in its own right.

It is important to note that mycoplasmal infection is still highly significant clinically in AIDS, even if it is merely one more example of an opportunistic infection. It is pathological to have an infectious agent growing in our organ systems such as liver, kidney, spleen, lung, or brain. After all, opportunistic infections are the direct cause of death in more than 80% of patients with AIDS. Needless to say, the findings of mycoplasmal infection become more significant if the microbe is acting as a disease-promoting cofactor or is itself responsible for certain pathogenic aspects of AIDS. In view of the complex disease process of AIDS, we believe that the mycoplasma may well have a role in all the above three processes.

Figure 9. Electron microscopic identification of *M. fermentans* (incognitus strain) in the liver of experimentally infected monkeys. (A) Low-magnification electron micrograph of the liver of monkey SL2. A degenerating cell with cytopathic changes is shown to be highly electron dense (right lower corner). An adjacent hepatocyte (left upper corner) appears to be unremarkable. Structures of mitochondria (M) and hemosiderin pigments (H) are identified in both cells. Numerous electron-dense polymorphic mycoplasmalike particles are seen between these two cells. Occasional branching structures (curved arrow) can be found among the pleomorphic mycoplasmalike structures. Many mycoplasmalike particles (arrowheads) which cannot be distinguished from the extracellular particles are also identified in the degenerating cell. Bar, 800 nm. (B) High magnification of the mycoplasmalike particles, many with identifiable outer limiting membrane (arrows), which are found in large numbers in some areas of the sinusoidal space. Bar, 100 nm.

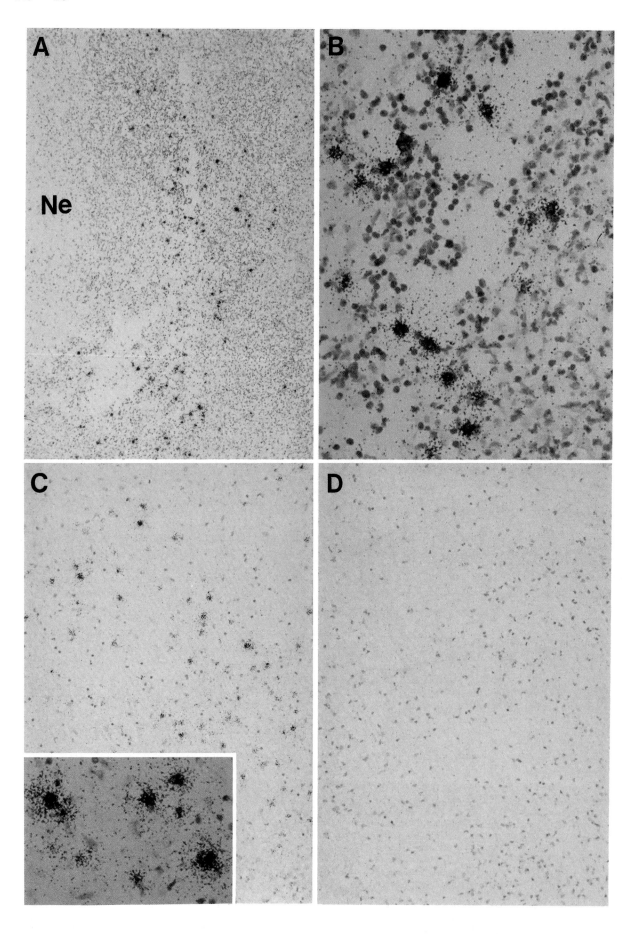

TREATMENT OF *M. FERMENTANS* INFECTION

Diseases associated with infections by the previously unrecognized procaryotic agents may potentially be amenable to proper antibiotic treatment. Thus, treatment of AIDS disease should also include treatment of the mycoplasmas. Quantitative assay of the susceptibility of *M. fermentans* (incognitus strain) in SP-4 broth cultures to representative antibiotics has revealed that the microbe is not susceptible to erythromycin, the most commonly used antibiotic for human mycoplasmal infections (30, 48). In vitro testing showed the incognitus strain to have various degrees of sensitivity to the antibiotics tetracycline, doxycycline, chloramphenicol, clindamycin, lincomycin, and ciprofloxacin (30, 48). Ciprofloxacin appeared to be the most effective. More recently, we have examined 24 different strains of *M. fermentans*, including 10 clinical isolates from either patients with AIDS or previously healthy non-AIDS patients having an acute fatal disease, for their antibiotic susceptibility in vitro. The findings are consistent with our earlier study of the incognitus strain. None of these isolates was found to be sensitive to erythromycin. They showed various degrees of susceptibility to tetracycline and doxycycline. The quinolones ciprofloxacin and ofloxacin had the best effect against all the isolates of *M. fermentans* in the assays (unpublished data). Quinolones were also found to be most effective against many other species of mycoplasma.

Appropriate reservation and caution is always necessary in extrapolating in vitro biological results to in vivo clinical conditions. It is well known that while mycoplasma infections can be suppressed by treatment with antibiotics, they are nonetheless extremely difficult to eradicate (66). Our report of successful treatment by antibiotics in a previously healthy non-AIDS patient with fulminant *M. fermentans* infection (39) may reflect a still intact immune system. Mycoplasma infections in patients with AIDS who lack a functional immune system could be very refractory to antibiotic treatments, even with high dose and a long course. Selection of resistant strains following prolonged treatment with antibiotics, without complete eradication of the mycoplasmas, in immune-compromised patients with AIDS is a major concern. The presence of bacterial IS-like elements in *M. fermentans* may provide an effective genetic mechanism to rapidly develop antibiotic-resistant traits. The true efficacy of antimicrobial treatments in immunocompromised AIDS patients infected by mycoplasmas is awaiting systematic clinical trials. It is also necessary to continue the search for more effective antibiotics which can eradicate the organisms from infected patients.

CONCLUSION

In an attempt to explain some of the complex disease processes, a few investigators cite indirect effects of mycoplasma infections as having a role in AIDS. Recently, a mitogenic antigen of *Mycoplasma arthritidis* (MAM) was found to act as a superantigen (14, 15). Montagnier reported that lymphocytes isolated from patients with AIDS appeared to undergo programmed cell death (apoptosis) in vitro, as compared with lymphocytes isolated from non-AIDS, normal subjects. The mechanism responsible for apoptosis is still not clear but is apparently not due to direct cell killing by HIV-1. Montagnier proposes that mycoplasmas, acting as superantigens, may trigger apoptosis of the CD4$^+$ lymphocytes in patients with AIDS, leading to immune suppression. To better understand the role of mycoplasma infections in AIDS, in the future we must continue to learn the fundamental biology of this group of unique organisms so that we may improve our diagnostic techniques in molecular genetics, serology, tissue diagnosis, and isolation techniques by culture. In addition, we may have to develop a convincing animal model to show evidence of immune suppression, wasting syndrome, and tumor development associated with infections with mycoplasma(s), to conclusively document their role in AIDS.

Mycoplasmas may be the only group of procaryotic organisms which are able to grow symbiotically with eucaryotic cells, in vitro as well as in vivo, without producing profound cytotoxicity or provoking marked host response. However, chronic persistent infection with the organisms in a eucaryotic system may gradually, yet significantly, alter the biology and physiology of mammalian cells in culture as well as affect the normal functions of various organs in infected patients. The previously unrecognized pathobiological effects of these hidden agents deserve further studies. Recent findings have already opened the exciting possibility that these long-ignored organisms may have an important role in human disease process. Because of the unusual features of these organisms, which in many ways are different from either viruses or bacteria, documentation of their infections in humans remains difficult. Although much has been learned, much more needs to be done before we can reach a conclusion. With the rapid development of new molecular techniques, scientists may now have a chance to

Figure 10. In situ hybridization for *M. fermentans* DNA in the necrotizing lesion of splenic tissue from a previously healthy non-AIDS patient having a fulminant systemic disease. (A) Strong labeling of cells is seen at the peripheral zone surrounding the area of necrosis (Ne). The labeling in this area is significantly higher than the background level of grains in the necrotic center or in outside areas where there is no necrosis. (×76.5.) (B) Higher magnification of panel A. Dense clusters of grains can be seen over numerous cells in this area. (×422.) (C) Occasional positive labeling can be seen in an area with diffuse necrosis in the spleen from the same patient as in panels A and B. Most of the labeling is associated with residual cells which are apparently still viable. (×150.) Insert shows a higher magnification of the positively labeled cells which contain dense cluster of grains. (×422.) (D) The same area as panel C in the consecutive tissue section, hybridized with ^{32}S-labeled cloning vector DNA which does not contain psb-2.2 *M. fermentans* DNA. (×150.) (From reference 40.)

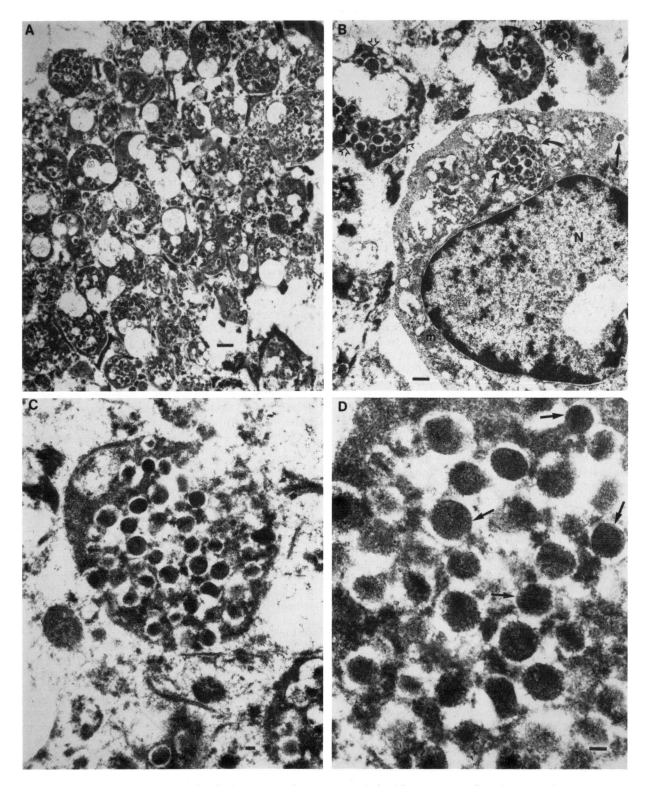

Figure 11. Electron micrographs of splenic tissues from a previously healthy, non-HIV-infected patient. There were extensive necrotizing lesions in the patient's liver and spleen. Immunohistochemical staining was highly positive for *M. fermentans*-specific antigen at the advancing margin of necrosis. (A) Margin of necrosis in spleen reveals numerous mycoplasmalike particles in fragments of cytoplasm from disrupted cells. Bar, 800 nm. (B) Clusters of typical mycoplasmalike particles (curved arrows) can be identified in the cytoplasm of intact mononuclear cells and in cytoplasmic fragments of disrupted cells (open arrows). The particles are also in membrane-bound vesicles (solid straight arrows) in the cells. Bar, 500 nm. (C and D) Higher magnification of electron micrographs showing the typical ultrastructure of *M. fermentans* particles. The limiting membrane (arrows) of some particles can still be recognized in specimens retrieved from Formalin-fixed, paraffin-embedded tissues. Bar, 100 nm. (From reference 39.)

unravel the significance of these extraordinary organisms in various human diseases, including the complex AIDS disease.

Acknowledgments. I thank my research associates in the laboratory, my scientific collaborators, and Douglas J. Wear for making possible the studies performed in my laboratory and described in this review. The work is supported in part by National Institute of Allergy and Infectious Diseases grant R01 AI-31830.

REFERENCES

1. **Barré-Sinoussi, F., J. C. Chermann, F. Rey, M. T. Nugeyre, S. Chamaret, J. Gruest, C. Dauguet, C. Axler-Blin, F. Vézinet-Brun, C. Rouzioux, W. Rozenbaum, and L. Montagnier.** 1983. Isolation of a T-lymphotrophic retrovirus from a patient at risk for acquired immune deficiency syndrome (AIDS). *Science* **220:**868–870.

2. **Baseman, J. B., S. F. Dallo, J. G. Tully, and D. L. Rose.** 1988. Isolation and characterization of *Mycoplasma genitalium* strains from the human respiratory tract. *J. Clin. Microbiol.* **26:**2266–2269.

3. **Bauer, F. A., D. J. Wear, P. Angritt, and S.-C. Lo.** 1991. *Mycoplasma fermentans* (incognitus strain) infection in the kidneys of patients with acquired immunodeficiency syndrome and associated nephropathy: a light microscopic, immunohistochemical and ultrastructural study. *Hum. Pathol.* **22:**63–69.

4. **Beecham, H. J., III, S.-C. Lo, D. E. Lewis, S. W. Comer, K. J. Riley, and E. C. Oldfield III.** 1991. Recovery from fulminant infection with *Mycoplasmas fermentans* (incognitus strain) in non-immunocompromised host. *Lancet* **338:**1014–1015.

5. **Biberfeld, G., and E. Nilsson.** 1978. Mitogenicity of *Mycoplasma fermentans* for human lymphocytes. *Infect. Immun.* **21:**48–54.

6. **Cassell, G. H., and B. C. Cole.** 1981. Mycoplasmas as agents of human disease. *N. Engl. J. Med.* **304:**80–89.

7. **Cassell, G. H., and A. Hill.** 1979. Murine and other small-animal mycoplasmas, p. 235–273. *In* J. G. Tully and R. F. Whitcomb (ed.), *The Mycoplasmas*, vol. 2. Academic Press, Inc., New York.

8. **Centers for Disease Control.** 1985. Revision of the case definition of acquired immunodeficiency syndrome for national reporting—United States. *Morbid. Mortal. Weekly Rep.* **34:**373–375.

9. **Centers for Disease Control.** 1987. Revision of the CDC surveillance case definition for acquired immunodeficiency syndrome. *JAMA* **258:**1143–1154.

10. **Chirgwin, K. D., M. C. Cummings, L. R. De Meol, M. Murphy, and W. M. McCormack.** Identification of mycoplasmas in urine of HIV-infected persons. *Clin. Infect. Dis.* (Suppl.) **16,** in press.

11. **Chowdhury, I. H., T. Munakata, Y. Koyanagi, S. Kobayashi, S. Arai, and N. Yamamoto.** 1990. Mycoplasma can enhance HIV replication *in vitro*: a possible cofactor responsible for the progression of AIDS. *Biochem. Biophys. Res. Commun.* **3:**1365–1370.

12. **Clyde, W. A., Jr.** 1979. *Mycoplasma pneumoniae* infections of man, p. 275–306. *In* J. G. Tully and R. F. Whitcomb (ed.), *The Mycoplasmas*, vol. 2. Academic Press, Inc., New York.

13. **Cole, B. C., and C. L. Atkin.** 1991. The *Mycoplasma arthritidis* T-cell mitogen, MAM: a model superantigen. *Immunol. Today* **12:**271–276.

14. **Cole, B. C., D. R. Kartchner, and D. J. Wells.** 1990. Stimulation of mouse lymphocytes by a mitogen derived from *Mycoplasma arthritidis* (MAM). VIII. Selective activation of T cells expressing distinct V_β T cell receptors from various strains of mice by the "superantigen" MAM. *J. Immunol.* **144:**425–431.

15. **Cole, B. C., and J. R. Ward.** 1979. Mycoplasmas as arthri-

togenic agents, p. 367–398. *In* J. G. Tully and R. F. Whitcomb (ed.), *The Mycoplasmas*, vol. 2. Academic Press, Inc., New York.

16. **D'Agati, V., J. I. Suh, L. Carbone, J. T. Cheng, and G. Appel.** 1989. Pathology of HIV-associated nephropathy: a detailed morphologic and comparative study. *Kidney Int.* **35:**1358–1370.

17. **Dallo, S. F., C. J. Su, J. R. Horton, and J. B. Baseman.** 1988. Identification of P1 gene domain containing epitope(s) mediating *Mycoplasma pneumoniae* cytadherence. *J. Exp. Med.* **167:**718–723.

18. **Dawson, M. S., M. M. Hayes, R. Y.-H. Wang, D. Armstrong, R. B. Kundsin, and S.-C. Lo.** Detection and isolation of *Mycoplasma fermentans* from urine of HIV-1 infected patients. *Arch. Pathol. Lab. Med.*, in press.

19. **Del Giudice, R. A., J. G. Tully, D. L. Rose, and R. M. Cole.** 1985. *Mycoplasma pirum* sp. nov., a terminal structured mollicute from cell cultures. *Int. J. Syst. Bacteriol.* **35:**285–291.

20. **Duesberg, P. H.** 1989. Human immunodeficiency virus and acquired immunodeficiency syndrome: correlation but not causation. *Proc. Natl. Acad. Sci. USA* **86:**755–764.

21. **Dular, R.** *Mycoplasma fermentans* disease in the respiratory tract of non-AIDS patients. *Clin. Infect. Dis.* (Suppl.) **16,** in press.

22. **Editorial.** 1991. Mycoplasma and AIDS—what connection? *Lancet* **337:**20–22.

23. **Fernald, G. W.** 1979. Humoral and cellular immune responses to mycoplasmas, p. 399–424. *In* J. G. Tully and R. F. Whitcomb (ed.), *The Mycoplasmas*, vol. 2. Academic Press, Inc., New York.

24. **Gabridge, M. G.** 1974. Role of gram-negative sepsis in lethal toxicity induced by *Mycoplasma. J. Infect. Dis.* **130:**529–533.

25. **Gabridge, M. G., G. D. Abrams, and W. H. Murphy.** 1972. Lethal toxicity of *Mycoplasma fermentans* for mice. *J. Infect. Dis.* **125:**153–160.

26. **Gabridge, M. G., and P. R. Schneider.** 1975. Cytotoxic effect of *Mycoplasma fermentans* on mouse thymocytes. *Infect. Immun.* **11:**460–465.

27. **Gallo, R. C., and F. Wong-Staal.** 1985. A human T-lymphotropic retrovirus (HTLV-III) as the cause of the acquired immunodeficiency syndrome. *Ann. Intern. Med* **103:**679–689.

28. **Gourlay, R. N., and C. J. Howard.** 1979. Bovine mycoplasmas, p. 49-102. *In* J. G. Tully and R. F. Whitcomb (ed.), *The Mycoplasmas*, vol. 2. Academic Press, Inc., New York.

29. **Hawkins, R. E., L. S. Rickman, S. H. Vermund, and M. Carl.** 1992. Association of mycoplasma and human immunodeficiency virus infection: detection of amplified-*Mycoplasma fermentans* DNA in blood. *J. Infect. Dis.* **165:**581–585.

30. **Hayes, M. M., D. J. Wear, and S.-C. Lo.** 1991. *In vitro* antimicrobial susceptibility testing for the newly identified AIDS-associated mycoplasma—*Mycoplasma fermentans* (incognitus strain). *Arch. Pathol. Lab. Med.* **115:**464–466.

31. **Hu, P. C., U. Schaper, A. M. Collier, W. A. Clyde, Jr., M. Horikawa, Y. S. Huang, and M. F. Barile.** 1987. A *Mycoplasma genitalium* protein resembling *Mycoplasma pneumoniae* attachment protein. *Infect. Immun.* **55:**1126–1131.

32. **Hu, W. S., R. Y.-H. Wang, R.-S. Liou, J. W.-K. Shih, and S.-C. Lo.** 1990. Identification of an insertion-sequence-like genetic element in the newly recognized human pathogen *Mycoplasma incognitus*. *Gene* **93:**67–72.

33. **Kenny, G. E.** 1985. Mycoplasmas, p. 407–411. *In* E. H. Lennette, A. Balows, W. J. Hausler, Jr., and H. J. Shadomy (ed.), *Manual of Clinical Microbiology*, 4th ed. American Society for Microbiology, Washington, D.C.

34. **Lane, H. C., and A. S. Fauci.** 1985. Immunologic abnormalities in the acquired immunodeficiency syndrome. *Annu. Rev. Immunol.* **3:**477–500.

35. **Leach, R. H., A. Hales, P. M. Furr, D. L. Mitchelmore, and D. Taylor-Robinson.** 1987. Problems in the identification of *Mycoplasma prium* isolated from human lyphoblastoid cell cultures. *FEMS Microbiol. Lett.* **44**:293–297.

36. **Lemaître, M., D. Guétard, Y. Hénin, L. Montagnier, and A. Zerial.** 1990. Protective activity of tetracycline analogs against the cytopathic effect of the human immunodeficiency viruses in CEM cells. *Res. Virol.* **141**:5–16.

37. **Lemaître, M., Y. Hénin, F. Destouesse, C. Ferrieux, L. Montagnier, and A. Blanchard.** 1992. Role of mycoplasma infection in the cytopathic effect induced by human immunodeficiency virus type 1 in infected cell lines. *Infect. Immun.* **60**:742–748.

38. **Lind, K.** 1983. Manifestations and complications of *Mycoplasma pneumoniae* disease: a review. *Yale J. Biol. Med.* **56**:461–468.

39. **Lo, S.-C., C. L. Buchholz, D. J. Wear, R. C. Hohm, and A. M. Marty.** 1991. Histopathology and doxycycline treatment in a previously healthy non-AIDS patient systemically infected by *Mycoplasma fermentans* (incognitus strain). *Mod. Pathol.* **6**:750–754.

40. **Lo, S.-C., M. S. Dawson, P. B. Newton III, M. A. Sonoda, J. W.-K. Shih, W. F. Engler, R. Y.-H. Wang, and D. J. Wear.** 1989. Association of the virus-like infectious agent originally reported in patients with AIDS with acute fatal disease in previously healthy non-AIDS patients. *Am. J. Trop. Med. Hyg.* **41**:364–376.

41. **Lo, S.-C., M. S. Dawson, D. M. Wong, P. B. Newton III, M. A. Sonoda, W. F. Engler, R. Y.-H. Wang, J. W.-K. Shih, H. J. Alter, and D. J. Wear.** 1989. Identification of *Mycoplasma incognitus* infection in patients with AIDS: an immunohistochemical, in situ hybridization and ultrastructural study. *Am. J. Trop. Med. Hyg.* **41**:601–616.

42. **Lo, S.-C., M. M. Hayes, J. G. Tully, R. Y.-H. Wang, H. Kotani, P. F. Pierce, D. L. Rose, and J. W.-K. Shih.** 1992. *Mycoplasma penetrans* sp. nov. from the urogenital tract of patients with AIDS. *Int. J. Syst. Bacteriol.* **42**:357–364.

43. **Lo, S.-C., M. M. Hayes, R. Y.-H. Wang, P. F. Pierce, H. Kotani, and J. W.-K. Shih.** 1991. Newly discovered mycoplasma isolated from patients infected with HIV. *Lancet* **338**:1415–1418.

44. **Lo, S.-C., J. W.-K. Shih, P. B. Newton III, D. M. Wong, M. M. Hayes, J. R. Benish, D. J. Wear, and R. Y.-H. Wang.** 1989. Virus-like infectious agent (VLIA) is a novel pathogenic mycoplasma: *Mycoplasma incognitus. Am. J. Trop. Med. Hyg.* **41**:586–600.

45. **Lo, S.-C., J. W.-K. Shih, N. Y. Yang, C. Y. Ou, and R. Y.-H. Wang.** 1989. A novel virus-like infectious agent in patients with AIDS. *Am. J. Trop. Med. Hyg.* **40**:213–226.

46. **Lo, S.-C., S. Tsai, J. R. Benish, J. W.-K. Shih, D. J. Wear, and D. M. Wong.** 1991. Enhancement of HIV-1 cytocidal effects in CD$_4$ $^+$ lymphocytes by the AIDS-associated mycoplasma. *Science* **251**:1074–1076.

47. **Lo, S.-C., R. Y.-H. Wang, P. B. Newton III, N. Y. Yang, M. A. Sonoda, and J. W.-K. Shih.** 1989. Fatal infection of silvered leaf monkeys with a virus-like infectious agent (VLIA) derived from a patient with AIDS. *Am. J. Trop. Med. Hyg.* **40**:399–409.

48. **Lo, S.-C., D. J. Wear, and M. M. Hayes.** 1990. *In vitro* antimicrobial susceptibility testing for the newly identified pathogenic human mycoplasma, *M. incognitus. The VI International Conference on AIDS*, abstr. no. Th.b 536.

49. **Loo, V. G., S. Richardson, and P. Quinn.** 1991. Isolation of *Mycoplasma pneumoniae* from pleural fluid. *Diagn. Microbiol. Infect. Dis.* **14**:443–445.

50. **Maddox, J.** 1991. News and views: AIDS research turned upside down. *Nature* (London) **353**:297.

51. **Madoff, S., and D. C. Hooper.** 1988. Nongenitourinary infections caused by *Mycoplasma hominis* in adults. *Rev. Infect. Dis.* **10**:602–611.

52. **Montagnier, L., D. Berneman, D. Guétard, A. Blanchard, S. Chamaret, V. Rame, J. Van Rietschoten, K. Mabrouk, and E. Bahraoui.** 1990. Inhibition of HIV prototype strains infectivity by antibodies directed against a peptidic sequence of mycoplasma. *C.R. Acad. Sci. Paris* **311**:425–430.

53. **Montagnier, L., A. Blanchard, D. Guétard, D. Berneman, M. Lemaître, A.-M. DiRienzo, S. Chamaret, Y. Hénin, E. Bahraoui, C. Dauguet, C. Axler, M. Kirstetter, R. Roue, G. Pialoux, and D. Dupont.** 1990. A possible role of mycoplasmas as co-factors in AIDS, p. 9–17. *In* M. Girard and L. Valette (ed.), *Retroviruses of Human AIDS and Related Animal Diseases: Proceedings of the Colloque des Cent Gardes.* Foundation M. Merieux, Lyons, France.

54. **Murphy, W. H., C. Bullis, L. Dabich, R. Heyn, and C. J. D. Zarafonetis.** 1970. Isolation of mycoplasma from leukemic and nonleukemic patients. *J. Natl. Cancer Inst.* **45**:243–251.

55. **Nagayama, Y., N. Sakurai, K. Tamai, A. Niwa, and K. Yamamoto.** 1987. Isolation of *Mycoplasma pneumoniae* from pleural fluid and/or cerebrospinal fluid: report of four cases. *Scand. J. Infect. Dis.* **19**:521–524.

56. **Nair, J. M. G., R. Bellevue, M. Bertoni, and H. Dosik.** 1988. Thrombotic thrombocytopenic purpura in patients with the acquired immunodeficiency syndrome (AIDS)-related complex. *Ann. Intern. Med.* **109**:209–212.

57. **Navia, B. A., B. D. Jordan, and R. W. Price.** 1986. The AIDS dementia complex. I. Clinical features. *Ann. Neurol.* **19**:517–524.

58. **O'Toole, C., and M. Lowdell.** 1990. Infection of human T cells with mycoplasma, inhibition of CD$_4$ expression and HIV-1 gp 120 glycoprotein binding, and infectivity. *Lancet* **336**:1067.

59. **Plata, E. J., M. R. Abell, and W. H. Murphy.** 1973. Induction of leukemoid disease in mice by *Mycoplasma fermentans. J. Infect. Dis.* **128**:588–597.

60. **Ponka, A.** 1979. The occurrence and clinical picture of serologically verified *Mycoplasma pneumoniae* infections with emphasis on central nervous system, cardiac and joint manifestations. *Ann. Clin. Res.* **11**(Suppl. 24):1–60.

61. **Reichert, C. M., T. J. O'Leary, D. L. Levens, C. R. Simrell, and A. M. Macher.** 1983. Autopsy pathology in the acquired immune deficiency syndrome. *Am. J. Pathol.* **112**:357–382.

62. **Root-Bernstein, R. S., and S. H. Hobbs.** 1991. Homologies between mycoplasma adhesion peptide, CD4 and class II MHC proteins: a possible mechanism for HIV-mycoplasma synergism in AIDS. *Res. Immunol.* **142**:519–523.

63. **Ruiter, M., and H. M. M. Wentholt.** 1950. A pleuropneumonia-like organism in primary fusospirochetal gangrene of the penis. *J. Invest. Dermatol.* **15**:301–304.

64. **Ruiter, M., and H. M. M. Wentholt.** 1953. Isolation of a pleuropneumonia-like organism (G-strain) in a case of fusospirillary vulvovaginitis. *Acta Derm. Venereol.* **33**:123–129.

65. **Salahuddin, S. Z., P. D. Markham, M. Popovic, M. G. Sarngadharan, S. Orndorff, A. Fladagar, A. Patel, J. Gold, and R. C. Gallo.** 1985. Isolation of infectious human T-cell leukemia/lymphotropic virus type III (HTLV-III) from patients with acquired immunodeficiency syndrome (AIDS) or AIDS-related complex (ARC) and from healthy carriers: a study of risk groups and tissue sources. *Proc. Natl. Acad. Sci. USA* **82**:5530–5534.

66. **Smith, C. B., W. T. Friedewald, and R. M. Chanock.** 1967. Shedding of *Mycoplasma pneumoniae* after tetracycline and erythromycin therapy. *N. Engl. J. Med.* **276**:1172–1175.

67. **Taylor-Robinson, D.** 1989. Genital mycoplasma infections. *Clin. Lab. Med.* **9**:501–523.

68. **Tully, J. G., D. Taylor-Robinson, R. M. Cole, and D. L. Rose.** 1981. A newly discovered mycoplasma in the human urogenital tract. *Lancet* **i**:1288–1291.

69. **Tully, J. G., D. Taylor-Robinson, D. L. Rose, P. M. Furr, and D. A. Hawkins.** 1983. Evaluation of culture media for recovery of *Mycoplasma hominis* from the human urogenital tract. *Sex. Transm. Dis.* (Suppl.) **10:**256–260.

70. **Wang, R. Y.-H., W. S. Hu, M. S. Dawson, J. W.-K. Shih, and S.-C. Lo.** 1992. Selective detection of *Mycoplasma fermentans* by the polymerase chain reaction and by using a nucleotide sequence within the insertion sequence-like element. *J. Clin. Microbiol.* **30:**245–248.

71. **Wang, R. Y.-H., and S.-C. Lo.** Detection of *Mycoplasma fermentans* infection in blood and urine by polymerase chain reaction. *In* D. H. Persing (ed.), *Diagnostic Molecular Microbiology,* in preparation. American Society for Microbiology, Washington, D.C.

72. **World Health Organization Workshop.** 1985. Leads from the MMWR: conclusion and recommendations on acquired immunodeficiency syndrome. *JAMA* **253:**3385–3386.

73. **Wright, K.** 1990. Research news: Mycoplasma in the AIDS spotlight. *Science* **248:**682–683.

VII. EVOLUTION

33. Phylogeny of Mycoplasmas

JACK MANILOFF

Nature will try anything once.... If you're dealing with organic compounds, then let them combine. If it works, if it quickens, set it clacking in the grass; there's always room for one more...

Annie Dillard (1974)

INTRODUCTION

Since the earliest studies of mycoplasmas, there have been questions about the nature of these small cells and their relationship to other microorganisms, such as free-living bacteria, obligate intracellular microbial parasites (e.g., the rickettsias), and viruses (reviewed in reference 15). The problems in understanding mycoplasmas reflected experimental difficulties in studying these organisms, absence of molecular methods for elaborating the physiology and genetics of both bacteria and mycoplasmas, and inability to apply evolutionary concepts to microbiology.

In the mid-1970s, as many of the details of bacterial biochemistry and physiology were being resolved, experimental methods for studying microbial molecular evolution were developed and reconstruction of the bacterial phylogenetic tree began. At that time, two models had been formulated for mycoplasma evolution. The first model, proposed by Neimark (45–47), was that mycoplasmas were polyphyletic and, presumably, had arisen by degenerate evolution. In this model, mycoplasmas would have arisen after evolution and diversification of the bacteria, with different mycoplasmas originating from different branches of the bacterial phylogenetic tree. Therefore, according to this model, different mycoplasma species are not phylogenetically related; instead, each mycoplasma species was thought to be a branch of a different part of the bacterial phylogenetic tree. This model was, in part, a variation on an idea going back to 1935, that mycoplasmas may be stable L-phase variants of bacteria (reviewed in references 15, 27, and 60).

The second model, proposed by Morowitz and Wallace (41, 69), was that mycoplasmas arose very early in the evolution of living forms on Earth and ancestral mycoplasmas were precursors of the bacteria. At the time this model was put forward, mycoplasma genomes were believed to be in two size ranges, 700 to 800 and 1,500 to 1,600 kb, and this model proposed that successive duplications of an ancestral 700 to 800-kb mycoplasma genome, with subsequent genome variation, led to the current distribution of microbial genome sizes. Hence, the 700- to 800-kb mycoplasma genome was postulated to be a primordial genome that duplicated to produce 1,500-kb mycoplasma genomes, and these in turn duplicated to produce bacterial genomes of several thousand kilobase pairs. Ancestral bacteria would have then arisen and diverged to form the present-day bacterial groups.

Since the late 1970s, it has been clear that neither of these models is correct. Instead, as described below, a different model of mycoplasma evolution was constructed by Woese, Maniloff, and coworkers from molecular evolution studies: the mycoplasma phylogenetic tree is monophyletic and arose from a branch of the gram-positive bacterial phylogenetic tree, and mycoplasma evolution has been by attrition, characterized by rapid evolution and decreasing genetic and physiological complexity.

Jack Maniloff • Department of Microbiology and Immunology, University of Rochester, Medical Center Box 672, Rochester, New York 14642.

549

EXPERIMENTAL APPROACHES TO MOLECULAR PHYLOGENY

In 1965, Zuckerkandl and Pauling (77) noted that cells contain a trace of their evolutionary history, their phylogeny, in their macromolecules. This is because physiological effects and errors inherent in DNA replication lead to base changes (mutations) in progeny DNA sequences, which provide a record of the organism's evolutionary history. Hence, comparison of DNA sequences gives a measure of the evolutionary distances of organisms from each other. Phylogenetic trees can then be reconstructed by analysis of these data (reviewed in references 12 and 44).

Although comparison of complete cell genome sequences was (and remains) an impractical project, several alternate sequence approaches have been used to obtain measures of molecular evolution. Since protein sequences represent transforms of specific gene base sequences, following the Zuckerkandl and Pauling paper, amino acid sequences of a few proteins (e.g., ferredoxin and cytochrome *c*) were determined and used to reconstruct phylogenetic trees. Unfortunately, this approach is limited to organisms containing the specific proteins chosen as phylogenetic measures. Finally, in the early 1970s, the advent of RNA sequencing and then DNA sequencing methods allowed base sequence information to be determined directly.

Woese and coworkers have delineated the criteria for phylogenetically useful genes or gene products (62, 63, 72): (i) the gene must be universally distributed, since every organism must contain the gene in order for it to be a universal phylogenetic measure, (ii) the gene product must have the same function in every organism, so that it has been under the same selective pressure in every organism, (iii) the gene must not be subject to significant lateral transfer, which would obviate its use as a phylogenetic measure, (iv) the gene base sequence must show clocklike behavior in terms of accumulating random base changes at a rate to allow changes over long genealogical times to be preserved, and (v) the gene or gene product must be readily isolated and sequenced for it to be an experimentally feasible phylogenetic measure.

The small ribosomal subunit rRNAs meet these requirements, and for the past two decades, Woese and coworkers have pioneered their use as phylogenetic measures and reconstructed increasingly detailed universal phylogenetic trees (reviewed in references 13 and 72). At first, oligonucleotide catalogs of 5S (62) and 16S (49) rRNAs were used; later, as sequencing methods developed, complete 5S (56) and 16S (31) rRNA sequences became the phylogenetic measures of choice. The 16S rRNA sequences have turned out to be the most useful phylogenetic tool because the longer 16S rRNA genes (about 1,540 bases) exhibit better clocklike behavior than do the smaller 5S rRNA genes (about 120 bases) and, quite serendipitously, 16S rRNAs contain two phylogenetic clocks (74). Some parts of the 16S rRNA sequence have evolved relatively slowly (i.e., have been conserved during microbial evolution), while other parts have evolved relatively rapidly. Hence, the slowly changing parts of the 16S rRNA sequence provide a phylogenetic measure of deep genealogical events, and the rapidly changing parts measure more recent genealogical events.

MYCOPLASMA PHYLOGENY

Construction of the Mycoplasma Phylogenetic Tree

In the 1970s, Woese, Maniloff, and coworkers began a series of collaborative studies of mycoplasma molecular phylogeny, in an attempt to choose between the two then current models of mycoplasma evolution (described above), i.e., that mycoplasmas were either polyphyletic degenerate bacteria or ancestors of a primitive microorganism that preceded the evolution of present-day bacteria. The former model predicts that different mycoplasma species are phylogenetically unrelated to each other and instead are related to different branches of the bacterial phylogenetic tree, and the latter model predicts that mycoplasma species are phylogenetically related to each other and are evolutionary precursors of all branches of the bacterial phylogenetic tree.

The earliest studies of Woese, Maniloff, and coworkers involved determination of 16S rRNA oligonucleotide catalogs of four mycoplasma species (representing the genera *Acholeplasma*, *Spiroplasma*, and *Mycoplasma*) and comparison of these data with those for other microorganisms. This effort led to publication of a preliminary report in 1978 (39) and a detailed paper in 1980 (75) presenting the first experimental description of the mycoplasma phylogenetic tree and showing that neither of the models previously proposed for mycoplasma evolution was correct. Instead, the results provided the outline of a new model for mycoplasma evolution, a model that has been confirmed and extended by subsequent studies (described below). The basic aspects of this model are as follows: (i) the mycoplasma phylogenetic tree is monophyletic, (ii) the mycoplasmas arose from a branch of the gram-positive eubacterial phylogenetic tree containing bacteria with DNAs having low G + C contents, and (iii) mycoplasma phylogeny has been characterized by a rapid rate of evolution (39, 75). This model had a significant impact on mycoplasma biology by providing a framework for organizing a variety of fragmentary data in the literature into a unified picture. It also explained the relationship of mycoplasmas to certain gram-positive bacteria that had been noted in studies of RNAs, enzymes, and lipids from diverse mycoplasma species (reviewed in reference 37).

Parenthetically, the 1980 phylogenetic study included *Thermoplasma acidophilum*, a wall-less, thermophilic, acidophilic microorganism, which was classified as a mycoplasma at that time. However, the phylogenetic results showed that *T. acidophilum* is an archaebacterium and not related to the mycoplasmas (75).

Subsequent studies by Woese, Maniloff, and coworkers confirmed their model, added additional mycoplasma species to the tree, and led to a more detailed picture of the mycoplasma phylogenetic tree. Improved mycoplasma phylogenetic trees based on complete 16S rRNA sequence data (70) were reported in 1985 for 10 mycoplasma species (representing the genera *Anaeroplasma*, *Acholeplasma*, *Spiroplasma*, *Mycoplasma*, and *Ureaplasma*) from complete 5S rRNA sequence data (51) and in 1989 for 45 mycoplasma species (representing all six mycoplasma genera [*Asteroplasma*, *Anaeroplasma*, *Acholeplasma*, *Spiro-*

plasma, Mycoplasma, and *Ureaplasma*]). An important recent addition to this tree, also based on 16S rRNA sequence data, has been location of a plant-pathogenic mycoplasmalike organism (MLO) on the *Acholeplasma* phylogenetic branch (35, 57). The current version of the mycoplasma phylogenetic tree is presented below.

Since the 1970s, a variety of data supporting this model for mycoplasma phylogeny have been reported by a number of different laboratories, each studying a few (generally only one) mycoplasma species and showing that some mycoplasma property was more similar to the same property in a gram-positive bacterium (e.g., *Bacillus subtilis*) than in a gram-negative bacterium (e.g., *Escherichia coli*). These properties have included lipid composition (17, 59, 61), 5S rRNA sequences (21, 67), tRNA sequences (2, 25, 26, 52–54, 68), tRNA gene organization (42, 52, 54), tRNA and rRNA methylation patterns (22), sensitivity to 6-(p-hydroxyphenylazo)-uracil (cited in reference 37), features of aromatic amino acid metabolism (4), specific transport systems (16), PP$_i$-dependent enzymes (50), and *tuf* gene copy number (58). In addition, sequence comparison of a tRNA from a single mycoplasma species (11, 32) and 5S rRNA from several mycoplasma species (8, 43) placed the mycoplasmas as a branch of the *B. subtilis* phylogenetic tree.

The Mycoplasma Phylogenetic Tree

The mycoplasma phylogenetic tree, based on currently available 16S rRNA sequence data, is shown in Fig. 1 to 9. This tree represents an improvement over the most recently published version of the mycoplasma phylogenetic tree (70) and was reconstructed

from 16S rRNA distance matrix data for these species (70, 73), wherein each matrix element is the number of base changes per 100 nucleotides between two microorganisms, corrected for multiple base changes and DNA base ratios (70). The tree topology was determined by the neighbor-joining method of Saitou and Nei (55), with branch lengths proportional to evolutionary distance (i.e., number of base changes).

Figure 1 is an overview of the mycoplasma phylogenetic tree, with closely related phylogenetic sublines grouped to facilitate visualization of the tree. These groupings, in part, reflect phenotypic similarities among phylogenetically related species and are different from those previously reported (70). The choice of species groupings used here allows biological implications of the mycoplasma phylogenetic tree to be more easily recognized, as discussed below. This tree is consistent with previously reported mycoplasma phylogenetic trees (37, 51, 70, 75), but the additional 16S rRNA sequence data and use of the neighbor-joining method to reconstruct the mycoplasma phylogenetic tree clarify a number of questions regarding tree topology, allow some questions about the phylogenetic order of the mycoplasmas to be resolved, and indicate apparent correlations between mycoplasma biology and phylogeny. On the basis of these data, the following conclusions regarding mycoplasma phylogeny can be stated.

Mycoplasma phylogeny is monophyletic, from the *Lactobacillus* group branch

The mycoplasma arose at a node on a branch of gram-positive bacteria having low G + C contents (Fig. 1), the *Lactobacillus* group. The *Lactobacillus* group

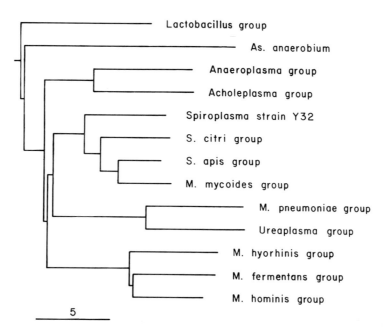

Figure 1. Mycoplasma phylogenetic tree reconstructed from 16S rRNA sequence comparisons, as described in the text. *E. coli* was used as an outgroup to establish the root of the tree. Closely related phylogenetic sublines have been grouped to facilitate visualization of the tree. Detailed phylogenetic trees of these groups are shown in Fig. 2 to 9. Branch lengths are proportional to evolutionary distance (i.e., number of base changes per 100 nucleotides). The scale at the bottom denotes the branch distance corresponding to five base changes per 100 nucleotides.

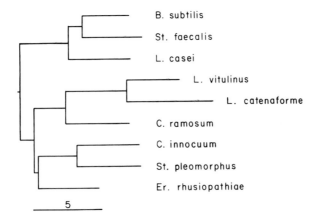

Figure 2. Detailed phylogenetic tree of the *Lactobacillus* group reconstructed from 16S rRNA sequence comparisons, as described in the text. This group contains *Bacillus*, *Lactobacillus*, and *Streptococcus* species, plus two unusual *Clostridium* species and *Erysipelothrix rhusiopathiae*. The scale at the bottom denotes the branch distance corresponding to five base changes per 100 nucleotides.

(Fig. 2) contains *Lactobacillus*, *Bacillus*, and *Streptococcus* species and two unusual *Clostridium* species, *Clostridium innocuum* and *C. ramosum*, which have been shown previously to be phylogenetically related to both the *Lactobacillus* group and the mycoplasmas (51, 70, 75).

Hence, the *Lactobacillus* group and the mycoplasmas had a common ancestor, represented by the node from which these two phylogenetic branches diverged. Mycoplasma phylogeny from this node must have been by degenerate evolution (i.e., evolution by attrition) from an organism having a *Lactobacillus* group type of bacterial cell wall and genome size (37, 75). Therefore, origin of the mycoplasma phylogenetic branch had to involve a significant reduction in genome size, presumably including loss of the genetic capability for cell wall synthesis. The question of whether loss of cell wall genes occurred as a single large deletion or under some type of selective pressure for sequential loss of these genes cannot be answered at present.

The mycoplasma phylogenetic order is *Asteroleplasma, Anaeroplasma* and *Acholeplasma, Spiroplasma, Mycoplasma,* and *Ureaplasma*

The phylogenetic tree (Fig. 1) suggests that mycoplasma genera arose to colonize new ecological niches as each became available during Earth's evolution. The deepest mycoplasma phylogenetic branch is to the sterol-nonrequiring, obligate anaerobic *Asteroleplasma* species (Fig. 1). Since the node of this branch is deeper than those of the aerobic eubacteria (13, 37), the *Asteroleplasma* branch must have originated while Earth still had a primitive reducing atmosphere. Hence, the *Asteroleplasma* branch clearly had an ecological niche different than the one it now occupies in animal rumens. The fact that *Asteroleplasma* is the deepest mycoplasma phylogenetic branch indicates that these organisms represent ancestral obligate anaerobic mycoplasmas rather than a more recent adap-

tation of mycoplasmas to anaerobic niches. This leaves unanswered the question of what niche *Asteroleplasma* species occupied between their origin on a planet with a reducing atmosphere and the evolution of ruminants.

The next phylogenetic branching was to the sterol-requiring, obligate anaerobic *Anaeroplasma* group and the sterol-nonrequiring, facultative anaerobic *Acholeplasma* group (Fig. 1 and 3). Present data cannot resolve the phylogenetic order of these two branches. The comments above about the *Asteroleplasma* niche also apply to the *Anaeroplasma* niche. The saprophytic *Acholeplasma* group presumably could have persisted in a variety of niches during the early stages of microbial evolution on Earth.

The question of whether origin of the mycoplasma requirement for sterol is monophyletic or polyphyletic cannot be resolved by the present tree. It has been suggested (37) that the sterol requirement in mycoplasmas arose by mutational loss of the capability for bacterial-type membrane polyterpenoid synthesis and adaptation to growth by incorporation of exogenous sterol. The bound sterol would be structurally and functionally equivalent to polyterpenoids and stabilize the cell membrane (48). If more recent mycoplasma phylogenetic lines arose from the *Anaeroplasma* branch, the most parsimonious explanation would be that the sterol requirement arose once, during *Anaeroplasma* evolution. However, if more recent mycoplasma phylogenetic lines arose from the *Acholeplasma* branch, the conclusion would be that the sterol requirement arose twice, once during *Anaeroplasma* evolution and once during *Spiroplasma* evolution. Whichever case turns out to be correct, origin of sterol-requiring mycoplasmas had to occur after formation of an oxygen-containing atmosphere on Earth (37), since sterol formation requires aerobic metabolism.

There is an additional subline on the *Acholeplasma* group phylogenetic branch that is not shown in Fig. 3.

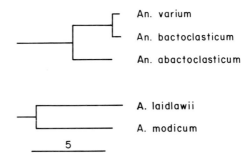

Figure 3. Detailed phylogenetic trees of the *Anaeroplasma* group (top) and *Acholeplasma* group (bottom) reconstructed from 16S rRNA sequence comparisons, as described in the text. The *Anaeroplasma* group tree also contains *Anaeroplasma intermedium* (71), which is not shown here. The *Acholeplasma* group tree also contains one of the plant-pathogenic MLOs (57), but (as described in text) the position of the MLO node on the *Acholeplasma* tree is unknown at present. Thus far, the only *Acholeplasma* species not found on the *Acholeplasma* group branch is *Acholeplasma entomophilum*, which is on the *M. mycoides* group tree (Fig. 5). The scale at the bottom denotes the branch distance corresponding to five base changes per 100 nucleotides.

Recent 16S rRNA sequence data show that one of the plant-pathogenic MLOs is a branch of the *Acholeplasma* group (35, 57). The lack of comparative sequence analysis data for this organism precludes its inclusion in the tree in Fig. 3 at present.

The remaining mycoplasma phylogenetic branches are to sterol-requiring facultative anaerobic genera: *Spiroplasma*, then *Mycoplasma*, and finally *Ureaplasma* (Fig. 1 and 4 to 9). *Spiroplasma* species colonize plants and insects, and *Mycoplasma* and *Ureaplasma* species colonize animals and humans. In view of the divergence of the *Ureaplasma* branch from the *Mycoplasma* tree (Fig. 1), *Ureaplasma* species represent biochemical (urea-requiring) variants of *Mycoplasma* species.

Mycoplasma species are polyphyletic

Although the mycoplasma phylogenetic tree is monophyletic, arising as a single branch from the *Lactobacillus* group branch, species currently included in the genus *Mycoplasma* are polyphyletic, having originated as three independent branches from the *Spiroplasma* branch (Fig. 1). The deepest *Mycoplasma* branch contains a diverse group of 16 *Mycoplasma* species, forming the *Mycoplasma hyorhinis* group (Fig. 7), *M. fermentans* group (Fig. 8), and *M. hominis* group (Fig. 9) branches. A more recent *Mycoplasma* branch consists of seven species forming the *M. pneumoniae* group and *Ureaplasma* group branches (Fig. 6). The most recent *Mycoplasma* branch is formed by the *M. mycoides* group, a group of seven species including one *Acholeplasma* species (Fig. 5). The phylogenetic distances between the three *Mycoplasma* branches suggest that species on these branches are members of different genera. However, a decision has recently been made not to change *Mycoplasma* taxonomy on the basis of phylogenetic data (23).

The position of *Acholeplasma entomophilum* on the *M. mycoides* phylogenetic branch (Fig. 5) is a puzzle-

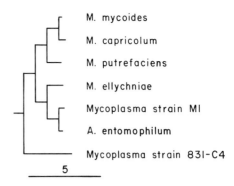

Figure 5. Detailed phylogenetic tree of the *M. mycoides* group reconstructed from 16S rRNA sequence comparisons, as described in the text. Note that at present, the *M. mycoides* tree contains one *Acholeplasma* species. The scale at the bottom denotes the branch distance corresponding to five base changes per 100 nucleotides.

ment, since *A. entomophilum* is a sterol-nonrequiring *Acholeplasma* species, has been isolated from a wide range of insects, and has a coccoid morphology different from that of the helical *Spiroplasma* species (67). The phylogeny and taxonomy of *A. entomophilum* need clarification.

Mycoplasmas are evolving more rapidly than are eubacteria

The original report of the mycoplasma phylogenetic tree noted that mycoplasmas had evolved at a more rapid rate than had the eubacteria (76). The latest mycoplasma phylogenetic tree (Fig. 1) provides more detailed information on that observation.

From the mycoplasma phylogenetic tree branch lengths (Fig. 1), it can be seen that mycoplasma branches have accumulated an average of about 50% more base changes (i.e., have evolved about 50% more rapidly) than has the *Lactobacillus* group. While each

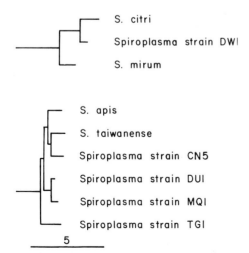

Figure 4. Detailed phylogenetic trees of the *Spiroplasma citri* group (top) and *S. apis* group (bottom) reconstructed from 16S rRNA sequence comparisons, as described in the text. The scale at the bottom denotes the branch distance corresponding to five base changes per 100 nucleotides.

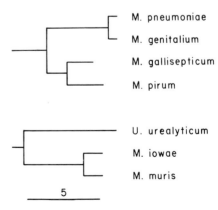

Figure 6. Detailed phylogenetic trees of the *M. pneumoniae* group (top) and *Ureaplasma* group (bottom) reconstructed from 16S rRNA sequence comparisons, as described in the text. Note that at present, the *Ureaplasma* group tree contains one *Ureaplasma* species and two *Mycoplasma* species. The scale at the bottom denotes the branch distance corresponding to five base changes per 100 nucleotides.

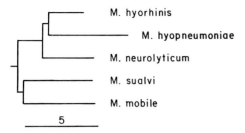

Figure 7. Detailed phylogenetic tree of the *M. hyorhinis* group reconstructed from 16S rRNA sequence comparisons, as described in the text. The scale at the bottom denotes the branch distance corresponding to five base changes per 100 nucleotides.

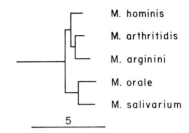

Figure 9. Detailed phylogenetic tree of the *M. hominis* group reconstructed from 16S rRNA sequence comparisons, as described in the text. The scale at the bottom denotes the branch distance corresponding to five base changes per 100 nucleotides.

of the mycoplasma phylogenetic branches has evolved more rapidly than has the *Lactobacillus* group branch, there is significant heterogeneity in the rate of evolution of the different mycoplasma branches. The *Asteroleplasma anaerobium* branch has evolved about 65% more rapidly, the *Anaeroplasma-Acholeplasma* group branch has evolved about 32% more rapidly, the *Spiroplasma-M. mycoides* group branch has evolved about 12% more rapidly, the *M. pneumoniae-Ureaplasma* group branch has evolved about 73% more rapidly, and the *M. hyorhinis-M. fermentans-M. hominis* group branch has evolved about 47% more rapidly than has the *Lactobacillus* group branch (36). These differences may reflect variations in DNA replication and/or repair fidelity in the major mycoplasma phylogenetic branches. The relationship between mycoplasma mutation and evolution rates will be discussed below. The detailed mycoplasma phylogenetic tree (Fig. 1) confirms the earlier conclusion (75) that the *M. pneumoniae-Ureaplasma* group branch is the most rapidly evolving microbial phylogenetic branch.

The small-genome mycoplasma species are on a few rapidly evolving mycoplasma phylogenetic branches

Recent measurements of mycoplasma genome sizes by pulsed-field gel electrophoresis (PFGE) and construction of genomic cleavage maps (see chapter 9) have found that many of the small genome sizes of *Mycoplasma* and *Ureaplasma* species determined by

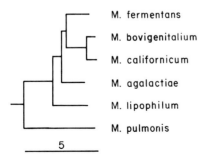

Figure 8. Detailed phylogenetic tree of the *M. fermentans* group reconstructed from 16S rRNA sequence comparisons, as described in the text. The scale at the bottom denotes the branch distance corresponding to five base changes per 100 nucleotides.

DNA renaturation kinetics are significant underestimates, while genome sizes of *Acholeplasma laidlawii* strains from DNA renaturation kinetics generally agree with PFGE data. The PFGE and cleavage map results have also shown that mycoplasma genome sizes range from about 600 to 1,700 kb, rather than falling into discrete 700- to 800-kb and 1,500- to 1,600-kb size classes (see chapter 9).

Genome sizes based on DNA renaturation kinetics measurements for *Asteroleplasma*, *Anaeroplasma*, *Acholeplasma*, and *Spiroplasma* species and from PFGE and cleavage maps for *Mycoplasma* and *Ureaplasma* species (references in chapter 9) are available for 22 species on the mycoplasma phylogenetic tree. Analysis of these data shows that mycoplasmas with small (<1,000-kb) genome sizes are on three of the most rapidly evolving mycoplasma phylogenetic branches: the *M. pneumoniae*, *Ureaplasma*, and *M. hominis* group branches (Fig. 1) (36). From the limited data available, the genome size ranges of the mycoplasma phylogenetic branches are as follows: *Asteroleplasma anaerobium*, *Anaeroplasma*, *Acholeplasma*, and *Spiroplasma* branches, 1,500 to 1,700 kb; *M. mycoides* group branch, 1,100 to 1,300 kb; *M. pneumoniae* group branch, 600 to 1,100 kb; *Ureaplasma* group branch, 900 to 1,300 kb; *M. hyorhinis* group branch, about 1,100 kb; *M. fermentans* group branch, 1,000 to 1,200 kb; and *M. hominis* group branch, 700 to 750 kb. These data suggest that a rapid rate of evolution is a necessary but not sufficient condition for genome size reductions extreme enough to approach what appears to be the minimal limit of cellular genetic complexity. A possible scenario for evolution of mycoplasmas with limiting genome sizes is discussed below.

The Direction of Time and Mycoplasma Evolution

In reconstructing the mycoplasma phylogenetic tree, determination of the root of the tree was critical in deducing the relationship between bacteria and mycoplasmas. By locating the root of a phylogenetic tree, the origin of the tree is identified, thereby allowing determination of ancestor-descendant relationships between the branches. Hence, establishing the root of a phylogenetic tree is equivalent to determining the direction of time on that tree.

However, Morowitz has noted (40) that, since in principle the direction of time on a phylogenetic tree cannot be determined with complete certainty, "[w]hether the mycoplasmas predate or are derived from bacteria cannot be determined solely from taxonomic trees." The implications of this concern are striking, because if an error has been made and the tree in Fig. 1 is backwards, then the universal phylogenetic tree for bacteria (72) is also backwards. In that case, mycoplasmas would be ancestral to all bacteria, including the phototrophs. Such a conclusion is contradicted by extensive experimental data showing that mycoplasmas are phylogenetically close to one branch of the gram-positive bacteria and distinct from other bacterial branches.

For perspective, about 10^{88} possible rooted trees can be drawn for the 56 species in Fig. 1 (6). Despite the fact that even with modern computers, one cannot examine all 10^{88} trees, Woese, Maniloff, and other workers used a variety of tree-building methods and derived similar trees (discussed above). This could be done because each group used tree-building algorithms based on the principle of either minimum evolution (i.e., minimizing pairwise sequence differences) or maximum parsimony (i.e., minimizing the number of base substitutions) (12, 44). Although these algorithms are not guaranteed to produce the correct tree, phylogenetic trees reconstructed by these methods have proven reliable. It should be noted that the alternative to a minimum evolution or maximum parsimony approach would be to allow as many base changes as needed to build any tree desired. Therefore, although one can never be absolutely positively sure, it seems reasonable to accept the most parsimonious explanation of the data available.

BIOLOGICAL CONSIDERATIONS RELATED TO MYCOPLASMA PHYLOGENY

Evolution of Limiting Genome Sizes

Analysis of mycoplasma genome sizes as a function of evolutionary distance from their origin on the *Lactobacillus* group branch suggests that mycoplasma genomes have evolved by attrition from an organism with a 2,200- to 2,500-kb genome (36). This ancestral genome size is similar to those currently found in a number of species in the *Lactobacillus* group (33).

The small *Mycoplasma* genome sizes may reflect the minimum amount of information needed for a living system. Consider a thought experiment asking the following question: "How many (and which) genes can be deleted from a microbial genome and still retain a living organism?" Nature appears to have done the experiment, and mycoplasmas are the answer. This conclusion, of course, leads to another question: "If mycoplasmas are the answer, what was the question?" *Mycoplasma* phylogeny tells us that on (at least) three occasions, organisms left the *Spiroplasma* phylogenetic branch and evolved to *Mycoplasma* and *Ureaplasma* species with even smaller genomes. The fact that the smallest genome sizes are all about 600 to 700 kb suggests that this amount of DNA represents the minimal genetic complexity for a living organism. Further loss of genetic information must have been lethal.

The Mycoplasma Genetic Balance Sheet

From this perspective, it is useful to examine which gene functions mycoplasmas have lost by attrition and which ones they have retained. Genes for cell processes can be grouped in terms of the three general classes of biochemical processes: intermediary metabolism and energy production, synthesis of small molecules, and synthesis of macromolecules.

Genes for intermediary metabolism and energy production

Mycoplasma intermediary metabolism involves pathways for the degradation of organic substrates to generate small molecules, for biosynthetic reactions, and for energy production via substrate-level phosphorylation (see chapters 11 to 14). Therefore, mycoplasmas have retained a variety of genes for the first class of reactions.

Genes for synthesis of small molecules

In their evolution by attrition from bacteria, mycoplasmas appear to have lost many of the enzymatic functions (and, therefore, presumably the genes) for synthesis of macromolecule precursors. This is seen in the loss of biochemical pathways for cell wall synthesis and in the nutritional requirements of mycoplasmas for amino acids, nucleotides, fatty acids, and vitamins (see chapters 2 and 11 to 14). The ecological niches in which mycoplasmas live (i.e., the surfaces of plant, insect, and animal tissues) provide a variety of small molecules and provide macromolecules for cleavage to small molecules. This environment seems to have allowed mycoplasmas to lose many of the genes needed for synthesis of macromolecule precursors and to compensate for this loss with a small number of genes for hydrolytic enzymes to degrade specific types of macromolecules. For example, rather than code for the enzymes for extensive amino acid and nucleotide biosynthesis, mycoplasmas code for extracellular proteases and nucleases that degrade proteins and nucleic acids to amino acids and nucleotides, for uptake and use as precursors in mycoplasma macromolecule synthesis. Parenthetically, as expected from the phylogenetic tree, many mycoplasma metabolic pathways and nutritional requirements resemble those found in streptococci and lactobacilli (37).

Genes for synthesis of macromolecules

Mycoplasmas have little or none of the redundancy for rRNA genes found in the bacteria. Bacteria generally have 5 to 10 copies of the rRNA genes (references in reference 29), while different mycoplasma species have either one or two copies (reviewed in reference 1; also see chapter 10).

This lack of redundancy is also seen in mycoplasma tRNAs. Unlike bacteria, mycoplasmas lack genes for many isoaccepting tRNAs (references in reference 37). Andachi and coworkers have shown that *M. capricolum* codes for only 29 tRNA species (3). Therefore, mycoplasmas make extensive use of wobble in translating mRNA; that is, anticodons of many mycoplasma tRNAs recognize more than one codon for a particular amino acid by non-Watson-Crick base pairing (see chapter 19).

An interesting aspect of the genetic code in mycoplasmas is that some mycoplasmas deviate from the universal genetic code by using the UGA termination codon, rather than the universal UGG tryptophan codon, to code for the amino acid tryptophan (see chapter 19). UGA also codes for tryptophan in mitochondria and ciliates (14). This variant usage seems to be an example of convergent evolution and may be a reverse evolutionary step in each case, since Jukes (24) has suggested UGA was originally a codon for tryptophan and subsequently evolved to function as a termination codon. *Acholeplasma* species retain the universal code, using UGA as a termination codon (36, 65), but phylogenetically more recent mycoplasma branches (*Spiroplasma*, *Mycoplasma*, and *Ureaplasma*) evolved to use UGA as a tryptophan codon (5; additional references in chapter 20). Hence, the change in codon usage, from UGA as a termination codon to UGA as a tryptophan codon, must have occurred after divergence of the *Spiroplasma* branch from the *Anaeroplasma-Acholeplasma* branch.

Mycoplasmas have conserved the bacterial gene functions for DNA replication, transcription of DNA to RNA, and translation of RNA to protein (see chapters 17 and 19). A number of bacterial DNA-related systems have been found in mycoplasmas, suggesting that functions such as DNA recombination and repair (see chapter 17), DNA restriction and modification (see chapter 18), heat shock proteins (see chapter 20), and *recA* genes (10) could not be readily deleted. It is particularly interesting that even with limited genetic complexity, mycoplasmas have retained restriction and modification systems. This fact implies that either DNA restriction and modification do more than protect a cell from infection by foreign DNA or such infectious DNA is a significant problem for mycoplasmas in nature.

A major remaining unanswered question is whether mycoplasma DNA replication has retained a proofreading capability. This question has implications for whether mycoplasmas are undergoing rapid evolution and is discussed below in terms of factors affecting the mycoplasma mutation rate.

An interesting feature of mycoplasma biology is that mycoplasmas have viruses. This property seems to be a supramolecular version of the early 18th century British satirist Jonathan Swift's line about little fleas having littler fleas: the smallest cells have viruses that grow on them. The first virus that could infect mycoplasms was isolated in 1970 by R. N. Gourlay, at the Agricultural Research Council Institute for Research on Animal Diseases in England (reviewed in chapter 3). Since then, many mycoplasma viruses have been isolated. Maniloff has noted that some mycoplasma viruses are probably bacteriophages that adapted to growth on wall-less bacteria and evolved from the bacteria in parallel with their mycoplasma host cells, while other mycoplasma viruses seem to be new viruses that evolved from mycoplasmas and are unlike any other viruses that have been reported (38; see also chapter 3).

From this review of mycoplasma biochemistry, the nature of most of the genetic information lost during mycoplasma evolution remains unknown. The gene functions that can be identified as functions that mycoplasmas have lost can account for only a small fraction of the deleted DNA. However, it should be remembered that even for *E. coli*, the most-studied bacterial genome, the approximately 1,400 genes mapped thus far are only about 25 to 30% of that organism's total genetic capacity. Until the function of most of the genetic material in bacteria is known, we cannot expect to define the genetic information lost during mycoplasma evolution.

Tempo and Mode of Mycoplasma Evolution

The rapid evolution and novel phenotypes that characterize the mycoplasmas suggest there has been coupling between the tempo or rate of evolution and the mode or quality of evolutionary changes during mycoplasma phylogeny (72, 76).

The rate of evolution of a species is the product of its mutation rate and mutation fixation probability (20). The rate of mycoplasma evolution can be estimated from the 16S rRNA sequence comparisons used to reconstruct the mycoplasma phylogenetic tree. These data (described above) indicate that the mycoplasma phylogenetic branch is evolving about 50% faster than the *Lactobacillus* group. The basis of this rapid evolution may be the mycoplasma mutation rate and/or the fixation probability.

It has been proposed that an organism's mutation rate is constrained between two limits (7, 9, 76). The lower limit may be determined by the need to maintain a sufficient number of mutations within a population to allow the species to adapt to fluctuations in its environment. The upper limit for the mutation rate may arise to prevent too large a fraction of the organisms in a population from having deleterious mutations. This upper limit may be a function of the organism's genome size, with larger-genome organisms having mutation rates higher than those of organisms with smaller genomes. The data available are consistent with this idea; the mutation rate for a variety of organisms has been found to be inversely related to genome size (9).

From these considerations, a possible scenario for mycoplasma evolution can be proposed. The ancestor of the mycoplasmas may have been a bacterial strain that, as a result of mutation, became error prone in DNA replication or repair. In either case, this mutant would have had a higher mutation rate than did its wild-type parent. Such a mutant, with a higher mutation rate, would be able to reduce its genome size and still replicate its genome with the same overall fidelity as the original bacterial genome. Hence, the genome size of this high-mutation-rate mutant subline might have decreased and finally stabilized at a size consistent with the mutation rate limits. A nucleotide bias in the mutational mechanism could have supplied the pressure leading to the low $G + C$ contents of mycoplasma DNAs (64).

Such a scenario pictures mycoplasmas as trapped in the type of hypervariable mutation state proposed by Hall (19) as a possible explanation for the Cairnsian "directed" mutations observed in bacteria under conditions of stress. As noted by Drake (9), "It seems likely that high mutation rates become profitable only when mutational adaptation can occur at many loci." Hence, mycoplasmas may be trapped in a hypervariable state by their limited genetic complexity and slow growth rate.

Direct measurements of mutation rates are inconclusive as to whether mycoplasmas, in general, have higher mutation rates than do eubacteria (28, 30, 34). The expected mycoplasma mutation rates would be less than twofold greater than those found in bacteria. It is difficult to measure such an incremental increase in overall mutation rates because of experimental problems in resolving small mutation rate differences and the large variation observed in mutation rates (i.e., the rate of amino acid substitutions) of different genes (reviewed in reference 44).

However, analysis of the types of base substitutions in mycoplasma and bacterial DNA sequences indicates mycoplasmas are less efficient than bacteria in repairing errors made during DNA replication. In a study of 5S rRNA and tRNA sequences, the ratio of transitions to transversions in mycoplasmas was found to be severalfold greater than in phylogenetically related bacteria (36). Transitions are a more common type of DNA replication error than are transversions, and DNA proofreading and repair systems are more efficient in correcting transitions than in correcting transversions (references in reference 72). Hence, the higher transition-to-transversion ratio in mycoplasma sequences than in *Lactobacillus* group sequences means that mycoplasmas are deficient in DNA proofreading and/or repair capability relative to phylogenetically related bacteria. This proofreading/repair deficiency should be expressed as an increased mycoplasma mutation rate. A more detailed analysis of the relationship of the transition-to-transversion ratio and the rate of evolution of mycoplasma phylogenetic branches is in progress (36).

Since the transition-to-transversion ratios suggest that mycoplasma mutation rates are several times greater than those of phylogenetically related bacteria, one must ask why mycoplasmas are not evolving even faster. The constraint on the survival of mycoplasmas with higher rates of evolution may be the fixation probability. Following evolution by attrition, most DNA in cells with limiting genome sizes must code for essential genes, and there is only a small probability that a base change will not adversely affect a gene function or that the mutated gene is not essential. There can probably be relatively few selectively neutral mutations in a genome-limited organism, particularly one that has only a limited set of isoaccepting tRNA species. Therefore, mycoplasmas must have a mutation rate that is greater, and a fixation probability that is smaller, than that of phylogenetically related bacteria to produce the product of these two, the rate of evolution, which is 50% faster for the mycoplasma phylogenetic branch than for the *Lactobacillus* group branch.

The higher mutation rate in mycoplasmas has important ramifications for mycoplasma evolution. A higher mutation rate allows an organism to explore evolutionary options requiring multiple compensating mutations—options effectively closed to organisms with lower mutation rates. The situation could arise when, in a single cell generation, a deleterious mutation is compensated for by one or more additional mutations, thereby rescuing the organism and perhaps producing saltatory evolution. These types of changes have been observed in the analyses of mycoplasma RNAs (51, 70, 75). Thus, organisms like mycoplasmas, with high mutation rates, appear to be able to access rare evolutionary possibilities.

PERSPECTIVES

The studies of Woese and Maniloff began as a effort to collect data to prove one of the two then accepted models for mycoplasma evolution. However, the data showed that neither model was correct and that mycoplasma evolution could be explained only by constructing an entirely new mycoplasma phylogenetic model. Since then, reaction to that model has progressed through the stages described by the 19th century embryologist von Baer (cited in reference 18): "Every triumphant theory passes through three stages: first it is dismissed as untrue; then it is rejected as contrary to religion; and finally it is accepted as dogma and each scientist claims he had long appreciated its truth."

The model of mycoplasma phylogeny constructed by Woese, Maniloff, and coworkers is now accepted in part because knowledge of the phylogenetic relationship between mycoplasmas and bacteria has produced a better understanding of mycoplasma biology, by allowing data on mycoplasma molecular and cellular biology to be explained in the broader context of bacteriology. The connection between mycoplasmas and gram-positive bacteria should also have clinical implications in considerations of chemotherapeutic approaches to pathogenic mycoplasmas.

Reconstruction of the mycoplasma phylogenetic tree has led to a new generation of questions regarding the nature of the mechanism driving the rapid evolutionary rate of the mycoplasmas, the conditions that have selected for rapidly evolving organisms with limited genetic complexity, and the organization and function of the limited mycoplasma genetic complexity. A measure of progress in mycoplasma biology is that these questions can be posed with some reasonable expectation that they are amenable to experimental answers.

Acknowledgments. I wish to acknowledge the role of Carl Woese in developing the philosophical and experimental approaches that have been so successful in elucidating microbial phylogeny, and I thank him for our long and productive collaboration in studying mycoplasma phylogeny.

REFERENCES

1. **Amikam, D., G. Glaser, and S. Razin.** 1984. Mycoplasmas (*Mollicutes*) have a low number of rRNA genes. *J. Bacteriol.* **158**:376–378.
2. **Andachi, Y., F. Yamao, M. Iwami, A. Muto, and S. Osawa.** 1987. Occurrence of unmodified adenine and uracil at the first position of anticodon in threonine tRNAs in *Mycoplasma capricolum. Proc. Natl. Acad. Sci. USA* **84**:7398–7402.
3. **Andachi, Y., F. Yamao, A. Muto, and S. Osawa.** 1989.

Codon recognition patterns as deduced from sequences of the complete set of transfer RNA species in *Mycoplasma capricolum*. *J. Mol. Biol.* **209:**37–54.

4. **Berry, A., S. Ahmad, A. Liss, and R. A. Jensen.** 1987. Enzymological features of aromatic amino acid biosynthesis reflect the phylogeny of mycoplasmas. *J. Gen. Microbiol.* **133:**2147–2154.

5. **Blanchard, A.** 1990. *Ureaplasma urealyticum* urease genes; use of a UGA tryptophan codon. *Mol. Microbiol.* **4:**669–676.

6. **Cavalli-Sforza, L. L., and A. W. F. Edwards.** 1967. Phylogenetic analysis: models and estimation procedures. *Am. J. Hum. Genet.* **19:**233–257.

7. **Crow, J. F.** 1986. *Basic Concepts in Population, Quantitative, and Evolutionary Genetics*, p. 206–207. W. H. Freeman & Co., New York.

8. **DeWachter, R., E. Huysmans, and A. Vandenberge.** 1985. 5S ribosomal RNA as a tool for studying evolution, p. 115–141. *In* K. H. Schleifer and E. Stackebrandt (ed.), *Evolution of Prokaryotes*. Academic Press, Inc., New York.

9. **Drake, J. W.** 1974. The role of mutation in microbial evolution. *Symp. Soc. Gen. Microbiol.* **24:**41–58.

10. **Dybvig, K.** Unpublished data.

11. **Eigen, M., W. Gardiner, P. Schuster, and R. Winkler-Oswatitsch.** 1981. The origin of genetic information. *Sci. Am.* **244:**88–118.

12. **Felsenstein, J.** 1988. Phylogenies from molecular sequences: inference and reliability. *Annu. Rev. Genet.* **22:**521–565.

13. **Fox, G. E., E. Stackebrandt, R. B. Hespell, J. Gibson, J. Maniloff, T. A. Dyer, R. S. Wolfe, W. E. Balch, R. S. Tanner, L. J. Magrum, L. B. Zablen, R. Blakemore, R. Gupta, L. Bonen, B. J. Lewis, D. A. Stahl, K. R. Luehrsen, K. N. Chen, and C. R. Woese.** 1980. The phylogeny of prokaryotes. *Science* **209:**457–463.

14. **Fox, T. D.** 1987. Natural variation in the genetic code. *Annu. Rev. Genet.* **21:**67–91.

15. **Freundt, A. A.** 1958. *The Mycoplasmataceae*, p. 90–117. Munksgaard, Copenhagen.

16. **Gilson, E., G. Alloing, T. Schmidt, J.-P. Claverys, R. Dudler, and M. Hofnung.** 1988. Evidence for high affinity binding-protein dependent transport systems in Gram-positive bacteria and in *Mycoplasma*. *EMBO J.* **7:**3971–3974.

17. **Goldfine, H.** 1982. Lipids of prokaryotes—structure and distribution. *Curr. Top. Membr. Transp.* **17:**1–43.

18. **Gould, S. J.** 1980. *Ever since Darwin*, p. 160. Penguin Books, Harmondsworth, England.

19. **Hall, B. G.** 1990. Spontaneous point mutations that occur more often when advantageous then when neutral. *Genetics* **126:**5–16.

20. **Hartl, D. L.** 1988. *A Primer of Population Genetics*, 2nd ed., p. 146. Sinauer Associates, Inc., Sunderland, Mass.

21. **Hori, H., M. Sawada, S. Osawa, K. Murao, and H. Ishikura.** 1981. The nucleotide sequence of 5S rRNA from *Mycoplasma capricolum*. *Nucleic Acids Res.* **9:**5407–5410.

22. **Hsuchen, C.-C., and D. T. Dubin.** 1980. Methylation patterns of mycoplasma transfer and ribosomal ribonucleic acid. *J. Bacteriol.* **144:**991–998.

23. **International Committee of Systematic Bacteriology Subcommittee on the Taxonomy of *Mollicutes*.** 1991. Minutes of the interim meetings, 7 and 8 July, 1990, Istanbul, Turkey. *Int. J. Syst. Bacteriol.* **41:**333–336.

24. **Jukes, T. H.** 1983. Evolution of the amino acid code: inferences from mitochondrial codes. *J. Mol. Evol.* **19:**219–225.

25. **Kilpatrick, M. W., and R. T. Walker.** 1980. The nucleotide sequence of glycine tRNA from Mycoplasma mycoides sp. capri. *Nucleic Acids Res.* **8:**2783–2786.

26. **Kimball, M. E., K. S. Szeto, and D. Soll.** 1974. The nucleotide sequence of phenylalanine tRNA from Mycoplasma sp. (Kid). *Nucleic Acids Res.* **1:**1721–1732.

27. **Klieneberger-Nobel, E.** 1962. *Pleuropneumonia-Like Organisms (PPLO): Mycoplasmataceae*, p. 75–89. Academic Press, Inc., New York.

28. **Krause, D. C., D. K. Leith, R. M. Wilson, and J. B. Baseman.** 1982. Identification of *Mycoplasma pneumoniae* proteins associated with hemadsorption and virulence. *Infect. Immun.* **35:**809–817.

29. **Krawiec, S., and M. Riley.** 1989. Organization of the bacterial chromosome. *Microbiol. Rev.* **54:**502–539.

30. **Labarère, J., and G. Barroso.** 1989. Lethal and mutation frequency responses of *Spiroplasma citri* cells to UV irradiation. *Mutat. Res.* **210:**135–141.

31. **Lane, D. J., B. Pace, G. J. Olsen, D. A. Stahl, M. L. Sogin, and N. R. Pace.** 1985. Rapid determination of 16S ribosomal RNA sequences for phylogenetic analysis. *Proc. Natl. Acad. Sci. USA* **82:**6955–6959.

32. **Larue, B., R. J. Cedergren, D. Sankoff, and H. Grosjean.** 1979. Evolution of methionine initiator and phenylalanine transfer RNAs. *J. Mol. Evol.* **14:**287–300.

33. **LeBourgeois, P., M. Mata, and P. Ritzenthaler.** 1989. Genome comparison of *Lactococcus* strains by pulsed-field gel electrophoresis. *FEMS Microbiol. Lett.* **59:**65–70.

34. **Lee, D. H., R. J. Miles, and J. R. M. Inal.** 1987. Antibiotic sensitivity and mutation rates to antibiotic resistance in *Mycoplasma mycoides* ssp. *mycoides*. *Epidemiol. Infect.* **98:**361–368.

35. **Lim, P.-O., and B. B. Sears.** 1989. 16S rRNA sequence indicates that plant-pathogenic mycoplasmalike organisms are evolutionarily distinct from animal mycoplasmas. *J. Bacteriol.* **171:**5901–5906.

36. **Maniloff, J.** Unpublished data.

37. **Maniloff, J.** 1983. Evolution of wall-less prokaryotes. *Annu. Rev. Microbiol.* **37:**477–499.

38. **Maniloff, J.** 1988. Mycoplasma viruses. *Crit. Rev. Microbiol.* **15:**339–389.

39. **Maniloff, J., L. Magrum, L. B. Zablen, and C. R. Woese.** 1978. Phylogenetic relationships of mycoplasmas as determined by 16S ribosomal RNA characterization. *Zentralbl. Bakteriol. Infektionskr. Parasitenkd. Hyg. Abt. I Orig. Reihe A* **241:**171–172.

40. **Morowitz, H. J.** 1984. The completeness of molecular biology. *Isr. J. Med. Sci.* **20:**750–753.

41. **Morowitz, H. J., and D. C. Wallace.** 1973. Genome size and life cycle of the mycoplasmas. *Ann. N.Y. Acad. Sci.* **225:**62–73.

42. **Muto, A., Y. Andachi, H. Yuzawa, F. Yamao, and S. Osawa.** 1990. The organization and evolution of transfer RNA genes in *Mycoplasma capricolum*. *Nucleic Acids Res.* **18:**5037–5043.

43. **Muto, A., H. Hori, M. Sawada, Y. Kawauchi, M. Iwami, F. Yamao, and S. Osawa.** 1983. The ribosomal genes of *Mycoplasma capricolum*. *Yale J. Biol. Med.* **56:**373–376.

44. **Nei, M.** 1987. *Molecular Evolutionary Genetics*, p. 50–53, 287–326. Columbia University Press, New York.

45. **Neimark, H.** 1973. Implications of the phylogenetic relationship between acholeplasmas and lactic acid bacteria. *Colloq. INSERM* **33:**71–78.

46. **Neimark, H.** 1979. Phylogenetic relationships between mycoplasmas and other prokaryotes, p. 43–61. *In* M. F. Barile and S. Razin (ed.), *The Mycoplasmas*, vol. 1. Academic Press, Inc., New York.

47. **Neimark, H., and J. London.** 1982. Origins of the mycoplasmas: sterol-nonrequiring mycoplasmas evolved from streptococci. *J. Bacteriol.* **150:**1259–1265.

48. **Ourisson, G., and M. Rohmer.** 1982. Prokaryotic polyterpenes: phylogenetic precursors of sterols. *Curr. Top. Membr. Transp.* **17:**153–182.

49. **Pechman, K. J., and C. R. Woese.** 1972. Characterization of the primary structural homology between the 16S ribosomal RNA's of *Escherichia coli* and *Bacillus megaterium* by oligomer cataloging. *J. Mol. Evol.* **1:**230–240.

50. **Petzel, J. P., P. A. Hartman, and M. J. Allison.** 1989. Pyrophosphate-dependent enzymes in walled bacteria phylo-

genetically related to the wall-less bacteria of the class *Mollicutes. Int. J. Syst. Bacteriol.* **39**:413–419.

51. **Rogers, M. J., J. Simmons, R. T. Walker, W. G. Weisburg, C. R. Woese, R. S. Tanner, I. M. Robinson, D. A. Stahl, G. Olsen, R. H. Leach, and J. Maniloff.** 1985. Construction of the mycoplasma evolutionary tree from 5S rRNA sequence data. *Proc. Natl. Acad. Sci. USA* **82**:1160–1164.

52. **Rogers, M. J., A. A. Steinmetz, and R. T. Walker.** 1984. A *Spiroplasma* tRNA gene cluster. *Isr. J. Med. Sci.* **20**:768–772.

53. **Rogers, M. J., A. A. Steinmetz, and R. T. Walker.** 1986. The nucleotide sequence of a tRNA gene cluster from *Spiroplasma melliferum. Nucleic Acids Res.* **14**:3145.

54. **Rogers, M. J., A. A. Steinmetz, and R. T. Walker.** 1987. Organization and structure of tRNA genes in *Spiroplasma melliferum. Isr. J. Med. Sci.* **23**:357–360.

55. **Saitou, N., and M. Nei.** 1987. The neighbor-joining method: a new method for reconstructing phylogenetic trees. *Mol. Biol. Evol.* **4**:406–425.

56. **Sankoff, D., C. Morel, and R. J. Cedergren.** 1973. Evolution of 5S rRNA and the non-randomness of base replacement. *Nature* (London) **245**:232–234.

57. **Sears, B. B., and C. R. Woese.** Unpublished data.

58. **Sela, S., D. Yogev, S. Razin, and H. Bercovier.** 1989. Duplication of the *tuf* gene: a new insight into the phylogeny of eubacteria. *J. Bacteriol.* **171**:581–584.

59. **Shaw, N.** 1974. Lipid composition as a guide to the classification of bacteria. *Adv. Appl. Microbiol.* **17**:63–108.

60. **Smith, P. F.** 1971. *The Biology of Mycoplasmas*, p. 16–34. Academic Press, Inc., New York.

61. **Smith, P. F.** 1979. The composition of membrane lipids and lipopolysaccharides, p. 231–257. *In* M. F. Barile and S. Razin (ed.), *The Mycoplasmas*, vol. 1. Academic Press, Inc., New York.

62. **Sogin, S. J., M. L. Sogin, and C. R. Woese.** 1972. Phylogenetic measurement in procaryotes by primary structural characterization. *J. Mol. Evol.* **1**:173–184.

63. **Stackebrandt, E., and C. R. Woese.** 1981. The evolution of prokaryotes. *Symp. Soc. Gen. Microbiol.* **32**:1–31.

64. **Sueoka, N.** 1988. Directional mutation pressure and neutral molecular evolution. *Proc. Natl. Acad. Sci. USA* **85**:2653–2657.

65. **Tanaka, R., A. Muto, and S. Osawa.** 1989. Nucleotide sequence of tryptophan tRNA gene in *Acholeplasma laidlawii. Nucleic Acids Res.* **17**:5842.

66. **Tully, J. G., D. L. Rose, P. Carle, J. M. Bove, K. J. Hackett, and R. F. Whitcomb.** 1988. *Acholeplasma entomophilum* sp. nov. from gut contents of a wide range of host insects. *Int. J. Syst. Bacteriol.* **38**:164–167.

67. **Walker, R. T., E. T. J. Chelton, M. W. Kilpatrick, M. J. Rogers, and J. Simmons.** 1982. The nucleotide sequence of the 5S rRNA from *Spiroplasma* species BC3 and *Mycoplasma mycoides* sp. *capri* PG3. *Nucleic Acids Res.* **10**:6363–6367.

68. **Walker, R. T., and U. L. RajBhandary.** 1978. The nucleotide sequence of formylmethionine tRNA from Mycoplasma mycoides sp. capri. *Nucleic Acids Res.* **5**:57–70.

69. **Wallace, D. C., and H. J. Morowitz.** 1973. Genome size and evolution. *Chromosoma* **40**:121–126.

70. **Weisburg, W. G., J. G. Tully, D. L. Rose, J. P. Petzel, H. Oyaizu, D. Yang, L. Mandelco, J. Sechrest, T. G. Lawrence, J. Van Etten, J. Maniloff, and C. R. Woese.** 1989. A phylogenetic analysis of the mycoplasmas: basis for their classification. *J. Bacteriol.* **171**:6455–6467.

71. **Wilson, A. C., R. L. Cann, S. M. Carr, M. George, U. B. Gyllensten, K. M. Helm-Bychowski, R. G. Higuchi, S. R. Palumbi, E. M. Prager, R. D. Sage, and M. Stoneking.** 1985. Mitochondrial DNA and two perspectives on evolutionary genetics. *Biol. J. Linnean Soc.* **26**:375–400.

72. **Woese, C. R.** 1987. Bacterial evolution. *Microbiol. Rev.* **51**:221–271.

73. **Woese, C. R. (University of Illinois).** Personal communication.

74. **Woese, C. R., G. E. Fox, L. Zablen, T. Uchida, L. Bonen, K. Pechman, B. J. Lewis, and D. Stahl.** 1975. Conservation of primary structure in 16S ribosomal RNA. *Nature* (London) **254**:83–86.

75. **Woese, C. R., J. Maniloff, and L. B. Zablen.** 1980. Phylogenetic analysis of the mycoplasmas. *Proc. Natl. Acad. Sci. USA* **77**:494–498.

76. **Woese, C. R., E. Stackebrandt, and W. Ludwig.** 1985. What are mycoplasmas: the relationship of tempo and mode in bacterial evolution. *J. Mol. Evol.* **21**:305–316.

77. **Zuckerkandl, E., and L. Pauling.** 1965. Molecules as documents of evolutionary history. *J. Theor. Biol.* **8**:357–366.

34. Genetic Variation in Natural Populations

GUNNA CHRISTIANSEN

INTRODUCTION

Analysis of genetic variation in natural populations of microorganisms is of importance not only because it tells us about the variability within a single species, eventually leading to population genetics of microbes, but also because it tells us about the mechanisms for genetic exchange and rearrangements involving conjugation, transduction and transformation, plasmids, phages, and transposable elements (85). Because of asexual reproduction in bacteria, these mechanisms play a major role in species diversity. Genetic variation has been studied most extensively in *Escherichia coli* (28, 62, 63). Analysis of enzyme polymorphisms (38, 41) indicated linkage disequilibrium due to insufficient genetic recombination. Genetic recombination is, however, important for evolution by increasing novel favorable combinations of alleles.

Mutation and selection can be studied by chemostat cultivation, whereby large populations can be cultivated under controlled conditions for many generations. In such experiments, it has been shown that selection for growth on a novel medium results in enzymatic mutations with altered substrate specificities (18) or activation of cryptic genes (27).

Woese and coworkers (82, 83) used variation in the DNA sequences of genes encoding 16S rRNAs of microorganisms to analyze bacterial evolution. These studies have shown that, as expected from their unusual phenotype and small genome size, mycoplasmas are rapidly evolving microorganisms (see chapter 33).

The high mutation rate may be responsible for adaptation of mycoplasmas to changing environments. The mutation rate also may be related to the reduction in genome size and the fact that some mycoplasmas are deficient in certain DNA repair mechanisms such as dark repair or photoreactivation (see chapter 17). There are only a few reports on transfer of genetic material in mycoplasmas by conjugation, transformation, and transfection and by plasmids, viruses, and transposable elements (see chapter 21). Therefore, studies of genetic variation in natural populations of mycoplasmas is of great interest and may result in an understanding of why some mycoplasma species are highly variable whereas others seem to be much more stable.

DETECTION OF HETEROGENEITY WITHIN MYCOPLASMA SPECIES

Species determination in the genus *Mycoplasma* is based primarily on serological tests. Some of these tests (growth inhibition, growth agglutination, and metabolic inhibition [39]) indicate antigenic heterogeneity in certain species. Genetic variation within mycoplasma species can be detected either as DNA heterogeneity or as protein heterogeneity. Protein heterogeneity is shown by a variety of methods, such as isoenzyme analysis (36, 56, 57), sodium dodecyl sulfate-polyacrylamide gel electrophoresis (SDS-PAGE) (2, 37, 46), immunoblotting analysis (2, 6), and two-dimensional (2-D) gel electrophoresis (2, 3, 31, 53, 54).

Various methods based on DNA analyses also indicate intraspecies heterogeneity. Variation in DNA base composition (G+C moles %) gives a rough estimate of heterogeneity. Identity in G+C content does not, however, guarantee homogeneity. DNA-DNA hybridization between heterologous DNAs, as compared with homologous hybridization, gives estimates of the genetic relationship of microorganisms (5, 11, 67, 68). This method is therefore recommended (82) as one of the tests for classification of new species (homology above 60%) or genera (homology above 20%) (61).

Newer methods, such as analysis of band patterns of restriction endonuclease-cleaved DNA fragments separated by gel electrophoresis (15, 48, 50, 51, 58), are important methods not only for analysis of intraspecies heterogeneity but also as epidemiological tools (33).

Gunna Christiansen • Institute of Medical Microbiology, University of Aarhus, DK-8000 Aarhus C, Denmark.

Restriction fragment length polymorphism (RFLP) analysis is a method in which restriction endonuclease-cleaved DNA fragments are separated by gel electrophoresis, transferred to nitrocellulose filters, and hybridized with a specific DNA probe. In mycoplasmas, only one or two copies of the conserved rRNA genes are present (1). Therefore, use of an rRNA gene fragment in RFLP analysis has been suggested as a tool in mycoplasma diagnostics (47, 84). Such RFLP analysis has also been used to describe intraspecies heterogeneity (14, 16).

Restriction enzyme cleavage maps constructed by pulsed-field gel electrophoresis (44), combined with construction of genetic maps (45), have been used to analyze intraspecies heterogeneity. By comparing such maps from different strains of a mycoplasma species, chromosomal rearrangements, gene duplications and deletions have been described (9, 34, 78).

The most accurate measure for genetic variability is, of course, comparison of specific DNA sequences. *Mycoplasma pneumoniae* strains, which appear to be homogeneous by RFLP analysis (70), have been shown to vary within the genomic region encoding the P1 protein. Sequence analysis showed that the P1 genes differed in two regions, leading to considerable amino acid changes (69). By use of the polymerase chain reaction and determination of the sequence of the amplified DNA, such sequence comparisons will probably be performed to a much greater extent in the future.

Antigenic variation, basically determined by serology, has been the basis for describing some mycoplasma species as heterogeneous (49). Much heterogeneity is seen in *M. hominis*, *M. capricolum*, *M. mycoides*, *M. pulmonis*, and *M. hyorhinis*.

GENETIC VARIABILITY WITHIN THE *M. MYCOIDES* CLUSTER

Phylogenetic and taxonomic studies have shown that *M. capricolum* and *M. mycoides* strains form a cluster (called the *M. mycoides* cluster) on the mycoplasma phylogenetic tree (20, 77). The *M. capricolum* group consists of *M. capricolum* (type strain California kid), serogroup 7 of Leach (type strain PG50), and the F38-like group (type strain F38); the *M. mycoides* group consists of *M. mycoides* subsp. *mycoides* SC (type strain PG1) and LC (type strain Y-goat) and subsp. *capri* (type

strain PG3). Some members of these groups are important pathogens for goats and cattle, while other members are less pathogenic. Interspecies relationships between members of the *M. mycoides* cluster show DNA-DNA hybridization values of 36 to 82% (Table 1). A high degree of serological cross-reactivity between members of the *M. mycoides* cluster has been observed (23, 64). Kibe et al. (32) demonstrated no cross-reactivity between F38 and *M. capricolum* California kid by enzyme-linked immunosorbent assay, but immunoblot analysis showed that the two strains were closely related. By immunoblotting, all strains of the *M. mycoides* cluster reacted with hyperimmune sera from F38 and PG50 (32). These results do not give a clear taxonomic classification (73).

Many studies have been carried out on members of the *M. mycoides* cluster because of the severe diseases caused by some of these strains and the diagnostic and taxonomic problems (19). Rodwell and Rodwell (53, 54) compared the protein patterns of *M. mycoides* strains by 2-D gel electrophoresis. They analyzed *M. mycoides* subsp. *mycoides* SC (PG1) and six isolates belonging to this group, *M. mycoides* subsp. *mycoides* LC (Y-goat) and eight isolates belonging to this group, *M. mycoides* subsp. *capri* (PG3), and two other isolates. By comparison of autoradiograms, the percentage of congruence between strains was calculated. The results showed that LC strains are more closely related to *M. mycoides* subsp. *capri* than to SC strains, but also that within each group there is a marked degree of heterogeneity. The SC group was the most homogeneous, with 64 to 71% congruence. This group showed the least relationship to Y-goat (21 to 33%) and to PG3 (28 to 38%). The *M. mycoides* subsp. *capri* strains and the LC strains showed a much wider range of intraspecies heterogeneity, with congruences of 42 to 88% and 47 to 90%, respectively. Pronounced interspecies relationships were observed when LC strains were compared with strain PG3 (congruence of 43 to 57%) and when the *M. mycoides* subsp. *capri* strains were compared with strain Y-goat (congruence of 40 to 64%). Thus, these studies show that the SC group is a relatively homogeneous group with low congruence to the other type strains, whereas the LC and *capri* groups not only are much more heterogeneous but also show substantial congruence to each other.

Rodwell (53) also calculated the congruence for the protein patterns of 10 strains belonging to serogroup

Table 1. Homology of strains within the *M. mycoides* cluster based on DNA-DNA hybridization

Organism	DNA-DNA hybridization (% of homologous hybridization)					
	PG1	Y-goat	PG3	California kid	PG50	F38
M. mycoides subsp. *mycoides* SC (PG1)	100					
M. mycoides subsp. *mycoides* LC (Y-goat)	82[a]	100				
M. mycoides subsp. *capri* (PG3)	70[a]	75[b]	100			
M. capricolum California kid	ND[c]	41[b]	40[b]			
Bovine serogroup 7 of Leach (PG50)			64[b]			
		72[a]	57[b]	55[a]	58[b]	100
Caprine F38 group strain F38	ND	36[b]	39[b]	80[b]	60[b]	100

[a] From Christiansen and Ernø (11).
[b] From Askaa et al. (4).
[c] ND, not determined.

7 of Leach. He found this group to be quite homogeneous, with congruence of 71 to 99% and with congruence to the *M. mycoides* group of about 20%. The *M. capricolum* group varied and seemed less related to the type strain California kid, with about 20% congruence. The F38 strain showed similarities of 20 to 30% to *M. mycoides* strains, serogroup 7 of Leach, and *M. capricolum*. These results were confirmed by Nascimento et al. (42).

By one-dimensional SDS-PAGE, the visual resolution of mycoplasma protein bands does not allow calculation of relatedness between strains. This method has, however, been used successfully for epidemiological studies and for confirmation of serological results (42). Using SDS-PAGE and computerized numerical analysis of protein patterns, Leach et al. (37) analyzed 25 strains classified by serology as *M. mycoides* subsp. *mycoides* LC or as *M. mycoides* subsp. *capri*. Their results showed that 23 of the 25 strains fell into one large phenon. At 85% similarity, six subphenons were formed. The largest contained four *M. mycoides* subsp. *capri* and five *M. mycoides* subsp. *mycoides* LC strains. These results confirmed those of Rodwell and Rodwell (53, 54). *M. mycoides* subsp. *mycoides* SC (PG1), serogroup 7 of Leach (PG50), *M. capricolum* California kid, and F38 were also included in the study of Leach et al. (37). None of these strains fell into the phenon containing the 23 strains from *M. mycoides* subsp. *mycoides* LC and *M. mycoides* subsp. *capri*.

Although genetic relationships between strains must be given by the results of DNA-DNA hybridization, only results from hybridization of type strains have been published so far (4, 11). The intraspecies heterogeneity seen within several of the groups belonging to the *M. mycoides* cluster makes the taxonomic classification difficult.

By comparing the cleavage patterns of different mycoplasma strains belonging to a specific species, heterogeneity or homogeneity between strains can be clearly demonstrated (50, 51). A simpler analysis can be performed by Southern blotting using a probe containing part of the conserved rRNA genes. In mycoplasmas, the number of rRNA genes is one or two (26, 59, 60). It is therefore possible to analyze RFLP in different strains.

We used this method to analyze RFLP in the *M. capricolum* group (16). From serogroup 7 of Leach (type strain PG50), five isolates serologically classified as serogroup 7 were analyzed; from *M. capricolum* (type

strain California kid), six other isolates were analyzed; and from the F38-like group, F38 and six other isolates were analyzed. Southern blots were probed with five different probes (Fig. 1), each containing part of the *rrnA* gene of PG50 (12). The results showed that all strains had identical restriction enzyme cleavage sites within both rRNA operons (16). Strains belonging to serogroup 7 of Leach all had identical but specific cleavage sites outside the rRNA genes. The *M. capricolum* group varied. Strain California kid had lost an *Eco*RI site outside the 16S rRNA gene in the *rrnA* operon; except for this site, the California kid strain and three other strains were identical. Three other strains all varied in the position of one or two restriction cleavage sites. The F38-like group was more similar to the *M. capricolum* group than to serogroup 7 (Fig. 2). F38 had a specific *Bgl*II site outside the 23S rRNA gene of *rrnB*; all other strains showed identical restriction sites. Outside the *rrnA* operon, the F38 group had two characteristic *Hin*dIII sites that separated this group from the two other groups (16).

The results obtained by RFLP analysis of the *M. capricolum* strains are in agreement with the results of Rodwell (53); i.e., by 2-D gel electrophoresis, serogroup 7 is more homogeneous than the *M. capricolum* group.

Preliminary results (16a) of 30 strains belonging to the *M. mycoides* cluster showed that all strains had identical restriction enzyme cleavage sites within their two rRNA operons. These sites differed slightly from the cleavage sites found in the *M. capricolum* group. Strains belonging to *M. mycoides* subsp. *mycoides* SC form an identical cluster, whereas strains belonging to *M. mycoides* subsp. *mycoides* LC and *M. mycoides* subsp. *capri* have more varying restriction sites outside the rRNA operons. On the basis of similarities with the type strains Y-goat and PG3, the other strains did not fall into two clusters. RFLP analysis of the *M. mycoides* cluster is thus in agreement with results of Rodwell (53).

GENETIC VARIABILITY WITHIN *M. HOMINIS* STRAINS

M. hominis is among the best studied of the heterogeneous mycoplasma groups (49; for a review, see reference 25). The first report on serological heterogeneity within the *M. hominis* group came from Nicol and

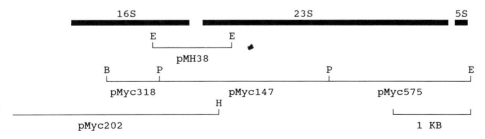

Figure 1. Recombinant plasmid probes from PG21 and the *rrnA* operon of strain PG50, containing mycoplasmal rRNA gene fragments. pMH38 contains a 1.2-kb *Eco*RI insert from *M. hominis* PG21 (E–E), pMYC probes contain inserts from the *rrnA* operon of serogroup 7 of Leach strain PG50, pMYC318 contains a 650-bp *Bgl*II-*Pst*I fragment (B–P), pMYC202 contains a 5.1-kb *Hin*dIII fragment (–H), pMYC147 contains a 2.7-kb *Pst*I fragment (P–P), and pMYC575 contains a 1.6-kb *Pst*I-*Eco*RI fragment (P–E). E, *Eco*RI; B, *Bgl*II; P, *Pst*I; H, *Hin*dIII.

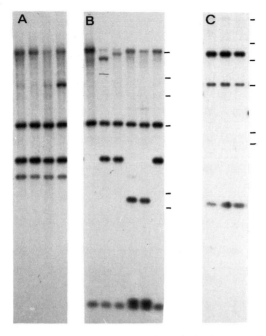

Figure 2. Autoradiogram of Southern hybridization of *M. mycoides* strains. (A) Four isolates from serogroup 7 of Leach. DNAs from strains C1888, C1889, C2097, and C2306 were cleaved with *Eco*RI and hybridized with pMYC202. (B) Six isolates from *M. capricolum*. DNAs from strains California kid, C1352, C1826, C2248, C2000, and C2255 were cleaved with *Eco*RI and hybridized with pMYC202. (C) Three isolates from the F38-like group; DNAs from strains C1849, C1848, and C1682 were cleaved with *Eco*RI and hybridized with pMYC318. Standard DNA was *Hind*III-digested bacteriophage lambda DNA (23.7, 9.5, 6.6, 4.3, 2.3, and 2.0 kb).

Edward in 1953 (43), who found that different strains classified as *M. hominis* type 1 differed in agglutination titers with antisera from four different strains classified as *M. hominis* type 1. Other serological methods confirmed this observation (30, 71). In 1974, Lin and Kass (39) published a study in which they selected seven strains of *M. hominis* against which they produced antisera. From the results of three serological methods (the complement-dependent mycoplasmacidal test, metabolic inhibition, and growth agglutination), they concluded that *M. hominis* consisted of at least seven serogroups and that the variable antigens probably were membrane antigens. A similar but more radical conclusion was reached by Somerson et al. (65), who investigated the relationship between eight *M. hominis* strains by DNA-RNA hybridization. Homology between strains was 17 to 90%. Only two strains were closely related, but they were not identical. Thus, all eight strains were genetically distinct and could not be divided into subgroups. Even though *M. hominis* is a heterogeneous group, there seems to exist no close correlation to other human mycoplasmas (13).

Because of questions concerning *M. hominis* heterogeneity, we analyzed these problems by molecular biological methods. We included the seven strains analyzed by Lin and Kass (39), three of the strains used in the study of Hollingdale and Lemcke (30), and three

strains isolated from the upper urinary tract (72). These strains presented a broad spectrum in terms of geographic origin and anatomical site of isolation (original strains). In some studies, we included 12 genital isolates collected in Denmark during a 3-month period (Table 2).

Andersen et al. (2) compared the proteins of 14 strains of *M. hominis* by using SDS-PAGE, immunoblot analysis, and 2-D gel electrophoresis. Results of the SDS-PAGE analysis showed congruence of 76 to 99% (Fig. 3). A more detailed analysis was obtained by 2-D gel electrophoresis and showed 41 to 72% congruence. The type strain, PG21, was most distant from other strains (congruence of 42 to 60%). No two strains were identical. The highest congruence was observed between strains 10 and W2 (72%). Higher congruence (60 to 68%) was seen between strains isolated from the upper urinary tract. The lower congruences found by 2-D gel electrophoresis analyses than by SDS-PAGE reflect the higher resolution obtained by the former method.

Immunoblot analysis (Fig. 4) seems more suitable than SDS-PAGE for comparison between strains because fewer bands are seen and differences are more pronounced (6). This is probably because many conserved cytoplasmic proteins are less antigenic than the more variable surface antigens. The number of bands seen in immunoblots by Andersen et al. (2) is much higher than the number of bands found by Brown et al. (8), who analyzed the heterogeneity of strains previously described by Lin and Kass (39) by immunoblot-

Table 2. *M. hominis* strains[a]

Strain designation	Source of isolation
PG21 (H50)[T]	Lower genital tract
M1449	Blood
93	Vagina
10	Vagina
4195	Vagina
183	Vagina
132	Vagina
W2	Wound
SC4	Male urethra
DC63	Oral cavity
V2785	Oral cavity
P71	Upper urinary tract
P7	Upper urinary tract
P2	Upper urinary tract
4076	Male urethra
7806	Female urethra
3849	Cervix
7488	Cervix
5941	Cervix
6188	Cervix
3105	Cervix
8264	Cervix
1893	Cervix
7357	Cervix
4712	Cervix
5503	Cervix

[a] PG21 through P2 are strains which present a broad spectrum in terms of geographic origin and anatomical site of isolation (original strains). 4076 through 5503 are genital isolates collected in Denmark during a 3-month period.

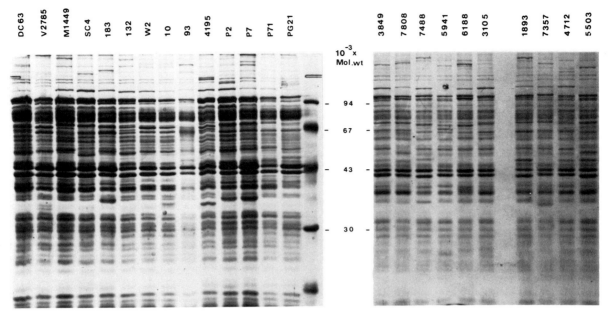

Figure 3. SDS-PAGE of Coomassie blue-stained proteins from *M. hominis* strains. Standards (kilodaltons) were phosphorylase *b* (94), bovine serum albumin (67), ovalbumin (43), carbonic anhydrase (30), and soybean trypsin inhibitor (20).

ting with rabbit hyperimmune serum against PG21. The substantial difference between the results of Brown et al. (8) and Andersen et al. (2) is presumably caused by differences in the immunization schemes used. Brown et al. (8) immunized rabbits with whole cells, so that the antibodies produced would probably be mainly against surface antigens, whereas Andersen et al. (2) immunized with sonicated cells, thus raising an immune response against a great number of cytoplasmic as well as membrane antigens. Except for the number of bands visualized by immunoblotting, the results were similar, confirming the heterogeneity and uniqueness of the strains.

Barile et al. (5) have suggested that strains isolated from the same anatomical region should be more similar to each other than to strains isolated from different anatomical sites. The three strains isolated from the upper urinary tract (P2, P7, and P71) indicated a somewhat greater similarity (60 to 68% congruence by 2-D gel electrophoresis) even though they were not identical. We therefore analyzed 12 genital isolates (Table 2) and compared them with the original 14 strains by immunoblotting. It was surprising that these strains varied as much from each other as the original strains did (Fig. 4).

Analysis of strain variation of single antigens was done by using monoclonal antibodies (MAbs). Ten MAbs against strain PG21 were produced. Characterization of the MAbs against PG21 has been reported by Ladefoged et al. (34). Eight of the MAbs reacted with epitopes localized at the surface of *M. hominis* PG21. Seven MAbs reacted with integral membrane proteins. Of these, only three reacted with all 26 strains (Table 3). It is characteristic that no MAb reacted with a protein of the same size in all strains, and no MAb reacted with only one protein in all strains. In contrast, the two MAbs against cytoplasmic, non-surface-exposed

polypeptide antigens showed identical reactions in all strains.

These results confirm the observation that surface antigens are more variable than cytoplasmic antigens. Furthermore, the results may explain why the complement fixation test, in which cytoplasmic as well as membrane antigens react, is the only serological test that does not demonstrate antigenic heterogeneity (39).

To study the genetic background for antigen variation, DNAs from the 26 strains were prepared, and selected strains were studied by DNA-DNA hybridization (15). This analysis confirmed the results obtained by Somerson et al. (65) and showed hybridization values of 51 to 91% between strains. The results of DNA-DNA hybridization agreed with the results of 2-D gel electrophoresis analyses and showed that type strain PG21 was more distantly related to most strains than was any other strain. A general impression of DNA heterogeneity from different strains was obtained by gel electrophoresis of restriction enzyme-cleaved DNA fragments (Fig. 5). As for 2-D gel electrophoresis analysis, the two strains most alike were W2 and 10.

Since antigenic variation of membrane proteins was pronounced compared with that of conserved cytoplasmic antigens (35), RFLP was analyzed for conserved genes and their flanking regions. All 26 strains were analyzed for RFLP within and outside the rRNA genes. Cloned fragments from the *rrnA* operon of strain PG50, as well as pMH38 with a 1.2-kb cloned *Eco*RI fragment from the gene library of PG21 (14), were used as probes. pMH38 contained the distal one-third of the 16S rRNA gene, the spacer, and the 5' end of the 23S rRNA gene (Fig. 1). Southern blot analysis of restriction enzyme-cleaved DNA from the 26 strains by using these probes showed variability of restriction enzyme cleavage sites outside the rRNA operons. However,

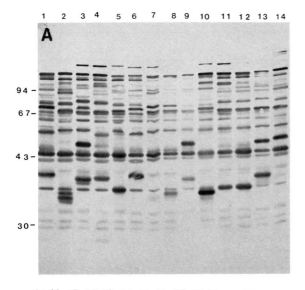

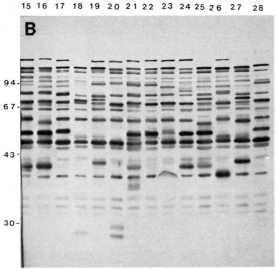

Figure 4. Immunoblotting from SDS-PAGE of *M. hominis* strains. (A) Original strains. Lanes: 1, DC63; 2, V2785; 3, M1449; 4, SC4; 5, 183; 6, 132; 7, W2; 8, 10; 9, 93; 10, 4195; 11, P2; 12, P7; 13, P71; 14, PG21. (B) Genital isolates. Lanes: 15, 3849; 16, 7808; 17, 7488; 18, 5941; 19, 6188; 20, 3105; 21, 8264; 22, 1893; 23, 7357; 24, 4712; 25, 5503; 26, 4076; 27, DC63; 28, PG21. Polyclonal PG21 hyperimmune rabbit serum was used as antibody. Standards were as for Fig. 3.

RFLP was also observed within the rRNA genes (Fig. 6). In two strains, DC63 and 10, the *Eco*RI sites within the 16S rRNA operons are missing (Fig. 6A and B). In strain SC4, a *Hin*dIII site within one of the 23S rRNA operons is missing (Fig. 6A and C).

M. hominis strains were classified on the basis of RFLP analysis (14). Six strains showed identical cleavage patterns (three of the original strains and three of the clinical isolates). Another class contained three strains, and a third class contained two strains. Fifteen strains showed unique restriction enzyme cleavage patterns. The classes obtained from RFLP analysis showed that strains from different anatomical regions belonged to the same class (upper urinary tract, blood,

and vagina and cervix). Two strains isolated from the upper urinary tract, P2 and P7 (2), fell into the same class, while the most similar strains, W2 and 10, which showed 72% congruence by 2-D gel electrophoresis analysis, were in different classes (Fig. 6A).

In microorganisms, the *atp* genes are also conserved (10). By using a probe containing the genes encoding the alpha and gamma subunits of the *atp* operon of bovine serogroup 7 of Leach (PG50), RFLP analysis was performed on the 14 original *M. hominis* strains (Table 2). This probe clearly detected RFLP in the *M. hominis* strains, but subdivision of the strains according to this RFLP was different from that of the classes obtained by RFLP of the rRNA genes (10). Therefore, we agree with the suggestion made by Somerson et al. (65) that *M. hominis* is composed of individual, unique strains that have more or less relationship to each other but that all possess the features characteristic of *M. hominis*, such as arginine hydrolysis and serological reaction with hyperimmune rabbit sera against *M. hominis* PG21.

Since surface antigens are the most variable *M. hominis* proteins, analysis of the genes encoding surface proteins and comparison of these genes from several strains would provide information on the genetic variability within *M. hominis*. A *Sau*3A library of *M. hominis* PG21 DNA was cloned into the expression vector system pEX1-3 (17, 66). In this system, recombinant DNA is inserted in the reading frame of the vector's β-galactosidase gene. Therefore, mycoplasma proteins are expressed as fusion proteins under control of the bacteriophage lambda promoter and, because of temperature-sensitive repressor, are inducible by a temperature shift.

Screening for recombinant bacteria expressing *M. hominis* antigens was performed by colony blotting with polyclonal PG21 hyperimmune rabbit serum as well as with the panel of MAbs (Table 3). Eighty-nine clones expressing *M. hominis* antigens were obtained. Three of the MAbs (552, 30.3.1 and 43.2) reacted with recombinant clones (29).

Recombinant plasmid DNAs were used to probe Southern blots containing restriction endonuclease-cleaved DNA from each of the 26 strains in order to analyze for RFLP in genes encoding surface antigens. As expected, RFLP was observed with all probes (17). The plasmid encoding the epitope for MAb 30.3.1 (containing a 0.3-kb insert) reacted with only strains harboring the epitope for MAb 30.3.1. In all cases, positively reacting strains showed that only one DNA fragment reacted with the probe. Lack of reactivity with this MAb is thus due to a chromosomal deletion. It is not known whether this deletion is identical in all strains.

The clone (containing a 1.2-kb insert) encoding the MAb 43.2 epitope hybridized to two or three bands in all strains regardless of the restriction enzyme used. RFLP was pronounced, and only a few strains showed identical hybridization patterns. Because the relatively small probe did not contain cleavage sites for the enzymes used and reacted with several DNA fragments, the DNA sequence or part of the DNA sequence homologous to the probe may be present more than once in the genome.

Ten recombinants with different insert sizes reacted with MAb 552. This MAb recognized surface epitopes

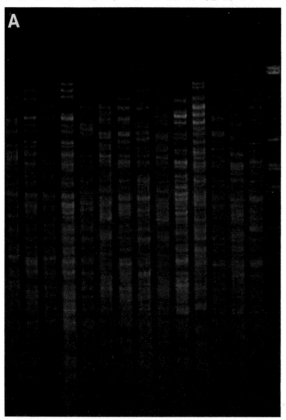

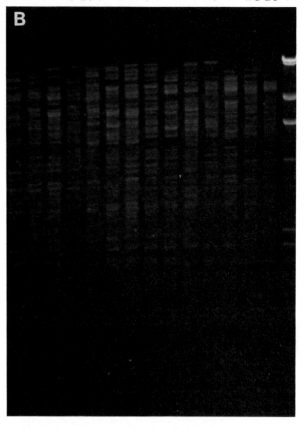

Figure 5. Cleavage patterns of DNA from *M. hominis* strains. (A) Original strains cleaved with *Hae*III. Lanes: 1, PG21; 2, DC63; 3, SC4; 4, 132; 5, 183; 6, 10; 7, P7; 8, 93; 9, W2; 10, V2785; 11, P71; 12, P2; 13, 4195; 14, M1449; 15, bacteriophage lambda DNA cleaved with *Eco*RI. (B) Genital strains cleaved with *Eco*RI. Lanes: 16, 3849; 17, 7807; 18, 7488; 19, 5941; 20, 6188; 21, 3105; 22, 8264; 23, 1893; 24, 7357; 25, 4712; 26, 5503; 27, 4076; 28, DC63; 29, PG21; 30, bacteriophage lambda DNA cleaved with *Hin*dIII.

in all 26 *M. hominis* strains. All recombinant plasmids gave identical hybridization patterns in the Southern blot analysis. When DNAs from the different *M. hominis* strains were cleaved with restriction enzyme *Eco*RI or *Bgl*II, the probes reacted with two bands in all strains. RFLP was pronounced. A much more complicated pattern was seen when the DNA was cleaved with *Hin*dIII. Further analysis showed that in PG21, two chromosomal regions each contained DNA encoding the epitope for MAb 552. In each region, a gene with a 124-kDa coding capacity was found by sequence analysis. Each gene contained internal repeats of 471 bp. In one of the genes, the repeats were identical except for two base pair substitutions, whereas in the other gene, the repeats were 87 to 99% identical. It is not known which of the genes is active during growth. None of the other strains showed this arrangement. Only a few strains had the *Hin*dIII repeat of 471 bp observed in PG21.

The genetic basis for antigenic strain variation thus seems to be very complicated. Deletions, repeated sequences, and base variations are part of the origin of mycoplasma heterogeneity. A clue to how antigenic variation might occur came from experiments by Ladefoged et al. (35a). *M. hominis* strains PG21 and 7488

were passaged continuously over a period of 3 months in media with or without addition of MAb 552. Twice during the cultivation, Southern analysis of the DNA was performed with a probe encoding the epitope specific for MAb 552. In PG21 cultivated in the presence of MAb 552, several deletion mutations were observed. The deletions were all located in the gene containing the perfect repeats and spanned a variable number of repeats. The other gene was unchanged. No other genomic alternations were observed. No changes were observed in strain 7488 or in strain PG21 cultivated without MAb.

Induction of intragenic deletions under selective pressure of an antibody added to the cultivation media has not previously been described. However, the possibility that antibodies play a role in the induction of antigenic variation was not unexpected because the 12 clinical isolates (Table 2) were all different and each sample contained only a single strain of *M. hominis*, as judged by RFLP analyses and analyses of single colonies after filter cloning.

M. hominis has usually been isolated from different anatomical sites as a commensal, but it sometimes causes infections (25). Strains isolated from the same anatomical site seem to vary as much as do strains

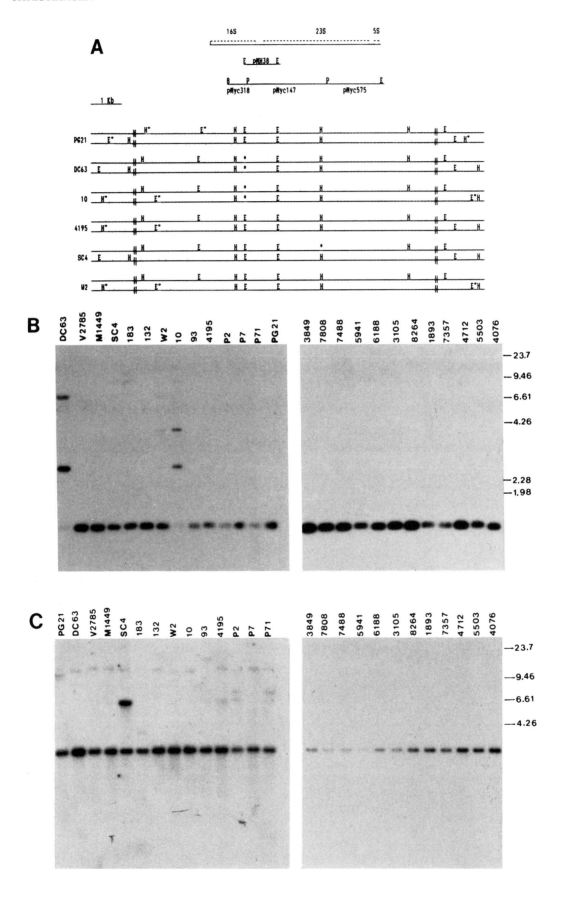

isolated from different sites. No pathogenicity factors have so far been detected. The strong genetic variability of these strains may help them survive in the human body by escaping attacks from the host immune system. Thus, genetic variability itself may be an important pathogenicity factor.

GENETIC VARIATION IN *M. PULMONIS*

M. pulmonis causes a chronic, naturally occurring respiratory disease in mice and rats. In the chronic stage of the infection, viable *M. pulmonis* can be isolated from the lungs of infected animals. Microbial antigen variation is often found in chronic infections. In *M. pulmonis*, variation in size and opacity of colonies of different pathogenic strains has been observed (40). Opacity is a stable character, and opaque cultures give rise to translucent colonies at a rate which suggests a single genetic event mutation. Comparison of DNA profiles of restriction enzyme-cleaved DNA showed some strain variation. Opaque and transparent colonies from specific strains were isolated, and the DNA and protein profiles were compared. Colony opacity seemed to be correlated with a specific restriction enzyme cleavage pattern. Protein analysis by SDS-PAGE showed variation in band patterns when different strains were compared, but minor variations were also seen when opaque and transparent colonies from the same strain were compared (40).

The major membrane antigen component in *M. pulmonis* is the V-1 antigen complex (21, 22, 74–76). Variability of the V-1 antigen complex has been hypothesized to be a potentially important pathogenicity factor for establishing chronic infections. Analysis of the V-1 antigen complex by SDS-PAGE and subsequent immunoblotting with monoclonal or monospecific antibodies show an unusual ladder pattern of protein bands of 150 to 200 kDa. The pattern differs between strains and between subclones of a single strain (76). Colony size variation correlated with changes in the band patterns of the V-1 antigen complex (22). Both constant and variable epitopes have been described (76). Watson et al. (74, 75) analyzed the structure of the V-1 antigen complex and found that phenol-H_2O-extracted material showed a regular 3.1-kDa spacing in the ladder pattern. Trypsin treatment resulted in a gradual collapse of the ladder to a single band. When the upper band of the phenol-H_2O-extracted material was eluted from the gel and analyzed again by SDS-PAGE and immunoblotting, a new ladder identical to the original pattern was generated. These results suggest that the V-1 antigen complex is composed of multiple, identical subunits. Triton X-114 extraction showed that low-molecular-weight material in the ladder partitioned into the hydrophobic phase, whereas high-molecular-weight material in the ladder pattern was found in the aqueous phase. Thus, high-molecular-weight material probably forms micelles with the hydrophobic material at the inner membrane surface, whereas hydrophilic regions are at the outer membrane surface (75). The variation of the V-1 antigen complex may affect the interaction between *M. pulmonis* and host cells, thereby mediating the difference in virulence observed by Davidson et al. (21) and the difference in clearance of *M. pulmonis* strains from the respiratory tract of mice (21).

The genetic background for the V-1 antigen complex variation is unknown. It is not known whether the antigen variation is correlated to the variation in DNA band patterns observed by Liss and Heiland (40).

GENETIC VARIATION IN *M. HYOPNEUMONIAE*

M. hyopneumoniae is the major cause of lung infections in swine and has not been described as a particularly variable species. However, several surface proteins have been shown to vary by the use of MAbs (80). In a comparison of two strains, one MAb recognized proteins of different sizes in the two strains, and another MAb failed to recognize an antigen in one of the strains (80).

Ferrell et al. (24) described the presence of two DNA repeats 1,550 bp in size, flanked by 28-bp inverted repeats. Two potential open reading frames are present within the sequence. The two repeats are present on an 8-kb *Eco*RI fragment. By using this fragment as a probe in Southern hybridization of five other strains of *M. hyopneumoniae*, it was found that the probe hybridized with two bands in four of the five strains, indicating that the repeated sequences were present on two different *Eco*RI fragments. The fifth strain did not react with the probe and thus did not contain the sequence.

GENETIC VARIATION IN *M. HYORHINIS*

M. hyorhinis is among the mycoplasma species known to be heterogeneous (79). This porcine mycoplasma is common in secondary pulmonary infections and is associated with arthritis and polyserositis. It is also commonly isolated from the nasal cavity of pigs and is frequently found to contaminate cell cultures (49).

Considerable serological variation between different isolates has been found (79), and reports on antigenic variation of surface-localized lipoproteins have been published (7, 52, 81). Rosengarten and Wise (55) described phenotypic switching in *M. hyorhinis* and showed that *M. hyorhinis* is capable of producing phenotypic changes in colony appearance (size, shape, and opacity) and of showing high-frequency phase transi-

---

Figure 6. Southern blot analysis of *M. hominis* strains. (A) Restriction maps of rRNA genes from *M. hominis* strains deduced from Southern blot analyses using the probes shown in Fig. 1. E, *Eco*RI; H, *Hin*dIII; *, no restriction enzyme cleavage sites. *E and *H indicate unique restriction enzyme cleavage sites. (B) Southern blotting of *M. hominis* DNA cleaved with *Eco*RI and hybridized with pMH38. (C) Southern blotting of *M. hominis* DNA cleaved with *Hin*dIII and hybridized with pMH38. Size standards (indicated in kilobases) were bacteriophage lambda DNA fragments cleaved with *Hin*dIII.

Table 3. Sizes of antigens to MAbs in *M. hominis* strains[a]

MAb	Size of antigen (kDa) in *M. hominis* strain:																									
	DC63	V2785	M1449	SC4	183	132	W2	10	93	4195	P2	P7	P71	PG21	3849	7808	7488	5941	6188	3105	8264	1893	7357	4712	5503	4076
552	138, 94	93	94	91	94	93	93	93	93	93	93	93	93	124, 96	96	153, 92	96, 92	93	90	90	144, 90	91	95	93	99	96
667		73	73	72									72, 44	72, 44		73	72									
434	91, 70	91, 70	93, 72	89, 71	92, 69	92, 71	92, 69	92, 69		91	92, 70	92, 70			92, 70	86, 70	70	70	70	70	70	70	70	70	70	70
21.1.6	72, 65	69, 65	68	69, 67	69	71, 65	69	69	69, 24	70	69	69	69, 65, 24	69, 65, 24	71, 64	71, 65	69	71	71, 64	68	69	69	69	69	71	68
43.2	72, 65	69, 65	68	69, 67	69	71, 65	69	69	69, 24	70	69	69	69, 65, 24	69, 65, 24	71, 64	71, 65	69	71	71, 64	68	69	69	69	69	71	68
54	36, 35	36, 35	47						47	36, 35			47	49	47	47	49				47	47		47	47	
46.2	39	36, 35	47, 38, 36	38	36	38		36	47, 38	35	36	36	47, 38	49	47, 38, 37	47, 38	49		39	38, 37	47, 38	47	36	47, 38	47, 38	36
522			47, 38, 36						47, 38, 36				47, 38, 36	49, 38	47, 38	47, 38	49, 38				47, 38	47		47, 38	37, 38	
30.3.1			47, 38, 36						47, 38, 36				47, 38, 36, 28, 27	49, 38	47, 38	47, 38	49, 38			28, 27	47, 38	47		47, 38	47, 38	

[a] For each MAb, similar size antigens are listed in the same row. For MAb 552, the vertical lines indicate the presence of antigens forming a reproducible ladder pattern between the upper and lower antigen sizes.

tion in expression of lipid-modified cell surface antigens.

CONCLUSION

There is a marked species-specific diversity in heterogeneity of mycoplasmas. *M. hominis* is probably the most heterogeneous, as reflected by serology, nucleic acid hybridization, and protein variability. *M. hyorhinis* strains, on the other hand, do not seem to vary by DNA hybridization, but they vary in serological tests and in antigen presentation.

Only a limited number of mycoplasma species have been analyzed for intraspecies diversity by serological methods, nucleic acid hybridization, and protein variability. Therefore, it is not possible to propose a general model for mycoplasma species diversity. From the data presented in this chapter, there seem to be several ways by which mycoplasmas are capable of producing intraspecies diversity. In *M. hominis*, DNA sequence variability, deletions, and duplications seem to be important for intraspecies heterogeneity. In *M. hyopneumoniae*, transposonlike elements may be involved in establishing heterogeneity. Use of variation in the number of repeated elements in surface-localized lipid-modified proteins is important in *M. pulmonis* and *M. hyorhinis* but is not observed in *M. hominis*.

Antigenic variability is probably necessary for many, if not all, mycoplasma species to avoid the host immune response. Since mycoplasmas are wall-less, they are particularly sensitive to immunological attack and must therefore have developed defense mechanisms to prevent their eradication.

It is characteristic of many of the heterogeneous mycoplasma species that they have a broad tissue tropism or host range and that some are involved in chronic disorders.

Species that are known as genetically stable mycoplasmas, such as *M. pneumoniae*, have developed a specialized tip structure for attachment to the host cell. They have also developed a specific way to modify the major adhesin protein (P1). Mycoplasmas without such a special adhesin structure probably need to be able to modify several membrane components, thereby inducing genetic variability. This variability seems not to be restricted to genes encoding surface proteins, even though these genes may vary more than other chromosomal regions.

REFERENCES

1. **Amikam, D., G. Glaser, and S. Razin.** 1984. Mycoplasmas (*Mollicutes*) have a low number of rRNA genes. *J. Bacteriol.* **158**:376–378.
2. **Andersen, H., S. Birkelund, G. Christiansen, and E. A. Freundt.** 1987. Electrophoretic analysis of proteins from *Mycoplasma hominis* strains detected by SDS-PAGE, two-dimensional gel electrophoresis and immunoblotting. *J. Gen. Microbiol.* **133**:181–191.
3. **Andersen, H., G. Christiansen, and C. Christiansen.** 1984. Electrophoretic analysis of proteins from *Mycoplasma capricolum* and related serotypes using extracts from infected cells and from minicells containing cloned *Mycoplasma* DNA. *J. Gen. Microbiol.* **130**:1409–1418.
4. **Askaa, G., H. Ernø, and M. O. Ojo.** 1978. Bovine mycoplasmas: classification of groups related to *Mycoplasma mycoides*. *Acta Vet. Scand.* **19**:166–178.
5. **Barile, M. F., M. W. Grabowski, E. B. Stephens, S. J. O'Brien, J. M. Simonson, K. Izumikawa, D. K. F. Chandler, D. Taylor-Robinson, and J. G. Tully.** 1983. *Mycoplasma hominis*-tissue cell interactions: a review with new observations on phenotypic and genotypic properties. *Sex. Transm. Dis.* **10**:345–354.
6. **Birkelund, S., and H. Andersen.** 1987. Comparative studies of mycoplasma antigens and corresponding antibodies, p. 25–33. *In* O. J. Bjerrum and N. H. H. Heegaard (ed.), *Handbook of Immunoblotting of Proteins*, vol. 11. CRC Press, Inc., Boca Raton, Fla.
7. **Boyer, M. J., and K. S. Wise.** 1989. Lipid-modified surface protein antigens expressing size variation within the species *Mycoplasma hyorhinis*. *Infect. Immun.* **57**:245–254.
8. **Brown, M. B., F. C. Minion, J. K. Davis, D. G. Pritchard, and G. H. Cassell.** 1983. Antigens of *Mycoplasma hominis*. *Sex. Transm. Dis.* **10**:247–255.
9. **Chen, X., and L. R. Finch.** 1989. Novel arrangement of rRNA genes in *Mycoplasma gallisepticum*: separation of the 16S gene of one set from the 23S and 5S genes. *J. Bacteriol.* **171**:2876–2878.
10. **Christiansen, C., G. Christiansen, and O. F. Rasmussen.** 1987. Heterogeneity of *Mycoplasma hominis* as detected by a probe for *atp* genes. *Isr. J. Med. Sci.* **23**:591–594.
11. **Christiansen, C., and H. Ernø.** 1982. Classification of the F38 group of caprine mycoplasma strains by DNA hybridization. *J. Gen. Microbiol.* **128**:2523–2526.
12. **Christiansen, C., J. Frydenberg, G. Christiansen, H. Andersen, and L. Hedegaard.** 1984. Analysis of the mycoplasma genome by recombinant DNA technology. *Isr. J. Med. Sci.* **20**:781–784.
13. **Christiansen, C., E. Hansen, and G. Christiansen.** 1983. The genetic relation between *Mycoplasma hominis* and other Mycoplasma species. *Sex. Transm. Dis.* **10**:230–231.
14. **Christiansen, G., and H. Andersen.** 1988. Heterogeneity among *Mycoplasma hominis* strains as detected by probes containing parts of ribosomal ribonucleic acid genes. *Int. J. Syst. Bacteriol.* **38**:108–115.
15. **Christiansen, G., H. Andersen, S. Birkelund, and E. A. Freundt.** 1987. Genomic and gene variation in *Mycoplasma hominis* strains. *Isr. J. Med. Sci.* **23**:595–602.
16. **Christiansen, G., and H. Ernø.** 1990. RFLP in rRNA genes of *Mycoplasma capricolum*, the caprine F38-like group and the bovine serogroup 7. *Zentralbl. Bakteriol. Suppl.* **20**:479–488.
16a. **Christiansen, G., and H. Ernø.** Unpublished data.
17. **Christiansen, G., S. Ladefoged, S. Hauge, S. Birkelund, and H. Andersen.** 1990. Use of monoclonal antibodies for detection of gene and antigen variation in *Mycoplasma hominis*. *Zentralbl. Bakteriol. Suppl.* **20**:535–545.
18. **Clark, P. H.** 1974. The evolution of enzymes for the utilization of novel substrates. *Symp. Soc. Gen. Microbiol.* **24**:183–217.
19. **Cottew, G. S.** 1979. Caprine-ovine mycoplasmas, p. 103–132. *In* J. G. Tully and R. F. Whitcomb (ed.), *The Mycoplasmas*, vol. 2. Academic Press, Inc., New York.
20. **Cottew, G. S., A. Breard, A. J. DaMassa, H. Ernø, R. H. Leach, P. C. Lefevre, A. W. Rodwell, and G. R. Smith.** 1987. Taxonomy of the *Mycoplasma mycoides* cluster. *Isr. J. Med. Sci.* **23**:632–635.
21. **Davidson, M. K., J. R. Lindsey, R. F. Parker, J. G. Tully, and G. H. Cassell.** 1988. Differences in virulence for mice among strains of *Mycoplasma pulmonis*. *Infect. Immun.* **56**:2156–2162.
22. **Dybvig, K., J. W. Simecka, H. L. Watson, and G. H. Cassell.** 1989. High-frequency variation in *Mycoplasma pulmonis* colony size. *J. Bacteriol.* **171**:5165–5168.
23. **Ernø, H., R. H. Leach, M. M. Salih, and K. J. MacOwan.** 1983. The F38-like group, a new group of caprine mycoplasmas? *Acta Vet. Scand.* **24**:275–286.
24. **Ferrell, R. V., M. B. Heidari, K. S. Wise, and M. A. McIn-**

tosh. 1989. A Mycoplasma genetic element resembling prokaryotic insertion sequences. *Mol. Microbiol.* **3**:957–967.

25. **Freundt, E. A.** 1983. Mycoplasma hominis: historical outline and taxonomy. *Sex. Transm. Dis.* **10**:226–229.

26. **Glaser, G., D. Amikam, and S. Razin.** 1984. Physical mapping of the ribosomal RNA genes of *Mycoplasma capricolum. Nucleic Acids Res.* **12**:2421–2426.

27. **Hall, B. G., and P. W. Betts.** 1987. Cryptic genes for cellobiose utilization in natural isolates of *Escherichia coli. Genetics* **115**:431–439.

28. **Hartl, D. L., and D. E. Dykhuizen.** 1984. The population genetics of *Escherichia coli. Annu. Rev. Genet.* **18**:31–68.

29. **Hauge, S., S. Ladefoged, S. Birkelund, and G. Christiansen.** 1990. Analysis of genes for *Mycoplasma hominis* antigens by use of recombinant DNA technique. *Zentralbl. Bakteriol. Suppl.* **20**:614–639.

30. **Hollingdale, M. R., and R. M. Lemcke.** 1970. Antigenic differences within the species *Mycoplasma hominis. J. Hyg.* (Cambridge) **68**:469–477.

31. **Kawauchi, Y., A. Muto, and S. Osawa.** 1982. The protein composition of *Mycoplasma capricolum. Mol. Gen. Genet.* **188**:7–11.

32. **Kibe, M. K., D. E. Bidwell, P. Turp, and G. R. Smith.** 1985. Demonstration of cross-reactive antigens in F38 and related mycoplasmas by enzyme-linked immunosorbent assay (ELISA) and immunoblotting. *J. Hyg.* (Cambridge) **95**:95–106.

33. **Kleven, S. H.** 1990. Epidemiological studies of *Mycoplasma gallisepticum* using restriction endonuclease analysis. *Zentralbl. Bakteriol. Suppl.* **20**:494–499.

34. **Ladefoged, F., B. Brock, and G. Christiansen.** 1990. Physical and genetic maps of the genome of five strains of *Mycoplasma hominis. IOM Lett.* **1**:253–354.

35. **Ladefoged, S., S. Hauge, H. Andersen, S. Birkelund, and G. Christiansen.** 1990. Use of monoclonal antibodies for detection of antigen variation in *Mycoplasma hominis. Zentralbl. Bakteriol. Suppl.* **20**:634–639.

35a.**Ladefoged, S., et al.** Unpublished data.

36. **Lanham, S. M., R. M. Lemcke, C. M. Scott, and J. M. Grendon.** 1980. Isoenzymes in two species of *Acholeplasma. J. Gen. Microbiol.* **117**:19–31.

37. **Leach, R. H., M. Costas, and D. L. Mitchelmore.** 1989. Relationship between *Mycoplasma mycoides* subsp. *mycoides* ('large-colony' strains) and *M. mycoides* subsp. *capri*, as indicated by numerical analysis of one-dimensional SDS-PAGE protein patterns. *J. Gen. Microbiol.* **135**:2993–3000.

38. **Levin, B. R.** 1981. Periodic selection, infectious gene exchange and the genetic structure of *E. coli* populations. *Genetics* **99**:1–23.

39. **Lin, J.-S., and E. H. Kass.** 1974. Serological reactions of *Mycoplasma hominis*: differences among mycoplasmacidal, metabolic inhibition, and growth agglutination tests. *Infect. Immun.* **10**:535–540.

40. **Liss, A., and R. A. Heiland.** 1983. Colonial opacity variation in *Mycoplasma pulmonis. Infect. Immun.* **41**:1245–1251.

41. **Milkman, R.** 1973. Electrophoretic variation in *Escherichia coli* from natural sources. *Science* **182**:1024–1026.

42. **Nascimento, E. R., M. da G. F. Nascimento, E. A. Freundt, and H. Andersen.** 1986. Isolation of *Mycoplasma mycoides* from outbreaks of caprine mycoplasmosis in Brazil. *Br. Vet. J.* **142**:246–257.

43. **Nicol, C. S., and D. G. ff. Edward.** 1953. Role of organisms of the pleuropneumonia group in human genital infections. *Br. J. Vener. Dis.* **29**:141–150.

44. **Pyle, L. E., and L. R. Finch.** 1988. Preparation and FIGE separation of infrequent restriction fragments from *Mycoplasma mycoides* DNA. *Nucleic Acids Res.* **16**:2263–2268.

45. **Pyle, L. E., and L. R. Finch.** 1988. A physical map of the genome of *Mycoplasma mycoides* subspecies mycoides Y

with some functional loci. *Nucleic Acids Res.* **16**:6027–6039.

46. **Razin, S.** 1968. Mycoplasma taxonomy studied by electrophoresis of cell proteins. *J. Bacteriol.* **96**:687–694.

47. **Razin, S., D. Amikam, and G. Glaser.** 1984. Mycoplasmal ribosomal RNA genes and their use as probes for detection and identification of *Mollicutes. Isr. J. Med. Sci.* **20**:758–761.

48. **Razin, S., M. F. Barile, R. Harasawa, D. Amikam, and G. Glaser.** 1983. Characterization of the Mycoplasma genome. *Yale J. Biol. Med.* **56**:357–366.

49. **Razin, S., and E. A. Freundt.** 1984. The mycoplasmas, p. 740–792. *In* N. R. Krieg and J. G. Holt (ed.), *Bergey's Manual of Systematic Bacteriology*, vol. 1. Williams & Wilkins, Baltimore.

50. **Razin, S., R. Harasawa, and M. F. Barile.** 1983. Cleavage patterns of the mycoplasma chromosome, obtained by using restriction endonucleases, as indicators of genetic relatedness among strains. *Int. J. Syst. Bacteriol.* **33**:201–206.

51. **Razin, S., J. G. Tully, D. L. Rose, and M. F. Barile.** 1983. DNA cleavage patterns as indicators of genotypic heterogeneity among strains of *Acholeplasma* and *Mycoplasma* species. *J. Gen. Microbiol.* **129**:1935–1944.

52. **Riethman, H. C., M. J. Boyer, and K. S. Wise.** 1987. Triton X-114 phase fractionation of an integral membrane surface protein mediating monoclonal antibody killing of *Mycoplasma hyorhinis. Infect. Immun.* **55**:1094–1100.

53. **Rodwell, A. W.** 1982. The protein fingerprints of mycoplasmas. *Rev. Infect. Dis.* **4**:S8–S17.

54. **Rodwell, A. W., and E. S. Rodwell.** 1978. Relationships between strains of *Mycoplasma mycoides* subspp. *mycoides* and *capri* studied by two-dimensional gel electrophoresis of cell proteins. *J. Gen. Microbiol.* **109**:259–263.

55. **Rosengarten, R., and K. S. Wise.** 1990. Phenotypic switching in Mycoplasmas: phase variation of diverse surface lipoproteins. *Science* **247**:315–318.

56. **Salih, M. M., H. Ernø, and V. Simonsen.** 1983. Electrophoresis analysis of isoenzymes of mycoplasma species. *Acta Vet. Scand.* **24**:14–33.

57. **Salih, M. M., V. Simonsen, and H. Ernø.** 1983. Electrophoretic analysis of isoenzymes of *Acholeplasma* species. *Int. J. Syst. Bacteriol.* **33**:166–172.

58. **Santha, M., K. Lukacs, K. Burg, S. Bernath, I. Rasko, and L. Stipkovits.** 1988. Intraspecies genotypic heterogeneity among *Mycoplasma gallisepticum* strains. *Appl. Environ. Microbiol.* **54**:607–609.

59. **Sawada, M., A. Muto, M. Iwami, F. Yamao, and S. Osawa.** 1984. Organization of ribosomal RNA genes in *Mycoplasma capricolum. Mol. Gen. Genet.* **196**:311–316.

60. **Sawada, M., S. Osawa, H. Kobayashi, H. Hori, and A. Muto.** 1981. The number of ribosomal RNA genes in *Mycoplasma capricolum. Mol. Gen. Genet.* **182**:502–504.

61. **Schleifer, K. H., and E. Stackebrandt.** 1983. Molecular systematics of prokaryotes. *Annu. Rev. Microbiol.* **37**:143–187.

62. **Selander, R. K., D. A. Caugant, H. Ochman, J. M. Musser, M. N. Gilmour, and T. S. Whittam.** 1986. Methods of multilocus enzyme electrophoresis for bacterial population genetics and systematics. *Appl. Environ. Microbiol.* **51**:873–884.

63. **Selander, R. K., D. A. Caugant, and T. S. Whittam.** 1987. Genetic structure and variation in natural populations of *Escherichia coli*, p. 1625–1648. *In* F. C. Neidhardt, J. L. Ingraham, K. B. Low, B. Magasanik, M. Schaechter, and H. E. Umbarger (ed.), *Escherichia coli and Salmonella typhimurium: Cellular and Molecular Biology*, vol. 2. American Society for Microbiology, Washington, D.C.

64. **Smith, G. R., and J. C. Oliphant.** 1983. Immunogenic variation among the so-called LC strains of *Mycoplasma mycoides* subspecies mycoides. *J. Hyg.* (Cambridge) **90**:441–449.

65. **Somerson, N. L., P. R. Reich, B. E. Walls, R. M. Chanock,**

and S. M. Weissman. 1966. Genetic differentiation by nucleic acid homology. II. Genotypic variations within two *Mycoplasma* species. *J. Bacteriol.* **92**:311–317.

66. Stanly, K. K., and J. P. Luzio. 1984. Construction of a new family of high efficiency bacterial expression vectors: identification of cDNA clones coding for human liver proteins. *EMBO J.* **3**:1429–1434.

67. Stehens, E. B., G. S. Aulakh, D. L. Rose, J. G. Tully, and M. F. Barile. 1983. Intraspecies genetic relatedness among strains of *Acholeplasma laidlawii* and *Acholeplasma axanthum* by nucleic acid hybridization. *J. Gen. Microbiol.* **129**:1929–1934.

68. Stehens, E. B., G. S. Aulakh, D. L. Rose, J. G. Tully, and M. F. Barile. 1983. Interspecies and intraspecies DNA homology among established species of *Acholeplasma*: a review. *Yale J. Biol. Med.* **56**:729–735.

69. Su, C. J., A Chavoya, S. F. Dallo, and J. B. Baseman. 1990. Sequence divergency of the cytadhesin gene of *Mycoplasma pneumoniae*. *Infect. Immun.* **58**:2669–2674.

70. Su, C. J., S. F. Dallo, and J. B. Baseman. 1990. Molecular distinctions among clinical isolates of *Mycoplasma pneumoniae*. *J. Clin. Microbiol.* **28**:1538–1540.

71. Taylor-Robinson, D., W. M. Ludwig, R. H. Purcell, M. A. Mufson, and R. M. Chanock. 1965. Significance of antibody to *Mycoplasma hominis* type 1 as measured by indirect hemagglutination. *Proc. Soc. Exp. Biol. Med.* **118**:1073–1083.

72. Thomsen, A. C. 1978. Mycoplasma in human pyelonephritis: demonstration of antibodies in serum and urine. *J. Clin. Microbiol.* **8**:197–202.

73. Tully, J. G. 1988. International Committee on Systematic Bacteriology Subcommittee on the Taxonomy of *Mollicutes*. Minutes of the interim meeting, 25 and 28 August 1986, Birmingham, Alabama. *Int. J. Syst. Bacteriol.* **38**:226–230.

74. Watson, H. L., D. K. Blalock, and G. H. Cassell. 1990. Characterization of the variable V-1 antigen of *Mycoplasma pulmonis*. *Zentralbl. Bakteriol. Suppl.* **20**:529–534.

75. Watson, H. L., K. Dybvig, D. K. Blalock, and G. H. Cassell. 1989. Subunit structure of the variable V-1 antigen of *Mycoplasma pulmonis*. *Infect. Immun.* **57**:1684–1690.

76. Watson, H. L., L. S. McDaniel, D. K. Blalock, M. T. Fallon, and G. H. Cassell. 1988. Heterogeneity among strains and a high rate of variation within strains of a major surface antigen of *Mycoplasma pulmonis*. *Infect. Immun.* **56**:1358–1363.

77. Weisburg, W. G., J. G. Tully, D. L. Rose, J. P. Petzel, H. Oyaizu, D. Yang, L. Mandelco, J. Sechrest, T. G. Lawrence, J. van Etten, J. Maniloff, and C. R. Woese. 1989. A phylogenetic analysis of the mycoplasmas: basis for their classification. *J. Bacteriol.* **171**:6455–6467.

78. Whitley, J. C., L. E. Pyle, T. Taylor, and L. R. Finch. 1990. Comparison of genomes within the *Mycoides* cluster. *IOM Lett.* **1**:68–69.

79. Whittlestone, P. 1979. Porcine mycoplasmas, p. 133–176. *In* J. G. Tully and R. F. Whitcomb (ed.), *The Mycoplasmas*, vol. 2. Academic Press, Inc., New York.

80. Wise, K. S., and M. F. Kim. 1987. Major membrane surface proteins of *M. hyopneumoniae* selectively modified by covalently bound lipid. *J. Bacteriol.* **169**:5546–5555.

81. Wise, K. S., and R. K. Watson. 1983. Monoclonal antibodies to *Mycoplasma hyorhinis* surface antigens: tools for analyzing mycoplasma-lymphoid cell interactions. *Yale J. Biol. Med.* **56**:623–629.

82. Woese, C. R. 1987. Bacterial evolution. *Microbiol. Rev.* **51**:221–271.

83. Woese, C. R., E. Stackebrandt, and W. Ludwig. 1985. What are mycoplasmas: the relationship of tempo and mode in bacterial evolution. *J. Mol. Evol.* **21**:305–316.

84. Yogev, D., D. Halachmi, G. E. Kenny, and S. Razin. 1988. Distinction of species and strains of mycoplasmas (Mollicutes) by genomic DNA fingerprints with an rRNA gene probe. *J. Clin. Microbiol.* **26**:1198–1201.

85. Young, J. P. W. 1989. The population genetics of bacteria, p. 417–440. *In* D. A. Hopwood and K. E. Chater (ed.), *Genetics of Bacterial Diversity*. Academic Press, London.

35. Evolution of Macromolecule Synthesis

TORE SAMUELSSON and THOMAS BORÉN

INTRODUCTION

The mycoplasmas are procaryotes with unusually small genomes, and all available phylogenetic data strongly support the notion that they evolved from ancestors that were common to gram-positive bacteria with a low content of G·C base pairs (see chapter 33). Since these ancestors presumably had genomes the size of typical bacterial genomes (approximately 4,000 kb), the evolution of the mycoplasmas must have involved a severe reduction in genome size. *Mycoplasma* and *Ureaplasma* species represent the most extreme evolution in this respect, as they have exceptionally small genomes of only 600 to 1,200 kb. The discussion in this chapter is to a large extent related to these general features of the evolution of the mycoplasmas.

When an organism has abandoned the majority of genetic information that is present in typical bacteria, this would obviously be reflected in the biochemical and physiological repertoire of the organism. For instance, the mycoplasmas lack the cell wall characteristic of other bacteria, and many species lack normal metabolic pathways such as the citric acid cycle and

many routes in nucleotide and amino acid metabolism. Mycoplasmas, therefore, seem to have retained only the essential functions and rely to a large extent on the availability of nutrients obtained from a host organism.

Evolution has affected not only many metabolic functions of these organisms but also, it would appear, their molecular genetic machinery. This chapter will deal with the synthesis of nucleic acids and protein—how it occurs in mycoplasmas as opposed to their larger-genome relatives and how the macromolecular synthetic apparatus could have evolved from the ancestral organisms. Also with respect to these processes, mycoplasmas seem to represent minimal systems and have preserved only the functions that are absolutely required. A difficulty when speculating on the evolution of mycoplasmas (and any other type of organism) is that the properties of the predecessors may not necessarily be very similar to those of the organisms that live today. Therefore, we may not be able to explain the mycoplasmas' mode of evolution by using as a starting point their present-day molecular machinery. We should perhaps also at this stage dis-

Tore Samuelsson and Thomas Borén • Department of Medical Biochemistry, University of Göteborg, Medicinareg. 9, S-413 90 Göteborg, Sweden.

criminate between two aspects of evolution. One is the evolution from the larger-genome ancestral bacteria to the small-genome mycoplasmas. In this respect, we must deal with questions like the following: what were the events in this early evolution that lead to the divergence to mycoplasmalike organisms, and why were genes lost? Another aspect is the more recent evolution within the group of mycoplasmas that exist today, with their small genome size and other aberrant properties.

Interesting information has accumulated in recent years on the macromolecules involved in *Mycoplasma* protein synthesis, in particular the tRNA molecules, which are found to differ significantly from those found in the protein-synthesizing apparatus in most other eubacteria. The emphasis in this chapter will be on protein synthesis, but we will first briefly comment on the evolution of nucleic acid synthesis. This evolution is tightly coupled to that of protein synthesis, and it is also more or less intimately associated with the unusual properties of mycoplasma chromosomes, such as their limited size and frequent use of adenine and thymine.

THE SYNTHESIS OF DNA AND THE UNUSUAL PROPERTIES OF MYCOPLASMA GENOMES

Why Were Genes Eliminated during the Evolution of Mycoplasma Genomes?

Mycoplasmas have exceptionally small genomes and yet are organisms that effectively occupy many different ecological niches and colonize a wide variety of organisms such as mammals, insects, and plants. When searching for a solution to the problem of why genes have been lost, we should first recall that economization of DNA content is a characteristic property of all procaryotes, and the small genome size observed in mycoplasmas may be thought of as an extreme application of this principle. All bacteria are streamlined organisms that probably during their evolution lost a large portion of noninformational DNA that was originally present, such as the introns and other noncoding nucleotide sequences that have been preserved by eucaryotic organisms (29, 30, 77, 87). Excess DNA is an energetic burden, and it is conceivable that under conditions such that the supply of metabolic energy is severely limited, small genomes that can be faithfully and efficiently replicated constitute a selective advantage. The organisms from which the mycoplasmas evolved may have from time to time suffered from such a lack of energy supply. The loss of genetic material was tolerable in mycoplasmas because they were, presumably even early in their evolution, parasitic in nature and able to obtain many complex organic molecules from their host organisms. Many genes involved in biosynthetic pathways could therefore be left out. Furthermore, the organisms were not dependent on the very high growth rate characteristic of many other bacteria. Rather, it may have been advantageous for mycoplasmas to restrict their growth ability in order to optimize the particular parasite-host relationship.

The reduction in genome size and the economization

of genes could also have been facilitated by a particular biochemical machinery, for instance, one giving rise to an elevated rate of mutations, such as point mutations, general recombination, or recombination mediated by transposons. For example, an increased rate of recombination could have been necessary to effectively eliminate genes, such as those encoding metabolic enzymes, that were no longer required in a parasitic mode of existence. This recombination system could fortuitously have also eliminated many noninformational sequences. Sladek (102) has proposed that mycoplasmas lost genes by recombination events in fusions between L forms of the mycoplasma ancestors.

A general aspect of evolution is that the genome size is related to the mutation rate, i.e., the number of mutations per base pair and cell generation (31, 67, 118). A high mutation rate is advantageous from an evolutionary point of view, but at the same time, the maximum level of errors must be restricted in order to avoid deleterious effects. With a given error frequently, the total number of errors introduced into a genome is roughly proportional to the size of genome. Therefore, an organism with a smaller genome can tolerate a comparatively high mutation rate. Consequently, as more and more genetic material was jettisoned from chromosomes during the evolution of mycoplasmas, it is likely that the mutation rate was gradually increased to finally reach the level observed in mycoplasmas today (66, 89, 117).

In conclusion, we have in this model of the reduction in genome size assumed that the driving force for this development is gene economy. It is also possible that a selective principle was instead an enhanced ability to adapt to changing environmental conditions and perhaps to express a high degree of variability in contact with the immune system of the host organism. This could have been accomplished by a high rate of mutational events such as recombination. A by-product of these mutational events was that a large amount of genetic material was lost, although this loss was not a selective advantage in itself.

It is a distinct feature of mycoplasma evolution that it is essentially at a dead end; the organisms cannot discard more genes, since the remaining genes are all essential for survival. In other words, mycoplasmas are truly minimal systems. At the same time, the mycoplasmas may have difficulties picking up genetic elements from other types of organisms such as their hosts or from other bacteria. This is because mycoplasma genes have, as a result of their high mutation rate, evolved rapidly and diverged strongly from other organisms. As noted below, they have a codon usage which deviates from that of most other bacteria, and some species have a different genetic code. Consequently, genes from most other species would be less functional in mycoplasmas. It would therefore seem that transfer of genes to mycoplasma genomes, if it occurs at all, is restricted to transfer from one mycoplasma to another.

The Preferential Use of Adenine and Thymine in Mycoplasma Genomes

Many organisms carry approximately equal proportions of the four bases in their genes; in other words, they have a G+C content which is close to 50%. A characteristic feature of mycoplasma genomes is a low G+C value; in certain *Mycoplasma* species, it may be as low as approximately 25%. These values, which are among the lowest recorded for a free-living organisms, pose two problems: what mechanism gives rise to the bias, and once the bias is established, what are its consequences for the biochemistry and physiology of the organism?

We do not know whether a selective advantage is directly associated with a low G+C content in myco-plasmas or whether mutations giving rise to a predom-inance of A·T base pairs have been more or less neutral events during evolution. What are the possible molec-ular mechanisms that could have promoted such a bias? First, a limitation of dGTP or dCTP nucleotide precursors could increase the level of errors intro-duced during DNA replication. This limitation could be the result of a mutation in a nucleotide biosynthetic enzyme. So far, there are no experimental data in sup-port of such a mechanism. Another possibility is that the DNA polymerase is of an unusual nature and in some way stimulates the enrichment in A·T base pairs. Another alternative is that DNA repair mechanisms are deficient or in some other way differ from those of bacteria with a higher G+C content. Mycoplasmas are in fact known to lack some of the repair systems of other eubacteria (35). Furthermore, an ineffective ura-cil-DNA glycosylase would result in a replacement of G·C base pairs by A·T base pairs in the DNA, and a mycoplasma enzyme with such properties has been identified (116).

The probability of finding A or T in a specific nucleo-tide position is dependent on the particular selective pressure. For instance, in noncoding sequences, the bias in favor of A·T base pairs is generally close to 80% (75, 80), whereas in coding regions, where a relatively high content of G·C base pairs is required (a typical example being a tRNA gene), the content of G+C is close to 50%. During the evolution of mycoplasmas, all genes that were not essential for survival would be sensitive to the AT bias so that a majority of G·C base pairs in these genes were replaced by A·T base pairs, thus converting a coding gene to a noncoding region with a predominance of A·T base pairs. Such regions in the chromosome might have had some specific property that facilitated their elimination from the ge-nome; they might, for instance, have stimulated re-combinational loss of genetic material.

The AT bias is reflected also in the codon usage in these organisms. Thus, codons with A or U in the third position predominate; in *Mycoplasma capricolum*, such codons make up approximately 90% of all codons (3, 74). Even the selection of amino acids during evolu-tion has been affected by the AT bias. Thus, in *M. capri-colum*, compared with the situation in *Escherichia coli*, lysine is preferred over arginine. This is because the A+U-rich lysine codons AAA and AAG are pre-ferred over the more G+C-rich arginine codons AGA, AGG, and CGN (74). Finally, it is likely that codon usage has been important also with respect to the evo-lutionary selection of tRNAs. This aspect will be dis-cussed further below in the context of the mycoplasma tRNAs.

When one considers the molecular mechanisms that give rise to the peculiar properties of mycoplasmas

and their genomes, it is clear that an important role is played by the macromolecular prerequisites of DNA replication, repair, and recombination. All of these systems may be relevant to the increased rate of muta-tion observed in mycoplasmas. The DNA replication apparatus appears to be simplified in some species of mycoplasmas in the sense that there seems to be only one DNA polymerase in these organisms, as opposed to the situation for bacteria with larger genomes (18, 69, 70). It is also possible that the DNA replication apparatus is more error prone in mycoplasmas than in normal bacteria such as *E. coli*. Recombination sys-tems may play an important part in the elimination of genes during evolution and may also be important for the evolution of mycoplasmas taking place today. It is clear that careful studies of DNA replication, repair, and recombination are required in order to under-stand many of the properties of mycoplasmas.

THE SYNTHESIS OF PROTEINS AND UNUSUAL PATTERNS OF CODON READING

In protein synthesis, many different macromole-cules are required and a large proportion of the total biochemical machinery of a bacterial cell is used. Among the molecules in mycoplasmas that are in-volved in protein synthesis, those that have been most carefully studied at the primary structure level are the tRNAs, rRNAs, and ribosomal proteins. However, we still lack information on the structure and function of many other macromolecule components involved in mycoplasma protein synthesis.

As noted previously, the evolution of mycoplasmas seems to be associated with a tendency to eliminate as many genes as possible. During this evolution, not only protein genes but also many tRNA and rRNA genes were discarded. For instance, it is known that in some *Mycoplasma* species, the genes for the rRNAs exist in only one copy each (109), whereas several copies are found in *E. coli* (53) and *Bacillus subtilis* (61). A ten-dency to eliminate genetic material may also explain why some RNAs and proteins seem to be somewhat smaller than those in typical bacteria. Examples are the 5S rRNAs, which in the gram-positive bacilli and clostridia have a size of 116 to 117 nucleotides (68, 86, 89), whereas the corresponding RNAs from mycoplas-mas contain 104 to 113 nucleotides (42, 89, 110). This difference in size is due mainly to a simplified E/E' helix and loop structure in mycoplasmas. Another ex-ample of an RNA that became reduced in size during evolution is a mycoplasma RNA related to the *E. coli* 4.5S RNA. This RNA from *M. mycoides* subsp. *capri* is only 77 nucleotides (97), whereas the corresponding molecule in *E. coli* is 114 nucleotides (44) and that in *B. sutilis* is 271 nucleotides (107) (Fig. 1).

Since the tRNAs in different *Mycoplasma* species have been carefully analyzed, the emphasis in this chapter will be on these molecules. The work on this group of molecules has revealed several interesting points that are also of importance to a discussion of evolutionary aspects. As discussed in more detail below, certain *Mycoplasma* species have a markedly reduced number of tRNAs in comparison with other free-living organisms. This fact is of consequence for the mechanism of recognition by these tRNAs of

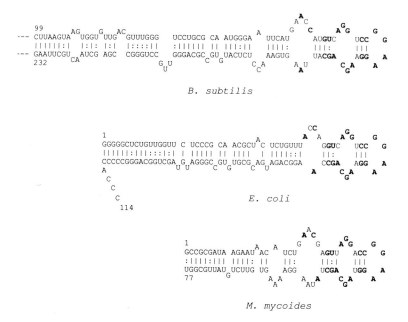

Figure 1. Comparison of RNAs related to *E. coli* 4.5S RNA. The sequences were obtained from Samuelsson et al. (97), Struck et al. (107), and Hsu et al. (44). The *B. subtilis* RNA is 217 nucleotides in size, and only the portion spanning nucleotide positions 99 to 232 is shown. The nucleotides that are shared among all three RNAs are in boldface. The *M. mycoides* and *B. subtilis* RNAs are probably functionally related to the 4.5S RNA of *E. coli*. This RNA is known to be essential for viability (19–21) and is part of a ribonucleoprotein complex that resembles the mammalian signal recognition particle (84).

mRNA codons. Important also for the codon-reading process is the fact that many *Mycoplasma* species are rich in A·T base pairs, as reflected in the use of codons in these organisms. Another striking property of certain species of mycoplasmas is that the codon UGA encodes tryptophan instead of being a termination codon as in the universal genetic code. Before discussing the relevance of these many aberrant properties of mycoplasmas and their evolutionary implications, we will briefly consider the genetic code and the common mode of codon reading that is utilized in normal protein synthesis.

Organization and Evolution of the Genetic Code

Figure 2 shows the universal genetic code. Its organization gives some clues as to the forces that were important for its evolution from a more primitive code. Thus, it appears to have been organized so as to minimize deleterious effects of mutations (113). Mutations in the first or second position of a codon will often give a similar (or the same) amino acid, and a majority of mutations in the third codon position will have no effect on the amino acid specified. Another principle of the code is that codons that have G or C in both of their first two positions are not randomly distributed. All such codons are found among the codon families, that is, the groups of four codons that specify the same amino acid (Fig. 2). This distribution could reflect the fact that such codons may be more prone to be read without discrimination in the third codon position, as discussed further below.

The Classic Concepts of Codon Reading

During protein synthesis, the anticodons of tRNA recognize codons on the mRNA in a highly specific manner. In most cells, there are no more than approximately 50 different tRNA anticodons that are responsible for reading the 61 different codons that specify amino acids. Clearly, the number of tRNA molecules is insufficient to enable the reading of codons strictly according to the Watson-Crick base-pairing rules. In 1966, Crick presented his wobble hypothesis (26) to explain the principles of codon-anticodon pairing. This hypothesis states that the first two nucleotides of the codon pair with the corresponding anticodon nucleotides according to Watson-Crick base-pairing rules; i.e., A pairs with U, while G pairs with C. Recognition of the third base, however, is less discriminating than recognition of the other two. Assuming some steric freedom (wobble) for the nucleotide in the first position in the tRNA anticodon, the pairs U·G, G·U, I·U, and I·A can be formed in addition to the standard Watson-Crick base pairs. Nevertheless, there are a number of interactions that are not allowed (Table 1). Since the time of the proposal of Crick, a large number of tRNAs have been investigated. For instance, a careful inventory of the tRNA genes of *E. coli* revealed 45 different tRNA species (54). The results of such investigations are compatible with the wobble hypothesis. Thus, many pairs of codons of the type XY(U/C) or XY(A/G) are read by a single tRNA species.

However, there are situations in which these rules do not provide a complete and accurate description of codon-anticodon pairing. One such situation, dis-

UUU	Phe	**UCU**	**Ser**	UAU	Tyr	UGU	Cys
UUC	Phe	**UCC**	**Ser**	UAC	Tyr	UGC	Cys
UUA	Leu	**UCA**	**Ser**	UAA	Stop	UGA	Stop
UUG	Leu	**UCG**	**Ser**	UAG	Stop	UGG	Trp
CUU	**Leu**	CCU	Pro	CAU	His	**CGU**	**Arg**
CUC	**Leu**	CCC	Pro	CAC	His	**CGC**	**Arg**
CUA	**Leu**	CCA	Pro	CAA	Gln	**CGA**	**Arg**
CUG	**Leu**	CCG	Pro	CAG	Gln	**CGG**	**Arg**
AUU	Ile	**ACU**	**Thr**	AAU	Asn	AGU	Ser
AUC	Ile	**ACC**	**Thr**	AAC	Asn	AGC	Ser
AUA	Ile	**ACA**	**Thr**	AAA	Lys	AGA	Arg
AUG	Met	**ACG**	**Thr**	AAG	Lys	AGG	Arg
GUU	**Val**	**GCU**	**Ala**	GAU	Asp	**GGU**	**Gly**
GUC	**Val**	**GCC**	**Ala**	GAC	Asp	**GGC**	**Gly**
GUA	**Val**	**GCA**	**Ala**	GAA	Glu	**GGA**	**Gly**
GUG	**Val**	**GCG**	**Ala**	GAG	Glu	**GGG**	**Gly**

Figure 2. The genetic code. In half of the codon groups, all four codons represent the same amino acid. These codons and their respective amino acids are in boldface.

cussed below, is the mode of codon-anticodon pairing that has been discovered in mycoplasmas. Crick based his hypothesis only on the nature of hydrogen bonding between bases in the opposing RNA strands. However, during many years of study of codon-anticodon pairing, information which strongly indicates that this interaction is highly complex has been collected. We now know that in order to predict the codon-reading properties of a particular tRNA anticodon, we must take into consideration many additional factors that influence the interaction between codon and anticodon. Such factors are the structure of the entire anticodon loop and stem (123), nucleotide modifications (13), and mRNA structural context (17, 103).

Codon Reading in Violation of the Classic Rules

In certain mycoplasmas, codons appear to be read in violation of the wobble rules. These codon readings will be discussed in detail below, but there are also experimental data that question the early classic rules of codon reading. For instance, the wobble rules have been tested in in vitro translational systems (32, 63, 71, 72, 93, 95, 104). In such studies, it was noted that tRNAs reading the family codons were unexpectedly efficient with respect to reading all codons. For instance, when the valine tRNA with anticodon UAC was the only source of that amino acid for protein synthe-

sis, the tRNA could read all four valine codons without difficulty (71, 72).

To explain these results, one could assume that the wobble restrictions are not valid; i.e., in the reading of the third codon position, base pairs may be formed in violation of the wobble rules, with a stability that is comparable to that of regular base pairs. However, it is difficult to see, from a structural point of view, how such base pairs could be formed. Furthermore, we know that translational errors would result if such stable base pairs were allowed in the reading of the third position of certain codons. To organize these observations into a concept, Lagerkvist proposed the "2-out-of-3" hypothesis (57–59).

This hypothesis suggests that a codon may be read by relying mainly on the Watson-Crick base pairs formed with the first two bases of the codon, while the mispaired bases in the third codon and anticodon wobble positions make a comparatively limited contribution to the total stability of the reading interaction. The hypothesis further assumes that the probability of 2-out-of-3 reading is a function of the strength of the interaction between the anticodon and the first two codon nucleotides and that a $G \cdot C$ interaction with three hydrogen bonds is stronger than an $A \cdot U$ interaction with only two. Therefore, the probability of such reading would be greatest for codons making only $G \cdot C$ interactions in these positions (G-C codons), intermediate for codons which make one $G \cdot C$ and one $A \cdot U$ interaction (mixed codons), and minimal for codons making only $A \cdot U$ interactions (A-U codons).

When the genetic code is examined for the distribution of the three codon categories, it is apparent, as noted above, that G-C codons are without exception restricted to the codon families, while the A-U codons are always outside the families (Fig. 2). This is the distribution to be expected as the result of an evolutionary process which selected for a code that minimized the probability that reading by the 2-out-of-3 principle could cause translational errors.

The hypothesis demands that family codons be eas-

Table 1. The wobble rules of codon-anticodon pairing

Wobble nucleotide	Watson-Crick base pair	Wobble base pair	Interaction(s) not allowed by wobble rules
U	A	G	U, C
C	G		U, C, A
I	C	U, A	G
G	C	U	A, G

ier to read by the 2-out-of-3 principle than are the non-family codons, and in vitro studies of the reading of the alanine, glycine, and valine codons compared with the glutamine and lysine codons show that this is indeed the case (63, 71, 93, 95). It may therefore be concluded that the hypothesis correctly predicts codon reading in vitro.

Unusual Modes of Codon Reading in Mitochondria and Chloroplasts

In its original version, the 2-out-of-3 hypothesis regards this type of reading mainly as a potential source of translational errors and attempts to explain how it could have acted as a restriction in the evolution of the genetic code. However, in the early 1980s, evidence that such reading could occur in vivo emerged through the analysis of tRNAs in mitochondria.

From the sequence information on mitochondrial tRNAs from a number of different organisms (4, 5, 9, 16, 27, 39), the following conclusions have been reached. There are fewer tRNAs than in normal cytoplasmic protein synthesis. For instance, the complete nucleotide sequence of the human mitochondrial genome revealed only 22 tRNA genes in the entire genome (4, 9). According to the wobble hypothesis, the minimum number of tRNAs required to read all codons would be substantially higher (at least 32). Since

no mitochondrial tRNAs are imported from the cytoplasm, it would seem that they must have codon-reading properties which are at variance with the wobble rules. For each codon family, there is only one tRNA in the mitochondrion (Table 2). For instance, there is only one glycine tRNA, and this tRNA must read all of the glycine codons. In contrast, an organism such as *E. coli* has three glycine tRNAs, each with a different anticodon (41, 88, 106). These findings indicate that a mechanism reminiscent of 2-out-of-3 reading operates in mitochondria from animals and yeasts. As a rule, the mitochondrial tRNAs that read family codons have an unsubstituted U as their wobble nucleotide (105). One exception is that the yeast arginine tRNA, which reads the family codons CGN, contains unmodified A in the wobble position (101).

The complete nucleotide sequences of chloroplast DNA from a liverwort (76) and from tobacco (100) have been determined, and these genomes are predicted to contain more than 120 genes, including 30 tRNA genes in tobacco chloroplasts and 32 tRNA genes in liverwort chloroplasts. Several family codon boxes seem to be read by an undiscriminating principle as in mitochondria, as there is only one tRNA for each of the leucine, alanine, and proline family boxes and, in the case of the tobacco chloroplasts, also the arginine family boxes (Table 2). All of these observations seem to support the conclusion that family codons are read

Table 2. tRNAs available to read family codons[a]

Amino acid	Codon family	tRNA anticodons			
		Mitochondria	*M. capricolum, M. mycoides*	Chloroplasts	*E. coli*
Leu	CUN	UAG	UAG	UA$\overset{*}{\text{G}}$	UAG GAG CAG
Val	GUN	UAC	UAC	UAC GAC	$\overset{*}{\text{U}}$AC GAC
Ser	UCN	UGA	UGA	UGA GGA	$\overset{*}{\text{U}}$GA GGA CGA
Pro	CCN	UGG	UGG	$\overset{*}{\text{U}}$GG (GGG)	$\overset{*}{\text{U}}$GG GGG CGG
Thr	ACN	UGU	UGU AGU	UGU GGU	$\overset{*}{\text{U}}$GU GGU CGU
Ala	GCN	UGC	UGC	$\overset{*}{\text{U}}$GC	$\overset{*}{\text{U}}$GC GGC
Arg	CGN	UCG (ACG)	ICG	ICG (GCG)	ICG CCG
Gly	GGN	UCC	UCC	UCC GCC	$\overset{*}{\text{U}}$CC GCC CCC

[a] The anticodons of tRNAs that read family codons in mitochondria (105), *M. mycoides* subsp. *capri* (37, 50, 94, 96, 98), *M. capricolum* (3), chloroplasts (76, 82, 100), and *E. coli* (54) are shown from left to right in order of increasing complexity with respect to the number of tRNA anticodons. Wobble nucleotides are in boldface, and posttranscriptionally modified nucleotides are marked with asterisks. The proline tRNA with anticodon GGG and the arginine tRNA with anticodon GCG are both present in chloroplasts from liverwort (76) but not from tobacco (100). An arginine tRNA with anticodon UCG is present in animal mitochondria (105), whereas yeast mitochondria have an arginine tRNA with anticodon ACG (101).

without discrimination in the third codon position in both mitochondria and chloroplasts.

A Restricted Number of tRNAs in Mycoplasmas

We now turn to the evidence that a codon family may be read by a single tRNA in certain *Mycoplasma* species. The first mycoplasma RNAs to be analyzed and sequenced were from *M. mycoides* and *M. capricolum* in the late 1970s and early 1980s (50, 51, 52, 111). These and other earlier studies (33, 91) suggested that the mycoplasmas were deficient in many isoaccepting tRNA species. Most notably, *M. mycoides* subsp. *capri* appeared to have only one glycine tRNA (50), and this tRNA contains an unmodified uridine in its wobble position.

The finding that *M. mycoides* seemed to have a single glycine tRNA suggested that the type of unconventional codon-reading mechanism that had been noted in mitochondria operated also in mycoplasmas. These indications led to the initiation of more thorough investigations of the population of tRNAs in *M. mycoides* subsp. *capri* (37, 94, 96, 98) and *M. capricolum* (2, 3, 73, 121).

The analyses of tRNAs genes and their products in these organisms reveal a number of interesting facts. There is a limited number of tRNAs; in *M. capricolum*, no more than 29 species have been detected (3), and in *M. mycoides* subsp. *capri*, the number is approximately the same (36a). Comparison of tRNA sequences between *M. capricolum* and *M. mycoides* shows that these sequences are all identical, indicating a very close evolutionary relationship between these two organisms. It has been suggested that three different tRNAs in *M. capricolum*, leucine tRNA(CAA), lysine tRNA(CUU), and tryptophan tRNA(CCA), are redundant and are not used significantly in protein synthesis (3). The number of tRNAs used in translation in *M. capricolum* may therefore actually be as low as 26.

With respect to the small number of tRNAs, therefore, these mycoplasmas are reminiscent of mitochondria and chloroplasts. Furthermore, family box codons are read by only one tRNA each, with the exception of the threonine codons, which are read by two different tRNAs (Table 2). All of these tRNAs have an unsubstituted U in the wobble position, with the exception of arginine tRNA, which has I (inosine), and one of the threonine isoacceptors, which has A. Finally, the mycoplasma tRNAs are relatively deficient in modified nucleosides. The properties of some of the individual mycoplasma tRNAs are discussed in more detail below.

The limited number of tRNAs observed in mycoplasmas may be a specific property of the small-genome mycoplasmas, as it has been shown that *Acholeplasma laidlawii* has a more complex set of tRNAs which is more like that of bacteria with larger genomes (72a).

There are important problems related to the limited number of tRNAs in mycoplasmas. We have already discussed the question of why the number of tRNAs has been reduced and have speculated that it was just a consequence of a general effort to reduce the amount of genetic material. Another problem is the following: what are the biochemical and physiological consequences of the reduction in the number of tRNAs?

Since the vast majority of organisms have at least 45 to 50 different tRNA species, one would imagine that these RNAs are required for an optimal rate and fidelity during protein synthesis. One could therefore speculate that mycoplasma protein synthesis suffers some kind of disadvantage from the lack of tRNAs; for instance, the rate of protein synthesis may be slow or translation may be less accurate. Unfortunately, none of these possibilities have so far been tested experimentally. Furthermore, we do not know whether the lack of tRNAs has any effect on the bacterial phenotype, such as growth rate. This is an essential problem that is worth more careful study.

EVOLUTION OF tRNAs

We will now take a closer look at some individual mycoplasma tRNAs and consider how they could have evolved from their ancestors and where they are heading today. We will first discuss the properties and evolution of the glycine and threonine tRNAs as examples of tRNAs reading family codons and then the turn to the tryptophan tRNAs and the change in the universal genetic code. It is interesting to observe that in the evolution of all of these RNAs, a central role is played by the wobble nucleotide of the tRNA anticodon, and we shall see as a recurring theme the adaptation of tRNAs and their wobble positions to the particular environmental pressure. This pressure is composed mainly of the force exerted to eliminiate genes on the one hand and the constraints with respect to the base composition in the genome, on the other hand.

Properties and Evolution of Mycoplasma Glycine tRNA

For the majority of amino acids that correspond to the family codons in *M. mycoides* and *M. capricolum*, there is, as already noted, only one tRNA for each amino acid. As a rule, these tRNAs have unmodified U in the wobble position. For instance, in both organisms, there is only one tRNA available to read the four glycine codons, and it has the anticodon UCC. In *M. capricolum*, all four glycine codons (GGN) are represented (3); although we have only very limited information on codon usage in *M. mycoides*, we may safely assume that all of the glycine codons are also used in this organism, since it is very closely related to *M. capricolum*. We must therefore assume that in both organisms, a single glycine tRNA is able to more or less effectively read all of the glycine codons. We must then ask how the tRNA is able to do this and whether it has any unique properties that make such reading possible.

The ability of the *M. mycoides* glycine tRNA to read the individual glycine codons has been tested experimentally by using a protein-synthesizing system derived from *E. coli* with the RNA from phage MS2 as message (62, 93). The codon-reading ability of the mycoplasma tRNA was compared with that of the three different glycine tRNAs of *E. coli* (anticodons NCC, GCC, and CCC, where N is an unidentified modification of U). The result of this investigation (Fig. 3) shows that the mycoplasma tRNA is remarkably efficient with respect to reading of the glycine codons GGU and GGC. These codons are read less effectively by the *E.*

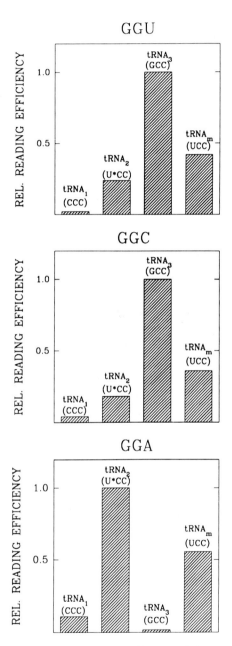

Figure 3. Relative codon-reading efficiency of glycine tRNAs during protein synthesis in vitro. Two different glycine tRNAs, esterified with [³H]- and [¹⁴C]glycine, respectively, were incubated together in an MS2 RNA-programmed in vitro system. The main product of this system, the MS2 coat protein, was purified and digested with proteolytic enzymes. Each of the peptides obtained corresponds to a specific glycine codon in the MS2 RNA. The relative efficiency of the competing tRNAs in the reading of a certain codon could be calculated by comparing the ratio of ³H to ¹⁴C in a peptide corresponding to the specific glycine codon with the isotopic ratio of the glycyl-tRNAs. Data are from Samuelsson et al. (93).

coli glycine tRNA₂, which has the same anticodon as does the mycoplasma tRNA except that the wobble uridine is modified. The glycine tRNA₁(CCC) from *E. coli* is extremely inefficient with respect to its unconventional reading of the codons GGU, GGC, and GGA, and the glycine tRNA₃(GCC) reads GGA and GGG only with difficulty. These data indicate that among the tRNAs tested in this experiment, the mycoplasma tRNA is the most efficient in reading all four codons, and it therefore appears to have been designed to read all glycine codons with comparable efficiency. This is, of course, what would be expected since it is the only glycine tRNA present in this organism.

One may now ask what makes the mycoplasma glycine tRNA able to effectively read the glycine codons in this unconventional manner. In an attempt to investigate the structural features of the tRNA that are important in this respect, *E. coli* glycine tRNA₁ with anticodon CCC was mutated so that it contained anticodon UCC, with an unmodified U in the wobble position (62). A tRNA was thus obtained which had exactly the same anticodon as did the mycoplasma tRNA but in another structural environment, that of *E. coli* tRNA₁. This RNA was found to be very inefficient in reading glycine codons GGC and GGU, which indicates that it is not only the anticodon UCC per se which is essential for the unconventional reading properties of the mycoplasma tRNA but, also, to a large extent, its structural environment in the tRNA molecule. The glycine tRNA₁(UCC) was further mutated to determine the structural elements that are important for its reading properties (61a). The resulting constructs are shown in Fig. 4. In glycine tRNA₁-ASL, the anticodon loop and stem are the same as in mycoplasma glycine tRNA. Another construct, tRNA₁-AS, has an anticodon stem identical with that of mycoplasma glycine tRNA, while in the last construct, glycine tRNA₁-C32, the only difference from glycine tRNA₁(UCC) is that the U in position 32 of the anticodon loop has been replaced by a C. These RNAs were tested for the ability to read glycine codons, and the results showed that the UCC, when present in tRNA₁-AS, discriminated between the glycine codons, while in the constructs glycine tRNA₁-ASL and glycine tRNA₁-C32, the same anticodon had lost its ability to discriminate; i.e., it behaved as in mycoplasma glycine tRNA. These results strongly suggest that the nature of the nucleotide in position 32 of the anticodon loop has a decisive influence on the reading properties of the anticodon UCC.

From what we know about the codon-reading properties of mycoplasma glycine tRNA, we may put forward a hypothesis for the evolutionary origin of this tRNA applicable to all mycoplasma tRNAs that read all four codons in a family. Mycoplasmas are believed to have originated from the gram-positive branch of eubacteria. The evolution of mycoplasmas led to a reduction in genome size and the elimination of genes. The predecessors of mycoplasmas therefore should have had more than one glycine tRNA isoacceptor and more than one glycine tRNA gene. Let us assume that the parent organism had two different glycine tRNAs with anticodons GCC and UCC, respectively (where U is possible modified). These two tRNAs are required by the classic wobble rules and are both found in typical bacteria such as *B. subtilis*. One or both of these tRNAs could have been encoded by multiple genes. A pressure

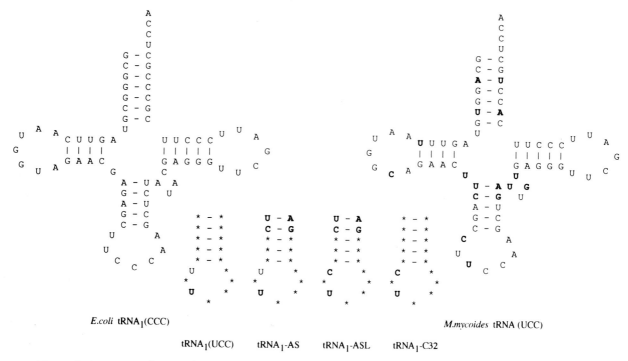

Figure 4. Sequences of mutated tRNA genes derived from the *E. coli* glycine tRNA₁(CCC) gene. Differences in the mutants and in *M. mycoides* glycine tRNA relative to *E. coli* glycine tRNA₁ are indicated by bold letters. Asterisks denote nucleotides in the mutant constructs that are identical to those of glycine tRNA₁(CCC).

is now exerted to remove tRNA genes, leaving only a single glycine tRNA gene. Assuming that all glycine codons are represented in the genome, the organism should retain the tRNA that is the most efficient when it comes to reading all of these codons. Anticodon GCC is very ineffective in its undiscriminating reading of codons GGA and GGG in protein synthesis in vitro (93), and anticodon UCC might therefore be the best choice as far as undiscriminating reading is concerned. An alternative explanation is that anticodon GCC, although equally effective as an unconventional reader, has some other disadvantage such as causing an intolerable number of translational errors (e.g., frameshift errors) when it is the only tRNA available to read the glycine codons.

The tRNA(UCC) present in the predecessors of mycoplasmas was probably not optimized for reading all glycine codons effectively. Therefore, it is likely that concomitant with the loss of the tRNA(GCC), a small number of point mutations in the tRNA(UCC) were necessary to change its properties to that of the present mycoplasma glycine tRNA. In other words, many different mutations must have occurred simultaneously in order to eliminate the tRNA(GCC). It is conceivable that such mutational events are allowed only in organisms like the mycoplasmas which are characterized by a high mutation rate. Therefore, the probability of this type of mechanism for gene elimination could be very low in typical bacteria.

In most organisms, the wobble uridine of glycine tRNA is posttranscriptionally modified. However, during mycoplasma evolution, the ability to modify this nucleotide was lost, possibly because of pressure to reduce the number of genes and because this partic-

ular modification was not essential for viability. We do not know when this modification was lost and what its effect on the codon reading process was. However, its loss might have influenced the evolution of the tRNA, leading to a structure optimized for efficient reading of glycine codons.

Evolution of Mycoplasma Threonine tRNAs

It has been demonstrated that in *M. mycoides* and *M. capricolum*, all codon families are read by only one tRNA each (Table 2). The only exception seems to be the threonine codons, which are read by two different tRNAs that have the anticodons UGU and AGU, respectively (2, 37, 98). There are a number of interesting points with respect to this finding. First, one has to search for an explanation of the fact that an additional tRNA with anticodon AGU is required. Furthermore, the threonine tRNA with anticodon AGU is the only tRNA, outside mitochondria, that is known to contain an unmodified adenosine in its wobble position. Finally, the two threonine tRNAs are interesting in terms of their evolutionary relationship.

Why are there two different tRNAs to read the threonine codons when all other family boxes, seven in all, are read by only one tRNA? The threonine tRNA with anticodon AGU presumably reads codon ACU, which is known to be abundant in *M. capricolum* (3). One could speculate that for some reason a threonine tRNA with anticodon UGU can read codon ACU only with difficulty and causes a pausing at these codons which is not tolerable. Another explanation could be that such decoding introduces translational errors and that therefore the development of a tRNA with anticodon AGU was a selective advantage. It should be possible to distinguish between these two possibilities by a careful analysis of the codon-reading properties of the two threonine tRNAs in an in vitro protein-synthesizing system.

It is very unusual for a tRNA to have an unmodified adenosine in its wobble position, and adenosine in this position in the primary RNA transcript is normally enzymatically modified to inosine (105). However, we have seen that one of the mycoplasma threonine tRNAs has an unmodified adenosine in its wobble position. The only other known example of such a tRNA is the yeast mitochondrial arginine tRNA, which has the anticodon ACG (101). According to the classic codon-reading rules, inosine is able to pair with U, A, and C but not with G. What are the codon-reading properties of a tRNA with unmodified adenosine in the wobble position? The arginine tRNA in yeast mitochondria should be able to read all codons CGN since it is the only tRNA in yeast mitochondria available to read these codons. On the other hand, we do not know precisely the codon-reading repertoire of the mycoplasma threonine tRNA(AGU). Why is unmodified adenosine avoided in "normal" tRNAs? Again, it is possible that a study of the mycoplasma threonine tRNAs could provide some clues to the resolution of this problem.

At this stage, it should be noted that while the threonine tRNA has an unmodified adenosine in its wobble position, the mycoplasma arginine tRNA has inosine. It may be concluded from this observation that the enzyme which modifies adenosine to inosine in the arginine tRNA is specific for this RNA and is not able to modify the wobble adenosine in the threonine tRNA.

Finally, what is the evolutionary origin of the two threonine tRNAs? The mycoplasmas are evolutionarily related to the gram-positive bacteria. The only threonine tRNAs that seem to be present in B. subtilis have the anticodons GGU and NGU, respectively, where N is 5-methoxyuridine. What then is the origin of the threonine tRNA in mycoplasmas with anticodon AGU? The following hypothesis has been put forward by Andachi et al. (2). The two different threonine tRNAs are 88% homologous, indicating a rather close evolutionary relationship. In addition, the tRNA(AGU) from mycoplasmas is 79% homologous to tRNA(NGU) in B. subtilis but only 64% homologous to tRNA(GGU) from the same organism. Furthermore, the threonine tRNA(AGU) gene in M. capricolum is part of a tRNA

gene cluster which seems be evolutionarily related to a cluster of tRNA genes in B. subtilis (114) that contains the threonine tRNA gene corresponding to anticodon NGU. These circumstances indicate that the mycoplasma tRNA(AGU) is evolutionarily related to the B. subtilis tRNA(NGU). One could therefore speculate that the tRNA with anticodon AGU evolved not from a tRNA with anticodon GGU but instead from a mutation of the gene encoding tRNA(NGU).

It is reasonable to assume that the early evolution of threonine tRNA occurred by a mechanism similar to that of the mycoplasma glycine tRNA. Thus, the pressure to lose tRNA genes led to loss of the gene(s) encoding the GGU anticodon, and the UGU anticodon was at one time the only tRNA to read the threonine codons. In order for a mutation from UGU to AGU to occur, there must have been at least two copies of the tRNA gene with UGU as the anticodon. If a single gene for tRNA(UGU) was originally present, an additional copy of this gene could have arisen by gene duplication. In an alternative model of the evolution of the threonine tRNAs, both anticodons UGU and AGU are required for viability, and the appearance of AGU must therefore have been a prerequisite for the disappearance of anticodon GGU.

Tryptophan tRNAs and Their Coevolution with the Genetic Code in Mycoplasmas

Although the genetic code was thought for a long time to be universal, a number of deviations from the code have been observed (Table 3). The majority of these deviations are found in mitochondria (4, 5, 10, 27, 34, 39, 60, 64, 65, 112, 119); for instance, in all animal and yeast mitochondria, UGA specifies tryptophan. Deviations from the universal scheme have been noted also in cytoplasmic protein synthesis; in the ciliated protozoa, UAA and UAG are glutamine codons (23, 40, 43, 56, 85). Certain species of mycoplasmas are known to use UGA as a tryptophan codon, and in this respect they are unique among free-living organisms (15, 24, 55, 121).

The codon UGG always specifies tryptophan (Fig. 2), and in organisms that make use of UGA as a stop codon (as in the normal code), UGG is read by a tryptophan tRNA with anticodon CCA (105). When, as in mitochondria and mycoplasmas, UGA is a tryptophan codon, this is made possible by the presence of another tryptophan tRNA with anticodon UCA. In mitochon-

Table 3. Variations of the genetic code[a]

| Codon | Universal code | Mitochondria | | | Ciliated protozoa | Mycoplasma, Ureaplasma, and Spiroplasma spp. |
		Mammals	D. melanogaster	Yeasts		
UGA	Stop	Trp	Trp	Trp		Trp
AUA	Ile	Met	Met	Met		
CUA	Leu			Thr		
AG(A/G)	Arg	Stop	Ser			
UA(A/G)	Stop				Gln	

[a] The normal genetic code is shown together with deviations from this scheme that occur in mitochondria from mammals (4, 5, 12), Drosophila melanogaster (27), and yeasts (39, 60, 64, 65, 112), in ciliated protozoa (23, 40, 43, 56, 85), and in Mycoplasma (121), Ureaplasma (15), and Spiroplasma (24) spp.

dria this is the only tryptophan tRNA, and it must therefore be able to read both UGG and UGA since both of these codons are used in mitochondrial genomes. In *M. capricolum* (120, 121) there are two different tryptophan tRNAs, one with anticodon UCA (where U is 2'-O methylated) and one with anticodon CCA (where C in the wobble position is partially 2'-O methylated). A corresponding pair of tryptophan tRNAs has been observed also in *M. gallisepticum* (46).

In *A. laidlawii*, UGA is probably a stop codon since a normal tRNA(CCA) is the only tryptophan tRNA present in this organism (108). The data available so far suggest that the use of UGA as a tryptophan codon is restricted to *Mycoplasma* (55, 120, 121), *Ureaplasma* (15), and *Spiroplasma* (24) species.

From an evolutionary point of view, there are interesting observations concerning the mycoplasma tryptophan tRNAs (120). One is that expression of the tRNAs in *M. capricolum* seems to be transcriptionally regulated so that tRNA(UCA) is more effectively transcribed, giving rise to a higher cellular concentration of this RNA than of the other isoacceptor. The intracellular concentration of tRNA(CCA) is only 10 to 20% of the tRNA(UCA) concentration. There is only one gene for each of these RNAs. These genes are located in tandem and have a common promoter. Between the two genes is a terminatorlike structure. The results of experiments with in vitro transcription of these genes reveal that tRNA(UCA) is produced in larger amounts than is tRNA(CCA), suggesting that transcription is arrested at the terminatorlike hairpin. A factor further reducing the physiological potential of the tryptophan tRNA(CCA) is the fact that it appears to be poorly aminoacylated in the cell (120).

The tRNA with anticodon UCA is probably able to read both UGA and UGG efficiently. This assumption is based on the facts that the corresponding mitochondrial tRNA reads these codons and that this type of reading is allowed according to the classic codon-reading rules. Therefore, tRNA(CCA) seems to be redundant in *M. capricolum* and *M. gallisepticum*. The fact that it is poorly expressed in these bacteria suggests that mutations that decrease the level of the tRNA with anticodon CCA are associated with a selective advantage or are at least neutral.

Another interesting observation is that *M. genitalium* and *M. pneumoniae* (46) lack the gene for the tryptophan tRNA(CCA) and have preserved only the tryptophan tRNA(UCA). One could therefore trace an evolution from larger-genome bacteria which have the normal code and only the tRNA with anticodon CCA to organisms with both anticodons CCA and UCA and finally to *M. pneumoniae* and *M. genitalium*, in which this evolution has proceeded one step further to retain only the UCA anticodon.

The situation regarding the tryptophan tRNA(CCA) is in a way reminiscent of that of the proline tRNA(GGG) gene in chloroplasts, which seems to be present as a pseudogene in liverwort since it lacks a portion of its amino acid stem (76). This proline tRNA gene is absent in the tobacco chloroplast genome (100). What we see in *M. capricolum* as well as in liverwort chloroplasts may be a stage in tRNA gene evolution at which a number of mutations have eliminated the function of a specific tRNA but the tRNA gene has not

yet been completely deleted as in *M. pneumoniae* and tobacco chloroplasts.

Why is the code altered in mycoplasma and mitochondria so that UGA specifies tryptophan? A hypothesis for the evolution of tryptophan tRNAs and the genetic code in mycoplasmas has been put forward by Jukes et al. (47–49, 78, 79, 81). An important element in this hypothesis is that a pressure is imposed on the organism to replace G·C base pairs by A·T base pairs in the genome. According to the hypothesis, one result of this AT pressure is that all UGA codons (originally stop codons) undergo a silent mutational change to UAA, another termination codon. Next, the gene encoding the tryptophan tRNA with anticodon CCA is duplicated, giving a tandem arrangement of the two tRNA genes. One of the copies is then mutated to have anticodon UCA, again as a result of the AT pressure. Then UGG codons are changed to UGA (again silent mutations), which are read by the tryptophan tRNA with anticodon UCA. The anticodon CCA may finally disappear, as there is no use for it. Ciliated protozoans also have a low content of G + C, and the fact that UAA and UAG are used as glutamine codons in these organisms (23, 40, 43, 56, 85) may be explained by the same type of hypothesis.

A complication with this hypothesis for the evolution of the code is introduced by the fact that UGA is also used as a tryptophan codon in genetic systems with only a modest AT bias. For instance, the content of G·C base pairs is 44% in human mitochondria (4) and 40% in *M. pneumoniae* (115). At the same time, other systems with a comparatively low G + C content, such as ciliated protozoa (49) and *B. cereus* (73), maintain the normal use of UGA as a stop codon. If the hypothesis is to be valid in these instances, one has to suppose that a very strong AT pressure is required for a change in the genetic code to occur and that such a strong pressure existed at an earlier stage in the evolution of mitochondria as well as some mycoplasmas. UGA then remained as a tryptophan codon at a later stage, when the AT pressure was diminished in these systems.

We have considered the reassignment of UGA as being caused by AT pressure on the genome. However, there may be other explanations for the reassignment of a codon. It has been suggested that certain changes in the genetic code that are observed in mitochondria have been caused by the pressure to use a minimum number of tRNAs. One such example is the change of the arginine AGA and AGG to termination codons in vertebrate mitochondria. This alteration in the code eliminates the need for the arginine tRNA normally required to read these codons (6, 22).

Organization of tRNA Genes and the Phylogeny of Mycoplasmas

An interesting pattern of evolution of the mycoplasma tRNA genes is noted in a comparison of the organization of these genes in different species of mollicutes with that in *B. subtilis*. A number of tRNA genes of various mollicute species have now been sequenced, and many of these genes appear to be organized in a way which is reminiscent of the tRNA gene organization in the gram-positive *B. subtilis* (Fig. 5).

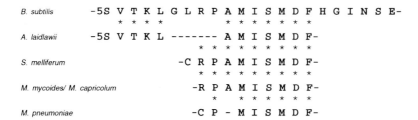

Figure 5. Organization of tRNA genes in mycoplasmas and *B. subtilis*. The organization of a tRNA gene cluster in *B. subtilis*, with 21 tRNA genes (36, 114), is compared with that of related tRNA gene clusters in the mycoplasmas *A. laidlawii* (72a), *S. melliferum* (90), *M. mycoides* subsp. *capri* (96), *M. capricolum* (73), and *M. pneumoniae* (101a). The individual tRNA genes are indicated by one-letter symbols for the specific amino acids. Upstream of the tRNA gene clusters in *B. subtilis* and *A. laidlawii* is a 5S rRNA gene. The homology of the mycoplasma gene clusters to that of *B. subtilis* is indicated by asterisks.

For instance, the *M. mycoides* (96) and *M. capricolum* (73) clusters of 9 tRNA genes that feature the tRNAs specific for the amino acids Arg, Pro, Ala, Met, Ile, Ser, fMet, Asp, and Phe seem to be related to a cluster in *B. subtilis* that has the same sequence of tRNAs but is part of a larger cluster with 21 tRNA genes (36, 114). Figure 5 shows a comparison of the gene organization in *B. subtilis*, *A. laidlawii* (72a), *Spiroplasma melliferum* (90), *M. mycoides* subsp. *capri*, *M. capricolum*, and *M. pneumoniae* (101a). Assuming an evolution from an ancestor common to *B. subtilis* and the mycoplasmas, it is tempting to speculate that a large tRNA gene cluster was present in the ancestral organism and that tRNA genes were discarded from this cluster during evolution. Among the organisms so far analyzed, *M. pneumoniae* seems to have suffered the most significant reductions in this cluster. This observation is consistent with the notion that *M. pneumoniae* is part of a branch of the mycoplasma evolutionary tree distinguished by a higher rate of evolution.

Evolutionary Aspects of Nucleotide Modifications in Mycoplasma RNAs

During the early studies of mycoplasma tRNAs, it was noted that these RNAs contain fewer modified nucleosides than do all other previously studied free-living organisms (50, 51), and we now have detailed information on this question through more recent investigations of tRNAs in *M. capricolum* and *M. mycoides* (2, 3, 37, 98, 121). Only 13 modified nucleosides have been identified in *M. capricolum*, compared with 23 in *E. coli* tRNAs (105). For instance, the ubiquitous 5-methyluridine in position 54 is lacking. Sequence analysis of several tRNAs in *M. mycoides* subsp. *capri* (37, 98) has failed to identify pseudouridine in nucleotide position 55 in the tRNA molecule, although this result is at variance with the results of other studies on tRNAs from this organism (50, 111). One explanation of this discrepancy is that different isolates of *M. mycoides* subsp. *capri* may differ as to the presence of this pseudouridine synthase.

As already noted, the majority of mycoplasma tRNAs that read family codons have an unmodified uridine as the wobble nucleotide. The corresponding wobble nucleotides in most other organisms are as a rule modified. For instance, the 5-oxyacetic acid deriv-

ative of uridine is present in *E. coli* tRNAs that read family codons, and it is believed to have a greater ability to wobble than does unmodified U (124). On the other hand, other uridine derivatives may restrict wobbling, and if such a modification was present in the ancestral glycine tRNA, it might have been selected against in mycoplasmas. However, as noted before, an unmodified uridine is probably not the only prerequisite for efficient undiscriminating reading, and we do not fully understand the functional significance of the unmodified wobble uridine in the mycoplasma tRNAs.

rRNAs of mycoplasmas are also known to be deficient in modification. For instance, the 23S RNA of *M. capricolum* contains only four methylated bases, all of which are ribose methylated (45), whereas the corresponding RNA in *E. coli* contains at least nine methylated bases (13).

It is tempting to interpret the absence of modified nucleosides merely as a consequence of the general tendency in mycoplasmas to reduce the number of genes or to reduce genome size as much as possible. The absence of modifying enzymes can thus be explained in the same way as can the absence of many other enzymes. The enzymes that have been disposed of would obviously be those that are not essential for viability or for a high growth rate. Indeed, some tRNA modification enzymes that have been studied in *E. coli* and yeasts, such as 5-methyluridine transferase (14) and dimethylguanosine transferase (83), are known not to be essential for viability. One may expect that the nucleotide modifications that are preserved in mycoplasmas are more or less essential for maintaining viability in other organisms as well.

The glycine tRNA from *M. mycoides* contains no more than three modified nucleosides (50, 98). Is a tRNA completely devoid of modifications able to sustain protein synthesis? We have no answer to this question as far as an in vivo situation is concerned. However, the in vitro properties of unmodified tRNAs have been tested (25, 38, 92, 94). An unmodified counterpart of the *M. mycoides* glycine tRNA was produced by in vitro T7 RNA polymerase transcription of the tRNA gene. This tRNA was shown to be fully active with respect to aminoacylation in vitro, and it was also able to effectively support protein synthesis in vitro. The outcome of this study further illustrates the relatively marginal effects of some nucleoside modifications; i.e., many modification reactions are not absolutely required in order for protein synthesis to proceed.

RESEMBLANCE OF MYCOPLASMAS TO OTHER GENETIC SYSTEMS

Knowing that the mycoplasmas have small genomes and many unique properties, we may consider other genetic systems that are comparable to the mycoplasmas in these respects. The rickettsiae and chlamydiae are known to have genomes roughly the size of the mycoplasma genomes, but so far we have only limited information on the molecular genetics of these organisms. The mitochondria and chloroplasts, however, which have been extensively studied, do share a number of properties with mycoplasmas, many of which have already been discussed. Before summarizing these similarities, we would like to point out that there are also some fundamental differences between these genetic systems. For example, the mycoplasmas can grow as free-living organisms, whereas the mitochondria and chloroplasts are intracellular organelles absolutely dependent on their cellular environment. Furthermore, the selective forces which guided the evolution of organelles have probably been different from those important for the development of the mycoplasmas. Organelles and mycoplasmas have entirely different evolutionary origins; mycoplasmas are believed to have originated from bacteria belonging to the gram-positive branch of the eubacterial tree and are most closely related to certain *Clostridium* species, whereas the mitochondria and chloroplasts originated from bacteria that were engulfed by a primitive eucaryotic organism. In the case of the mitochondria, the ancestral bacteria were most closely related to the purple bacteria; examples of such bacteria are agrobacteria, rhizobacteria, and rickettsiae (122). The chloroplasts are derived from cyanobacteria, i.e., primitive photosynthetic bacteria (99).

These important differences notwithstanding, there are some interesting properties that the organelles have in common with mycoplasmas. We have already seen that the population of tRNAs is very unusual and remarkably similar in all of these systems, and the mechanisms of codon reading must therefore be similar. Furthermore, many members of the mycoplasmas as well as mitochondria (particularly those of yeasts) and chloroplasts have a bias toward A·T base pairs in their genomes. There are exceptions, however; genomes such as those of *M. pneumoniae* and mammalian mitochondria do not have a particularly strong bias. Apparently, there is no obvious correlation between AT bias and the other properties shared by the organelles and mycoplasmas. Another property shared by some mycoplasmas and mitochondria from yeasts and animals is that UGA specifies tryptophan. However, plant mitochondria and chloroplasts seem to make use of the normal genetic code.

A significant similarity between organelles and mycoplasmas is that they both evolved from bacteria with larger genomes and during their evolution lost a large amount of genetic material. *Mycoplasma* and *Ureaplasma* species have chromosomes of 600 to 1,200 kbp, the smallest size recorded for a free-living organism. Mitochondrial DNAs range in size from 16 kbp (as in mammalian mitochondria) to 78 kbp (as in *Saccharomyces* mitochondria). Plant mitochondrial DNAs are exceptionally large, although much of this DNA may be noncoding material. Chloroplast genomes are also limited in size; the tobacco and liverwort chloroplasts have genomes of 155 and 120 kbp, respectively.

As a consequence of their small size, the organelle and mycoplasma genomes evolve rapidly. Again, mitochondria represent the most extreme case; one example is the marked divergence of the mitochondrial protein synthetic machinery from that of procaryote systems (11). Even some tRNAs have aberrant properties, such as the serine-accepting tRNA in both yeast and animal mitochondria that lacks the D loop commonly found in tRNAs (28). Clearly, mitochondria have evolved even more rapidly than mycoplasmas.

What were the driving forces for the elimination of genes from organellar genomes, and were they to some extent the same as for mycoplasmas? Again, we can only speculate on this subject. In the case of the mycoplasmas, we have hypothesized that these forces were gene economization and/or increased adaptability through an elevated rate of mutation. Both of these forces could have been important for the evolution of organelle genomes. For instance, an extreme case of gene economization is observed in the genomes of animal mitochondria (7). Adaptability may have been important in order for a free-living bacterium to become part of the eucaryotic cell. Another principle could be that the evolution of organelles was guided by the nucleus so that all genes originally present in the organelle ancestor that were not essential for mitochondrial function were eliminated. This gene loss may have been necessary to construct a highly efficient organelle. In any case, it is likely that the selective pressures imposed upon the organelle genomes must have been different from those of free-living bacteria. Why were the genetic systems of the organelles not eliminated completely? The organelle genomes as they exist today could have arisen by the following scheme (1). A reduction in genome size by the transfer of genes to the nucleus was concomitant with changes in codon usage, tRNA population, and the protein synthetic apparatus as a whole. Eventually the gene expression mechanisms in the organelle were so different from those specified by the nucleus that genes could not easily be transferred to the nucleus and expressed there. For instance, the change in the genetic code in mitochondria so that UGA codes for tryptophan would have made expression of a mitochondrial gene by the nucleus-encoded apparatus difficult. In addition, the elimination of RNA genes from the organelle genome may be difficult, as nucleic acids are not readily transported into mitochondria. Therefore, transfer of genes from the organelle to the nucleus ceased during evolution, and a dead end was reached. The genome of the organelle could not be reduced further, and consequently its genetic apparatus could not be eliminated completely.

This model of organelle evolution is clearly not immediately applicable to the mycoplasmas. For instance, there is no evidence that mycoplasma genes interacted with or were transferred to another genome during evolution. Even if the mechanism of evolution was entirely different in mycoplasmas than in mitochondria and chloroplasts, it is an interesting observation that the evolution of organelles resulted in genetic systems with properties very similar to those of the mycoplasmas.

CONCLUDING REMARKS

The analysis of mycoplasmas at a molecular level has provided a large body of information that is of interest in many respects. First, this information has made it possible to trace an evolution from a larger-genome ancestor that belonged to the branch of gram-positive bacteria. This evolution was associated with a loss of genetic material and resulted in what appears to be a minimal genetic system. The analyses of tRNAs and tRNA genes in mycoplasmas are one example of studies that have revealed details about the evolutionary changes of the protein synthetic machinery from the larger-genome ancestor to the mycoplasmas of today. As more information on the molecular biology of different mycoplasmas becomes available, we will see more clearly the paths of evolution that are related to macromolecule synthesis. Furthermore, mycoplasmas are interesting systems for evolutionary studies since they evolve rapidly as a result of their high mutation rate. Through the studies of these bacteria, we will certainly learn more about evolution in general. The evolution of mycoplasmas is also associated with a number of interesting problems that as yet have no obvious solution. For instance, what are the principles underlying the elimination of genetic material that gave mycoplasmas many of their unusual phenotypic properties?

The small-genome members of the mollicutes are minimal genetic systems and employ a scheme for the synthesis of macromolecules with a reduced number of components. For instance, the DNA replication and repair machinery appears to be less complex than in most other free-living organisms, and the protein-synthesizing apparatus uses a simplified scheme for the translation of mRNA, since only a restricted number of tRNAs are available in this process. Being minimal systems, the mycoplasmas are obviously attractive as model systems for living organisms, since a thorough examination of their cellular machinery is more feasible than studies of counterpart systems in other free-living organisms. Such an analysis would require, among many other tasks, the sequence analysis of an entire mycoplasma genome. It is important to note that the information obtained from such an enterprise would be of substantial biochemical, biological, and medical interest.

Acknowledgment. We thank Ulf Lagerkvist for introducing us to important principles of codon reading and for support and encouragement during our studies of the translational machinery in mycoplasmas.

REFERENCES

1. **Alberts, B., D. Bray, J. Lewis, M. Raff, K. Roberts, and J. D. Watson.** 1989. *Molecular Biology of the Cell*, 2nd ed. Garland Publishing, Inc., New York.
2. **Andachi, Y., F. Yamao, M. Iwami, A. Muto, and S. Osawa.** 1987. Occurrence of unmodified adenine and uracil at the first position of anticodon in threonine tRNAs in *Mycoplasma capricolum. Proc. Natl. Acad. Sci. USA* **84**:7398–7402.
3. **Andachi, Y., F. Yamao, A. Muto, and S. Osawa.** 1989. Codon recognition patterns as deduced from sequences of the complete set of transfer RNA species in *Mycoplasma capricolum*. Resemblance to mitochondria. *J. Mol. Biol.* **209**:37–54.
4. **Anderson, S., A. T. Bankier, B. G. Barrell, M. H. L. de Bruijn, A. R. Coulson, J. Drouin, I. C. Eperon, D. P. Nierlich, B. A. Roe, F. Sanger, P. H. Schreier, A. J. H. Smith, R. Staden, and I. G. Young.** 1981. Sequence and organization of the human mitochondrial genome. *Nature* (London) **290**:457–464.
5. **Anderson, S., M. H. L. de Bruijn, A. R. Coulson, I. C. Eperon, F. Sanger, and I. G. Young.** 1982. Complete sequence of bovine mitochondrial DNA. Conserved features of the mammalian mitochondrial genome. *J. Mol. Biol.* **156**:683–717.
6. **Andersson, S. G. E., and C. G. Kurland.** 1990. Codon preferences in free-living microorganisms. *Microbiol. Rev.* **54**:198–210.
7. **Attardi, G.** 1985. Animal mitochondrial DNA: an extreme example of genetic economy. *Int. Rev. Cytol.* **93**:93–145.
8. **Ayer, D., and M. Yarus.** 1986. The context effect does not require a fourth base pair. *Science* **231**:393–395.
9. **Barrell, B. G., S. Anderson, A. T. Bankier, M. H. L. de Bruijn, E. Chen, A. R. Coulson, J. Drouin, I. C. Eperon, D. P. Nierlich, B. A. Roe, F. Sanger, P. H. Schreier, A. J. H. Smith, R. Staden, and I. G. Young.** 1980. Different pattern of codon recognition by mammalian mitochondrial tRNAs. *Proc. Natl. Acad. Sci. USA* **77**:3164–3166.
10. **Barrell, B. G., A. T. Bankier, and J. Drouin.** 1979. A different genetic code in human mitochondria. *Nature* (London) **282**:189–193.
11. **Benne, R., and P. Sloof.** 1987. Evolution of the mitochondrial protein synthetic machinery. *BioSystems* **21**:51–68.
12. **Bibb, M. J., R. A. Van Etten, C. T. Wright, M. W. Walberg, and D. A. Clayton.** 1981. Sequence and gene organization of mouse mitochondrial DNA. *Cell* **26**:167–180.
13. **Björk, G. R.** 1987. Modification of stable RNA, p. 719–731. *In* F. C. Neidhardt, J. L. Ingraham, K. B. Low, B. Magasanik, M. Schaechter, and H. E. Umbarger (ed.), *Escherichia coli and Salmonella typhimurium: Cellular and Molecular Biology*. American Society for Microbiology, Washington, D.C.
14. **Björk, G. R., and F. C. Neidhardt.** 1975. Physiological and biochemical studies on the function of 5-methyluridine in the transfer ribonucleic acid of *Escherichia coli. J. Bacteriol.* **124**:99–111.
15. **Blanchard, A.** 1990. Urease genes in *Ureaplasma urealyticum. IOM Lett.* **1**:87.
16. **Bonitz, S. G., R. Berlani, G. Coruzzi, M. Li, G. Marcino, F. G. Nobrega, M. P. Nobrega, B. E. Thalenfeld, and A. Tzagoloff.** 1980. Codon recognition rules in yeast mitochondria. *Proc. Natl. Acad. Sci. USA* **77**:3167–3170.
17. **Bossi, L, and J. R. Roth.** 1980. The influence of codon context on genetic code translation. *Nature* (London) **286**:123–127.
18. **Boxer, L. M., and D. Korn.** 1979. Structural and enzymological characterization of the homogenous deoxyribonucleic acid polymerase from *Mycoplasma orale. Biochemistry* **18**:4742–4749.
19. **Brown, S.** 1989. Time of action of 4.5 S RNA in *Escherichia coli* translation. *J. Mol. Biol.* **209**:79–90.
20. **Brown, S., and M. J. Fournier.** 1984. The 4.5 S RNA gene of *Escherichia coli* is essential for cell growth. *J. Mol. Biol.* **178**:533–550.
21. **Brown, S., G. Thon, and E. Tolentino.** 1989. Genetic

selection and DNA sequences of 4.5S RNA homologs. *J. Bacteriol.* **171**:6517–6520.

22. **Bulmer, M.** 1988. Evolutionary aspects of protein synthesis. *Oxford Surv. Evol. Biol.* **5**:1–40.

23. **Caron, F., and E. Myer.** 1985. Does *Paramecium primaurelia* use a different genetic code in its macronucleus? *Nature* (London) **314**:185–188.

24. **Citti, C., C. Saillard, and J. M. Bové.** 1990. UGA-UGG tryptophan tRNA genes in *Spiroplasma citri*. *IOM Lett.* **1**:88–89.

25. **Claesson, C., T. Samuelsson, T. Borén, and F. Lustig.** 1990. Codon reading properties of an unmodified transfer RNA. *FEBS Lett.* **273**:173–176.

26. **Crick, F. H. C.** 1966. Codon-anticodon pairing: the wobble hypothesis. *J. Mol. Biol.* **19**:548–555.

27. **de Bruijn, M. H. L.** 1983. *Drosophila melanogaster* mitochondrial DNA, a novel organization and genetic code. *Nature* (London) **304**:234–240.

28. **de Bruijn, M. H. L., P. H. Schreier, I. C. Eperon, B. G. Barell, E. Y. Chen, P. W. Armstrong, J. F. H. Wong, and B. A. Roe.** 1980. A mammalian mitochondrial serine transfer RNA lacking the "dihydrouridine" loop and stem. *Nucleic Acids Res.* **8**:5213–5222.

29. **Doolittle, W. F.** 1978. Genes in pieces: were they ever together? *Nature* (London) **272**:581–582.

30. **Doolittle, W. F., and C. Sapienza.** 1980. Selfish genes, the phenotype paradigm and genome evolution. *Nature* (London) **284**:601–603.

31. **Drake, J. W.** 1974. The role of mutation in microbial evolution. *Symp. Soc. Gen. Microbiol.* **24**:41–58.

32. **Elias, P., F. Lustig, T. Axberg, B. Åkesson, and U. Lagerkvist.** 1979. Reading of the lysine codons in the MS2 coat protein cistron during protein synthesis *in vitro*. *FEBS Lett.* **98**:145–151.

33. **Feldman, H., and H. Falter.** 1971. Transfer ribonucleic acid from *Mycoplasma laidlawii* A. *Eur. J. Biochem.* **18**:573–581.

34. **Fox, T. D.** 1987. Natural variation in the genetic code. *Annu. Rev. Genet.* **21**:67–91.

35. **Ghosh, A., J. Das, and J. Maniloff.** 1977. Lack of repair of ultraviolet light damage in *Mycoplasma gallisepticum*. *J. Mol. Biol.* **116**:337–344.

36. **Green, C. J., and B. S. Vold.** 1983. Sequence analysis of a cluster of twenty-one tRNA genes in *Bacillus subtilis*. *Nucleic Acids Res.* **11**:5673–5774.

36a.**Guindy, Y.** Personal communication.

37. **Guindy, Y. S., T. Samuelsson, and T.-I. Johansen.** 1989. Unconventional codon reading by *M. mycoides* tRNAs as revealed by partial sequence analysis. *Biochem. J.* **258**:869–873.

38. **Hall, K. B., J. R. Sampson, O. C. Uhlenbeck, and A. G. Redfield.** 1989. Structure of an unmodified tRNA molecule. *Biochemistry* **28**:5794–5801.

39. **Heckman, J. E., J. Sarnoff, B. Alzner-DeWeerd, S. Yin, and U. L. RajBandary.** 1980. Novel features in the genetic code and codon reading patterns in *Neurospora crassa* mitochondria based on sequences of six mitochondrial tRNAs. *Proc. Natl. Acad. Sci. USA* **77**:3159–3163.

40. **Helftenbein, E.** 1985. Nucleotide sequence of a macronuclear DNA molecule for α-tubulin from the ciliate *Stylonychia lemnae*. Special codon usage: TAA is not a translation termination codon. *Nucleic Acids Res.* **13**:415–433.

41. **Hill, C. W., G. Combriato, W. Steinhart, D. L. Riddle, and J. Carbon.** 1973. The nucleotide sequence of the GGG-specific glycine transfer ribonucleic acid of *Escherichia coli* and of *Salmonella typhimurium*. *J. Biol. Chem.* **248**:4252–4262.

42. **Hori, H., M. Sawada, S. Osawa, K. Murao, and H. Ishikura.** 1981. The nucleotide sequence of 5S rRNA from *Mycoplasma capricolum*. *Nucleic Acids Res.* **9**:5407–5410.

43. **Horowitz, S., and M. A. Gorovsky.** 1985. An unusual genetic code in nuclear genes of *Tetrahymena*. *Proc. Natl. Acad. Sci. USA* **82**:2452–2455.

44. **Hsu, L. M., J. Zagorski, and M. J. Fournier.** 1984. Cloning and sequence analysis of the *Escherichia coli* 4.5S RNA gene. *J. Mol. Biol.* **178**:509–531.

45. **Hsuchen, C.-C., and D. T. Dubin.** 1980. Methylation patterns of mycoplasma transfer and ribosomal ribonucleic acid. *J. Bacteriol.* **144**:991–998.

46. **Inamine, J., K.-C. Ho, S. Loechel, and P. C. Hu.** 1990. Evidence that UGA is read as a tryptophan codon rather than as a stop codon by *Mycoplasma pneumoniae*, *Mycoplasma genitalium*, and *Mycoplasma gallisepticum*. *J. Bacteriol.* **172**:504–506.

47. **Jukes, T. H.** 1985. A change in the genetic code in *Mycoplasma capricolum*. *J. Mol. Evol.* **22**:361–362.

48. **Jukes, T. H., S. Osawa, and A. Muto.** 1987. Divergence and directional mutation pressures. *Nature* (London) **325**:668.

49. **Jukes, T. H., S. Osawa, A. Muto, and N. Lehman.** 1987. Evolution of anticodons: variations in the genetic code. *Cold Spring Harbor Symp. Quant. Biol.* **52**:769–776.

50. **Kilpatrick, M. W., and R. T. Walker.** 1980. The nucleotide sequence of glycine tRNA from Mycoplasma mycoides sp. capri. *Nucleic Acids Res.* **8**:2783–2786.

51. **Kimball, M. E., and D. Söll.** 1974. The phenylalanine tRNA from *Mycoplasma* sp. (kid): a tRNA lacking hypermodified nucleosides functional in protein synthesis. *Nucleic Acids Res.* **1**:1713–1720.

52. **Kimball, M. E., K. S. Szeto, and D. Söll.** 1974. The nucleotide sequence of phenylalanine tRNA from *Mycoplasma* sp. (kid). *Nucleic Acids Res.* **1**:1721–1732.

53. **Kiss, A., B. Sain, and R. Venetianer.** 1977. The number of rRNA genes in *Escherichia coli*. *FEBS Lett.* **79**:7–79.

54. **Komine, Y., T. Andachi, H. Inokuchi, and H. Ozeki.** 1990. Genomic organization and physical mapping of the transfer RNA genes in *Escherichia coli* K12. *J. Mol. Biol.* **212**:579–598.

55. **Kondo, K., H. Sone, H. Yoshida, T. Toida, K. Kanatani, Y.-M. Hong, N. Nishino, J.-J. Tanaka.** 1990. Cloning and sequence analysis of the arginine deiminase gene from *Mycoplasma arginini*. *Mol. Gen. Genet.* **221**:81–86.

56. **Kuchino, Y., N. Hanyu, F. Tashiro, and S. Nishimura.** 1985. *Tetrahymena thermophila* glutamine tRNA and its gene that corresponds to UAA termination codon. *Proc. Natl. Acad. Sci. USA* **82**:4758–4762.

57. **Lagerkvist, U.** 1978. "Two out of three": an alternative method for codon reading. *Proc. Natl. Acad. Sci. USA* **75**:1759–1762.

58. **Lagerkvist, U.** 1981. Unorthodox codon reading and the evolution of the genetic code. *Cell* **23**:305–306.

59. **Lagerkvist, U.** 1986. Evolutionary aspects of unconventional codon reading. *Chem. Scr.* **26B**:85–89.

60. **Li, M., and A. Tzagoloff.** 1979. Assembly of the mitochondrial membrane system: sequences of yeast mitochondrial valine and an unusual threonine tRNA gene. *Cell* **18**:47–53.

61. **Loughney, K., E. Lund, and J. E. Dahlberg.** 1982. tRNA genes are found between the 16S and 23S rRNA genes in *Bacillus subtilis*. *Nucleic Acids Res.* **10**:1607–1623.

61a.**Lustig, F., T. Borén, C. Claesson, M. Barciszewska and U. Lagerkvist.** Unpublished data.

62. **Lustig, F., T. Borén, Y. S. Guindy, P. Elias, T. Samuelsson, C. W. Gehrke, K. C. Kuo, and U. Lagerkvist.** 1989. Codon discrimination and anticodon structural context. *Proc. Natl. Acad. Sci. USA* **86**:6873–6877.

63. **Lustig, F., P. Elias, T. Axberg, T. Samuelsson, I. Tittawella, and U. Lagerkvist.** 1981. Codon reading and translational error. Reading of the glutamine and lysine codons during protein synthesis *in vitro*. *J. Biol. Chem.* **256**:2635–2643.

64. **Macino, G., G. Coruzzi, F. G. Nobrega, M. Li, and A. Tzagoloff.** 1979. Use of the UGA terminator as a trypto-

phan codon in yeast mitochondria. *Proc. Natl. Acad. Sci. USA* **76**:3784–3785.

65. **Macino, G., and A. Tzagoloff.** 1979. Assembly of the mitochondrial membrane system: partial sequence of a mitochondrial ATPase gene in *Saccharomyces cerevisiae*. *Proc. Natl. Acad. Sci. USA* **76**:131–135.

66. **Maniloff, J.** 1978. Molecular biology of mycoplasma, p. 390–393. *In* D. Schlessinger (ed.), *Microbiology—1978.* American Society for Microbiology, Washington, D.C.

67. **Maniloff, J.** 1983. Evolution of wall-less prokaryotes. *Annu. Rev. Microbiol.* **37**:477–499.

68. **Marotta, C. A., F. Varricchio, I. Smith, S. M. Weissman, M. L. Sogin, and N. R. Pace.** 1976. The primary structure of *Bacillus subtilis* and *Bacillus stearothermophilus* 5 S ribonucleic acid. *J. Biol. Chem.* **251**:3122–3127.

69. **Maurel, D., A. Charron, and C. Bébéar.** 1989. Mollicutes DNA polymerases: characterization of a single enzyme from *Mycoplasma mycoides* and *Ureaplasma urealyticum* and of three enzymes from *Acholeplasma laidlawii*. *Res. Microbiol.* **140**:191–205.

70. **Mills, L. B., E. J. Stanbridge, W. D. Sedwick, and D. Korn.** 1977. Purification and partial characterization of the principle deoxyribonucleic acid polymerase from *Mycoplasmatales. J. Bacteriol.* **132**:641–649.

71. **Mitra, S. K., F. Lustig, B. Åkesson, T. Axberg, P. Elias, and U. Lagerkvist.** 1979. Relative efficiency of anticodons in reading the valine codons during protein synthesis *in vitro. J. Biol. Chem.* **254**:6397–6401.

72. **Mitra, S. K., F. Lustig, B. Åkesson, L. Strid, and U. Lagerkvist.** 1977. Codon-anticodon recognition in the valine family. *J. Biol. Chem.* **252**:471–478.

72a. **Muto, A.** Personal communication.

73. **Muto, A., Y. Andachi, H. Yuzawa, F. Yamao, and S. Osawa.** 1990. The organization and evolution of transfer RNA genes in *Mycoplasma capricolum. Nucleic Acids Res.* **18**:5037–5043.

74. **Muto, A., Y. Kawauchi, F. Yamao, and S. Osawa.** 1984. Preferential use of A- and U-rich codons for *Mycoplasma capricolum* ribosomal proteins S8 and L6. *Nucleic Acids Res.* **12**:8209–8217.

75. **Muto, A., and S. Osawa.** 1987. The guanine and cytosine content of genomic DNA and bacterial evolution. *Proc. Natl. Acad. Sci. USA* **84**:166–169.

76. **Ohyama, K., H. Fukuzawa, T. Kohchi, H. Shirai, T. Sano, S. Sano, K. Umesono, Y. Shiki, M. Takeuchi, Z. Chang, S.-I. Aota, H. Inokuchi, and H. Ozeki.** 1986. Chloroplast gene organization deduced from complete sequence of liverwort *Marchantia polymorpha* chloroplast DNA. *Nature* (London) **322**:572–574.

77. **Orgel, L. E., and F. H. C. Crick.** 1980. Selfish DNA: the ultimate parasite. *Nature* (London) **284**:604–607.

78. **Osawa, S., and T. H. Jukes.** 1988. Evolution of the genetic code as affected by anticodon content. *Trends Genet.* **4**:191–198.

79. **Osawa, S., and T. H. Jukes.** 1989. Codon reassignment (codon capture) in evolution. *J. Mol. Biol.* **28**:271–278.

80. **Osawa, S., T. H. Jukes, A. Muto, F. Yamao, T. Ohama, and Y. Andachi.** 1987. Role of directional mutation pressure in the evolution of the eubacterial genetic code. *Cold Spring Harbor Symp. Quant. Biol.* **52**:777–789.

81. **Osawa, S., T. Ohama, F. Yamao, A. Muto, T. H. Jukes, H. Ozeki, and K. Umesono.** 1988. Directional mutation pressure and transfer RNA in choice of the third nucleotide of synonymous two-codon sets. *Proc. Natl. Acad. Sci. USA* **85**:1124–1128.

82. **Pfitzinger, H., J. H. Weil, D. T. N. Pillay, and P. Guillemaut.** 1990. Codon recognition mechanisms in plant chloroplasts. *Plant Mol. Biol.* **14**:805–814.

83. **Phillips, S. H., and K. Kjellin-Stråby.** 1967. Studies on microbial ribonucleic acid. IV. Two mutants of *Saccharomyces cerevisiae* lacking N²-dimethylguanine in soluble ribonucleic acid. *J. Mol. Biol.* **26**:509–518.

84. **Poritz, M. A., H. D. Bernstein, K. Strub, D. Zopf, H. Wilhelm, and P. Walter.** 1990. An *E. coli* ribonucleoprotein containing 4.5S RNA resembles mammalian signal recognition particle. *Science* **250**:1111–1117.

85. **Preer, J. R., Jr., L. B. Preer, B. M. Rudman, and A. J. Barnett.** 1985. Deviation from the universal code shown by the gene for surface protein 51A in *Paramecium. Nature* (London) **314**:188–190.

86. **Pribula, C. D., G. E. Fox, and C. R. Woese.** 1976. Nucleotide sequence of *Clostridium pasteurianum* 5S RNA. *FEBS Lett.* **64**:350–352.

87. **Reanney, D.** 1974. On the origin of prokaryotes. *J. Theor. Biol.* **48**:243–251.

88. **Roberts, J. W., and J. Carbon.** 1975. Nucleotide sequence studies of normal and genetically altered glycine transfer ribonucleic acids from *Escherichia coli. J. Biol. Chem.* **250**:5530–5541.

89. **Rogers, M. J., J. J. Simmons, R. T. Walker, W. G. Weisburg, C. R. Woese, R. S. Tannar, I. M. Robinson, D. A. Stahl, G. Olsen, R. L. Leach, and J. Maniloff.** 1985. Construction of the mycoplasma evolutionary tree from 5S rRNA sequence data. *Proc. Natl. Acad. Sci. USA* **82**:1160–1164.

90. **Rogers, M. J., A. A. Steimetz, and R. T. Walker.** 1986. The nucleotide sequence of a tRNA gene cluster from *Spiroplasma melliferum. Nucleic Acids Res.* **14**:3145.

91. **Ryan, J. L., and H. J. Morowitz.** 1969. Partial purification of native rRNA and tRNA cistrons from *Mycoplasma* sp. (kid). *Proc. Natl. Acad. Sci. USA* **63**:1282–1289.

92. **Sampson, J. R., and O. C. Uhlenbeck.** 1988. Biochemical and physical characterization of an unmodified yeast phenylalanine transfer RNA transcribed *in vitro. Proc. Natl. Acad. Sci. USA* **85**:1033–1037.

93. **Samuelsson, T., T. Axberg, T. Borén, and U. Lagerkvist.** 1983. Unconventional reading of the glycine codons. *J. Biol. Chem.* **258**:13178–13184.

94. **Samuelsson, T., T. Borén, and T.-I. Johansen.** 1988. Properties of a transfer RNA lacking modified nucleosides. *J. Biol. Chem.* **263**:13692–13699.

95. **Samuelsson, T., P. Elias, F. Lustig, T. Axberg, G. Fölsch, B. Åkesson, and U. Lagerkvist.** 1980. Aberrations of the classic codon reading scheme during protein synthesis in vitro. *J. Biol. Chem.* **255**:4583–4588.

96. **Samuelsson, T., P. Elias, F. Lustig, and Y. S. Guindy.** 1985. Cloning and nucleotide sequence analysis of tRNA genes from *Mycoplasma mycoides. Biochem. J.* **232**:223–228.

97. **Samuelsson, T., and Y. S. Guindy.** 1990. Nucleotide sequence of a *Mycoplasma mycoides* RNA which is homologous to *E. coli* 4.5S RNA. *Nucleic Acids Res.* **18**:4938.

98. **Samuelsson, T., Y. S. Guindy, F. Lustig, T. Borén, and U. Lagerkvist.** 1987. Apparent lack of discrimination in the reading of certain codons in *Mycoplasma mycoides. Proc. Natl. Acad. Sci. USA* **84**:3166–3170.

99. **Schwartz, R. M., and M. O. Dayhoff.** 1978. Origins of prokaryotes, eukaryotes, mitochondria and chloroplasts. *Science* **199**:395–403.

100. **Shinozaki, K., M. Ohme, M. Tanaka, T. Wakasugi, N. Hayashido, T. Matsubayashi, N. Zaita, J. Chunwongse, J. Obokata, K. Yamaguchi-Shinozaki, C. Ohto, K. Torazawa, B. Y. Meng, M. Sugita, H. Deno, T. Kamogashira, K. Yamada, J. Kusuda, F. Takaiwa, A. Kato, N. Tohdoh, H. Shimada, and M. Sugiura.** 1986. The complete nucleotide sequence of the tobacco chloroplast genome: its gene organization and expression. *EMBO J.* **5**:2043–2049.

101. **Sibler, A.-P., G. Dirheimer, and R. P. Martin.** 1986. Codon reading patterns in *Saccharomyces cerevisiae* mitochondria based on sequences of mitochondrial tRNAs. *FEBS Lett.* **194**:131–138.

101a. **Simoneau, P., and P.-C. Hu.** Personal communication.

102. **Sladek, T. L.** 1986. A hypothesis for the mechanism of mycoplasma evolution. *J. Theor. Biol.* **120**:457–465.

103. **Smith, D., and M. Yarus.** 1989. tRNA-tRNA interactions within cellular ribosomes. *Proc. Natl. Acad. Sci. USA* **86**:4397–4401.

104. **Smith, D. W. E., and D. L. Hatfield.** 1986. Effects of post-transcriptional base modifications on the site-specific function of transfer RNA in eukaryotic translation. *J. Mol. Biol.* **189**:663–671.

105. **Sprinzl, M., T. Hartmann, J. Weber, J. Blank, and R. Zeidler.** 1989. Compilation of tRNA sequences and sequences of tRNA genes. *Nucleic Acids Res. Seq. Suppl.* **17**:1–172.

106. **Squires, C., and J. Carbon.** 1971. Normal and mutant glycine transfer RNAs. *Nature* (London) *New Biol.* **233**:274–277.

107. **Struck, J. C. R., D. W. Vogel, N. Ulbrich, and V. A. Erdmann.** 1988. The *Bacillus subtilis* scRNA is related to the 4.5S RNA from *Escherichia coli*. *Nucleic Acids Res.* **16**:2719.

108. **Tanaka, R., A. Muto, and S. Osawa.** 1989. Nucleotide sequence of tryptophan tRNA gene in *Acholeplasma laidlawii*. *Nucleic Acids Res.* **17**:5842.

109. **Taschke, C. T., M.-Q. Klinkert, J. Wolters, and R. Herrmann.** 1986. Organization of the ribosomal RNA genes in *Mycoplasma hyopneumoniae*: the 5S rRNA gene is separated from the 16S and 23S rRNA genes. *Mol. Gen. Genet.* **205**:428–433.

110. **Walker, R. T., E. T. J. Chelton, M. W. Kilpatrich, M. J. Rogers, and J. Simmons.** 1982. The nucleotide sequence of the 5S rRNA from *Spiroplasma* species BC3 and *Mycoplasma mycoides* sp. *capri* PG. *Nucleic Acids Res.* **10**:6363–6367.

111. **Walker, R. T., and U. L. RajBhandary.** 1978. Nucleotide sequence of formylmethionine tRNA from *Mycoplasma mycoides* subsp *capri*. *Nucleic Acids Res.* **5**:57–70.

112. **Waring, R. B., R. W. Davies, S. Lee, E. Grisi, M. McPhail Berks, and C. Scazzocchio.** 1981. The mosaic organization of the apocytochrome b gene of *Aspergillus nidulans* revealed by DNA sequencing. *Cell* **27**:4–11.

113. **Watson, J. D., N. H. Hopkins, J. D. Roberts, J. A. Steitz, and A. M. Weiner.** 1987. *Molecular Biology of the Gene*, 4th ed. The Benjamin-Cummings Publishing Company, Inc., Menlo Park, Calif.

114. **Wawrousek, E. F., N. Narasimhan, and J. N. Hansen.** 1984. Two large clusters with thirty-seven transfer RNA genes adjacent to ribosomal RNA gene sets in *Bacillus subtilis*. *J. Biol. Chem.* **259**:3694–3702.

115. **Weisburg, W. G., J. G. Tully, D. L. Rose, J. P. Petzel, H. Oyaizu, D. Yang, L. Mandelco, J. Sechrest, T. G. Lawrence, J. Van Etten, J. Maniloff, and C. R. Woese.** 1989. A phylogenetic analysis of the mycoplasmas: basis for their classification. *J. Bacteriol.* **171**:6455–6467.

116. **Williams, M. V., and J. D. Pollack.** 1990. A mollicute (mycoplasma) DNA repair enzyme: purification and characterization of uracil-DNA glycosylase. *J. Bacteriol.* **172**:2979–2985.

117. **Woese, C. R., J. Maniloff, and L. B. Zahlen.** 1980. Phylogenetic analysis of the mycoplasmas. *Proc. Natl. Acad. Sci. USA* **77**:494–498.

118. **Woese, C. R., E. Stackebrandt, and W. Ludwig.** 1985. What are mycoplasmas: the relationship of tempo and mode in bacterial evolution. *J. Mol. Evol.* **21**:305–316.

119. **Wolstenholme, D. R., J. L. Macfarlane, R. Okimoto, D. O. Clary, and J. A. Wahleithner.** 1987. Bizarre tRNAs inferred from DNA sequences of mitochondrial genomes of nematode worms. *Proc. Natl. Acad. Sci. USA* **84**:1324–1328.

120. **Yamao, F., S. Iwagami, Y. Azumi, A. Muto, S. Osawa, N. Fujita, and A. Ishihama.** 1988. Evolutionary dynamics of tryptophan tRNAs in *Mycoplasma capricolum*. *Mol. Gen. Genet.* **212**:364–369.

121. **Yamao, F., A. Muto, Y. Kawauchi, M. Iwami, S. Iwagami, Y. Azumi, and S. Osawa.** 1985. UGA is read as tryptophan in *Mycoplasma capricolum*. *Proc. Natl. Acad. Sci. USA* **82**:2306–2309.

122. **Yang, D., Y. Oyaizu, H. Oyaizu, G. J. Olsen, and C. R. Woese.** 1985. Mitochondrial origins. *Proc. Natl. Acad. Sci. USA* **82**:4443–4447.

123. **Yarus, M.** 1982. Translational efficiency of transfer RNAs: uses of an extended anticodon. *Science* **218**:646–652.

124. **Yokoyama, S., T. Watanabe, K. Murao, H. Ishikura, Z. Yamaizumi, S. Nishimura, and T. Miyazawa.** 1985. Molecular mechanism of codon recognition by tRNA species with modified uridine in the first position of the anticodon. *Proc. Natl. Acad. Sci. USA* **82**:4905–4909.

INDEX

593